The American Medical Association
Home Health Library

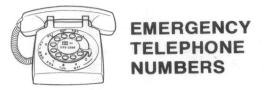 **EMERGENCY TELEPHONE NUMBERS**

Doctor —————————————————

Doctor —————————————————

Doctor —————————————————

Poison control center —————————————————

Hospital emergency room —————————————————

Paramedics —————————————————

Fire department —————————————————

Police department —————————————————

Ambulance —————————————————

Parents at work —————————————————

Neighborhood pharmacy —————————————————

24-Hour pharmacy —————————————————

Electric company —————————————————

Gas company —————————————————

Neighbor —————————————————

Relative —————————————————

—————————————————

THE
AMERICAN MEDICAL
ASSOCIATION
FAMILY MEDICAL GUIDE

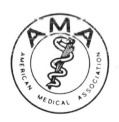

Editor-in-Chief
Jeffrey R.M. Kunz, MD

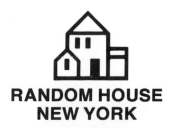

RANDOM HOUSE
NEW YORK

The recommendations and information in this book are appropriate in most
cases. For specific information concerning your personal medical condition,
however, the AMA suggests that you consult a physician. The names of
organizations appearing in the book are given for informational purposes
only. Their inclusion implies neither approval nor disapproval by the AMA.

Library of Congress Cataloging in Publication Data
Main entry under title:

The American Medical Association family
medical guide.

Includes index.
1. Medicine, Popular. I. Kunz, Jeffrey R. M.
RC81.A543   1982   610   82–3873
ISBN 0–394–51015–1   AACR2

Manufactured in the United States of America

4689753

Preface

It has often been said that the greatest gift of life is life itself. Surely this is true, but today we are also concerned with the *quality* of life, and the cornerstone of a quality life is good health.

No one can guarantee us good health, but by adopting prudent habits and a sensible lifestyle, each of us can prevent unnecessary illness, needless loss of vitality, and premature old age. You are the person best equipped to maintain your health, but as doctors, we feel a responsibility to work with you in achieving this goal, as well as to treat you for illness if the need should arise. It is this philosophy, with its emphasis on preventive care, that has motivated the American Medical Association, in collaboration with Random House, to publish this *Family Medical Guide*.

The original concept for the *Guide* was developed by Dorling/Kindersley Limited of London and presented to us by Random House. The AMA prepared and edited the content of the book specifically for an American audience, in accordance with the practices of the American medical-care system. The book is one of a series of volumes cumulatively entitled the *American Medical Association Home Health Library*.

In the economic climate of the 1980s, there is a special urgency about the responsible maintenance of health and the sensible treatment of disease. Inflation has pushed medical costs – and family medical bills – to unprecedented levels. Certainly one of the best ways to combat this debilitating inflation is for all of us to avoid the avoidable and prevent the preventable. When illness does afflict us, surely the best prospect for early recovery lies in the effective partnership of patient and physician.

The *Family Medical Guide* shows you how your body is structured, how it functions and what you must do to keep it healthy. It answers your questions about all the most common diseases and their symptoms. Then, too, there are the Self-Diagnosis Charts that will help you decide whether an ache or pain you have is simply a temporary annoyance or something more serious about which you should seek prompt medical advice.

We physicians firmly believe that if you are given the facts about your body and how it functions, and the professional guidance necessary to put those facts appropriately to use in your daily life, you will act wisely in your own behalf. We believe that you will find much useful information on a wide range of medical subjects in this *Guide*, and that this knowledge will help you maintain your well-being and make you and your doctor more effective partners in responding to your physical and emotional needs.

The best of health to you!

James H. Sammons, M.D.
Executive Vice President
American Medical Association

Contents

Consultants

How to use this book

The *AMA Family Medical Guide* is designed to help you both in sickness and in health. The book has four parts: The Healthy Body; Symptoms and Self-diagnosis; Diseases and Other Disorders and Problems; and Caring for the Sick. Since it includes a great deal of health information, it is cross-referenced and indexed to help you find what you want. The following additional suggestions should help you take full advantage of the *Guide*.

Questionnaires to help determine how healthy you are
You might begin by checking the current state of your health and the ways in which your lifestyle, including eating and drinking habits, may affect it. These factors can have an impact on your health. The questionnaires in the first part of the book can help you learn more about your health (see, for example, How good are your chances for staying healthy? on p.13). They also lead you into relevant sections of Part I, where you will find advice on how you can improve your general health. For a better understanding of all aspects of health and illness, Part I contains a detailed atlas of the body (pp.49–64), in color, which you can consult for the positions and names of almost every organ, bone and muscle in the body.

If you have a health problem
A large portion of the book is concerned with diagnosis and disease, and here the emphasis is on problem solving. The best way for you to use this material is to begin with the self-diagnosis symptom charts in Part II (see pp.66–232). These charts provide a unique method of finding out what a particular symptom (or set of symptoms) may signify.

The symptom charts have been specifically compiled for people who do not know what is wrong with them or whether something actually *is* wrong. To use the charts, look up the symptom that is troubling you in the Chartfinder on p.68, turn to the correct symptom chart and follow through. The introduction to Part II gives you thorough instructions for finding the relevant symptom chart for your problem. The chart may indicate the necessity for medical help either immediately or within a few days, or it may suggest that your problem is not serious enough to require the services of a physician. In most cases you will be referred to an article in Part III of the book for more information on your tentative self-diagnosis. The article will describe in some detail the disease or disorder that is probably causing your present problem, and the treatment you are likely to need if your diagnosis is correct. You may also be directed to a color photograph in the section containing Visual Aids to Diagnosis (see pp.233–48).

Diseases and disorders

If you are already seeing a physician about a specific disorder and would like to know more about it, you can look it up in the General Index and turn directly to the relevant article in Part III. In other cases, you may be referred to an article from one of the self-diagnosis symptom charts in Part II. Another possibility is referral from the first part of the book, where you may have learned that an aspect of your current lifestyle could cause you to develop a particular disease.

The articles in Part III are organized to anticipate questions and to answer them frankly and as nontechnically as possible. Once the disease or problem has been defined, further information about each disorder is arranged to provide answers to four basic questions, in this order:

What are the symptoms?
What are the risks?
What should be done?
What is the treatment?

In certain cases additional questions such as *What are the long-term prospects?* may arise, and these questions are answered where appropriate. Diseases that are extremely rare, that cannot be treated or that are minor are covered briefly or not at all.

The first two questions are self-explanatory. A word about the last two, however: *What should be done?* involves both what you yourself should do (for example, see your physician right away or simply spend a few days in bed), and what you can expect the doctor to do to make a firm diagnosis of your condition. Note, also, that in *What is the treatment?*, specific drugs are not identified. This is because, while it may be possible to specify a type of medication for a disorder, the exact choice of a drug can only be made by your physician. Additional information about drugs, however, is given in the Drug Index (see next column).

Most articles in Part III deal with health problems common to both sexes and all ages. There are also articles that concentrate on diseases and problems that mainly affect certain population groups. The health problems of men, women, couples, infants and children, adolescents and the elderly are given special treatment. In addition, a group of articles covers pregnancy and childbirth.

Caring for the sick

In the last part of the *Guide*, Part IV, you will find information about general problems of health care that everyone must face from time to time. The articles cover both professional medical care and self-help. The complexities of the American health-care system are explained in simple terms. This section provides suggestions on how to choose a family physician, definitions of various medical specialties, and information about hospital services and about care of the sick at home. There are also suggestions about matters that are seldom discussed, such as ways of coping with terminal illness and death.

Drugs

The Drug Index (pp.776–87) provides information on the uses of various drugs, the way they are administered and some of their possible side effects. The most commonly used drugs in the United States are included in that index under both generic and trade names. General information about broad categories of drugs is also provided.

Words you may not understand

In reading about medicine and disease, you will probably come across occasional words or phrases that are unfamiliar or are used in a particular medical way. These words are italicized, explained briefly in the text and further defined in the Glossary (pp.788–99).

First aid for accidents and emergencies

Before you need to take immediate action to safeguard your health or the health of others, turn to the quick-reference section on Accidents and Emergencies (pp.801–16). Then, if an emergency does arise, you will be better prepared to deal with it. In addition to providing information on lifesaving measures, these pages also give practical instructions for treating minor problems.

A prescription for health

As a physician, I urge you to use this book to help maintain and improve your health and that of your family. No book, however, should be considered a substitute for professional medical care. Even a text as comprehensive as the *AMA Family Medical Guide* cannot replace that.

There is no stronger medicine than an informed patient and a dedicated physician. To this alliance we dedicate this book.

Jeffrey R. M. Kunz, M.D.
Editor-in-Chief

Part I

The healthy body

The healthy body

Introduction

Are you in good health? It may be several years since you last saw your physician or were ill enough to stay in bed for a week, but of course that is no guarantee of future good health. Physical and mental breakdowns may occur at any age. Many breakdowns are due to years of unhealthy living and are therefore avoidable.

Unless you are one of the relatively few really health-conscious individuals, your current life style is almost certainly less healthy than it could be. Now is the time to modify it. You will benefit, first of all, by lowering the risks of preventable illness. And as you become increasingly fit, you will feel better all around and will find that you are more able to enjoy life. Certain basic guidelines for healthy living are simple, and medical research shows convincingly that they improve your chances for a long healthy life. These guidelines are set out below, as five basic rules for healthy living.

Following the guidelines will help you retain your health and vigor and increase your life expectancy. Even if you are middle-aged and overweight and last exercised regularly when you were a teenager, you can move gradually into a healthier living pattern. First, however, check on the present state of your health and the advisability of various aspects of your current life style. The series of questionnaires in this part of the book will help you to evaluate your fitness, and the accompanying articles should serve as a guide to staying healthy.

Certain aspects of life style, behavior and personal medical history are especially important in assessing the current state of your health. The questionnaire on the opposite page entitled How good are your chances for staying healthy? identifies the most significant factors, as indicated by many recent medical studies. Try this questionnaire as a starting point for a health program.

Our society's current emphasis on diet, exercise and other aspects of life style is not just a passing fashion or fad. The major diseases of adult life are serious and often fatal, but many of them are easier to prevent than to cure. There is no mystery about what to do. Your life is largely in your own hands.

Five basic rules for healthy living

1 If you smoke, give it up. Now! There is no longer any doubt about the link between smoking tobacco and the development of serious illnesses such as lung cancer and some forms of heart disease.

2 If you drink alcohol, drink in moderation – no more than an average of two bottles of beer (or two cocktails or two glasses of wine) each day.

3 Exercise strenuously at least twice, and preferably three times, each week.

4 Eat sensibly. You need a balanced diet with plenty of fruit and vegetables, but go easy on cream, butter, fatty foods, sugar, cakes and other sweet things.

5 Do not let yourself get overweight. If you are already obese (see the Weight chart, p.28), go on a reducing diet until you are healthily slim.

The health questionnaires

The questionnaires included here have been compiled mainly for the use of adults, but most of the questions are applicable to any age group. You may find them helpful as a starting point in evaluating your physical and mental well-being and that of all members of your family. Evaluation is only the first step, however. Where possible, you should go on to take further steps to improve your chances of avoiding illness by reading and acting on the information given in the articles that accompany each questionnaire.

Two of the questionnaires, those that deal with drinking alcohol and smoking, may not concern you directly. However, they may concern others in your family who can test themselves, and who should read the relevant articles. It is important for each person to answer honestly. If you cheat on the questions, you are cheating only yourself.

How good are your chances for staying healthy?

Answer YES or NO to the following questions

1 Are you within desirable weight limits for your height (see the Weight chart, p.28)?
YES ☐   NO ☐

2 When walking briskly with people of your own age group, can you match their pace and carry on casual conversation without becoming short of breath?
YES ☐   NO ☐

3 Can you walk up three flights of stairs (each including about 15 to 20 steps) without having to pause for breath?
YES ☐   NO ☐

4 Do you exercise vigorously enough to make you breathless and sweaty at least three times a week?
YES ☐   NO ☐

5 Do you ordinarily sleep soundly and wake up feeling energetic and ready for the day ahead?
YES ☐   NO ☐

6 At the end of a working day do you usually feel energetic enough to go out and enjoy a social evening?
YES ☐   NO ☐

7 Do you drink, on average, less than two bottles of beer (or two cocktails, or two glasses of wine) a day?
YES ☐   NO ☐

8 Are you, and have you been for at least the last 15 years, a non-smoker?
YES ☐   NO ☐

9 Are you happy with your life, and do you generally have a positive outlook?
YES ☐   NO ☐

10 Do you drive defensively and always wear seat belts?
YES ☐   NO ☐

EVALUATION
If you can answer YES to all of the above questions, you are at this moment maximizing your chances of staying healthy. The more NO answers the more the need for serious consideration of some sort of change in life style. You should try the more detailed questionnaires in the following pages, and adopt any suggestions in the accompanying articles that may apply in your case. In addition, all readers will do well to examine the list of symptoms included under Early warning signs of possible serious illness (see p.48).

Keeping physically fit

It is no accident that the words "fit" and "healthy" are often linked. Your level of physical fitness reflects the state of your general health, and your body's fitness is largely determined by the amount of physical work that you do. Physical work includes all movements, even such routine activities as walking, eating, sitting and breathing. But the quantity and quality of vigorous exercise you get is most important from the standpoint of fitness. In these pages you will find an explanation of why exercise can improve your health, well-being and life expectancy, along with some tips on how to become physically fit by devising your own exercise program. As a starting point, assess your present approximate level of fitness by trying the "step test" recommended below.

How fit are you?

The following test is designed to assess the approximate efficiency of heart, lungs and muscles in response to exercise. The result gives an indication of almost anyone's general level of fitness. Note: if you answered NO to question 3 in the questionnaire How good are your chances for staying healthy? (see previous page) you should *not* attempt this test. See your physician first.

Before you try the step test . . .
This exercise separates the unfit from those of average or just-below average fitness. Walk steadily up three flights of stairs (each including 15 to 20 steps). Do you have to pause for breath, or are you so breathless when you reach the top that you cannot talk normally? If you answer YES, you are not fit and should consult your physician before you attempt to do any vigorous exercise.

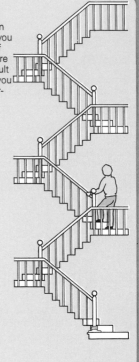

The step test
Choose a bottom stair or any fixed platform about 20 cm (8 in) high. Step onto it with one foot, bring up the other, and then step back down onto the floor (below left). Repeat the up-and-down process at a rate of 24 times a minute for 3 minutes. A test run will help you get the rhythm right.

WARNING: Do not continue the exercise if you begin to feel unpleasantly out of breath, dizzy, nauseated, or in any way uncomfortable.
   Stop after 3 minutes and wait for exactly 1 minute. Then count your heartbeats by counting your pulse over the next 15 seconds, and read off your fitness rating on the table below.

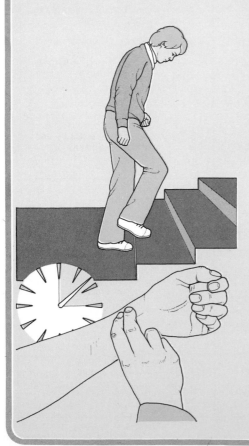

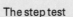

Pulses (heartbeats) counted in 15 seconds				Fitness rating
MEN		WOMEN		
Under 45 years	Over 45 years	Under 45 years	Over 45 years	
Below 18	Below 19	Below 20	Below 21	Excellent
18–20	19–21	20–22	21–23	Good
21–25	22–26	23–28	24–29	Average
Above 25	Above 26	Above 28	Above 29	Poor

Why exercise is good for you

In the context of physical fitness, "exercise" refers to any activity involving a fairly high degree of physical movement that makes you breathless and sweaty if you do it vigorously. Gardening or walking can be as much exercise as a game of tennis or an hour of bicycling, provided it is done vigorously enough.

There is a sound medical reason why physical activity is good for you. Any work that muscles must do increases their need for oxygen. During physical exercise, you must breathe more deeply to get more oxygen into your lungs, and your heart (which is itself almost all muscle) must beat harder and faster to pump blood to the muscles. Heart disease accounts for almost a third of all deaths and a high proportion of serious illness in North America. So an efficient, resilient heart, not to mention strong lungs, means you are less likely to have major health problems compared to a non-exercising contemporary. One medical study has shown that middle-aged people with desk jobs who do not exercise are twice as susceptible to heart attacks as those people who exercise regularly.

Up to a reasonable point, the more you work your muscles and the larger the number of muscles and joints you use, the greater the physical gain. The most beneficial kind of exercise is known as "dynamic." Dynamic exercise such as swimming or jogging strengthens the heart, lungs and body muscles when it makes you breathless and sweaty. It also keeps joints supple, and your mind and body active. The alternative, "static" exercise such as weight lifting, can build specific muscles to excessive degrees, does less to improve your heart and lungs and may not raise your general level of fitness.

Lack of exercise can contribute to development of various disorders. Anyone who has had an illness or injury and was forced to lie in bed for a time knows how weak their muscles become. The same disuse also affects the bones and can affect the heart and lungs. Unexercised, weak muscles can also put extra strain on other structures such as joints and ligaments by overloading them.

The physical benefits of dynamic exercise are apparent, but there are psychological benefits as well. Many people sleep better after exercise, wake up more refreshed, and are more alert and better able to concentrate than they were when they did not exercise. And exercise helps, to some extent, to keep you healthily slim. To sum up, exercise of the right type should make you feel better, look better, live longer and have less illness.

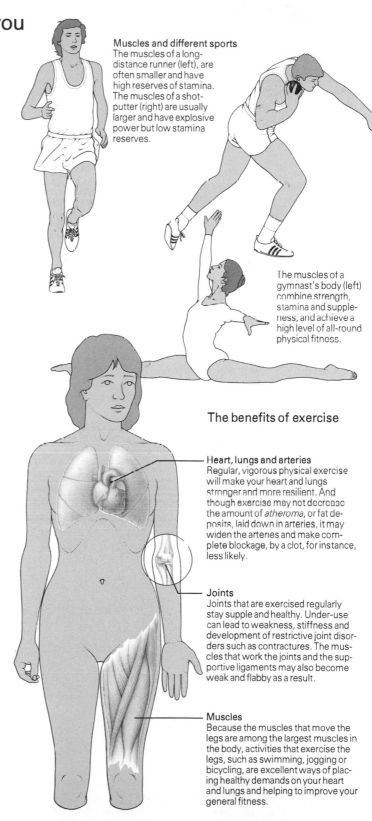

Muscles and different sports
The muscles of a long-distance runner (left), are often smaller and have high reserves of stamina. The muscles of a shot-putter (right) are usually larger and have explosive power but low stamina reserves.

The muscles of a gymnast's body (left) combine strength, stamina and suppleness, and achieve a high level of all-round physical fitness.

The benefits of exercise

Heart, lungs and arteries
Regular, vigorous physical exercise will make your heart and lungs stronger and more resilient. And though exercise may not decrease the amount of *atheroma*, or fat deposits, laid down in arteries, it may widen the arteries and make complete blockage, by a clot, for instance, less likely.

Joints
Joints that are exercised regularly stay supple and healthy. Under-use can lead to weakness, stiffness and development of restrictive joint disorders such as contractures. The muscles that work the joints and the supportive ligaments may also become weak and flabby as a result.

Muscles
Because the muscles that move the legs are among the largest muscles in the body, activities that exercise the legs, such as swimming, jogging or bicycling, are excellent ways of placing healthy demands on your heart and lungs and helping to improve your general fitness.

The essentials of a good exercise program

The right kind of exercise for you is exercise that will benefit your own body in its current state of fitness. The following recommendations are based on three sets of guidelines that apply to almost everyone who wants to embark on a successful exercise program.

1. Have at least three, and possibly more, exercise sessions every week, preferably at regular intervals and stated times. Make each session 20 minutes or longer, with little or no pause for rest. Choose a level of activity high enough to make you breathless, sweaty and aware of your heart beating, but not so violent that you get dizzy or nauseated, or risk straining muscles or joints. Do warm-up exercises before the main exercise session and cool-down exercises at the end.

2. Choose forms of exercise that you enjoy and that you can fit into your schedule. If you dislike sports, energetic gardening or do-it-yourself work around the house can be good purposeful ways to stay active. Bicycling or brisk walking to and from work will often fit into everyday routines. The goal is to develop a habit of physical fitness, and enjoyment will be an extra incentive.

3. Do not attempt to get into shape too rapidly. Start gently, exercising just hard enough to become aware of mild strain, and increase your efforts gradually over the first four weeks. If you start a new sport, beware of early over-competitiveness. If you take up a potentially very strenuous game such as racquetball or handball, try to improve on your last performance rather than competing with your opponent's.

A final note of warning. If you belong to one of the following groups, ask your physician for advice before you take up any sort of strenuous activity:
- People over 60 years of age, or those over 45 who have had little or no hard exercise since early adulthood.
- Heavy smokers (anyone who smokes more than 20 cigarettes a day).
- People who are seriously overweight (see the Weight chart, p.28).
- People under treatment or supervision for a long-term health problem such as high blood pressure; heart, lung or kidney disease; or diabetes.
- People with a rating of "poor" according to the fitness test described in How fit are you? (see p.14).

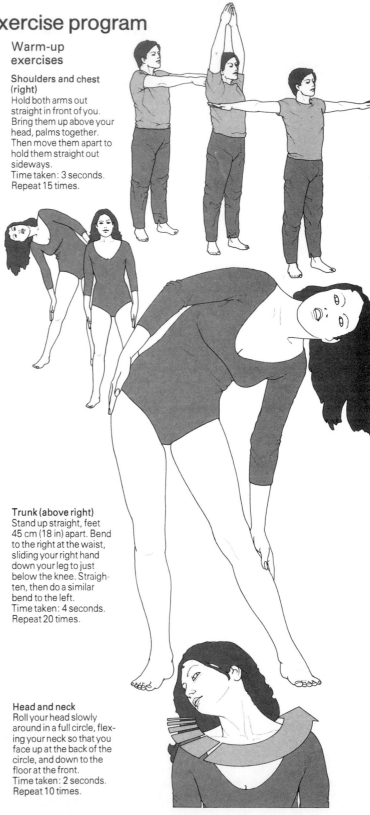

Warm-up exercises

Shoulders and chest (right)
Hold both arms out straight in front of you. Bring them up above your head, palms together. Then move them apart to hold them straight out sideways.
Time taken: 3 seconds.
Repeat 15 times.

Trunk (above right)
Stand up straight, feet 45 cm (18 in) apart. Bend to the right at the waist, sliding your right hand down your leg to just below the knee. Straighten, then do a similar bend to the left.
Time taken: 4 seconds.
Repeat 20 times.

Head and neck
Roll your head slowly around in a full circle, flexing your neck so that you face up at the back of the circle, and down to the floor at the front.
Time taken: 2 seconds.
Repeat 10 times.

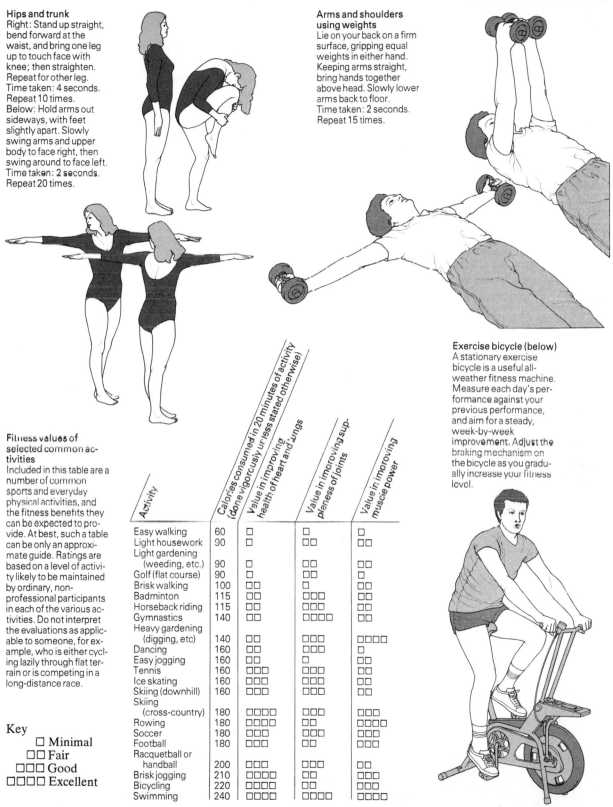

Hips and trunk

Right: Stand up straight, bend forward at the waist, and bring one leg up to touch face with knee; then straighten. Repeat for other leg. Time taken: 4 seconds. Repeat 10 times.
Below: Hold arms out sideways, with feet slightly apart. Slowly swing arms and upper body to face right, then swing around to face left. Time taken: 2 seconds. Repeat 20 times.

Arms and shoulders using weights

Lie on your back on a firm surface, gripping equal weights in either hand. Keeping arms straight, bring hands together above head. Slowly lower arms back to floor. Time taken: 2 seconds. Repeat 15 times.

Exercise bicycle (below)

A stationary exercise bicycle is a useful all-weather fitness machine. Measure each day's performance against your previous performance, and aim for a steady, week-by-week improvement. Adjust the braking mechanism on the bicycle as you gradually increase your fitness level.

Fitness values of selected common activities

Included in this table are a number of common sports and everyday physical activities, and the fitness benefits they can be expected to provide. At best, such a table can be only an approximate guide. Ratings are based on a level of activity likely to be maintained by ordinary, non-professional participants in each of the various activities. Do not interpret the evaluations as applicable to someone, for example, who is either cycling lazily through flat terrain or is competing in a long-distance race.

Key
☐ Minimal
☐☐ Fair
☐☐☐ Good
☐☐☐☐ Excellent

Activity	Calories consumed in 20 minutes of activity (done vigorously unless stated otherwise)	Value in improving health of heart and lungs	Value in improving suppleness of joints	Value in improving muscle power
Easy walking	60	☐	☐	☐
Light housework	90	☐	☐☐	☐☐
Light gardening (weeding, etc.)	90	☐	☐☐	☐☐
Golf (flat course)	90	☐	☐☐	☐
Brisk walking	100	☐☐	☐	☐☐
Badminton	115	☐☐	☐☐☐	☐☐
Horseback riding	115	☐☐	☐☐☐	☐☐
Gymnastics	140	☐☐	☐☐☐☐	☐☐
Heavy gardening (digging, etc)	140	☐☐	☐☐☐	☐☐☐☐
Dancing	160	☐☐	☐☐☐	☐
Easy jogging	160	☐☐	☐	☐☐
Tennis	160	☐☐☐	☐☐☐	☐☐
Ice skating	160	☐☐☐	☐☐☐	☐☐
Skiing (downhill)	160	☐☐☐	☐☐☐	☐☐
Skiing (cross-country)	180	☐☐☐☐	☐☐☐	☐☐☐
Rowing	180	☐☐☐☐	☐☐	☐☐☐☐
Soccer	180	☐☐☐	☐☐☐	☐☐☐
Football	180	☐☐☐	☐☐	☐☐☐
Racquetball or handball	200	☐☐☐	☐☐☐	☐☐
Brisk jogging	210	☐☐☐☐	☐☐	☐☐☐
Bicycling	220	☐☐☐☐	☐☐	☐☐☐
Swimming	240	☐☐☐☐	☐☐☐☐	☐☐☐☐

Keeping mentally fit

As indicated in the section of this book that deals with mental and emotional problems (see p.294), most people, though they may be on a fairly even keel most of the time, must undergo occasional periods of great stress. Bereavement, financial difficulties, ill-health and worry are all part of life, but it is often when several such events occur together that mental health suffers. Although these times of excessive stress may not literally cause mental (and physical) disease, they can play an important part in making you more susceptible to illness (see Are you under too much stress?, p.23).

So, since you cannot always avoid stress, study the following pages for advice about how you can develop an attitude of mind that will protect your mental (and also your physical) health. Some people, because they are not able to cope when they are subjected to extreme stress, develop mental illness. To withstand the tensions of difficult periods in life, everyone needs the resource of a healthy frame of mind as well as a healthy body. The questionnaire entitled How good is your mental health? (below) will help you to assess the current state of your mental well-being and resilience.

How good is your mental health?

Answer YES or NO to the following questions:

1 Are you sleeping poorly?
YES ☐ NO ☐

2 Do you feel generally tired and lacking in energy?
YES ☐ NO ☐

3 Do you find it hard to concentrate on something even when you intensely want to do so?
YES ☐ NO ☐

4 Are you so discontented with your job that you suspect you are not doing it as well as you should?
YES ☐ NO ☐

5 Do you have a few or no interests and activities other than your work?
YES ☐ NO ☐

6 Do you usually try to avoid meeting new people because of the strain of having to think of something to say to them?
YES ☐ NO ☐

7 Do you usually find it difficult to get along with people?
YES ☐ NO ☐

8 Do trivial setbacks and inconveniences make you irritable or bad-tempered even when you know they are trivial?
YES ☐ NO ☐

9 Do you feel really close to nobody, not even members of your immediate family?
YES ☐ NO ☐

10 Do you view life as a continual uphill struggle?
YES ☐ NO ☐

11 Do you tend to neglect your personal appearance?
YES ☐ NO ☐

12 Do you often have headaches?
YES ☐ NO ☐

13 When you think about the future, do you become extremely depressed?
YES ☐ NO ☐

EVALUATION
The more questions you answer with YES, the more important it is that you study the following articles, and seriously consider accepting some of the advice they offer. This is especially important if external events are already producing a stressful period in your life. To estimate the possible impact of current external events on your ability to cope, see the questionnaire entitled Are you under too much stress? (see p.23).

How to relieve tension

Some people manage to appear easy-going and relaxed no matter what the stresses and pressures on them. For others, even a small problem becomes a major disaster, a source of constant worry or anger. If you are in the latter group, try to remember that strong emotions affect the body physically by releasing the hormone adrenalin into the bloodstream. Adrenalin increases breathing and heartbeat rates, can make the stomach queasy and the muscles tense, and raises blood pressure. If excessive stress is not reduced, the body's reactions may become harmful, especially to people with heart disease, but also to people who are physically healthy. The procedures that are recommended below and on the next page should help to dissipate the tension that can build up, before it becomes harmful.

Muscle relaxation exercises
There are many ways to relax. Often the problem seems to center around finding the time to "get away from it all." The following simple exercises do not take very much time, and can be done on your own, without going anywhere. Try to do them regularly, not just when you feel you must either relax or burst. A gradually acquired ability to relax may help you if trouble comes.

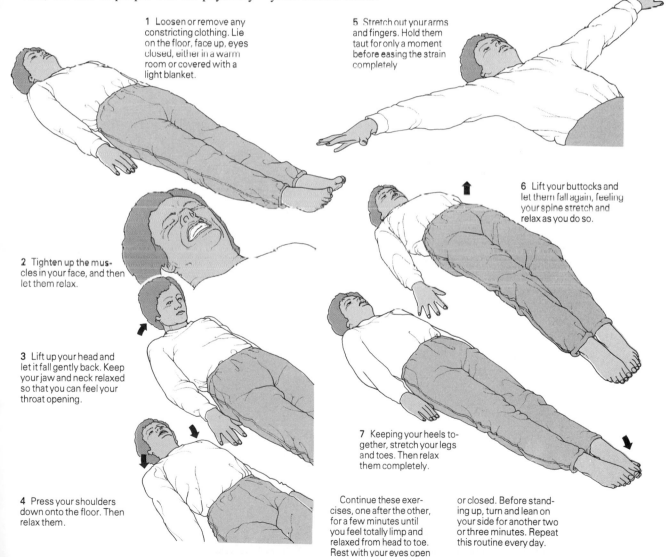

1 Loosen or remove any constricting clothing. Lie on the floor, face up, eyes closed, either in a warm room or covered with a light blanket.

2 Tighten up the muscles in your face, and then let them relax.

3 Lift up your head and let it fall gently back. Keep your jaw and neck relaxed so that you can feel your throat opening.

4 Press your shoulders down onto the floor. Then relax them.

5 Stretch out your arms and fingers. Hold them taut for only a moment before easing the strain completely

6 Lift your buttocks and let them fall again, feeling your spine stretch and relax as you do so.

7 Keeping your heels together, stretch your legs and toes. Then relax them completely.

Continue these exercises, one after the other, for a few minutes until you feel totally limp and relaxed from head to toe. Rest with your eyes open or closed. Before standing up, turn and lean on your side for another two or three minutes. Repeat this routine every day.

Breathing exercises
Deep breathing helps the heart and lungs function efficiently, and a habit of taking deep rather than shallow breaths can help to reduce tension. To develop the habit, sit or lie in a comfortable position, and breathe deeply and slowly, timing the breaths so that you take about half as many as usual in the course of one minute. Continue this rhythmic activity for five minutes, but stop if you begin to feel dizzy. Try to do this twice a day every day. If at other times you begin to feel a build-up of tension, make a point of breathing slowly and deeply for a few minutes. One result should be some easing of your sensation of mental strain.

Meditation
There are many meditation techniques, all of which have the same goal: To achieve tranquility by emptying the mind of distracting thoughts and worries.

A number of organizations teach meditation methods, but you do not have to take a course or join a group to learn to meditate. Most people are able to acquire the necessary skills for meditation on their own. Try using the following simple method:

1. With your eyes closed and your back straight, sit in an upright but comfortable chair in a quiet room. Choose a place where you are unlikely to be disturbed. Put your feet flat on the floor and unhurriedly take as relaxed a position as you can.

2. Choose a word or phrase that has no emotional overtones for you, such as "oak" or "bring." Without moving your lips, repeat the word silently to yourself, giving your full attention to the word as a word, not to its meaning. If any thought or image enters your mind, do not actively try to banish it, but do not focus on that thought. Instead, concentrate on the unspoken sound of the word that you have chosen.

3. Do this regularly for five minutes twice a day for a week, or until you have become skilled at emptying your mind of all thoughts for an extended period. Then gradually increase the meditation period. Soon you will be able to meditate for about 20 minutes at each session.

Some people find it easier to focus their attention on something visual, such as a wall pattern or a candle, instead of a word. The important thing is to decrease thought (and also your worries) by using this relaxing form of concentration.

How to get a good night's sleep

The "average" person gets between seven and eight hours of sleep in a usual day. But, in fact, sleep requirements differ widely. If you always wake up after only five or six hours and find it impossible to drop off again, do not worry; this is probably as much sleep as you need. And there is generally no cause for concern if you usually wake up once or twice during the night. Many people tend not only to over-estimate their need for sleep but also to under-estimate the amount they get during a restless night. Research into sleep-time behavior and electrical brainwaves indicates that most people who think they get "hardly a wink" of sleep, really get more rest in those nights than they realize.

A few days, or even a fairly regular diet, of skimpy sleep will do you no harm as long as you remain energetic and healthily alert during waking hours. If, however, you feel over-tired or too tense to relax into sleep when you go to bed, try some of the following suggestions. If you continue to suffer from some form of insomnia and it appears to be affect-

How to cope with a crisis

No matter how healthy your normal state of mind and body, you probably will have an occasional crisis brought on by stress throughout your life. At such times, the best way to remain on an even keel is to adopt the following attitudes and behavior:

1 Concentrate on things as they are now. Do not increase your mental burdens by brooding about the past. Think about future events only to the extent that you can help to shape them. Do not worry about a future that you cannot control.

2 Consider your problems one at a time. Sometimes lumping them together can make them seem overwhelming, but if you look at them individually you may be able to see that each one is not as serious as you thought. Then you can begin to look for solutions.

3 Talk things over with your family and friends. Do not always complain or burden them with your troubles, but seek, and listen to, their opinions and advice.

ing your daily routine, consult your physician. Though prolonged spells of sleeplessness may not damage health by themselves, insomnia is sometimes a warning symptom of mental illness such as anxiety (see p.300) or depression (see p.297). For other possible causes of difficulty in sleeping, see Self-diagnosis symptom chart 4, p.76.

1. Do not take work to bed with you. If you like to read in bed, do some light reading that is not filled with suspense or vivid descriptions of other people's problems.

2. Have at least some physical exercise during the day so that your body feels tired enough to want rest at bedtime. If you do not get enough exercise, try taking a walk before bedtime. Also read Keeping physically fit (see p.14).

3. A warm bath, not a brisk shower, just before bedtime may help you relax.

4. Although an emotional upset or strenuous exercise just before going to bed is likely to retard sleep, satisfactory sexual intercourse is apt to have a sedative effect.

5. Make sure that your bed is comfortable and that you are neither too hot nor too cold. Most people sleep best in a room temperature of 60 to 65°F (16 to 18°C).

6. Use the relaxation techniques described on the preceding pages.

7. If all else fails, rather than trying to sleep and turning and tossing restlessly in bed, get out of bed and stay up until you are tired. Then go to bed and try to sleep. Be sure to get up at your normal time and try to make it through the day. Take a short nap only if you must to keep going.

Sleep patterns
The diagram below shows how the brain's activity changes during a night's sleep. Periods of "REM" (rapid eye movement) sleep, during which dreams are thought to occur, alternate with sessions of deep sleep. As morning approaches, sleep becomes gradually more shallow until you awaken.

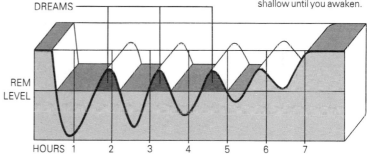

4 Once you have decided what you want to do about a problem that you can do something about, act promptly and firmly. Positive action is usually healthier than passive brooding.

5 Occupy yourself and your mind as much as possible. Social activities such as sports, volunteer work or discussion groups are often preferable to solitude during a time of strain.

6 Do not hold grudges or blame other people for your current problems. Even if you have been wronged in some way, a constant sense of frustrated hostility will accomplish nothing except further damage to your mental health.

7 Make a point of devoting some time every day to physical relaxation that temporarily frees your mind from its preoccupations. If you go for a walk, for instance, concentrate on what you see around you instead of thinking about your problems.

8 Apart from being more sociable and more physically active than usual, it is especially important to stick as closely as you can to your daily routine. At times of crisis a familiar pattern of regular meals and activities at specified hours can encourage a sense of security by providing an orderly outer environment.

9 To avoid taking your worries to bed with you, try not to think about them after 8 pm. You will probably sleep better if you can wind down a few hours before going to bed. Also, if you wake up during the night, you are more likely to be relaxed enough to go back to sleep if you were not occupied with problem-solving when you first fell asleep.

10 Learn to recognize a crisis, and do not be too proud to admit that you are overwhelmed by anxiety and can no longer manage on your own. Consult a physician sooner rather than later. Alternatively (or in addition), ask for help from a community mental health agency or a religious organization. You may find that when you talk about your problems and fears with an objective but sympathetic professional, your worries no longer seem insurmountable.

The effects of stress

Any substantial change in your routine, including changes for the better as well as changes for the worse, will make demands on mental and emotional resources. Research has shown that as stresses accumulate, an individual becomes increasingly susceptible to physical illness, mental and emotional problems and accidental injuries as well. Shown here are the parts of the body that are susceptible to stress-related diseases, though the exact cause-and-effect relationship is often unclear.

Brain
Many mental and emotional problems, among them anxiety and depression, may be triggered off by stress.

Hair
Some forms of baldness, among them alopecia areata, have been linked to high levels of stress.

Mouth
Certain mouth problems such as aphthous ulcers (mouth ulcers) and oral lichen planus often seem to crop up under stress.

Lungs
Asthmatics often find that their condition worsens when they are subjected to high levels of mental or emotional stress.

Heart
Attacks of angina and disturbances of heart rate and rhythm often occur at the same time as, or shortly after, a period of stress.

Muscles
Various minor muscular twitches and "nervous tics" become more noticeable when the individual is under stress, and the muscular tremor of Parkinson's disease is also more marked at such times.

Digestive tract
Diseases of the digestive tract that may be either caused or aggravated by stress include gastritis, stomach and duodenal ulcers, ulcerative colitis and irritable colon.

Reproductive organs
Stress-related problems in this part of the body include menstrual disorders such as absence of periods in women, and impotence and premature ejaculation in men.

Bladder
The bladders of many people react to stress by becoming "irritable."

Skin
Some people have outbreaks of skin problems such as eczema and psoriasis when subjected to abnormal stress.

Pulse rate during the day
The graph on the right shows how a person's pulse rate may vary throughout a varied day. Each peak, whether it is caused by physical or mental stress, places increased demands on the heart, blood vessels, and other body organs. In some cases, such as playing a game of racquetball, the increase in pulse rate is linked to healthy physical exercise. In other cases, such as driving through rush-hour traffic, or making an important telephone call, external events help increase stress.

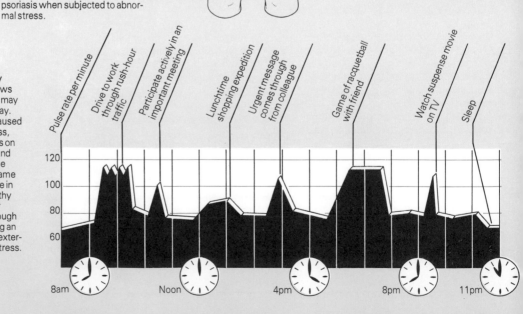

Pulse rate per minute

Drive to work through rush-hour traffic

Participate actively in an important meeting

Lunchtime shopping expedition

Urgent message comes through from colleague

Game of racquetball with friend

Watch suspense movie on TV

Sleep

120
100
80
60

8am   Noon   4pm   8pm   11pm

Are you under too much stress?

To assess the current level of stress in your life, answer the following questions and add up the number of points indicated for each YES answer.

Note: The words "wife" and "husband" apply to any partner, providing the relationship is close and has lasted for some time.

During the past six months:

1 Has your wife or husband died?
20 points

2 Have you become divorced or separated from your partner?
15 points

3 Has a close relative (other than husband or wife) died?
13 points

4 Have you been hospitalized because of injury or illness?
11 points

5 Have you married or had a reconciliation with your husband or wife after a separation?
10 points

6 Have you found out you are soon to become a parent?
9 points

7 Has there been a major change, whether for better or worse, in the health of a close member of your family?
9 points

8 Have you lost your job or retired?
9 points

9 Are you experiencing any sexual difficulties?
8 points

10 Has a new member been born or married into your immediate family?
8 points

11 Has a close friend died?
8 points

12 Have your finances become markedly better or worse?
8 points

13 Have you changed your job?
8 points

14 Have any of your children moved out of the family home or started or finished school?
8 points

15 Is trouble with in-laws causing tension within your family?
6 points

16 Is there anyone at home or at work whom you dislike strongly?
6 points

17 Do you frequently have premenstrual tension?
6 points

18 Have you had an important personal success, such as a rapid promotion at work?
6 points

19 Have you had "jet lag" (travel fatigue) at least twice?
6 points

20 Has there been a major domestic upheaval such as a move or extensive remodeling of your house (though not a change in family relationships)?
5 points

21 Have you had problems at work that may be putting your job at risk?
5 points

22 Have you taken on a substantial debt or mortgage?
3 points

23 Have you had a minor brush with the law, such as being ticketed for a traffic violation?
2 points

EVALUATION

The higher your total score, the more stressful your life. As a general guide, a score of under 30 suggests that you are not very likely to have a stress-related illness or accidental injury now or in the near future. If your score is 60 or more, the pressures on you are substantial. This means you are at a higher risk from one or more stress-related problems as described on the previous page.

Eating and drinking sensibly

If you eat a balanced diet – if, in other words, you do not eat too much or too little of certain kinds of food, or miss out on essential vitamins and other essential food elements – you are obeying the first rule of sensible eating. Too many people, however, tend to disregard the second rule, which is: Do not eat more than you need. All other factors being equal, a balanced but just adequate diet helps to promote good health.

The following articles explain which foods contain which nutrients, and provide guidelines you can follow to maintain a balanced diet that will help keep your body working efficiently.

Are you eating and drinking sensibly?

This questionnaire tests the prudence of your current eating and drinking habits. For a questionnaire that deals specifically with drinking alcohol, read Are you drinking too much alcohol? (see p.32).

Answer YES or NO to the following questions

1 Is your weight within the normal range for your height (see the weight chart on p.28)?
YES ☐　NO ☐

2 Do you generally have two or three medium-sized meals a day rather than occasional snacks and one big meal?
YES ☐　NO ☐

3 Do you make a point of setting aside specific times for leisurely meals instead of eating hastily while continuing your other activities?
YES ☐　NO ☐

4 Do you limit your use of fats and use mainly polyunsaturated cooking oil and margarine?
YES ☐　NO ☐

5 Do you eat fried foods sparingly, and limit yourself to no more than three or four helpings of fried food a week?
YES ☐　NO ☐

6 Do you eat no more than four eggs a week?
YES ☐　NO ☐

7 Do you drink, on average, several glasses of water or skim milk each day?
YES ☐　NO ☐

8 Do you have a generous portion of at least two high-fiber foods every day?
YES ☐　NO ☐

9 Do you often choose to eat fish or poultry rather than red or fatty meats such as beef or pork?
YES ☐　NO ☐

10 For between-meal snacks and desserts do you eat fresh fruit rather than cakes, pies and cookies?
YES ☐　NO ☐

11 Do you avoid lavish use of salty foods such as pickles, pretzels and potato chips?
YES ☐　NO ☐

12 Do you limit your use of salt and always taste foods before salting them?
YES ☐　NO ☐

13 Do you drink tea or coffee without sugar, and do you avoid sweet soft drinks?
YES ☐　NO ☐

14 Do you limit your intake of coffee to five cups a day?
YES ☐　NO ☐

EVALUATION
The more YES answers you gave, the healthier your diet and the more sensible your eating habits. The following pages explain why. The more NO answers you gave, the more important it is that you consider a change in your eating habits.

The components of a healthy diet

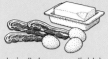

A healthy diet contains adequate quantities of six groups of substances: proteins, carbohydrates and fats, all of which contain calories (that is, produce energy); and fibers (roughage), vitamins and minerals, which, though they are essential, do not contain calories. In addition, you need water, without which life is impossible. A human being deprived of both food and drink usually can survive for only four or five days, but can live for up to two months on liquids alone.

To see the part that each of these dietary components plays in keeping your body alive and healthy, see the accompanying material.

Proteins

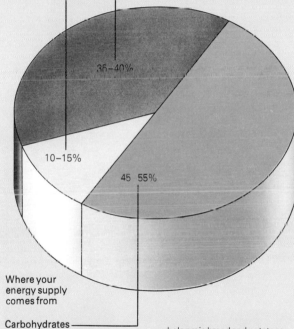

Where your energy supply comes from

Carbohydrates

Proteins

Proteins are the chemical compounds that form the basis of the structural framework of living matter. You need a regular daily intake of protein for the repair, replacement and growth of body tissues. Animal proteins (meat, fish, eggs, cheese) can provide much essential protein in the form your body needs. A wide variety of vegetable proteins is also necessary. These are found most abundantly in peas, beans and other legumes, but also are present in grains, and therefore in bread. A lack of variety in the diet can cause malnutrition in strict vegetarians. Also, protein adds taste and interest to meals. It is satisfying, yet not bulky. If you eat more of it than your body needs, the rest provides extra energy or is converted to fat and stored.

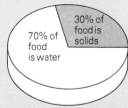

Water
Your body is approximately half water. You lose about 2 liters (up to 4 pints) every day in breathed-out moisture, urine, bowel movements and sweat. The lost fluid must be replaced. Since about 70 per cent of most foods is water, you do not need to drink 2 liters of liquid to replace what is lost.

These are chemicals that contain carbon, hydrogen and oxygen. All the foods that we think of as being either "starchy" or "sugary" contain a high proportion of carbohydrates. Some examples are sugar, bread, biscuits, pasta, potatoes and cereals. These foods are good sources of energy, and some are useful because they contribute other elements of a balanced diet. For example,

Fats
Fats (technically known as lipids) are found in plant foods such as olives and peanuts as well as in animals. Fats provide energy, and minute quantities are also used for growth and repair. In addition, they make food more palatable and filling. Excess fat is laid down in the body as fatty tissue. Though it may have some insulating properties, this fat can cause serious health problems (see Obesity, p.492).

Depending on chemical composition, fats are either *saturated* or *unsaturated*—a distinction that matters chiefly in that saturated whole grain bread and potatoes contain fiber, cereals contain protein, and whole grain bread is a good source of iron.

Sugar, however, is not an especially valuable dietary ingredient even though it is a quick producer of energy. Most overweight people take in too many calories, often in the form of sugar or high-sugar foods. Moreover, sugar encourages tooth decay. It is not an essential source of energy, since other, more nutritionally useful carbohydrates, and also proteins and fats, can produce energy. In a balanced reducing diet, a lack of sugar can force the body to use up stored fat for energy without depriving it of essential foods.

fats are thought to increase the amount of *cholesterol* (see p.27) in the blood. Animal fats, especially those in milk, butter, cheese and meat, are mostly highly saturated, and an excess intake of such foods may be partly responsible for the development of *atheroma*, which causes atherosclerosis (see p.372). The fat in fish, chicken, turkey and most vegetable oils is largely unsaturated. In chicken and turkey most of the fat is in the skin, which you need not eat. From the standpoint of health the best fats are *polyunsaturated*.

Vitamins and minerals
Vitamins are chemicals, usually complex ones. Your body cannot make vitamins, but it requires them to function well. There are many types of vitamins, but anyone who eats a reasonably balanced diet is virtually certain to get them all (for fuller information see Vitamin deficiency, p.494).

The minerals needed in a healthy diet are mostly metals and salts such as iron, phosphorus, calcium and sodium chloride (table salt). Like vitamins, they are needed only in minute quantities, and you are unlikely to have a mineral deficiency if you eat a fairly well-balanced diet. In the case of salt, however, too much can be bad for you, especially if you have high blood pressure (see p.382). You may be surprised at how easily you can adapt to eating food that has not been salted, either during cooking or at the table.

Fiber (roughage)
The human digestive tract is unable to digest fiber, or plant materials such as cellulose and pectin that are found in unrefined flour, cereals, fruit, leafy vegetables, and legumes such as lentils. Fiber is, however, of great importance to your diet. It provides bulk to help the large intestine efficiently carry away body wastes, and it may also help prevent diverticular disease (see p.479) and cancer of the large intestine (see p.481). Some physicians believe that because fiber affects the way the body uses fats, a high-fiber diet may even help to reduce the development of *atheroma* by lowering the levels of fats (including cholesterol) in the blood.

What is a balanced diet?

Failure to eat sensibly does not stem from eating the "wrong" foods, but from eating too much of one particular ingredient or not enough of another. If you consume a variety of food, and most people do so automatically, you are probably getting the essential nutrients. On the other hand, if you subsist on only a few foods, your health may suffer.

Surplus energy from too much fatty or sugary food is stored in the body as fat and can become a serious health problem (see Obesity, p.492). A balanced diet should give you all the nutrients and energy you need, but no more. Here are some pointers to help you maintain a balanced diet.

1. Eat meat no more than once a day. Fish and poultry are less fattening than red meat, sausages and processed meats.

2. Bake or broil food rather than frying it. If you do fry, use *polyunsaturated* oils (such as corn oil) rather than butter, lard or saturated margarines.

3. Cut down on salt and other sodium-containing substances such as meat tenderizers (monosodium glutamate or MSG). Do not salt your food without tasting it first. You may be surprised at how easy it is to reduce the amount of sodium in your diet.

4. Get your daily quota of fiber by eating plenty of leafy vegetables and fruit. Eat them raw or lightly cooked, because prolonged cooking destroys essential vitamins. Another good source of fiber is potato skins. A food does not have to have a tough or stringy texture in order to contain fiber.

5. Do not eat more than a total of four eggs a week. Although they are low in saturated fats, eggs have a very high cholesterol content.

6. For dessert or a snack choose fresh fruit (without cream) rather than cookies, cakes or puddings.

Finally, remember that the saying "everything in moderation" has a great deal of merit. Too much of anything, whether it be the number of calories you consume or a certain kind of food, is unwise. A balanced diet taken in moderation along with adequate exercise cannot guarantee good health, but it is a big help in maintaining your health.

A moderate but balanced day's eating

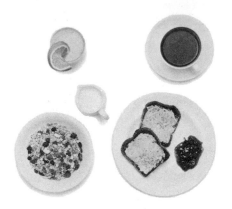

Breakfast
Whole grain cereal with milk (high fiber and vitamins); natural orange juice (high vitamins); 2 slices whole grain toast with low-fat margarine and marmalade (medium protein, high carbohydrate and fiber); coffee, tea, skim milk or water.

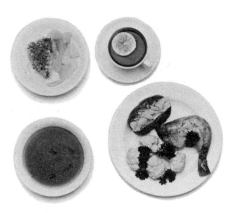

Midday meal
Clear soup (medium carbohydrate); roast chicken (high protein, medium fat); baked potato (high carbohydrate, medium fiber and vitamins); cauliflower (high fiber); apple crumble and custard (medium carbohydrate, fat and fiber); coffee, tea, skim milk or water.

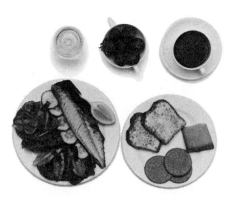

Evening meal
Boiled fish (high protein, medium fat); green salad (medium fiber and vitamins); 2 slices whole grain bread with low-fat margarine (medium protein and carbohydrate); fresh raspberries (medium fiber and vitamins); cheese and whole grain crackers (high protein, medium fat and fiber); glass of white wine; coffee, tea, skim milk or water.

Cholesterol

Cholesterol, a *steroid* chemical, is present in certain foods; mainly, though not exclusively, fatty foods. Small amounts of cholesterol are essential for making and maintaining nerve cells and for synthesizing natural hormones. But you do not have to eat cholesterol-rich foods such as fatty meat and dairy products in order to have your daily quota of the substance. Your liver can utilize other foods to manufacture all the cholesterol you need. If you cut all cholesterol-rich foods out of your diet, you could lower the cholesterol content of your blood by about 15 per cent. That 15 per cent, however, might make all the difference between the healthy functioning of your system and the development of a life-threatening disorder. High cholesterol levels in the blood may lead to a narrowing of the arteries as a result of the formation of large deposits of *atheroma*, a type of fatty tissue, in arteries (see Atherosclerosis, p.372). So if you include only small quantities of saturated fats and other high-cholesterol foods such as eggs in your normal diet, you may significantly lower your blood cholesterol level, and also lower your risk of atherosclerosis.

Counting calories

A calorie is a measurement of energy. If you burn a piece of coal, you can measure the resultant energy (released as heat) in calories. Similarly, your body burns a given quantity of food to release a certain number of calories. The three basic dietary components – proteins, carbohydrates and fats – produce varying amounts of energy. Weight for weight, protein-rich foods have fewer calories than carbohydrate-rich foods, and have far fewer calories than fats.

Note that "calorie" spelled with a small "c" specifies a relatively small unit of energy. A Calorie (with a capital "C") is equal to 1,000 calories (with a small "c"). Most articles about diet (including the ones in this book) speak in terms of large Calories rather than small calories. Thus, when we say that there are 10 Calories in a few lettuce leaves, we mean that the lettuce contains 10,000 calories. The number of Calories you need depends largely on how physically active you are (some examples of average daily requirements are shown to the right). You will probably gain weight each day if you have a few hundred Calories more than your average requirements, unless you move on to a job that involves more physical exertion or take up an activity that burns up more Calories. If you are in the later stages of pregnancy or are a breast-feeding mother, you may need up to an extra 800 Calories each day to feed your growing baby.

A few people are able to eat more than their daily energy (calorie) requirement without putting on weight. This is because their bodies are somehow able to burn up the extra calories without putting the excess energy to specific use. As you get older, you may find that it becomes harder to keep your weight down even when your calorie intake remains theoretically "correct" (see Age and increasing weight, p.29). The ability to gain or lose weight depends, at least partly, on factors that are more difficult to measure than the number of Calories you eat.

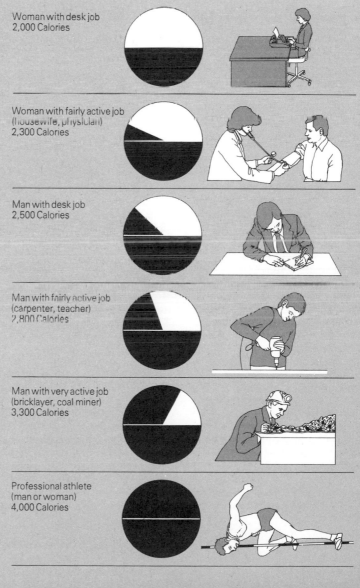

Woman with desk job
2,000 Calories

Woman with fairly active job
(housewife, physician)
2,300 Calories

Man with desk job
2,500 Calories

Man with fairly active job
(carpenter, teacher)
2,800 Calories

Man with very active job
(bricklayer, coal miner)
3,300 Calories

Professional athlete
(man or woman)
4,000 Calories

How to lose weight

Fat ordinarily accounts for about 10 to 20 per cent of the weight of an adult male, and about 25 per cent of the weight of a female. Any more than this is unnecessary and unhealthy. The weight chart below shows the "desirable" weight range for someone of your height. Ideally, your weight should remain roughly constant after the age of 25. Most people do gain a little as they grow older, and reach their heaviest weight at about 50, but there is no obvious physiological reason for this. It is usually due to a combination of a less active life style and an over-adequate diet (see Age and increasing weight, next page).

If you are in the "overweight" category on the weight chart, you should read the article on obesity (see p.492). If you are not convinced that you are unhealthily fat, take a critical look at yourself naked in front of a full-length mirror, and jump up and down. If you are seriously overweight, accumulated fat will shake noticeably. Are you still unconvinced? Try pinching a fold of skin from your stomach, just above your navel. If the fold is more than about 25 mm (1 in) thick, examine your diet now!

Fat-fold thickness
The most telling site to measure the thickness of a fold of fat for both men and women is the stomach. If the fold is thicker than about 25 mm (1 in), then you are probably overweight.

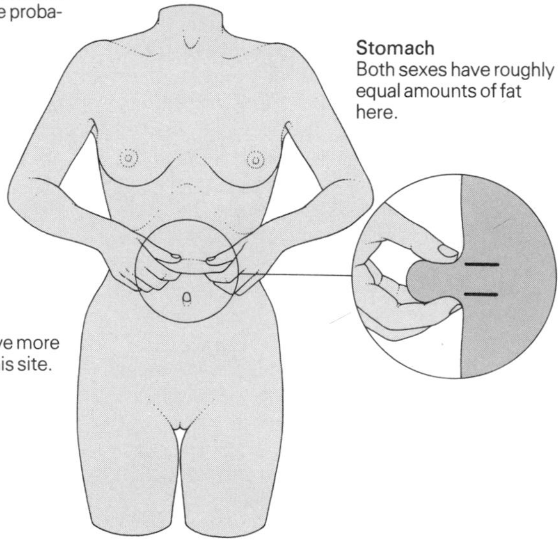

Upper arm
Women usually have more fat than men at this site.

Thigh
Most women have more fat than men at this site.

Stomach
Both sexes have roughly equal amounts of fat here.

Weight chart
To check your actual weight against the acceptable weight range for your height and sex, first find your height under the appropriate sex on the chart. Then look at the range for your height. If you weigh more than the highest figure in the range, you are more susceptible than thinner people to coronary artery disease, diabetes, osteoarthritis and many other disorders. If you weigh less than the lowest figure, you may be seriously underweight. This too may be cause for concern, so consult your physician.

Height (ft, in. without shoes)	MEN Acceptable weight (lbs. without clothing)	WOMEN Acceptable weight (lbs. without clothing)
4 10		92 — 119
4 11		94 — 122
5 0		96 — 125
5 1		99 — 128
5 2	112 — 141	102 — 131
5 3	115 — 144	105 — 134
5 4	118 — 148	108 — 138
5 5	121 — 152	111 — 142
5 6	124 — 156	114 — 146
5 7	128 — 161	118 — 150
5 8	132 — 166	122 — 154
5 9	136 — 170	126 — 158
5 10	140 — 174	130 — 163
5 11	144 — 179	134 — 168
6 0	148 — 184	138 — 173
6 1	152 — 189	
6 2	156 — 194	
6 3	160 — 199	
6 4	164 — 204	

The step-by-step diet

This diet is not designed to bring quick, dramatic results. It is suitable for people who simply want to remain healthily slim as well as for those who want to lose weight. The goal is to help you lose weight slowly but steadily, modifying your diet so that once you have reached a desirable weight, you can keep it fairly constant.

Fattening foods and drinks are those that, weight for weight, are the highest in calories and yet have the least nutritional value. The "step-by-step" reducing diet is based on the principle that the surest way to lose weight is to limit your intake of such foods while eating virtually all you want of non-fattening foods that you like. Foods listed in group 1 are mainly sweet or rich in fats, and can easily add on weight. Those in group 2, though they are also fattening if eaten in quantity, provide more bulk and contain more of the essential ingredients of a nourishing diet. Group 3 is a selection of foods that contain comparatively few calories, yet provide hunger-satisfying bulk along with a variety of useful nutrients. Proceed as follows:

Step 1 Cut out (or cut down on) all foods listed in group 1. In addition, limit your daily intake of alcoholic beverages to no more than one beer (or the equivalent in wine or spirits – see How much alcohol is in your favorite drink?, p.35). Eat normal portions of any food from groups 2 and 3. If you feel hungry at any time, satisfy your hunger with something from group 3 rather than group 2.

Step 2 If you have not lost any weight after two weeks, stop having any group 1 foods that you have continued to eat, and reduce your consumption of alcohol. Cut your helpings of group 2 foods in half. Eat as much as you want of group 3 foods.

Step 3 If you still fail to lose weight after two more weeks, halve your helpings of group 3 foods, and eat as little as you can of the things listed in group 2.

This program permits you to enjoy varied, flexible and pleasant meals while you are on a reducing diet. When you have reached your desired weight, you can either remain on the same diet or gradually modify it. If you find yourself putting on weight again, you should then be able to pinpoint foods that add weight and cut back on them. Follow these dieting steps and choose foods that you like, but also be sure to maintain a balanced diet as outlined on p.26.

MEAT	VEGETABLES	DAIRY FOODS	FISH	OTHER
Group 1 foods				
Visible fat on any meat Bacon Duck, goose Sausages, salami Pates		Butter Cream Ice cream		Thick gravies or sauces Sugar and chocolates Cakes, pies, pastries, cookies Puddings, custards Dried fruits Nuts Jams, honey, syrups Canned fruits in syrup
Group 2 foods				
Lean beef, lamb, pork	Beans	Eggs Cheese (other than cottage cheese) Whole milk	Oily fish such as herring, mackerel, sardines and tuna packed in oil	Pasta Rice Thick soups Bread and crackers Cereals (unsweetened) Margarine Polyunsaturated vegetable oils
Group 3 foods				
Poultry (not including the skin) other than duck or goose Veal, liver, soy meat extenders	Potatoes Vegetables (raw or lightly cooked) Clear or vegetarian soups	Skim milk Yogurt Cottage cheese	Non-oily fish such as cod, haddock and salmon canned in water Shellfish such as shrimp, crab	Bran Fresh fruit Unsweetened fruit juice

Age and increasing weight

As you grow older, your body seems to need less energy, partly because you become less active, and partly for other reasons not yet clear. But many people do not reduce their food intake to correspond with their decreasing energy requirements. In addition, some people drink more alcohol than they did when younger, and alcoholic drinks contain calories in abundance. The end result is a calorie surplus that shows up as increasing deposits of fat as you age. The gray area in the graph shows how excess calories mount up, causing many people to gain weight over the years.

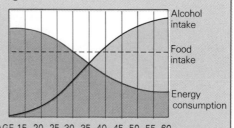

Mealtimes

If you lead a busy life and are short of time, you may find that you are eating a full meal only about once a day. From the standpoint of health this is a bad practice. You would be treating your body with more consideration if you had several small meals instead of a single big one. A given amount of food is used more efficiently by the body if it is spaced throughout the day rather than eaten at one sitting. People who have large, infrequent meals tend to gain more weight and to have a higher level of fat in the blood than do those who eat smaller quantities (but the same total) at regular intervals. Frequent small meals also help prevent peptic ulcers. And because they play a part in keeping blood sugar at a fairly constant level, they prevent hunger from making you tired and irritable. Many people who feel edgy for no evident reason simply are hungry without knowing it.

Sit down and relax at mealtimes. If you eat absent-mindedly while doing something else, whether working or watching television, you are likely to eat more than you realize. Take time to thoroughly chew and savor your food; time aids the digestive process. Finish off each meal with fruit such as an apple – or better still, a piece of cheese – rather than sweet puddings. Apples are not quite as good as cheese; they are slightly acidic, contain sugar, and bits of the fruit tend to get stuck between the teeth. All of this predisposes you to tooth decay. Finally, be sure to clean your teeth thoroughly after eating.

Caffeine

Caffeine, a drug found in coffee, tea, cocoa and certain soft drinks such as cola, stimulates your central nervous system and makes you feel more energetic. It also increases urination. Although the effects of the drug vary from person to person, one or two cups of either tea or coffee will generally be enough to produce the stimulant effect. Very large doses of caffeine – 1,000 mgs (about 1/30 oz) or more – can lead to restlessness, sleeplessness, trembling, palpitations and diarrhea. Such symptoms are apt to occur in people who drink more than about five cups of strong black coffee in a single day. An average sized cup of coffee contains about 100 mg of caffeine. Weak, milky or instant coffee contains less caffeine. There is much less in tea and cocoa, and even less in cola beverages. You should try to keep your average consumption below five cups of coffee daily.

Although habitual tea or coffee drinkers may become emotionally dependent on the drug, actual addiction (physical dependence, with withdrawal symptoms) seems to be rare (see Drug addiction, p.305). Emotional dependence is unlikely to become a major health problem. Still, it is worth remembering that there are no vitamins or minerals in coffee, tea or cola. Fruit juice and water are better alternatives.

Food hygiene

Poorly prepared, cooked or stored food is a health hazard because of the risk of food poisoning. Keep your food clean and free of infectious agents by following this advice:

1 Store food in clean, covered containers. To discourage infection keep foods either refrigerated or piping hot.

2 Minimize the need to reheat left-overs or pre-prepared foods. If you must re-heat something, make sure it is thoroughly cooked before serving it.

3 Make sure you and your family always wash your hands (*not* in the kitchen sink) after using the toilet and before handling food.

4 Cover cuts and sores on your hands with a clean, waterproof dressing, or wear gloves, when preparing food.

5 Clean working surfaces with hot, soapy water before placing unwrapped food on them.

6 Rinse dishes before actually washing them. Use hot, soapy water and *clean* dishcloths for washing. Rinse off soap with hot water and dry with a clean towel.

7 Keep lids on garbage cans, and empty and clean them regularly.

8 Do not keep cream cakes, custards and other milky foods, even when refrigerated, for longer than 48 hours.

9 Let frozen food thaw out in the refrigerator before cooking it, and then do not refreeze it.

10 Cook poultry thoroughly, especially if you are cooking a pre-frozen bird.

Calorie index

The following table shows a sampling of approximate Calorie values of some foods. If you are trying to lose weight by counting Calories, you will need a more complete index, but this one can give you a rough idea of how foods compare to each other. Simply look up each food you eat, note the number of Calories it contains, and total the Calories for a day's meals. Be sure to include each pat of butter and spoonful of sugar; they can make a difference!

Food or drink	Amount	Calories
Almonds	25 g (2 tbsp)	150
Apple	25 g (small)	40
Apple juice	240 ml (8 oz)	125
Apple pie	240 g (⅙ of medium pie)	400
Apricot	100 g (4, canned)	100
Asparagus	150 g (6 spears, boiled)	15
Avocado	120 g (½ pear)	250
Bacon (middle cut)	50 g (2 rashers, fried)	225
Banana	150 g (average)	65
Beans (baked)	100 g (4 tbsp, canned)	60
Beans (green)	100 g (4 tbsp, boiled)	20
Beef (lean)	100 g (4 thin slices, roast)	210
Beef (steak)	240 g (average, broiled)	400
Beef (steak)	240 g (average, fried)	500
Beer	360 ml (12 oz)	170
Bran	10 g (1 tbsp)	15
Bread (white)	25 g (small slice)	60
Bread (whole grain)	25 g (small slice)	55
Broccoli	100 g (medium stalk)	20
Butter	5 g (pat)	35
Cabbage	100 g (4 tbsp, boiled)	15
Carrots	100 g (4 tbsp, boiled)	20
Candied peel	25 g (1 tbsp)	80
Cauliflower	100 g (4 tbsp)	10
Celery	25 g (5 cm or 2 inch stalk)	2
Cheese (cheddar)	25 g (25 mm or 1 inch cube)	100
Cheese (cottage)	120 g (4 oz serving)	100
Cheesecake	100 g (small serving)	400
Cherries (canned in syrup)	100 g (3½ oz serving)	100
Chicken	100 g (drumstick, broiled)	140
Chocolate cake	100 g (small portion)	300
Chocolate candy	28 g (1 oz)	152
Chocolate malt	240 ml (8 oz)	500
Cocoa (milk and sugar)	170 ml (5½ oz cup)	155
Cod	200 g (fillet, steamed)	155
Coffee (black, no sugar)	170 ml (5½ oz cup)	0
Cola soft drink	360 ml (12 oz)	160
Cooking oil	14 g (1 tbsp)	126
Corn (canned)	100 g (4 tbsp)	70
Corn (on cob)	100 g (4 inch ear)	100
Crab	100 g (small, dressed)	100
Cream	25 g (1 tbsp)	60
Cream (sour)	25 g (1 tbsp)	45
Croissant	75 g (average)	260
Cucumber	50 g (25 mm or 1 inch slice)	5
Doughnut (plain)	100 g (average)	150
Duck	120 g (breast, roasted)	380
Egg	54 g (large, raw)	88
Egg, fried	50 g (medium)	108
Egg white	31 g (medium)	16
Egg yolk	17 g (medium)	60
Flour (white)	25 g (1 tbsp)	85
Grapes	25 g (5)	10
Ham	90 g (3 slices, boiled)	230
Hamburger	120 g (large, broiled)	300
Herring	150 g (fillet, fried)	330
Honey	5 g (1 tsp)	15
Hot dog	50 g (average)	124
Ice cream	60 g (average scoop)	100
Jam or jelly	5 g (1 tsp)	60
Lamb chop	100 g (3½ oz, broiled)	350
Lemon	100 g (average)	30
Lettuce	5 g (1 leaf)	5
Mackerel	200 g (small, fried)	380
Margarine	5 g (pat)	35
Melon	200 g (slice)	25
Milk (whole)	200 ml (6½ oz glass)	130
Milk (skim)	200 ml (6½ oz glass)	70
Muffin, English	(large)	280
Mushroom	25 g (large)	5
Oats (rolled)	25 g (1 tbsp)	105
Olives (with pits)	25 g (8 small)	25
Onion	150 g (medium)	40
Orange	150 g (medium)	60
Orange juice (fresh)	200 ml (6½ oz glass)	100
Pancakes	100 g (3½ oz serving)	225
Pasta	25 g (1 tbsp)	10
Pate	25 g (25 mm or 1 inch cube)	90
Peas (fresh)	100 g (4 tbsp, boiled)	55
Peas (canned)	100 g (4 tbsp, cooked)	70
Pear	150 g (average)	50
Peanuts (roasted, unsalted)	20 g (20 to 22 nuts)	114
Peanut butter	20 g (1 rounded tbsp)	115
Pepper (sweet)	100 g (small)	15
Pineapple (fresh)	100 g (slice)	40
Pineapple (canned in syrup)	100 g (slice with syrup)	75
Popcorn (no butter)	100 g	30
Pork chop	100 g (3½ oz, broiled)	357
Potato (boiled)	100 g (medium)	80
Potato (french fries)	50 g (10 large)	140
Potato chips	10 g (5–2 inch chips)	54
Potato (sweet)	100 g (medium, baked)	155
Raisins (seedless)	40 g (¼ cup)	116
Raspberries	100 g (4 tbsp)	25
Rice	25 g (1 tbsp)	100
Salami	25 g (4 slices)	130
Salmon (fresh)	150 g (serving, poached)	280
Salmon (canned in water)	100 g (3½ oz serving)	150
Sausages (pork)	25 g (small, broiled)	55
Shrimp	100 g (10, peeled, boiled)	95
Shrimp (french fried)	100 g (4 large, breaded, fried)	260
Spinach	100 g (4 tbsp, boiled)	35
Sugar (white)	5 g (1 tsp)	25
Tangerine (fresh)	75 g (average)	25
Tea (no sugar)	170 ml (5½ oz cup)	0
Tomato	25 g (small)	5
Trout	240 g (small, fried)	300
Tuna (canned in oil)	100 g (¾ cup)	300
Tuna (canned in water)	100 g (¾ cup)	160
Turkey	100 g (2 slices, roasted)	150
Veal cutlet	100 g (3½ oz)	275
Vinegar	25 g (2 tbsp)	1
Whiskey, bourbon	30 ml (1 oz)	85
Wine	140 ml (4½ oz glass)	125
Yogurt (low fat, plain)	244 g (8 oz)	122
Yogurt (low fat, fruit)	244 g (8 oz)	250

The dangers of alcohol

What is generally called "social" or "occasional" drinking is a habit in which millions of adults indulge. Moderate drinking, whether of beer, wine or cocktails, is not generally harmful to the health of adults, but it can evolve almost imperceptibly into excessive, damaging consumption of alcohol. Remember that alcohol is a drug, and any drug consumed in excess, or at the wrong time, can be harmful. Your answers to the questions below will help determine whether you are, or are in danger of becoming, dependent on alcohol. The next few pages look at the harm that excessive consumption of alcohol can cause to your body and mind. For information on alcohol addiction, read the article on Alcoholism (see p.304).

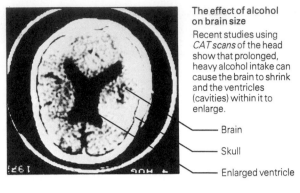

The effect of alcohol on brain size
Recent studies using *CAT scans* of the head show that prolonged, heavy alcohol intake can cause the brain to shrink and the ventricles (cavities) within it to enlarge.

— Brain

— Skull

— Enlarged ventricle

Are you drinking too much alcohol?

Answer YES or NO to the following questions

1 When you are holding an empty glass at a party, do you always actively look for a refill instead of waiting to be offered one?

YES ☐   NO ☐

2 If given the chance, do you frequently pour out a more generous drink for yourself than seems to be the "going" amount for others?

YES ☐   NO ☐

3 Do you often have a drink or two when you are alone, either at home or in a bar?

YES ☐   NO ☐

4 Is your drinking ever the direct cause of a family quarrel, or do quarrels often seem to occur, if only by coincidence, when you have had a drink or two?

YES ☐   NO ☐

5 Do you feel that you *must* have a drink at a specific time every day – right after work, for instance?

YES ☐   NO ☐

6 When worried or under unusual stress, do you almost automatically take a stiff drink to "settle your nerves"?

YES ☐   NO ☐

7 Are you untruthful about how much you have had to drink when questioned on the subject?

YES ☐   NO ☐

8 Does drinking ever cause you to take time off work, or to miss scheduled meetings or appointments?

YES ☐   NO ☐

9 Do you feel physically deprived if you cannot have at least one drink every day?

YES ☐   NO ☐

10 Do you sometimes crave a drink in the morning?

YES ☐   NO ☐

11 Do you sometimes have "mornings after" when you cannot remember what happened the night before?

YES ☐   NO ☐

EVALUATION
You should regard a YES answer to any one of the above questions as a warning sign. Do not increase your consumption of alcohol. Two YES answers suggest that you may already be becoming dependent on alcohol. Three or more YES answers indicate that you may have a serious drinking problem, and you should get professional help.

The effects of alcohol

The main effect of alcohol – and a major reason why many people enjoy moderate drinking – is a gradual dulling of the reactions of the brain and nervous system. One or two drinks act as a tranquilizer or relaxant. Even in small quantities alcohol is *not* a stimulant, as many people believe. However, alcohol sometimes causes a noticeable loss of inhibitions, and this may lead to an appearance of creativity or sometimes to actual aggressiveness. Temporarily, alcohol can make some drinkers feel unusually alert and witty, even if those around them do not see it that way.

Alcohol is also a *vasodilator*. The rush of blood into the skin from widened blood vessels can make it seem as if warmth is flowing into a chilled body. This is misleading. Alcohol is also a *diuretic*, which means that it causes increased urination.

Heavy drinking causes the level of sugar in the blood to fall rapidly. This may lead, a few hours after a drinking session, to hypo-

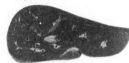
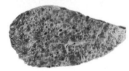

The effects of alcohol on the liver
A slice of healthy liver (upper photograph) shows a smooth, even texture. A slice of cirrhotic liver (lower photograph) shows a diseased organ riddled with non-functioning scar tissue.

glycemia (see p.522), in which the drinker feels weak, dizzy, confused and abnormally hungry. (If this happens to you, eat or drink something sweet.) Drinking tends to increase sexual desire, but it also decreases a man's ability to maintain an erection, possibly because the drug dulls the nerves that control erection and ejaculation. Some of the major alcohol-related diseases are shown below.

Although alcoholic drinks contain plenty of calories in the form of carbohydrates, they have no other nutritional value. This is why even overweight heavy drinkers may develop symptoms of nutritional deficiency (see Vitamin deficiency, p.494).

Finally, regular, heavy drinking leads almost inevitably to problems at work, with your family and with the law. Alcohol is an important factor in roughly half of all automobile accidents. If you drink and drive, you risk doing serious injury both to yourself and to others.

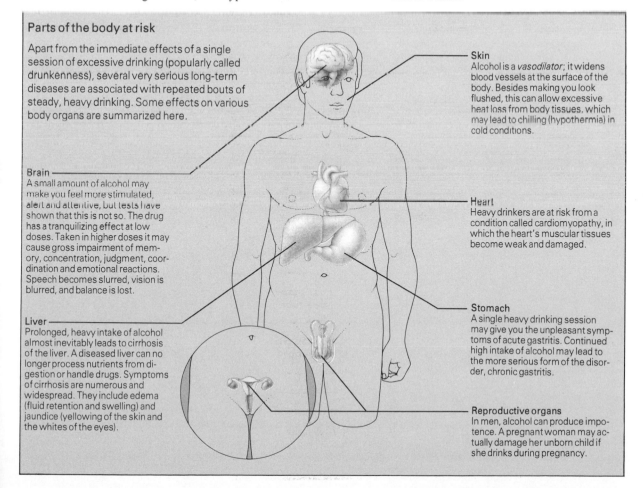

Parts of the body at risk

Apart from the immediate effects of a single session of excessive drinking (popularly called drunkenness), several very serious long-term diseases are associated with repeated bouts of steady, heavy drinking. Some effects on various body organs are summarized here.

Skin
Alcohol is a *vasodilator*; it widens blood vessels at the surface of the body. Besides making you look flushed, this can allow excessive heat loss from body tissues, which may lead to chilling (hypothermia) in cold conditions.

Brain
A small amount of alcohol may make you feel more stimulated, alert and attentive, but tests have shown that this is not so. The drug has a tranquilizing effect at low doses. Taken in higher doses it may cause gross impairment of memory, concentration, judgment, coordination and emotional reactions. Speech becomes slurred, vision is blurred, and balance is lost.

Heart
Heavy drinkers are at risk from a condition called cardiomyopathy, in which the heart's muscular tissues become weak and damaged.

Stomach
A single heavy drinking session may give you the unpleasant symptoms of acute gastritis. Continued high intake of alcohol may lead to the more serious form of the disorder, chronic gastritis.

Liver
Prolonged, heavy intake of alcohol almost inevitably leads to cirrhosis of the liver. A diseased liver can no longer process nutrients from digestion or handle drugs. Symptoms of cirrhosis are numerous and widespread. They include edema (fluid retention and swelling) and jaundice (yellowing of the skin and the whites of the eyes).

Reproductive organs
In men, alcohol can produce impotence. A pregnant woman may actually damage her unborn child if she drinks during pregnancy.

How much is too much?

The real question is, how much is too much *for you?* The effect that alcohol has on the body and mind depends on its concentration in the blood. The drug is absorbed into the blood from the digestive system and remains in the blood until it is broken down by the liver or excreted in the urine. The rate at which the alcohol level in the blood falls is fairly constant. It follows that, whatever the circumstances and however long it may take for you to be affected, once you have reached a certain blood-alcohol peak it will take the drug about the same time to leave your system as it takes to leave the system of someone who is affected more slowly or more quickly than you. However, the rate at which the alcohol level in the blood rises is variable, depending on the circumstances. So if you want to prevent the amount of alcohol in your blood from rising too high, do your drinking with the following factors in mind.

Body size Because there is more blood in a large person than in a small person, the concentration of alcohol in a larger person's blood tends to rise more slowly and to reach lower levels overall when the same amounts of alcohol are consumed.

Eating while drinking Food in the stomach and intestines slows the rate at which alcohol is absorbed into the bloodstream. If you eat while drinking (or "line your stomach" with food before going to a party), you temporarily slow down the absorption of alcohol. Of course, you also consume more calories.

Type of drink and speed of drinking The more slowly you drink, the less drastic the effects. If you drink whiskey, the high alcohol content produces a high concentration of alcohol in your blood more quickly than does beer. If you gulp down a shot of whiskey, the alcohol is quickly absorbed into your system. If you slowly sip a stein of beer, much of the alcoholic content may have dissipated by the time you have emptied your glass.

Physical tolerance Regular doses of alcohol induce a gradual "acclimatization" to a substantial quantity in the blood. The brain gets "used to" being bathed in alcohol. As a result, if you have drunk heavily for years, you may be able to look normal and behave in an apparently normal fashion even though your blood level would make a less hardened drinker seem drunk. Appearances are, however, deceptive. Heavy drinkers may talk plausibly and coherently, but their ability to drive a car will still be impaired and damage to the brain and body continues.

An unfortunate result of increased tolerance is that you can come to be dependent on having a concentration of alcohol in your blood. Also, you gradually need greater and greater amounts of the drug to give you whatever effects you require from drinking. In some people this dependence degenerates into addiction (see Alcoholism, p.304).

Another point to remember is that the level of alcohol in the blood is cumulative over time (see The cumulative effects of a day's drinking, below).

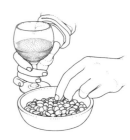

Eating while drinking
Consuming food, even snacks at a party, helps slow the rate of alcohol absorption, so the level in the blood rises more slowly and peaks at a lower level than if the digestive tract remained empty of food.

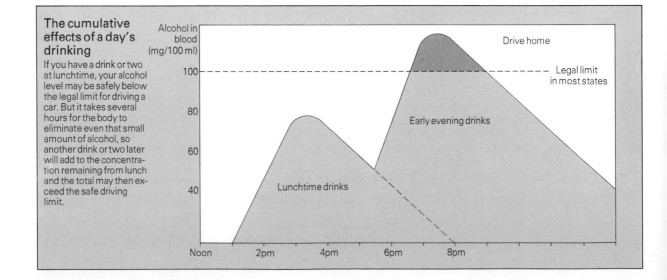

The cumulative effects of a day's drinking

If you have a drink or two at lunchtime, your alcohol level may be safely below the legal limit for driving a car. But it takes several hours to eliminate even that small amount of alcohol, so another drink or two later will add to the concentration remaining from lunch and the total may then exceed the safe driving limit.

Alcohol in blood (mg/100 ml)

Lunchtime drinks
Early evening drinks
Drive home
Legal limit in most states

100
80
60
40

Noon 2pm 4pm 6pm 8pm

How much alcohol is there in your favorite drink?

In its pure form alcohol is a colorless liquid too strong for the mouth and stomach to tolerate undiluted. There are many types of alcohol, but the type present in varying proportions in alcoholic drinks is known as ethyl alcohol or ethanol. Another common type is what chemists call methyl alcohol. It is sometimes called wood alcohol because it can be distilled from wood. This is a dangerous poison that should not be drunk. Shown below is a summary of the approximate alcohol content of various kinds of drinks. This will give you a rough guide to use in estimating your actual intake of alcohol.

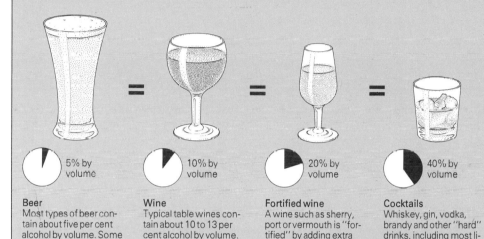

5% by volume

10% by volume

20% by volume

40% by volume

Beer
Most types of beer contain about five per cent alcohol by volume. Some so-called "real ales" are stronger and may contain up to eight or nine per cent.

Wine
Typical table wines contain about 10 to 13 per cent alcohol by volume. The alcohol content of a wine is not necessarily related to its taste or bouquet; a "powerful, full-bodied" vintage may be less alcoholic than a "light, fragrant" wine.

Fortified wine
A wine such as sherry, port or vermouth is "fortified" by adding extra quantities of alcohol. These wines may contain up to 20 per cent by volume.

Cocktails
Whiskey, gin, vodka, brandy and other "hard" drinks, including most liqueurs, contain from 40 to 50 per cent alcohol by volume.

Equivalent sizes
The size of the glass in which each of the various types of drink is conventionally served will naturally determine the quantity of alcohol in normal drinks at parties or in a bar. So although there is a much smaller proportion of alcohol in beer than in sherry, for example, a single glass of beer is ordinarily many times the size of a single glass of sherry. The following equivalents are based on typical sizes of drinks served in bars. The approximate alcohol content of a 12 oz glass of beer *equals* one glass of wine, which *equals* one glass of sherry, which *equals* one shot of whiskey.

Teenage drinking

In recent years, there has been an increase in the number of teenagers who drink alcohol, and some researchers report that as many as 27 per cent of teenagers misuse alcohol. This means that alcohol use affects their physical health; their school-work or job performance; their ability to deal with feelings such as anger, anxiety or depression; and/or their ability to relate to family and friends. A person who begins to drink at an early age may become so accustomed to having alcohol in his or her system that being "high" may seem normal. Alcohol dependence may follow. Teenagers are also apt to try using alcohol with other drugs, and this can be very dangerous. Instead of simply adding to the effects of other drugs, alcohol can multiply those effects and cause an overdose.

Another danger for teenagers who drink is the possibility of being in an accident. Alcohol use is related to more than half of traffic accidents and 90 per cent of boating accidents.

Use of alcohol is often part of a period of rebelliousness that is common in adolescence (see Psychological and behavioral problems of adolescence, p.712). It should not be ignored, because of the possible dangers. Some parents make the mistake of thinking that teenage use of alcohol is better than use of other drugs, perhaps because they drink themselves, or because alcohol can be obtained legally while other drugs cannot. Remember that alcohol *is* a drug, and that, like many other drugs, it is a poison when taken in excess. A good parental example and a clear understanding of the possibility of being involved in a serious or even fatal accident may help to discourage teenagers from drinking excessively. It is important to convince them that, if they do drink, they should not drive a car. It is also important to avoid riding in a car being driven by someone else who has been drinking.

If you think your teenager, or anyone else in your family, may have a drinking problem, consult your physician or contact the local chapter of Alcoholics Anonymous.

How to cut down your drinking

If you gave two or more YES answers on the questionnaire on p.32, you may be jeopardizing your health through excessive consumption of alcohol. Now is the time to start limiting your intake of alcohol. For many people who are determined to control the problem, it is not that hard to do. The first and most important step is to *want* to cut down. If you want to cut down but find you cannot, you had better accept the probability that drink is becoming a serious problem for you, and you should seek guidance from your physician or from an organization such as Alcoholics Anonymous. The next page gives some additional suggestions on how you can cut down your intake of alcohol.

Effects of alcohol at rising levels

Using results obtained from blood tests, and after observing the behavior of representative samples of people with alcohol in their blood, medical researchers have produced the following guide to the likely effects of various alcohol levels on an average individual. For the purposes of the guide, it is assumed that stated quantities are drunk by a person who weighs about 70 kg (154 lb). If you weigh less than this, you should modify the amount you drink accordingly.

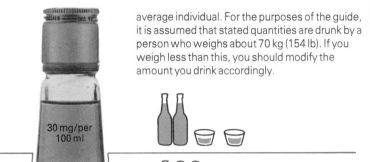
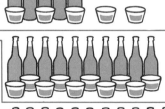
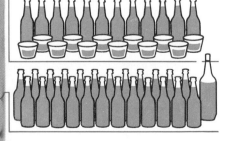

2 bottles of beer (2 shots of whiskey)
Effects may seem negligible, but judgement becomes slightly impaired and reactions slightly slowed.

30 mg/per 100 ml

3 bottles of beer (3 whiskies)
A feeling of cheerfulness and warmth; judgement is noticeably impaired as inhibitions start to disappear.

50 mg/per 100 ml

80 mg/per 100 ml

5 bottles of beer (5 whiskies)
At this level, the risk of having an accident is increased fourfold.

150 mg/per 100 ml

10 bottles of beer (10 whiskies)
Exuberance and aggressive tendencies magnified; impairments including slurred speech along with marked loss of self-control. Chances of an auto accident are 25 times greater than normal.

200 mg/per 100 ml

12 bottles of beer (12 whiskies)
Blurred or double vision, loss of balance, greatly impaired mental competence.

400 mg/per 100 ml

24 bottles of beer (¾ bottle whiskey)
Loss of consciousness.

600 mg/per 100 ml

1 bottle whiskey
Death from alcohol poisoning becomes increasingly probable.

Note: All drinks are consumed during a single drinking session (a few hours).

Blood alcohol level (approximate figures)

Set reasonable limits for yourself

Decide not to exceed a certain number of drinks on a given occasion, and stick to your decision. No more than two beers or two cocktails a day is a reasonable limit. You have proved to yourself that you can control your drinking if you set such a target and regularly do not exceed it.

Learn to say no

Many people have "just one more" drink because others in the group are having one or because someone puts pressure on them, not because they really want a drink. When you reach the sensible limit you have set for yourself, politely but firmly refuse to exceed it. If you are being the generous host, pour yourself a glass of water or juice "on the rocks." Nobody will notice the difference.

Drink slowly

Never gulp down a drink. Choose your drinks for their flavor, not their "kick," and savor the taste of each sip.

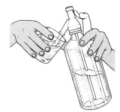

Dilute your drinks
Adding non-alcoholic liquid mixers to strong drinks is one way to decrease your alcohol intake.

Dilute your drinks

If you prefer cocktails to beer, try having long drinks. Instead of downing your gin or whiskey neat, or nearly so, drink it diluted with a mixer such as tonic, water or soda water, in a tall glass. That way, you can enjoy the flavor as well as the act of drinking, but it will take longer to finish each drink. Also, you can make your two-drink limit last all evening or switch to the mixer by itself.

Do not drink on your own

Make a point of confining your drinking to social gatherings. It is sometimes hard to resist the urge to pour yourself a relaxing drink at the end of a hard day, but many formerly heavy drinkers have found that a cup of coffee or a soft drink satisfies the need as well as alcohol did, and that it was just a habit. What may help you really to unwind, even with no drink at all, is a comfortable chair, loosened clothing, and perhaps a soothing record, a television program or a good book to read.

Hangovers and alcohol folklore

How bad you feel after an evening's drinking depends partly on your constitution, which you cannot greatly modify, but also on what and how much you have drunk. Most alcoholic drinks contain substances called congeners, which are added for color and flavor. It is the different congeners in different drinks that combine with the amount of alcohol to give a drinking bout its "hangover potential." Brandy, bourbon and red wines produce the worst hangovers. Gin and vodka contain few congeners and are therefore least likely to cause a hangover. With all drinks, smoking seems to contribute to the severity of the hangover.

When prevention fails, rest is the best cure. Because alcohol is a *diuretic* drug, and causes an increased rate of urination, you should try to compensate for the loss of body fluid by drinking as much water as you can after a drinking spree. And if you have a bad headache, take aspirin (or an aspirin substitute if your stomach is upset).

Alcohol folklore

There are a number of traditional beliefs associated with drinking, and many people tend to assume that they are true. Personal experience may have "proved" to you that the following familiar statements are true. But is there medical evidence for their validity?

1 "It is risky to mix your drinks (for instance, to have beer after whiskey or wine after gin)." There is no evidence that mixing drinks will do more damage to the system than sticking to one type. It does seem to be true, however, that a hangover is more likely when you mix drinks.

2 "Drinking black coffee sobers you up." This is only partly true. Any non-alcoholic liquid helps to counteract the diuretic effect of alcohol, and a mild stimulant such as coffee, which contains caffeine (see p.30), may compensate for the depressant effect of alcohol to some extent. In any event, the coffee is unlikely to do you any harm. But no drug can speed the rate at which alcohol is removed from the bloodstream.

3 "A hair of the dog that bit you eases a hangover." If you pour yourself a drink on the morning after a spree, it may make you feel better for two reasons. First, the additional liquid helps to reverse the *dehydrating* effects of alcohol, which is a contributing cause of the hangover. Second, the characteristic headache of a hangover may be due in part to the sudden change in the alcohol level in your body, and a morning-after drink can add just enough alcohol to make the change more gradual. But if you find that you are frequently forced to rely on this method of curing your hangovers, the hangovers themselves are probably withdrawal symptoms of alcohol addiction. This is a clear warning that you have a drinking problem and should seek help immediately.

4 "The best medicine for a badly chilled body is a stiff drink." This is false. Because alcohol is a *vasodilator*, a comfortable feeling of warmth does follow the rush of blood to the surface tissues of the body. But this diversion of blood from vital inner organs actually increases the risks of exposure, including chilling and its more serious consequence, hypothermia (see p.723).

The dangers of smoking

If you are a regular smoker, you are probably losing about $5\frac{1}{2}$ minutes of life expectancy for each cigarette you smoke. Up to age 65, people who smoke 20 or more cigarettes a day die at almost twice the rate for non-smokers in the same age group, according to government statistics. Yet, despite the vast medical evidence supporting such statistics, and the publicity given to them, most heavy smokers continue to smoke. And thousands of adolescents every year begin to smoke occasionally, often on the assumption that "everybody does." Research indicates that about 85 per cent of these occasional smokers eventually become regular, full-time smokers.

The following pages outline the health problems associated with smoking, discuss the dangerous substances contained in tobacco, and suggest ways that you can break the life-threatening habit.

How much is smoking affecting your health?

Smoking in any form is harmful, but the extent of the damage tobacco does to your body depends on several factors: whether you smoke pipes, cigars or cigarettes; the amount of smoke that you regularly take into your lungs; and the length of time you have been smoking. The numerical weight assigned to each YES answer in the questionnaire below roughly reflects the hazard to health presented by that particular facet of smoking.

If you used to be a smoker but have given up, your chances of having a tobacco-related disease diminish with each successive year. For an indication of where you now stand, see How your chances improve, p.41.

1 Do you smoke a pipe?
2 points

2 On average, do you smoke:
a) 1 to 4 cigars a day?
2 points
b) 5 to 9 cigars a day?
4 points
c) more than 10 cigars a day?
7 points

3 On average, do you smoke:
a) 1 to 9 cigarettes a day?
10 points
b) 10 to 19 cigarettes a day?
15 points
c) 20 to 39 cigarettes a day?
18 points
d) more than 39 cigarettes a day?
24 points

4 Have you been a regular smoker for:
a) less than 15 years?
2 points
b) 15 to 25 years?
7 points
c) 25 to 35 years?
9 points
d) more than 35 years?
13 points

5 If you smoke cigarettes, are they mostly "high tar" ones?
4 points

6 Do you smoke your cigarette or cigar right down to the butt?
7 points

7 Regardless of what or how much you smoke, do you usually inhale (breathe tobacco smoke into your lungs)?
10 points

EVALUATION
There is slight reason for concern if your total score in response to the above questions is under 10 points. Note, however, that if you smoke cigarettes you cannot possibly score less than 10. For a discussion of why cigarette smoking is the most harmful form, read Cigarettes vs cigars and pipes (see p.40). A score between 10 and 25 indicates that you are seriously jeopardizing your chances for health and long life. And remember that if you are relatively young and do not "kick" the habit, your score will rise quickly as time passes. If you already score over 25 points, you are in an extremely high-risk category. Remember, though, that however high your score, it is always worth giving up smoking. Your chances of getting a smoking-associated disease begin to diminish as soon as you stop.

Smoking can seriously damage your health

Tobacco contains at least three dangerous chemicals: tar, nicotine and carbon monoxide. Tar is a mixture of several substances that condense into a sticky substance in the lungs. Nicotine is an addictive drug that is absorbed from the lungs and acts mainly on the nervous system. And carbon monoxide lessens the ability of red blood cells to carry oxygen throughout the body.

Consider the average smoker, a person who smokes 15 to 20 cigarettes a day. Compared with non-smokers he or she is approximately 14 times more likely to die from cancer of the lung, throat or mouth; four times more likely to die from cancer of the esophagus; twice as likely to die from cancer of the bladder; and twice as likely to die from a heart attack. Cigarettes are a principal cause of chronic bronchitis and emphysema, and chronic lung disease itself increases the risks of pneumonia and heart failure. Smoking also increases the risks of high blood pressure.

The usually minor risks of oral contraceptives are greater among women smokers (see p.608). Also, a pregnant woman who smokes 15 to 20 cigarettes a day is twice as likely as a non-smoker to have a miscarriage, and more likely to have a premature, and therefore vulnerable, baby. In the immediate post-natal period the mortality rate for babies born to women who smoke is almost 30 per cent higher than the rate for babies born to non-smokers. Furthermore, "passive smoking," or breathing in air contaminated by smoke from other people's tobacco, has been reported to increase the risk of lung cancer in non-smokers.

Some brands of cigarette contain less tar and nicotine than others, but there is no such thing as an entirely "safe" cigarette. Neither does switching to "mild" cigarettes always help. Habitually heavy smokers usually adapt their smoking habits to the switch by taking longer puffs, lighting up more often and inhaling more deeply.

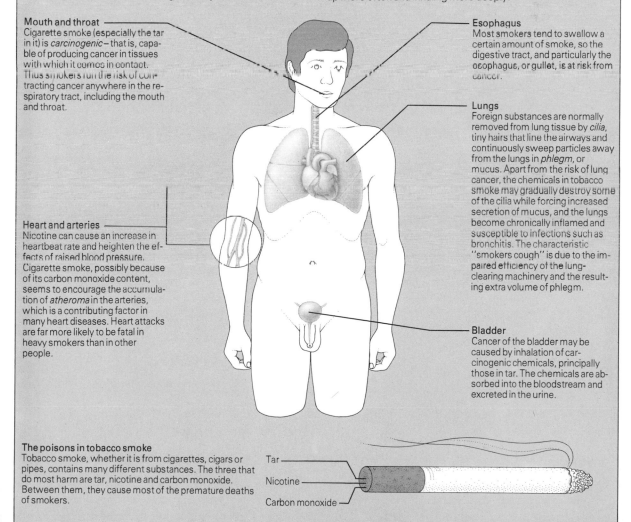

Mouth and throat
Cigarette smoke (especially the tar in it) is *carcinogenic* – that is, capable of producing cancer in tissues with which it comes in contact. Thus smokers run the risk of contracting cancer anywhere in the respiratory tract, including the mouth and throat.

Heart and arteries
Nicotine can cause an increase in heartbeat rate and heighten the effects of raised blood pressure. Cigarette smoke, possibly because of its carbon monoxide content, seems to encourage the accumulation of *atheroma* in the arteries, which is a contributing factor in many heart diseases. Heart attacks are far more likely to be fatal in heavy smokers than in other people.

Esophagus
Most smokers tend to swallow a certain amount of smoke, so the digestive tract, and particularly the esophagus, or gullet, is at risk from cancer.

Lungs
Foreign substances are normally removed from lung tissue by *cilia*, tiny hairs that line the airways and continuously sweep particles away from the lungs in *phlegm*, or mucus. Apart from the risk of lung cancer, the chemicals in tobacco smoke may gradually destroy some of the cilia while forcing increased secretion of mucus, and the lungs become chronically inflamed and susceptible to infections such as bronchitis. The characteristic "smokers cough" is due to the impaired efficiency of the lung-clearing machinery and the resulting extra volume of phlegm.

Bladder
Cancer of the bladder may be caused by inhalation of carcinogenic chemicals, principally those in tar. The chemicals are absorbed into the bloodstream and excreted in the urine.

The poisons in tobacco smoke
Tobacco smoke, whether it is from cigarettes, cigars or pipes, contains many different substances. The three that do most harm are tar, nicotine and carbon monoxide. Between them, they cause most of the premature deaths of smokers.

Tar

Nicotine

Carbon monoxide

Why do smokers smoke?

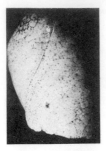

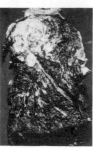

Consider these two pictures. Top: a normal human lung. Bottom: a lung in the advanced stage of cancer.

Many smokers regret their inability to stop, although some are eager to blame their hacking cough on a persistent summer cold, or their high blood pressure on the stresses of daily life. Such smokers cannot face the fact that their real problem is smoking. The percentage of cigarette smokers in the United States dropped from approximately 42 per cent of adults in 1965 to around 33 per cent in 1978. Though the number of men who smoke declined during that time, there was an increase in the number of women who smoke.

Most smokers begin in adolescence, when the possibilities of ill health and death may appear too remote to be real. The teenager lights up occasionally because his or her friends do. Cigarettes have become a symbol of swaggering maturity, and also a support against outward signs of shyness or awkwardness in social situations. The progression from an occasional cigarette without inhaling to heavy smoking usually occurs so gradually that young people never quite realize when they actually became "hooked."

If you are a smoker and have adolescent or pre-adolescent children, you can at least set them a good example by stopping now. But remember that adolescents are by nature rebels, and that moralizing or preaching is not likely to be productive. Tell them the facts: smoking is an expensive habit, in terms of both money and health.

Warning to parents

Tobacco contains poisonous substances. Never leave cigarettes, cigars or loose tobacco where an inquisitive toddler might find it. If you suspect a child has eaten tobacco, contact your physician, the local poison center or a hospital emergency room.

If you smoke you are probably also damaging the health of your children. They are inhaling tobacco smoke (so-called "passive smoking"). Children whose parents smoke have more diseases of the respiratory tract than do the children of non-smokers.

How to stop smoking

Almost all health risks associated with smoking decrease as soon as you give it up, no matter how long you have smoked. Your chances of having a heart attack, for example, drop rapidly. After five non-smoking years, the risk of premature death from smoking-related diseases is almost halved. After 15 years the risk has all but disappeared (see How your chances improve, next page).

Cigarettes vs cigars and pipes

Though the smoke from a cigar or pipe contains a higher concentration of both tar and nicotine than does cigarette smoke, even a few cigarettes a day pose a greater risk to health than a number of cigars or pipes of tobacco would. This may be because, while it is extremely difficult to smoke cigarettes without inhaling, it is more difficult to inhale cigar or pipe smoke voluntarily. Cigarette smokers tend to inhale actively, deeply and constantly. But because the smoke from burning cigar or pipe tobacco is very harsh, it is more difficult to breathe it directly into healthy lungs.

However, simply switching to a pipe or cigars from cigarettes is likely to increase your risk instead of lessening it. This is because you have probably become accustomed to inhaling. You may find yourself retaining the habit, and you will then be inhaling even more harmful smoke than before.

Research about smoking indicates that while nearly four out of five smokers want to stop, only about a quarter of those who try manage to do so. However, many of those who fail to give it up are those who are not willing to put up with the inconvenience and withdrawal symptoms that giving up smoking almost inevitably involves. A method such as hypnotism, group therapy or acupuncture may help to ease those symptoms. If you want to stop and have been unable to succeed on your own, consult your physician. He or she may be able to suggest ways to stop or refer you to a stop-smoking program if there is one in your community.

Most smokers who really want to stop can, in fact, do it by themselves. The following step-by-step procedure has proved effective for thousands of people who have been able to quit smoking.

Step one: Analyze your smoking habits. Prepare a chart of every cigarette you usually smoke in a 24-hour period, along with the times when you almost automatically light up, such as with every cup of coffee, after every meal, or as you begin the day's work. Give yourself two or three weeks in which to study when and why you "need" cigarettes,

If you really cannot stop smoking

Are you unable to stop smoking cigarettes no matter how hard you try? If so, you can at least reduce the health risks by adopting the following measures:

1 Choose a low-tar brand of cigarettes.

2 Smoke fewer cigarettes.

3 Take fewer puffs per cigarette, and smoke it only halfway down its length.

4 When you are not puffing, keep the cigarette out of your mouth.

5 Do your best not to breathe smoke into your lungs.

6 Be wary of changing to cigars or a pipe. If you do switch, try as hard as you can *never* to inhale.

so that you actually pay attention to every puff you take. This increasing concern with the act of smoking is a good way to prepare for the task of giving up the habit.

Step two: Make up your mind that there can be no turning back. List all the reasons why you want to stop, including all the good things that will happen when you have stopped. For instance, you will probably be better able to taste your food, and you may have no more morning cough. Convince yourself that the effort is worth making before you do it.

Step three: Name the day, circle it on your calendar, and give up totally on that day. This is the most successful and, in the long run, least painful way to break the smoking habit. It helps if family members or close friends can act together, giving up on the same date and sustaining one another through the difficult early days. It may help to choose a time when your usual routine is being changed for another reason (for example, just as you go on a vacation). Some smokers have found that it helps to make a great show of stopping by announcing it to the world at large. This makes it a matter of pride not to succumb to temptation in a weak moment.

Step four: Feel free to use any device you can as a cigarette substitute during the difficult early days. It may help to chew gum or use some of the anti-smoking tablets that can be

bought without a prescription. If your hand seems empty without a cigarette between your fingers, hold a pencil or pen. In addition, practice one of the relaxation exercises recommended in this book (see How to relieve tension, p.19) to ease the tensions that smoking seemed to relieve for you. It often helps to give up, at least temporarily, some of the activities that you associate with smoking. For instance, if you habitually smoked while having a drink at the neighborhood bar, stay away for a while. Avoid situations that encourage smoking; for example, it may help to travel in the no-smoking sections of trains, buses and airplanes.

Step five: Enjoy not smoking! Do not forget that you are saving several dollars a week. You can give yourself a positive reward by saving up the unspent money to buy something you could not otherwise afford.

Step six: During the difficult early weeks, eat as much as you want of low-calorie food and drink. Your appetite is almost certain to increase, and when you are feeling tense and restless (the natural result of trying to overcome an addictive habit), you may often be impelled to nibble at something, so you will probably put on a few pounds. Remember that the first four weeks are the hardest. You can expect to lose your intense craving for tobacco after about eight weeks, and you can then begin to eat more sparingly if necessary.

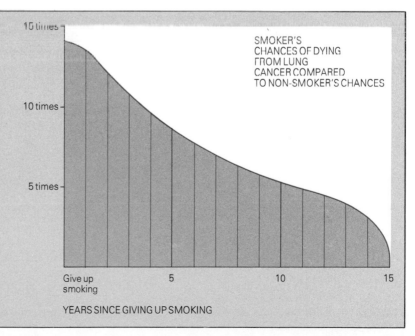

How your chances improve

When you stop smoking, you automatically reduce your chances of dying from a smoking-related disease. The longer you abstain, the less likely you are to succumb, until after about 15 years of non-smoking your chances of unnecessary early death are just about the same as for someone who has never smoked. How long you smoked makes little difference to the general trend, so it is *always* worth giving up. The graph (right) shows how the average smoker's chances of dying from lung cancer (compared to a non-smoker) decrease from the time he or she stops smoking. This tendency, though less marked than for lung cancer, applies to all the illnesses associated with smoking.

SMOKER'S CHANCES OF DYING FROM LUNG CANCER COMPARED TO NON-SMOKER'S CHANCES

15 times

10 times

5 times

Give up smoking

5

10

15

YEARS SINCE GIVING UP SMOKING

Safety and environmental health

Accidents account for about five per cent of deaths in the United States, and are the fourth most common cause of death. These figures could be considerably reduced if each person paid more attention to basic safety precautions. Health-consciousness should also include safety-consciousness.

The work that you do may expose you to a particular set of hazards. But if you (and your employers) take reasonable precautions, your chances of getting an occupational disease such as a lung disorder or skin disorder can be kept to a minimum. As for possible risks from the environment, such as from air or water, in most situations they are small in comparison with the innumerable other risks of just being alive. For a more detailed discussion of occupational and environmental risks see the article on p.45.

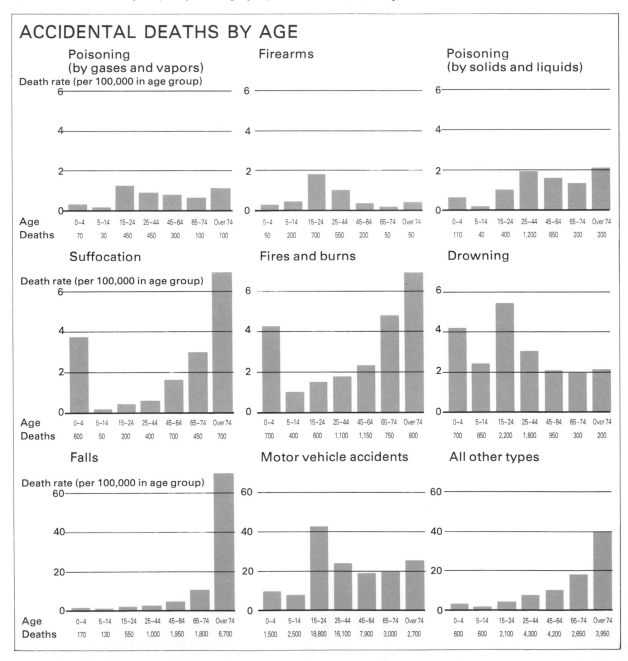

ACCIDENTAL DEATHS BY AGE

Poisoning (by gases and vapors)
Death rate (per 100,000 in age group)

Age	0–4	5–14	15–24	25–44	45–64	65–74	Over 74
Deaths	70	30	450	450	300	100	100

Firearms

Age	0–4	5–14	15–24	25–44	45–64	65–74	Over 74
Deaths	50	200	700	550	200	50	50

Poisoning (by solids and liquids)

Age	0–4	5–14	15–24	25–44	45–64	65–74	Over 74
Deaths	110	40	400	1,200	650	200	200

Suffocation
Death rate (per 100,000 in age group)

Age	0–4	5–14	15–24	25–44	45–64	65–74	Over 74
Deaths	600	50	200	400	700	450	700

Fires and burns

Age	0–4	5–14	15–24	25–44	45–64	65–74	Over 74
Deaths	700	400	600	1,100	1,150	750	800

Drowning

Age	0–4	5–14	15–24	25–44	45–64	65–74	Over 74
Deaths	700	850	2,200	1,800	950	300	200

Falls
Death rate (per 100,000 in age group)

Age	0–4	5–14	15–24	25–44	45–64	65–74	Over 74
Deaths	170	130	550	1,000	1,950	1,800	6,700

Motor vehicle accidents

Age	0–4	5–14	15–24	25–44	45–64	65–74	Over 74
Deaths	1,500	2,500	18,800	16,100	7,900	3,000	2,700

All other types

Age	0–4	5–14	15–24	25–44	45–64	65–74	Over 74
Deaths	600	600	2,100	4,300	4,200	2,650	3,950

Are you doing enough to prevent accidents?

Accidents very often cause serious injury, and accidents cause a large number of deaths (see chart, previous page). The following questions are designed to test how well you protect yourself and your family from accidental injury. The first group of questions concentrates on guarding against possible hazards in and around your house or apartment. The second group deals with safety measures that should be taken against accidents that might happen to you or your family on the road, whether in a vehicle or as pedestrians. The third and last group is mainly concerned with safety on vacations, when unfamiliar surroundings and activities present special hazards.

Basic safety at home

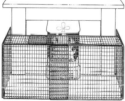

Always make sure that any fireplace is surrounded by a screen.

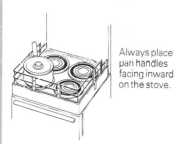

Always place pan handles facing inward on the stove.

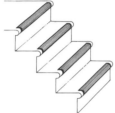

Always be sure that stair carpets are secure. Use tread grips if you can.

Group 1 Safety at home

Answer YES or NO to the following questions:

1 Do you make it a point never to smoke in bed?
YES ☐   NO ☐

2 Do all your fireplaces have screens around them?
YES ☐   NO ☐

3 When cooking, do you guard against accidental tipping by positioning pan handles so that they do not extend outwards?
YES ☐   NO ☐

4 Do you keep electric cords out of the reach of children and avoid overloading the outlets?
YES ☐   NO ☐

5 Are you careful never to leave small children unsupervised in the kitchen or bathroom?
YES ☐   NO ☐

6 Are your children's nightclothes and soft toys labeled to show they are made of non-flammable materials?
YES ☐   NO ☐

7 Are medicines in your house kept in a secure place out of children's reach, and away from beds?
YES ☐   NO ☐

8 Are you careful never to store drugs or dangerous chemicals (bleach, paint-stripper etc.) within children's reach or in incorrectly labelled containers?
YES ☐   NO ☐

9 Do you make a point of preventing your children from playing with objects small enough to be swallowed or inhaled?
YES ☐   NO ☐

10 Do you keep plastic bags away from your children?
YES ☐   NO ☐

11 When working around the house, do you wear safety glasses, ear plugs and protective clothing such as sturdy shoes?
YES ☐   NO ☐

12 Are your carpets firmly fixed, with no ragged spots or edges, and are loose rugs placed to minimize the risk of sliding or tripping?
YES ☐   NO ☐

13 Are your stairs, halls, and other passages well lit (brightly enough to read a newspaper)?
YES ☐   NO ☐

14 Is it a rule in your house that nothing is left on the stairs?
YES ☐   NO ☐

15 If you spill or drop something that might be slippery on the floor, do you always clean it up right away?
YES ☐   NO ☐

16 Do you keep non-slip mats both in and alongside the bath or shower?
YES ☐   NO ☐

(Continued on next page)

Group 2 **Safety on the road** Answer YES or NO to the following questions:

17 Have you taught your children exactly how, when and where to cross streets safely?
YES ☐ NO ☐

18 Have your children been taught the basic rules of the road to use when bicycling?
YES ☐ NO ☐

19 When walking in streets or open roads at twilight or in the dark, do all members of your family carry a light, or wear a markedly visible outer garment such as a white or luminous jacket?
YES ☐ NO ☐

20 Do you always drive within the speed limit and drive defensively?
YES ☐ NO ☐

21 Are you always careful to drink very little alcohol or none at all if you are going to drive a car soon afterwards?
YES ☐ NO ☐

22 Do you avoid driving when you feel unusually tired or ill, or if you are taking drugs (such as antihistamines) that are known to impair alertness?
YES ☐ NO ☐

23 Do you have your car fully serviced, including lights, tires, windshield washer and wipers, brakes and steering, either every 10,000 km (6,000 miles) or at least every 6 months?
YES ☐ NO ☐

24 Do you check at least once a week to make sure that your car windows, lights, mirrors and reflectors are clean?
YES ☐ NO ☐

25 When driving, do you always try to keep a gap of at least a meter (yard) for each mile-per-hour of speed between your car and the one in front?
YES ☐ NO ☐

26 Do you always make sure that you and all passengers in your car use available seat belts?
YES ☐ NO ☐

27 Are any infants or toddlers riding in your car securely strapped into infant car seats?
YES ☐ NO ☐

Group 3 **Safety on vacations** Answer YES or NO to the following questions:

28 Are all members of your family able to swim, or in the process of learning how to swim?
YES ☐ NO ☐

29 Do you test the depth of the water and go in feet first?
YES ☐ NO ☐

30 In a boat, does everyone always wear a life-jacket?
YES ☐ NO ☐

31 If you do any skiing, hiking or climbing, do you always go properly prepared with the right clothing and equipment?
YES ☐ NO ☐

32 When going on an excursion for a day or longer, do you tell someone what your route is and when you expect to be back?
YES ☐ NO ☐

33 Do you and your family take full safety precautions and have the proper equipment when you engage in contact and other possibly dangerous sports?
YES ☐ NO ☐

34 Before taking up a new and potentially dangerous activity such as hang-gliding, do you make sure you get proper instruction?
YES ☐ NO ☐

35 During a vacation, do you make sure you get adequate rest and relaxation?
YES ☐ NO ☐

EVALUATION
A NO answer to any of the above questions indicates that you are not doing all you can to minimize the risk of accidents. You can and should take all the protective steps suggested in the questions. For a discussion of some less obvious risks, which may or may not be preventable, see Occupational and environmental risks, next page. For precautions against accidental falls, to which the elderly are particularly susceptible, see p.719.

Occupational and environmental risks

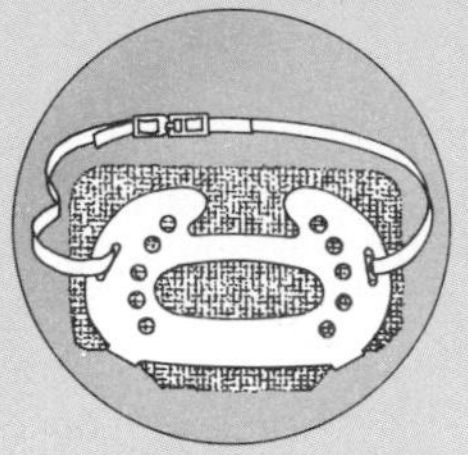

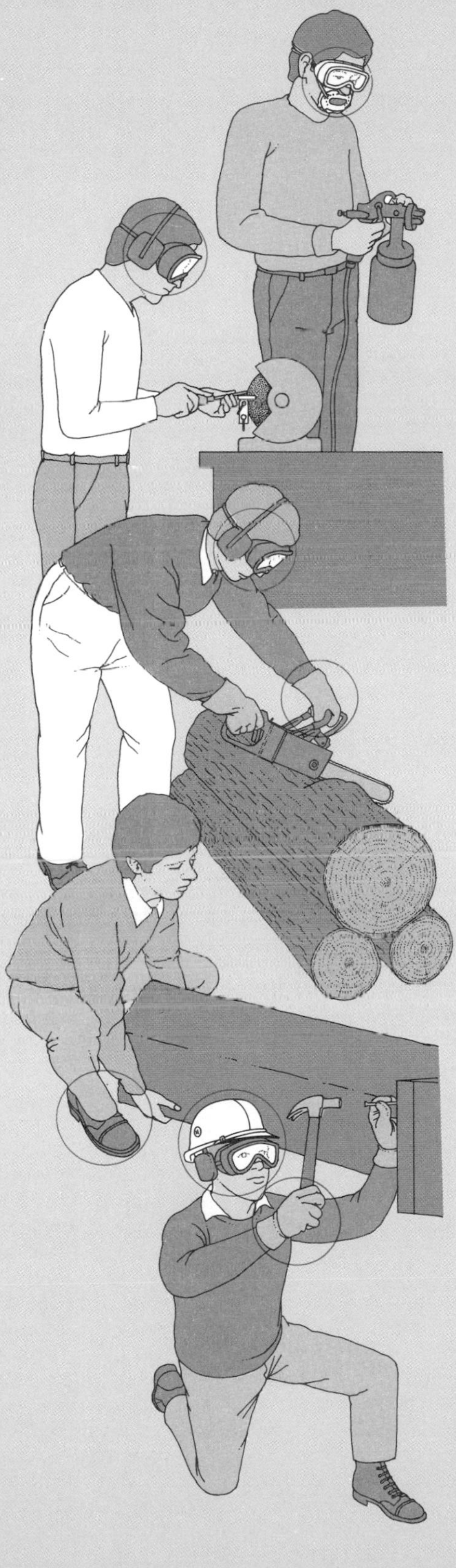

Direct causal links between occupation and disease are becoming better understood. This is particularly true of respiratory-system disorders that are caused by years of exposure to certain chemicals or dusty substances. Examples are pneumoconiosis, and related dust diseases such as asbestosis and silicosis (see p.365). Miners, stone masons, quarry workers, asbestos handlers, and people who smelt or grind aluminum, iron, and similar metals are susceptible to these disorders. Less obvious are complaints such as farmer's lung (see p.365), which sometimes affects people who work on the land. Another example of such diseases is anthrax, an infection that attacks dock workers or handlers who come into contact with contaminated pelts or other animal products. This disease is very rare in the United States. Craftsmen who grind or polish metal are especially susceptible to eye injuries from airborne particles of metal. The prolonged handling of vibrating machinery can lead to Raynaud's disease (see p.412), and working in extremely noisy conditions can lead to occupational hearing loss (see p.338). And, of course, there is always a risk of accidental injury in manual labor, whether on a farm or in the city, and whether the work is skilled or unskilled. There are many very dangerous jobs. One of the most hazardous is deep-sea diving. Also the risk of death as a direct result of servicing off-shore oil-drilling equipment is very high.

Are you at risk?

No list of potential hazards can cover all the possibilities. For one thing, there are always new industries developing that create different types of work, and these jobs may lead to disorders of the body or mind. Then, too, unsuspected links between certain jobs and diseases may still be discovered. There is recent evidence, for instance, that workers

Air-filter mask

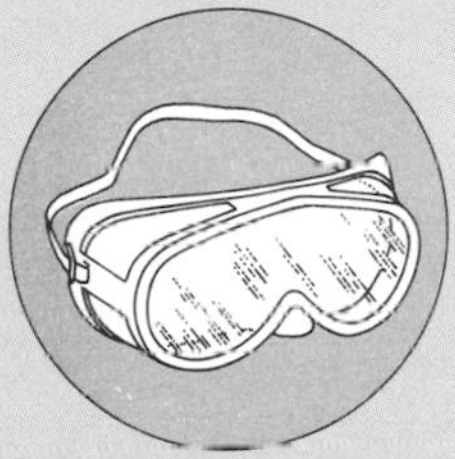

Eye protectors

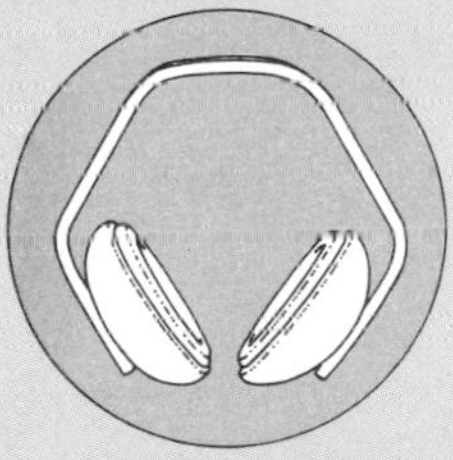

Ear protectors

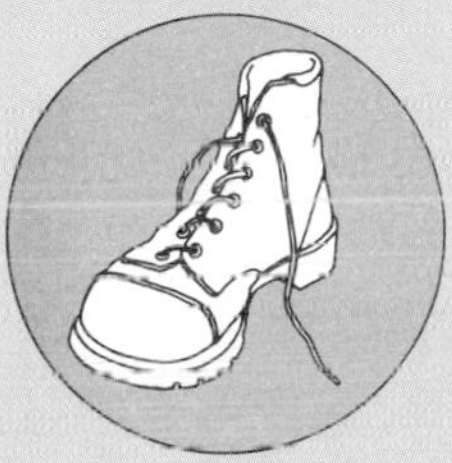

Reinforced footwear

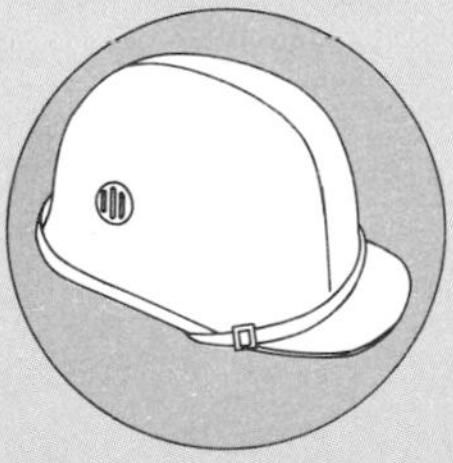

Protective headgear

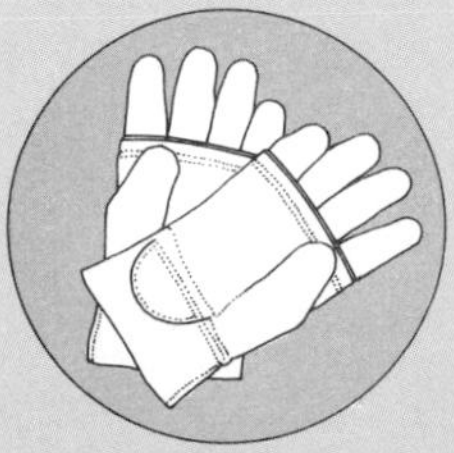

Heavy gloves

Safety at work and at home
In the United States there are regulations that require safe working conditions for employees, especially where machinery is concerned. It is a good idea to observe safety rules at home as well, particularly as more and more people become "do-it-yourselfers" and use power tools for gardening and house and car maintenance. The six examples given here suggest ways to protect yourself from injury or illness while using potentially dangerous tools or chemicals. Never leave safety guards off power tools, and make sure you follow instruction leaflets carefully.

exposed to certain chemicals used in the industrial manufacture of polyvinyl chloride (PVC) are susceptible to cancer of the liver. In fact, virtually every job has its health risks. If you are safely seated at a desk all day, you are more likely than others to develop coronary artery disease. In general, however, you are most at risk of a specific job-related disorder if your occupation:

• Exposes your respiratory system to chemicals, floating particles or gases;
• Exposes your skin to a chemical (especially in concentrated form);
• Exposes your ears to loud noise; or
• Exposes you to machinery of any sort.

What should be done?

Today most of the obvious occupational hazards are recognized and publicized, and employers are legally required to take steps to safeguard health and minimize accidents. If your job is even slightly risky, be sure you understand what the hazards are. Your employer or union representative should have leaflets or other information on the subject. Then make sure you take all recommended safety precautions and wear approved protective clothing. Use the ear plugs or muffs provided if you work with noisy machinery, to protect your ears from occupational hearing loss (see p.338). Never trust your luck instead of wearing a hard hat on a construction site. In short, take advantage of every safety precaution that is available to you.

If you are concerned about the adequacy of health-protection measures at your place of work, do not hesitate to bring up the subject. A representative of your employer or union is an obvious person to see. Otherwise, get in touch with the nearest branch of the Occupational Safety and Health Administration (OSHA), which is a federal agency, or a similar state or local agency. Remember that a major characteristic of job-related illnesses other than those caused by direct injury is that early symptoms are barely noticeable, but they develop relentlessly over months or years. Be sure to take all possible precautions now to safeguard your future health.

Environmental hazards

The quality of the air, land and water of North America is a precious asset. As industries try to contribute to a strong economy by making a profit and providing the consumer goods that have become an important part of life in North America, it is important to realize that, while there are certainly benefits from these things, there can be a cost in terms of damage to the environment. Thanks to concerned citizen, business and government groups, these environmental problems are being examined and, in some cases, solved.

As a result of anti-air-pollution laws, the industrial smoke that once caused many cases of bronchitis and emphysema is now largely under control. The greatest modern sources of air pollution, however, are the carbon monoxide and lead in motor-vehicle exhaust fumes. Still, these very real health risks must be put into perspective. It is less risky, for example, to breathe the air in heavy traffic than it is to smoke cigarettes. Lead is certainly a powerful poison, and workers who are exposed to high concentrations of the metal may develop damage to their kidneys or nerves. But there is no clear evidence that the concentration of air-borne lead is great enough anywhere in North America to damage health. There is, however, a real danger of lead poisoning from lead-based paint, which is most often found in older homes and buildings.

Water pollution can occur through natural mechanisms as well as individual, agricultural or industrial practices. Polluted air can affect rainwater, and both construction and use of pesticides in farming can pollute streams, rivers and lakes as soil washes into them. Chemical pollutants in water have not been directly related to disease in humans, except in incidents when leakage or dumping of a concentrated chemical has contaminated a specific water supply. However, cancers and chronic diseases may take years to develop, so the effects of these pollutants may yet be felt. Bacterial and viral pollutants, which often come from sewage containing human and animal wastes, are rare in North America because municipal water is purified and sewage is treated. Several diseases have been virtually eliminated in the United States due to public health measures including sewage treatment. Examples are cholera (see p. 462), typhoid (see p. 462) and amebic dysentery (see p. 461).

You can help ensure that water supplies remain as pure as possible. Have your septic tank, well or cistern inspected regularly for leakage. Dispose of garbage and sewage properly, and learn about the sources, treatment and safety of your municipal water supply. Also, have well or spring water tested periodically, to be sure it remains pure.

Except for those people who, physicians believe, are particularly susceptible to risks from environmental hazards, there is virtually no reason for most people to "escape" environmental risks by moving away or installing so-called water purifiers. Changing locations is advisable chiefly for people who have chronic bronchitis (see p. 354), and therefore may do better in a warm, dry climate. Some people who have lung diseases such as emphysema (see p. 358), however, are advised against moving to an area where the altitude is high, because the low oxygen content of the air can cause shortness of breath and difficulty with sleeping. And if you move to a sunny area, remember that heavy doses of sunlight can cause skin cancer, especially in light-skinned people.

The facts about cancer

One reason why the early-warning signs of possible serious illness listed on the next page should not be ignored is that most of them suggest the possibility of cancer. Since fear of the unknown can be far more frightening than fear of the known, here for your information are some basic facts about this dreaded disease.

To begin with, cancer is not a single disease. It is the name of a group of diseases in which body cells multiply and spread uncontrollably. This can happen in virtually any part of the body. Except in blood cancers such as leukemia, the unchecked spread of cells develops into a *malignant* tumor, which generally keeps growing and is likely to invade neighboring tissues, with potentially fatal consequences. Non-cancerous tumors are known as *benign*. Although such tumors may grow, their cells do not multiply and spread. A cancer that occurs in bone or muscle tissue is technically called a *sarcoma*. One that occurs in the skin, a gland, or the lining of an organ such as the lung, liver, bladder or brain is called a *carcinoma*. But physicians also use many other words as labels for specific types of cancer. Of the approximately 550 physical disorders covered in this book, about 50 deal with some kind of malignant growth.

What causes cancer?

Medical scientists have identified many of the causes of cancer; smoking is associated with lung cancer, for example. They believe that about 80 per cent of all cancers are due to contamination of the environment by chemicals called *carcinogens*. But exactly how these substances cause cells to become malignant is still not known. Among possible carcinogens are industrial substances such as asbestos, tar and chromium, and nuclear radiation. But even some of the things you eat and drink may make you more or less susceptible to malignancy. And although there is no evidence that cancer is contagious or can be inherited, it does seem to occur more often in some families. The implication is that your home environment and diet may affect your susceptibility to malignant tumors. For this reason most physicians advise their patients not only to give up smoking and heavy drinking, but also to eat certain foods, animal fats in particular, in moderation.

What are the chances for cure?

Many cancers, including those of the cervix, rectum and skin, can be detected early. If they are treated promptly, before malignant cells have spread very far, they can often be completely cured. Once cells have *metastasized*, or spread, from the original tumor, however, and have formed secondary growths in other parts of the body, the chances for cure are lessened. This is why early detection is so important, and why medical professionals are constantly working to develop new techniques for discovering malignancy in its very early stages. Fortunately, progress is being made all the time, and there are now successful screening tests for early detection of several kinds of bowel and bladder cancer as well as cancer of the cervix and breast. Moreover, painless diagnostic procedures such as *ultra-sound* and *radioisotope scanning* have largely replaced the often unpleasant investigative techniques of a few years ago.

Cancer is still a killer, of course. It accounts for about one in every five deaths in the United States. It is the second most common cause of death; the first is heart disease. In the decade of the 1970s, an estimated 3.5 million people died of cancer in the United States. Although these figures may be disturbing, the general outlook is improving. In recent years the rate of cure in treating many forms of cancer has been steadily increasing, as the following examples show.

● Early surgical removal of a cancer of the cervix now has an almost 100 per cent rate of cure.
● Hodgkin's disease, if treated in the early stages, can be cured in more than 80 per cent of cases.
● Surgical removal of cancer of the colon or of the type of skin cancer called malignant melanoma now has a cure rate of more than 50 per cent
● In acute lymphocytic leukemia, which used to be considered a hopeless childhood disease, modern drugs can clear up the disease in nearly 50 per cent of the cases.

So remember, you should not assume that cancer is incurable. Instead, be alert for early symptoms, and see your physician promptly if any develop.

Early warning signs of possible serious illness

Many serious illnesses begin with apparently minor or localized symptoms that, if they are recognized early, can alert you to act in time for the disease to be cured or controlled. In most cases, of course, nothing is seriously wrong. Even so, if you experience any of the following symptoms, you should consult the relevant self-diagnosis chart in this book. You should also discuss the problem with your physician without delay.

1	Rapid loss of weight – more than about 4 kg (10 lbs) in 10 weeks – without apparent cause.		**13**	A bluish tinge to the lips, the insides of the eyelids, or the nail-beds.
2	A sore, scab or ulcer, either in the mouth or on the body, that fails to heal within a period of about three weeks.		**14**	Extreme shortness of breath for no apparent reason.
3	A skin blemish or mole that begins to bleed or itch, or that changes color, size or shape.		**15**	Vomiting of blood or a substance that resembles coffee-grounds.
			16	Persistent indigestion or abdominal pain.
4	Severe headaches that develop for no obvious reason.		**17**	A marked change in normal bowel habits, such as alternating attacks of diarrhea and constipation.
5	Sudden attacks of vomiting, without preceding nausea.		**18**	Bowel movements that look black and tarry.
6	Fainting spells for no apparent reason.		**19**	Rectal bleeding.
7	Visual problems such as seeing "haloes" around lights, or intermittently blurred vision, especially in dim light.		**20**	Unusually cloudy, pink, red or smoky-looking urine.
8	Increasing difficulty with swallowing.		**21**	In men, discomfort or difficulty when urinating.
9	Hoarseness without apparent cause that lasts for a week or more.		**22**	In men, discharge from the tip of the penis.
10	A "smoker's" cough or any other nagging cough that has been getting worse.		**23**	In women, a lump or unusual thickening of a breast or any alteration in breast shape such as flattening, bulging or puckering of skin.
11	Blood in coughed-up *phlegm*, or sputum.		**24**	In women, bleeding or unusual discharge from the nipple.
12	Constantly swollen ankles.		**25**	In women, vaginal bleeding or "spotting" that occurs between usual menstrual periods or after menopause.

Atlas of the body

Introduction

Until the Middle Ages, medicine was based almost entirely on the teaching of the Ancient Greek physicians Hippocrates and Galen. Their advice on the treatment of common illnesses and injuries sprang soundly from practical experience, but they had little understanding of the structure and functioning of the human body. Medieval medicine was still rooted in such concepts as the "four humors" – blood, phlegm, yellow bile and black bile.

The science of medicine began in the 16th century with the careful dissection and detailed study of corpses by the Italian artist and inventor Leonardo da Vinci. In 1543 the Belgian scientist Andreas Vesalius produced the first comprehensive anatomical textbook, *de humani corporis fabrica* ("The Structure of the Human Body"). Vesalius was able to correct many of the misconceptions in the teachings of the Ancients, and he laid the foundations for modern anatomy (the structure of the body), and physiology (the functioning of the body). The next major landmark came in 1628 when the English physician William Harvey explained for the first time the true nature of how blood circulates throughout the body.

The twin studies of anatomy and physiology have developed steadily since Harvey's day. They have provided the essential foundations for the scientific study of diseases by pathologists and microbiologists and their treatment by drugs and surgery. But the pace of discovery has accelerated with the recent development of new techniques for studying the body – for example, *CAT scans, ultrasound scans, radioisotope scans,* and *endoscopy.*

This section of the book deals with the anatomy of the body. It illustrates the major divisions of the body's structure and shows how new techniques have helped us to visualize the structures of internal organs. (Descriptions of how the various parts and systems of the body function are given in the section introductions in Part III.)

Historical beliefs about the body
Until the 16th century, religious and other constraints prevented dissection of corpses – whether healthy or diseased – to study how the human body is put together. As a result, there grew up a number of beliefs about anatomy and physiology that we know are misconceptions. They seem to us surprising and bizarre; but it is likely that in another hundred years some of the beliefs held today will be exposed in the same way.

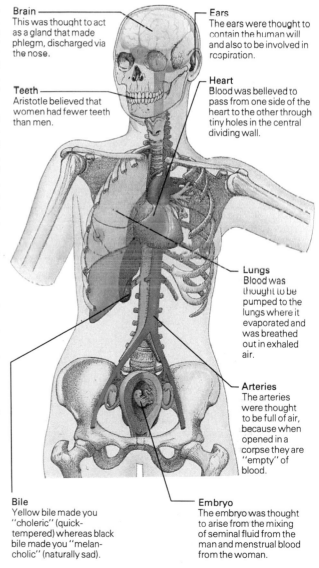

Brain
This was thought to act as a gland that made phlegm, discharged via the nose.

Teeth
Aristotle believed that women had fewer teeth than men.

Ears
The ears were thought to contain the human will and also to be involved in respiration.

Heart
Blood was believed to pass from one side of the heart to the other through tiny holes in the central dividing wall.

Lungs
Blood was thought to be pumped to the lungs where it evaporated and was breathed out in exhaled air.

Arteries
The arteries were thought to be full of air, because when opened in a corpse they are "empty" of blood.

Bile
Yellow bile made you "choleric" (quick-tempered) whereas black bile made you "melancholic" (naturally sad).

Embryo
The embryo was thought to arise from the mixing of seminal fluid from the man and menstrual blood from the woman.

The skeleton

The average human skeleton has 206 bones. There are 32 in each arm, 31 in each leg, 29 in the skull, 26 in the spine, and 25 in the chest. In some skeletons the number of bones varies slightly from the norm – for example, you may have a few extra bones in your hands or feet, or one or more bones may be missing.

The separate bones of the skeleton are connected by joints. There are several types of joint. Fixed joints (*sutures*) hold the bones firmly together, as in the skull. Partly movable joints allow some flexibility, as in the bones of the spine. And freely movable joints provide great flexibility in several planes of movement, as in the shoulder.

The male and female skeletons differ very little. One difference is that male bones are generally slightly larger and heavier than their female counterparts. Also, the cavity in the male pelvis, surrounded by the hip bones and sacrum, is narrower than that of the female pelvis, through which the baby's head and body have to pass during childbirth.

Ossification (bone formation)

In the early months before birth, very little of the skeleton contains actual bone. Most of the bones that eventually form are made of cartilage. As the child grows, the cartilage turns into true bone in a process known as "ossification." The areas of ossification appear at set times during the growth of a healthy child. On an X-ray the only areas that show up are those formed of bone (cartilage is pretty much invisible); therefore, it is easy to detect ossification on an X-ray. The series of X-ray photographs below shows how the ankle and foot "bones" of a child gradually appear and grow to replace the "invisible" cartilage until, by the mid-teen years, the bones have assumed their mature, adult configuration.

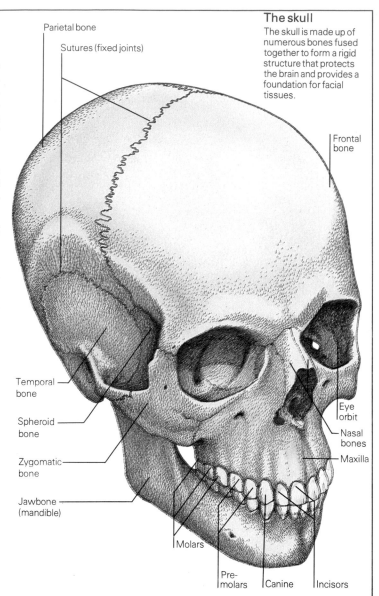

Parietal bone

Sutures (fixed joints)

The skull
The skull is made up of numerous bones fused together to form a rigid structure that protects the brain and provides a foundation for facial tissues.

Frontal bone

Temporal bone

Spheroid bone

Zygomatic bone

Jawbone (mandible)

Molars

Pre-molars

Canine

Incisors

Eye orbit

Nasal bones

Maxilla

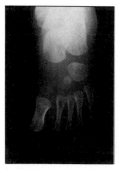

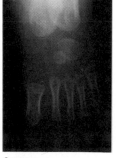

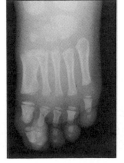

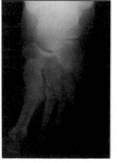

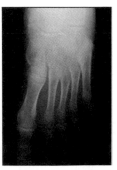

1 year

2 years

4 years

9 years

15 years

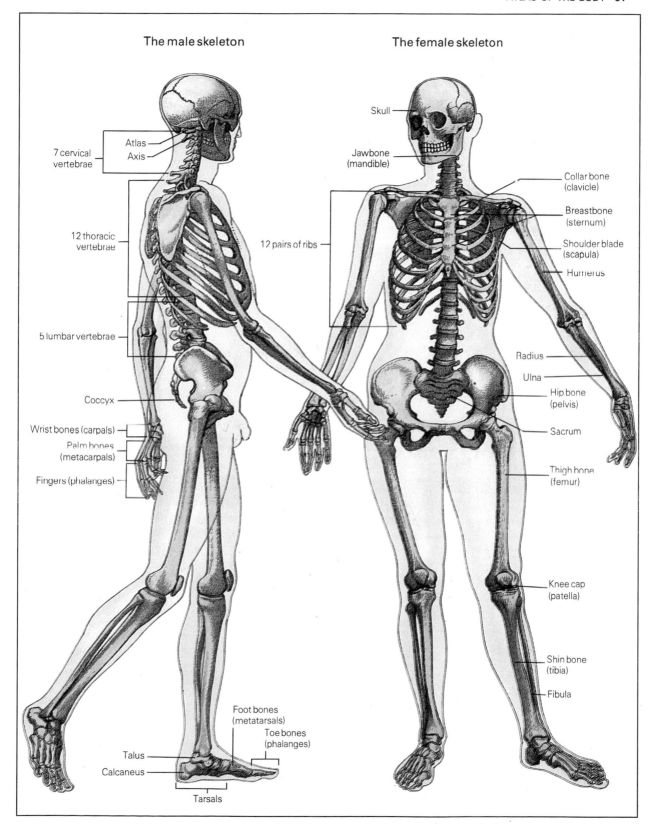

The male skeleton

The female skeleton

7 cervical vertebrae

Atlas

Axis

12 thoracic vertebrae

5 lumbar vertebrae

12 pairs of ribs

Coccyx

Wrist bones (carpals)

Palm bones (metacarpals)

Fingers (phalanges)

Talus

Calcaneus

Foot bones (metatarsals)

Toe bones (phalanges)

Tarsals

Skull

Jawbone (mandible)

Collar bone (clavicle)

Breastbone (sternum)

Shoulder blade (scapula)

Humerus

Radius

Ulna

Hip bone (pelvis)

Sacrum

Thigh bone (femur)

Knee cap (patella)

Shin bone (tibia)

Fibula

The muscles

There are well over 600 named muscles in the normal body. Each muscle is made up of bundles of closely interlocking muscle fibers, which vary in length from a few millimeters, as in the muscles that move the eyeball, to about 30 cm (1 ft), as in the buttock muscles. Some of these muscle fibers contract and relax very quickly; others are designed for the long-term contraction that is required to maintain body posture.

Each end of skeletal muscle is attached to a bone (except in the case of a few muscles in the face, which are attached to skin or other tissue), either directly or by means of a tendon. The tendon may be long and tapering or a flat sheet of tissue. Besides the skeletal muscles shown here, there are many other muscles in the body; the heart, for instance, and the digestive-tract walls, contain large quantities of muscular tissue.

The muscles of the head and neck (right)

These produce the various movements associated with eating and with positioning of the head. In addition, they are responsible for the vast range of facial expressions that we use to communicate our moods and emotions to others.

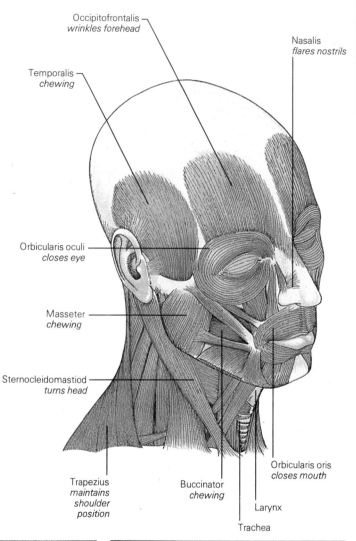

Occipitofrontalis
wrinkles forehead

Nasalis
flares nostrils

Temporalis
chewing

Orbicularis oculi
closes eye

Masseter
chewing

Sternocleidomastiod
turns head

Orbicularis oris
closes mouth

Trapezius
maintains shoulder position

Buccinator
chewing

Larynx

Trachea

Muscle biopsies

A muscle biopsy is a laboratory examination of a small sample of muscle tissue for signs of disease. The photographs shown here are of very thin slices of healthy muscle, magnified 8,000 times. Each fiber is made of many tiny dark stripes (myosin molecules) and light stripes (actin molecules). In a relaxed muscle (right) the stripes overlap only slightly. In a contracted muscle (far right) they slide over each other, shortening the length of the muscle.

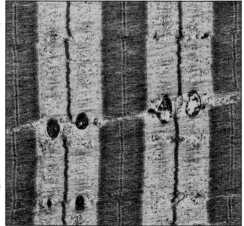

Relaxed muscle fiber

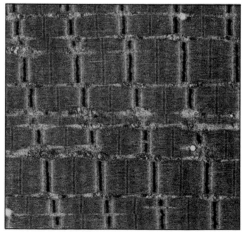

Contracted muscle fiber

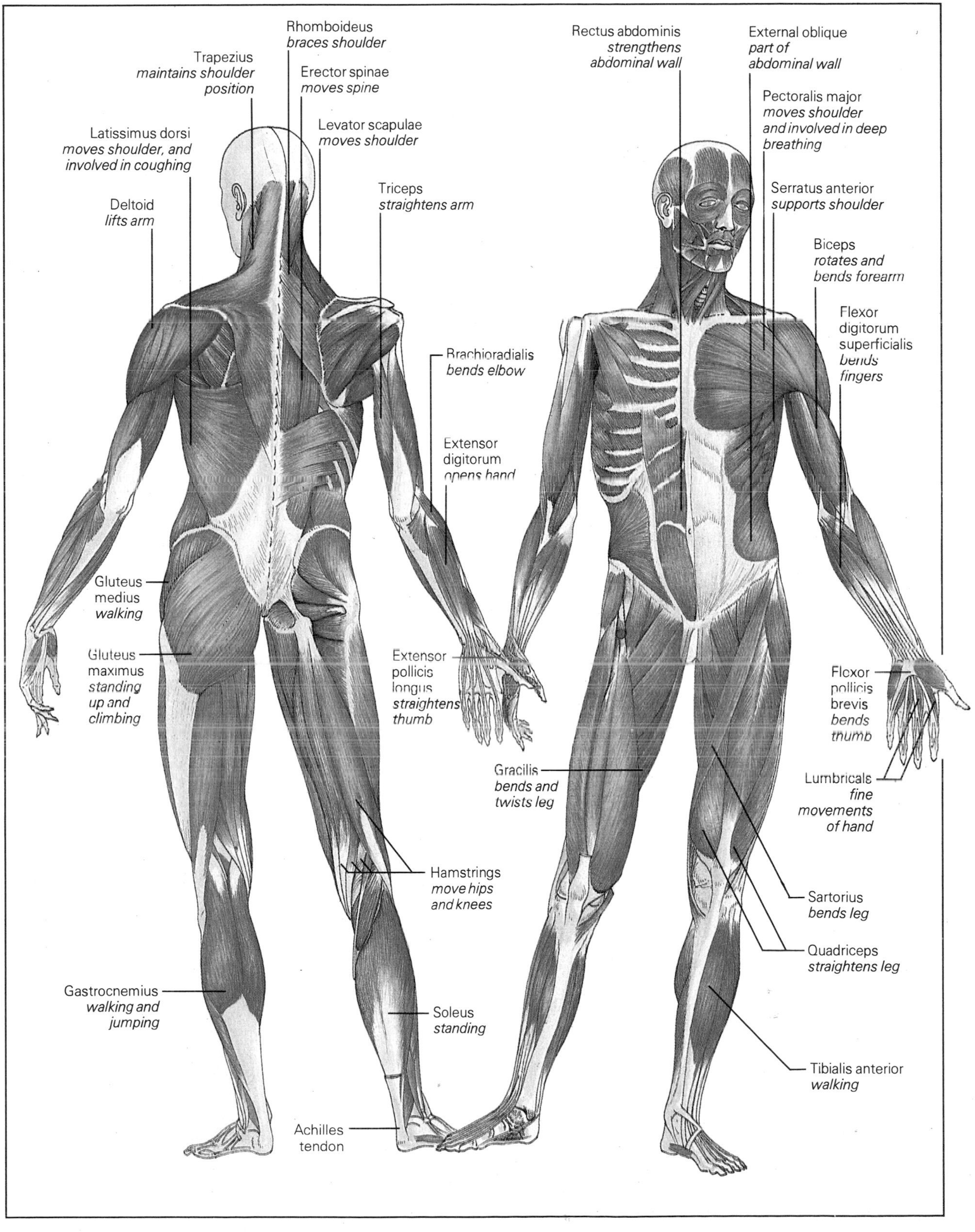

Trapezius
maintains shoulder position

Rhomboideus
braces shoulder

Erector spinae
moves spine

Levator scapulae
moves shoulder

Latissimus dorsi
moves shoulder, and involved in coughing

Triceps
straightens arm

Deltoid
lifts arm

Brachioradialis
bends elbow

Extensor digitorum
opens hand

Gluteus medius
walking

Gluteus maximus
standing up and climbing

Extensor pollicis longus
straightens thumb

Hamstrings
move hips and knees

Gastrocnemius
walking and jumping

Soleus
standing

Achilles tendon

Rectus abdominis
strengthens abdominal wall

External oblique
part of abdominal wall

Pectoralis major
moves shoulder and involved in deep breathing

Serratus anterior
supports shoulder

Biceps
rotates and bends forearm

Flexor digitorum superficialis
bends fingers

Flexor pollicis brevis
bends thumb

Lumbricals
fine movements of hand

Gracilis
bends and twists leg

Sartorius
bends leg

Quadriceps
straightens leg

Tibialis anterior
walking

The brain and nerves

Lying well protected within the rigid, bony box formed by the skull bones is the brain. The main components of the brain are the two cerebral hemispheres, the cerebellum and the brain stem.

The cerebral hemispheres comprise nearly 90 per cent of brain tissue. Each hemisphere is about 15 cm (6 in) from the front to back, and together they are about 11 cm (4½ in) across. They are made up of intricate folds of nerve tissues whose total surface area is approximately the same as the area of a large sheet of newspaper.

The cerebellum, which is concerned with muscular coordination, lies beneath the rear part of the cerebral hemispheres. The cerebellum also consists of nerve cells and is divided into two hemispheres.

The brain stem, which is about 75 mm (3 in) long, connects the rest of the brain to the spinal cord and contains the nerve centers that control "automatic" functions.

The brain is a hollow organ. Within it are four interconnected cavities, called ventricles, filled with a fluid called cerebrospinal fluid. The ventricles are connected to the long, thin cavity that runs down the middle of the spinal cord. The cavity is also filled with cerebrospinal fluid.

The cranial nerves

There are 12 pairs of cranial nerves (below) that run from the underside of the brain to various organs and body parts. Some of the more important nerves carry information from the main sense organs. For example, the optic nerves transmit visual information from the eyes to the brain, where it is coordinated and interpreted.

Nerve junctions

Shown below are two small parts of the nervous system, the brachial plexus (upper diagram) in the lower neck, and the lumbosacral plexus (lower diagram) in the lower back. These junctions illustrate the tremendous complexity of the nervous system as a whole.

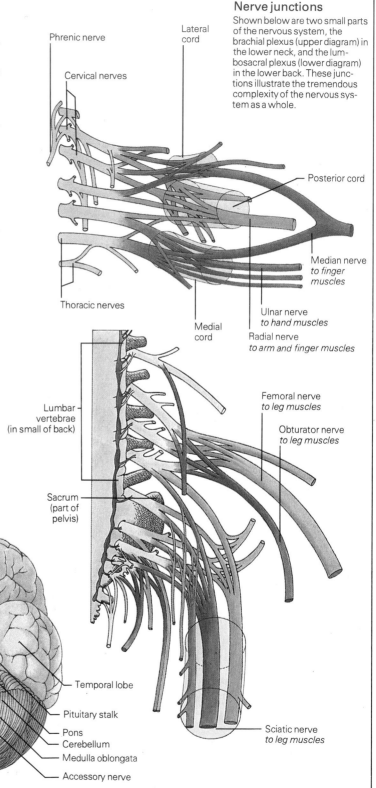

Phrenic nerve

Cervical nerves

Lateral cord

Posterior cord

Median nerve *to finger muscles*

Ulnar nerve *to hand muscles*

Radial nerve *to arm and finger muscles*

Thoracic nerves

Medial cord

Lumbar vertebrae (in small of back)

Sacrum (part of pelvis)

Femoral nerve *to leg muscles*

Obturator nerve *to leg muscles*

Sciatic nerve *to leg muscles*

Frontal lobe

Olfactory nerve

Optic nerve

Oculomotor nerve

Trochlear nerve

Abducent nerve

Trigeminal nerve

Facial nerve

Auditory nerve

Glossopharyngeal nerve

Vagus nerve

Hypoglossal nerve

Temporal lobe

Pituitary stalk

Pons

Cerebellum

Medulla oblongata

Accessory nerve

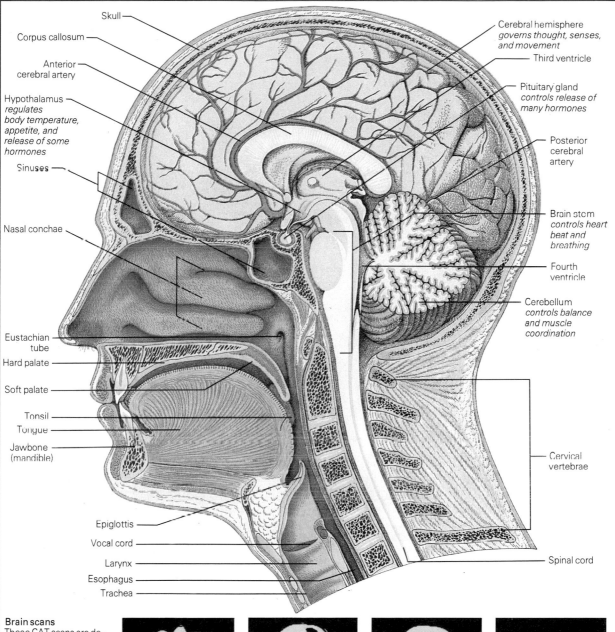

Skull

Corpus callosum

Anterior cerebral artery

Hypothalamus *regulates body temperature, appetite, and release of some hormones*

Sinuses

Nasal conchae

Eustachian tube

Hard palate

Soft palate

Tonsil

Tongue

Jawbone (mandible)

Epiglottis

Vocal cord

Larynx

Esophagus

Trachea

Cerebral hemisphere *governs thought, senses, and movement*

Third ventricle

Pituitary gland *controls release of many hormones*

Posterior cerebral artery

Brain stem *controls heart beat and breathing*

Fourth ventricle

Cerebellum *controls balance and muscle coordination*

Cervical vertebrae

Spinal cord

Brain scans
These CAT scans are derived from a series of X-ray pictures taken as a camera moves around the head. A computer integrates this information into pictures of horizontal "slices" through the head. The darker areas are less dense tissues. The light parts are dense tissues such as the skull bones (see also the body scans on p.58).

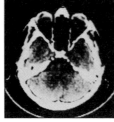

At eye level the skull and nasal bones and the bones of the eye sockets are clearly visible.

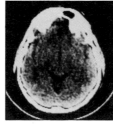

At eyebrow level an airfilled asymmetrical sinus appears as a well-defined dark patch.

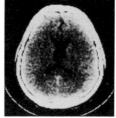

At mid-forehead level the dark, fluid-filled cavities (ventricles) within the brain can be seen.

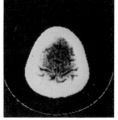

At hair-line level the convolutions on the surface of the brain begin to come into view.

The heart, lungs and blood vessels

The heart is a cone-shaped organ, made almost entirely of muscle, about the size of your clenched fist. It lies roughly in the center of the chest. Two-thirds of it is to the left of the breast bone, the other third to the right.

The lungs, also cone-shaped, lie on either side of the heart. The left lung is slightly smaller than the right one, to accommodate the heart. Between them, the lungs contain about 300 million tiny air sacs (alveoli), whose combined surface area equals that of a tennis court. The tops of the lungs come right up to the collar line, at the base of the neck. When you breathe in deeply, the bases of the lungs extend to the depth of the tenth pair of ribs. When you breathe out, they retract to the level of the eighth pair of ribs.

Bronchogram of the lungs
A small amount of liquid visible on X-rays is trickled down the throat into the lungs, and outlines the branching pattern of the trachea and bronchi (airways).

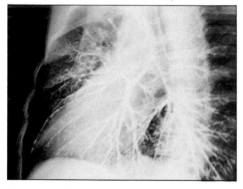

Endoscopic picture of the lungs
The inside of the lungs can be viewed directly by a bronchoscope, a type of endoscope. This picture shows the trachea dividing into the two main bronchi (see also the pictures on p.60).

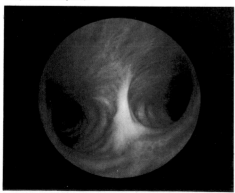

The circulatory system
The circulatory system carries blood to and from every part of the body. Arteries carry blood away from the heart. Veins return blood to the heart.

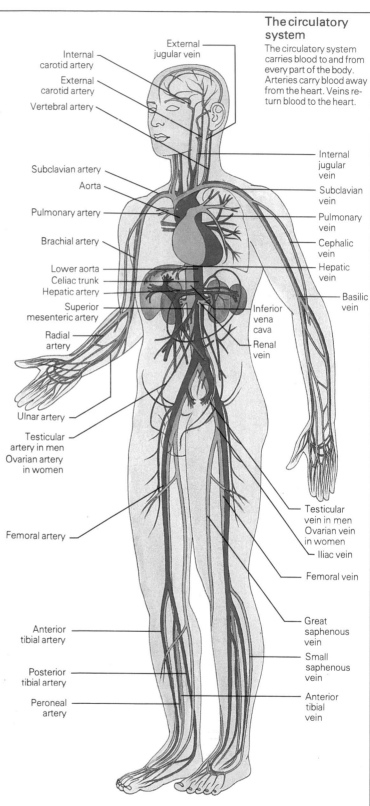

External jugular vein
Internal carotid artery
External carotid artery
Vertebral artery
Subclavian artery
Aorta
Pulmonary artery
Brachial artery
Lower aorta
Celiac trunk
Hepatic artery
Superior mesenteric artery
Radial artery
Ulnar artery
Testicular artery in men
Ovarian artery in women
Femoral artery
Anterior tibial artery
Posterior tibial artery
Peroneal artery

Internal jugular vein
Subclavian vein
Pulmonary vein
Cephalic vein
Hepatic vein
Basilic vein
Inferior vena cava
Renal vein
Testicular vein in men
Ovarian vein in women
Iliac vein
Femoral vein
Great saphenous vein
Small saphenous vein
Anterior tibial vein

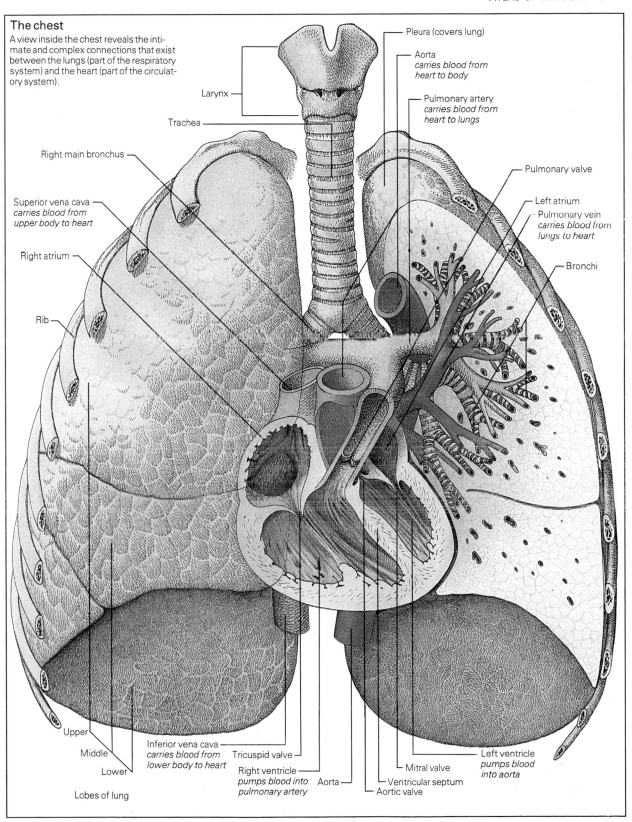

The chest

A view inside the chest reveals the intimate and complex connections that exist between the lungs (part of the respiratory system) and the heart (part of the circulatory system).

Larynx

Trachea

Right main bronchus

Superior vena cava
carries blood from upper body to heart

Right atrium

Rib

Pleura (covers lung)

Aorta
carries blood from heart to body

Pulmonary artery
carries blood from heart to lungs

Pulmonary valve

Left atrium

Pulmonary vein
carries blood from lungs to heart

Bronchi

Upper

Middle

Lower

Lobes of lung

Inferior vena cava
carries blood from lower body to heart

Tricuspid valve

Right ventricle
pumps blood into pulmonary artery

Aorta

Ventricular septum

Aortic valve

Mitral valve

Left ventricle
pumps blood into aorta

The torso

The upper part of the torso is the chest, which contains the heart and lungs (see also the previous page). The chest is separated from the lower part of the torso – the abdomen – by the diaphragm, a dome-shaped sheet of muscle. The edge of the diaphragm is attached to the bottom of the ribcage. Because of its domed shape, its middle reaches to only 25 mm (1 in) below the level of the nipples.

Packed into the abdomen are the organs of the digestive and urinary systems. The lower part of the abdomen, cradled within the hip bone, is often called the pelvis. In the female, the pelvis contains the reproductive organs.

Body scans

Pictures of horizontal "slices" through the body can be taken by the CAT scanner (see also the brain scans on p.55). The denser the tissue that is pictured, the lighter it appears on the scan.

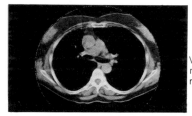

At mid-chest level, the palest areas are the backbone and ribs, the heart appears slightly darker, and the air-filled lungs look black.

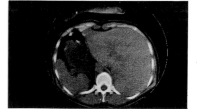

At a level just below the breastbone, the large light area on the right is the liver and the similar, smaller area to the left is the spleen. The darker patch is the stomach.

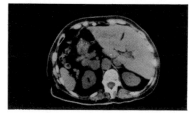

Just above the navel, the liver shows up as a large light area to the right. The light circles on either side of the backbone are the kidneys. The patchy areas toward the left are loops of intestine.

The female torso

The right lung and part of the liver have been omitted to show the heart and abdominal organs. The main blood vessels and nerves in the chest are visible, but those in the abdomen are hidden by the intestines.

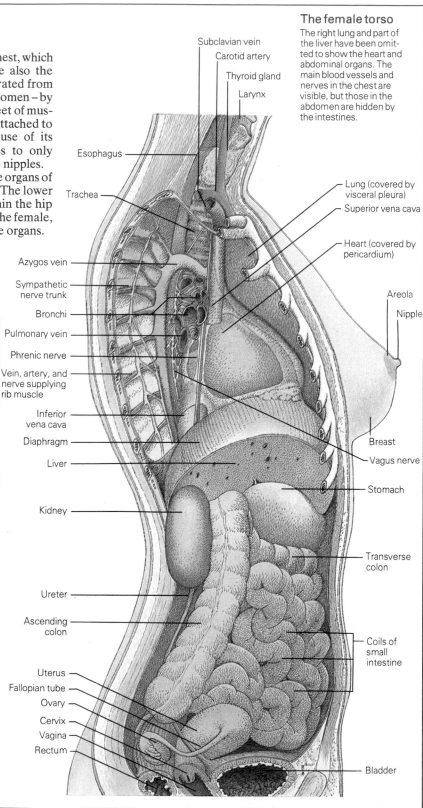

Labels (clockwise):
Subclavian vein
Carotid artery
Thyroid gland
Larynx
Esophagus
Trachea
Lung (covered by visceral pleura)
Superior vena cava
Heart (covered by pericardium)
Areola
Nipple
Azygos vein
Sympathetic nerve trunk
Bronchi
Pulmonary vein
Phrenic nerve
Vein, artery, and nerve supplying rib muscle
Inferior vena cava
Diaphragm
Liver
Kidney
Breast
Vagus nerve
Stomach
Transverse colon
Ureter
Ascending colon
Coils of small intestine
Uterus
Fallopian tube
Ovary
Cervix
Vagina
Rectum
Bladder

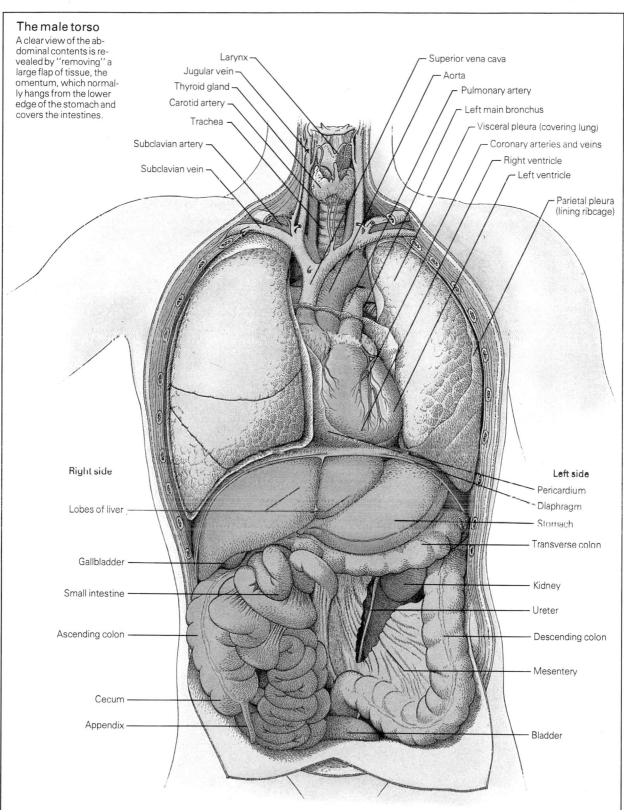

The male torso

A clear view of the abdominal contents is revealed by "removing" a large flap of tissue, the omentum, which normally hangs from the lower edge of the stomach and covers the intestines.

Larynx

Jugular vein

Thyroid gland

Carotid artery

Trachea

Subclavian artery

Subclavian vein

Superior vena cava

Aorta

Pulmonary artery

Left main bronchus

Visceral pleura (covering lung)

Coronary arteries and veins

Right ventricle

Left ventricle

Parietal pleura (lining ribcage)

Right side

Lobes of liver

Gallbladder

Small intestine

Ascending colon

Cecum

Appendix

Left side

Pericardium

Diaphragm

Stomach

Transverse colon

Kidney

Ureter

Descending colon

Mesentery

Bladder

The digestive organs

The digestive tract is basically one long tube extending from the mouth to the anus. Food passes from the mouth down the esophagus, a section of the tube about 25 cm (10 in) long, to the stomach, which holds about 1.5 liters (2½ pints) when fairly full. After the stomach comes the duodenum, a C-shaped tube about the same length as the esophagus. Small ducts carry digestive juices from the liver and pancreas into the duodenum. The next section of the tract is about 5 m (about 16 ft) of coiled small intestine, followed by 1.5 m (about 5 ft) of large intestine, which leads into the rectum and, finally, the anus.

The lengths of the various portions of digestive tract vary markedly from person to person. They also vary depending on whether the tissues are alive or not. After death, the muscles in the digestive-tract walls lose their tone and relax, and the tract becomes considerably longer.

The digestive system
The digestive system includes the digestive tract – the tube from mouth to anus – plus two organs, the liver and pancreas, that manufacture digestive juices.

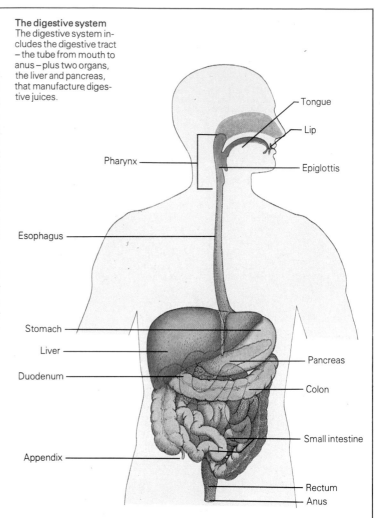

Endoscopy
Modern endoscopes (long, flexible tubes that transmit visual images) can reach and view virtually all parts of the digestive tract. Most regions of the tract are normally flattened and contain murky semi-liquids. So, to obtain a clear view, air is pumped down the endoscope into the tract to hold its wall apart while the photograph is being taken. Below left is a photograph of the stomach lining with its shiny, ridged surface. Below right is the lining of the duodenum. It has a smooth interior on which an abnormality – an ulcer, for instance – would be clearly visible (see also the picture on p.56).

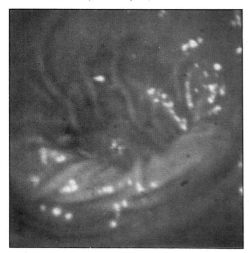

Endoscopic view of stomach

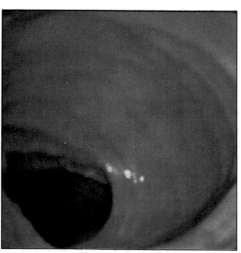

Endoscopic view of duodenum

The abdominal digestive organs

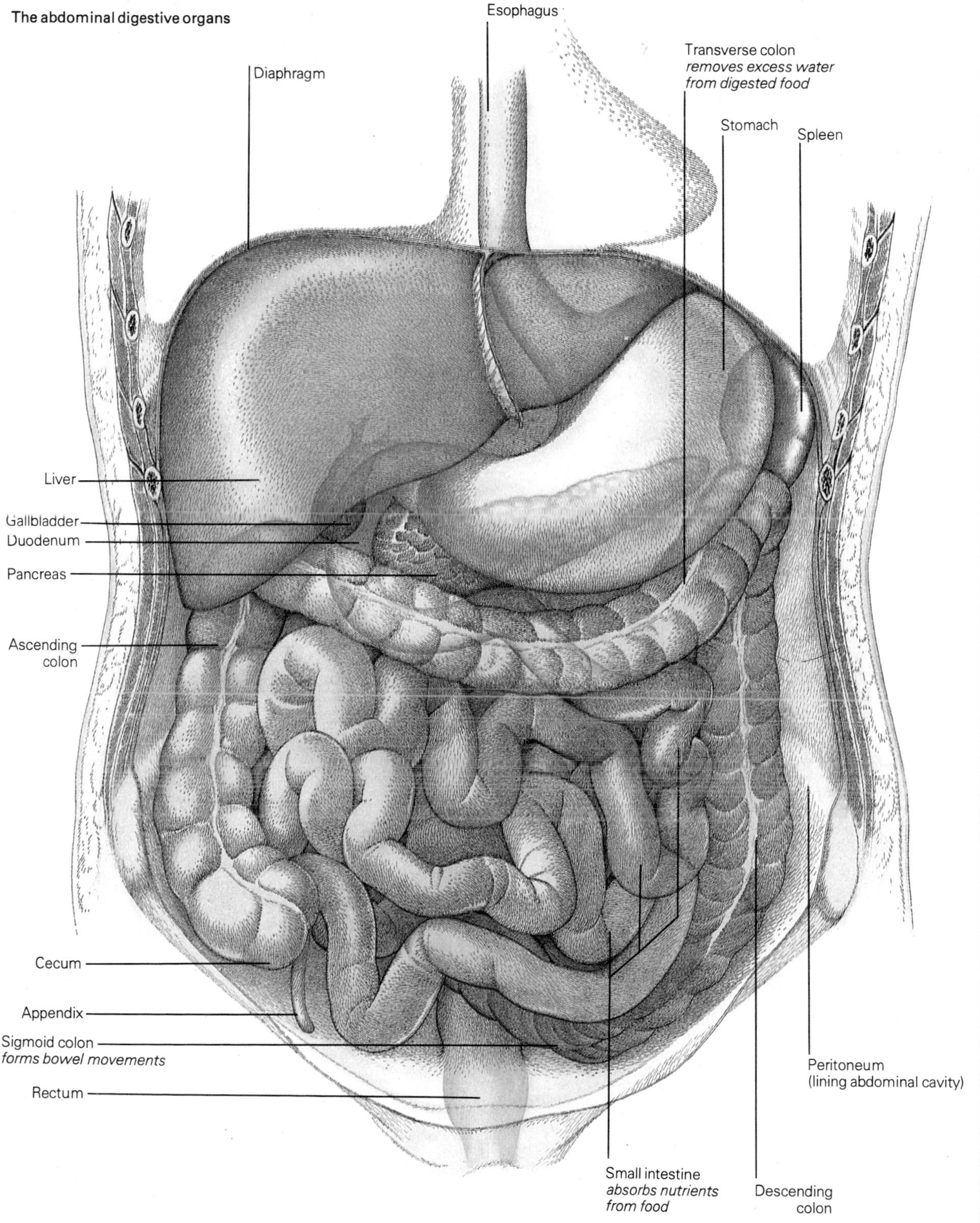

Esophagus

Diaphragm

Transverse colon
*removes excess water
from digested food*

Stomach

Spleen

Liver

Gallbladder

Duodenum

Pancreas

Ascending
colon

Cecum

Appendix

Sigmoid colon
forms bowel movements

Rectum

Small intestine
*absorbs nutrients
from food*

Descending
colon

Peritoneum
(lining abdominal cavity)

The organs of the lower abdomen

The lower abdominal organs are concerned principally with removal of wastes, in the form of urine and bowel movements, and with reproduction (see below). The bladder stores urine from the kidneys. It is a muscular sac about 75 mm (3 in) in diameter when full. The urine is passed to the outside along a tube called the urethra, which in the male is 25 cm (about 10 in) long but in the female only 25 mm (approximately 1 in) long. The lower abdominal organs are sometimes called the pelvic organs because they are situated within the cup-shaped hip bone, or pelvis.

The male reproductive organs
In addition to the visible male genitalia – two testes in their pouch (the scrotum) and the penis – there are glands and ducts inside the abdomen. These internal organs are the prostate gland, two seminal vesicles, and the two tubes that are called the vas deferens.

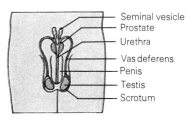

Seminal vesicle
Prostate
Urethra
Vas deferens
Penis
Testis
Scrotum

The female reproductive organs
The female genital organs are all situated within the abdomen, except for the vagina, which leads from the abdominal area to the external genitals, the vulva. Inside the abdomen are two ovaries connected by the two fallopian tubes to the uterus (commonly called the womb).

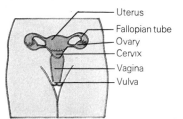

Uterus
Fallopian tube
Ovary
Cervix
Vagina
Vulva

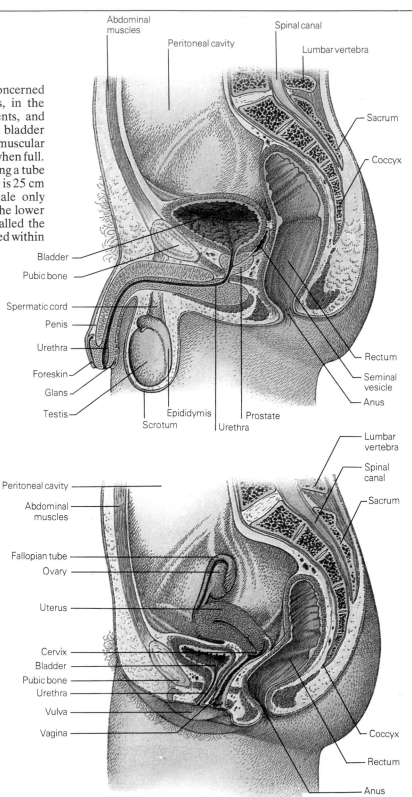

Abdominal muscles
Peritoneal cavity
Spinal canal
Lumbar vertebra
Sacrum
Coccyx
Bladder
Pubic bone
Spermatic cord
Penis
Urethra
Foreskin
Glans
Testis
Scrotum
Epididymis
Urethra
Prostate
Rectum
Seminal vesicle
Anus

Peritoneal cavity
Abdominal muscles
Fallopian tube
Ovary
Uterus
Cervix
Bladder
Pubic bone
Urethra
Vulva
Vagina
Lumbar vertebra
Spinal canal
Sacrum
Coccyx
Rectum
Anus

The fetus

A fetus (baby within the uterus) is almost ready for birth and in the typical birth position – head down and the back of the head towards the mother's abdomen.

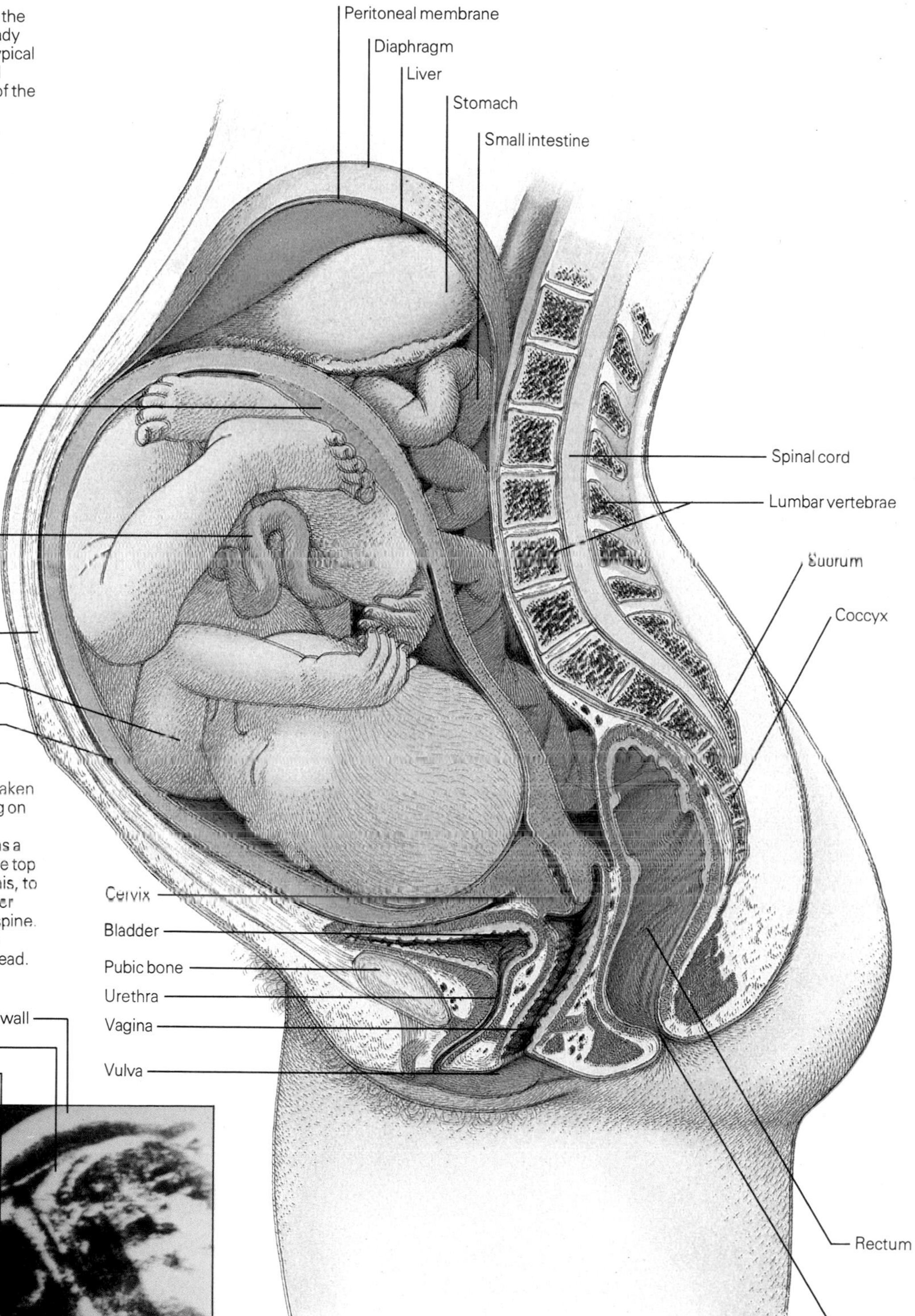

Peritoneal membrane
Diaphragm
Liver
Stomach
Small intestine

Placenta
supplies oxygen and nutrients to fetus

Spinal cord

Lumbar vertebrae

Umbilical cord
carries fetus' blood to and from placenta

Sacrum

Coccyx

Abdominal muscles

Fetus

Uterus

Fetal scan

An ultrasound scan taken with the mother lying on her back reveals the mother's abdomen as a thick light curve at the top of the scan. Below this, to the right, is the thinner light curve of fetus' spine. The light circle in the center is the fetus' head.

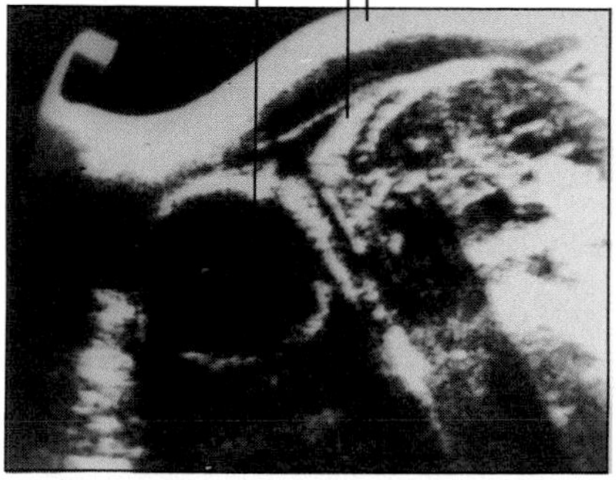

Cervix
Bladder
Pubic bone
Urethra
Vagina
Vulva

Rectum

Anus

Mother's abdominal wall
Fetus' spine
Fetus' head

The special sense organs

The two senses that provide most information about the world around us are sight and hearing. The eyes and ears are delicate and sensitive structures of great complexity, but they lie well protected inside shaped cavities within the skull bones. The eye is "directional" in that six separate muscles swivel it to look at objects in various locations, and this directional information is passed to the brain. The human ear does not have this ability, though many animals are able to pinpoint the direction a sound comes from by moving the external ear, or pinna.

Ophthalmoscope view of the retina
The pale disc is the optic disc, where all the nerves come together and leave the eye on their way to the brain. Arteries can be seen radiating from the disc to supply the retina and other structures in the eye with blood.

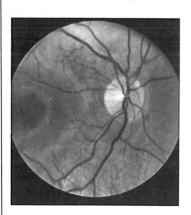

The ear
The outer ear canal, which is about 2 cm (¾ in) long, leads through the skull bone to the middle and inner ear. Connecting the middle ear to the back of the throat is another tube about 4 cm (approximately 1½ in) long, the eustachian tube. Besides enabling you to hear, the ear also contains the semicircular canals, which function to help you to keep your balance.

The eye
The eyeball is about 25 mm (1 in) in diameter. The socket for it in the skull bone is appreciably larger, to allow room for the muscles that control eye movement.

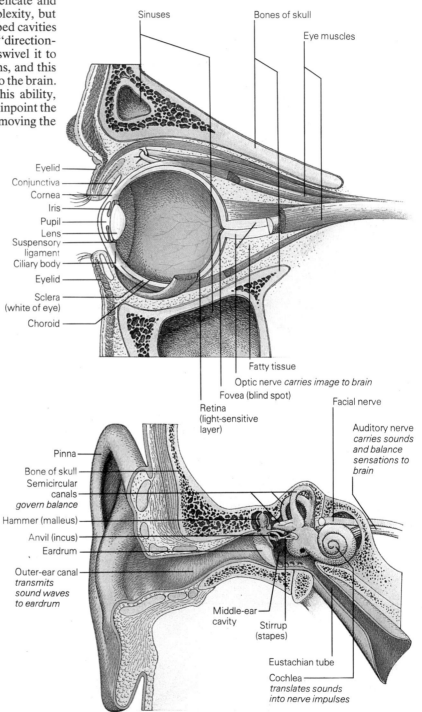

Sinuses

Bones of skull

Eye muscles

Eyelid
Conjunctiva
Cornea
Iris
Pupil
Lens
Suspensory ligament
Ciliary body
Eyelid
Sclera (white of eye)
Choroid

Fatty tissue
Optic nerve *carries image to brain*
Fovea (blind spot)
Retina (light-sensitive layer)

Facial nerve

Auditory nerve *carries sounds and balance sensations to brain*

Pinna
Bone of skull
Semicircular canals *govern balance*
Hammer (malleus)
Anvil (incus)
Eardrum
Outer-ear canal *transmits sound waves to eardrum*

Middle-ear cavity
Stirrup (stapes)
Eustachian tube
Cochlea *translates sounds into nerve impulses*

Part II

Symptoms and self-diagnosis

Self-diagnosis symptom charts
Visual aids to diagnosis

Self-diagnosis symptom charts

How to use the charts

Each of the self-diagnosis symptom charts in this section is aimed at helping you to track down the possible significance of a particular symptom, either on its own or combined with other symptoms. Every chart has a common symptom as its starting point, from which you are led by a series of questions and answers to a logical conclusion. The end point you reach will probably refer you elsewhere in this book, and may also tell you to seek professional help either routinely or urgently. First find the chart you want by consulting the Chart-finder (see p.68), which gives you the appropriate *chart number*. Then, turn to the chart itself, and check its relevance by noting the *definition* and *chart group*.

As shown on the two samples on these pages, each chart consists of a series of simple YES or NO *questions*. Begin at the first question, and follow through to the *diagnosis*

Chart number
Each chart has a number that accompanies all references to it.

Chart group
This indicates what segment of the population the chart is designed to help. Before using a chart, make sure you have chosen one for the right sex and age group.

Chart title
A short descriptive term for the symptom heads each chart.

Definition
To avoid confusion, the named symptom is defined in simple, non-technical terms.

The questions
Each question is phrased so that it requires either a YES or NO reply. Follow your yes or no answer to the appropriate next question, and continue until, in most cases, you reach a diagnosis.

The diagnosis
Possible reasons for your problem appear in the diagnosis. For further information you are usually referred elsewhere in this book. If you probably need urgent medical attention, this is emphasized. Exact meanings of the instructions are explained on p.67.

Visual aids to diagnosis
A number of disorders are illustrated in full color in a special section of the book. If there is such an illustration, the page and illustration number will be given.

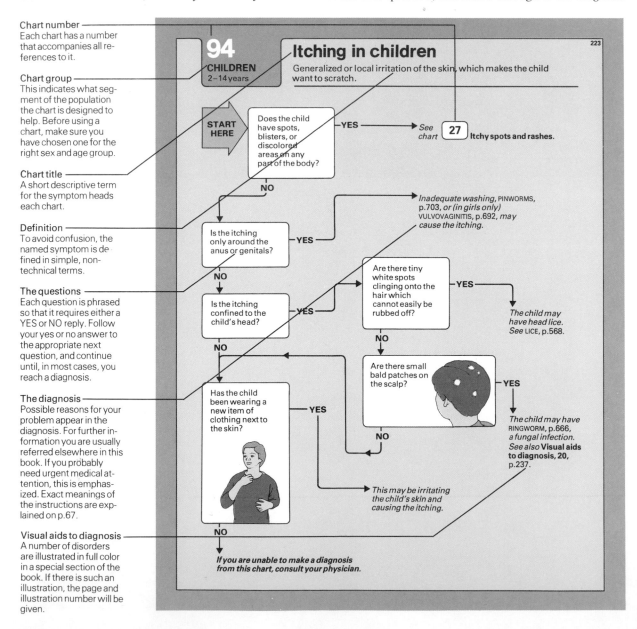

94
CHILDREN
2–14 years

Itching in children

Generalized or local irritation of the skin, which makes the child want to scratch.

223

START HERE

Does the child have spots, blisters, or discolored areas on any part of the body? — YES → *See chart* **27** Itchy spots and rashes.

NO

Is the itching only around the anus or genitals? — YES → *Inadequate washing*, PINWORMS, p.703, *or (in girls only)* VULVOVAGINITIS, p.692, *may cause the itching.*

NO

Is the itching confined to the child's head? — YES → Are there tiny white spots clinging onto the hair which cannot easily be rubbed off? — YES → *The child may have head lice.* See LICE, p.568.

NO

Are there small bald patches on the scalp? — YES → *The child may have* RINGWORM, p.666, *a fungal infection.* See also **Visual aids to diagnosis, 20,** p.237.

NO

NO

Has the child been wearing a new item of clothing next to the skin? — YES → *This may be irritating the child's skin and causing the itching.*

NO

If you are unable to make a diagnosis from this chart, consult your physician.

that fits your case. Here you will usually find one – or sometimes more than one – likely explanation of your problem, along with *instructions* on what steps to take. Except in urgent cases, be sure to follow through on all cross-references to get as much information as possible.
Important: Remember that the charts give only tentative diagnoses. For firm diagnosis, and for treatment, consult your physician.

What the instructions mean

Call your physician now!
Seek medical advice within a few hours at the most. Telephone your physician immediately. If your physician is not available, telephone or visit the nearest hospital emergency room.

EMERGENCY
Get medical help now!
The problem may be life-threatening and needs immediate attention. If you fail to reach your own physician within minutes, call for an ambulance, or take the person to the nearest hospital emergency room if he or she can be moved safely.

Consult your physician.
Do not delay!
Get medical advice within a day or two. Ask your doctor's receptionist for an appointment or discuss the problem with your physician by telephone.

If your problem is not identified as one requiring immediate attention, you can assume that an urgent consultation is not vital. Turn to the page(s) indicated for further information.

First aid
Wherever first-aid measures are applicable, a cross-reference to the Accidents and emergencies section is provided.

134

39
GENERAL
all ages

Coughing up blood
Coughing up phlegm that is colored or streaked bright red or rusty brown, or that is pink and frothy.

START HERE → Is your temperature 102°F (39°C) or above?

— YES → **Call your physician now!**
These symptoms suggest that you may have PNEUMONIA, *p.359, especially if your phlegm is rusty brown.*

— NO →

Are you short of breath even though you have not been exercising?
— YES → Is your phlegm pink and frothy?
— YES → **EMERGENCY**
Get medical help now!
You may have a build-up of fluid in the lungs.
See PULMONARY EDEMA, p.368.

— NO (from phlegm question) ↓

— NO (from short of breath) ↓

Have you recently had an operation, or been confined to bed by an injury or prolonged illness?
— YES → **EMERGENCY**
Get medical help now!
You may have a blood clot in the lung.
See PULMONARY EMBOLISM, p.406.

— NO ↓

Has a cold or bout of flu within the past month left you with a persistent cough?
— YES → *Consult your physician. Coughing may have ruptured a small blood vessel.*

— NO ↓

Have you had a cough for many weeks or months?
— YES → *Consult your physician.*
Do not delay!
These symptoms indicate the possibility of LUNG CANCER, p.366, *or* TUBERCULOSIS, p.563.

— NO ↓

If you are unable to make a diagnosis from this chart, consult your physician without further delay.

Cancer watch
Coughing up blood may be a sign of lung cancer if you have had a cough for many weeks or months. This diagnosis is particularly likely if you smoke.

Consult your physician without delay!

Boxed information
Some charts contain boxes giving important additional information such as self-help advice or, more often, warnings about possibly dangerous symptoms. Whenever there is a possibility of cancer the box will be headed **Cancer watch.**

How to find the chart you need

The special *Chart-finder* index (below) directs you to the number of the chart that deals with your problem. To find the chart you want, follow these steps:

1. Single out your major problem. If you have two or more symptoms (a high fever, a cough and a runny nose, for example), select the one that bothers you the most.

2. Find the symptom in the chart-finder. For your convenience the charts are indexed according to a variety of key words. Irregular vaginal bleeding, for instance, is listed in three places, under the letters B, I, and V.

3. If you cannot find your main symptom in the chart-finder, look for a chart dealing with a secondary symptom (if you have one).

4. When you have found the correct chart, turn to the chart number (*not* the page number) indicated and proceed with your diagnosis. For a full explanation of how to use the charts, see p.66.

CHART-FINDER

1

GENERAL
all ages

Feeling under the weather

A vague, generalized feeling of being ill.

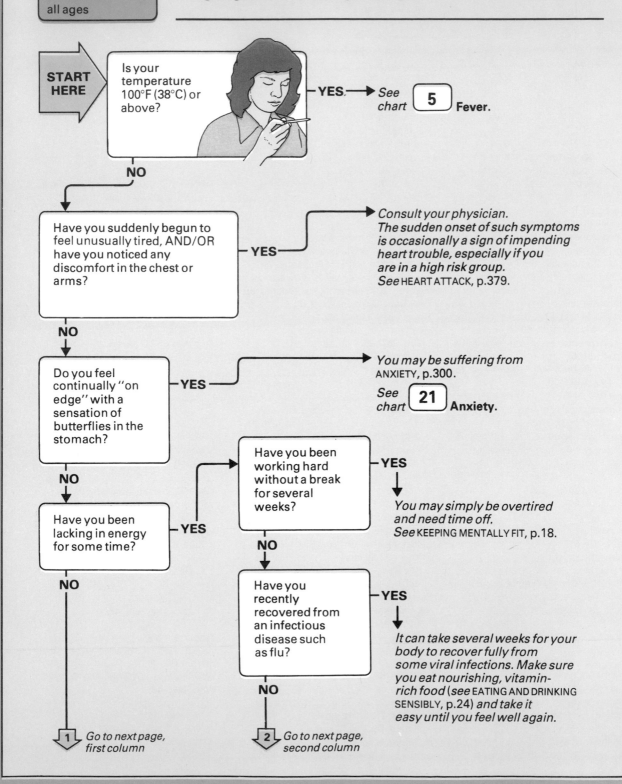

START HERE → Is your temperature 100°F (38°C) or above?

YES → *See chart* **5** *Fever.*

NO ↓

Have you suddenly begun to feel unusually tired, AND/OR have you noticed any discomfort in the chest or arms?

YES → *Consult your physician. The sudden onset of such symptoms is occasionally a sign of impending heart trouble, especially if you are in a high risk group. See* HEART ATTACK, p.379.

NO ↓

Do you feel continually "on edge" with a sensation of butterflies in the stomach?

YES → *You may be suffering from* ANXIETY, p.300. *See chart* **21** *Anxiety.*

NO ↓

Have you been lacking in energy for some time?

YES → Have you been working hard without a break for several weeks?

YES → *You may simply be overtired and need time off. See* KEEPING MENTALLY FIT, p.18.

NO ↓

Have you recently recovered from an infectious disease such as flu?

YES → *It can take several weeks for your body to recover fully from some viral infections. Make sure you eat nourishing, vitamin-rich food (see* EATING AND DRINKING SENSIBLY, p.24) *and take it easy until you feel well again.*

NO ↓

NO ↓

1 *Go to next page, first column*

2 *Go to next page, second column*

1 *Continued from previous page, first column*

2 *Continued from previous page, second column*

Do you have one or more of the following symptoms?
☐ difficulty in sleeping
☐ inability to concentrate or make decisions
☐ lack of interest in sex
☐ recurrent headaches,
☐ Feeling in low spirits

YES → *You may be anemic or depressed. See* ANEMIA, p.419, *and* chart **20** **Depression**

NO

Are you overweight according to the chart on p.28?

YES → *Being overweight puts a strain on your whole body. You may feel better if you lose weight. See* OBESITY, p.492, *and* HOW TO LOSE WEIGHT, p.28.

NO

Do you get little or no regular exercise?

YES → *Physical exercise is necessary to keep the body functioning efficiently. See* KEEPING PHYSICALLY FIT, p.14.

NO

Are you currently taking any medicines?

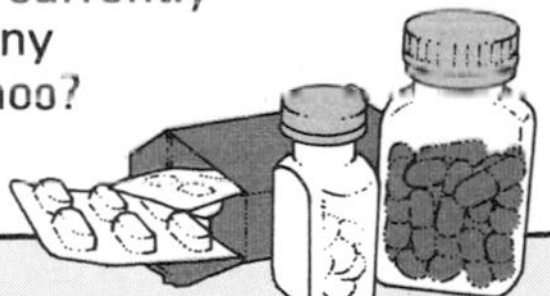

YES → *Some drugs can make you feel vaguely ill. Discuss with your physician.*

NO

Have you lost weight (more than 4kg, or 10lb, in 10 weeks) without trying?

YES → *See* chart **2** **Loss of weight.**

NO

If you are unable to make a diagnosis from this chart, consult your physician.

2

GENERAL
all ages

Loss of weight

Loss of 10lb (4kg) or more over a period of 10 weeks or less, without a deliberate change in eating habits.

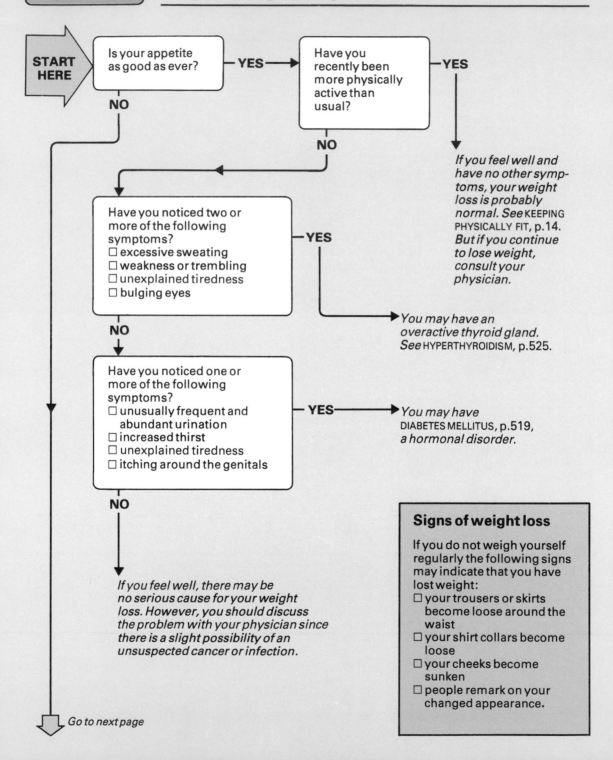

START HERE

Is your appetite as good as ever?

— YES →

Have you recently been more physically active than usual?

— YES →

If you feel well and have no other symptoms, your weight loss is probably normal. See KEEPING PHYSICALLY FIT, p.14. But if you continue to lose weight, consult your physician.

NO

NO

Have you noticed two or more of the following symptoms?
☐ excessive sweating
☐ weakness or trembling
☐ unexplained tiredness
☐ bulging eyes

— YES →

You may have an overactive thyroid gland. See HYPERTHYROIDISM, p.525.

NO

Have you noticed one or more of the following symptoms?
☐ unusually frequent and abundant urination
☐ increased thirst
☐ unexplained tiredness
☐ itching around the genitals

— YES →

You may have DIABETES MELLITUS, p.519, a hormonal disorder.

NO

If you feel well, there may be no serious cause for your weight loss. However, you should discuss the problem with your physician since there is a slight possibility of an unsuspected cancer or infection.

Signs of weight loss

If you do not weigh yourself regularly the following signs may indicate that you have lost weight:
☐ your trousers or skirts become loose around the waist
☐ your shirt collars become loose
☐ your cheeks become sunken
☐ people remark on your changed appearance.

Go to next page

⬇ *Continued from previous page*

Have you been having recurrent bouts of diarrhea?

— **YES** → **Are your bowel movements unusually pale, bulky and difficult to flush away?** — **YES** →

You may have faulty digestion.
See MALABSORPTION, p.475.

NO ↓

NO ↓ (from bowel movements box)

Have you been constipated AND/OR have you noticed blood in your bowel movements?

— **YES** →

Consult your physician.
Do not delay!
You may have inflammation of the small intestine (see CROHN'S DISEASE, p.473*), but there is also a chance of* CANCER OF THE LARGE INTESTINE, p.481.

NO ↓

Have you been having re-current attacks of upper abdominal pain?

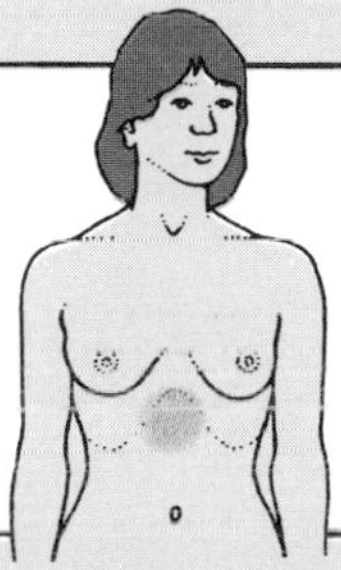

— **YES** →

Consult your physician.
Do not delay!
You may have a STOMACH ULCER, p.465, *but there is also a possibility of* CANCER OF THE STOMACH, p.466.

NO ↓

Have you noticed two or more of the following symptoms?
☐ sweating at night
☐ recurrent fever
☐ unexplained tiredness
☐ general feeling of ill health
☐ persistent cough
☐ blood in phlegm

— **YES** →

Consult your physician.
Do not delay!
You may have a chronic infection such as TUBERCULOSIS, p.563.

NO ↓

If you are unable to make a diagnosis from this chart, consult your physician.

Cancer watch

There is a possibility of cancer if weight loss and loss of appetite are combined with abdominal pain OR a change in bowel habits.

Consult your physician without delay!

Overweight

The chart on p.28 indicates the optimum weight for your height. If you are heavier, you are overweight and may be endangering your health.

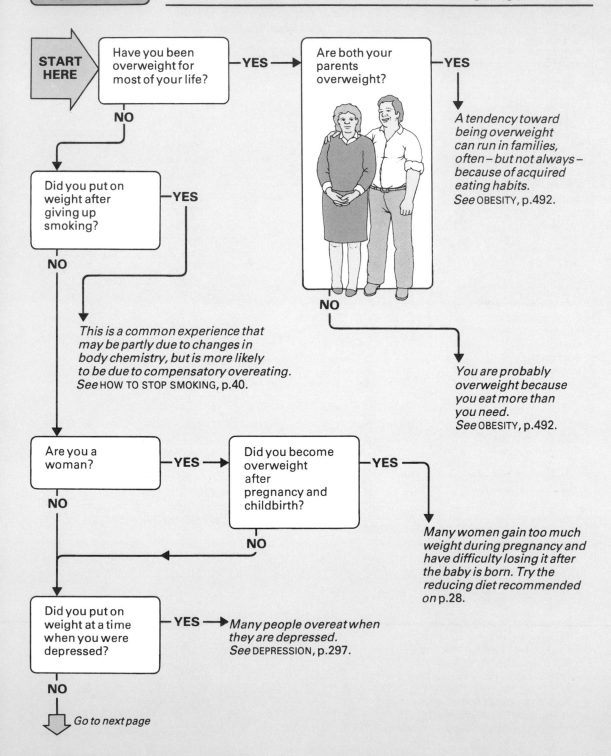

START HERE

Have you been overweight for most of your life? — **YES** → Are both your parents overweight? — **YES** →

A tendency toward being overweight can run in families, often – but not always – because of acquired eating habits.
See OBESITY, p.492.

NO ↓

Did you put on weight after giving up smoking? — **YES**

NO ↓

This is a common experience that may be partly due to changes in body chemistry, but is more likely to be due to compensatory overeating.
See HOW TO STOP SMOKING, p.40.

NO (from parents box)

You are probably overweight because you eat more than you need.
See OBESITY, p.492.

Are you a woman? — **YES** → Did you become overweight after pregnancy and childbirth? — **YES** →

Many women gain too much weight during pregnancy and have difficulty losing it after the baby is born. Try the reducing diet recommended on p.28.

NO ↓ **NO** ←

Did you put on weight at a time when you were depressed? — **YES** → *Many people overeat when they are depressed.*
See DEPRESSION, p.297.

NO ↓

Go to next page

⬇ *Continued from previous page*

Did the weight gain follow a change from a physically strenuous job to sedentary work?

YES → *In your former job you probably needed more calories than you do now. You should adjust your eating habits accordingly.* See COUNTING CALORIES, p.27.

NO ↓

Have you noticed any of the following symptoms since you began to put on weight?
☐ feeling the cold more than you used to
☐ thinning or brittle hair
☐ dry skin

YES → *You may have an underactive thyroid gland.* See HYPOTHYROIDISM, p.526.

NO ↓

Have you been taking steroid drugs for a problem such as asthma or rheumatoid arthritis?

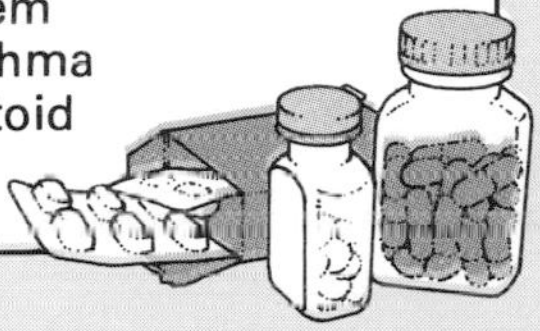

YES → *Such drugs can cause weight gain. Discuss with your physician.*

NO ↓

Are you over 40?

YES → *Weight gain as you grow older may be a result of such factors as a decline in the amount of exercise you get and changes in the rate that your body burns up food.* See AGE AND INCREASING WEIGHT, p.29.

NO ↓

If you are unable to make a diagnosis from this chart, your excess weight is probably due only to overeating. If after a month of following the recommended reducing diet, you fail to lose weight, consult your physician.

Losing excess weight

Whatever the cause of your weight gain, following the balanced reducing diet described on p.28 will help you achieve and maintain a healthy weight.

4

GENERAL
all ages

Difficulty in sleeping

Frequent difficulty in either falling asleep or staying asleep during the night (often called insomnia).

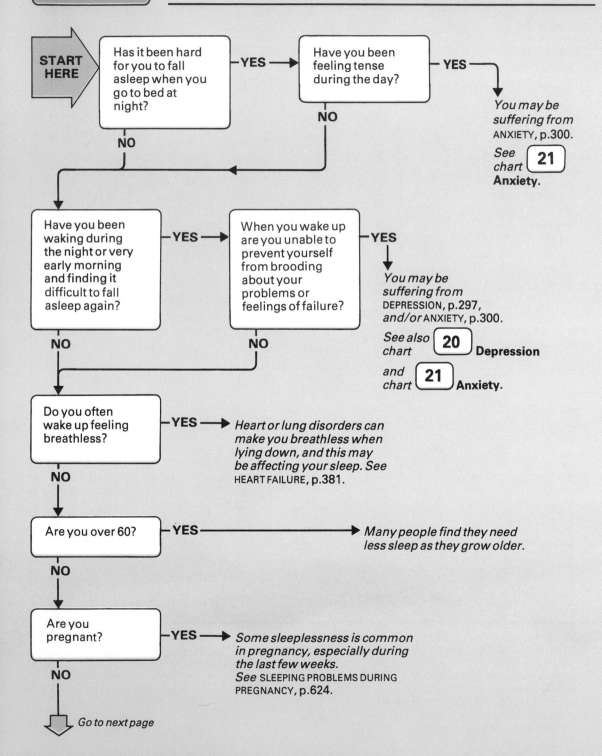

START HERE

Has it been hard for you to fall asleep when you go to bed at night? — **YES** → Have you been feeling tense during the day? — **YES** →

You may be suffering from ANXIETY, p.300.

See chart **21** **Anxiety**.

NO

NO

Have you been waking during the night or very early morning and finding it difficult to fall asleep again? — **YES** → When you wake up are you unable to prevent yourself from brooding about your problems or feelings of failure? — **YES** →

You may be suffering from DEPRESSION, p.297, *and/or* ANXIETY, p.300.

See also chart **20** **Depression**

and chart **21** **Anxiety**.

NO

NO

Do you often wake up feeling breathless? — **YES** → *Heart or lung disorders can make you breathless when lying down, and this may be affecting your sleep. See* HEART FAILURE, p.381.

NO

Are you over 60? — **YES** → *Many people find they need less sleep as they grow older.*

NO

Are you pregnant? — **YES** → *Some sleeplessness is common in pregnancy, especially during the last few weeks.* See SLEEPING PROBLEMS DURING PREGNANCY, p.624.

NO

Go to next page

⬇ *Continued from previous page*

On nights when you have difficulty sleeping, have you drunk more tea, cola or coffee than usual?

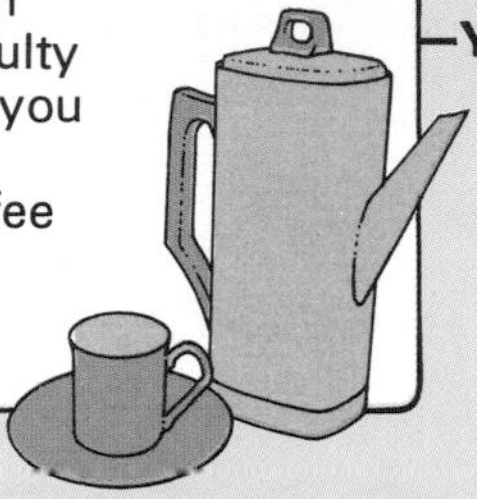

YES → *The caffeine in tea, cola and coffee is a stimulant and could be the cause of your problem. Try to avoid or cut down on these drinks in the late afternoon and evening. If you still have trouble sleeping, try drinking decaffeinated products or cutting out tea, cola and coffee altogether.* See CAFFEINE, p.30.

NO ↓

On nights when you have difficulty in sleeping, have you eaten a late, heavy meal, or drunk a lot of alcohol?

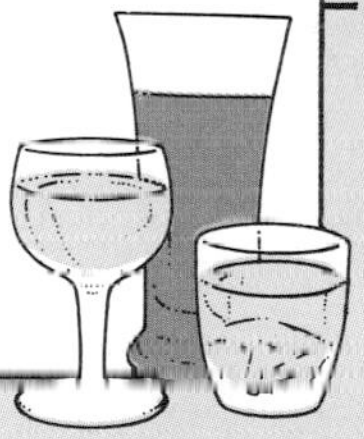

YES → *These are common causes of difficulty in sleeping. Try eating your evening meals earlier and/or reducing your alcohol intake.*

NO ↓

Have you recently stopped taking sleeping pills or tranquilizers?

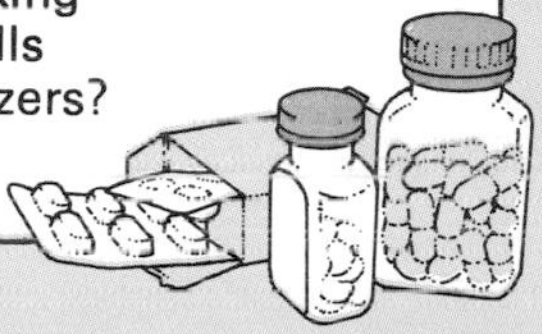

YES → *It can take several weeks for your sleeping pattern to return to normal after using these drugs.*

NO ↓

Do you have a sedentary job and do you get little physical exercise on most days?

YES → *Your body may not be tired enough to allow you to sleep easily. Try exercising in the fresh air if possible before bedtime.* See WHY EXERCISE IS GOOD FOR YOU, p.15.

NO ↓

If you are unable to make a diagnosis from this chart, and self-help suggestions do not work, consult your physician.

Self-help

If you have difficulty in sleeping for any reason, try the following self-help measures:
☐ reduce your consumption of tea, coffee, cola and alcohol
☐ avoid large, late evening meals.
☐ take a walk in the fresh air before bedtime
☐ have a warm drink before going to bed.

See also HOW TO GET A GOOD NIGHT'S SLEEP, p.20.

Fever

Temperature of about 100°F (38°C) or above.
For children see chart 90, **Fever in infants**, or chart 91, **Fever in children**.

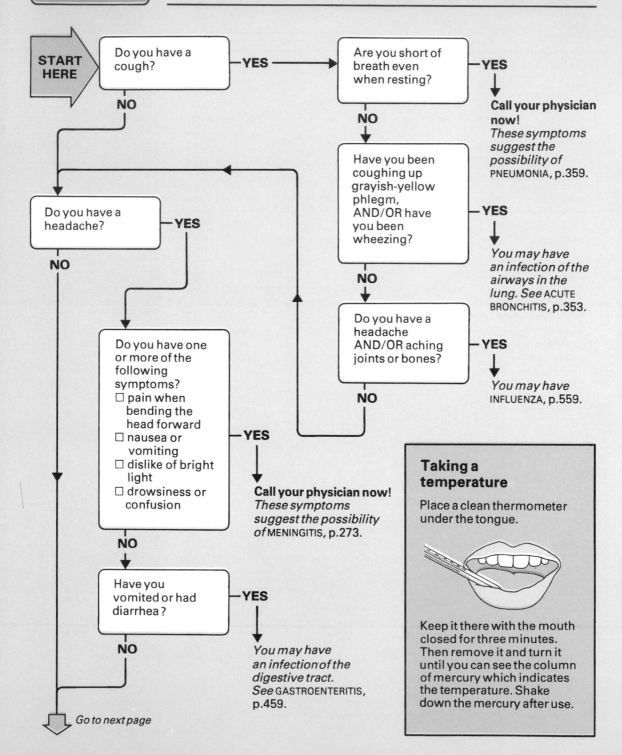

START HERE

Do you have a cough? — **YES** → Are you short of breath even when resting? — **YES** ↓

Call your physician now! *These symptoms suggest the possibility of* PNEUMONIA, p.359.

NO ↓

Have you been coughing up grayish-yellow phlegm, AND/OR have you been wheezing? — **YES** ↓

You may have an infection of the airways in the lung. See ACUTE BRONCHITIS, p.353.

NO ↓

Do you have a headache AND/OR aching joints or bones? — **YES** ↓

You may have INFLUENZA, p.559.

NO

Do you have a headache? — **YES** ↓

NO ↓

Do you have one or more of the following symptoms?
☐ pain when bending the head forward
☐ nausea or vomiting
☐ dislike of bright light
☐ drowsiness or confusion

— **YES** ↓

Call your physician now! *These symptoms suggest the possibility of* MENINGITIS, p.273.

NO ↓

Have you vomited or had diarrhea? — **YES** ↓

You may have an infection of the digestive tract. See GASTROENTERITIS, p.459.

NO ↓

Go to next page

Taking a temperature

Place a clean thermometer under the tongue.

Keep it there with the mouth closed for three minutes. Then remove it and turn it until you can see the column of mercury which indicates the temperature. Shake down the mercury after use.

⬇ *Continued from previous page*

Do you have aching joints or bones? — **YES** ⟶ *You may have* INFLUENZA, p.559.

NO ↓

Do you have a rash? — **YES** ⟶ *See chart* **28** **Rash with fever.**

NO ↓

Do you have a sore throat? — **YES** ⟶ *You may have a throat infection. See* PHARYNGITIS, *p.350, and* TONSILLITIS, *p.351.*

NO ↓

Do you have pain in the small of your back on one side just above the waist? — **YES** ⟶ *You may have a kidney infection. See* ACUTE PYELONEPHRITIS, *p.502.*

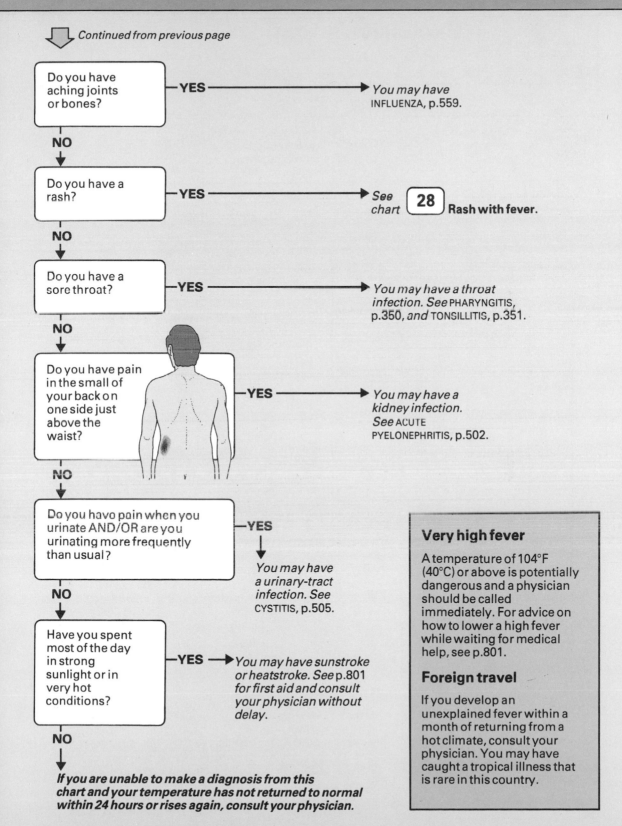

NO ↓

Do you have pain when you urinate AND/OR are you urinating more frequently than usual? — **YES** ↓ *You may have a urinary-tract infection. See* CYSTITIS, *p.505.*

NO ↓

Have you spent most of the day in strong sunlight or in very hot conditions? — **YES** ⟶ *You may have sunstroke or heatstroke. See p.801 for first aid and consult your physician without delay.*

NO ↓

If you are unable to make a diagnosis from this chart and your temperature has not returned to normal within 24 hours or rises again, consult your physician.

Very high fever

A temperature of 104°F (40°C) or above is potentially dangerous and a physician should be called immediately. For advice on how to lower a high fever while waiting for medical help, see p.801.

Foreign travel

If you develop an unexplained fever within a month of returning from a hot climate, consult your physician. You may have caught a tropical illness that is rare in this country.

6

GENERAL
all ages

Excessive sweating

Sweating that is not associated with heat or exercise.

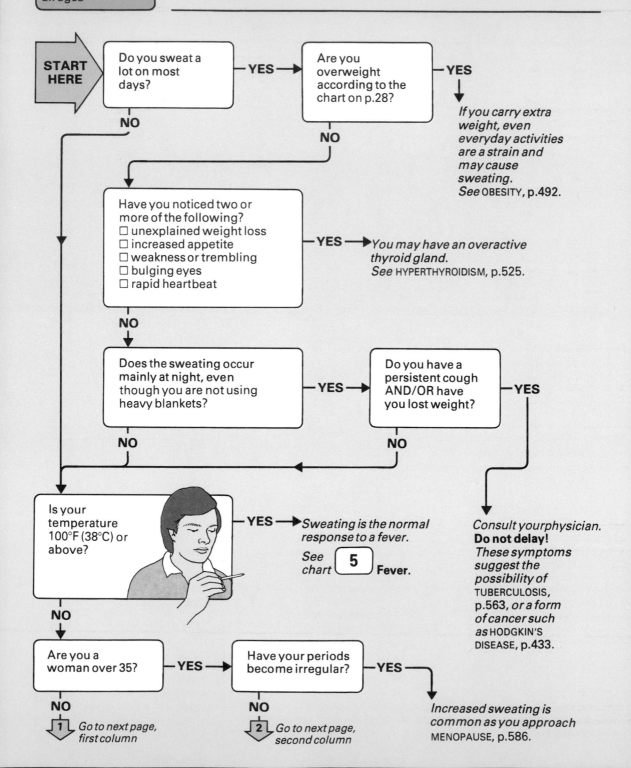

START HERE

Do you sweat a lot on most days? — **YES** → **Are you overweight according to the chart on p.28?** — **YES** →

If you carry extra weight, even everyday activities are a strain and may cause sweating. See OBESITY, p.492.

NO ↓ (from "Do you sweat a lot")

NO ↓ (from "overweight")

Have you noticed two or more of the following?
☐ unexplained weight loss
☐ increased appetite
☐ weakness or trembling
☐ bulging eyes
☐ rapid heartbeat

— **YES** → *You may have an overactive thyroid gland.* See HYPERTHYROIDISM, p.525.

NO ↓

Does the sweating occur mainly at night, even though you are not using heavy blankets? — **YES** → **Do you have a persistent cough AND/OR have you lost weight?** — **YES** →

NO ↓ **NO** ↓

Is your temperature 100°F (38°C) or above? — **YES** → *Sweating is the normal response to a fever.*

See chart **5** **Fever.**

Consult your physician. **Do not delay!** *These symptoms suggest the possibility of* TUBERCULOSIS, p.563, *or a form of cancer such as* HODGKIN'S DISEASE, p.433.

NO ↓

Are you a woman over 35? — **YES** → **Have your periods become irregular?** — **YES** →

NO ↓ **NO** ↓

⬇ **1** *Go to next page, first column*

⬇ **2** *Go to next page, second column*

Increased sweating is common as you approach MENOPAUSE, p.586.

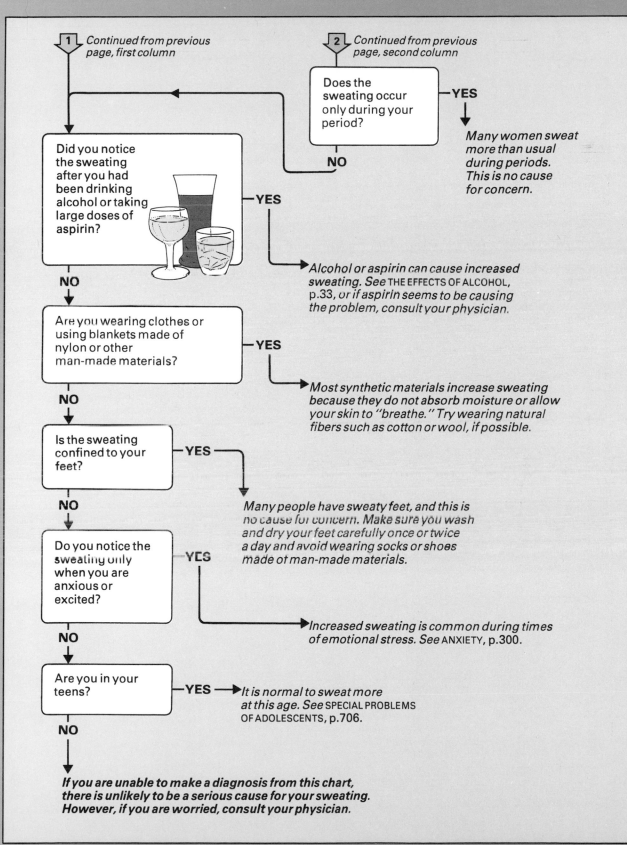

1 *Continued from previous page, first column*

2 *Continued from previous page, second column*

Does the sweating occur only during your period? — **YES**

↓

Many women sweat more than usual during periods. This is no cause for concern.

NO

Did you notice the sweating after you had been drinking alcohol or taking large doses of aspirin? — **YES**

Alcohol or aspirin can cause increased sweating. See THE EFFECTS OF ALCOHOL, *p.33, or if aspirin seems to be causing the problem, consult your physician.*

NO

Are you wearing clothes or using blankets made of nylon or other man-made materials? — **YES**

Most synthetic materials increase sweating because they do not absorb moisture or allow your skin to "breathe." Try wearing natural fibers such as cotton or wool, if possible.

NO

Is the sweating confined to your feet? — **YES**

Many people have sweaty feet, and this is no cause for concern. Make sure you wash and dry your feet carefully once or twice a day and avoid wearing socks or shoes made of man-made materials.

NO

Do you notice the sweating only when you are anxious or excited? — **YES**

Increased sweating is common during times of emotional stress. See ANXIETY, *p.300.*

NO

Are you in your teens? — **YES** → *It is normal to sweat more at this age. See* SPECIAL PROBLEMS OF ADOLESCENTS, *p.706.*

NO

↓

If you are unable to make a diagnosis from this chart, there is unlikely to be a serious cause for your sweating. However, if you are worried, consult your physician.

7

GENERAL
over 14 years

Swellings under the skin

Any new lump or swollen area that can be seen or felt under your skin.
For children see chart 96, **Swellings in children**.

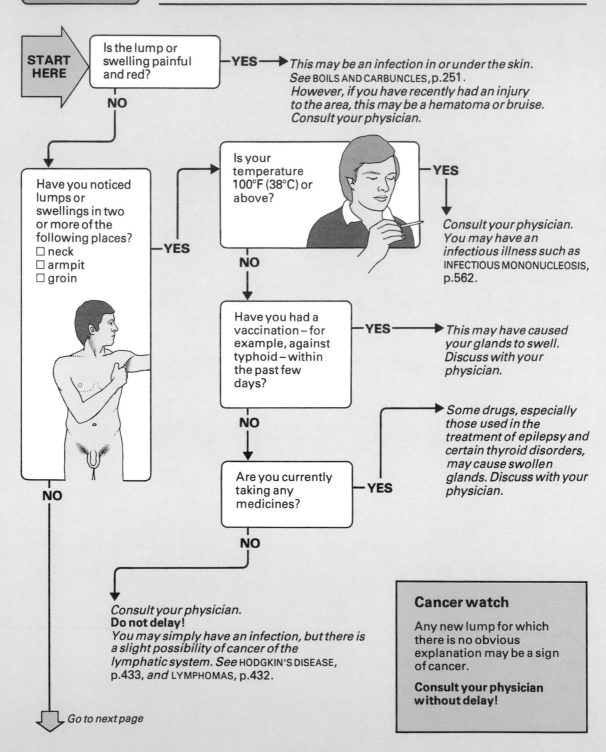

START HERE

Is the lump or swelling painful and red? — **YES** → *This may be an infection in or under the skin. See* BOILS AND CARBUNCLES, p.251. *However, if you have recently had an injury to the area, this may be a hematoma or bruise. Consult your physician.*

NO

Have you noticed lumps or swellings in two or more of the following places?
☐ neck
☐ armpit
☐ groin

— **YES** → Is your temperature 100°F (38°C) or above? — **YES** → *Consult your physician. You may have an infectious illness such as* INFECTIOUS MONONUCLEOSIS, p.562.

NO

Have you had a vaccination – for example, against typhoid – within the past few days? — **YES** → *This may have caused your glands to swell. Discuss with your physician.*

NO

Are you currently taking any medicines? — **YES** → *Some drugs, especially those used in the treatment of epilepsy and certain thyroid disorders, may cause swollen glands. Discuss with your physician.*

NO

NO

Consult your physician.
Do not delay!
You may simply have an infection, but there is a slight possibility of cancer of the lymphatic system. See HODGKIN'S DISEASE, p.433, *and* LYMPHOMAS, p.432.

⬇ *Go to next page*

Cancer watch

Any new lump for which there is no obvious explanation may be a sign of cancer.

Consult your physician without delay!

Continued from previous page

Is the swelling on your face between the ear and the angle of your jaw? —**YES**→ Is the swelling on both sides? 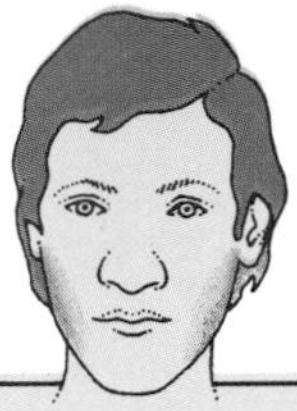 —**YES**→ This may be MUMPS, p.700.

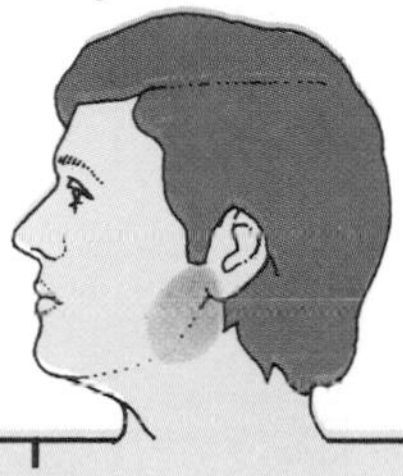

NO ↓

NO ↓ (from "both sides")

Consult your physician.
Do not delay!
One-sided swelling of the face is likely to be due to MUMPS, p.700, a tooth abscess (see ABSCESSES IN TEETH, p.439), or a salivary gland problem such as a SALIVARY DUCT STONE, p.453.
However, there is a slight chance of a SALIVARY GLAND TUMOR, p.454.

Is there a swelling on both sides of the back of your neck? —**YES**→

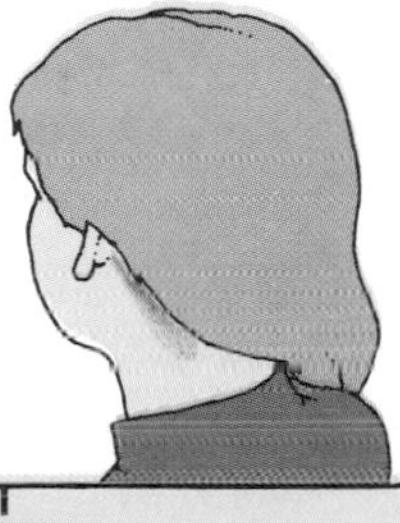

NO ↓

Do you have a pink rash AND/OR is your temperature 100°F (38°C) or above? —**YES**→ You may have GERMAN MEASLES, p.699.

NO ↓

Are there swellings on both sides of your neck? —**YES**→ Is your throat sore? —**YES**→ You may have a throat infection (see PHARYNGITIS, p.350, and TONSILLITIS, p.351) or INFECTIOUS MONONUCLEOSIS, p.562.

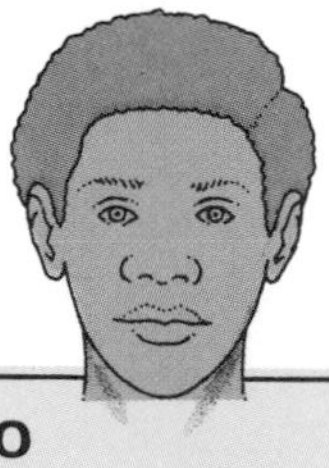

NO ↓ (throat sore)

NO ↓

Go to next page

Consult your physician.
Do not delay!
You may simply have an infection, but there is a slight possibility of cancer of the lymphatic system.
See HODGKIN'S DISEASE, p.433, and LYMPHOMAS, p.432.

Swellings under the skin
continued from previous page

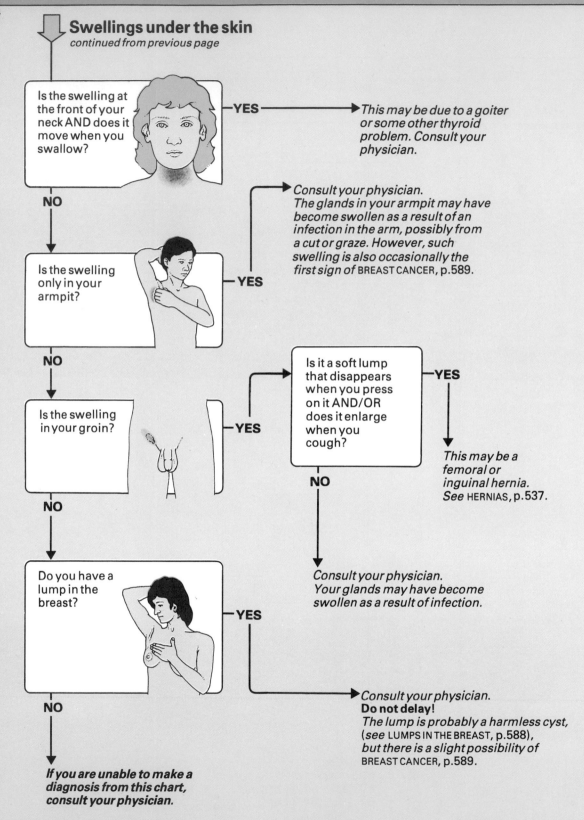

Is the swelling at the front of your neck AND does it move when you swallow?

YES → *This may be due to a goiter or some other thyroid problem. Consult your physician.*

NO

Is the swelling only in your armpit?

YES → *Consult your physician. The glands in your armpit may have become swollen as a result of an infection in the arm, possibly from a cut or graze. However, such swelling is also occasionally the first sign of* BREAST CANCER, p.589.

NO

Is the swelling in your groin?

YES → Is it a soft lump that disappears when you press on it AND/OR does it enlarge when you cough?

YES → *This may be a femoral or inguinal hernia. See* HERNIAS, p.537.

NO → *Consult your physician. Your glands may have become swollen as a result of infection.*

NO

Do you have a lump in the breast?

YES → *Consult your physician.* **Do not delay!** *The lump is probably a harmless cyst, (see* LUMPS IN THE BREAST, p.588), *but there is a slight possibility of* BREAST CANCER, p.589.

NO

If you are unable to make a diagnosis from this chart, consult your physician.

8

GENERAL
over 14 years

Itching without a rash

Irritation of the skin without any change in its appearance.
For children see chart 94, **Itching in children**.

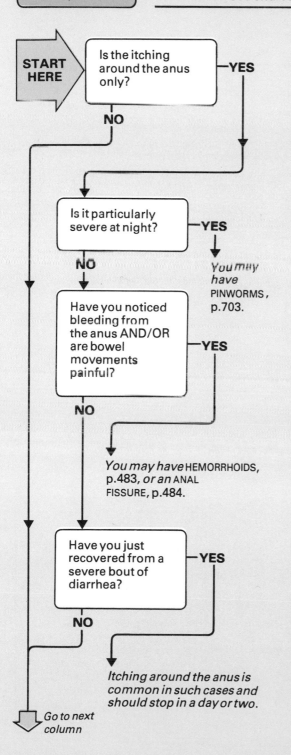

START HERE

Is the itching around the anus only? —**YES**

NO

Is it particularly severe at night? —**YES**

You may have PINWORMS, p.703.

NO

Have you noticed bleeding from the anus AND/OR are bowel movements painful? —**YES**

NO

You may have HEMORRHOIDS, p.483, *or an* ANAL FISSURE, p.484.

Have you just recovered from a severe bout of diarrhea? —**YES**

NO

Itching around the anus is common in such cases and should stop in a day or two.

Go to next column

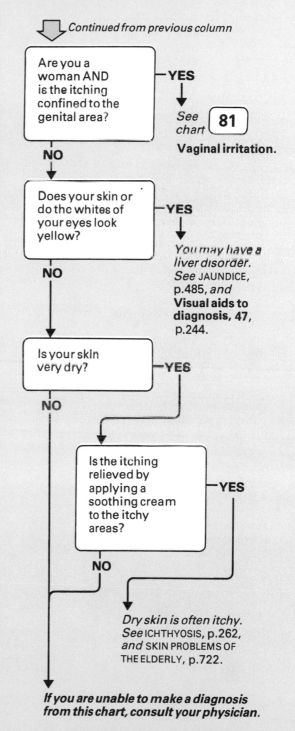

Continued from previous column

Are you a woman AND is the itching confined to the genital area? —**YES**

See chart **81**

Vaginal irritation.

NO

Does your skin or do the whites of your eyes look yellow? —**YES**

You may have a liver disorder. See JAUNDICE, p.485, *and* **Visual aids to diagnosis, 47**, p.244.

NO

Is your skin very dry? —**YES**

NO

Is the itching relieved by applying a soothing cream to the itchy areas? —**YES**

NO

Dry skin is often itchy. See ICHTHYOSIS, p.262, *and* SKIN PROBLEMS OF THE ELDERLY, p.722.

If you are unable to make a diagnosis from this chart, consult your physician.

9

GENERAL
all ages

Feeling faint and fainting

A sudden feeling of weakness and unsteadiness that may result in brief loss of consciousness.

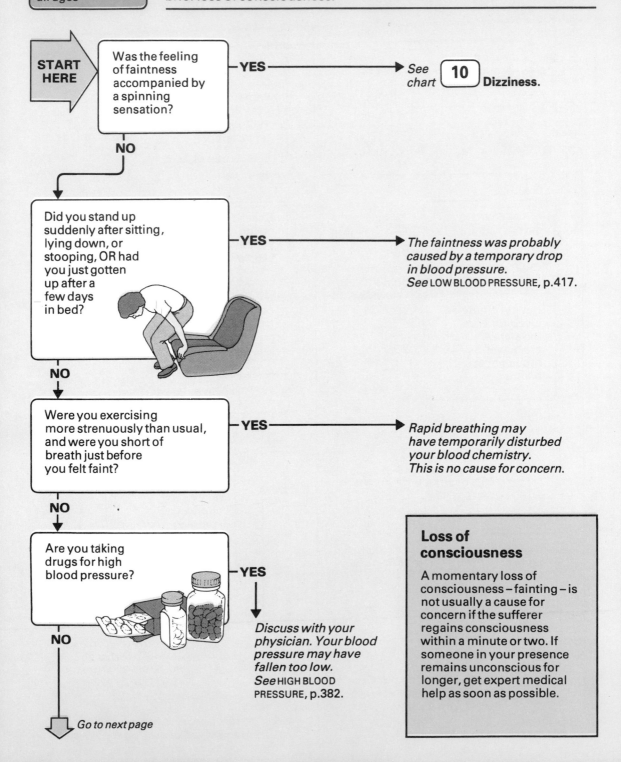

START HERE

Was the feeling of faintness accompanied by a spinning sensation? — **YES** → *See* chart **10** Dizziness.

NO

Did you stand up suddenly after sitting, lying down, or stooping, OR had you just gotten up after a few days in bed? — **YES** → *The faintness was probably caused by a temporary drop in blood pressure. See* LOW BLOOD PRESSURE, p.417.

NO

Were you exercising more strenuously than usual, and were you short of breath just before you felt faint? — **YES** → *Rapid breathing may have temporarily disturbed your blood chemistry. This is no cause for concern.*

NO

Are you taking drugs for high blood pressure? — **YES** → *Discuss with your physician. Your blood pressure may have fallen too low. See* HIGH BLOOD PRESSURE, p.382.

NO

Go to next page

Loss of consciousness

A momentary loss of consciousness – fainting – is not usually a cause for concern if the sufferer regains consciousness within a minute or two. If someone in your presence remains unconscious for longer, get expert medical help as soon as possible.

Continued from previous page

Are you a diabetic OR is it an unusually long time since you last ate something?

—**YES** →

Low blood sugar is probably causing your faintness. A sweet drink or something sugary or starchy to eat will probably make you feel better. If you are diabetic and have had several such attacks, consult your physician. (See HYPOGLYCEMIA, p.522.)

NO

Had you spent several hours in strong sunshine or in very hot or stuffy conditions before you felt faint?

—**YES**

→ *You may have heat exhaustion. For first aid see p.801.*

NO

Have you noticed one or more of the following symptoms since the attack of faintness?
- ☐ numbness and/or tingling in any part of the body
- ☐ blurred vision
- ☐ confusion
- ☐ difficulty in speaking
- ☐ loss of movement in arms or legs

—**YES**—→ *Consult your physician.*
Do not delay!
You may have had a mild STROKE, p.268, *or a* TRANSIENT ISCHEMIC ATTACK, p.270.

NO

Do you have any form of heart disease AND/OR did you notice your heartbeat speeding up or slowing down before you felt faint?

—**YES**→ **Did you lose consciousness?** —**YES**—

NO

Discuss with your physician. You may have a disorder of HEART RATE OR RHYTHM, p.388.

Consult your physician.
Do not delay!
You may have had a Stokes-Adams attack, which indicates a disorder of heart rhythm. See HEART BLOCK, p.390.

NO

Go to next page

Dealing with faintness

If you feel faint, lie down with your legs raised

or, if this is not possible, sit with your head between your knees until you feel better.

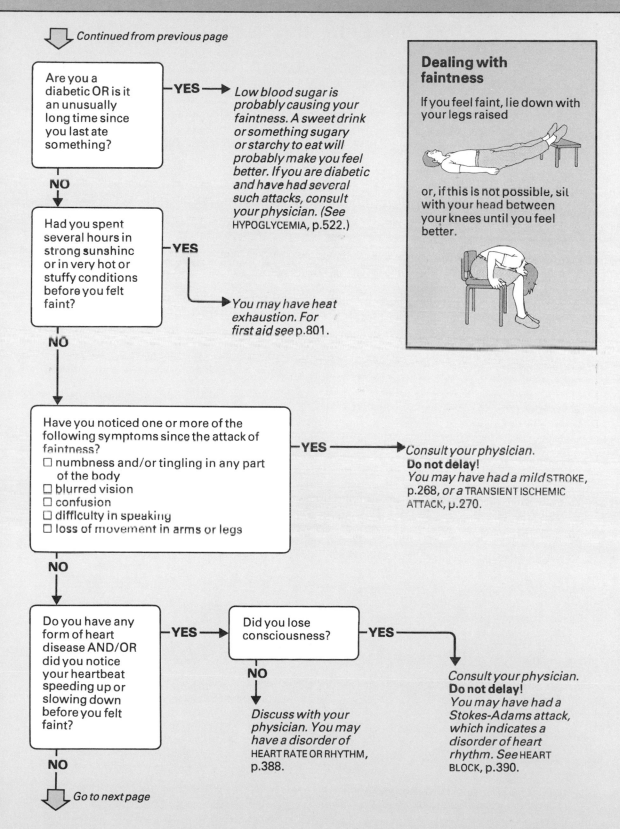

Feeling faint and fainting
Continued from previous page

Were you breathing very deeply or rapidly before you felt faint?

— **YES** → *The faintness was probably caused by hyperventilation, or "overbreathing," possibly as a result of anxiety or stress. See* ANXIETY, *p.300.*

NO ↓

Did you feel faint after an emotional shock?

— **YES** → *Emotional upsets can easily affect the nerves that control blood pressure, and this may cause faintness.*

NO ↓

Did you feel faint while you were doing any of the following?
☐ coughing
☐ urinating
☐ stretching
☐ holding your breath

— **YES** → *Any of these activities will sometimes affect the supply of oxygen to the brain, and cause faintness. This is usually no cause for concern. But if it happens more than once, consult your physician.*

NO ↓

Are you over 50? — **YES** → **Does turning your head slowly make you feel faint?** — **YES** → *These symptoms suggest a disorder that affects the nerves and bones in the neck. See* CERVICAL SPONDYLOSIS, *p.280.*

NO ↓ (from "Are you over 50?")

NO (from "Does turning your head slowly make you feel faint?")

Do you feel inexplicably tired AND/OR are you often short of breath?

— **YES** → *You may be suffering from a form of* ANEMIA, *p.419, or from* HEART FAILURE, *p.381.*

NO ↓

If you are unable to make a diagnosis from this chart, consult your physician.

10

GENERAL
all ages

Dizziness

A sense of being dazed and unsteady accompanied by a sensation of spinning.

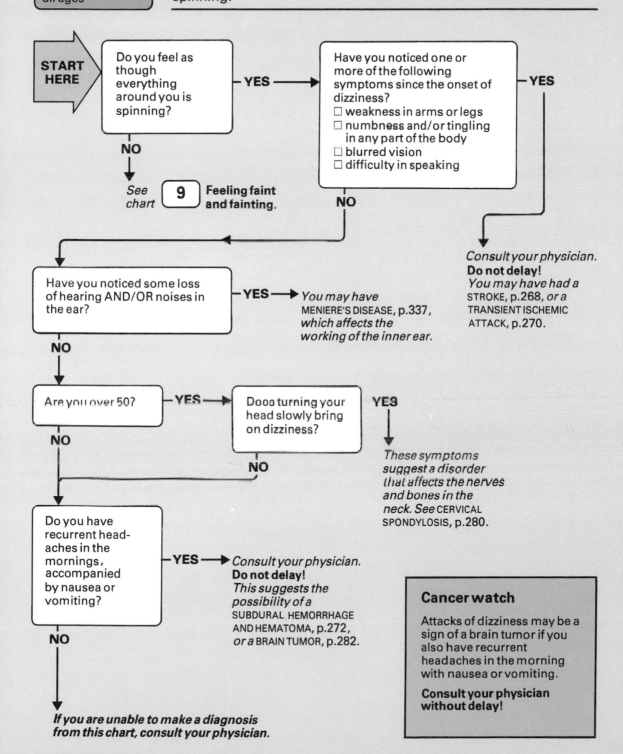

START HERE

Do you feel as though everything around you is spinning?

YES →

Have you noticed one or more of the following symptoms since the onset of dizziness?
- ☐ weakness in arms or legs
- ☐ numbness and/or tingling in any part of the body
- ☐ blurred vision
- ☐ difficulty in speaking

YES →

Consult your physician. **Do not delay!** *You may have had a* STROKE, p.268, *or a* TRANSIENT ISCHEMIC ATTACK, p.270.

NO ↓

See chart **9** **Feeling faint and fainting.**

NO ↓

Have you noticed some loss of hearing AND/OR noises in the ear?

YES → *You may have* MENIERE'S DISEASE, p.337, *which affects the working of the inner ear.*

NO ↓

Are you over 50?

YES →

Does turning your head slowly bring on dizziness?

YES ↓

These symptoms suggest a disorder that affects the nerves and bones in the neck. See CERVICAL SPONDYLOSIS, p.280.

NO ↓

NO →

Do you have recurrent headaches in the mornings, accompanied by nausea or vomiting?

YES → *Consult your physician.* **Do not delay!** *This suggests the possibility of a* SUBDURAL HEMORRHAGE AND HEMATOMA, p.272, *or a* BRAIN TUMOR, p.282.

NO ↓

If you are unable to make a diagnosis from this chart, consult your physician.

Cancer watch

Attacks of dizziness may be a sign of a brain tumor if you also have recurrent headaches in the morning with nausea or vomiting.

Consult your physician without delay!

11

GENERAL
all ages

Headache

Pain in the head that may be anything from mild to severe and incapacitating.

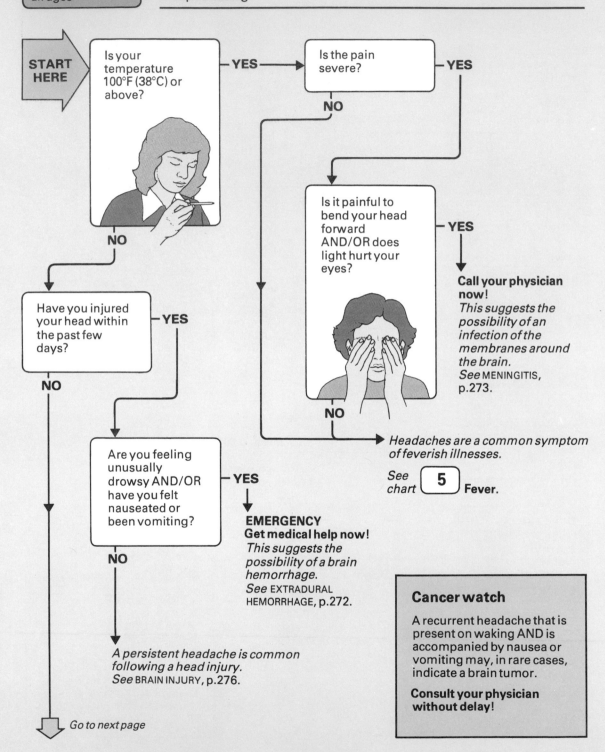

START HERE

Is your temperature 100°F (38°C) or above?

— **YES** → Is the pain severe? — **YES**

NO

NO

Is it painful to bend your head forward AND/OR does light hurt your eyes? — **YES**

Call your physician now!
This suggests the possibility of an infection of the membranes around the brain.
See MENINGITIS, p.273.

NO

Have you injured your head within the past few days? — **YES**

NO

Headaches are a common symptom of feverish illnesses.

See chart **5** *Fever.*

Are you feeling unusually drowsy AND/OR have you felt nauseated or been vomiting? — **YES**

EMERGENCY
Get medical help now!
This suggests the possibility of a brain hemorrhage.
See EXTRADURAL HEMORRHAGE, p.272.

NO

A persistent headache is common following a head injury.
See BRAIN INJURY, p.276.

Cancer watch

A recurrent headache that is present on waking AND is accompanied by nausea or vomiting may, in rare cases, indicate a brain tumor.

Consult your physician without delay!

Go to next page

Continued from previous page

Have you felt nauseated or been vomiting? — **YES** → **Do you have severe pain in and around one eye AND is your vision in that eye blurred?** — **YES** →

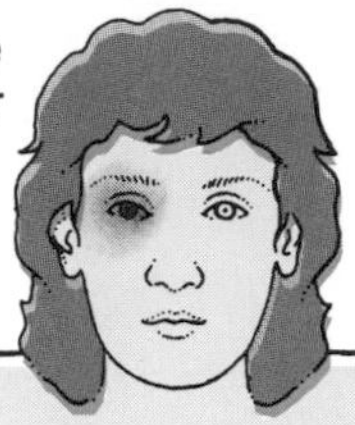

Call your physician now! *This suggests the possibility of raised pressure inside the eye.* See ACUTE GLAUCOMA, p.320.

NO (from nauseated)

NO (from severe pain)

Do you have one or more of the following symptoms?
☐ pain when you bend your head forward
☐ dislike of bright light
☐ drowsiness or confusion

— **YES** → **EMERGENCY Get medical help now!** *These symptoms suggest the possibility of a brain hemorrhage.* See SUBARACHNOID HEMORRHAGE, p.271.

NO

Was the pain preceded by disturbed vision or relieved by vomiting? — **YES** → *You may have a* MIGRAINE, p.285.

NO

Have you had a similar headache on waking several days out of the past week or more? — **YES** → **Do the headaches only occur when you have drunk a lot of alcohol the night before?** — **YES** →

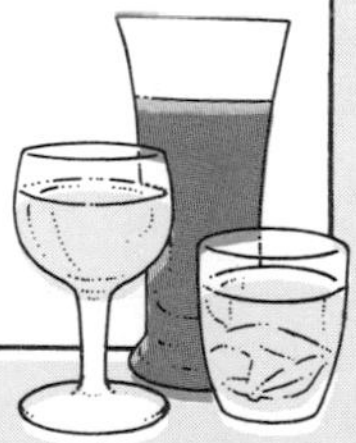

You probably have a "hangover". See HEADACHE, p.284.

NO (from similar headache)

NO (from headaches only occur)

Are you currently taking any medicines? — **YES** → *Some drugs can cause headaches. Discuss with your physician.*

NO

Go to next page

Consult your physician. **Do not delay!** *Such headaches may be a symptom of tension or* HIGH BLOOD PRESSURE, p.382, *but in very rare cases may indicate a* BRAIN TUMOR, p.282.

Headache
Continued from previous page

Have you recently had or do you now have a runny or stuffy nose?

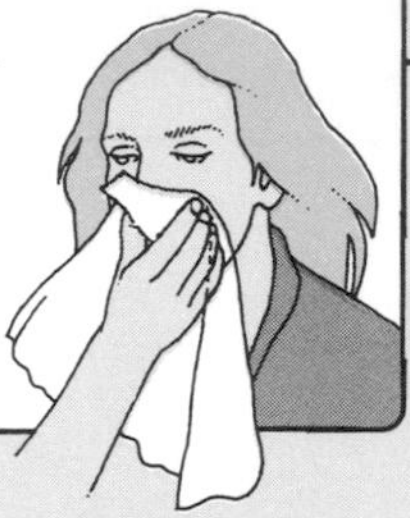

YES →

Do you have dull pain and tenderness around the eyes and cheek-bones that worsens when you bend forwards?

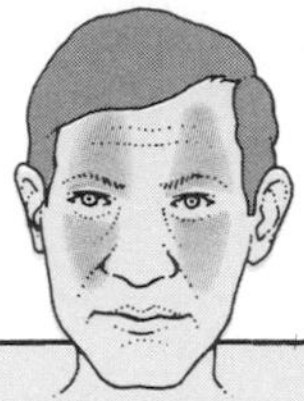

YES

NO

NO

Headache is a common symptom of a COLD, p.342.

You may have an infection of the sinuses. See SINUSITIS, p.347.

Are you feeling tense or under stress AND/OR are you sleeping poorly?

YES

NO

Anxiety often causes headaches. See ANXIETY, p.300, *and* HEADACHE, p.284.

Did the headache occur after you had been reading or doing close work such as sewing?

YES

NO

Strain on your neck muscles may have caused the headache. See HEADACHE, p.284.

Did any of the following apply in the 12 hours before the headache started?
☐ you were exposed to strong sunlight
☐ you were in stuffy, smoky or noisy surroundings
☐ you drank more alcohol than usual
☐ you missed a meal

YES

NO

Headaches are often brought on by such circumstances, and are usually no cause for concern. See HEADACHE, p.284.

If you are unable to make a diagnosis from this chart and the headache persists overnight or if you develop other symptoms, consult your physician.

12

GENERAL
all ages

Numbness and/or tingling

Loss of feeling and/or a prickling sensation ("pins and needles") in any part of the body.

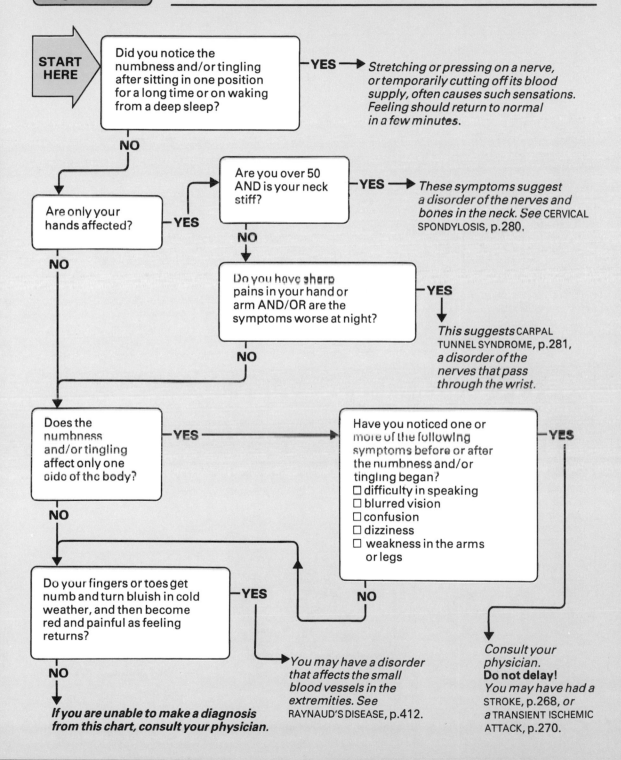

START HERE

Did you notice the numbness and/or tingling after sitting in one position for a long time or on waking from a deep sleep?

YES → *Stretching or pressing on a nerve, or temporarily cutting off its blood supply, often causes such sensations. Feeling should return to normal in a few minutes.*

NO

Are only your hands affected?

YES

Are you over 50 AND is your neck stiff?

YES → *These symptoms suggest a disorder of the nerves and bones in the neck. See* CERVICAL SPONDYLOSIS, p.280.

NO

Do you have sharp pains in your hand or arm AND/OR are the symptoms worse at night?

— YES

This suggests CARPAL TUNNEL SYNDROME, p.281, *a disorder of the nerves that pass through the wrist.*

NO

NO

Does the numbness and/or tingling affect only one side of the body?

— YES —

Have you noticed one or more of the following symptoms before or after the numbness and/or tingling began?
☐ difficulty in speaking
☐ blurred vision
☐ confusion
☐ dizziness
☐ weakness in the arms or legs

— YES

NO

NO

Do your fingers or toes get numb and turn bluish in cold weather, and then become red and painful as feeling returns?

— YES

You may have a disorder that affects the small blood vessels in the extremities. See RAYNAUD'S DISEASE, p.412.

NO

Consult your physician.
Do not delay!
You may have had a STROKE, p.268, *or a* TRANSIENT ISCHEMIC ATTACK, p.270.

If you are unable to make a diagnosis from this chart, consult your physician.

13

GENERAL
all ages

Twitching and trembling

Any involuntary movements during consciousness, including persistent trembling and shaking or sudden twitching.

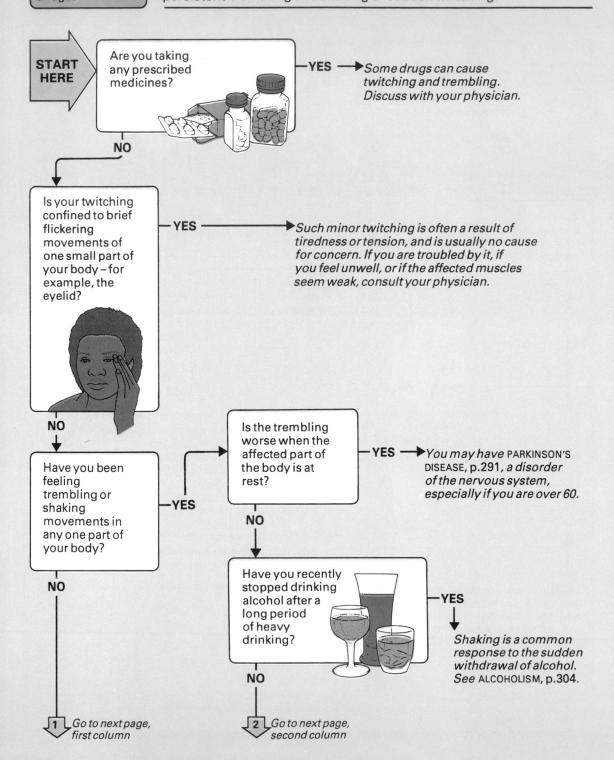

START HERE

Are you taking any prescribed medicines?

YES → *Some drugs can cause twitching and trembling. Discuss with your physician.*

NO

Is your twitching confined to brief flickering movements of one small part of your body – for example, the eyelid?

YES → *Such minor twitching is often a result of tiredness or tension, and is usually no cause for concern. If you are troubled by it, if you feel unwell, or if the affected muscles seem weak, consult your physician.*

NO

Have you been feeling trembling or shaking movements in any one part of your body?

YES

Is the trembling worse when the affected part of the body is at rest?

YES → *You may have* PARKINSON'S DISEASE, p.291, *a disorder of the nervous system, especially if you are over 60.*

NO

Have you recently stopped drinking alcohol after a long period of heavy drinking?

YES

Shaking is a common response to the sudden withdrawal of alcohol. See ALCOHOLISM, p.304.

NO

NO

1 *Go to next page, first column*

2 *Go to next page, second column*

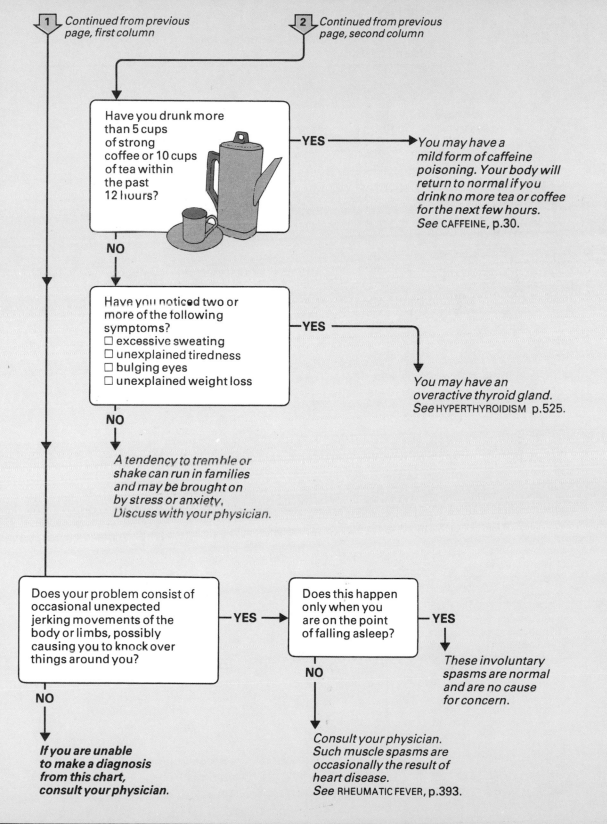

1 Continued from previous page, first column

2 Continued from previous page, second column

Have you drunk more than 5 cups of strong coffee or 10 cups of tea within the past 12 hours?

YES → You may have a mild form of caffeine poisoning. Your body will return to normal if you drink no more tea or coffee for the next few hours. *See* CAFFEINE, p.30.

NO

Have you noticed two or more of the following symptoms?
☐ excessive sweating
☐ unexplained tiredness
☐ bulging eyes
☐ unexplained weight loss

YES → You may have an overactive thyroid gland. *See* HYPERTHYROIDISM p.525.

NO

A tendency to tremble or shake can run in families and may be brought on by stress or anxiety. Discuss with your physician.

Does your problem consist of occasional unexpected jerking movements of the body or limbs, possibly causing you to knock over things around you?

YES → Does this happen only when you are on the point of falling asleep?

YES → These involuntary spasms are normal and are no cause for concern.

NO (below first box)

If you are unable to make a diagnosis from this chart, consult your physician.

NO (below second box)

Consult your physician. Such muscle spasms are occasionally the result of heart disease. *See* RHEUMATIC FEVER, p.393.

14

GENERAL
all ages

Pain in the face

Pain in one or both sides of the face or forehead that may be dull and throbbing or intense and stabbing.

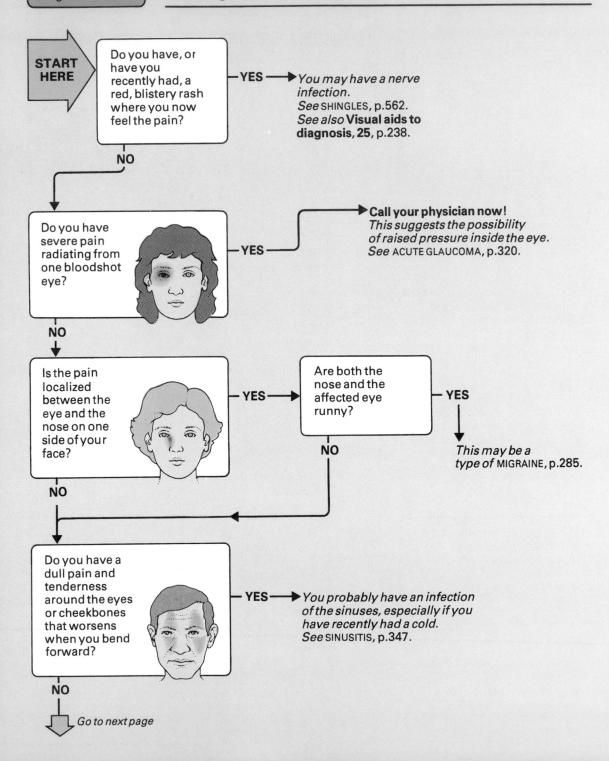

START HERE → Do you have, or have you recently had, a red, blistery rash where you now feel the pain? — **YES** → *You may have a nerve infection.*
See SHINGLES, p.562.
See also **Visual aids to diagnosis, 25**, p.238.

NO

Do you have severe pain radiating from one bloodshot eye? — **YES** → **Call your physician now!**
This suggests the possibility of raised pressure inside the eye.
See ACUTE GLAUCOMA, p.320.

NO

Is the pain localized between the eye and the nose on one side of your face? — **YES** → Are both the nose and the affected eye runny? — **YES** → *This may be a type of* MIGRAINE, p.285.

NO (from "Are both the nose and the affected eye runny?")

NO

Do you have a dull pain and tenderness around the eyes or cheekbones that worsens when you bend forward? — **YES** → *You probably have an infection of the sinuses, especially if you have recently had a cold.*
See SINUSITIS, p.347.

NO

Go to next page

Continued from previous page

Do you have a continuous, throbbing pain on one side of your face?

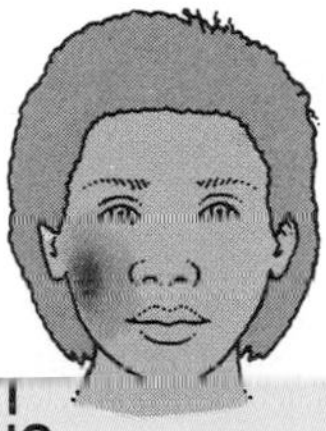

YES → Is the pain worse at night, when you eat, or when you touch a particular tooth?

YES →

Consult your physician or dentist.
Do not delay!
You may have a tooth abscess.
See ABSCESSES IN TEETH, p.439

NO

NO

Have you suddenly begun to have a severe throbbing pain in one or both temples?

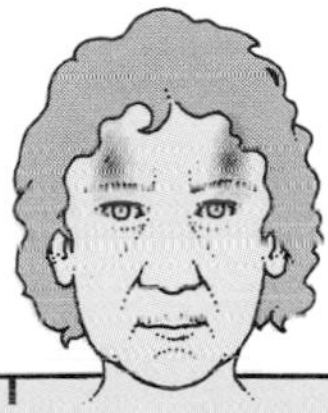

YES → Have you been feeling generally unwell AND/OR is your scalp sensitive to touch?

YES →

Consult your physician.
Do not delay!
You may have inflammation of the arteries in your head.
See TEMPORAL ARTERITIS, p.414.

NO

NO

Do you have a severe, stabbing pain on one side of the face, brought on by touching your face or by chewing?

YES → *The pain is probably caused by a damaged nerve.*
See TRIGEMINAL NEURALGIA, p.722.

NO

If you are unable to make a diagnosis from this chart, consult your physician.

15

GENERAL
all ages

Confusion

Confusion may vary from a muddling of times, places, and events, to an alarming loss of contact with reality, such as delirium or psychosis.

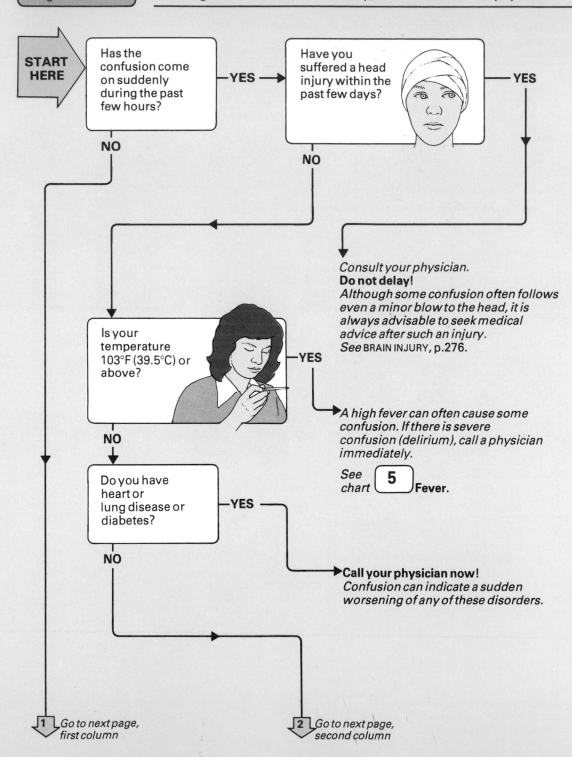

START HERE

Has the confusion come on suddenly during the past few hours? — **YES** →

Have you suffered a head injury within the past few days? — **YES**

NO

NO

Consult your physician.
Do not delay!
Although some confusion often follows even a minor blow to the head, it is always advisable to seek medical advice after such an injury.
See BRAIN INJURY, p.276.

Is your temperature 103°F (39.5°C) or above? — **YES**

NO

▶ *A high fever can often cause some confusion. If there is severe confusion (delirium), call a physician immediately.*

See chart **5** *Fever.*

Do you have heart or lung disease or diabetes? — **YES**

NO

▶**Call your physician now!**
Confusion can indicate a sudden worsening of any of these disorders.

1 *Go to next page, first column*

2 *Go to next page, second column*

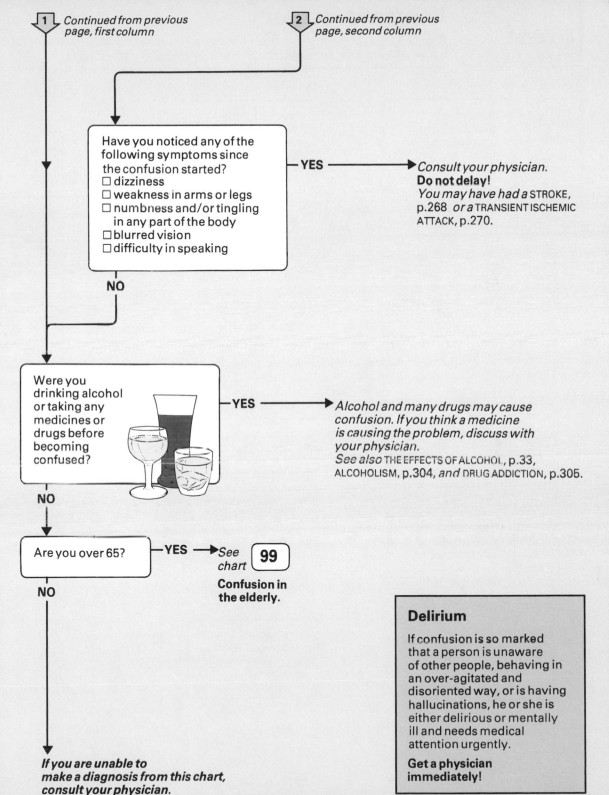

1 Continued from previous page, first column

2 Continued from previous page, second column

Have you noticed any of the following symptoms since the confusion started?
☐ dizziness
☐ weakness in arms or legs
☐ numbness and/or tingling in any part of the body
☐ blurred vision
☐ difficulty in speaking

YES → *Consult your physician.* **Do not delay!** *You may have had a* STROKE, p.268 *or a* TRANSIENT ISCHEMIC ATTACK, p.270.

NO

Were you drinking alcohol or taking any medicines or drugs before becoming confused?

YES → *Alcohol and many drugs may cause confusion. If you think a medicine is causing the problem, discuss with your physician. See also* THE EFFECTS OF ALCOHOL, p.33, ALCOHOLISM, p.304, *and* DRUG ADDICTION, p.305.

NO

Are you over 65?

YES → *See chart* **99** **Confusion in the elderly.**

NO

If you are unable to make a diagnosis from this chart, consult your physician.

Delirium

If confusion is so marked that a person is unaware of other people, behaving in an over-agitated and disoriented way, or is having hallucinations, he or she is either delirious or mentally ill and needs medical attention urgently.

Get a physician immediately!

16

GENERAL
all ages

Impaired memory

Difficulty in remembering either individual events and facts (often called absent-mindedness), or whole periods of time (amnesia).

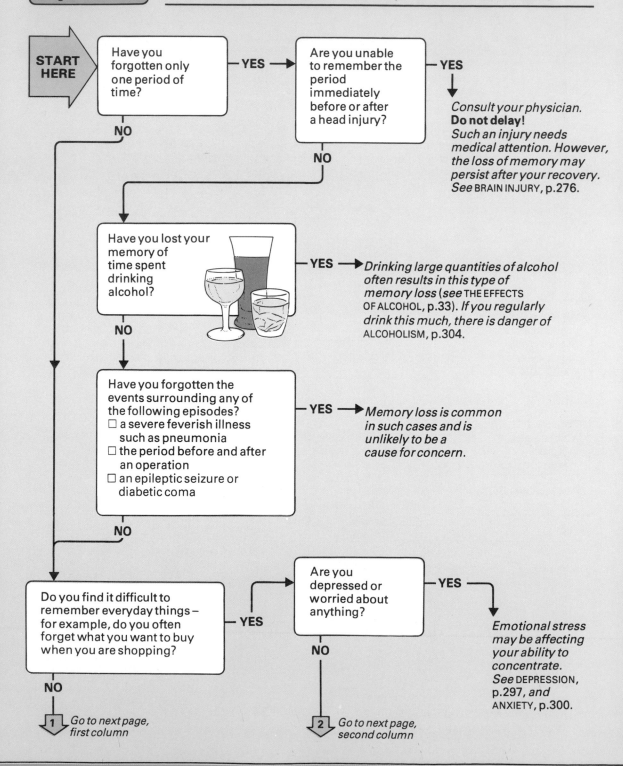

START HERE

Have you forgotten only one period of time? — **YES** → **Are you unable to remember the period immediately before or after a head injury?** — **YES** ↓

Consult your physician. **Do not delay!** *Such an injury needs medical attention. However, the loss of memory may persist after your recovery.* See BRAIN INJURY, p.276.

NO ↓ (from first box)

NO (from head injury box)

Have you lost your memory of time spent drinking alcohol? — **YES** → *Drinking large quantities of alcohol often results in this type of memory loss (see* THE EFFECTS OF ALCOHOL, p.33). *If you regularly drink this much, there is danger of* ALCOHOLISM, p.304.

NO ↓

Have you forgotten the events surrounding any of the following episodes?
☐ a severe feverish illness such as pneumonia
☐ the period before and after an operation
☐ an epileptic seizure or diabetic coma

— **YES** → *Memory loss is common in such cases and is unlikely to be a cause for concern.*

NO ↓

Do you find it difficult to remember everyday things – for example, do you often forget what you want to buy when you are shopping? — **YES** → **Are you depressed or worried about anything?** — **YES** ↓

Emotional stress may be affecting your ability to concentrate. See DEPRESSION, p.297, *and* ANXIETY, p.300.

NO ↓

1 *Go to next page, first column*

NO ↓

2 *Go to next page, second column*

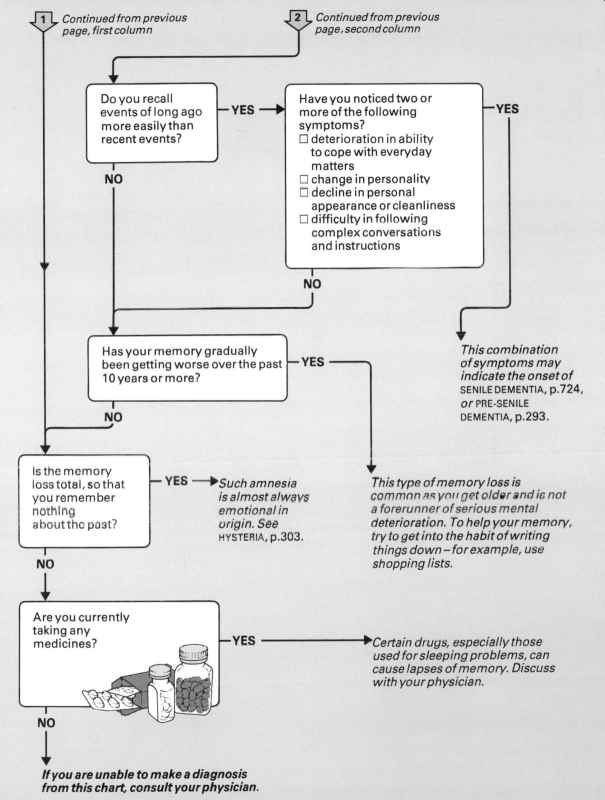

1 *Continued from previous page, first column*

2 *Continued from previous page, second column*

Do you recall events of long ago more easily than recent events?

YES →

Have you noticed two or more of the following symptoms?
- ☐ deterioration in ability to cope with everyday matters
- ☐ change in personality
- ☐ decline in personal appearance or cleanliness
- ☐ difficulty in following complex conversations and instructions

YES

NO ↓

NO ↓

Has your memory gradually been getting worse over the past 10 years or more?

YES →

This combination of symptoms may indicate the onset of SENILE DEMENTIA, p.724, *or* PRE-SENILE DEMENTIA, p.293.

NO ↓

Is the memory loss total, so that you remember nothing about the past?

YES → *Such amnesia is almost always emotional in origin. See* HYSTERIA, p.303.

This type of memory loss is common as you get older and is not a forerunner of serious mental deterioration. To help your memory, try to get into the habit of writing things down – for example, use shopping lists.

NO ↓

Are you currently taking any medicines?

YES → *Certain drugs, especially those used for sleeping problems, can cause lapses of memory. Discuss with your physician.*

NO ↓

If you are unable to make a diagnosis from this chart, consult your physician.

17
GENERAL
all ages

Difficulty in speaking

A deterioration in the ability to choose, use, or pronounce words.

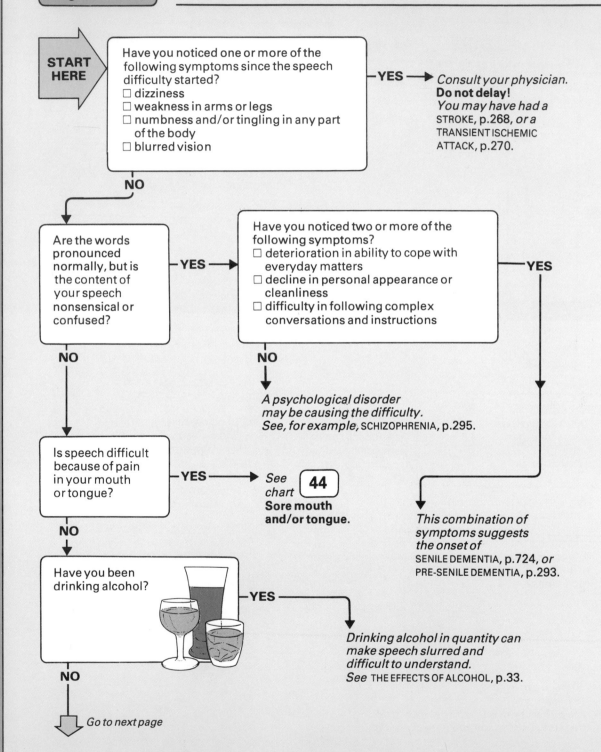

START HERE → Have you noticed one or more of the following symptoms since the speech difficulty started?
☐ dizziness
☐ weakness in arms or legs
☐ numbness and/or tingling in any part of the body
☐ blurred vision

YES → *Consult your physician.* **Do not delay!** *You may have had a* STROKE, p.268, *or a* TRANSIENT ISCHEMIC ATTACK, p.270.

NO

Are the words pronounced normally, but is the content of your speech nonsensical or confused?

YES → Have you noticed two or more of the following symptoms?
☐ deterioration in ability to cope with everyday matters
☐ decline in personal appearance or cleanliness
☐ difficulty in following complex conversations and instructions

YES

NO

A psychological disorder may be causing the difficulty. See, for example, SCHIZOPHRENIA, p.295.

NO

Is speech difficult because of pain in your mouth or tongue?

YES → *See chart* **44** **Sore mouth and/or tongue.**

This combination of symptoms suggests the onset of SENILE DEMENTIA, p.724, *or* PRE-SENILE DEMENTIA, p.293.

NO

Have you been drinking alcohol?

YES → *Drinking alcohol in quantity can make speech slurred and difficult to understand. See* THE EFFECTS OF ALCOHOL, p.33.

NO

Go to next page

Continued from previous page

Are you currently taking any medicines?

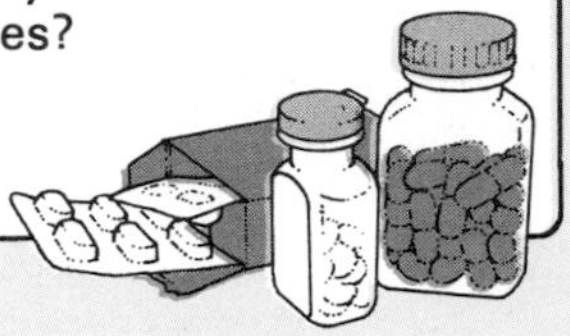

—**YES** → *Some drugs can affect speech. Discuss with your physician.*

NO

Is speech difficult because you are unable to move the muscles on one side of your face?

—**YES** → *You may have* BELL'S PALSY, p.280, *a disorder of the facial nerves.*

NO

Does your speech lack normal intonation and pauses, so that it sounds expressionless?

—**YES** → **Do your hands tremble?**

—**YES**

NO

These symptoms suggest PARKINSON'S DISEASE, p.291, *a degenerative disorder of the nervous system.*

NO

Are you sometimes unable to speak even though you know what you want to say, AND/OR do you sometimes get stuck at the beginning of a word and find yourself repeating the first consonant for several seconds before you can get the whole word out?

—**YES** → *Discuss with your physician. This stammering or stuttering often develops in early childhood and may recur in an adult under stress.*

NO

If you are unable to make a diagnosis from this chart, consult your physician.

18

GENERAL
all ages

Disturbing thoughts and feelings

Any thoughts or feelings that may seem (whether to other people or to you) to be abnormal or unhealthy.

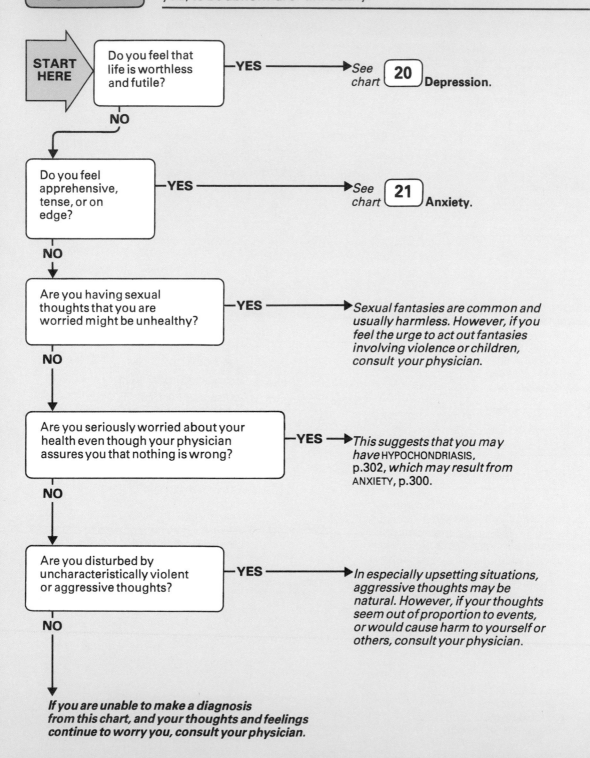

START HERE

Do you feel that life is worthless and futile? — **YES** → *See chart* **20** Depression.

NO

Do you feel apprehensive, tense, or on edge? — **YES** → *See chart* **21** Anxiety.

NO

Are you having sexual thoughts that you are worried might be unhealthy? — **YES** → *Sexual fantasies are common and usually harmless. However, if you feel the urge to act out fantasies involving violence or children, consult your physician.*

NO

Are you seriously worried about your health even though your physician assures you that nothing is wrong? — **YES** → *This suggests that you may have* HYPOCHONDRIASIS, *p.302, which may result from* ANXIETY, *p.300.*

NO

Are you disturbed by uncharacteristically violent or aggressive thoughts? — **YES** → *In especially upsetting situations, aggressive thoughts may be natural. However, if your thoughts seem out of proportion to events, or would cause harm to yourself or others, consult your physician.*

NO

If you are unable to make a diagnosis from this chart, and your thoughts and feelings continue to worry you, consult your physician.

19

GENERAL
all ages

Strange behavior

Any behavior, whether it develops suddenly or gradually, that seems out of keeping with previous behavior patterns.

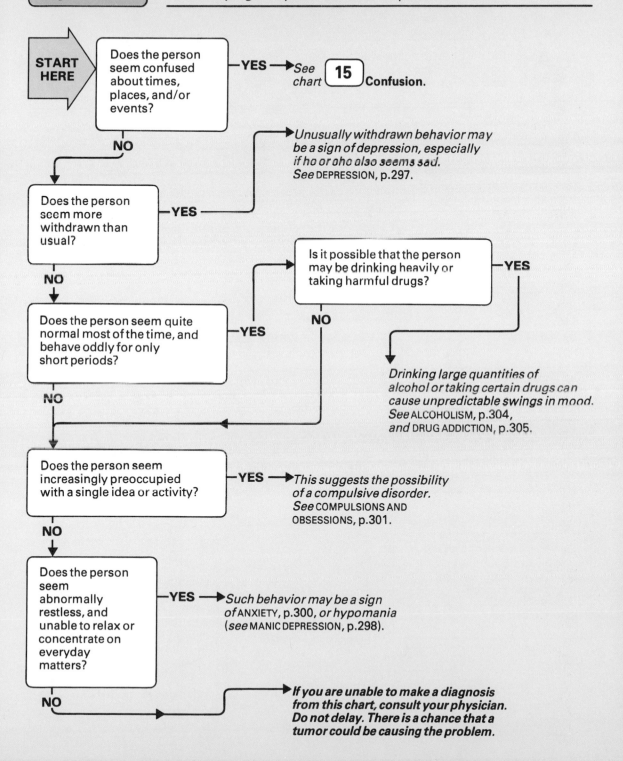

START HERE → Does the person seem confused about times, places, and/or events? — **YES** → *See chart* **15** *Confusion.*

NO

Does the person seem more withdrawn than usual? — **YES** → *Unusually withdrawn behavior may be a sign of depression, especially if he or she also seems sad. See DEPRESSION, p.297.*

NO

Does the person seem quite normal most of the time, and behave oddly for only short periods? — **YES** → Is it possible that the person may be drinking heavily or taking harmful drugs? — **YES** → *Drinking large quantities of alcohol or taking certain drugs can cause unpredictable swings in mood. See ALCOHOLISM, p.304, and DRUG ADDICTION, p.305.*

NO (from drinking question)

NO

Does the person seem increasingly preoccupied with a single idea or activity? — **YES** → *This suggests the possibility of a compulsive disorder. See COMPULSIONS AND OBSESSIONS, p.301.*

NO

Does the person seem abnormally restless, and unable to relax or concentrate on everyday matters? — **YES** → *Such behavior may be a sign of ANXIETY, p.300, or hypomania (see MANIC DEPRESSION, p.298).*

NO → *If you are unable to make a diagnosis from this chart, consult your physician. Do not delay. There is a chance that a tumor could be causing the problem.*

20

GENERAL
all ages

Depression

A feeling of sadness, futility, unworthiness, and/or despair that may make you feel unable to cope with normal life.

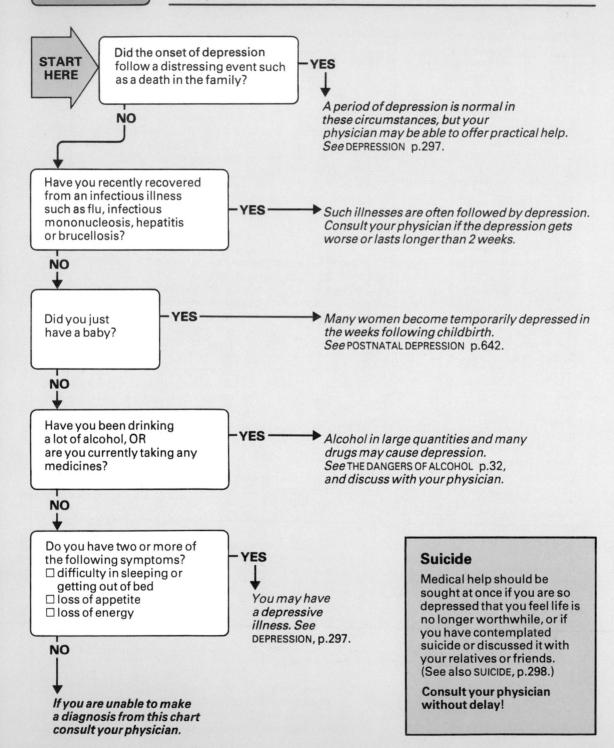

START HERE

Did the onset of depression follow a distressing event such as a death in the family? — **YES**

A period of depression is normal in these circumstances, but your physician may be able to offer practical help. See DEPRESSION p.297.

NO

Have you recently recovered from an infectious illness such as flu, infectious mononucleosis, hepatitis or brucellosis? — **YES**

Such illnesses are often followed by depression. Consult your physician if the depression gets worse or lasts longer than 2 weeks.

NO

Did you just have a baby? — **YES**

Many women become temporarily depressed in the weeks following childbirth. See POSTNATAL DEPRESSION p.642.

NO

Have you been drinking a lot of alcohol, OR are you currently taking any medicines? — **YES**

Alcohol in large quantities and many drugs may cause depression. See THE DANGERS OF ALCOHOL p.32, *and discuss with your physician.*

NO

Do you have two or more of the following symptoms?
☐ difficulty in sleeping or getting out of bed
☐ loss of appetite
☐ loss of energy
— **YES**

You may have a depressive illness. See DEPRESSION, p.297.

NO

If you are unable to make a diagnosis from this chart consult your physician.

Suicide

Medical help should be sought at once if you are so depressed that you feel life is no longer worthwhile, or if you have contemplated suicide or discussed it with your relatives or friends. (See also SUICIDE, p.298.)

Consult your physician without delay!

21

GENERAL
all ages

Anxiety

A feeling of tension, apprehension, or edginess, which may be accompanied by physical symptoms such as palpitations or diarrhea.

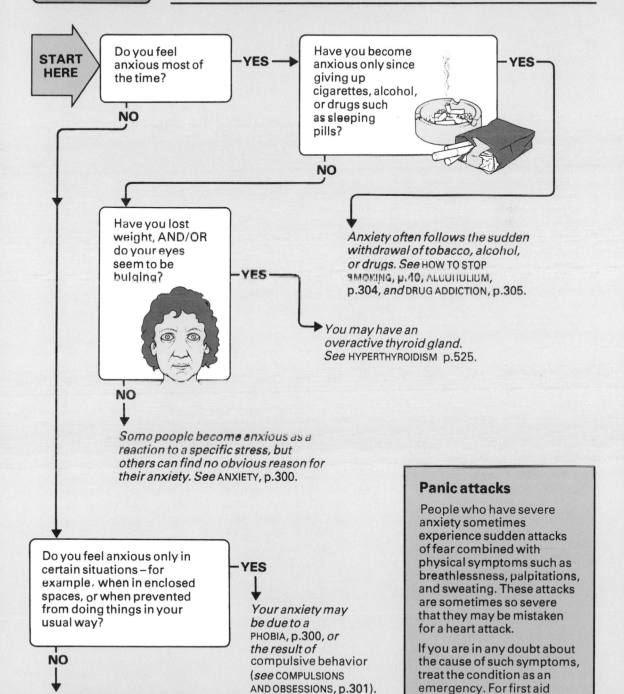

START HERE

Do you feel anxious most of the time?

— **YES** →

Have you become anxious only since giving up cigarettes, alcohol, or drugs such as sleeping pills?

— **YES**

NO

NO

Have you lost weight, AND/OR do your eyes seem to be bulging?

— **YES** —

Anxiety often follows the sudden withdrawal of tobacco, alcohol, or drugs. See HOW TO STOP SMOKING, p.40, ALCOHOLISM, p.304, *and* DRUG ADDICTION, p.305.

→ *You may have an overactive thyroid gland. See* HYPERTHYROIDISM p.525.

NO

Some people become anxious as a reaction to a specific stress, but others can find no obvious reason for their anxiety. See ANXIETY, p.300.

Do you feel anxious only in certain situations – for example, when in enclosed spaces, or when prevented from doing things in your usual way?

— **YES**

Your anxiety may be due to a PHOBIA, p.300, *or the result of compulsive behavior (see* COMPULSIONS AND OBSESSIONS, p.301).

NO

If you are unable to make a diagnosis from this chart, consult your physician.

Panic attacks

People who have severe anxiety sometimes experience sudden attacks of fear combined with physical symptoms such as breathlessness, palpitations, and sweating. These attacks are sometimes so severe that they may be mistaken for a heart attack.

If you are in any doubt about the cause of such symptoms, treat the condition as an emergency. For first aid see p.801.

22

GENERAL
all ages

Hallucinations

Mistakenly and repeatedly hearing, feeling, smelling or seeing things
that are not heard, felt, smelled, or seen by other people.

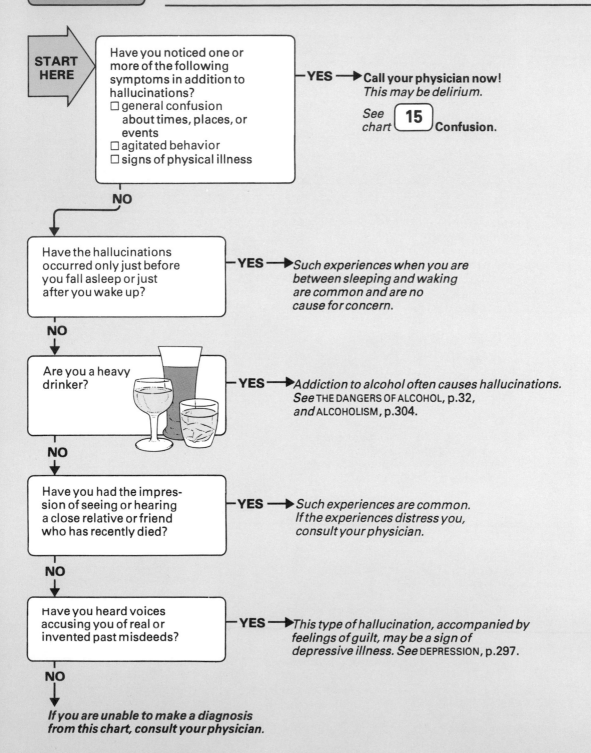

START HERE

Have you noticed one or
more of the following
symptoms in addition to
hallucinations?
☐ general confusion
about times, places, or
events
☐ agitated behavior
☐ signs of physical illness

— **YES** ➔ **Call your physician now!**
This may be delirium.

See chart **15** **Confusion.**

NO

Have the hallucinations
occurred only just before
you fall asleep or just
after you wake up?

— **YES** ➔ *Such experiences when you are
between sleeping and waking
are common and are no
cause for concern.*

NO

Are you a heavy
drinker?

— **YES** ➔ *Addiction to alcohol often causes hallucinations.
See* THE DANGERS OF ALCOHOL, p.32,
and ALCOHOLISM, p.304.

NO

Have you had the impres-
sion of seeing or hearing
a close relative or friend
who has recently died?

— **YES** ➔ *Such experiences are common.
If the experiences distress you,
consult your physician.*

NO

Have you heard voices
accusing you of real or
invented past misdeeds?

— **YES** ➔ *This type of hallucination, accompanied by
feelings of guilt, may be a sign of
depressive illness. See* DEPRESSION, p.297.

NO

*If you are unable to make a diagnosis
from this chart, consult your physician.*

23
GENERAL
all ages

Nightmares
Frightening dreams that may be disturbing enough to wake you up.

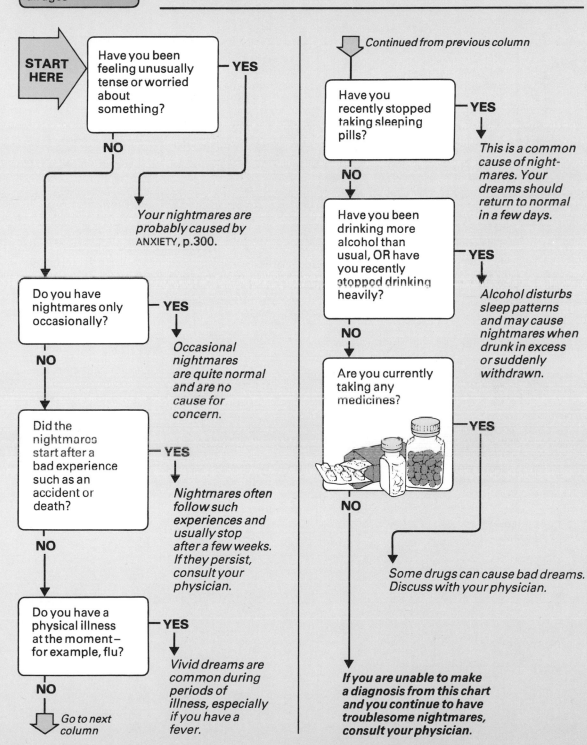

START HERE

Have you been feeling unusually tense or worried about something? — **YES**

NO

Your nightmares are probably caused by ANXIETY, p.300.

Do you have nightmares only occasionally? — **YES**

NO

Occasional nightmares are quite normal and are no cause for concern.

Did the nightmares start after a bad experience such as an accident or death? — **YES**

NO

Nightmares often follow such experiences and usually stop after a few weeks. If they persist, consult your physician.

Do you have a physical illness at the moment — for example, flu? — **YES**

NO

Go to next column

Vivid dreams are common during periods of illness, especially if you have a fever.

Continued from previous column

Have you recently stopped taking sleeping pills? — **YES**

NO

This is a common cause of nightmares. Your dreams should return to normal in a few days.

Have you been drinking more alcohol than usual, OR have you recently stopped drinking heavily? — **YES**

NO

Alcohol disturbs sleep patterns and may cause nightmares when drunk in excess or suddenly withdrawn.

Are you currently taking any medicines? — **YES**

NO

Some drugs can cause bad dreams. Discuss with your physician.

If you are unable to make a diagnosis from this chart and you continue to have troublesome nightmares, consult your physician.

24

GENERAL
all ages

Hair loss

Thinning or loss of hair on all or part of the head.

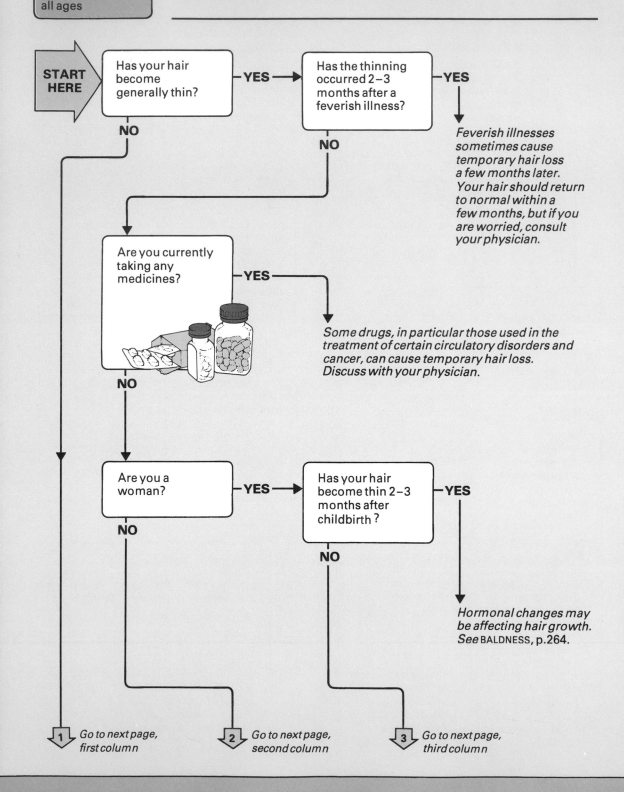

START HERE

Has your hair become generally thin?

NO

YES → Has the thinning occurred 2–3 months after a feverish illness?

NO

YES →

Feverish illnesses sometimes cause temporary hair loss a few months later. Your hair should return to normal within a few months, but if you are worried, consult your physician.

Are you currently taking any medicines?

NO

YES →

Some drugs, in particular those used in the treatment of certain circulatory disorders and cancer, can cause temporary hair loss. Discuss with your physician.

Are you a woman?

NO

YES → Has your hair become thin 2–3 months after childbirth?

NO

YES →

Hormonal changes may be affecting hair growth. See BALDNESS, p.264.

1 *Go to next page, first column*

2 *Go to next page, second column*

3 *Go to next page, third column*

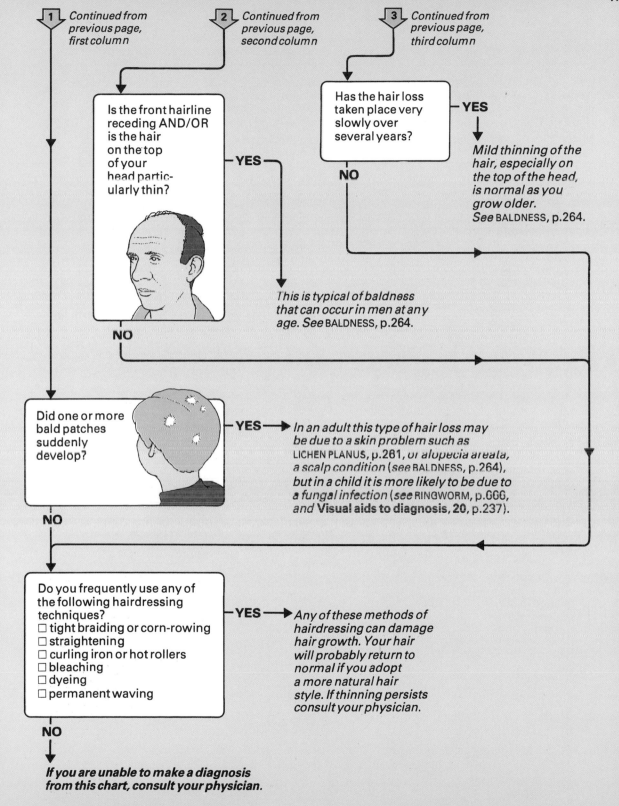

1 Continued from previous page, first column

2 Continued from previous page, second column

3 Continued from previous page, third column

Is the front hairline receding AND/OR is the hair on the top of your head particularly thin?

Has the hair loss taken place very slowly over several years?

YES

Mild thinning of the hair, especially on the top of the head, is normal as you grow older. See BALDNESS, p.264.

NO

YES

This is typical of baldness that can occur in men at any age. See BALDNESS, p.264.

NO

Did one or more bald patches suddenly develop?

YES ➤ *In an adult this type of hair loss may be due to a skin problem such as* LICHEN PLANUS, p.261, *or alopecia areata, a scalp condition (see* BALDNESS, p.264), *but in a child it is more likely to be due to a fungal infection (see* RINGWORM, p.666, *and* Visual aids to diagnosis, **20**, p.237).

NO

Do you frequently use any of the following hairdressing techniques?
☐ tight braiding or corn-rowing
☐ straightening
☐ curling iron or hot rollers
☐ bleaching
☐ dyeing
☐ permanent waving

YES ➤ *Any of these methods of hairdressing can damage hair growth. Your hair will probably return to normal if you adopt a more natural hair style. If thinning persists consult your physician.*

NO

If you are unable to make a diagnosis from this chart, consult your physician.

25
GENERAL
over 2 years

General skin problems
Any change in the skin, including rashes and spots.
For babies under 2 see chart 89, **Skin problems in infants**.

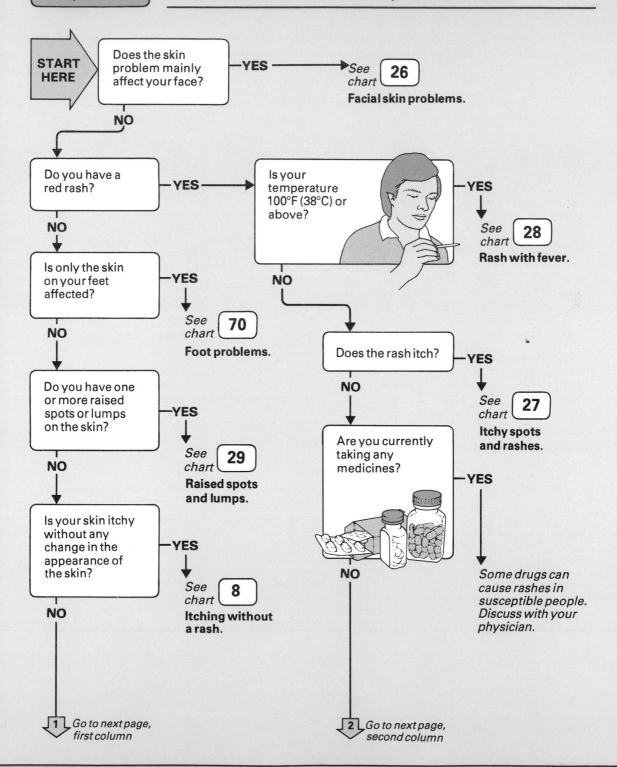

START HERE

Does the skin problem mainly affect your face? — **YES** → See chart **26** **Facial skin problems.**

NO

Do you have a red rash? — **YES** → Is your temperature 100°F (38°C) or above? — **YES** → See chart **28** **Rash with fever.**

NO

Is only the skin on your feet affected? — **YES** → See chart **70** **Foot problems.**

NO (temperature question) → Does the rash itch? — **YES** → See chart **27** **Itchy spots and rashes.**

NO

Do you have one or more raised spots or lumps on the skin? — **YES** → See chart **29** **Raised spots and lumps.**

NO

Are you currently taking any medicines? — **YES** → Some drugs can cause rashes in susceptible people. Discuss with your physician.

Is your skin itchy without any change in the appearance of the skin? — **YES** → See chart **8** **Itching without a rash.**

NO

NO

1 Go to next page, first column

2 Go to next page, second column

113

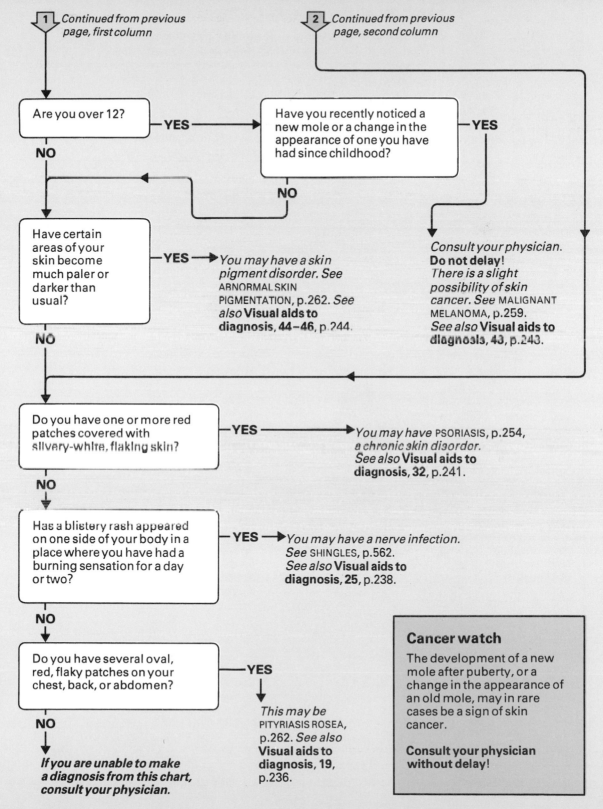

1 Continued from previous page, first column

2 Continued from previous page, second column

Are you over 12? — **YES** → **Have you recently noticed a new mole or a change in the appearance of one you have had since childhood?** — **YES**

NO ↓   **NO** ↓

Have certain areas of your skin become much paler or darker than usual? — **YES** → *You may have a skin pigment disorder. See* ABNORMAL SKIN PIGMENTATION, p.262. *See also* **Visual aids to diagnosis, 44–46,** p.244.

Consult your physician. **Do not delay!** *There is a slight possibility of skin cancer. See* MALIGNANT MELANOMA, p.259. *See also* **Visual aids to diagnosis, 43,** p.243.

NO ↓

Do you have one or more red patches covered with silvery-white, flaking skin? — **YES** → *You may have* PSORIASIS, p.254, *a chronic skin disorder. See also* **Visual aids to diagnosis, 32,** p.241.

NO ↓

Has a blistery rash appeared on one side of your body in a place where you have had a burning sensation for a day or two? — **YES** → *You may have a nerve infection. See* SHINGLES, p.562. *See also* **Visual aids to diagnosis, 25,** p.238.

NO ↓

Do you have several oval, red, flaky patches on your chest, back, or abdomen? — **YES** ↓ *This may be* PITYRIASIS ROSEA, p.262. *See also* **Visual aids to diagnosis, 19,** p.236.

NO ↓

If you are unable to make a diagnosis from this chart, consult your physician.

Cancer watch

The development of a new mole after puberty, or a change in the appearance of an old mole, may in rare cases be a sign of skin cancer.

Consult your physician without delay!

26

GENERAL
over 2 years

Facial skin problems

Any rash, spots or change in the skin on the face.
For babies under 2 see chart 89, **Skin problems in infants**.

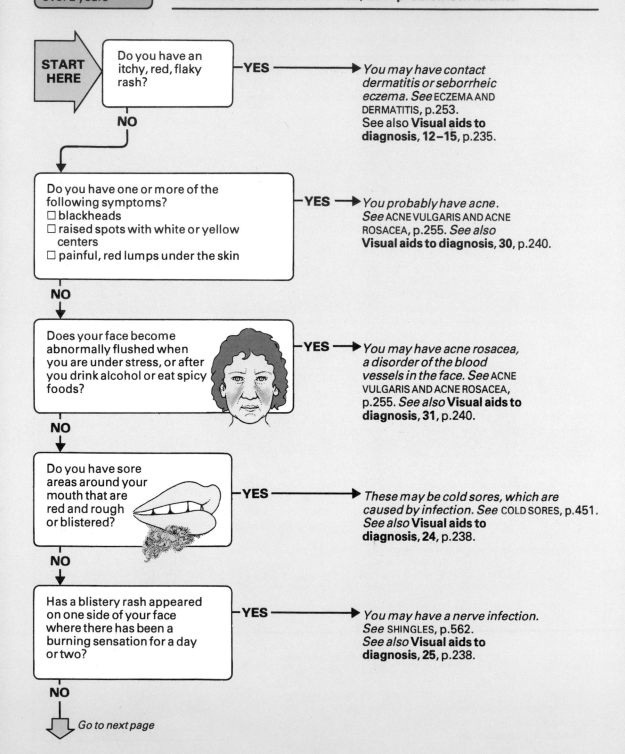

START HERE →

Do you have an itchy, red, flaky rash? — **YES** → *You may have contact dermatitis or seborrheic eczema. See* ECZEMA AND DERMATITIS, p.253. See also **Visual aids to diagnosis, 12–15**, p.235.

NO

Do you have one or more of the following symptoms?
☐ blackheads
☐ raised spots with white or yellow centers
☐ painful, red lumps under the skin
— **YES** → *You probably have acne. See* ACNE VULGARIS AND ACNE ROSACEA, p.255. *See also* **Visual aids to diagnosis, 30**, p.240.

NO

Does your face become abnormally flushed when you are under stress, or after you drink alcohol or eat spicy foods? — **YES** → *You may have acne rosacea, a disorder of the blood vessels in the face. See* ACNE VULGARIS AND ACNE ROSACEA, p.255. *See also* **Visual aids to diagnosis, 31**, p.240.

NO

Do you have sore areas around your mouth that are red and rough or blistered? — **YES** → *These may be cold sores, which are caused by infection. See* COLD SORES, p.451. *See also* **Visual aids to diagnosis, 24**, p.238.

NO

Has a blistery rash appeared on one side of your face where there has been a burning sensation for a day or two? — **YES** → *You may have a nerve infection. See* SHINGLES, p.562. *See also* **Visual aids to diagnosis, 25**, p.238.

NO

Go to next page

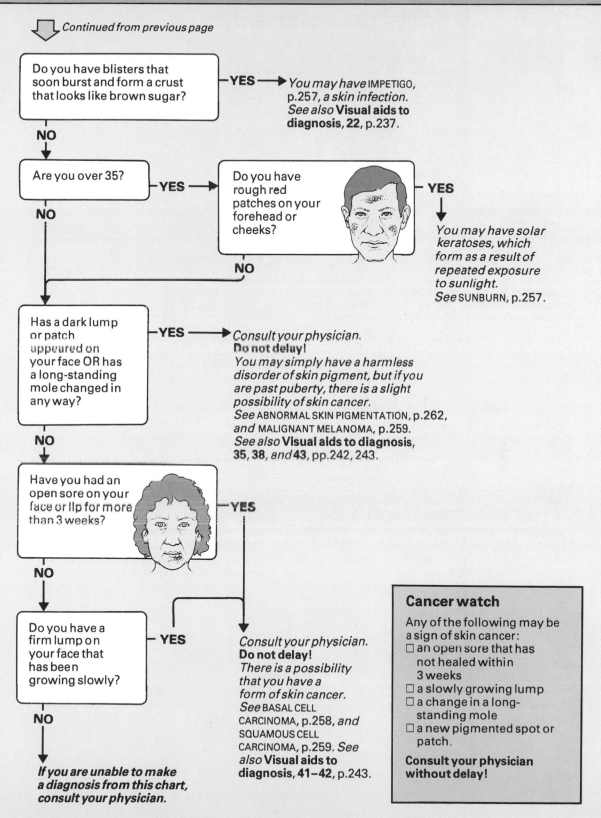

Continued from previous page

Do you have blisters that soon burst and form a crust that looks like brown sugar? — **YES** → *You may have* IMPETIGO, p.257, *a skin infection. See also* **Visual aids to diagnosis, 22,** p.237.

NO

Are you over 35? — **YES** → **Do you have rough red patches on your forehead or cheeks?** — **YES** → *You may have solar keratoses, which form as a result of repeated exposure to sunlight. See* SUNBURN, p.257.

NO

NO

Has a dark lump or patch appeared on your face OR has a long-standing mole changed in any way? — **YES** → *Consult your physician.* **Do not delay!** *You may simply have a harmless disorder of skin pigment, but if you are past puberty, there is a slight possibility of skin cancer. See* ABNORMAL SKIN PIGMENTATION, p.262, *and* MALIGNANT MELANOMA, p.259. *See also* **Visual aids to diagnosis, 35, 38,** *and* **43,** pp.242, 243.

NO

Have you had an open sore on your face or lip for more than 3 weeks? — **YES**

NO

Do you have a firm lump on your face that has been growing slowly? — **YES** → *Consult your physician.* **Do not delay!** *There is a possibility that you have a form of skin cancer. See* BASAL CELL CARCINOMA, p.258, *and* SQUAMOUS CELL CARCINOMA, p.259. *See also* **Visual aids to diagnosis, 41–42,** p.243.

NO

If you are unable to make a diagnosis from this chart, consult your physician.

Cancer watch

Any of the following may be a sign of skin cancer:
- ☐ an open sore that has not healed within 3 weeks
- ☐ a slowly growing lump
- ☐ a change in a long-standing mole
- ☐ a new pigmented spot or patch.

Consult your physician without delay!

27
GENERAL
over 2 years

Itchy spots and rashes
Discolored and/or raised areas of itchy skin.
For babies under 2 years see chart 89, **Skin problems in infants**.

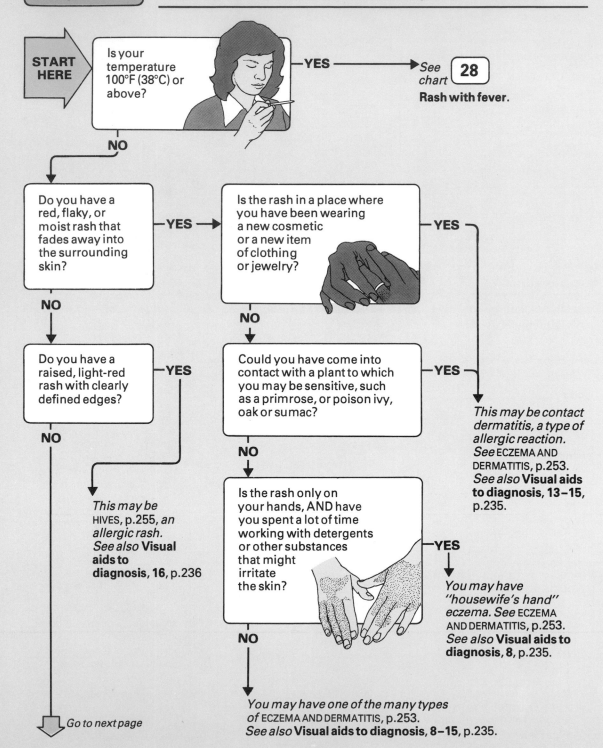

START HERE

Is your temperature 100°F (38°C) or above?

YES → *See chart* **28** **Rash with fever.**

NO

Do you have a red, flaky, or moist rash that fades away into the surrounding skin?

YES → Is the rash in a place where you have been wearing a new cosmetic or a new item of clothing or jewelry?

YES →

This may be contact dermatitis, a type of allergic reaction. See ECZEMA AND DERMATITIS, p.253. *See also* **Visual aids to diagnosis, 13–15,** p.235.

NO

NO

Do you have a raised, light-red rash with clearly defined edges?

YES →

Could you have come into contact with a plant to which you may be sensitive, such as a primrose, or poison ivy, oak or sumac?

YES →

NO

This may be HIVES, p.255, *an allergic rash. See also* **Visual aids to diagnosis, 16,** p.236

NO

Is the rash only on your hands, AND have you spent a lot of time working with detergents or other substances that might irritate the skin?

YES

You may have "housewife's hand" eczema. See ECZEMA AND DERMATITIS, p.253. *See also* **Visual aids to diagnosis, 8,** p.235.

NO

You may have one of the many types of ECZEMA AND DERMATITIS, p.253. *See also* **Visual aids to diagnosis, 8–15,** p.235.

Go to next page

⬇ *Continued from previous page*

Have you started to take any medicines recently? — **YES** → *Some drugs can cause an itchy rash. Discuss with your physician.*

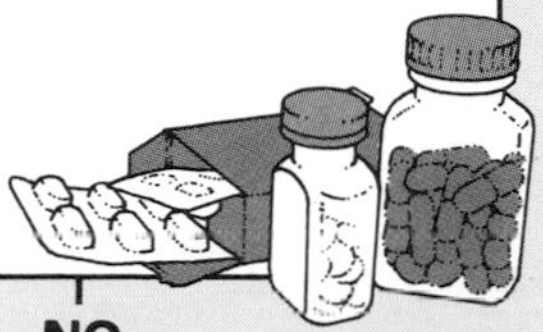

NO ↓

Do you have one or more red, scaly patches spreading out in a ring? — **YES** → *This may be a fungal infection. See* RINGWORM, p.666. *See also* **Visual aids to diagnosis, 20**, p.237.

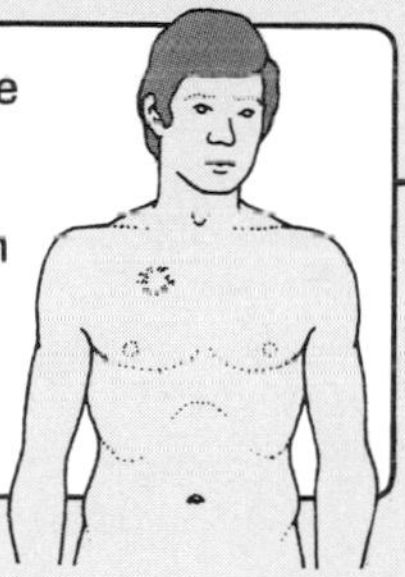

NO ↓

Do you have a widespread red rash that is particularly itchy at night? — **YES** → Have you noticed tiny gray lines or red, infected-looking spots between your fingers or on your wrists? — **YES** ↓

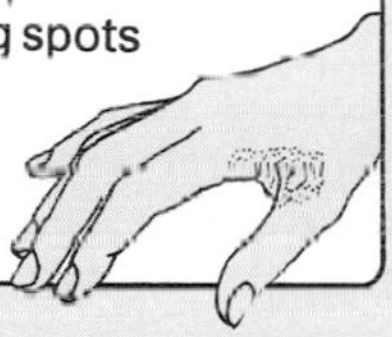

You may have SCABIES, p.568, *a parasitic infection, especially if someone you are in close physical contact with has the same problem. See also* **Visual aids to diagnosis, 67**, p.248.

NO (from scabies box) →

NO ↓ (from widespread red rash box)

Do you have one or more raised red spots in a small area? — **YES** → *You may have been bitten by an insect. For first aid see p.801. See also* **Visual aids to diagnosis, 68**, p.248.

NO ↓

If you are unable to make a diagnosis from this chart, consult your physician.

28
GENERAL
all ages

Rash with fever

Any spots, discolored areas, or blisters on the skin combined with a temperature of 100°F (38°C) or above.

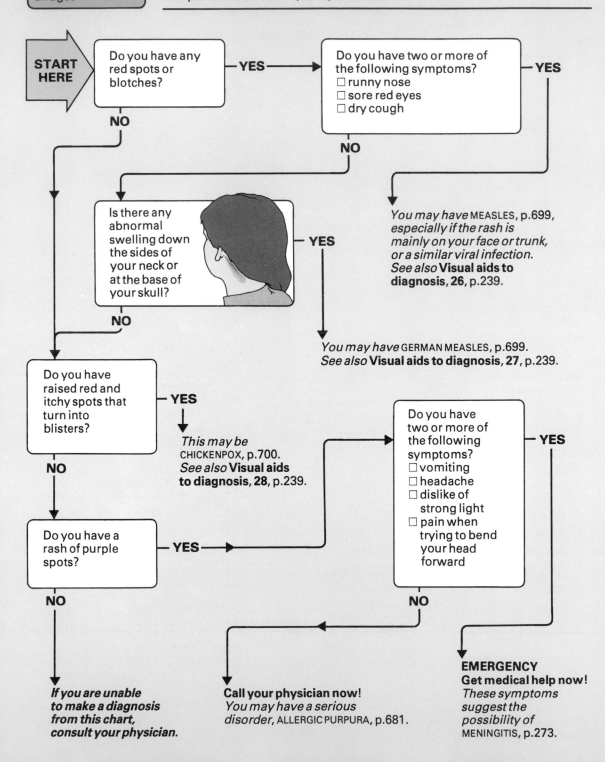

START HERE

Do you have any red spots or blotches?

— YES → **Do you have two or more of the following symptoms?**
☐ runny nose
☐ sore red eyes
☐ dry cough

— YES →

NO ↓

NO ↓

Is there any abnormal swelling down the sides of your neck or at the base of your skull?

— YES →

NO ↓

You may have MEASLES, p.699, *especially if the rash is mainly on your face or trunk, or a similar viral infection. See also* **Visual aids to diagnosis, 26**, p.239.

You may have GERMAN MEASLES, p.699. *See also* **Visual aids to diagnosis, 27**, p.239.

Do you have raised red and itchy spots that turn into blisters?

— YES →

NO ↓

This may be CHICKENPOX, p.700. *See also* **Visual aids to diagnosis, 28**, p.239.

Do you have two or more of the following symptoms?
☐ vomiting
☐ headache
☐ dislike of strong light
☐ pain when trying to bend your head forward

— YES →

NO ↓

Do you have a rash of purple spots?

— YES →

NO ↓

If you are unable to make a diagnosis from this chart, consult your physician.

Call your physician now!
You may have a serious disorder, ALLERGIC PURPURA, p.681.

EMERGENCY
Get medical help now!
These symptoms suggest the possibility of MENINGITIS, p.273.

29

GENERAL
all ages

Raised spots and lumps

Any raised spots or lumps on the surface of the skin that may be inflamed, dark, or the same color as the surrounding skin.

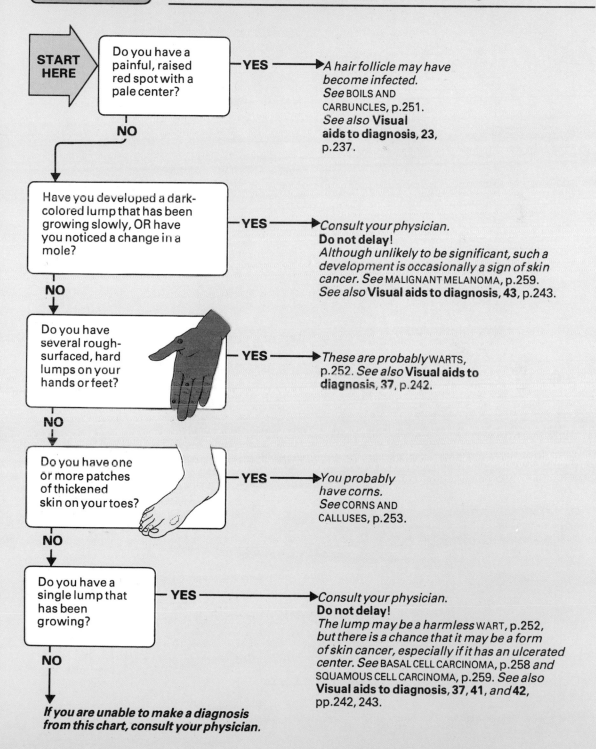

START HERE

Do you have a painful, raised red spot with a pale center?

— **YES** —

A hair follicle may have become infected. See BOILS AND CARBUNCLES, p.251. *See also* **Visual aids to diagnosis, 23,** p.237.

NO

Have you developed a dark-colored lump that has been growing slowly, OR have you noticed a change in a mole?

— **YES** —

Consult your physician. **Do not delay!** *Although unlikely to be significant, such a development is occasionally a sign of skin cancer.* See MALIGNANT MELANOMA, p.259. *See also* **Visual aids to diagnosis, 43,** p.243.

NO

Do you have several rough-surfaced, hard lumps on your hands or feet?

— **YES** —

These are probably WARTS, p.252. *See also* **Visual aids to diagnosis, 37,** p.242.

NO

Do you have one or more patches of thickened skin on your toes?

— **YES** —

You probably have corns. See CORNS AND CALLUSES, p.253.

NO

Do you have a single lump that has been growing?

— **YES** —

Consult your physician. **Do not delay!** *The lump may be a harmless* WART, p.252, *but there is a chance that it may be a form of skin cancer, especially if it has an ulcerated center.* See BASAL CELL CARCINOMA, p.258 *and* SQUAMOUS CELL CARCINOMA, p.259. *See also* **Visual aids to diagnosis, 37, 41,** *and* **42,** pp.242, 243.

NO

If you are unable to make a diagnosis from this chart, consult your physician.

30

GENERAL
all ages

Painful eye

Pain may be continuous or intermittent and may be felt in or around the eye.

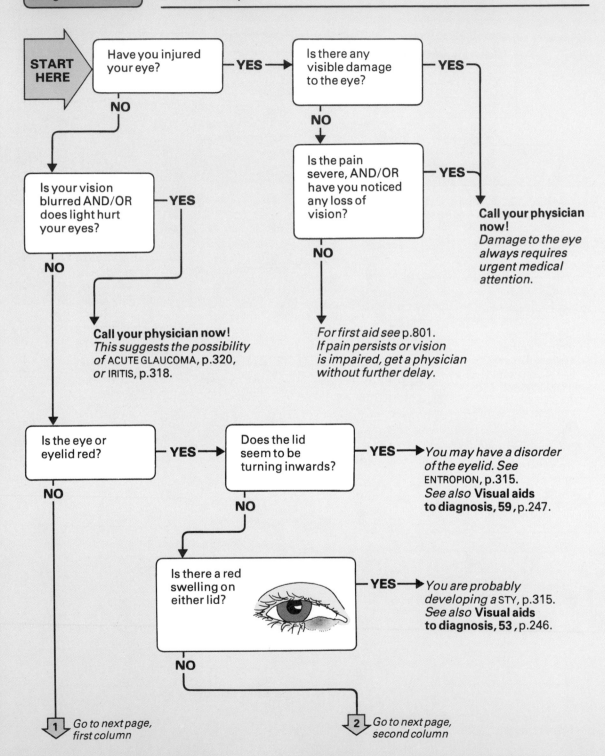

START HERE → Have you injured your eye?

— **YES** → Is there any visible damage to the eye? — **YES** →

NO ↓

Is your vision blurred AND/OR does light hurt your eyes? — **YES** →

NO ↓

Is there any visible damage to the eye?
NO ↓

Is the pain severe, AND/OR have you noticed any loss of vision? — **YES** →

NO ↓

Call your physician now!
Damage to the eye always requires urgent medical attention.

Call your physician now!
This suggests the possibility of ACUTE GLAUCOMA, p.320, *or* IRITIS, p.318.

For first aid see p.801. If pain persists or vision is impaired, get a physician without further delay.

Is the eye or eyelid red? — **YES** → Does the lid seem to be turning inwards? — **YES** → *You may have a disorder of the eyelid. See* ENTROPION, p.315. *See also* **Visual aids to diagnosis, 59,** p.247.

NO ↓

NO ↓

Is there a red swelling on either lid? — **YES** → *You are probably developing a* STY, p.315. *See also* **Visual aids to diagnosis, 53,** p.246.

NO ↓

1 ↓ *Go to next page, first column*

2 ↓ *Go to next page, second column*

1 Continued from previous page, first column

2 Continued from previous page, second column

Does the eye feel gritty? — **YES** → **Is the eye sticky?** — **YES** →

You may have CONJUNCTIVITIS, p.317. *See also* **Visual aids to diagnosis, 55**, p.246.

↓ **NO** (from "Is the eye sticky?")

You may have DRY EYE, p.316.

↓ **NO** (from "Does the eye feel gritty?")

Is the eye watering? — **YES** →

You may have a foreign body in the eye. *See* WATERING EYE, p.316. For first aid, see p.801.

↓ **NO**

Does the pain seem to come from behind the eye? — **YES** → **Do you have two or more of the following symptoms?**
- ☐ severe headache
- ☐ dislike of bright light
- ☐ pain when you bend your head forwards
- ☐ drowsiness or confusion

— **YES** →

EMERGENCY Get medical help now! *You may have* MENINGITIS, p.273, *or a* SUBARACHNOID HEMORRHAGE, p.271.

↓ **NO**

Is there an area of tenderness in the temple above the affected eye? — **YES** →

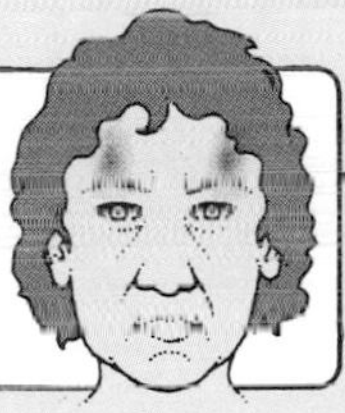

Consult your physician. **Do not delay!** *You may have inflammation of the arteries in your forehead. See* TEMPORAL ARTERITIS, p.414.

↓ **NO**

Is there an area of tenderness over your nose and/or in your cheekbones? — **YES** →

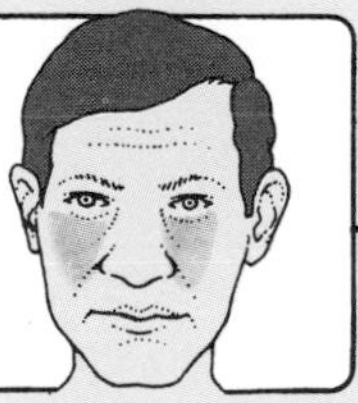

You may have an infection of the sinuses, especially if you have recently had a cold. See SINUSITIS, p.347.

↓ **NO** (from "Does the pain seem to come from behind the eye?")

↓ **NO** (from "Is there an area of tenderness over your nose")

If you are unable to make a diagnosis from this chart, consult your physician.

Disturbed or impaired vision

Any reduction in your ability to see, including blurring, double vision, and/or seeing flashing lights or floating spots.

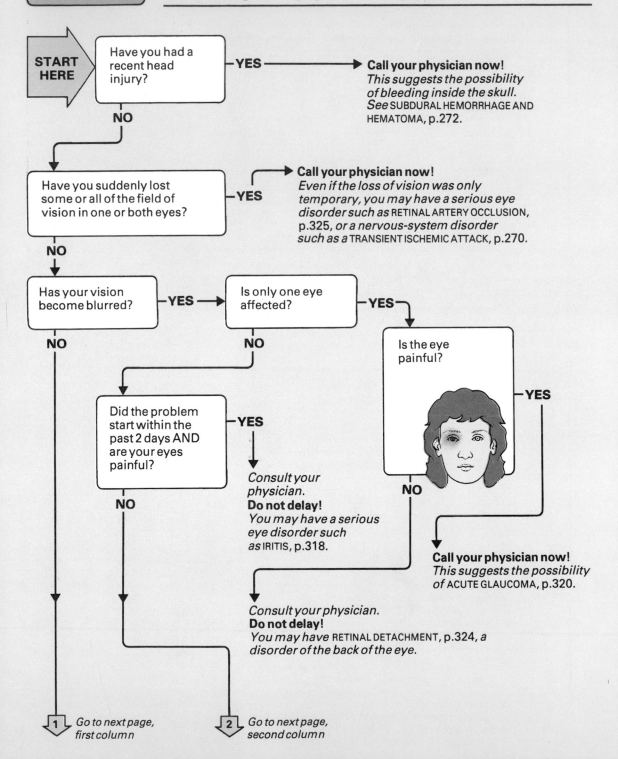

START HERE

Have you had a recent head injury? —**YES**—

Call your physician now!
This suggests the possibility of bleeding inside the skull. See SUBDURAL HEMORRHAGE AND HEMATOMA, p.272.

NO

Have you suddenly lost some or all of the field of vision in one or both eyes? —**YES**—

Call your physician now!
Even if the loss of vision was only temporary, you may have a serious eye disorder such as RETINAL ARTERY OCCLUSION, *p.325, or a nervous-system disorder such as a* TRANSIENT ISCHEMIC ATTACK, *p.270.*

NO

Has your vision become blurred? —**YES**→ **Is only one eye affected?** —**YES**→ **Is the eye painful?** —**YES**—

NO ... **NO** ... **NO**

Did the problem start within the past 2 days AND are your eyes painful? —**YES**—

Consult your physician.
Do not delay!
You may have a serious eye disorder such as IRITIS, p.318.

NO

Consult your physician.
Do not delay!
You may have RETINAL DETACHMENT, p.324, *a disorder of the back of the eye.*

Call your physician now!
This suggests the possibility of ACUTE GLAUCOMA, p.320.

1 *Go to next page, first column*

2 *Go to next page, second column*

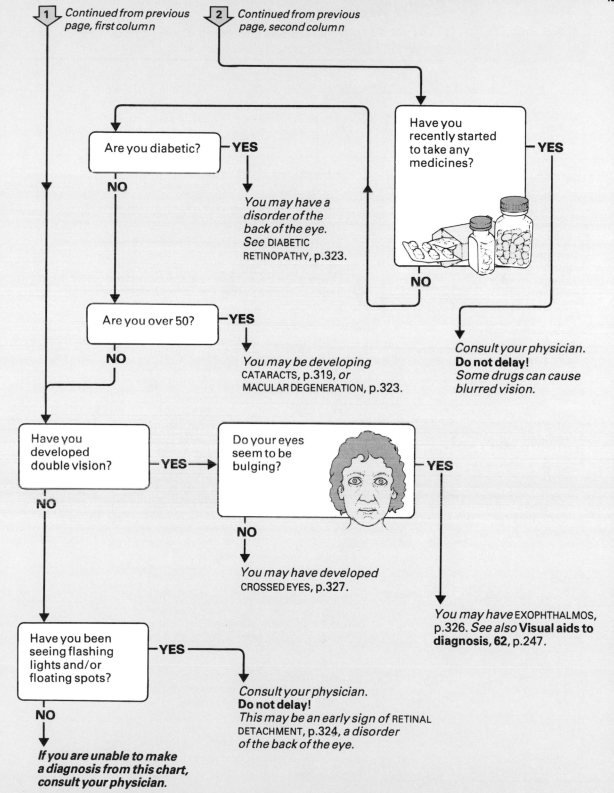

1 *Continued from previous page, first column*

2 *Continued from previous page, second column*

Are you diabetic? — **YES**

NO

You may have a disorder of the back of the eye. See DIABETIC RETINOPATHY, p.323.

Have you recently started to take any medicines? — **YES**

NO

Are you over 50? — **YES**

NO

You may be developing CATARACTS, p.319, *or* MACULAR DEGENERATION, p.323.

Consult your physician. **Do not delay!** *Some drugs can cause blurred vision.*

Have you developed double vision? — **YES**

NO

Do your eyes seem to be bulging? — **YES**

NO

You may have developed CROSSED EYES, p.327.

You may have EXOPHTHALMOS, p.326. *See also* **Visual aids to diagnosis, 62**, p.247.

Have you been seeing flashing lights and/or floating spots? — **YES**

NO

Consult your physician. **Do not delay!** *This may be an early sign of* RETINAL DETACHMENT, p.324, *a disorder of the back of the eye.*

If you are unable to make a diagnosis from this chart, consult your physician.

32
GENERAL
all ages

Earache
Pain in one or both ears, either sharp and stabbing or dull and throbbing.

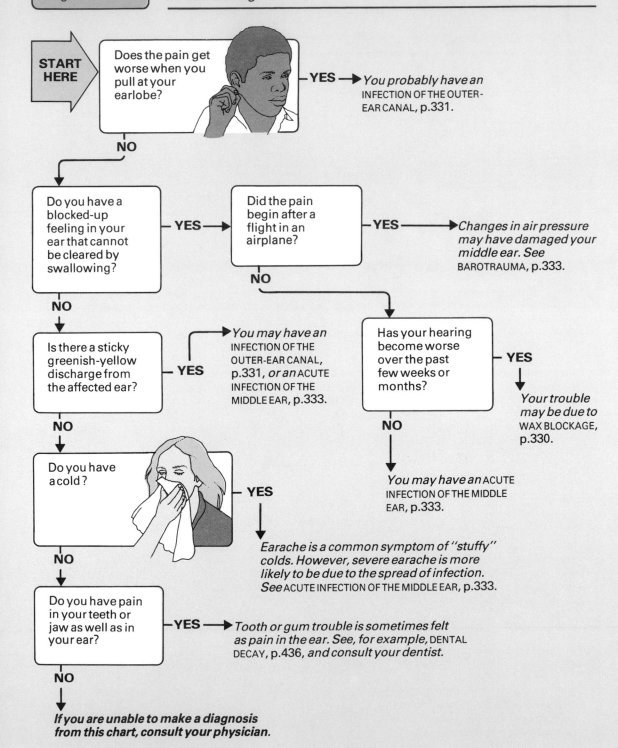

START HERE

Does the pain get worse when you pull at your earlobe?

YES → *You probably have an* INFECTION OF THE OUTER-EAR CANAL, p.331.

NO

Do you have a blocked-up feeling in your ear that cannot be cleared by swallowing?

YES →

Did the pain begin after a flight in an airplane?

YES → *Changes in air pressure may have damaged your middle ear. See* BAROTRAUMA, p.333.

NO

NO

Is there a sticky greenish-yellow discharge from the affected ear?

YES → *You may have an* INFECTION OF THE OUTER-EAR CANAL, p.331, *or an* ACUTE INFECTION OF THE MIDDLE EAR, p.333.

Has your hearing become worse over the past few weeks or months?

YES → *Your trouble may be due to* WAX BLOCKAGE, p.330.

NO

NO

Do you have a cold?

YES →

You may have an ACUTE INFECTION OF THE MIDDLE EAR, p.333.

Earache is a common symptom of "stuffy" colds. However, severe earache is more likely to be due to the spread of infection. See ACUTE INFECTION OF THE MIDDLE EAR, p.333.

NO

Do you have pain in your teeth or jaw as well as in your ear?

YES → *Tooth or gum trouble is sometimes felt as pain in the ear. See, for example,* DENTAL DECAY, p.436, *and consult your dentist.*

NO

If you are unable to make a diagnosis from this chart, consult your physician.

33

GENERAL
all ages

Noises in the ear

Any ringing, buzzing, or hissing (but not speech or music) that only you can hear.

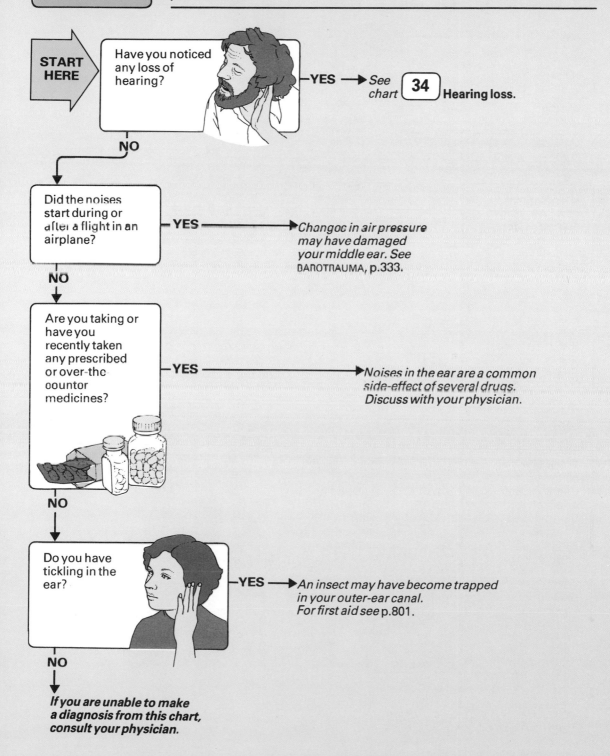

START HERE

Have you noticed any loss of hearing?

YES → *See chart* **34** **Hearing loss.**

NO

Did the noises start during or after a flight in an airplane?

YES → *Changes in air pressure may have damaged your middle ear. See* BAROTRAUMA, p.333.

NO

Are you taking or have you recently taken any prescribed or over-the-counter medicines?

YES → *Noises in the ear are a common side-effect of several drugs. Discuss with your physician.*

NO

Do you have tickling in the ear?

YES → *An insect may have become trapped in your outer-ear canal. For first aid see p.801.*

NO

If you are unable to make a diagnosis from this chart, consult your physician.

34
GENERAL
all ages

Hearing loss

Deterioration in the ability to hear some or all sounds in one or both ears.

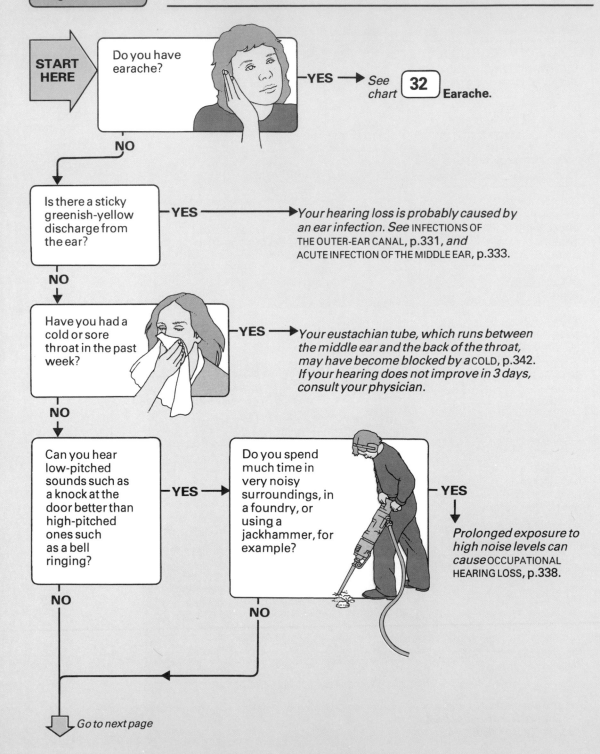

START HERE

Do you have earache?

YES → *See chart* **32** **Earache.**

NO

Is there a sticky greenish-yellow discharge from the ear?

YES → *Your hearing loss is probably caused by an ear infection. See* INFECTIONS OF THE OUTER-EAR CANAL, p.331, *and* ACUTE INFECTION OF THE MIDDLE EAR, p.333.

NO

Have you had a cold or sore throat in the past week?

YES → *Your eustachian tube, which runs between the middle ear and the back of the throat, may have become blocked by a* COLD, p.342. *If your hearing does not improve in 3 days, consult your physician.*

NO

Can you hear low-pitched sounds such as a knock at the door better than high-pitched ones such as a bell ringing?

YES →

Do you spend much time in very noisy surroundings, in a foundry, or using a jackhammer, for example?

YES ↓

Prolonged exposure to high noise levels can cause OCCUPATIONAL HEARING LOSS, p.338.

NO   **NO**

Go to next page

⬇ *Continued from previous page*

Have you recently taken any prescribed or over-the-counter medicines?

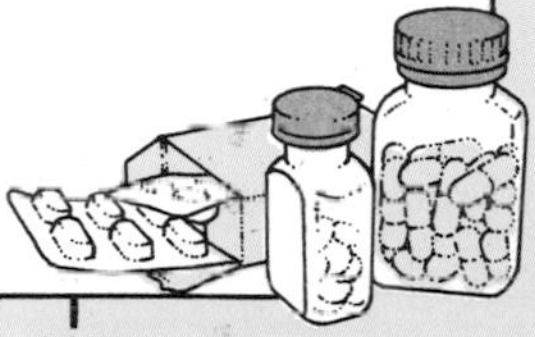

YES ➡ *Hearing loss is a common side-effect of several drugs. Discuss with your physician.*

NO ⬇

Do you have occasional attacks of dizziness when everything around you seems to spin?

YES ➡ *You may have* MENIERE'S DISEASE, p.337, *which affects the balance mechanism of the inner ear.*

NO ⬇

Are you over 60?

YES ➡ *Some hearing loss is common in later life, but it often can be treated. See* AGING AND THE SENSES, p.721.

NO ⬇

Has your hearing been getting worse over a period of several weeks or more?

YES ➡ **Have other members of your family suffered from gradual loss of hearing?**

YES ➡ *You may have* OTOSCLEROSIS, p.332 , *which affects the working of the middle ear.*

NO ⬇

Your problem may be due to WAX BLOCKAGE, p.330.

NO ⬇

If you are unable to make a diagnosis from this chart, consult your physician.

35

GENERAL
all ages

Runny nose

Completely or partially blocked nose, with a liquid discharge.

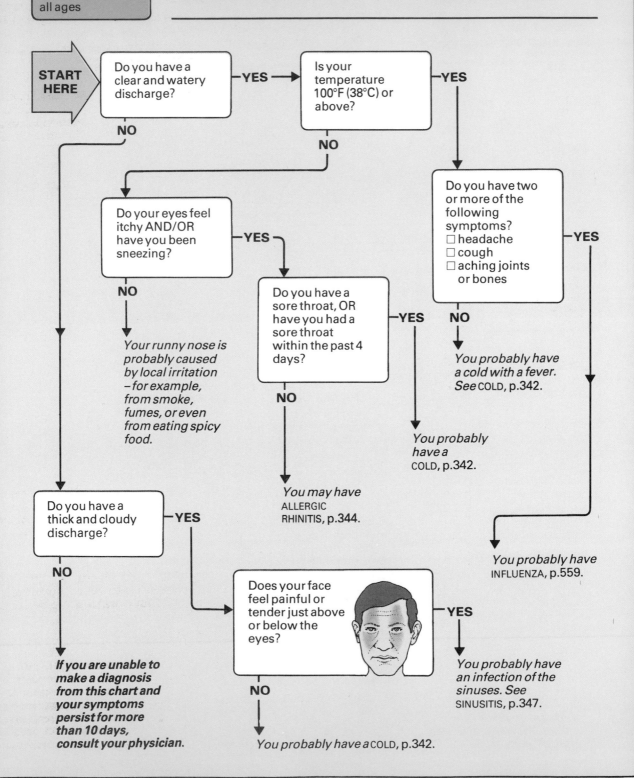

START HERE

Do you have a clear and watery discharge?

— **YES** → **Is your temperature 100°F (38°C) or above?**

NO ↓

NO ↓

— **YES** → **Do you have two or more of the following symptoms?**
☐ headache
☐ cough
☐ aching joints or bones

Do your eyes feel itchy AND/OR have you been sneezing?

— **YES** → **Do you have a sore throat, OR have you had a sore throat within the past 4 days?**

NO ↓

Your runny nose is probably caused by local irritation – for example, from smoke, fumes, or even from eating spicy food.

— **YES** →

NO ↓

You may have ALLERGIC RHINITIS, p.344.

NO ↓

You probably have a cold with a fever. See COLD, p.342.

— **YES** →

You probably have a COLD, p.342.

You probably have INFLUENZA, p.559.

Do you have a thick and cloudy discharge?

— **YES** →

NO ↓

If you are unable to make a diagnosis from this chart and your symptoms persist for more than 10 days, consult your physician.

Does your face feel painful or tender just above or below the eyes?

— **YES** ↓

You probably have an infection of the sinuses. See SINUSITIS, p.347.

NO ↓

You probably have a COLD, p.342.

36

GENERAL
all ages

Sore throat

Any rough or raw feeling in the back of the throat that causes discomfort, especially when you swallow.

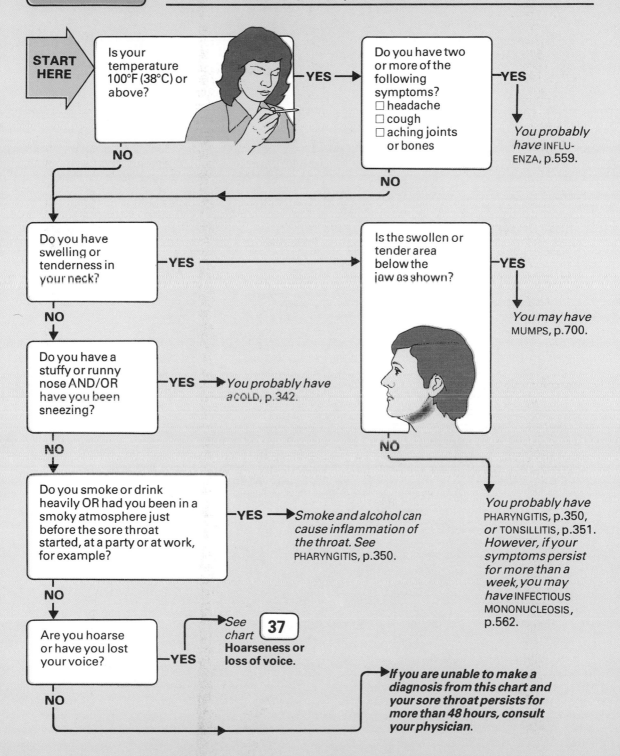

START HERE

Is your temperature 100°F (38°C) or above?

NO →

YES → Do you have two or more of the following symptoms?
☐ headache
☐ cough
☐ aching joints or bones

YES → *You probably have* INFLUENZA, p.559.

NO

Do you have swelling or tenderness in your neck?

NO

YES → Is the swollen or tender area below the jaw as shown?

YES → *You may have* MUMPS, p.700.

Do you have a stuffy or runny nose AND/OR have you been sneezing?

YES → *You probably have a* COLD, p.342.

NO

NO → *You probably have* PHARYNGITIS, p.350, *or* TONSILLITIS, p.351. *However, if your symptoms persist for more than a week, you may have* INFECTIOUS MONONUCLEOSIS, p.562.

Do you smoke or drink heavily OR had you been in a smoky atmosphere just before the sore throat started, at a party or at work, for example?

YES → *Smoke and alcohol can cause inflammation of the throat. See* PHARYNGITIS, p.350.

NO

Are you hoarse or have you lost your voice?

YES → *See chart* **37** **Hoarseness or loss of voice.**

NO

If you are unable to make a diagnosis from this chart and your sore throat persists for more than 48 hours, consult your physician.

37

GENERAL
all ages

Hoarseness or loss of voice

Any abnormal huskiness in the voice that may be so severe that you can make little or no sound.

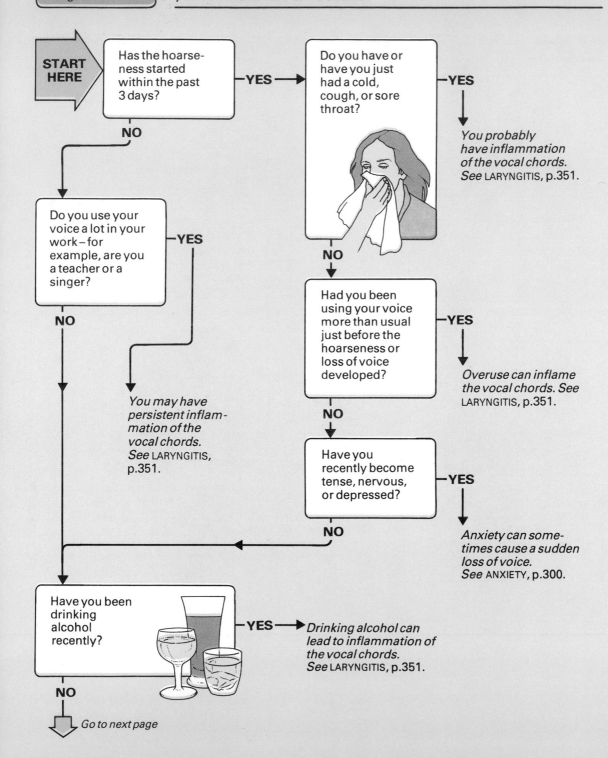

START HERE → Has the hoarseness started within the past 3 days?

— **YES** → Do you have or have you just had a cold, cough, or sore throat?

— **YES** → *You probably have inflammation of the vocal chords. See* LARYNGITIS, p.351.

NO ↓ (from first box)

Do you use your voice a lot in your work – for example, are you a teacher or a singer?

— **YES** → *You may have persistent inflammation of the vocal chords. See* LARYNGITIS, p.351.

NO ↓

NO ↓ (from cold/cough box)

Had you been using your voice more than usual just before the hoarseness or loss of voice developed?

— **YES** → *Overuse can inflame the vocal chords. See* LARYNGITIS, p.351.

NO ↓

Have you recently become tense, nervous, or depressed?

— **YES** → *Anxiety can sometimes cause a sudden loss of voice. See* ANXIETY, p.300.

NO →

Have you been drinking alcohol recently?

— **YES** → *Drinking alcohol can lead to inflammation of the vocal chords. See* LARYNGITIS, p.351.

NO ↓

Go to next page

↓ *Continued from previous page*

Do you smoke?

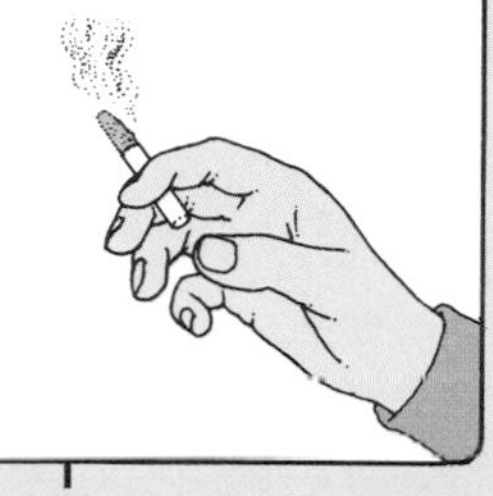

— **YES** ——————→ *Smoking can lead to inflammation of the vocal chords.* See LARYNGITIS, p.351.

NO ↓

Do you have two or more of the following symptoms?
☐ feeling the cold more than you used to
☐ dry skin or hair
☐ weight increase without overeating
☐ unexplained tiredness

— **YES** ——→ *You may have an under-active thyroid gland.* See HYPOTHYROIDISM, p.526.

NO ↓

Has your hoarse-ness or loss of voice lasted for more than a week?

— **YES** ———→ *Consult your physician.* **Do not delay!** *Although there is probably a simple explanation for your hoarseness or loss of voice, there is a slight possibility of a growth on the larynx. See* TUMORS OF THE LARYNX, p.352.

NO ↓

Have you had several attacks of hoarseness or loss of voice in the past 6 months?

— **YES** ———↑

NO ↓

If you are unable to make a diagnosis from this chart and your hoarseness persists for more than a week, consult your physician.

Cancer watch

Hoarseness or loss of voice that is recurrent or lasts for more than a week may indicate cancer of the larynx.

Consult your physician without delay!

38

GENERAL
over 14 years

Coughing

A noisy expulsion of air from the lungs, that may produce phlegm or be "dry." For children see chart 95, **Coughing in children.**

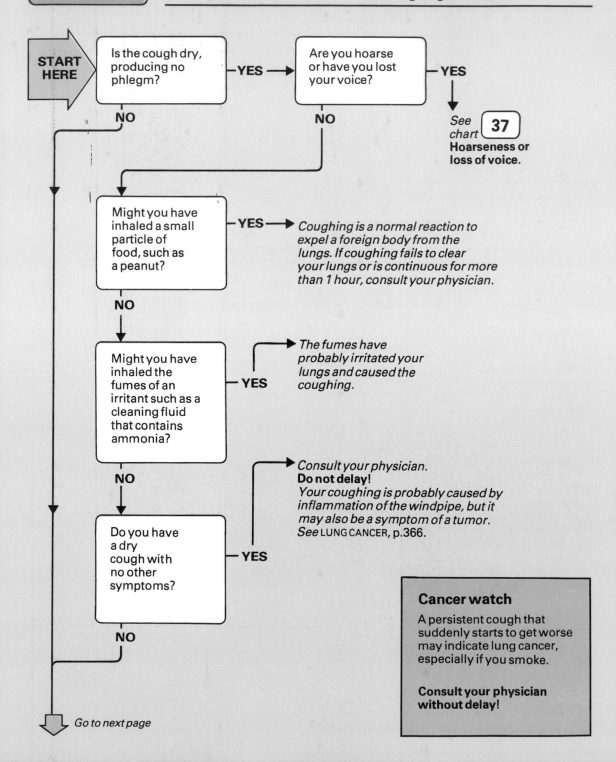

START HERE

Is the cough dry, producing no phlegm? — **YES** → Are you hoarse or have you lost your voice? — **YES**

NO

NO

↓

See chart **37** Hoarseness or loss of voice.

Might you have inhaled a small particle of food, such as a peanut? — **YES** → *Coughing is a normal reaction to expel a foreign body from the lungs. If coughing fails to clear your lungs or is continuous for more than 1 hour, consult your physician.*

NO

Might you have inhaled the fumes of an irritant such as a cleaning fluid that contains ammonia? — **YES** → *The fumes have probably irritated your lungs and caused the coughing.*

NO

Do you have a dry cough with no other symptoms? — **YES** → *Consult your physician.* **Do not delay!** *Your coughing is probably caused by inflammation of the windpipe, but it may also be a symptom of a tumor. See* LUNG CANCER, p.366.

NO

Cancer watch

A persistent cough that suddenly starts to get worse may indicate lung cancer, especially if you smoke.

Consult your physician without delay!

⇩ *Go to next page*

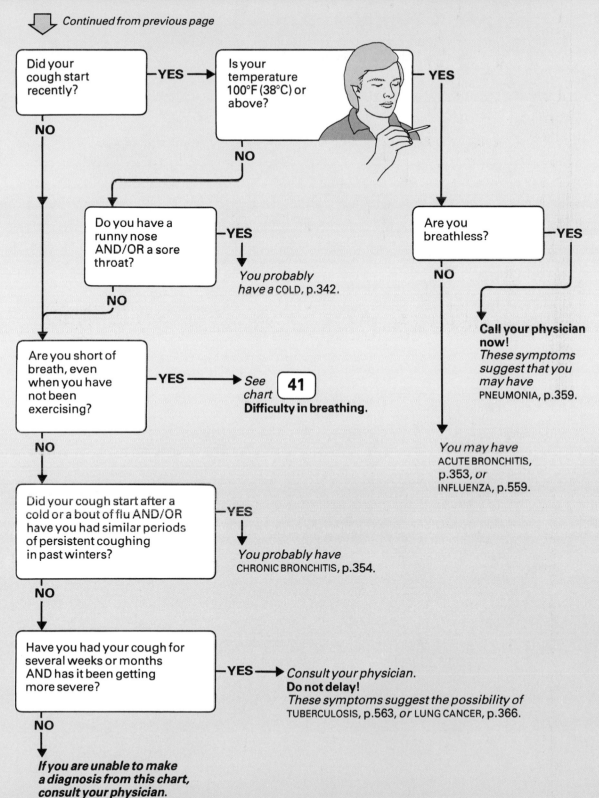

Continued from previous page

Did your cough start recently? —YES→ **Is your temperature 100°F (38°C) or above?** —YES→

NO

NO

Do you have a runny nose AND/OR a sore throat? —YES↓

You probably have a COLD, p.342.

NO

Are you short of breath, even when you have not been exercising? —YES→ *See chart* **41** **Difficulty in breathing.**

NO

Did your cough start after a cold or a bout of flu AND/OR have you had similar periods of persistent coughing in past winters? —YES↓

You probably have CHRONIC BRONCHITIS, p.354.

NO

Have you had your cough for several weeks or months AND has it been getting more severe? —YES→ *Consult your physician.* **Do not delay!** *These symptoms suggest the possibility of* TUBERCULOSIS, p.563, *or* LUNG CANCER, p.366.

NO

If you are unable to make a diagnosis from this chart, consult your physician.

Are you breathless? —YES→

NO

Call your physician now! *These symptoms suggest that you may have* PNEUMONIA, p.359.

You may have ACUTE BRONCHITIS, p.353, *or* INFLUENZA, p.559.

39

GENERAL
all ages

Coughing up blood

Coughing up phlegm that is colored or streaked bright red or rusty brown, or that is pink and frothy.

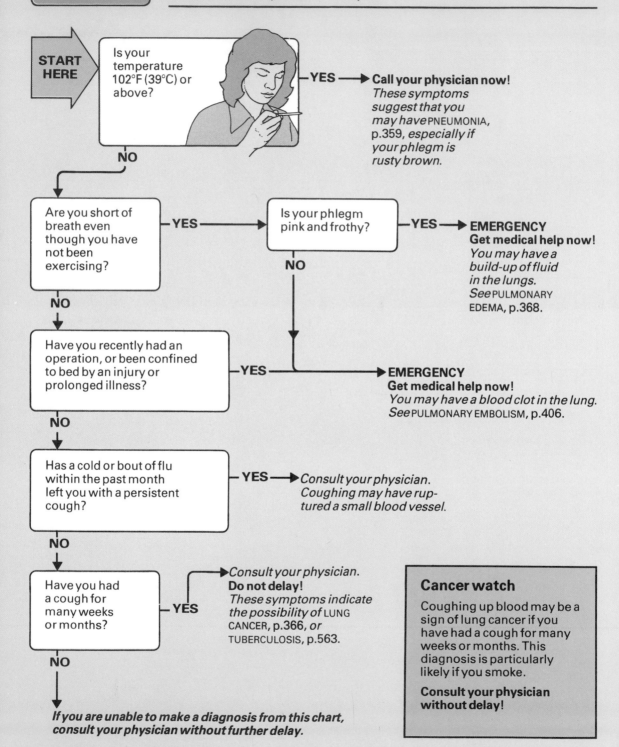

START HERE → Is your temperature 102°F (39°C) or above?

— **YES** → **Call your physician now!** *These symptoms suggest that you may have* PNEUMONIA, p.359, *especially if your phlegm is rusty brown.*

NO ↓

Are you short of breath even though you have not been exercising?

— **YES** → Is your phlegm pink and frothy?

— **YES** → **EMERGENCY Get medical help now!** *You may have a build-up of fluid in the lungs. See* PULMONARY EDEMA, p.368.

NO ↓

Have you recently had an operation, or been confined to bed by an injury or prolonged illness?

— **YES** → **EMERGENCY Get medical help now!** *You may have a blood clot in the lung. See* PULMONARY EMBOLISM, p.406.

NO ↓

Has a cold or bout of flu within the past month left you with a persistent cough?

— **YES** → *Consult your physician. Coughing may have ruptured a small blood vessel.*

NO ↓

Have you had a cough for many weeks or months?

— **YES** → *Consult your physician.* **Do not delay!** *These symptoms indicate the possibility of* LUNG CANCER, p.366, *or* TUBERCULOSIS, p.563.

NO ↓

If you are unable to make a diagnosis from this chart, consult your physician without further delay.

Cancer watch

Coughing up blood may be a sign of lung cancer if you have had a cough for many weeks or months. This diagnosis is particularly likely if you smoke.

Consult your physician without delay!

40

GENERAL
all ages

Wheezing

Noisy, difficult breathing, particularly when breathing out.

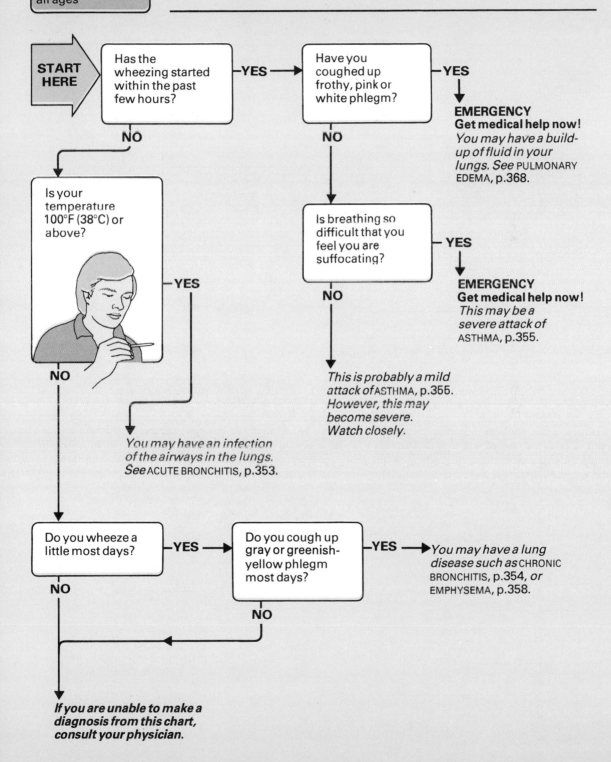

START HERE → Has the wheezing started within the past few hours? —**YES**→ Have you coughed up frothy, pink or white phlegm? —**YES**→

NO ↓

EMERGENCY
Get medical help now!
You may have a build-up of fluid in your lungs. See PULMONARY EDEMA, p.368.

Is your temperature 100°F (38°C) or above?

Have you coughed up frothy, pink or white phlegm? → **NO** ↓

Is breathing so difficult that you feel you are suffocating? —**YES**→

EMERGENCY
Get medical help now!
This may be a severe attack of ASTHMA, p.355.

NO ↓

YES →

This is probably a mild attack of ASTHMA, p.355. *However, this may become severe. Watch closely.*

NO ↓

You may have an infection of the airways in the lungs. See ACUTE BRONCHITIS, p.353.

Do you wheeze a little most days? —**YES**→ Do you cough up gray or greenish-yellow phlegm most days? —**YES**→ *You may have a lung disease such as* CHRONIC BRONCHITIS, p.354, *or* EMPHYSEMA, p.358.

NO ↓

NO ↓

If you are unable to make a diagnosis from this chart, consult your physician.

41

GENERAL
all ages

Difficulty in breathing

Breathlessness or tightness in the chest that makes you aware of your breathing.

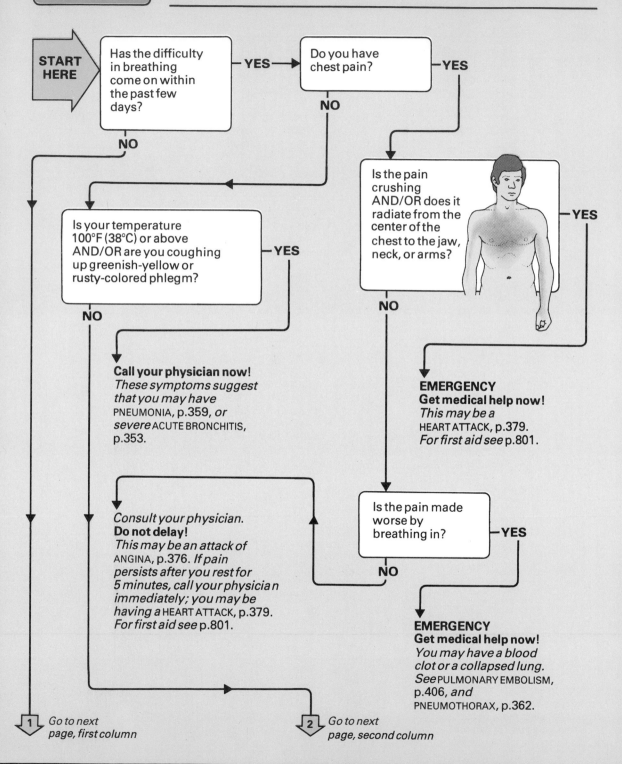

START HERE → Has the difficulty in breathing come on within the past few days?

— **YES** → Do you have chest pain?

— **YES** → Is the pain crushing AND/OR does it radiate from the center of the chest to the jaw, neck, or arms?

— **YES** →

Has the difficulty in breathing come on within the past few days? — **NO** →

Do you have chest pain? — **NO** →

Is your temperature 100°F (38°C) or above AND/OR are you coughing up greenish-yellow or rusty-colored phlegm?

— **YES** →

Is your temperature... — **NO** →

Call your physician now!
These symptoms suggest that you may have PNEUMONIA, p.359, *or severe* ACUTE BRONCHITIS, p.353.

Is the pain crushing... — **NO** →

EMERGENCY
Get medical help now!
This may be a HEART ATTACK, p.379. *For first aid see* p.801.

Consult your physician.
Do not delay!
This may be an attack of ANGINA, p.376. *If pain persists after you rest for 5 minutes, call your physician immediately; you may be having a* HEART ATTACK, p.379. *For first aid see* p.801.

Is the pain made worse by breathing in?

— **YES** →

Is the pain made worse by breathing in? — **NO** →

EMERGENCY
Get medical help now!
You may have a blood clot or a collapsed lung. See PULMONARY EMBOLISM, p.406, *and* PNEUMOTHORAX, p.362.

1 *Go to next page, first column*

2 *Go to next page, second column*

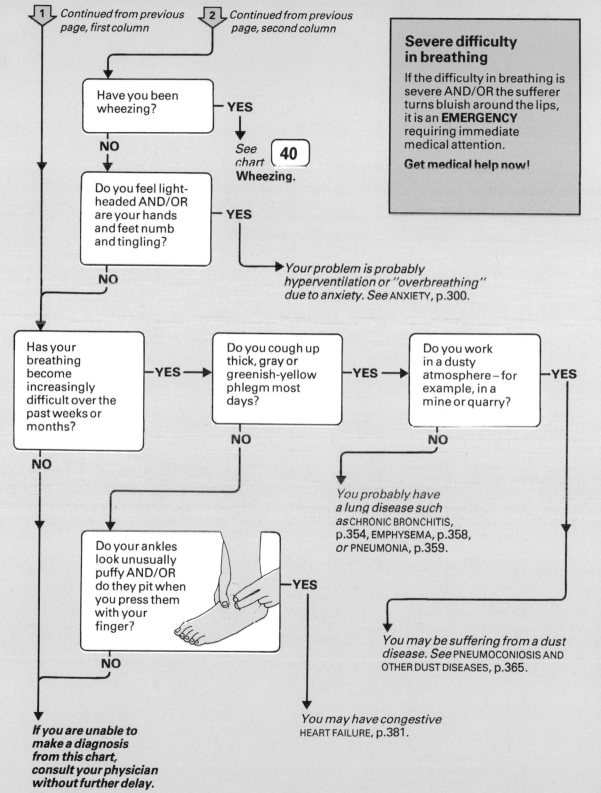

1 Continued from previous page, first column

2 Continued from previous page, second column

Have you been wheezing? — YES → See chart **40** Wheezing.

NO

Do you feel light-headed AND/OR are your hands and feet numb and tingling? — YES → *Your problem is probably hyperventilation or "overbreathing" due to anxiety. See* ANXIETY, p.300.

NO

Severe difficulty in breathing

If the difficulty in breathing is severe AND/OR the sufferer turns bluish around the lips, it is an **EMERGENCY** requiring immediate medical attention.

Get medical help now!

Has your breathing become increasingly difficult over the past weeks or months? — YES → **Do you cough up thick, gray or greenish-yellow phlegm most days?** — YES → **Do you work in a dusty atmosphere – for example, in a mine or quarry?** — YES →

NO (breathing) / NO (phlegm) / NO (dusty)

You probably have a lung disease such as CHRONIC BRONCHITIS, p.354, EMPHYSEMA, p.358, *or* PNEUMONIA, p.359.

Do your ankles look unusually puffy AND/OR do they pit when you press them with your finger? — YES → *You may have congestive* HEART FAILURE, p.381.

NO

You may be suffering from a dust disease. See PNEUMOCONIOSIS AND OTHER DUST DISEASES, p.365.

If you are unable to make a diagnosis from this chart, consult your physician without further delay.

42

GENERAL
all ages

Toothache

Pain in one tooth, or in the teeth and gums generally, felt either as a dull throb or a sharp twinge.

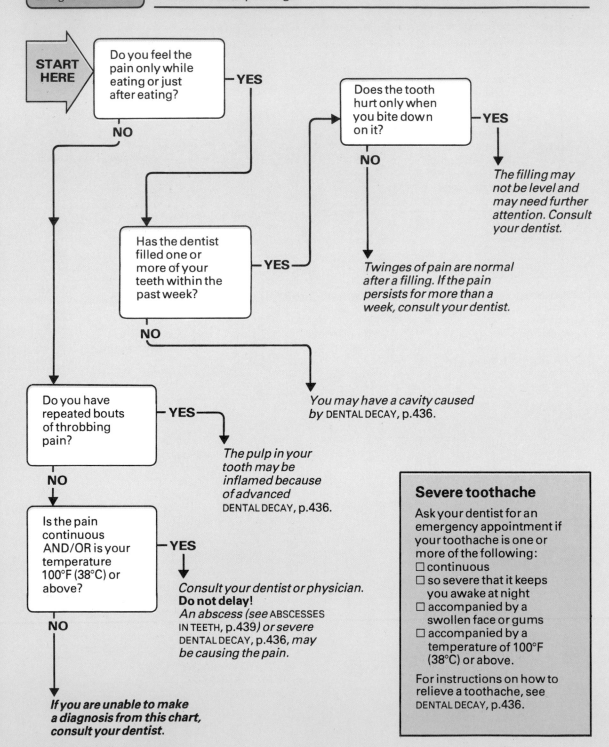

START HERE

Do you feel the pain only while eating or just after eating? — **YES**

NO

Does the tooth hurt only when you bite down on it? — **YES**

NO

The filling may not be level and may need further attention. Consult your dentist.

Has the dentist filled one or more of your teeth within the past week? — **YES**

NO

Twinges of pain are normal after a filling. If the pain persists for more than a week, consult your dentist.

You may have a cavity caused by DENTAL DECAY, p.436.

Do you have repeated bouts of throbbing pain? — **YES**

NO

The pulp in your tooth may be inflamed because of advanced DENTAL DECAY, p.436.

Is the pain continuous AND/OR is your temperature 100°F (38°C) or above? — **YES**

NO

Consult your dentist or physician. **Do not delay!** *An abscess (see* ABSCESSES IN TEETH, p.439*) or severe* DENTAL DECAY, p.436, *may be causing the pain.*

If you are unable to make a diagnosis from this chart, consult your dentist.

Severe toothache

Ask your dentist for an emergency appointment if your toothache is one or more of the following:
☐ continuous
☐ so severe that it keeps you awake at night
☐ accompanied by a swollen face or gums
☐ accompanied by a temperature of 100°F (38°C) or above.

For instructions on how to relieve a toothache, see DENTAL DECAY, p.436.

43

GENERAL
all ages

Difficulty in swallowing

Discomfort or pain when swallowing, or difficulty in making food go down at all.

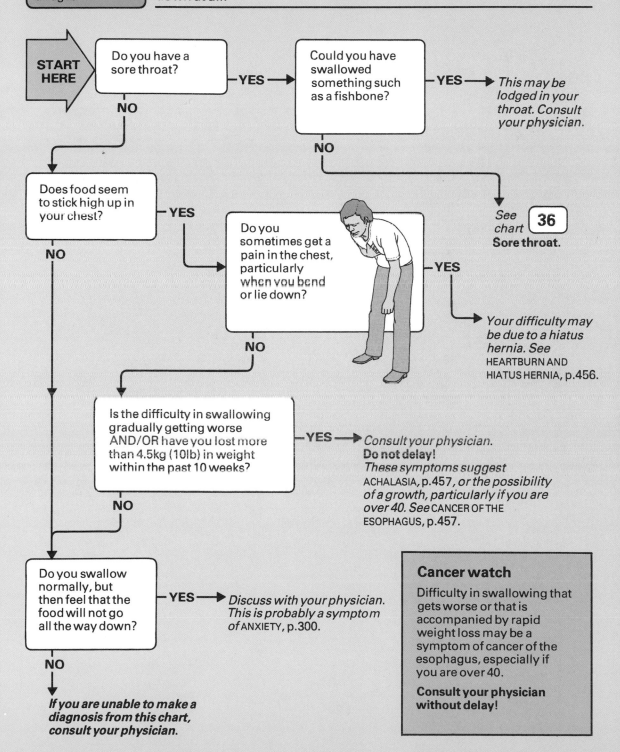

START HERE → **Do you have a sore throat?**

YES → **Could you have swallowed something such as a fishbone?**

YES → *This may be lodged in your throat. Consult your physician.*

NO ↓

Does food seem to stick high up in your chest?

YES → **Do you sometimes get a pain in the chest, particularly when you bend or lie down?**

YES → *Your difficulty may be due to a hiatus hernia. See* HEARTBURN AND HIATUS HERNIA, p.456.

From "fishbone" box: **NO** → See chart **36** **Sore throat.**

NO (from chest box) ↓

Is the difficulty in swallowing gradually getting worse AND/OR have you lost more than 4.5kg (10lb) in weight within the past 10 weeks?

YES → *Consult your physician.* **Do not delay!** *These symptoms suggest* ACHALASIA, p.457, *or the possibility of a growth, particularly if you are over 40. See* CANCER OF THE ESOPHAGUS, p.457.

NO ↓

Do you swallow normally, but then feel that the food will not go all the way down?

YES → *Discuss with your physician. This is probably a symptom of* ANXIETY, p.300.

NO ↓

If you are unable to make a diagnosis from this chart, consult your physician.

Cancer watch

Difficulty in swallowing that gets worse or that is accompanied by rapid weight loss may be a symptom of cancer of the esophagus, especially if you are over 40.

Consult your physician without delay!

44
GENERAL
all ages

Sore mouth and/or tongue

Soreness anywhere inside the mouth and/or on or around the tongue and lips.

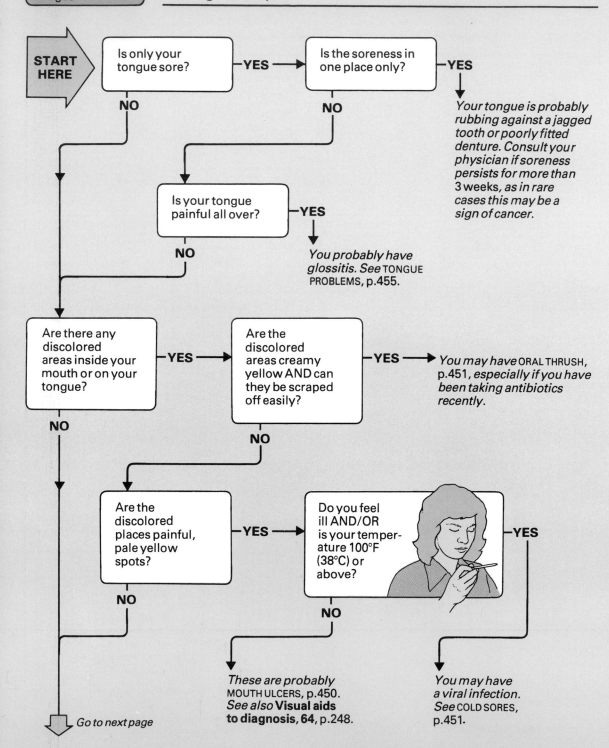

START HERE

Is only your tongue sore? — NO → (down)

Is only your tongue sore? — YES → **Is the soreness in one place only?** — YES →

Your tongue is probably rubbing against a jagged tooth or poorly fitted denture. Consult your physician if soreness persists for more than 3 weeks, as in rare cases this may be a sign of cancer.

Is the soreness in one place only? — NO → **Is your tongue painful all over?** — NO → (down)

Is your tongue painful all over? — YES → *You probably have glossitis. See* TONGUE PROBLEMS, p.455.

Are there any discolored areas inside your mouth or on your tongue? — YES → **Are the discolored areas creamy yellow AND can they be scraped off easily?** — YES → *You may have* ORAL THRUSH, p.451, *especially if you have been taking antibiotics recently.*

Are there any discolored areas inside your mouth or on your tongue? — NO → (down)

Are the discolored areas creamy yellow AND can they be scraped off easily? — NO → (down)

Are the discolored places painful, pale yellow spots? — YES → **Do you feel ill AND/OR is your temperature 100°F (38°C) or above?** — YES → *You may have a viral infection. See* COLD SORES, p.451.

Are the discolored places painful, pale yellow spots? — NO → (down)

Do you feel ill AND/OR is your temperature 100°F (38°C) or above? — NO → *These are probably* MOUTH ULCERS, p.450. *See also* **Visual aids to diagnosis, 64**, p.248.

Go to next page

Continued from previous page

Are your gums painful, red and swollen? —**YES**→ **Does your breath smell bad AND/OR do you have a foul taste in your mouth?** —**YES**→ *Consult your dentist. You may have* TRENCH MOUTH, p.452, *an infection of the gums.*

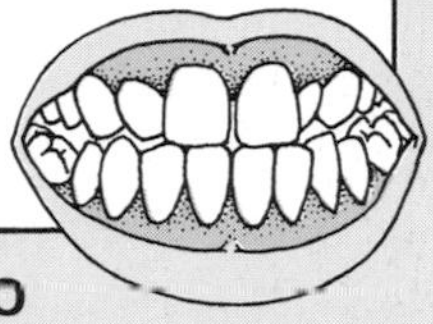

NO (down)

(breath box) **NO** ↓ *You may have severe* GINGIVITIS, p.445, *or a viral infection. See* COLD SORES, p.451.

Do you have sore places on or around the lips? —**YES**→ **Are the sores red, rough, AND/OR blistered?** —**YES**→ *You probably have a* COLD SORE, p.451. *See also* **Visual aids to diagnosis, 24,** p.238.

NO (down)

NO ↓

Are there cracks at the corners of your mouth? —**YES**→ *This soreness may be caused by dentures poorly fitted. See* DENTURE PROBLEMS, p.443. *Or you may have a vitamin B$_{12}$ deficiency, see* VITAMIN DEFICIENCY, p.494.

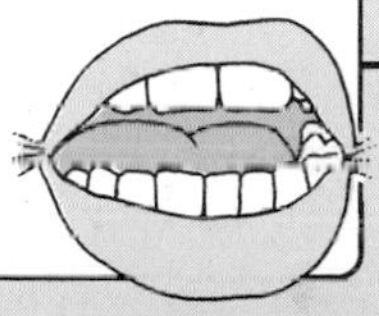

NO ↓

Have you recently started to use any new creams or cosmetics on your lips? —**YES**↓ *The soreness may be an allergic reaction to one of the ingredients. See* ECZEMA AND DERMATITIS, p.253.

NO

If you are unable to make a diagnosis from this chart, consult your physician.

Cancer watch
Any sore area in the mouth or on the tongue may indicate cancer if it fails to heal within 3 weeks.

Consult your physician without delay!

45
GENERAL
all ages

Bad breath
Offensive-smelling breath of which you may be unaware unless it is mentioned by somebody else.

START HERE → Do your gums ever bleed? —**YES**→ *Bad breath is often due to inflammation of the gums.* See GINGIVITIS, p.445.

NO ↓

Is your tongue or the inside of your mouth sore or painful? —**YES**→ *Infection or ulceration of the mouth and tongue can cause bad breath.*

See chart **44** **Sore mouth and tongue.**

NO ↓

Is it more than 6 months since you last visited your dentist, AND/OR do you have a toothache? —**YES**→ *Tooth decay may be causing your bad breath.* See DENTAL DECAY, p.436.

NO ↓

Do you often fail to clean your teeth twice a day, or do you clean them inadequately (for less than 3 minutes morning and evening)? —**YES**→ *Decaying food particles lodged between the teeth can affect the breath.* See KEEPING YOUR TEETH AND GUMS HEALTHY, p.438.

NO ↓

Do you wear a denture? —**YES**→ Do you sometimes fail to clean it thoroughly on both sides once a day? —**YES**↓

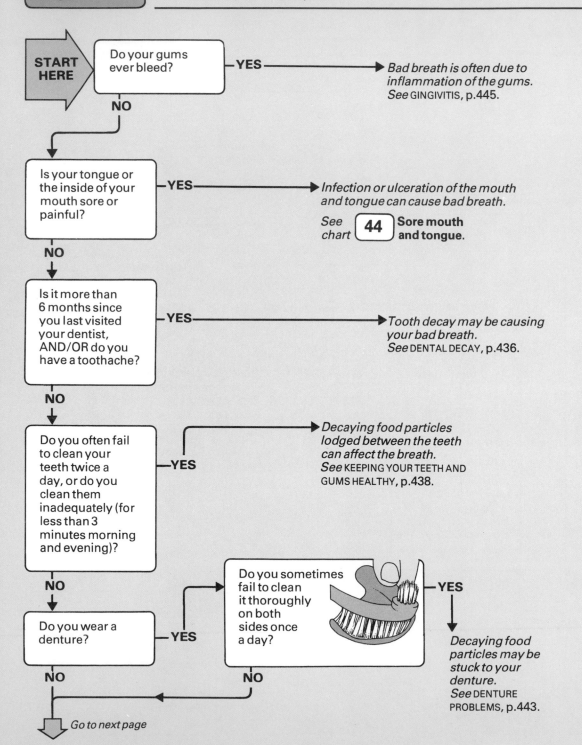

Decaying food particles may be stuck to your denture. See DENTURE PROBLEMS, p.443.

NO ↓   **NO** ↓

Go to next page

Continued from previous page

Have you eaten garlic or onions, or drunk alcohol within the past 24 hours?

YES → *These things contain volatile substances that are absorbed into the bloodstream and then released into the lungs. These substances may cause bad breath. Your breath should be back to normal in 24 hours.*

NO

Do you smoke?

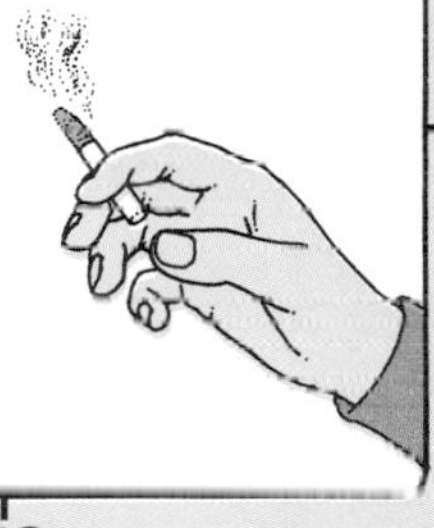

YES → *Smoking almost always causes bad breath.* See THE DANGERS OF SMOKING, p.38.

NO

Is your temperature 100°F (38°C) or above?

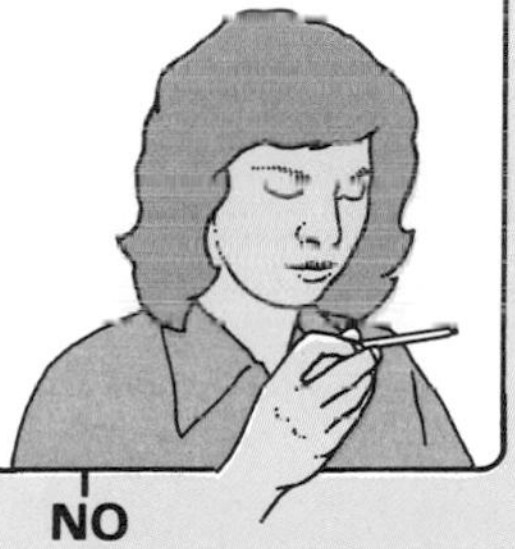

YES → *Bad breath often occurs with feverish illnesses.*

See chart **5** *Fever.*

For children

see chart **91** *Fever in infants*

or chart **92** *Fever in children.*

NO

Do you have a persistent cough that produces foul-smelling phlegm?

YES → *You may have* BRONCHIECTASIS, *p.363, a chronic lung disease.*

NO

Your bad breath is unlikely to be a symptom of an underlying disease. However, if it persists for more than 3 days, consult your physician or dentist.

46

GENERAL
over 6 months

Vomiting

Throwing-up of stomach contents that may be preceded by nausea.
For babies under 6 months see chart 87, **Vomiting in infants.**

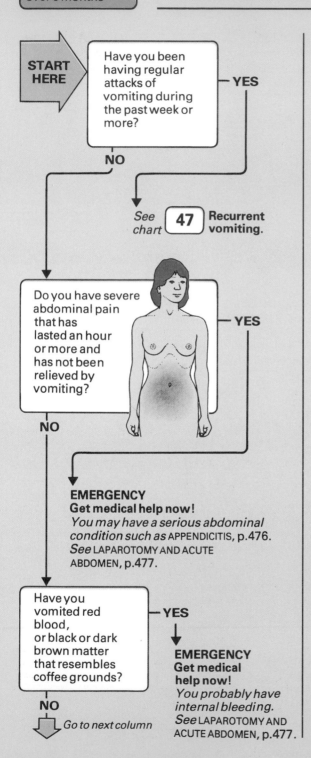

START HERE

Have you been having regular attacks of vomiting during the past week or more?

YES → *See chart* **47** **Recurrent vomiting.**

NO ↓

Do you have severe abdominal pain that has lasted an hour or more and has not been relieved by vomiting?

YES →

EMERGENCY
Get medical help now!
You may have a serious abdominal condition such as APPENDICITIS, p.476.
See LAPAROTOMY AND ACUTE ABDOMEN, p.477.

NO ↓

Have you vomited red blood, or black or dark brown matter that resembles coffee grounds?

YES →

EMERGENCY
Get medical help now!
You probably have internal bleeding.
See LAPAROTOMY AND ACUTE ABDOMEN, p.477.

NO ↓ *Go to next column*

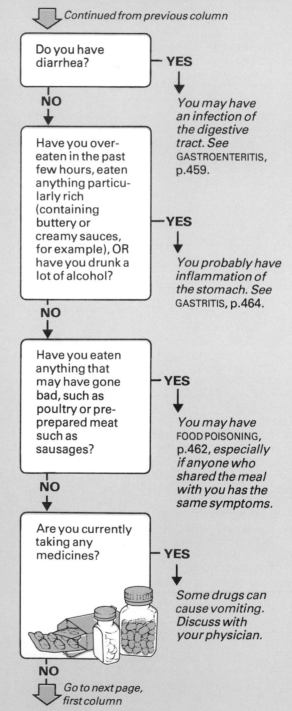

↓ *Continued from previous column*

Do you have diarrhea?

YES →

You may have an infection of the digestive tract. See GASTROENTERITIS, p.459.

NO ↓

Have you over-eaten in the past few hours, eaten anything particularly rich (containing buttery or creamy sauces, for example), OR have you drunk a lot of alcohol?

YES →

You probably have inflammation of the stomach. See GASTRITIS, p.464.

NO ↓

Have you eaten anything that may have gone bad, such as poultry or pre-prepared meat such as sausages?

YES →

You may have FOOD POISONING, p.462, *especially if anyone who shared the meal with you has the same symptoms.*

NO ↓

Are you currently taking any medicines?

YES →

Some drugs can cause vomiting. Discuss with your physician.

NO ↓ *Go to next page, first column*

Continued from previous page

Do you have severe pain in or around one eye AND is your vision blurred? — **YES**

→ **Call your physician now!** *This suggests the possibility of* ACUTE GLAUCOMA, p.320.

NO

Do you have a headache? — **YES**

NO

Before you vomited, did you feel so dizzy that everything around you seemed to spin? — **YES**

→ *You may have a disorder of the inner ear such as* LABYRINTHITIS, p.338, *or* MENIERE'S DISEASE, p.337.

NO

Does your skin or do the whites of your eyes look yellow? — **YES**

NO

You may have a disorder of the liver or gallbladder. See ACUTE HEPATITIS A, p.486, *and* GALLSTONES, p.489.

If you are unable to make a diagnosis from this chart and your vomiting persists for more than 24 hours, consult your physician.

Go to next column

Continued from previous column

Have you had a head injury within the past 24 hours? — **YES**

→ **EMERGENCY Get medical help now!** *You may have a* BRAIN INJURY, p.276.

NO

Do you have one or more of the following symptoms?
☐ pain when you bend your head forwards
☐ dislike of bright light
☐ drowsiness or confusion
— **YES**

→ **EMERGENCY Get medical help now!** *These symptoms suggest the possibility of* MENINGITIS, p.273, *or a* SUBARACHNOID HEMORRHAGE, p.271.

NO

See chart **11** *Headache.*

Persistent vomiting

If you have vomited several times in the course of one day, you may have lost a dangerous amount of body fluid.

Consult your physician without delay!

Red or black blood in vomit

If your vomit contains red blood or black or dark brown matter that resembles coffee grounds (partly digested blood), it is an **EMERGENCY** indicating an acute abdominal condition.

Get medical help now!

47

GENERAL
over 6 months

Recurrent vomiting

Throwing up of stomach contents several times in a week.
For babies under 6 months see chart 87, **Vomiting in infants**.

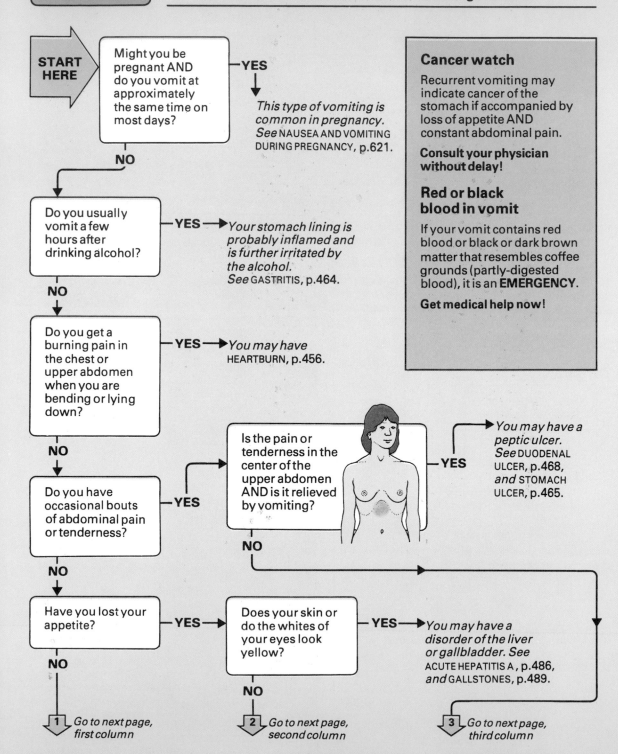

START HERE

Might you be pregnant AND do you vomit at approximately the same time on most days?

— YES

This type of vomiting is common in pregnancy. See NAUSEA AND VOMITING DURING PREGNANCY, p.621.

NO

Do you usually vomit a few hours after drinking alcohol?

— YES →

Your stomach lining is probably inflamed and is further irritated by the alcohol. See GASTRITIS, p.464.

NO

Do you get a burning pain in the chest or upper abdomen when you are bending or lying down?

— YES →

You may have HEARTBURN, p.456.

NO

Do you have occasional bouts of abdominal pain or tenderness?

— YES

Is the pain or tenderness in the center of the upper abdomen AND is it relieved by vomiting?

— YES →

You may have a peptic ulcer. See DUODENAL ULCER, p.468, *and* STOMACH ULCER, p.465.

NO

NO

Have you lost your appetite?

— YES →

Does your skin or do the whites of your eyes look yellow?

— YES →

You may have a disorder of the liver or gallbladder. See ACUTE HEPATITIS A , p.486, *and* GALLSTONES, p.489.

NO

NO

1 *Go to next page, first column*

2 *Go to next page, second column*

3 *Go to next page, third column*

Cancer watch

Recurrent vomiting may indicate cancer of the stomach if accompanied by loss of appetite AND constant abdominal pain.

Consult your physician without delay!

Red or black blood in vomit

If your vomit contains red blood or black or dark brown matter that resembles coffee grounds (partly-digested blood), it is an **EMERGENCY**.

Get medical help now!

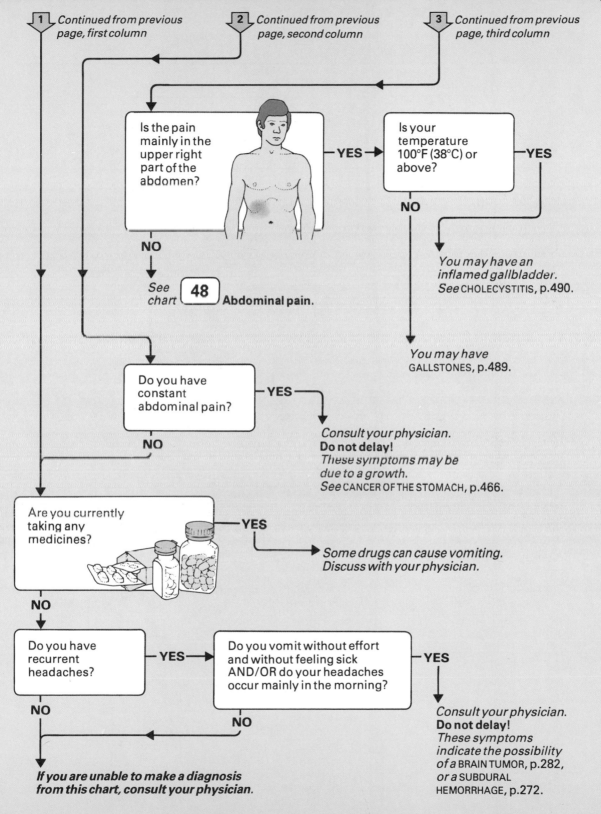

1 Continued from previous page, first column

2 Continued from previous page, second column

3 Continued from previous page, third column

Is the pain mainly in the upper right part of the abdomen?

YES → Is your temperature 100°F (38°C) or above?

YES → You may have an inflamed gallbladder. See CHOLECYSTITIS, p.490.

NO (temperature) → You may have GALLSTONES, p.489.

NO (upper right pain) → See chart **48** Abdominal pain.

Do you have constant abdominal pain?

YES → Consult your physician. **Do not delay!** These symptoms may be due to a growth. See CANCER OF THE STOMACH, p.466.

NO

Are you currently taking any medicines?

YES → Some drugs can cause vomiting. Discuss with your physician.

NO

Do you have recurrent headaches?

YES → Do you vomit without effort and without feeling sick AND/OR do your headaches occur mainly in the morning?

YES → Consult your physician. **Do not delay!** These symptoms indicate the possibility of a BRAIN TUMOR, p.282, or a SUBDURAL HEMORRHAGE, p.272.

NO (recurrent headaches)

NO (vomit without effort) →

If you are unable to make a diagnosis from this chart, consult your physician.

48

GENERAL
over 14 years

Abdominal pain

General or localized pain between the bottom of the ribcage and the groin. For children see chart 93, **Abdominal pain in children**.

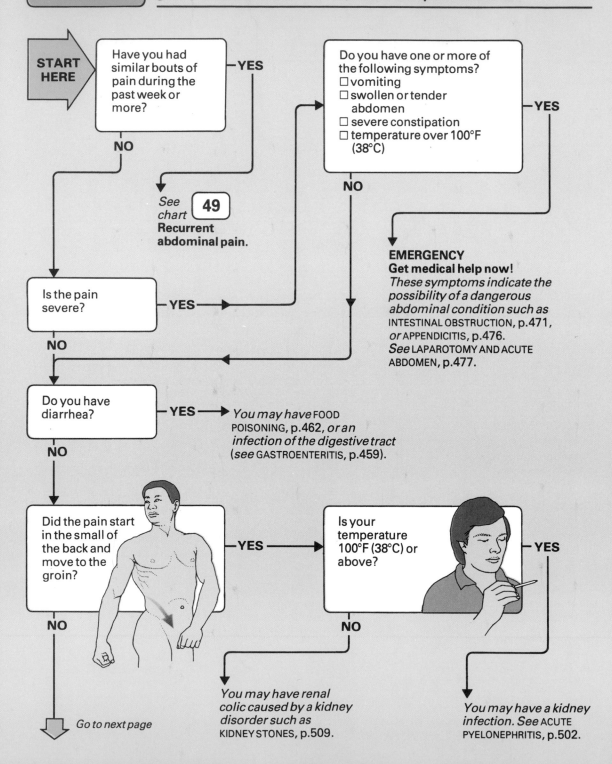

START HERE

Have you had similar bouts of pain during the past week or more?

YES → See chart **49** **Recurrent abdominal pain.**

NO

Do you have one or more of the following symptoms?
☐ vomiting
☐ swollen or tender abdomen
☐ severe constipation
☐ temperature over 100°F (38°C)

YES →

NO

Is the pain severe?

YES →

NO

**EMERGENCY
Get medical help now!**
These symptoms indicate the possibility of a dangerous abdominal condition such as INTESTINAL OBSTRUCTION, p.471, *or* APPENDICITIS, p.476. *See* LAPAROTOMY AND ACUTE ABDOMEN, p.477.

Do you have diarrhea?

YES → *You may have* FOOD POISONING, p.462, *or an infection of the digestive tract* (*see* GASTROENTERITIS, p.459).

NO

Did the pain start in the small of the back and move to the groin?

YES →

NO

Is your temperature 100°F (38°C) or above?

YES →

NO

Go to next page

You may have renal colic caused by a kidney disorder such as KIDNEY STONES, p.509.

You may have a kidney infection. See ACUTE PYELONEPHRITIS, p.502.

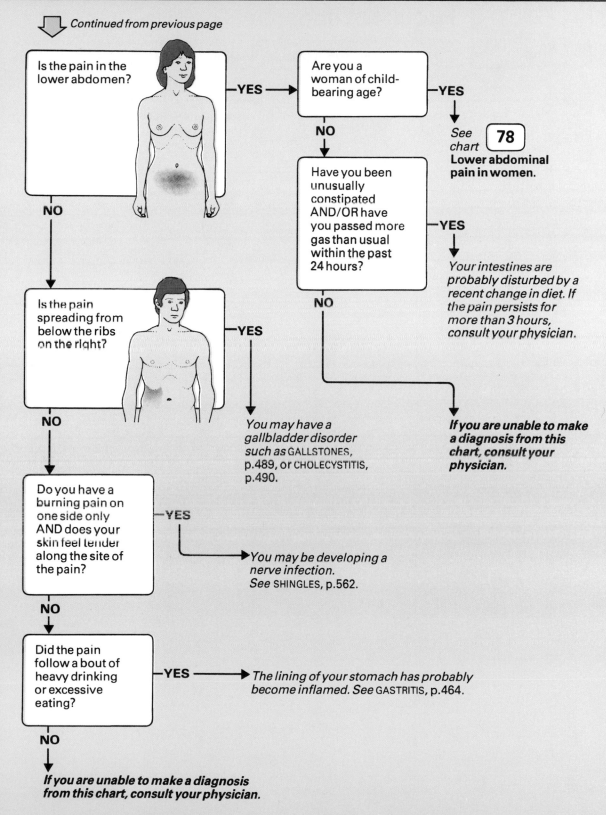

Continued from previous page

Is the pain in the lower abdomen?

YES → Are you a woman of child-bearing age?

YES → See chart **78** Lower abdominal pain in women.

NO ↓

Have you been unusually constipated AND/OR have you passed more gas than usual within the past 24 hours?

YES → *Your intestines are probably disturbed by a recent change in diet. If the pain persists for more than 3 hours, consult your physician.*

NO →

NO ↓

Is the pain spreading from below the ribs on the right?

YES → *You may have a gallbladder disorder such as* GALLSTONES, *p.489, or* CHOLECYSTITIS, *p.490.*

If you are unable to make a diagnosis from this chart, consult your physician.

NO ↓

Do you have a burning pain on one side only AND does your skin feel tender along the site of the pain?

YES → *You may be developing a nerve infection. See* SHINGLES, *p.562.*

NO ↓

Did the pain follow a bout of heavy drinking or excessive eating?

YES → *The lining of your stomach has probably become inflamed. See* GASTRITIS, *p.464.*

NO ↓

If you are unable to make a diagnosis from this chart, consult your physician.

49

GENERAL
over 14 years

Recurrent abdominal pain

Abdominal pain that has recurred on several days over a week or more. For children see chart 93, **Abdominal pain in children.**

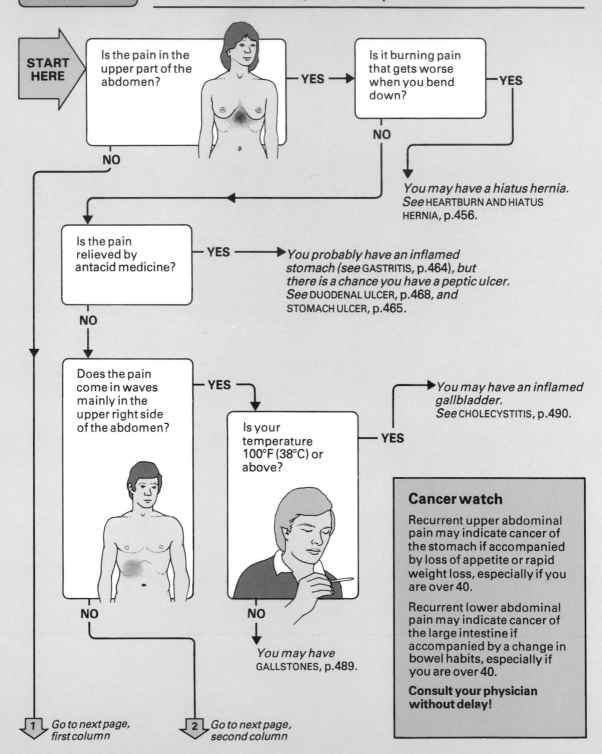

START HERE

Is the pain in the upper part of the abdomen?

YES → Is it burning pain that gets worse when you bend down?

YES →

NO ↓

NO ↓

You may have a hiatus hernia. See HEARTBURN AND HIATUS HERNIA, p.456.

Is the pain relieved by antacid medicine?

YES → *You probably have an inflamed stomach (see GASTRITIS, p.464), but there is a chance you have a peptic ulcer.* See DUODENAL ULCER, p.468, *and* STOMACH ULCER, p.465.

NO ↓

Does the pain come in waves mainly in the upper right side of the abdomen?

YES → Is your temperature 100°F (38°C) or above?

YES → *You may have an inflamed gallbladder.* See CHOLECYSTITIS, p.490.

NO ↓

NO ↓

You may have GALLSTONES, p.489.

Cancer watch

Recurrent upper abdominal pain may indicate cancer of the stomach if accompanied by loss of appetite or rapid weight loss, especially if you are over 40.

Recurrent lower abdominal pain may indicate cancer of the large intestine if accompanied by a change in bowel habits, especially if you are over 40.

Consult your physician without delay!

1 *Go to next page, first column*

2 *Go to next page, second column*

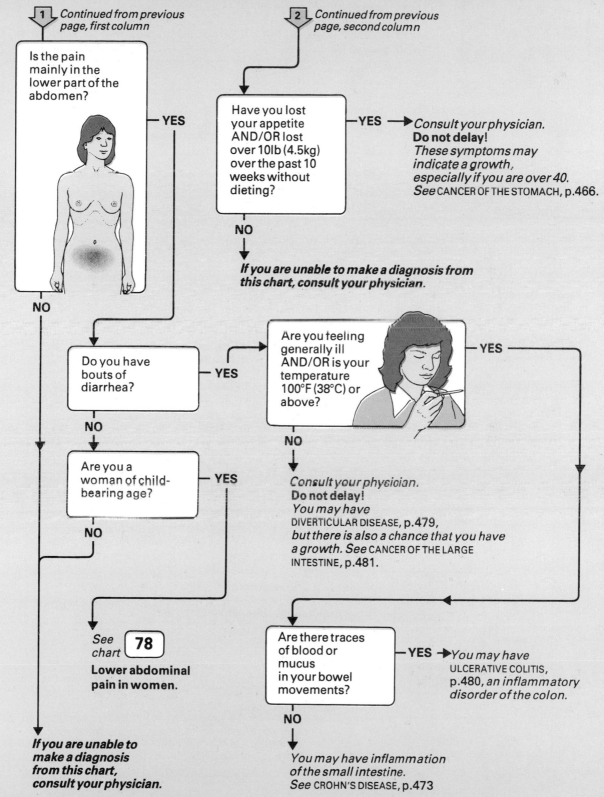

1 Continued from previous page, first column

Is the pain mainly in the lower part of the abdomen?

YES →

NO ↓

2 Continued from previous page, second column

Have you lost your appetite AND/OR lost over 10lb (4.5kg) over the past 10 weeks without dieting?

YES → Consult your physician. **Do not delay!** These symptoms may indicate a growth, especially if you are over 40. See CANCER OF THE STOMACH, p.466.

NO ↓

If you are unable to make a diagnosis from this chart, consult your physician.

Do you have bouts of diarrhea?

YES →

NO ↓

Are you feeling generally ill AND/OR is your temperature 100°F (38°C) or above?

YES →

NO ↓

Consult your physician. **Do not delay!** You may have DIVERTICULAR DISEASE, p.479, but there is also a chance that you have a growth. See CANCER OF THE LARGE INTESTINE, p.481.

Are you a woman of child-bearing age?

YES →

NO ↓

See chart **78**
Lower abdominal pain in women.

Are there traces of blood or mucus in your bowel movements?

YES → You may have ULCERATIVE COLITIS, p.480, an inflammatory disorder of the colon.

NO ↓

You may have inflammation of the small intestine. See CROHN'S DISEASE, p.473

If you are unable to make a diagnosis from this chart, consult your physician.

50

GENERAL
all ages

Swollen abdomen

Generalized swelling over the whole abdomen between the bottom of the ribcage and the groin.

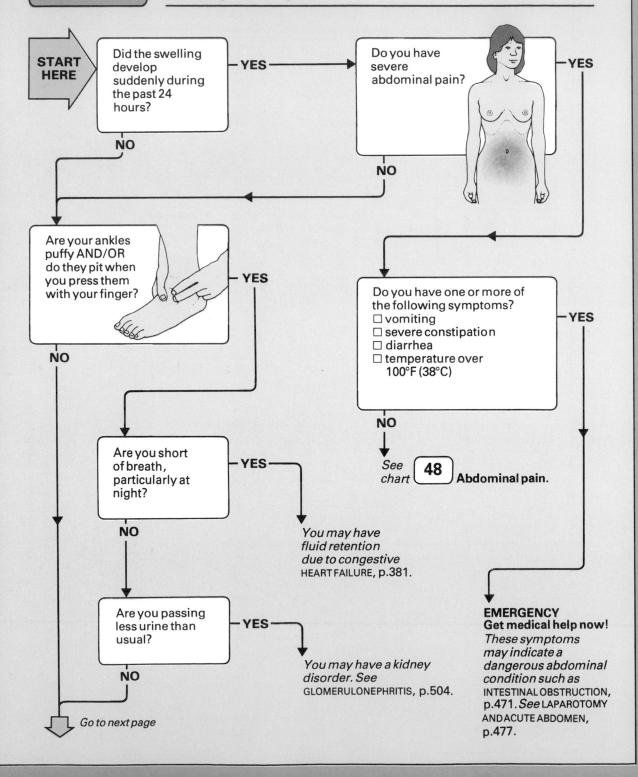

START HERE → Did the swelling develop suddenly during the past 24 hours? — **YES** → Do you have severe abdominal pain? — **YES**

NO ↓

Are your ankles puffy AND/OR do they pit when you press them with your finger? — **YES**

NO ↓

Are you short of breath, particularly at night? — **YES**

NO ↓

Are you passing less urine than usual? — **YES**

NO ↓

Go to next page

Do you have one or more of the following symptoms?
☐ vomiting
☐ severe constipation
☐ diarrhea
☐ temperature over 100°F (38°C) — **YES**

NO ↓

See chart **48** **Abdominal pain.**

You may have fluid retention due to congestive HEART FAILURE, p.381.

You may have a kidney disorder. See GLOMERULONEPHRITIS, p.504.

EMERGENCY
Get medical help now!
These symptoms may indicate a dangerous abdominal condition such as INTESTINAL OBSTRUCTION, p.471. *See* LAPAROTOMY AND ACUTE ABDOMEN, p.477.

⬇ *Continued from previous page*

Does your skin or do the whites of your eyes look yellow?

→ **YES** → *Consult your physician.* **Do not delay!** *This suggests a liver disorder such as* CIRRHOSIS OF THE LIVER, p.487.

NO

Are you a woman of child-bearing age?

→ **YES** → **Might you be more than 3 months pregnant?**

→ **YES** → *Consult your physician, who will be able to determine whether you are pregnant. See* GENERAL PROBLEMS OF PREGNANCY, p.620.

NO

NO

Did the swelling develop just before, or during your period?

→ **YES** → *Many women get a swollen abdomen at this time. See* PREMENSTRUAL TENSION, p.585.

NO

Do you have persistent constipation?

→ **YES** → *Constipation sometimes causes a swollen abdomen See* CONSTIPATION AND DIARRHEA, p.474.

NO

Are you over-weight according to the chart on p.28 AND is your navel deeply sunken?

→ **YES** → *Your problem is probably* OBESITY, p.492.

NO

If you are unable to make a diagnosis from this chart, and your abdomen remains swollen for more than 24 hours, consult your physician.

Painful swollen abdomen

It is an **EMERGENCY** requiring immediate hospital treatment, if a swollen abdomen is accompanied by severe pain AND one or more of the following symptoms:
☐ vomiting
☐ severe constipation
☐ temperature over 100°F (38°C)
☐ diarrhea.

51

GENERAL
all ages

Gas and belching

The expulsion of air from the digestive tract through the mouth or anus (also called flatulence).

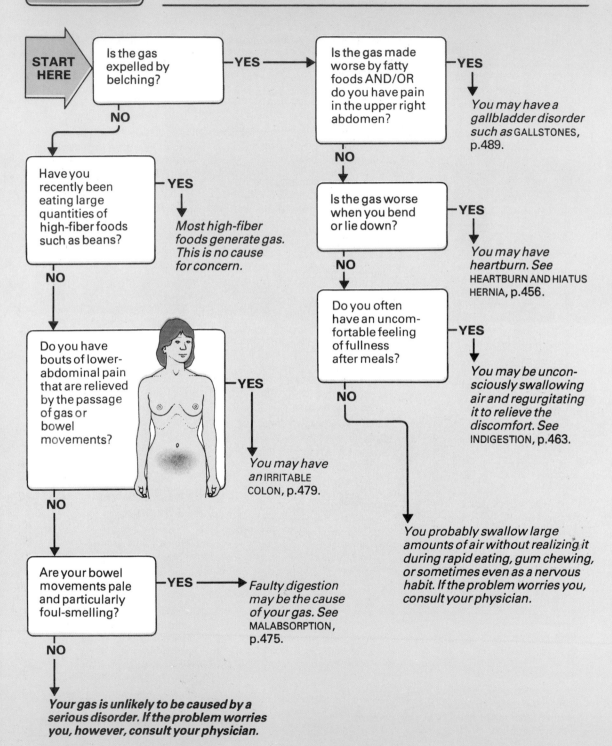

START HERE → Is the gas expelled by belching?

— **YES** → Is the gas made worse by fatty foods AND/OR do you have pain in the upper right abdomen?

— **YES** → *You may have a gallbladder disorder such as* GALLSTONES, *p.489.*

NO ↓ (from belching)

Have you recently been eating large quantities of high-fiber foods such as beans?

— **YES** → *Most high-fiber foods generate gas. This is no cause for concern.*

NO ↓

Do you have bouts of lower-abdominal pain that are relieved by the passage of gas or bowel movements?

— **YES** → *You may have an* IRRITABLE COLON, *p.479.*

NO ↓

Are your bowel movements pale and particularly foul-smelling?

— **YES** → *Faulty digestion may be the cause of your gas. See* MALABSORPTION, *p.475.*

NO ↓

Your gas is unlikely to be caused by a serious disorder. If the problem worries you, however, consult your physician.

NO ↓ (from "made worse by fatty foods")

Is the gas worse when you bend or lie down?

— **YES** → *You may have heartburn. See* HEARTBURN AND HIATUS HERNIA, *p.456.*

NO ↓

Do you often have an uncomfortable feeling of fullness after meals?

— **YES** → *You may be unconsciously swallowing air and regurgitating it to relieve the discomfort. See* INDIGESTION, *p.463.*

NO ↓

You probably swallow large amounts of air without realizing it during rapid eating, gum chewing, or sometimes even as a nervous habit. If the problem worries you, consult your physician.

52

GENERAL
over 6 months

Diarrhea

Frequent passing of unusually loose and runny bowel movements.
For babies under 6 months see chart 88, **Diarrhea in infants.**

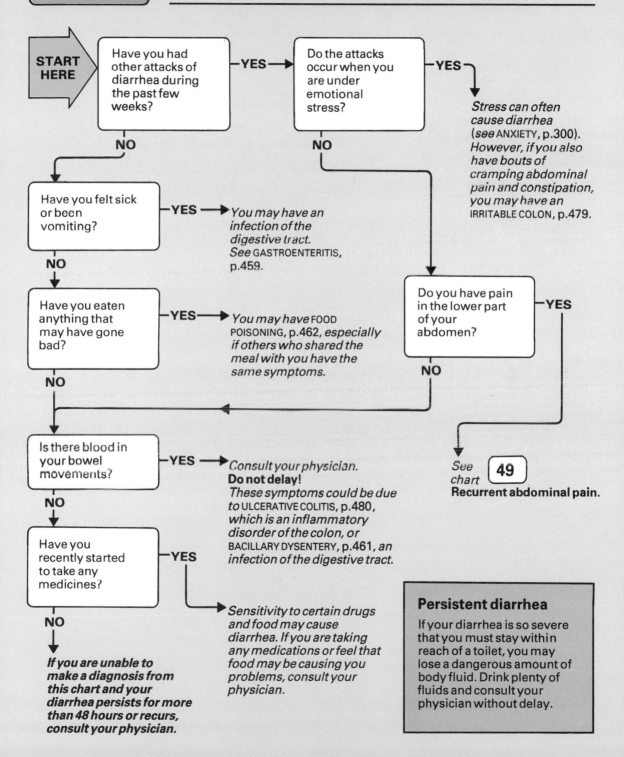

START HERE

Have you had other attacks of diarrhea during the past few weeks? — **YES** → Do the attacks occur when you are under emotional stress? — **YES** →

Stress can often cause diarrhea (see ANXIETY, p.300). However, if you also have bouts of cramping abdominal pain and constipation, you may have an IRRITABLE COLON, p.479.

NO (from first box)

Have you felt sick or been vomiting? — **YES** → *You may have an infection of the digestive tract. See GASTROENTERITIS, p.459.*

NO

Have you eaten anything that may have gone bad? — **YES** → *You may have FOOD POISONING, p.462, especially if others who shared the meal with you have the same symptoms.*

NO

NO (from stress box)

Do you have pain in the lower part of your abdomen? — **YES**

NO

Is there blood in your bowel movements? — **YES** → *Consult your physician.* **Do not delay!** *These symptoms could be due to ULCERATIVE COLITIS, p.480, which is an inflammatory disorder of the colon, or BACILLARY DYSENTERY, p.461, an infection of the digestive tract.*

NO

Have you recently started to take any medicines? — **YES** → *Sensitivity to certain drugs and food may cause diarrhea. If you are taking any medications or feel that food may be causing you problems, consult your physician.*

NO

If you are unable to make a diagnosis from this chart and your diarrhea persists for more than 48 hours or recurs, consult your physician.

See chart **49** **Recurrent abdominal pain.**

Persistent diarrhea

If your diarrhea is so severe that you must stay within reach of a toilet, you may lose a dangerous amount of body fluid. Drink plenty of fluids and consult your physician without delay.

53

GENERAL
all ages

Constipation

Infrequent or difficult passing of hard bowel movements.

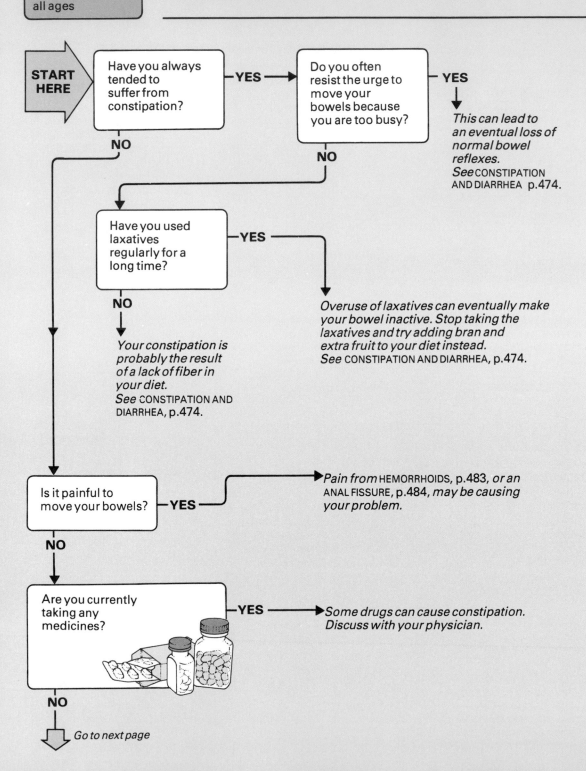

START HERE

Have you always tended to suffer from constipation? — **YES** → **Do you often resist the urge to move your bowels because you are too busy?** — **YES** ↓

This can lead to an eventual loss of normal bowel reflexes.
See CONSTIPATION AND DIARRHEA p.474.

NO ↓

NO ↓

Have you used laxatives regularly for a long time? — **YES** ↓

Overuse of laxatives can eventually make your bowel inactive. Stop taking the laxatives and try adding bran and extra fruit to your diet instead.
See CONSTIPATION AND DIARRHEA, p.474.

NO ↓

Your constipation is probably the result of a lack of fiber in your diet.
See CONSTIPATION AND DIARRHEA, p.474.

Is it painful to move your bowels? — **YES** →

Pain from HEMORRHOIDS, p.483, *or an* ANAL FISSURE, p.484, *may be causing your problem.*

NO ↓

Are you currently taking any medicines? — **YES** →

Some drugs can cause constipation. Discuss with your physician.

NO ↓

Go to next page

Continued from previous page

Are you on a diet, or could your diet be short of water or high-fiber foods such as fruit, vegetables, and wholegrain bread?

YES → There may be insufficient water or bulk in your diet to stimulate proper bowel action. *See* EATING AND DRINKING SENSIBLY, p.24.

NO

Are you pregnant?

YES → This problem is common in pregnancy. *See* CONSTIPATION DURING PREGNANCY, p.623.

NO

Do you have two or more of the following symptoms?
☐ feeling the cold more than you used to
☐ dry skin or hair
☐ unexplained weight gain
☐ inexplicable tiredness

YES → You may have an underactive thyroid gland. *See* HYPOTHYROIDISM, p.526.

NO

Do you have lower abdominal pain?

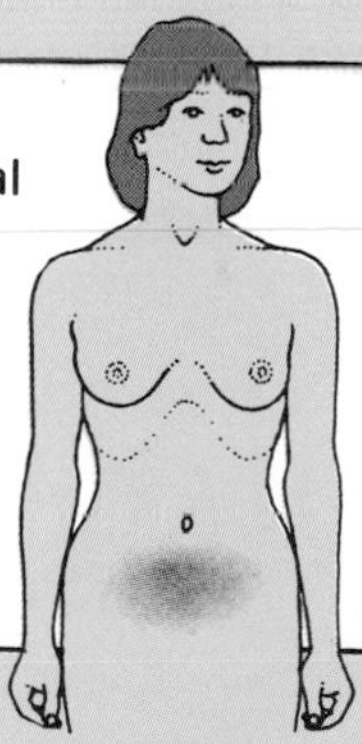

YES → Have you had similar episodes of pain and constipation for many years?

YES → You probably have an IRRITABLE COLON, p.479.

NO → Consult your physician. **Do not delay!** You may have DIVERTICULAR DISEASE, p.479, but there is a chance that you may have a growth. *See* CANCER OF THE LARGE INTESTINE, p.481.

NO

If you are unable to make a diagnosis from this chart and your constipation persists for more than 2 weeks, or if you do not have any bowel movements for 3 days or more, consult your physician.

Cancer watch

Prolonged attacks of constipation after years of regularity, especially in those over 40, may indicate cancer of the large intestine.

Consult your physician without delay!

54

Abnormal-looking bowel movements
Passing bowel movements that are unusually colored.

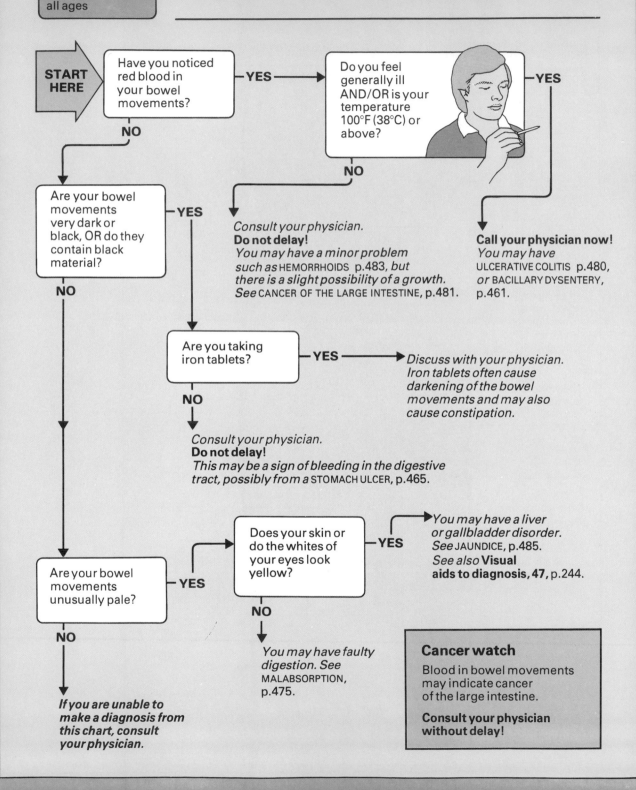

START HERE

Have you noticed red blood in your bowel movements?

YES →

Do you feel generally ill AND/OR is your temperature 100°F (38°C) or above?

YES →

NO (below, left)

Are your bowel movements very dark or black, OR do they contain black material?

YES →

NO

Consult your physician.
Do not delay!
You may have a minor problem such as HEMORRHOIDS p.483, *but there is a slight possibility of a growth.*
See CANCER OF THE LARGE INTESTINE, p.481.

Call your physician now!
You may have
ULCERATIVE COLITIS p.480,
or BACILLARY DYSENTERY,
p.461.

Are you taking iron tablets?

YES →

Discuss with your physician. Iron tablets often cause darkening of the bowel movements and may also cause constipation.

NO

Consult your physician.
Do not delay!
This may be a sign of bleeding in the digestive tract, possibly from a STOMACH ULCER, p.465.

Does your skin or do the whites of your eyes look yellow?

YES →

You may have a liver or gallbladder disorder.
See JAUNDICE, p.485.
See also **Visual aids to diagnosis, 47,** p.244.

NO

Are your bowel movements unusually pale?

YES →

NO

You may have faulty digestion. See MALABSORPTION, p.475.

If you are unable to make a diagnosis from this chart, consult your physician.

Cancer watch

Blood in bowel movements may indicate cancer of the large intestine.

Consult your physician without delay!

55

GENERAL
all ages

Palpitations

A feeling that your heart is beating irregularly, more strongly, or more rapidly than normal.

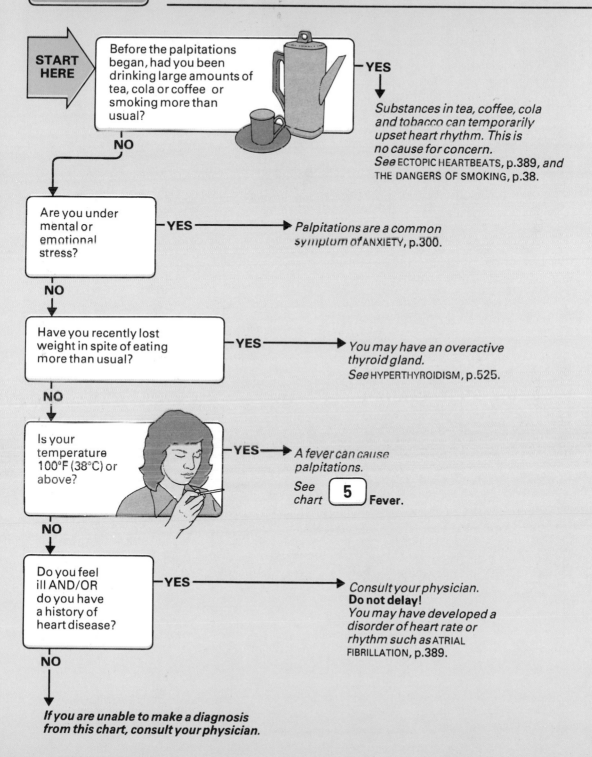

START HERE

Before the palpitations began, had you been drinking large amounts of tea, cola or coffee or smoking more than usual?

YES → *Substances in tea, coffee, cola and tobacco can temporarily upset heart rhythm. This is no cause for concern.* See ECTOPIC HEARTBEATS, p.389, *and* THE DANGERS OF SMOKING, p.38.

NO

Are you under mental or emotional stress?

YES → *Palpitations are a common symptom of* ANXIETY, p.300.

NO

Have you recently lost weight in spite of eating more than usual?

YES → *You may have an overactive thyroid gland.* See HYPERTHYROIDISM, p.525.

NO

Is your temperature 100°F (38°C) or above?

YES → *A fever can cause palpitations.* See chart **5** Fever.

NO

Do you feel ill AND/OR do you have a history of heart disease?

YES → *Consult your physician.* **Do not delay!** *You may have developed a disorder of heart rate or rhythm such as* ATRIAL FIBRILLATION, p.389.

NO

If you are unable to make a diagnosis from this chart, consult your physician.

56

GENERAL
all ages

Chest pain

Pain anywhere between the neck and the bottom of the ribcage, which may be dull and persistent, stabbing, burning, or crushing.

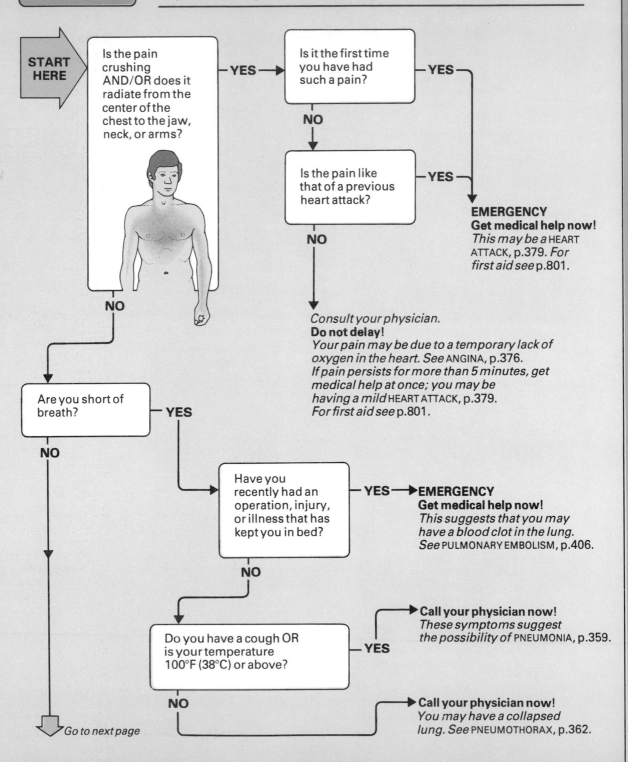

START HERE

Is the pain crushing AND/OR does it radiate from the center of the chest to the jaw, neck, or arms?

— YES → **Is it the first time you have had such a pain?** — YES —

NO ↓

Is the pain like that of a previous heart attack? — YES —

NO ↓

**EMERGENCY
Get medical help now!**
This may be a HEART ATTACK, p.379. *For first aid see* p.801.

Consult your physician.
Do not delay!
Your pain may be due to a temporary lack of oxygen in the heart. See ANGINA, p.376.
If pain persists for more than 5 minutes, get medical help at once; you may be having a mild HEART ATTACK, p.379.
For first aid see p.801.

NO ↓

Are you short of breath? — YES →

NO ↓

Have you recently had an operation, injury, or illness that has kept you in bed? — YES → **EMERGENCY
Get medical help now!**
*This suggests that you may have a blood clot in the lung.
See* PULMONARY EMBOLISM, p.406.

NO ↓

Do you have a cough OR is your temperature 100°F (38°C) or above? — YES → **Call your physician now!**
These symptoms suggest the possibility of PNEUMONIA, p.359.

NO ↓

Call your physician now!
You may have a collapsed lung. See PNEUMOTHORAX, p.362.

Go to next page

Continued from previous page

Have you coughed up grayish-yellow phlegm?

YES → *You may have an infection of the airways in the lung. See* ACUTE BRONCHITIS, p.353.

NO

Is it a burning pain that worsens when you bend or lie down?

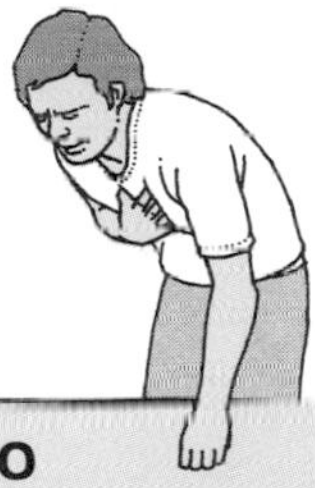

YES → *You may have heartburn. See* HEARTBURN AND HIATUS HERNIA, p.456.

NO

Is the pain worse when you swallow?

YES → *See chart* **43** **Difficulty in swallowing.**

NO

Is the pain on one side only?

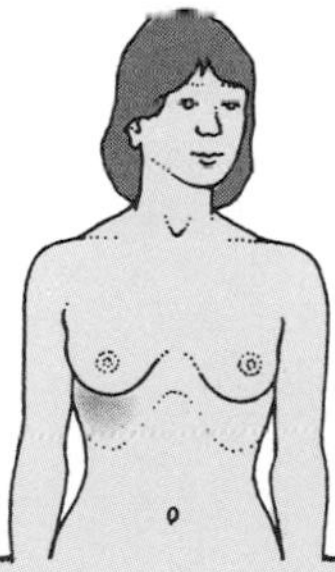

YES → Have you recently had a chest injury, chest surgery OR a severe cough?

YES ↓ *You may have a* PULLED MUSCLE, p.532, *or a broken rib* (see FRACTURES, p.534).

NO ↓

Does the pain cause a burning feeling in the skin AND is it unaffected by breathing?

YES ↓ *You may have a nerve infection. See* SHINGLES, p.562.

NO

NO

If you are unable to make a diagnosis from this chart, consult your physician without further delay.

57

GENERAL
all ages

Abnormally frequent urination

Feeling the urge to urinate and doing so more often than usual, even though little urine may be produced.

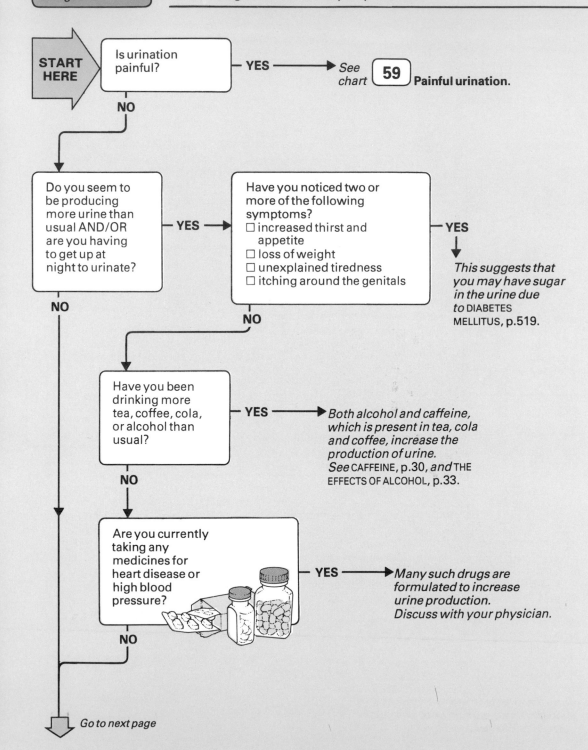

START HERE

Is urination painful?

YES → *See chart* **59** **Painful urination.**

NO

Do you seem to be producing more urine than usual AND/OR are you having to get up at night to urinate?

YES →

Have you noticed two or more of the following symptoms?
☐ increased thirst and appetite
☐ loss of weight
☐ unexplained tiredness
☐ itching around the genitals

YES ↓

This suggests that you may have sugar in the urine due to DIABETES MELLITUS, p.519.

NO

NO

Have you been drinking more tea, coffee, cola, or alcohol than usual?

YES → *Both alcohol and caffeine, which is present in tea, cola and coffee, increase the production of urine.*
See CAFFEINE, p.30, *and* THE EFFECTS OF ALCOHOL, p.33.

NO

Are you currently taking any medicines for heart disease or high blood pressure?

YES → *Many such drugs are formulated to increase urine production.*
Discuss with your physician.

NO

Go to next page

⬇ *Continued from previous page*

Is the weather very cold OR are you unusually anxious or excited? —— **YES** ——▶ *Cold or excitement can cause frequent urination. This is no cause for concern.*

NO ↓

Are you a woman? —— **YES** ▶ **Are you pregnant?** —— **YES** ——▶ *Increased frequency of urination is common in the first three and the last three months of pregnancy. This is probably not a cause for concern.*

NO ↓   **NO** ↓

Are you over 50? — **YES**

NO ↓

Do you have two or more of the following symptoms?
☐ waking to urinate at night
☐ difficulty in starting to urinate
☐ weak stream
☐ leakage of urine after urination
—— **YES** ↓ *You may have a disorder of the prostate gland. See* ENLARGED PROSTATE, p.574.

Do you sometimes have a strong urge to urinate followed quickly by an uncontrollable leakage of urine? — **YES**

NO ↓

NO ↓

This is probably "urge incontinence" caused by an IRRITABLE BLADDER, p.601.

Do you have difficulty in controlling your bladder? — **YES** ▶ *See chart* **60** **Lack of bladder control.**

NO ↓

If you are unable to make a diagnosis from this chart, the increased frequency of urination may be a cause for concern. Consult your physician if the increase becomes enough to wake you at night or if it continues for more than a week.

58

GENERAL
all ages

Abnormal-looking urine

Urine that differs from the usual straw color, or that is cloudy or blood-tinged.

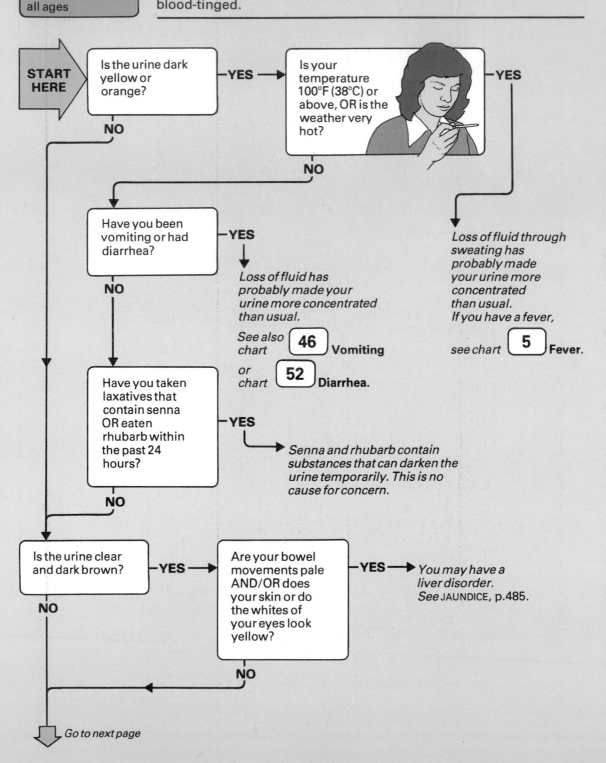

START HERE

Is the urine dark yellow or orange?

— **YES** →

Is your temperature 100°F (38°C) or above, OR is the weather very hot?

— **YES**

NO

NO

Have you been vomiting or had diarrhea?

— **YES**

NO

Loss of fluid has probably made your urine more concentrated than usual.

See also chart **46** *Vomiting*
or chart **52** *Diarrhea.*

Loss of fluid through sweating has probably made your urine more concentrated than usual.
If you have a fever, see chart **5** *Fever.*

Have you taken laxatives that contain senna OR eaten rhubarb within the past 24 hours?

— **YES**

Senna and rhubarb contain substances that can darken the urine temporarily. This is no cause for concern.

NO

Is the urine clear and dark brown?

— **YES** →

Are your bowel movements pale AND/OR does your skin or do the whites of your eyes look yellow?

— **YES** → *You may have a liver disorder.*
See JAUNDICE, p.485.

NO

NO

Go to next page

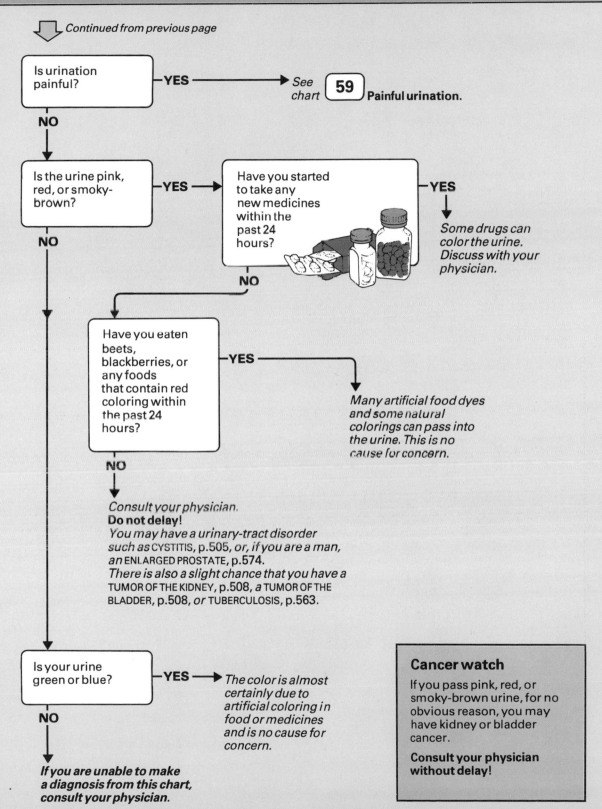

Continued from previous page

Is urination painful? — YES → *See chart* **59** **Painful urination.**

NO

Is the urine pink, red, or smoky-brown? — YES → **Have you started to take any new medicines within the past 24 hours?** — YES ↓ *Some drugs can color the urine. Discuss with your physician.*

NO

NO ↓

Have you eaten beets, blackberries, or any foods that contain red coloring within the past 24 hours? — YES → *Many artificial food dyes and some natural colorings can pass into the urine. This is no cause for concern.*

NO ↓

Consult your physician.
Do not delay!
You may have a urinary-tract disorder such as CYSTITIS, p.505, *or, if you are a man, an* ENLARGED PROSTATE, p.574.
There is also a slight chance that you have a TUMOR OF THE KIDNEY, p.508, *a* TUMOR OF THE BLADDER, p.508, *or* TUBERCULOSIS, p.563.

Is your urine green or blue? — YES → *The color is almost certainly due to artificial coloring in food or medicines and is no cause for concern.*

NO ↓

If you are unable to make a diagnosis from this chart, consult your physician.

Cancer watch

If you pass pink, red, or smoky-brown urine, for no obvious reason, you may have kidney or bladder cancer.

Consult your physician without delay!

59

GENERAL
all ages

Painful urination

Discomfort when urinating, which may be accompanied by pain in the lower abdomen or urinary passage.

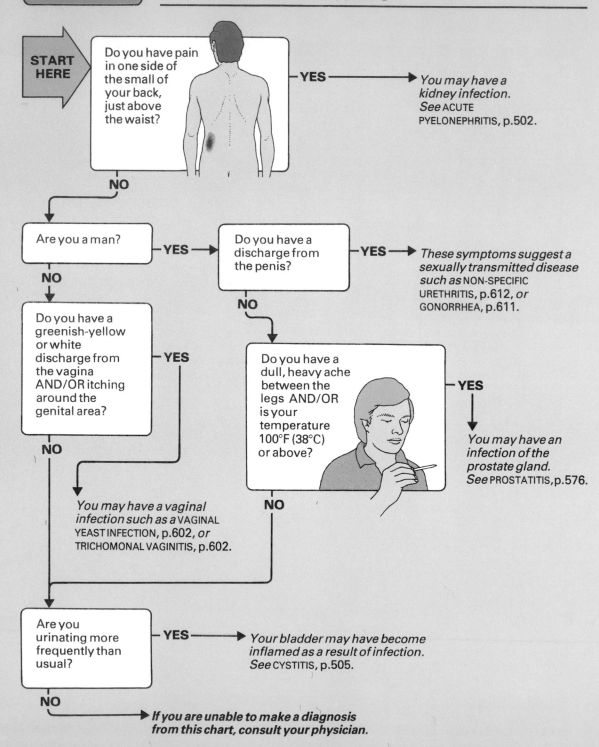

START HERE

Do you have pain in one side of the small of your back, just above the waist? — **YES** → *You may have a kidney infection.* See ACUTE PYELONEPHRITIS, p.502.

NO

Are you a man? — **YES** → Do you have a discharge from the penis? — **YES** → *These symptoms suggest a sexually transmitted disease such as* NON-SPECIFIC URETHRITIS, p.612, *or* GONORRHEA, p.611.

NO

Do you have a greenish-yellow or white discharge from the vagina AND/OR itching around the genital area? — **YES** → *You may have a vaginal infection such as a* VAGINAL YEAST INFECTION, p.602, *or* TRICHOMONAL VAGINITIS, p.602.

NO

Do you have a dull, heavy ache between the legs AND/OR is your temperature 100°F (38°C) or above? — **YES** → *You may have an infection of the prostate gland.* See PROSTATITIS, p.576.

NO

Are you urinating more frequently than usual? — **YES** → *Your bladder may have become inflamed as a result of infection.* See CYSTITIS, p.505.

NO

If you are unable to make a diagnosis from this chart, consult your physician.

60

GENERAL
0–65 years

Lack of bladder control

Involuntary urination.
For those over 65 see chart 98, **Incontinence in the elderly**.

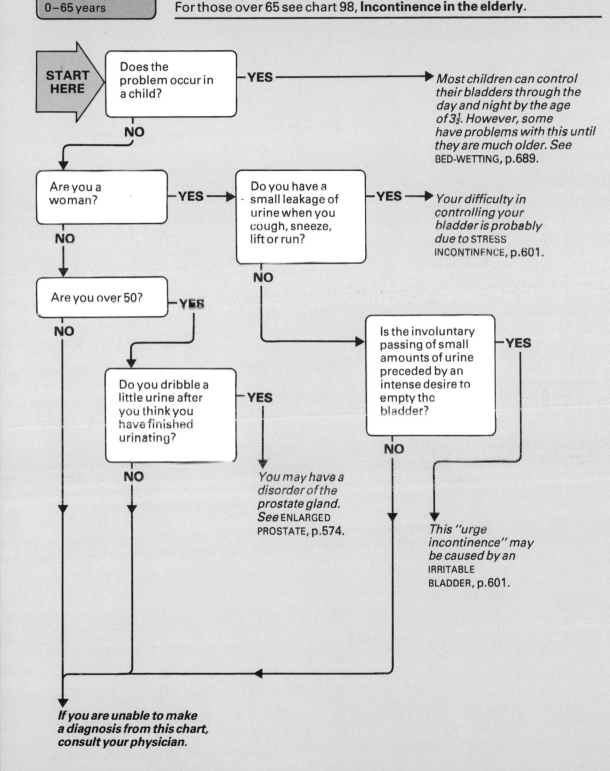

START HERE → **Does the problem occur in a child?**

— **YES** → *Most children can control their bladders through the day and night by the age of 3½. However, some have problems with this until they are much older. See* BED-WETTING, p.689.

NO ↓

Are you a woman?

— **YES** → **Do you have a small leakage of urine when you cough, sneeze, lift or run?**

— **YES** → *Your difficulty in controlling your bladder is probably due to* STRESS INCONTINENCE, p.601.

NO ↓ (from woman)

Are you over 50?

— **YES** →

NO ↓

Do you dribble a little urine after you think you have finished urinating?

— **YES** → *You may have a disorder of the prostate gland. See* ENLARGED PROSTATE, p.574.

NO ↓

Is the involuntary passing of small amounts of urine preceded by an intense desire to empty the bladder?

— **YES** → *This "urge incontinence" may be caused by an* IRRITABLE BLADDER, p.601.

NO ↓

If you are unable to make a diagnosis from this chart, consult your physician.

61

GENERAL
all ages

Backache

Pain and/or stiffness in the back that may be continuous or intermittent.

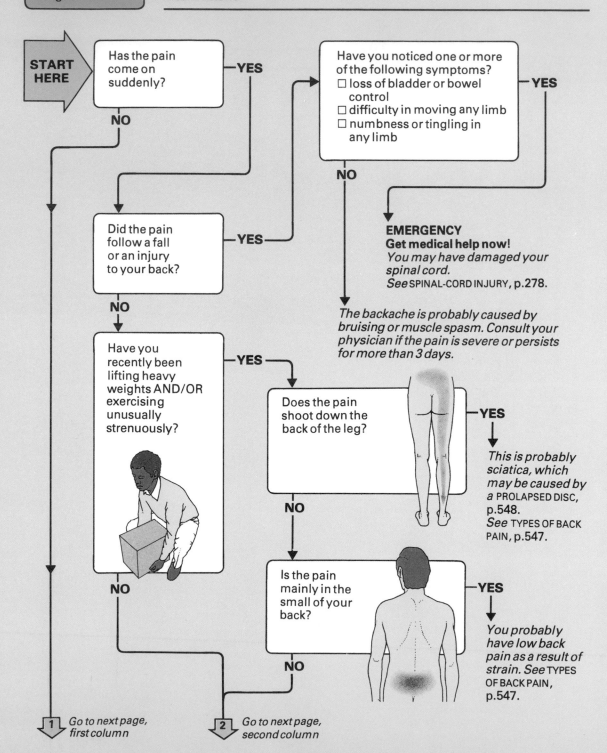

START HERE

Has the pain come on suddenly? — **YES** →

Have you noticed one or more of the following symptoms?
☐ loss of bladder or bowel control
☐ difficulty in moving any limb
☐ numbness or tingling in any limb

— **YES** →

NO

EMERGENCY
Get medical help now!
You may have damaged your spinal cord.
See SPINAL-CORD INJURY, p.278.

NO

Did the pain follow a fall or an injury to your back? — **YES** →

The backache is probably caused by bruising or muscle spasm. Consult your physician if the pain is severe or persists for more than 3 days.

NO

Have you recently been lifting heavy weights AND/OR exercising unusually strenuously? — **YES** →

Does the pain shoot down the back of the leg? — **YES** →

This is probably sciatica, which may be caused by a PROLAPSED DISC, p.548.
See TYPES OF BACK PAIN, p.547.

NO

Is the pain mainly in the small of your back? — **YES** →

You probably have low back pain as a result of strain. See TYPES OF BACK PAIN, p.547.

NO

NO

1 *Go to next page, first column***

2 *Go to next page, second column***

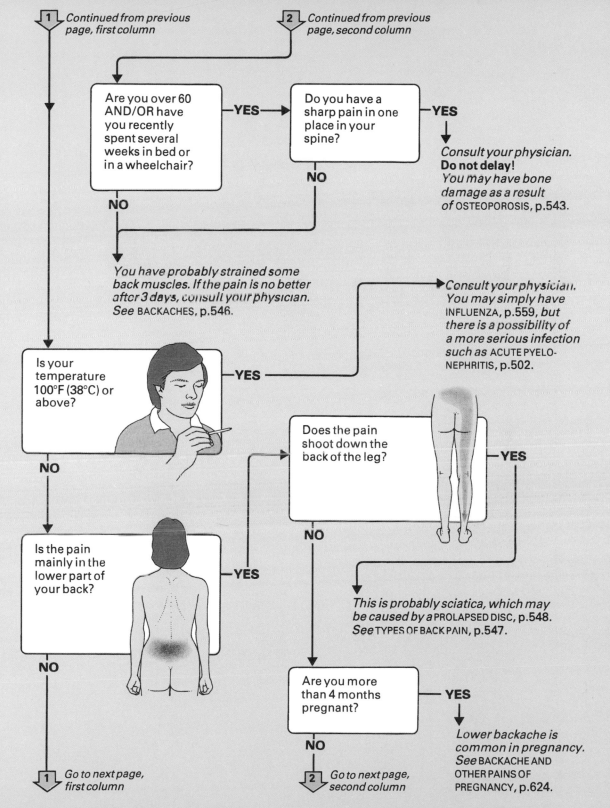

1 *Continued from previous page, first column*

2 *Continued from previous page, second column*

Are you over 60 AND/OR have you recently spent several weeks in bed or in a wheelchair? — **YES** → Do you have a sharp pain in one place in your spine? — **YES**

↓ *Consult your physician.* **Do not delay!** *You may have bone damage as a result of* OSTEOPOROSIS, p.543.

NO (from first box)

NO (from spine box)

You have probably strained some back muscles. If the pain is no better after 3 days, consult your physician. See BACKACHES, p.546.

Is your temperature 100°F (38°C) or above? — **YES** → *Consult your physician. You may simply have* INFLUENZA, p.559, *but there is a possibility of a more serious infection such as* ACUTE PYELO-NEPHRITIS, p.502.

NO

Is the pain mainly in the lower part of your back? — **YES** → Does the pain shoot down the back of the leg? — **YES**

NO (does the pain shoot box)

This is probably sciatica, which may be caused by a PROLAPSED DISC, p.548. *See* TYPES OF BACK PAIN, p.547.

NO (lower part of back)

Are you more than 4 months pregnant? — **YES**

↓ *Lower backache is common in pregnancy. See* BACKACHE AND OTHER PAINS OF PREGNANCY, p.624.

NO

1 *Go to next page, first column*

2 *Go to next page, second column*

Backache

1 Continued from previous page, first column

2 Continued from previous page, second column

Are you overweight according to the chart on p.28?

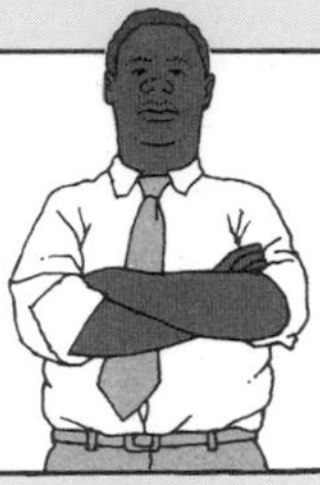

YES → *Carrying too much weight can strain your back. See* BACKACHES, p.546, *and* OBESITY, p.492.

NO

Is the pain worse when you get up in the morning?

YES → *Your bed may not be giving your back enough support (see* BACKACHES, p.546), *but there is a possibility of chronic inflammation of the joints, (see* ANKYLOSING SPONDYLITIS, p.553) *especially if you are a man under 40.*

NO

Are you over 60?

YES → **Do you have pain in other joints, for example the hip, knee, or ankle?**

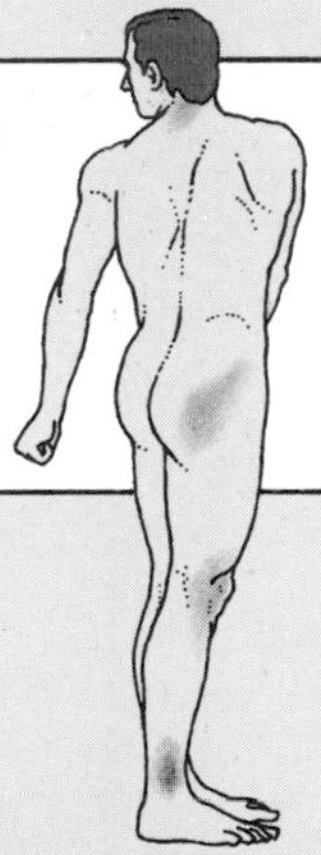

YES → *You may have* OSTEOARTHRITIS, p.550, *a degenerative condition of the joints.*

NO

NO

Could your working conditions, for example, sitting in a chair the wrong height for your desk or using a jackhammer, be straining your back muscles?

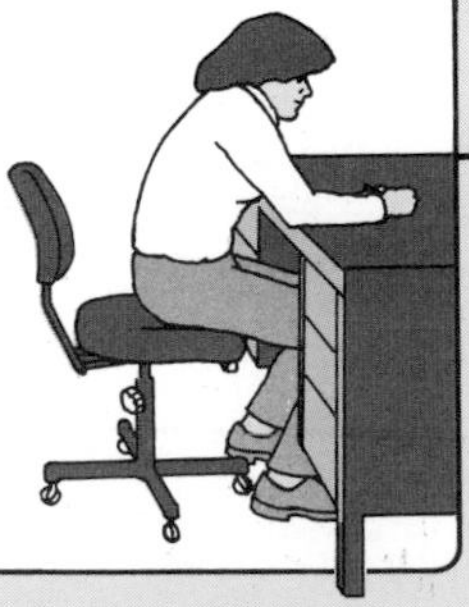

YES → *Backache often results from such strain. See* BACKACHES, p.546.

NO

If you are unable to make a diagnosis from this chart, consult your physician.

62

GENERAL
all ages

Cramp

Involuntary, painful tightening of muscles other than abdominal muscles. For abdominal cramps see chart 48, **Abdominal pain**.

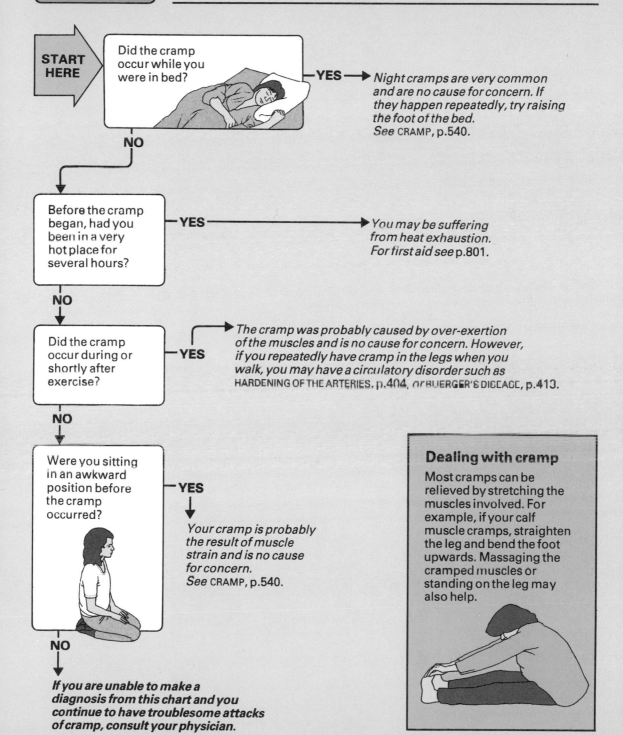

START HERE → Did the cramp occur while you were in bed?

YES → *Night cramps are very common and are no cause for concern. If they happen repeatedly, try raising the foot of the bed. See CRAMP, p.540.*

NO

Before the cramp began, had you been in a very hot place for several hours?

YES → *You may be suffering from heat exhaustion. For first aid see p.801.*

NO

Did the cramp occur during or shortly after exercise?

YES → *The cramp was probably caused by over-exertion of the muscles and is no cause for concern. However, if you repeatedly have cramp in the legs when you walk, you may have a circulatory disorder such as HARDENING OF THE ARTERIES, p.404, or BUERGER'S DISEASE, p.413.*

NO

Were you sitting in an awkward position before the cramp occurred?

YES

↓

Your cramp is probably the result of muscle strain and is no cause for concern. See CRAMP, p.540.

NO

↓

If you are unable to make a diagnosis from this chart and you continue to have troublesome attacks of cramp, consult your physician.

Dealing with cramp

Most cramps can be relieved by stretching the muscles involved. For example, if your calf muscle cramps, straighten the leg and bend the foot upwards. Massaging the cramped muscles or standing on the leg may also help.

63

GENERAL
all ages

Painful and/or stiff neck

Pain (or discomfort) that may or may not be accompanied by a slight headache.

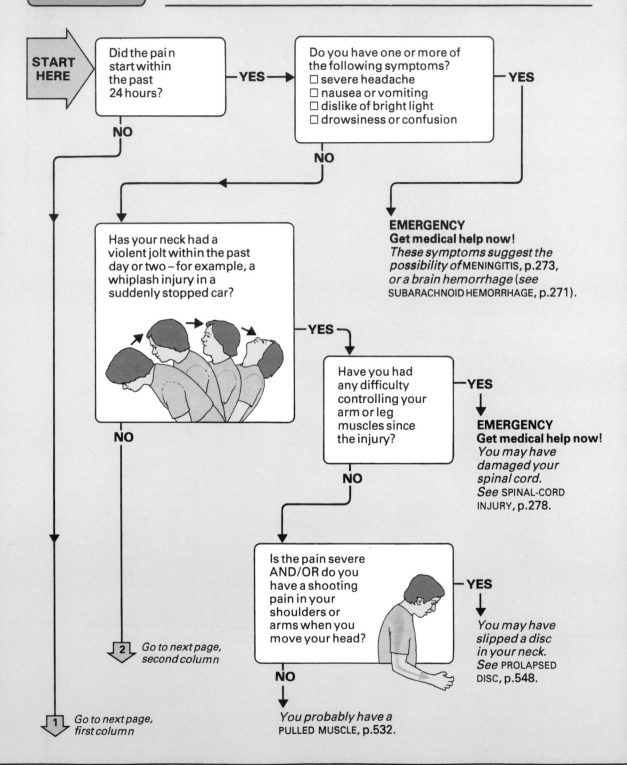

START HERE

Did the pain start within the past 24 hours?

YES →

Do you have one or more of the following symptoms?
☐ severe headache
☐ nausea or vomiting
☐ dislike of bright light
☐ drowsiness or confusion

YES

NO

NO

EMERGENCY
Get medical help now!
These symptoms suggest the possibility of MENINGITIS, p.273, *or a brain hemorrhage (see* SUBARACHNOID HEMORRHAGE, p.271).

Has your neck had a violent jolt within the past day or two – for example, a whiplash injury in a suddenly stopped car?

YES

Have you had any difficulty controlling your arm or leg muscles since the injury?

YES

EMERGENCY
Get medical help now!
You may have damaged your spinal cord.
See SPINAL-CORD INJURY, p.278.

NO

NO

Is the pain severe AND/OR do you have a shooting pain in your shoulders or arms when you move your head?

YES

You may have slipped a disc in your neck.
See PROLAPSED DISC, p.548.

NO

2 *Go to next page, second column*

You probably have a PULLED MUSCLE, p.532.

1 *Go to next page, first column*

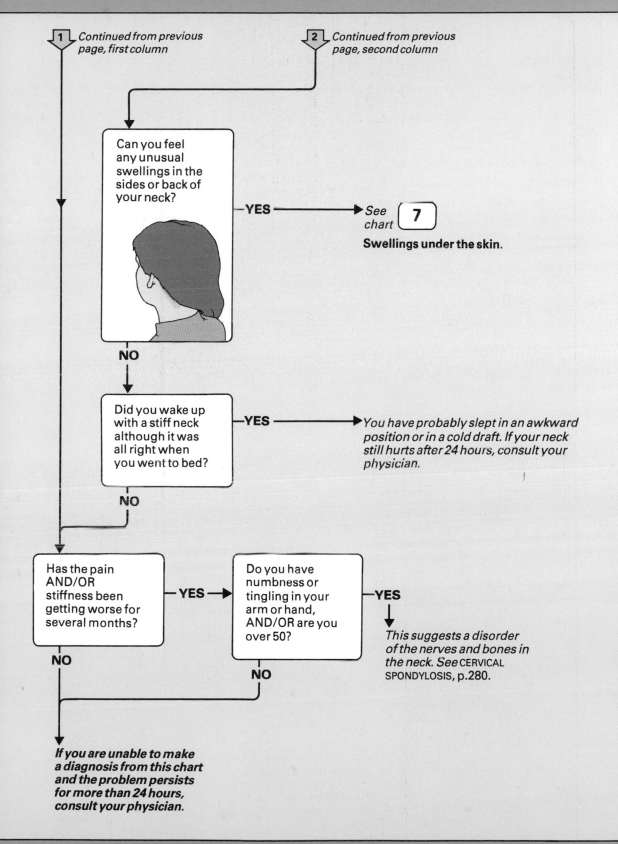

1 ⌐ *Continued from previous page, first column*

2 ⌐ *Continued from previous page, second column*

Can you feel any unusual swellings in the sides or back of your neck?

—YES——→ *See chart* **7**

Swellings under the skin.

NO

Did you wake up with a stiff neck although it was all right when you went to bed?

—YES——→ *You have probably slept in an awkward position or in a cold draft. If your neck still hurts after 24 hours, consult your physician.*

NO

Has the pain AND/OR stiffness been getting worse for several months?

—YES—→ **Do you have numbness or tingling in your arm or hand, AND/OR are you over 50?**

—YES

This suggests a disorder of the nerves and bones in the neck. See CERVICAL SPONDYLOSIS, p.280.

NO

NO

If you are unable to make a diagnosis from this chart and the problem persists for more than 24 hours, consult your physician.

64

GENERAL
all ages

Painful arm or hand

Pain in the arm, elbow, wrist, or hand, but not including the shoulder.

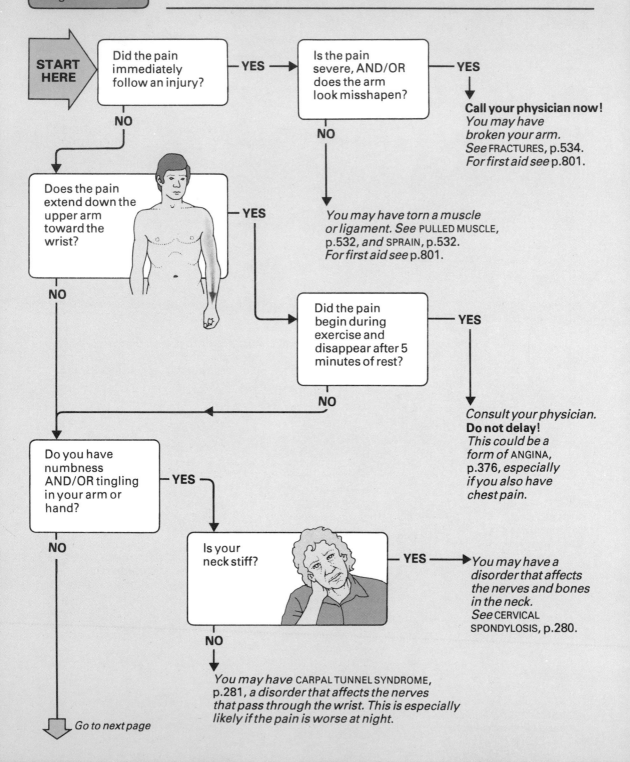

START HERE →

Did the pain immediately follow an injury?
→ **YES** → **Is the pain severe, AND/OR does the arm look misshapen?** → **YES** ↓

Call your physician now! *You may have broken your arm. See* FRACTURES, *p.534. For first aid see p.801.*

NO ↓

NO ↓

You may have torn a muscle or ligament. See PULLED MUSCLE, *p.532, and* SPRAIN, *p.532. For first aid see p.801.*

Does the pain extend down the upper arm toward the wrist? → **YES** →

NO ↓

Did the pain begin during exercise and disappear after 5 minutes of rest? → **YES** ↓

NO ↓

Consult your physician. **Do not delay!** *This could be a form of* ANGINA, *p.376, especially if you also have chest pain.*

Do you have numbness AND/OR tingling in your arm or hand? → **YES** ↓

NO ↓

Is your neck stiff? → **YES** → *You may have a disorder that affects the nerves and bones in the neck. See* CERVICAL SPONDYLOSIS, *p.280.*

NO ↓

You may have CARPAL TUNNEL SYNDROME, *p.281, a disorder that affects the nerves that pass through the wrist. This is especially likely if the pain is worse at night.*

⬇ *Go to next page*

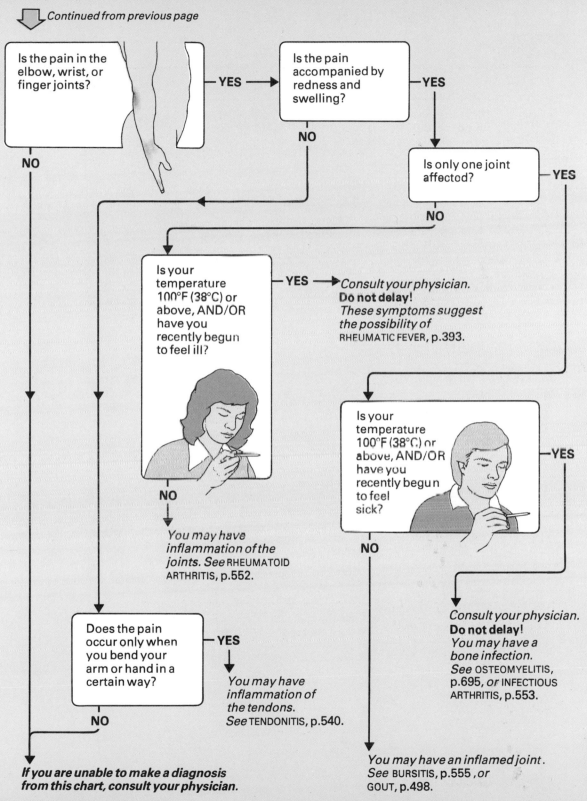

Continued from previous page

Is the pain in the elbow, wrist, or finger joints?

→ YES → **Is the pain accompanied by redness and swelling?**

→ YES → **Is only one joint affected?** → YES

Is the pain accompanied by redness and swelling? — NO

Is only one joint affected? — NO

Is your temperature 100°F (38°C) or above, AND/OR have you recently begun to feel ill?

→ YES → *Consult your physician.* **Do not delay!** *These symptoms suggest the possibility of* RHEUMATIC FEVER, p.393.

Is your temperature 100°F (38°C) or above, AND/OR have you recently begun to feel ill? — NO

You may have inflammation of the joints. See RHEUMATOID ARTHRITIS, p.552.

Is your temperature 100°F (38°C) or above, AND/OR have you recently begun to feel sick? → YES

Is your temperature 100°F (38°C) or above, AND/OR have you recently begun to feel sick? — NO

Consult your physician. **Do not delay!** *You may have a bone infection. See* OSTEOMYELITIS, p.695, *or* INFECTIOUS ARTHRITIS, p.553.

Does the pain occur only when you bend your arm or hand in a certain way? → YES

You may have inflammation of the tendons. See TENDONITIS, p.540.

Does the pain occur only when you bend your arm or hand in a certain way? — NO

If you are unable to make a diagnosis from this chart, consult your physician.

You may have an inflamed joint. See BURSITIS, p.555, *or* GOUT, p.498.

65

GENERAL
all ages

Painful leg

Pain in the thigh and/or calf that may be fleeting or continuous.

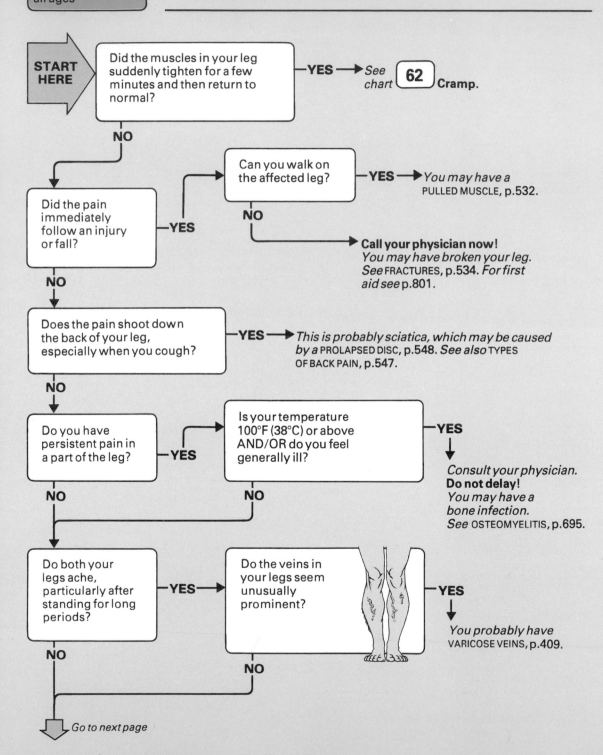

START HERE → Did the muscles in your leg suddenly tighten for a few minutes and then return to normal? —**YES**→ *See chart* **62** *Cramp.*

NO

Did the pain immediately follow an injury or fall? —**YES**→ Can you walk on the affected leg? —**YES**→ *You may have a* PULLED MUSCLE, p.532.

NO (from "Can you walk")
→ **Call your physician now!** *You may have broken your leg. See* FRACTURES, p.534. *For first aid see* p.801.

NO (injury)

Does the pain shoot down the back of your leg, especially when you cough? —**YES**→ *This is probably sciatica, which may be caused by a* PROLAPSED DISC, p.548. *See also* TYPES OF BACK PAIN, p.547.

NO

Do you have persistent pain in a part of the leg? —**YES**→ Is your temperature 100°F (38°C) or above AND/OR do you feel generally ill? —**YES**→ *Consult your physician.* **Do not delay!** *You may have a bone infection. See* OSTEOMYELITIS, p.695.

NO / **NO**

Do both your legs ache, particularly after standing for long periods? —**YES**→ Do the veins in your legs seem unusually prominent? —**YES**→ *You probably have* VARICOSE VEINS, p.409.

NO / **NO**

Go to next page

Continued from previous page

Is the hip painful and/or stiff on the same side as the affected leg? —**YES**→ *A disorder of the hip such as* OSTEOARTHRITIS, p.550, *may cause pain in the leg.*

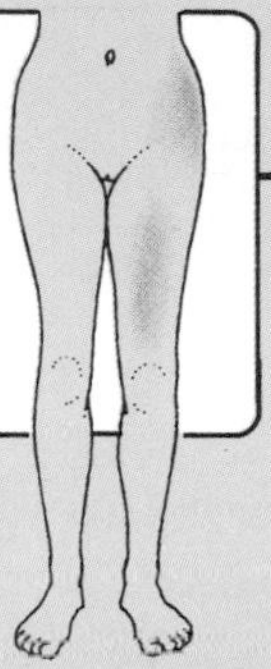

NO

Is the pain mainly in the calf? —**YES**→ Is the calf swollen and tender? 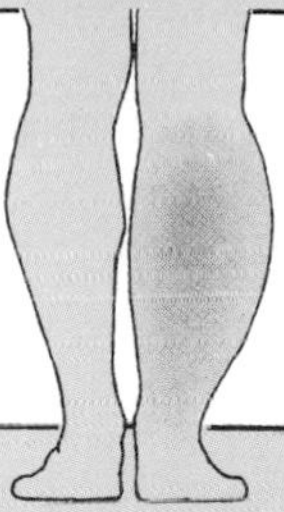 —**YES**→

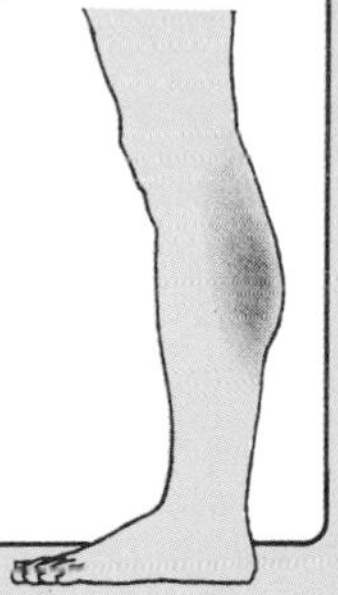

Call your physician now! *You may have a blood clot in your leg. See* DEEP-VEIN THROMBOSIS, p.405.

NO

Is one of your veins red and inflamed? —**YES**→

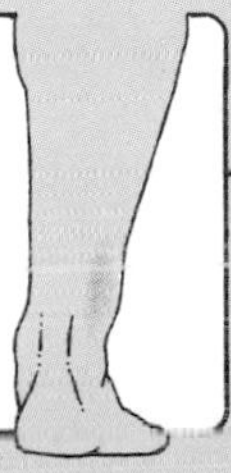

This may be THROMBO-PHLEBITIS, p.407.

NO

NO

Did your leg become painful following unusually strenuous exercise? —**YES**→

NO

You may have a PULLED MUSCLE, p.532.

Does the leg begin to hurt when you are walking and does the pain disappear with rest? —**YES**→

Recurrent pain in the calf during exercise may be a sign of a circulatory problem such as HARDENING OF THE ARTERIES, p.404, *or* BUERGER'S DISEASE, p.413, *or a sports injury. See* SPORTS INJURIES, p.536.

NO

If you are unable to make a diagnosis from this chart, and the pain persists for more than 48 hours or gets worse, consult your physician.

66

GENERAL
all ages

Painful knee

Pain in or around the knee joint that may be accompanied by swelling.

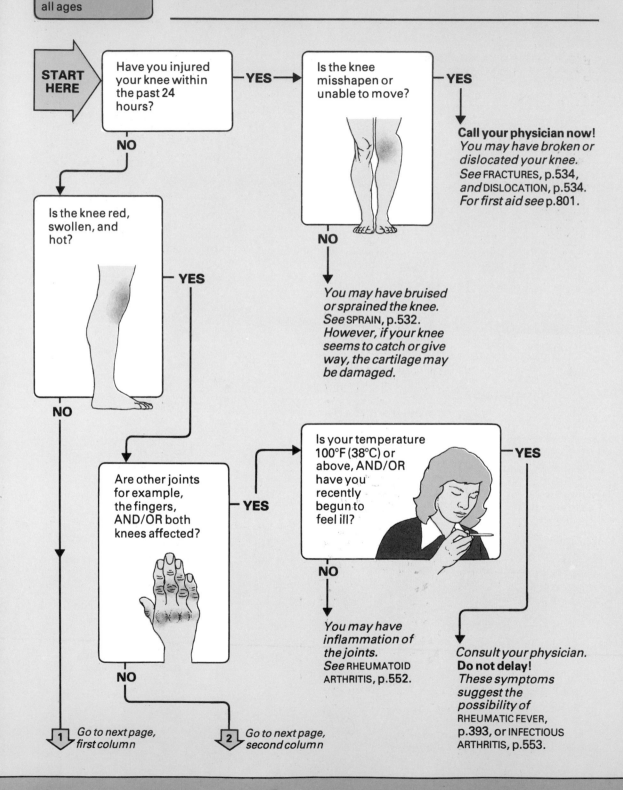

START HERE

Have you injured your knee within the past 24 hours?

NO

YES →

Is the knee misshapen or unable to move?

YES →

Call your physician now!
*You may have broken or dislocated your knee.
See* FRACTURES, p.534, *and* DISLOCATION, p.534.
For first aid see p.801.

NO

*You may have bruised or sprained the knee.
See* SPRAIN, p.532.
However, if your knee seems to catch or give way, the cartilage may be damaged.

Is the knee red, swollen, and hot?

YES

NO

Are other joints for example, the fingers, AND/OR both knees affected?

YES

Is your temperature 100°F (38°C) or above, AND/OR have you recently begun to feel ill?

YES

NO

*You may have inflammation of the joints.
See* RHEUMATOID ARTHRITIS, p.552.

Consult your physician.
Do not delay!
These symptoms suggest the possibility of RHEUMATIC FEVER, p.393, *or* INFECTIOUS ARTHRITIS, p.553.

NO

1 *Go to next page, first column*

2 *Go to next page, second column*

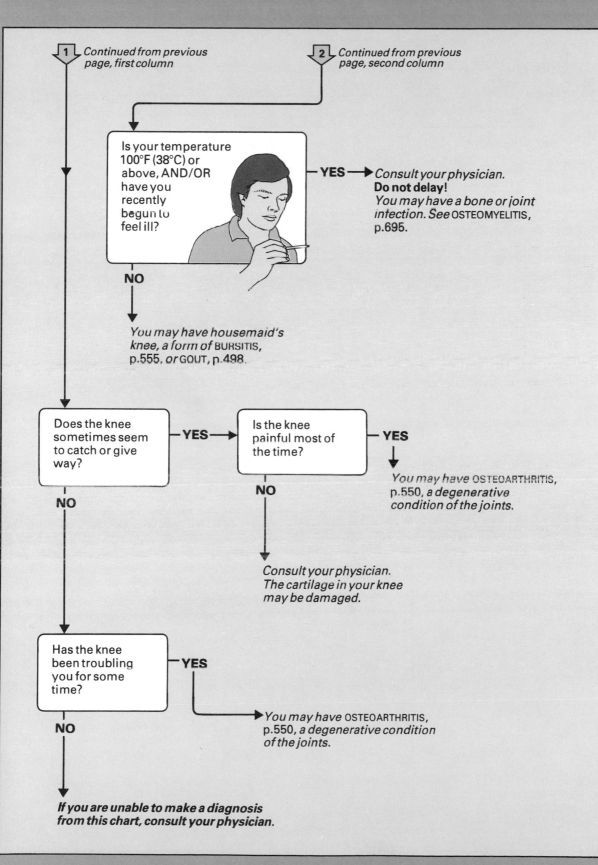

1 Continued from previous page, first column

2 Continued from previous page, second column

Is your temperature 100°F (38°C) or above, AND/OR have you recently begun to feel ill?

YES → Consult your physician. **Do not delay!** You may have a bone or joint infection. See OSTEOMYELITIS, p.695.

NO

You may have housemaid's knee, a form of BURSITIS, p.555, or GOUT, p.498.

Does the knee sometimes seem to catch or give way?

YES → Is the knee painful most of the time?

YES
↓
You may have OSTEOARTHRITIS, p.550, a degenerative condition of the joints.

NO
↓
Consult your physician. The cartilage in your knee may be damaged.

NO

Has the knee been troubling you for some time?

YES
→ You may have OSTEOARTHRITIS, p.550, a degenerative condition of the joints.

NO

If you are unable to make a diagnosis from this chart, consult your physician.

67
GENERAL
all ages

Painful shoulder

Pain in the shoulder, which may be accompanied by stiffness that limits upper-arm movements.

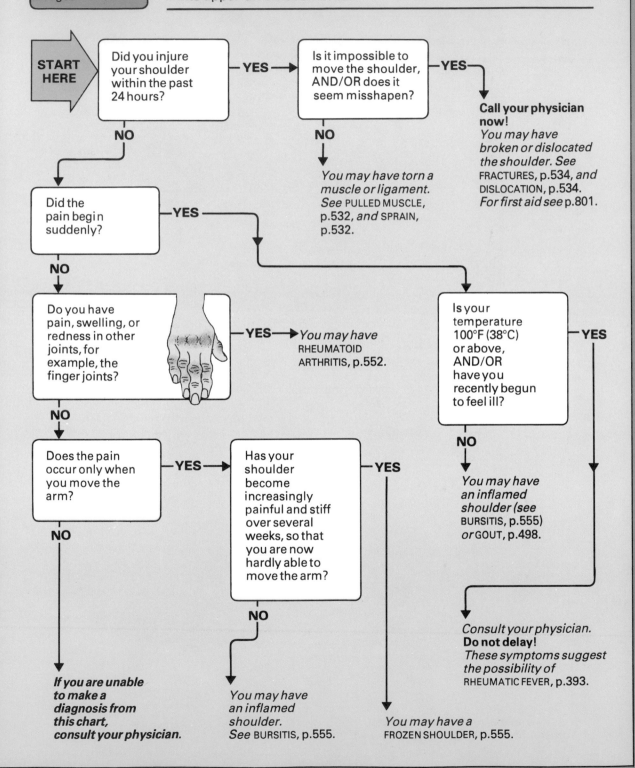

START HERE

Did you injure your shoulder within the past 24 hours? — **YES** → **Is it impossible to move the shoulder, AND/OR does it seem misshapen?** — **YES** →

Call your physician now!
You may have broken or dislocated the shoulder. See FRACTURES, p.534, *and* DISLOCATION, p.534. *For first aid see* p.801.

NO (from injure question) ↓

NO (from misshapen question) ↓
You may have torn a muscle or ligament. See PULLED MUSCLE, p.532, *and* SPRAIN, p.532.

Did the pain begin suddenly? — **YES** →

NO ↓

Do you have pain, swelling, or redness in other joints, for example, the finger joints? — **YES** → *You may have* RHEUMATOID ARTHRITIS, p.552.

NO ↓

Is your temperature 100°F (38°C) or above, AND/OR have you recently begun to feel ill? — **YES** →

NO ↓
You may have an inflamed shoulder (see BURSITIS, p.555) *or* GOUT, p.498.

Does the pain occur only when you move the arm? — **YES** → **Has your shoulder become increasingly painful and stiff over several weeks, so that you are now hardly able to move the arm?** — **YES** →

NO ↓

NO ↓

If you are unable to make a diagnosis from this chart, consult your physician.

You may have an inflamed shoulder. See BURSITIS, p.555.

You may have a FROZEN SHOULDER, p.555.

Consult your physician. **Do not delay!** *These symptoms suggest the possibility of* RHEUMATIC FEVER, p.393.

68

GENERAL
all ages

Painful ankles

Pain, with or without swelling, in or around one or both ankles.

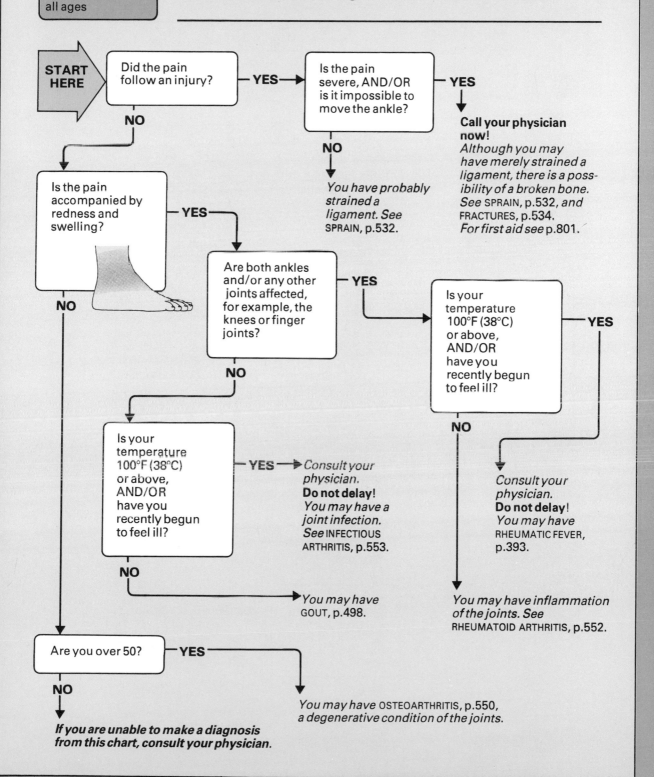

START HERE

Did the pain follow an injury? — **YES** → **Is the pain severe, AND/OR is it impossible to move the ankle?** — **YES** →

Call your physician now!
Although you may have merely strained a ligament, there is a possibility of a broken bone. See SPRAIN, p.532, *and* FRACTURES, p.534. *For first aid see* p.801.

NO (from severe question) → *You have probably strained a ligament. See* SPRAIN, p.532.

NO (did pain follow injury) ↓

Is the pain accompanied by redness and swelling? — **YES** → **Are both ankles and/or any other joints affected, for example, the knees or finger joints?** — **YES** → **Is your temperature 100°F (38°C) or above, AND/OR have you recently begun to feel ill?** — **YES** →

Consult your physician. **Do not delay!** *You may have* RHEUMATIC FEVER, p.393.

NO (temperature) → *Consult your physician.* **Do not delay!** *You may have* RHEUMATIC FEVER, p.393.

You may have inflammation of the joints. See RHEUMATOID ARTHRITIS, p.552.

NO (both ankles affected) ↓

Is your temperature 100°F (38°C) or above, AND/OR have you recently begun to feel ill? — **YES** → *Consult your physician.* **Do not delay!** *You may have a joint infection. See* INFECTIOUS ARTHRITIS, p.553.

NO → *You may have* GOUT, p.498.

NO (redness and swelling) ↓

Are you over 50? — **YES** → *You may have* OSTEOARTHRITIS, p.550, *a degenerative condition of the joints.*

NO ↓

If you are unable to make a diagnosis from this chart, consult your physician.

69

GENERAL
all ages

Swollen ankles

Swelling that may affect one or both ankles.

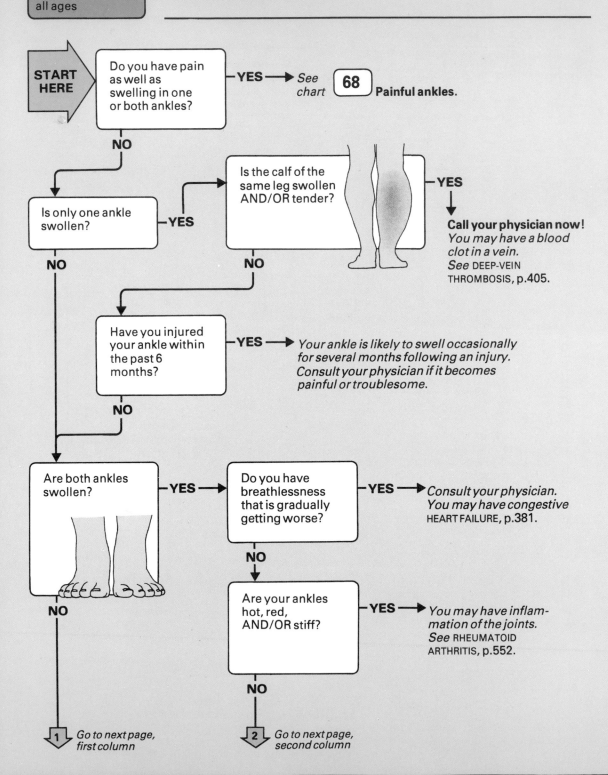

START HERE → **Do you have pain as well as swelling in one or both ankles?** — **YES** → *See chart* **68** **Painful ankles.**

NO ↓

Is only one ankle swollen? — **YES** → **Is the calf of the same leg swollen AND/OR tender?** — **YES** ↓

Call your physician now! *You may have a blood clot in a vein.* *See* DEEP-VEIN THROMBOSIS, p.405.

NO ↓ (Is only one ankle swollen?)

NO ↓ (Is the calf of the same leg swollen AND/OR tender?)

Have you injured your ankle within the past 6 months? — **YES** → *Your ankle is likely to swell occasionally for several months following an injury. Consult your physician if it becomes painful or troublesome.*

NO ↓

Are both ankles swollen? — **YES** → **Do you have breathlessness that is gradually getting worse?** — **YES** → *Consult your physician. You may have congestive* HEART FAILURE, p.381.

NO ↓ (breathlessness)

Are your ankles hot, red, AND/OR stiff? — **YES** → *You may have inflammation of the joints. See* RHEUMATOID ARTHRITIS, p.552.

NO ↓ (Are both ankles swollen?)

NO ↓ (Are your ankles hot, red, AND/OR stiff?)

1 *Go to next page, first column*

2 *Go to next page, second column*

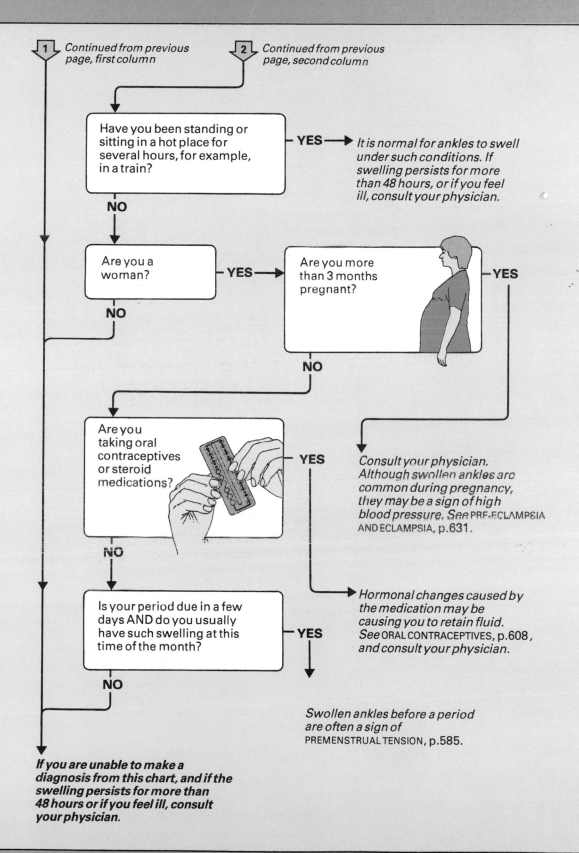

1 *Continued from previous page, first column*

2 *Continued from previous page, second column*

Have you been standing or sitting in a hot place for several hours, for example, in a train?

YES → *It is normal for ankles to swell under such conditions. If swelling persists for more than 48 hours, or if you feel ill, consult your physician.*

NO

Are you a woman?

YES → Are you more than 3 months pregnant?

YES

NO

NO

Are you taking oral contraceptives or steroid medications?

YES

NO

Consult your physician. Although swollen ankles are common during pregnancy, they may be a sign of high blood pressure. See PRE-ECLAMPSIA AND ECLAMPSIA, p.631.

Is your period due in a few days AND do you usually have such swelling at this time of the month?

YES

NO

Hormonal changes caused by the medication may be causing you to retain fluid. See ORAL CONTRACEPTIVES, p.608, and consult your physician.

Swollen ankles before a period are often a sign of PREMENSTRUAL TENSION, p.585.

If you are unable to make a diagnosis from this chart, and if the swelling persists for more than 48 hours or if you feel ill, consult your physician.

70

GENERAL
all ages

Foot problems

Pain, irritation, or swelling anywhere in one or both feet, but not including the ankles.

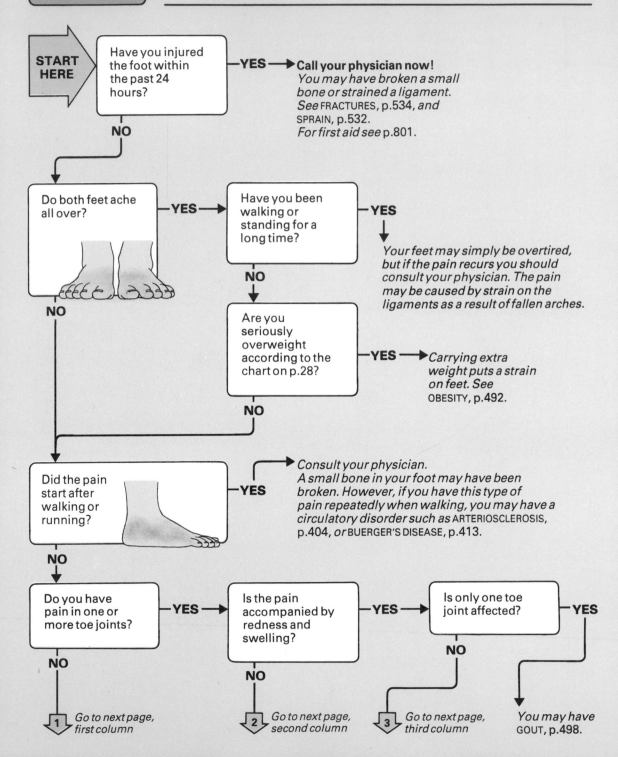

START HERE

Have you injured the foot within the past 24 hours?

— **YES** → **Call your physician now!** *You may have broken a small bone or strained a ligament. See* FRACTURES, p.534, *and* SPRAIN, p.532. *For first aid see* p.801.

NO

Do both feet ache all over?

— **YES** → **Have you been walking or standing for a long time?**

— **YES** → *Your feet may simply be overtired, but if the pain recurs you should consult your physician. The pain may be caused by strain on the ligaments as a result of fallen arches.*

NO

Are you seriously overweight according to the chart on p.28?

— **YES** → *Carrying extra weight puts a strain on feet. See* OBESITY, p.492.

NO

NO

Did the pain start after walking or running?

— **YES** → *Consult your physician. A small bone in your foot may have been broken. However, if you have this type of pain repeatedly when walking, you may have a circulatory disorder such as* ARTERIOSCLEROSIS, p.404, *or* BUERGER'S DISEASE, p.413.

NO

Do you have pain in one or more toe joints?

— **YES** → **Is the pain accompanied by redness and swelling?**

— **YES** → **Is only one toe joint affected?**

— **YES**

NO

NO

NO

1 *Go to next page, first column*

2 *Go to next page, second column*

3 *Go to next page, third column*

You may have GOUT, p.498.

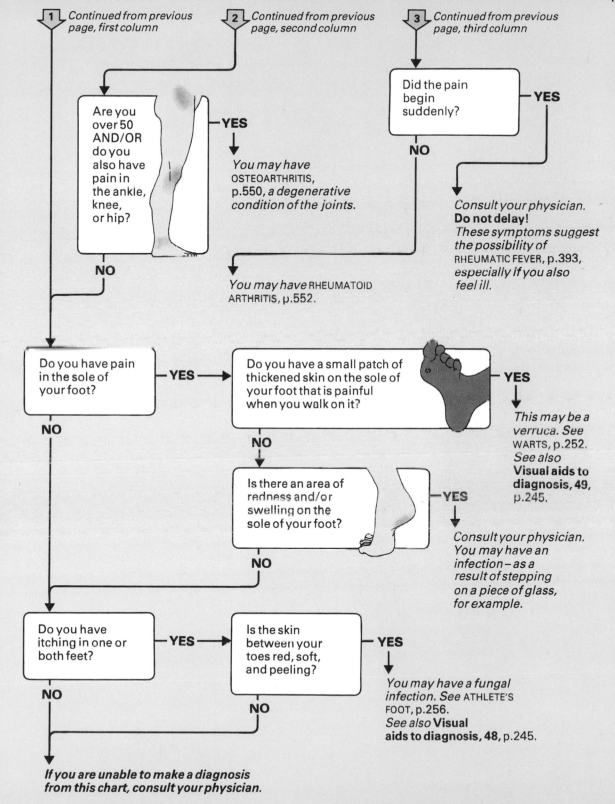

1 *Continued from previous page, first column*

2 *Continued from previous page, second column*

3 *Continued from previous page, third column*

Are you over 50 AND/OR do you also have pain in the ankle, knee, or hip?

YES → *You may have* OSTEOARTHRITIS, p.550, *a degenerative condition of the joints.*

NO → *You may have* RHEUMATOID ARTHRITIS, p.552.

Did the pain begin suddenly?

YES → *Consult your physician.* **Do not delay!** *These symptoms suggest the possibility of* RHEUMATIC FEVER, p.393, *especially if you also feel ill.*

NO

Do you have pain in the sole of your foot?

YES → **Do you have a small patch of thickened skin on the sole of your foot that is painful when you walk on it?**

YES → *This may be a verruca. See* WARTS, p.252. *See also* **Visual aids to diagnosis, 49,** p.245.

NO → **Is there an area of redness and/or swelling on the sole of your foot?**

YES → *Consult your physician. You may have an infection – as a result of stepping on a piece of glass, for example.*

NO

NO

Do you have itching in one or both feet?

YES → **Is the skin between your toes red, soft, and peeling?**

YES → *You may have a fungal infection. See* ATHLETE'S FOOT, p.256. *See also* **Visual aids to diagnosis, 48,** p.245.

NO

NO

If you are unable to make a diagnosis from this chart, consult your physician.

71
MEN

Painful or enlarged testicles

Pain or swelling that may affect one or both testicles, or the whole area within the scrotum (the supportive bag).

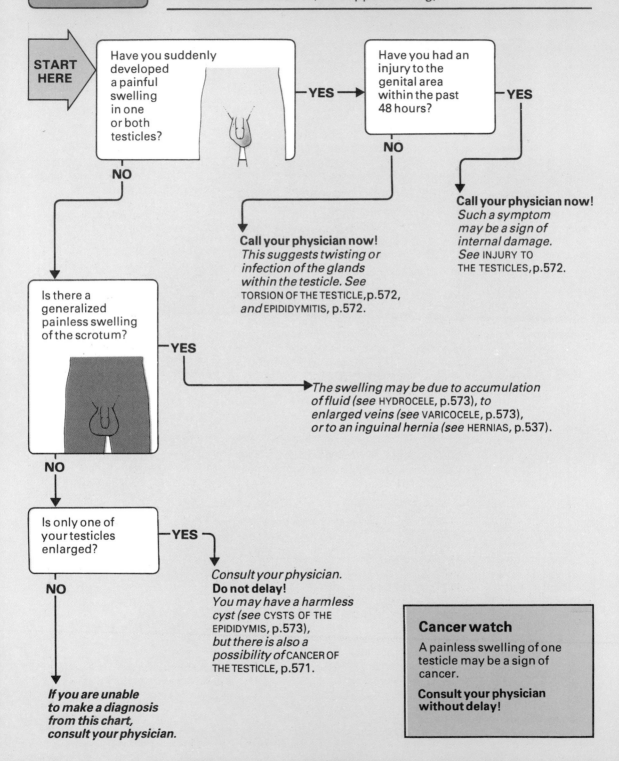

START HERE

Have you suddenly developed a painful swelling in one or both testicles?

YES →

Have you had an injury to the genital area within the past 48 hours?

YES →

NO

NO

Call your physician now!
This suggests twisting or infection of the glands within the testicle. See TORSION OF THE TESTICLE, p.572, *and* EPIDIDYMITIS, p.572.

Call your physician now!
Such a symptom may be a sign of internal damage. See INJURY TO THE TESTICLES, p.572.

Is there a generalized painless swelling of the scrotum?

YES

The swelling may be due to accumulation of fluid (see HYDROCELE, p.573), *to enlarged veins (see* VARICOCELE, p.573), *or to an inguinal hernia (see* HERNIAS, p.537).

NO

Is only one of your testicles enlarged?

YES

Consult your physician.
Do not delay!
You may have a harmless cyst (see CYSTS OF THE EPIDIDYMIS, p.573), *but there is also a possibility of* CANCER OF THE TESTICLE, p.571.

NO

If you are unable to make a diagnosis from this chart, consult your physician.

Cancer watch

A painless swelling of one testicle may be a sign of cancer.

Consult your physician without delay!

72
MEN

Painful intercourse in men
Pain or discomfort during or just after intercourse.

START HERE → Is the pain brought on by ejaculation? — **YES** → Do you have a burning feeling when you urinate, AND/OR any unusual discharge from the penis? — **YES**

Is the pain brought on by ejaculation? — **NO**

Do you have a burning feeling when you urinate, AND/OR any unusual discharge from the penis? — **NO**

You may have an infection such as URETHRITIS, p.578, *or* PROSTATITIS, p.576.

Do you have pain in the penis during intercourse? — **YES** → Can you see any redness, swelling, lumps, or sores on the skin or tip of the penis? — **YES**

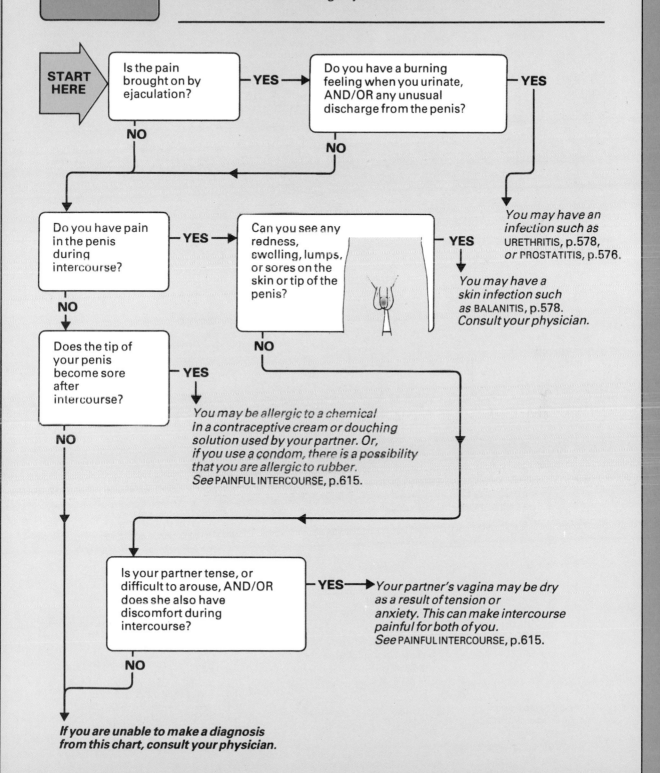

You may have a skin infection such as BALANITIS, p.578. *Consult your physician.*

Do you have pain in the penis during intercourse? — **NO**

Can you see any redness, swelling, lumps, or sores on the skin or tip of the penis? — **NO**

Does the tip of your penis become sore after intercourse? — **YES**

You may be allergic to a chemical in a contraceptive cream or douching solution used by your partner. Or, if you use a condom, there is a possibility that you are allergic to rubber. See PAINFUL INTERCOURSE, p.615.

Does the tip of your penis become sore after intercourse? — **NO**

Is your partner tense, or difficult to arouse, AND/OR does she also have discomfort during intercourse? — **YES** → *Your partner's vagina may be dry as a result of tension or anxiety. This can make intercourse painful for both of you. See* PAINFUL INTERCOURSE, p.615.

Is your partner tense, or difficult to arouse, AND/OR does she also have discomfort during intercourse? — **NO**

If you are unable to make a diagnosis from this chart, consult your physician.

73

WOMEN

Pain or lumps in the breast

Pain, tenderness, or lumps in one or both breasts that may be noticed when you examine yourself as described on p.589.

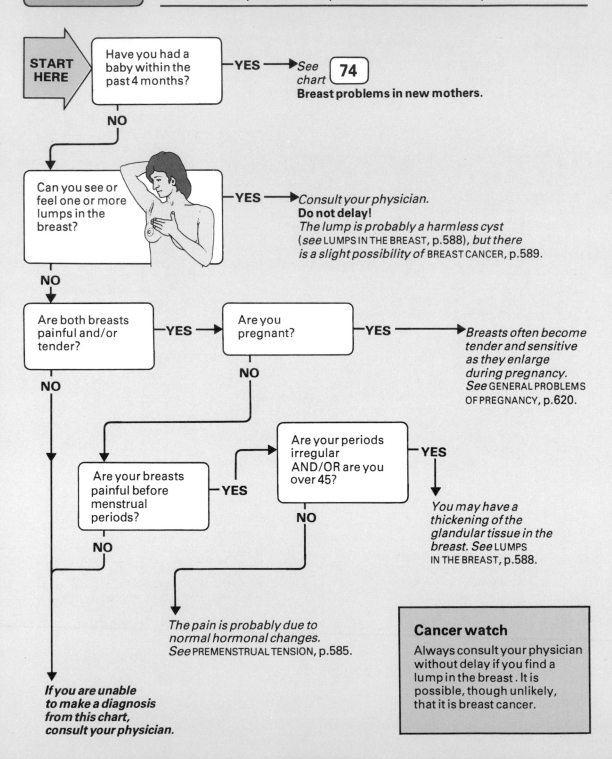

START HERE

Have you had a baby within the past 4 months? — **YES** → *See chart* **74**
Breast problems in new mothers.

NO

Can you see or feel one or more lumps in the breast? — **YES** → *Consult your physician.*
Do not delay!
The lump is probably a harmless cyst (*see* LUMPS IN THE BREAST, p.588), *but there is a slight possibility of* BREAST CANCER, p.589.

NO

Are both breasts painful and/or tender? — **YES** → **Are you pregnant?** — **YES** → *Breasts often become tender and sensitive as they enlarge during pregnancy. See* GENERAL PROBLEMS OF PREGNANCY, p.620.

NO

NO

Are your breasts painful before menstrual periods? — **YES** → **Are your periods irregular AND/OR are you over 45?** — **YES** →

NO

NO

You may have a thickening of the glandular tissue in the breast. See LUMPS IN THE BREAST, p.588.

The pain is probably due to normal hormonal changes. See PREMENSTRUAL TENSION, p.585.

If you are unable to make a diagnosis from this chart, consult your physician.

Cancer watch

Always consult your physician without delay if you find a lump in the breast. It is possible, though unlikely, that it is breast cancer.

74
WOMEN

Breast problems in new mothers

Pain, tenderness, or lumps in the breasts of women who have had a baby within the past 4 months.

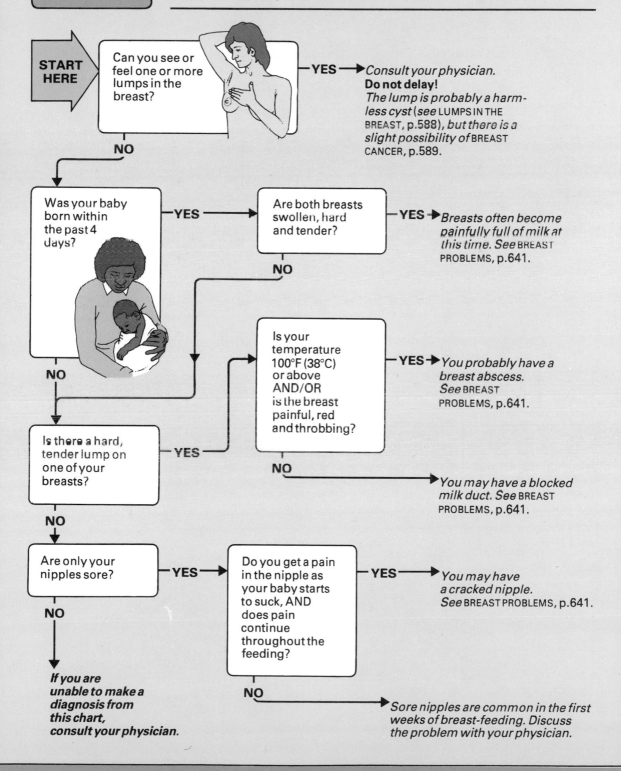

START HERE → Can you see or feel one or more lumps in the breast?

YES → *Consult your physician.* **Do not delay!** *The lump is probably a harmless cyst (see* LUMPS IN THE BREAST, p.588), *but there is a slight possibility of* BREAST CANCER, p.589.

NO

Was your baby born within the past 4 days?

YES → Are both breasts swollen, hard and tender?

YES → *Breasts often become painfully full of milk at this time. See* BREAST PROBLEMS, p.641.

NO

NO

Is there a hard, tender lump on one of your breasts?

YES → Is your temperature 100°F (38°C) or above AND/OR is the breast painful, red and throbbing?

YES → *You probably have a breast abscess. See* BREAST PROBLEMS, p.641.

NO

You may have a blocked milk duct. See BREAST PROBLEMS, p.641.

NO

Are only your nipples sore?

YES → Do you get a pain in the nipple as your baby starts to suck, AND does pain continue throughout the feeding?

YES → *You may have a cracked nipple. See* BREAST PROBLEMS, p.641.

NO

If you are unable to make a diagnosis from this chart, consult your physician.

NO → *Sore nipples are common in the first weeks of breast-feeding. Discuss the problem with your physician.*

Absent periods

Absence of periods for at least 2 weeks after a period was due.

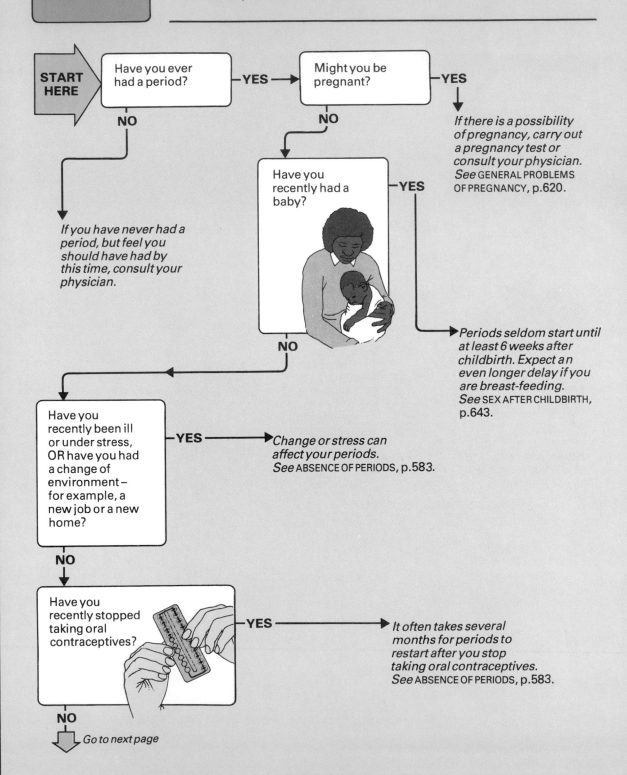

START HERE →

Have you ever had a period? — **YES** → **Might you be pregnant?** — **YES** ↓

If there is a possibility of pregnancy, carry out a pregnancy test or consult your physician. See GENERAL PROBLEMS OF PREGNANCY, p.620.

NO ↓ (from "Have you ever had a period?")

If you have never had a period, but feel you should have had by this time, consult your physician.

NO ↓ (from "Might you be pregnant?")

Have you recently had a baby? — **YES** →

Periods seldom start until at least 6 weeks after childbirth. Expect an even longer delay if you are breast-feeding. See SEX AFTER CHILDBIRTH, p.643.

NO ↓

Have you recently been ill or under stress, OR have you had a change of environment – for example, a new job or a new home? — **YES** →

Change or stress can affect your periods. See ABSENCE OF PERIODS, p.583.

NO ↓

Have you recently stopped taking oral contraceptives? — **YES** →

It often takes several months for periods to restart after you stop taking oral contraceptives. See ABSENCE OF PERIODS, p.583.

NO ↓ Go to next page

Continued from previous page

Have you lost
a lot of weight in
a short time
through a strict
reducing diet
or vigorous
exercise?

YES → *Sudden loss of weight often results in an absence of periods.* See ABSENCE OF PERIODS, p.583.

NO

Are you over 45?

YES → *It is common for women over 45 to begin skipping periods.* See MENOPAUSE, p.586.

NO

Do you have two or more of
the following symptoms?
☐ increased hairiness
☐ deepening of the voice
☐ unexplained weight gain

YES → *The delay may be caused by disruption in the production of hormones.* See ABNORMALITIES OF THE HYPOTHALAMUS, PITUITARY AND OVARIES, p.587.

NO

Are you currently
taking any
medicines?

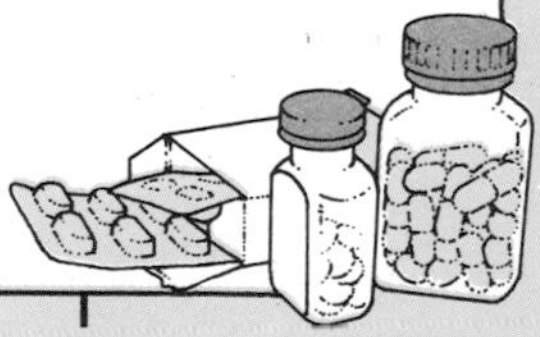

YES → *Some drugs can cause periods to stop. Discuss with your physician.*

NO

If you are unable to make a diagnosis from this chart, consult your physician.

76

WOMEN

Heavy periods

Menstrual periods that either last more than 7 days or have recently become longer or begun to produce more blood than usual.

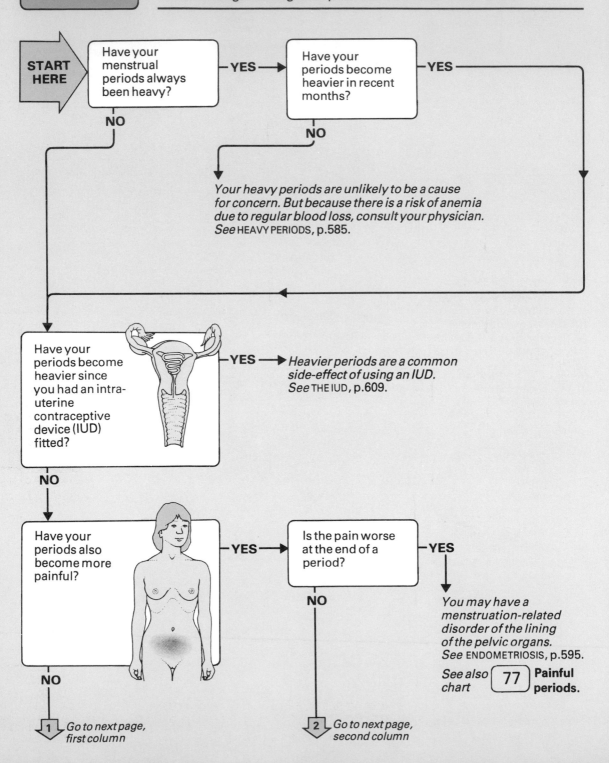

START HERE → Have your menstrual periods always been heavy?

— **YES** → Have your periods become heavier in recent months?

— **YES** →

NO (from first box) ↓

NO (from second box) ↓

Your heavy periods are unlikely to be a cause for concern. But because there is a risk of anemia due to regular blood loss, consult your physician. See HEAVY PERIODS, p.585.

Have your periods become heavier since you had an intra-uterine contraceptive device (IUD) fitted?

— **YES** → *Heavier periods are a common side-effect of using an IUD. See* THE IUD, p.609.

NO ↓

Have your periods also become more painful?

— **YES** → Is the pain worse at the end of a period?

— **YES** ↓

You may have a menstruation-related disorder of the lining of the pelvic organs. See ENDOMETRIOSIS, p.595.

See also chart 77 **Painful periods.**

NO (from painful box) ↓

NO (from pain worse box) ↓

1 *Go to next page, first column*

2 *Go to next page, second column*

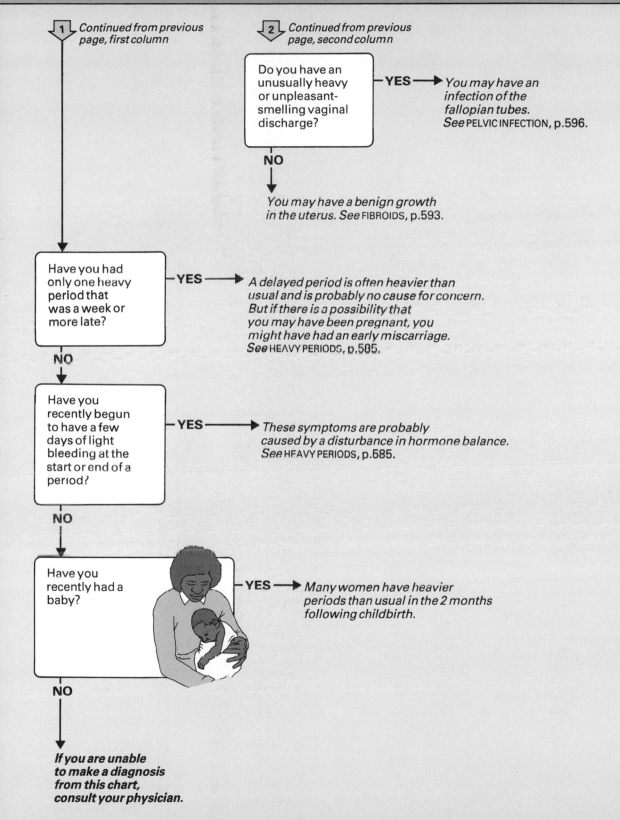

1 *Continued from previous page, first column*

2 *Continued from previous page, second column*

Do you have an unusually heavy or unpleasant-smelling vaginal discharge?

YES → *You may have an infection of the fallopian tubes.* See PELVIC INFECTION, p.596.

NO ↓

You may have a benign growth in the uterus. See FIBROIDS, p.593.

Have you had only one heavy period that was a week or more late?

YES → *A delayed period is often heavier than usual and is probably no cause for concern. But if there is a possibility that you may have been pregnant, you might have had an early miscarriage.* See HEAVY PERIODS, p.585.

NO ↓

Have you recently begun to have a few days of light bleeding at the start or end of a period?

YES → *These symptoms are probably caused by a disturbance in hormone balance.* See HEAVY PERIODS, p.585.

NO ↓

Have you recently had a baby?

YES → *Many women have heavier periods than usual in the 2 months following childbirth.*

NO ↓

If you are unable to make a diagnosis from this chart, consult your physician.

77
WOMEN

Painful periods

Pain associated with menstruation, usually felt as a dull ache or cramps in the lower abdomen.

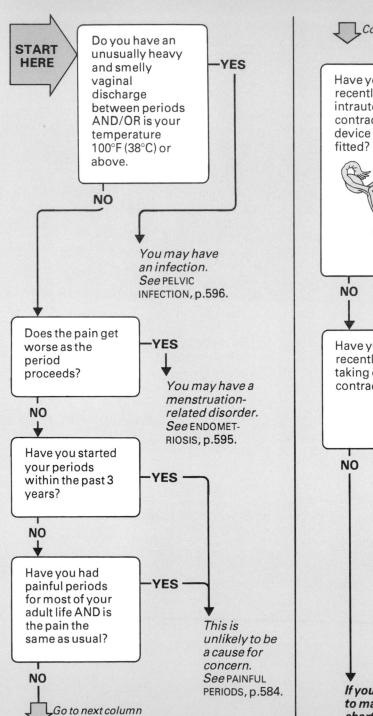

START HERE

Do you have an unusually heavy and smelly vaginal discharge between periods AND/OR is your temperature 100°F (38°C) or above.

YES →

You may have an infection. See PELVIC INFECTION, p.596.

NO ↓

Does the pain get worse as the period proceeds?

YES →

You may have a menstruation-related disorder. See ENDOMET-RIOSIS, p.595.

NO ↓

Have you started your periods within the past 3 years?

YES →

NO ↓

Have you had painful periods for most of your adult life AND is the pain the same as usual?

YES →

This is unlikely to be a cause for concern. See PAINFUL PERIODS, p.584.

NO ↓

Go to next column

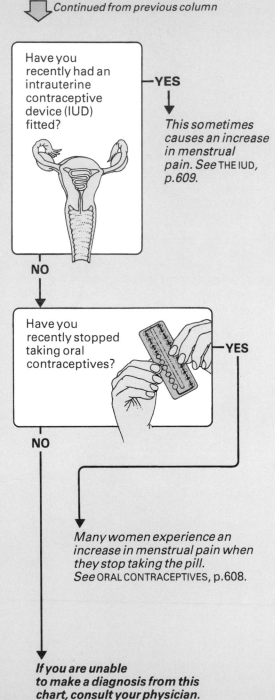

↓ *Continued from previous column*

Have you recently had an intrauterine contraceptive device (IUD) fitted?

YES →

This sometimes causes an increase in menstrual pain. See THE IUD, p.609.

NO ↓

Have you recently stopped taking oral contraceptives?

YES →

NO ↓

Many women experience an increase in menstrual pain when they stop taking the pill. See ORAL CONTRACEPTIVES, p.608.

If you are unable to make a diagnosis from this chart, consult your physician.

78

WOMEN

Lower abdominal pain in women

Pain below the waist in women of childbearing age.
Use this chart only after consulting chart 48, **Abdominal pain**.

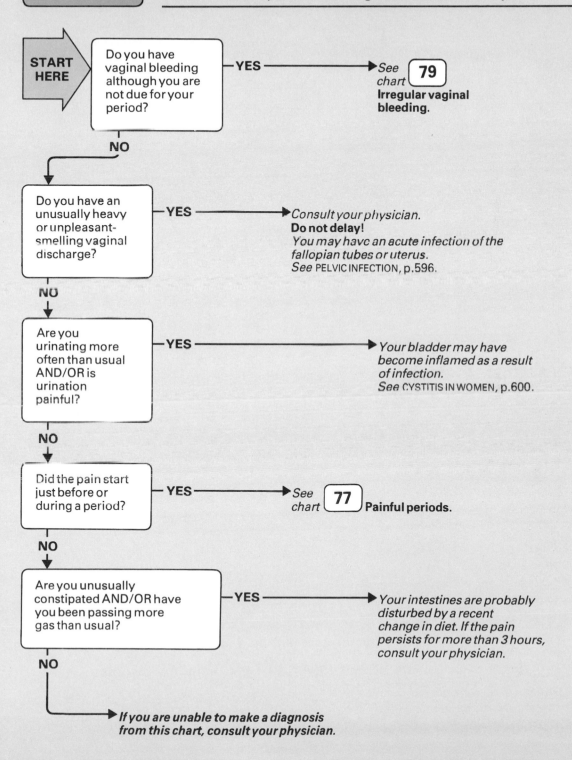

START HERE

Do you have vaginal bleeding although you are not due for your period?
— YES → *See chart* **79** **Irregular vaginal bleeding.**

NO ↓

Do you have an unusually heavy or unpleasant-smelling vaginal discharge?
— YES → *Consult your physician.* **Do not delay!** *You may have an acute infection of the fallopian tubes or uterus.* *See* PELVIC INFECTION, p.596.

NO ↓

Are you urinating more often than usual AND/OR is urination painful?
— YES → *Your bladder may have become inflamed as a result of infection.* *See* CYSTITIS IN WOMEN, p.600.

NO ↓

Did the pain start just before or during a period?
— YES → *See chart* **77** **Painful periods.**

NO ↓

Are you unusually constipated AND/OR have you been passing more gas than usual?
— YES → *Your intestines are probably disturbed by a recent change in diet. If the pain persists for more than 3 hours, consult your physician.*

NO ↓

If you are unable to make a diagnosis from this chart, consult your physician.

79

WOMEN

Irregular vaginal bleeding

Any bleeding that occurs between normal menstrual periods, during pregnancy, or after menopause.

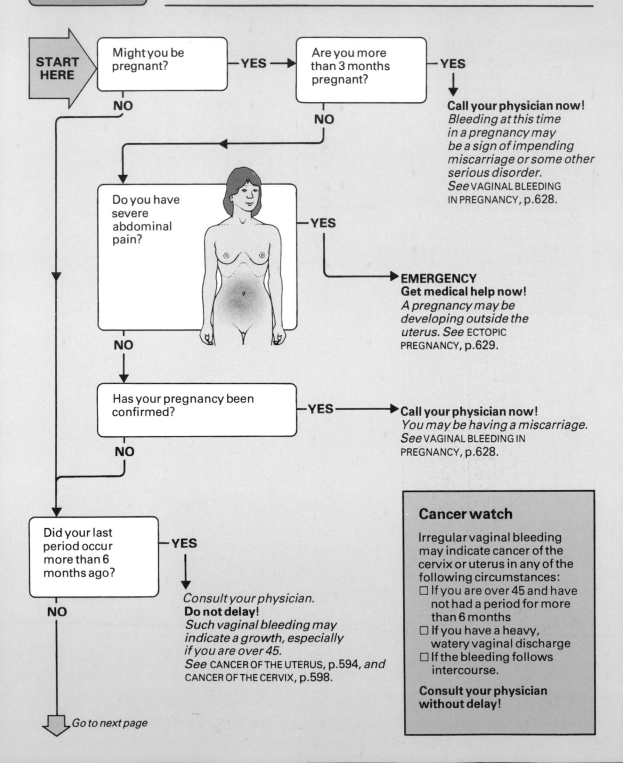

START HERE

Might you be pregnant? — YES → **Are you more than 3 months pregnant?** — YES ↓

NO ↓

NO ↓

Call your physician now!
Bleeding at this time in a pregnancy may be a sign of impending miscarriage or some other serious disorder.
See VAGINAL BLEEDING IN PREGNANCY, p.628.

Do you have severe abdominal pain? — YES →

NO ↓

EMERGENCY
Get medical help now!
A pregnancy may be developing outside the uterus. See ECTOPIC PREGNANCY, p.629.

Has your pregnancy been confirmed? — YES →

NO ↓

Call your physician now!
You may be having a miscarriage.
See VAGINAL BLEEDING IN PREGNANCY, p.628.

Did your last period occur more than 6 months ago? — YES

NO

Consult your physician.
Do not delay!
Such vaginal bleeding may indicate a growth, especially if you are over 45.
See CANCER OF THE UTERUS, p.594, *and* CANCER OF THE CERVIX, p.598.

⬇ *Go to next page*

Cancer watch

Irregular vaginal bleeding may indicate cancer of the cervix or uterus in any of the following circumstances:

☐ If you are over 45 and have not had a period for more than 6 months

☐ If you have a heavy, watery vaginal discharge

☐ If the bleeding follows intercourse.

Consult your physician without delay!

Continued from previous page

Do you have a heavy, watery vaginal discharge OR does the bleeding occur immediately after intercourse? — **YES** → *Consult your physician.* **Do not delay!** *The bleeding is probably caused by* CERVICAL EROSION, p.597, *but there is a chance that you have* CANCER OF THE CERVIX, p.598, *or* CANCER OF THE UTERUS, p.594.

NO

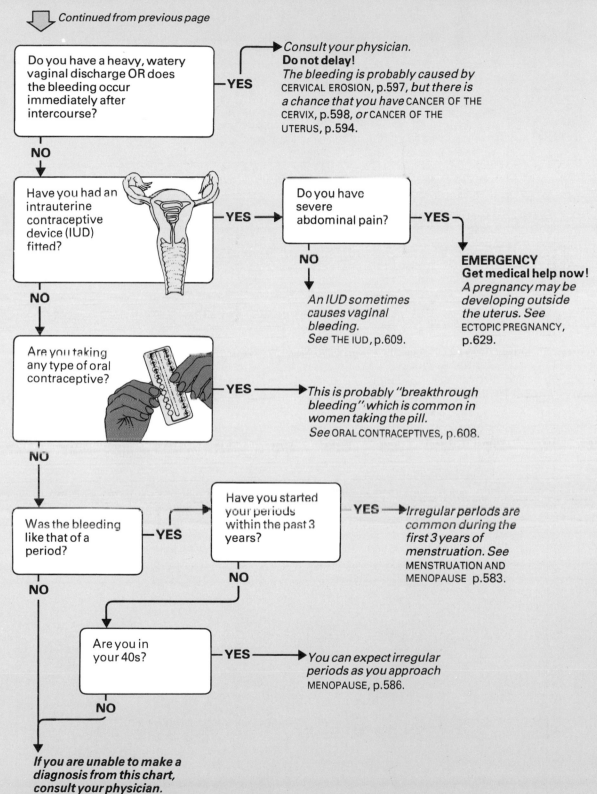

Have you had an intrauterine contraceptive device (IUD) fitted? — **YES** → Do you have severe abdominal pain? — **YES** →

NO

An IUD sometimes causes vaginal bleeding. *See* THE IUD, p.609.

EMERGENCY
Get medical help now!
A pregnancy may be developing outside the uterus. See ECTOPIC PREGNANCY, p.629.

NO

Are you taking any type of oral contraceptive? — **YES** → *This is probably "breakthrough bleeding" which is common in women taking the pill.* See ORAL CONTRACEPTIVES, p.608.

NO

Was the bleeding like that of a period? — **YES** → Have you started your periods within the past 3 years? — **YES** → *Irregular periods are common during the first 3 years of menstruation. See* MENSTRUATION AND MENOPAUSE p.583.

NO

NO

Are you in your 40s? — **YES** → *You can expect irregular periods as you approach* MENOPAUSE, p.586.

NO

If you are unable to make a diagnosis from this chart, consult your physician.

80
WOMEN

Abnormal vaginal discharge

Discharge from the vagina that differs in color, consistency, and/or quantity from what you normally have between periods.

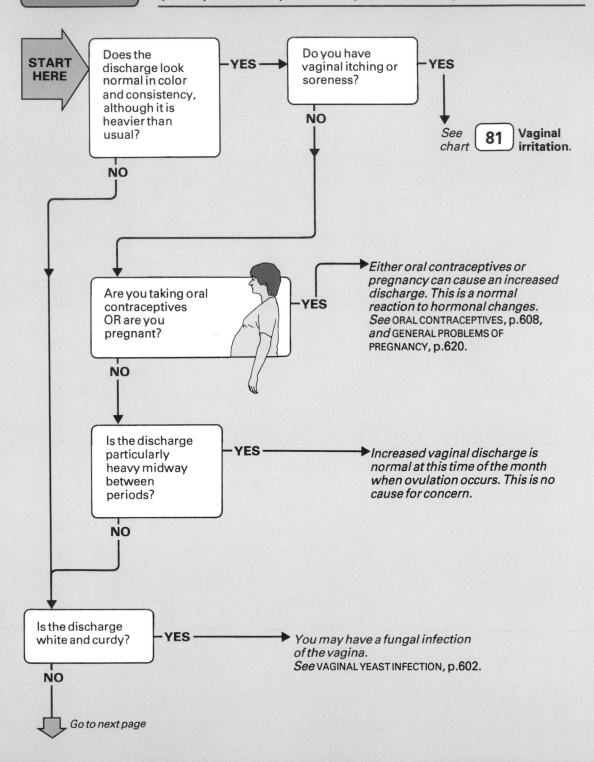

START HERE

Does the discharge look normal in color and consistency, although it is heavier than usual? —**YES**→ **Do you have vaginal itching or soreness?** —**YES**→

↓ **NO**

↓ **NO**

See chart **81** **Vaginal irritation.**

Are you taking oral contraceptives OR are you pregnant? —**YES**→ *Either oral contraceptives or pregnancy can cause an increased discharge. This is a normal reaction to hormonal changes. See* ORAL CONTRACEPTIVES, p.608, *and* GENERAL PROBLEMS OF PREGNANCY, p.620.

↓ **NO**

Is the discharge particularly heavy midway between periods? —**YES**→ *Increased vaginal discharge is normal at this time of the month when ovulation occurs. This is no cause for concern.*

↓ **NO**

Is the discharge white and curdy? —**YES**→ *You may have a fungal infection of the vagina. See* VAGINAL YEAST INFECTION, p.602.

↓ **NO**

Go to next page

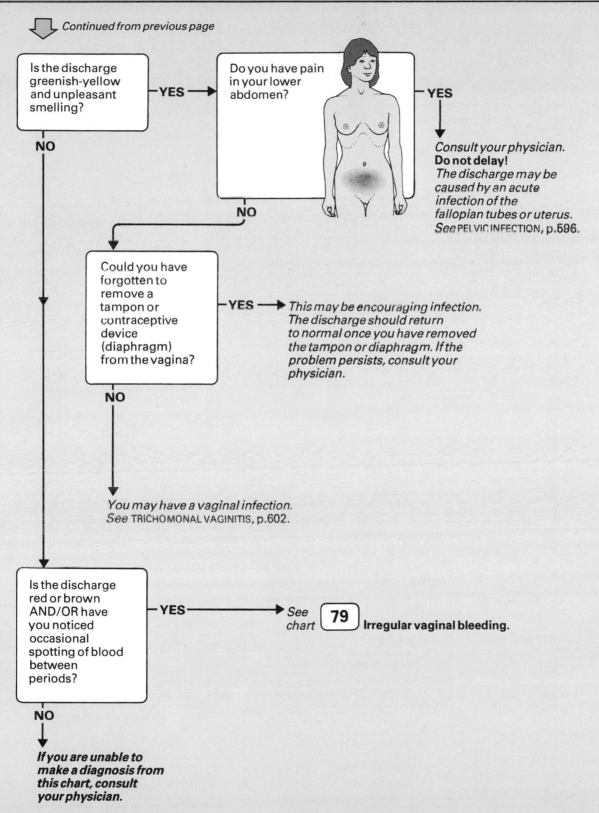

⬇ *Continued from previous page*

Is the discharge greenish-yellow and unpleasant smelling?

YES → **Do you have pain in your lower abdomen?**

YES ↓

Consult your physician. **Do not delay!** *The discharge may be caused by an acute infection of the fallopian tubes or uterus.* *See* PELVIC INFECTION, p.596.

NO (from pain question)

NO (from discharge question)

Could you have forgotten to remove a tampon or contraceptive device (diaphragm) from the vagina?

YES → *This may be encouraging infection. The discharge should return to normal once you have removed the tampon or diaphragm. If the problem persists, consult your physician.*

NO ↓

You may have a vaginal infection. *See* TRICHOMONAL VAGINITIS, p.602.

Is the discharge red or brown AND/OR have you noticed occasional spotting of blood between periods?

YES → *See chart* **79** **Irregular vaginal bleeding.**

NO ↓

If you are unable to make a diagnosis from this chart, consult your physician.

Vaginal irritation
Itching or soreness in the vagina or around the genital area.

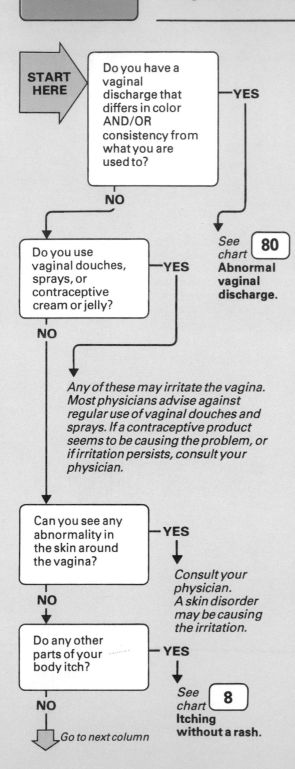

START HERE → Do you have a vaginal discharge that differs in color AND/OR consistency from what you are used to?

YES → See chart **80** **Abnormal vaginal discharge.**

NO ↓

Do you use vaginal douches, sprays, or contraceptive cream or jelly?

YES → *Any of these may irritate the vagina. Most physicians advise against regular use of vaginal douches and sprays. If a contraceptive product seems to be causing the problem, or if irritation persists, consult your physician.*

NO ↓

Can you see any abnormality in the skin around the vagina?

YES → *Consult your physician. A skin disorder may be causing the irritation.*

NO ↓

Do any other parts of your body itch?

YES → See chart **8** **Itching without a rash.**

NO ↓ Go to next column

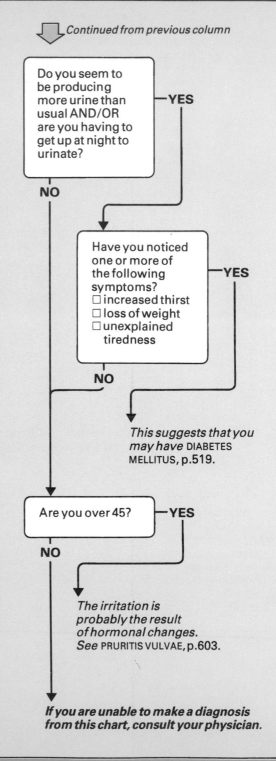

Continued from previous column ↓

Do you seem to be producing more urine than usual AND/OR are you having to get up at night to urinate?

YES ↓

NO ↓

Have you noticed one or more of the following symptoms?
☐ increased thirst
☐ loss of weight
☐ unexplained tiredness

YES ↓

NO ↓

This suggests that you may have DIABETES MELLITUS, p.519.

Are you over 45? **YES** ↓

NO ↓

The irritation is probably the result of hormonal changes. See PRURITIS VULVAE, p.603.

If you are unable to make a diagnosis from this chart, consult your physician.

82
WOMEN

Abnormal hairiness in women
Any excessive hair growth on the face, limbs, or torso.

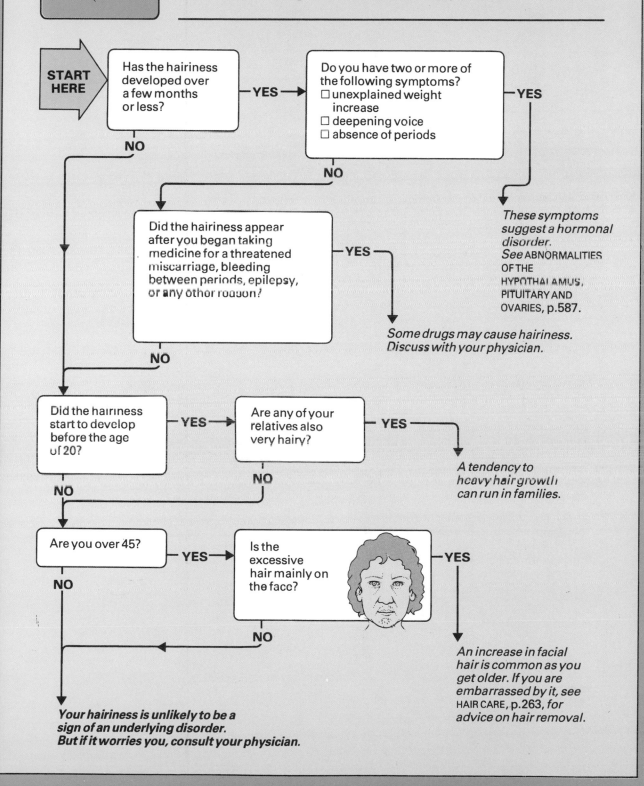

START HERE →

Has the hairiness developed over a few months or less?

— **YES** → **Do you have two or more of the following symptoms?**
☐ unexplained weight increase
☐ deepening voice
☐ absence of periods

— **YES** → *These symptoms suggest a hormonal disorder. See* ABNORMALITIES OF THE HYPOTHALAMUS, PITUITARY AND OVARIES, *p.587.*

NO (from hairiness question)

NO (from symptoms question) → **Did the hairiness appear after you began taking medicine for a threatened miscarriage, bleeding between periods, epilepsy, or any other reason?**

— **YES** → *Some drugs may cause hairiness. Discuss with your physician.*

NO → **Did the hairiness start to develop before the age of 20?**

— **YES** → **Are any of your relatives also very hairy?**

— **YES** → *A tendency to heavy hair growth can run in families.*

NO (relatives)

NO (before age 20) → **Are you over 45?**

— **YES** → **Is the excessive hair mainly on the face?**

— **YES** → *An increase in facial hair is common as you get older. If you are embarrassed by it, see* HAIR CARE, *p.263, for advice on hair removal.*

NO (over 45)

NO (excessive hair on face)

Your hairiness is unlikely to be a sign of an underlying disorder. But if it worries you, consult your physician.

83
WOMEN

Painful intercourse in women
Pain or discomfort during or just after sexual intercourse.

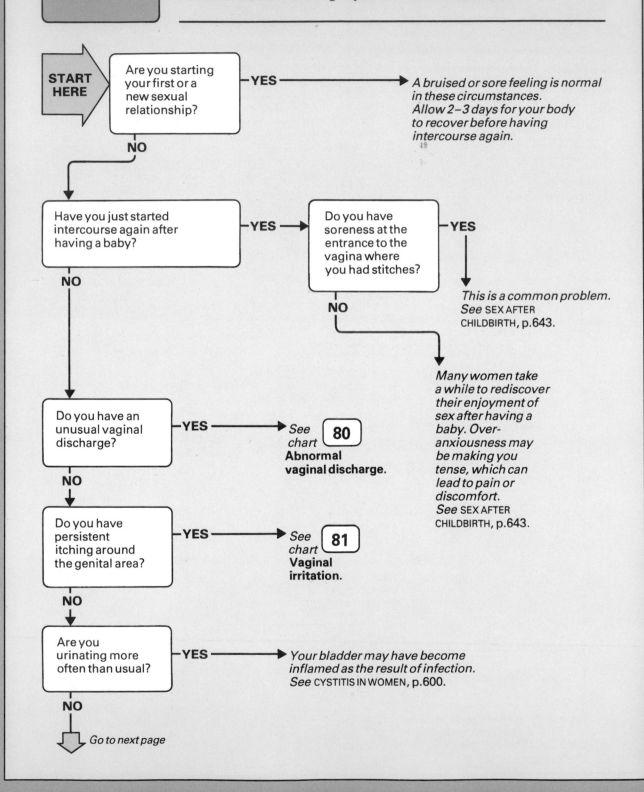

START HERE

Are you starting your first or a new sexual relationship? — **YES** → *A bruised or sore feeling is normal in these circumstances. Allow 2–3 days for your body to recover before having intercourse again.*

NO

Have you just started intercourse again after having a baby? — **YES** → **Do you have soreness at the entrance to the vagina where you had stitches?** — **YES** → *This is a common problem. See* SEX AFTER CHILDBIRTH, p.643.

NO (from "Have you just started...")

NO (from "Do you have soreness...") → *Many women take a while to rediscover their enjoyment of sex after having a baby. Over-anxiousness may be making you tense, which can lead to pain or discomfort. See* SEX AFTER CHILDBIRTH, p.643.

Do you have an unusual vaginal discharge? — **YES** → *See chart* **80 Abnormal vaginal discharge.**

NO

Do you have persistent itching around the genital area? — **YES** → *See chart* **81 Vaginal irritation.**

NO

Are you urinating more often than usual? — **YES** → *Your bladder may have become inflamed as the result of infection. See* CYSTITIS IN WOMEN, p.600.

NO

⬇ *Go to next page*

⬇ *Continued from previous page*

Is your vagina so dry that penetration is uncomfortable and difficult? —**YES**→ **Are you over 45?** —**YES**→ *Some dryness is common during and after* MENOPAUSE, p.586. *See also* PAINFUL INTERCOURSE, p.615.

NO (from "Are you over 45?")

↓

If you do not become aroused, this may account for your dryness. *See* PAINFUL INTERCOURSE, p.615.

NO (from "Is your vagina so dry...")

↓

When your partner penetrates deeply, does it feel as though he is hitting a tender place? —**YES**→ **Have your periods become more painful than they used to be?** —**YES**→ *You may have a menstruation-related disorder of the lining of the pelvic organs.* *See* ENDOMETRIOSIS, p.595.

NO (from "Have your periods...")

↓

Do you have pain only when you have intercourse in certain positions? —**YES**→ *The pain may be caused by pressure on an ovary during intercourse.* *See* RETROVERSION OF THE UTERUS, p.597, *and* PAINFUL INTERCOURSE, p.615.

NO (from "Do you have pain only...")

NO (from "When your partner penetrates deeply...")

↓

Does your vagina seem too small, so that penetration is difficult? —**YES**→ *Your problem is probably due to involuntary tightening of the muscles in the vagina.* *See* PAINFUL INTERCOURSE, p.615.

NO

↓

If you are unable to make a diagnosis from this chart, consult your physician.

84
COUPLES

Failure to conceive

Failure to conceive after more than 12 months without contraception. In order to make a diagnosis, each partner should read the chart in turn.

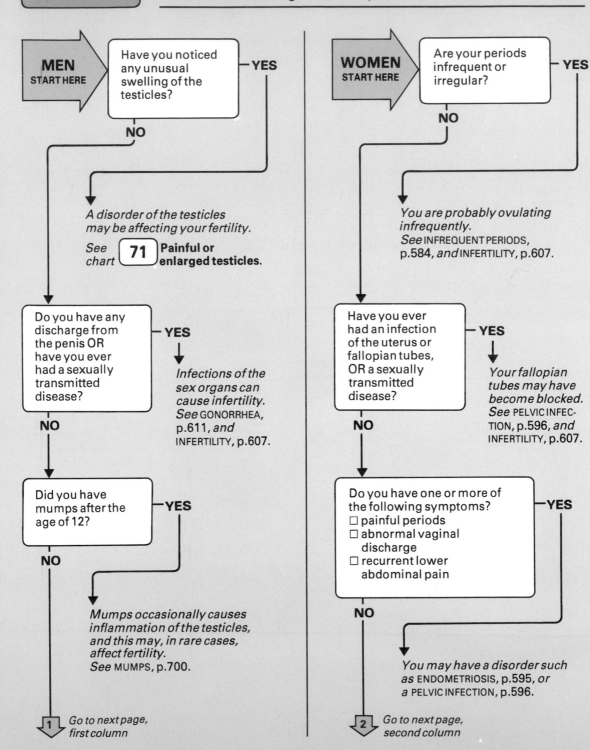

MEN START HERE

Have you noticed any unusual swelling of the testicles? — **YES**

NO

A disorder of the testicles may be affecting your fertility.
See chart **71** **Painful or enlarged testicles**.

Do you have any discharge from the penis OR have you ever had a sexually transmitted disease? — **YES**

Infections of the sex organs can cause infertility. See GONORRHEA, p.611, *and* INFERTILITY, p.607.

NO

Did you have mumps after the age of 12? — **YES**

NO

Mumps occasionally causes inflammation of the testicles, and this may, in rare cases, affect fertility. See MUMPS, p.700.

1 *Go to next page, first column*

WOMEN START HERE

Are your periods infrequent or irregular? — **YES**

NO

You are probably ovulating infrequently. See INFREQUENT PERIODS, p.584, *and* INFERTILITY, p.607.

Have you ever had an infection of the uterus or fallopian tubes, OR a sexually transmitted disease? — **YES**

Your fallopian tubes may have become blocked. See PELVIC INFECTION, p.596, *and* INFERTILITY, p.607.

NO

Do you have one or more of the following symptoms?
☐ painful periods
☐ abnormal vaginal discharge
☐ recurrent lower abdominal pain
— **YES**

NO

You may have a disorder such as ENDOMETRIOSIS, p.595, *or a* PELVIC INFECTION, p.596.

2 *Go to next page, second column*

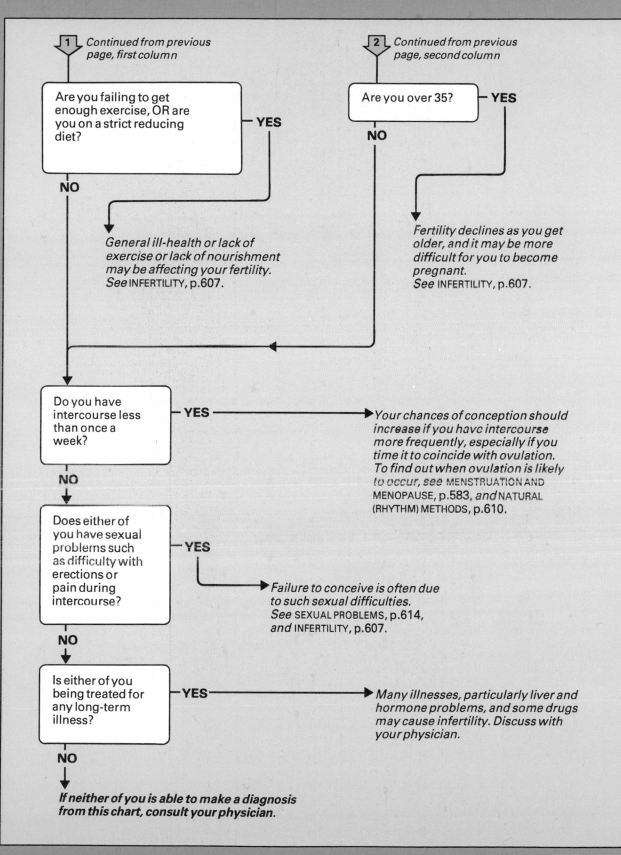

1 *Continued from previous page, first column*

Are you failing to get enough exercise, OR are you on a strict reducing diet?

— **YES**

NO

General ill-health or lack of exercise or lack of nourishment may be affecting your fertility. See INFERTILITY, p.607.

2 *Continued from previous page, second column*

Are you over 35? — **YES**

NO

Fertility declines as you get older, and it may be more difficult for you to become pregnant. See INFERTILITY, p.607.

Do you have intercourse less than once a week?

— **YES** →

Your chances of conception should increase if you have intercourse more frequently, especially if you time it to coincide with ovulation. To find out when ovulation is likely to occur, see MENSTRUATION AND MENOPAUSE, p.583, *and* NATURAL (RHYTHM) METHODS, p.610.

NO

Does either of you have sexual problems such as difficulty with erections or pain during intercourse?

— **YES**

→ *Failure to conceive is often due to such sexual difficulties. See* SEXUAL PROBLEMS, p.614, *and* INFERTILITY, p.607.

NO

Is either of you being treated for any long-term illness?

— **YES** →

Many illnesses, particularly liver and hormone problems, and some drugs may cause infertility. Discuss with your physician.

NO

If neither of you is able to make a diagnosis from this chart, consult your physician.

Waking at night

Any waking after the child has gone to sleep for the night that may cause the child to cry or call out.

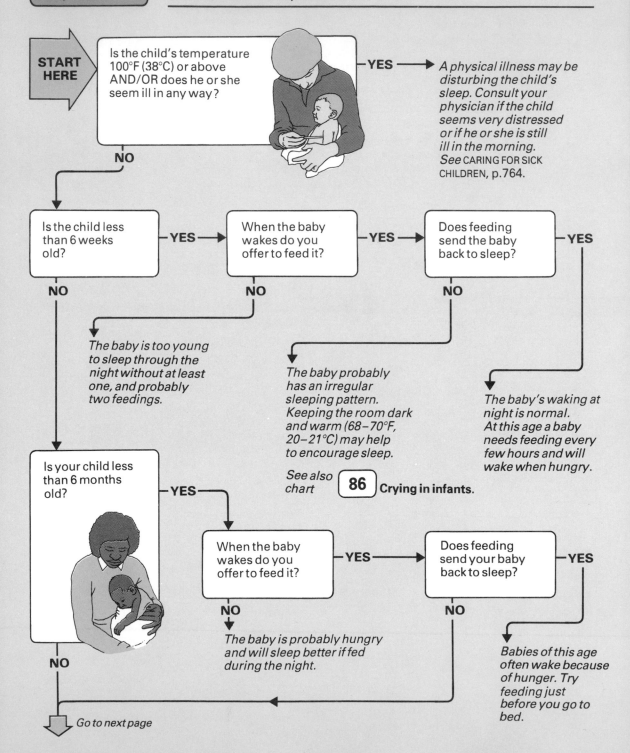

START HERE → Is the child's temperature 100°F (38°C) or above AND/OR does he or she seem ill in any way? — **YES** → A physical illness may be disturbing the child's sleep. Consult your physician if the child seems very distressed or if he or she is still ill in the morning. *See* CARING FOR SICK CHILDREN, p.764.

NO

Is the child less than 6 weeks old? — **YES** → When the baby wakes do you offer to feed it? — **YES** → Does feeding send the baby back to sleep? — **YES**

NO — The baby is too young to sleep through the night without at least one, and probably two feedings.

NO — The baby probably has an irregular sleeping pattern. Keeping the room dark and warm (68–70°F, 20–21°C) may help to encourage sleep.

See also chart **86** *Crying in infants.*

NO — The baby's waking at night is normal. At this age a baby needs feeding every few hours and will wake when hungry.

Is your child less than 6 months old? — **YES** → When the baby wakes do you offer to feed it? — **YES** → Does feeding send your baby back to sleep? — **YES**

NO — The baby is probably hungry and will sleep better if fed during the night.

NO — Babies of this age often wake because of hunger. Try feeding just before you go to bed.

NO

↓ *Go to next page*

⬇ *Continued from previous page*

Is the child less than a year old?

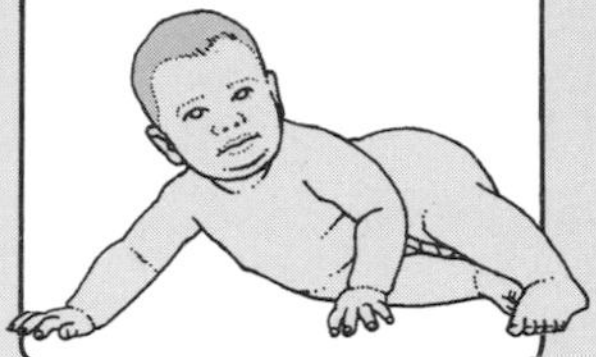

→ **YES** → **When you go to the baby in the night, do you find that the bedclothes have been kicked off?**

→ **YES** → *The baby is probably awakened by the cold. A sleeping bag or a warmer room may solve the problem.*

NO (from bedclothes question)

NO (from less than a year old)

Does the baby's bottom look red, sore, or spotty?

— **YES** → *The baby probably has* DIAPER RASH, *p.650, which stings when the baby's diaper is wet. This may cause the baby to wake.* See also **Visual aids to diagnosis, 4**, p.234.

NO

Does the baby usually sleep through most of the night, but wake early in the morning?

— **YES** → *The baby probably does not need any more sleep. Change the baby's diaper, give him or her a drink, and put a few toys in the crib. This may enable you to get some more sleep.*

NO → *The baby probably has in irregular sleeping pattern. See* SLEEPING PROBLEMS IN CHILDREN, p.671.

Does the child seem upset or frightened on waking?

— **YES** → *Nightmares may be waking the child. See* SLEEPING PROBLEMS IN CHILDREN, p.671. *A dim light in the room may help if the child is afraid of the dark.*

NO

Does the child have any cause for worry, such as the arrival of a new baby, starting a new school or tension in the home?

— **YES** → *Anxiety may be making the child wakeful. Extra reassurance and affection during the day may help to solve the problem.* See SLEEPING PROBLEMS IN CHILDREN, p.671.

NO → ***The child's wakefulness is probably due to an irregular sleeping pattern, and is unlikely to be a sign of any disorder. However, if you are worried by it, consult your physician.***

86

CHILDREN
0–6 months

Crying in infants

Any sobbing, whimpering, or wailing that indicates your baby is not content.

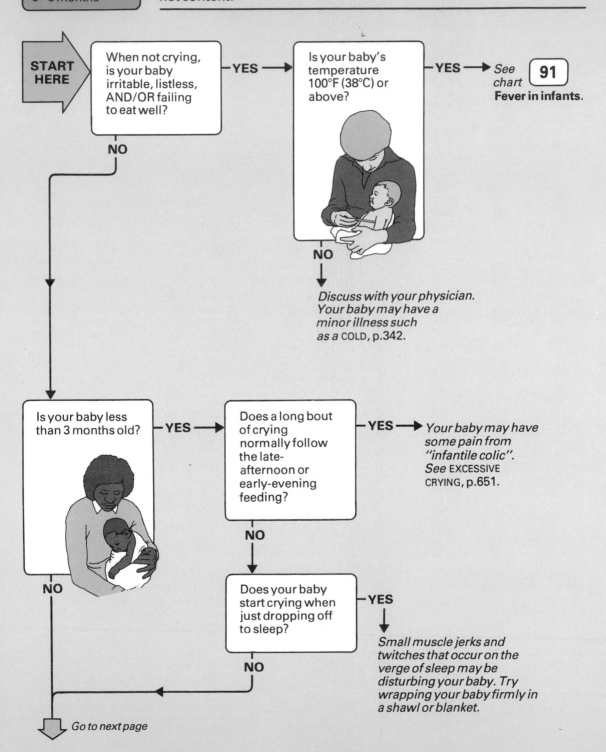

START HERE

When not crying, is your baby irritable, listless, AND/OR failing to eat well? — **YES** →

Is your baby's temperature 100°F (38°C) or above? — **YES** → *See chart* **91** **Fever in infants**.

NO ↓

Discuss with your physician. Your baby may have a minor illness such as a COLD, p.342.

NO ↓

Is your baby less than 3 months old? — **YES** →

Does a long bout of crying normally follow the late-afternoon or early-evening feeding? — **YES** → *Your baby may have some pain from "infantile colic". See* EXCESSIVE CRYING, p.651.

NO ↓

Does your baby start crying when just dropping off to sleep? — **YES** ↓

Small muscle jerks and twitches that occur on the verge of sleep may be disturbing your baby. Try wrapping your baby firmly in a shawl or blanket.

NO ↓

NO ↓

Go to next page

⬇ *Continued from previous page*

Is your baby in a cool room, or outside in a buggy on a chilly day? ——**YES**——➤ *Your baby may simply be too cold. Moving into a warm room will probably help.*

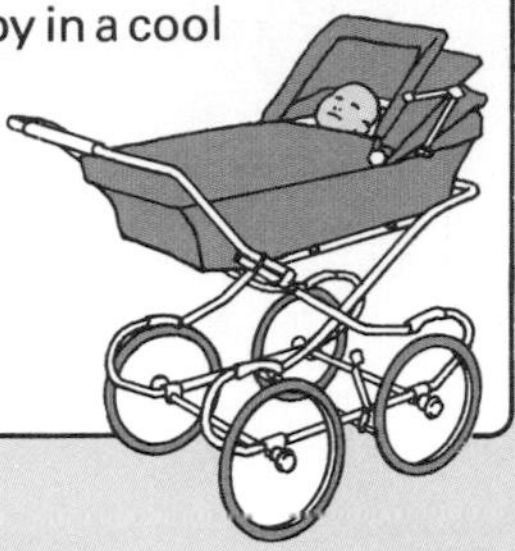

NO
⬇

Does your baby generally stop crying when picked up? ——**YES**——➤ *Your baby is probably bored or lonely. Try giving a little more attention or placing the baby where he or she can see you.*

NO
⬇

Does your baby's bottom look red, sore, or spotty? ——**YES**——➤ DIAPER RASH, p.650, *may be making your baby uncomfortable. See also* **Visual aids to diagnosis, 4,** p.234.

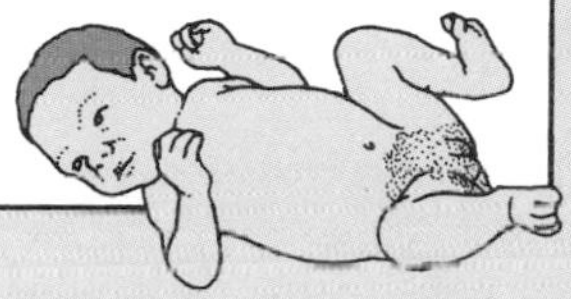

NO
⬇

Does your baby stop crying after being fed? ——**YES**——➤ **Does your baby start crying again less than 2 hours after a feeding?** ——**YES**——

NO
⬇

Your baby probably cries simply because of hunger. Try offering a feeding whenever he or she seems hungry.

⬇

You may not be giving enough food. If you are breast-feeding, allow your baby to suck more often and longer. If you are bottle-feeding, increase the amount offered. Remember that babies also get thirsty. Giving water between feedings may help to reduce crying. See FEEDING PROBLEMS, p.648, *and* EXCESSIVE CRYING, p.651.

NO
⬇

If you are unable to make a diagnosis from this chart and the crying is worrying you, consult your physician.

87

Vomiting in infants

Bringing back or throwing up stomach contents.

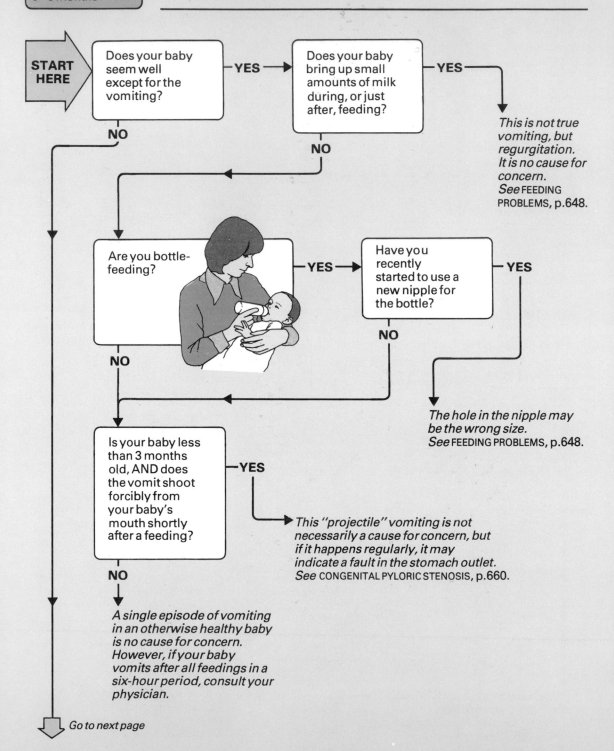

START HERE

Does your baby seem well except for the vomiting?

— **YES** → Does your baby bring up small amounts of milk during, or just after, feeding?

— **YES** → *This is not true vomiting, but regurgitation. It is no cause for concern. See* FEEDING PROBLEMS, p.648.

NO

NO

Are you bottle-feeding?

— **YES** → Have you recently started to use a new nipple for the bottle?

— **YES** → *The hole in the nipple may be the wrong size. See* FEEDING PROBLEMS, p.648.

NO

NO

Is your baby less than 3 months old, AND does the vomit shoot forcibly from your baby's mouth shortly after a feeding?

— **YES** → *This "projectile" vomiting is not necessarily a cause for concern, but if it happens regularly, it may indicate a fault in the stomach outlet. See* CONGENITAL PYLORIC STENOSIS, p.660.

NO

A single episode of vomiting in an otherwise healthy baby is no cause for concern. However, if your baby vomits after all feedings in a six-hour period, consult your physician.

Go to next page

⬇ *Continued from previous page*

Is your baby having frequent, watery bowel movements? — **YES** → *Consult your physician.*
Do not delay!
Your baby may have an infection of the digestive tract.
See GASTROENTERITIS IN INFANTS, p.649.

NO

Is your baby's temperature 100°F (38°C) or above? — **YES** → *See chart* **91** **Fever in infants.**

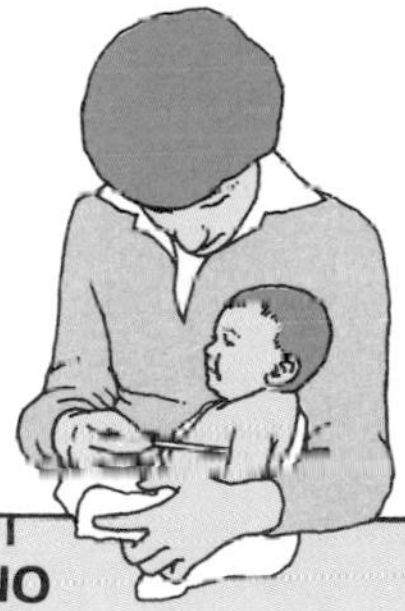

NO

Does your baby have a cough or a runny nose? — **YES** → *A* COLD, p.342, *is probably causing the vomiting. This is no cause for concern unless your baby vomits all feedings in a six-hour period, in which case you should consult your physician.*

NO

Is your baby having bouts of loud, uncontrollable crying as if in great pain? — **YES** →

EMERGENCY
Get medical help now!
Your baby may have an acute abdominal condition such as INTUSSUSCEPTION, p.683, *or* INTESTINAL OBSTRUCTION, p.471.

NO

If you are unable to make a diagnosis from this chart, consult your physician.

Persistent vomiting

If your baby's vomiting is persistent (after all feedings in a six-hour period) and severe, a dangerous amount of body fluid may be lost.

Consult your physician without delay!

88
CHILDREN
0–6 months

Diarrhea in infants
Having runny, watery bowel movements abnormally frequently.

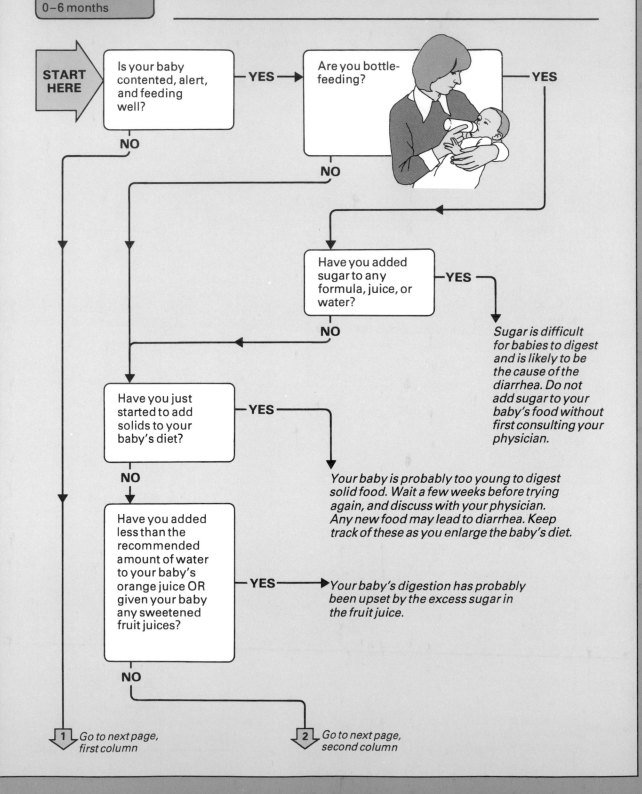

START HERE → Is your baby contented, alert, and feeding well? — **YES** → Are you bottle-feeding? — **YES**

NO (from "Is your baby contented...")

NO (from "Are you bottle-feeding?")

Have you added sugar to any formula, juice, or water? — **YES**

NO

Sugar is difficult for babies to digest and is likely to be the cause of the diarrhea. Do not add sugar to your baby's food without first consulting your physician.

Have you just started to add solids to your baby's diet? — **YES**

NO

Your baby is probably too young to digest solid food. Wait a few weeks before trying again, and discuss with your physician. Any new food may lead to diarrhea. Keep track of these as you enlarge the baby's diet.

Have you added less than the recommended amount of water to your baby's orange juice OR given your baby any sweetened fruit juices? — **YES** →

Your baby's digestion has probably been upset by the excess sugar in the fruit juice.

NO

1 Go to next page, first column

2 Go to next page, second column

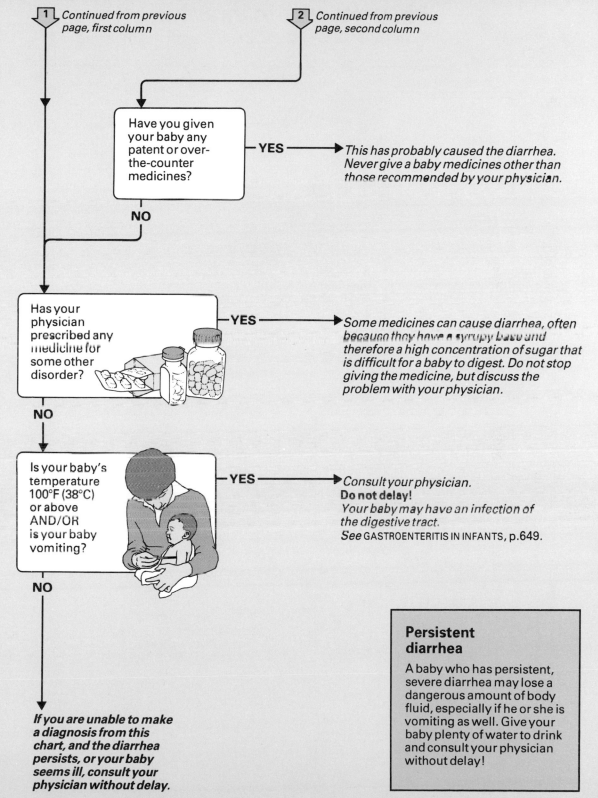

1 Continued from previous page, first column

2 Continued from previous page, second column

Have you given your baby any patent or over-the-counter medicines?

YES → *This has probably caused the diarrhea. Never give a baby medicines other than those recommended by your physician.*

NO

Has your physician prescribed any medicine for some other disorder?

YES → *Some medicines can cause diarrhea, often because they have a syrupy base and therefore a high concentration of sugar that is difficult for a baby to digest. Do not stop giving the medicine, but discuss the problem with your physician.*

NO

Is your baby's temperature 100°F (38°C) or above AND/OR is your baby vomiting?

YES → *Consult your physician.* **Do not delay!** *Your baby may have an infection of the digestive tract.* See GASTROENTERITIS IN INFANTS, p.649.

NO

If you are unable to make a diagnosis from this chart, and the diarrhea persists, or your baby seems ill, consult your physician without delay.

Persistent diarrhea

A baby who has persistent, severe diarrhea may lose a dangerous amount of body fluid, especially if he or she is vomiting as well. Give your baby plenty of water to drink and consult your physician without delay!

89
CHILDREN
0–2 years

Skin problems in infants

Any skin spots, discolored areas, or blisters that may be sore or itchy.

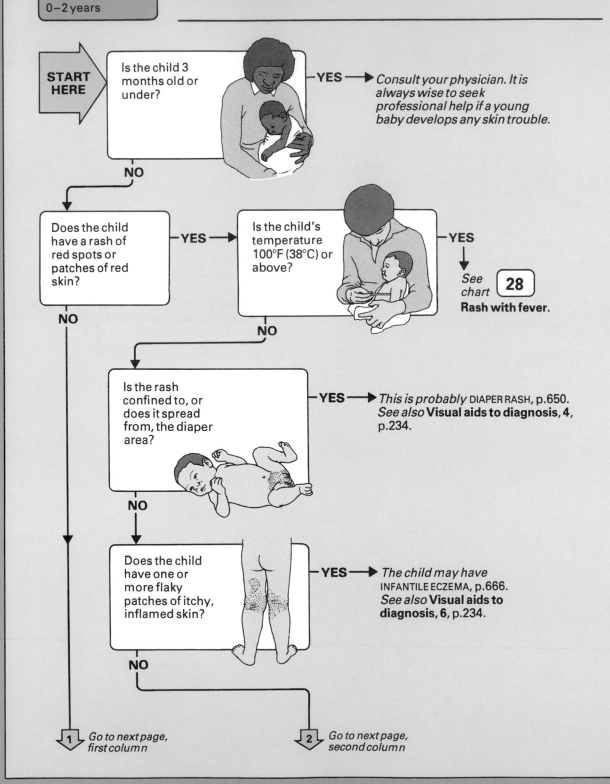

START HERE

Is the child 3 months old or under? —**YES**→ *Consult your physician. It is always wise to seek professional help if a young baby develops any skin trouble.*

NO

Does the child have a rash of red spots or patches of red skin? —**YES**→ **Is the child's temperature 100°F (38°C) or above?** —**YES** → *See chart* **28** **Rash with fever.**

NO

NO

Is the rash confined to, or does it spread from, the diaper area? —**YES**→ *This is probably* DIAPER RASH, p.650. *See also* **Visual aids to diagnosis, 4,** p.234.

NO

Does the child have one or more flaky patches of itchy, inflamed skin? —**YES**→ *The child may have* INFANTILE ECZEMA, p.666. *See also* **Visual aids to diagnosis, 6,** p.234.

NO

1 *Go to next page, first column*

2 *Go to next page, second column*

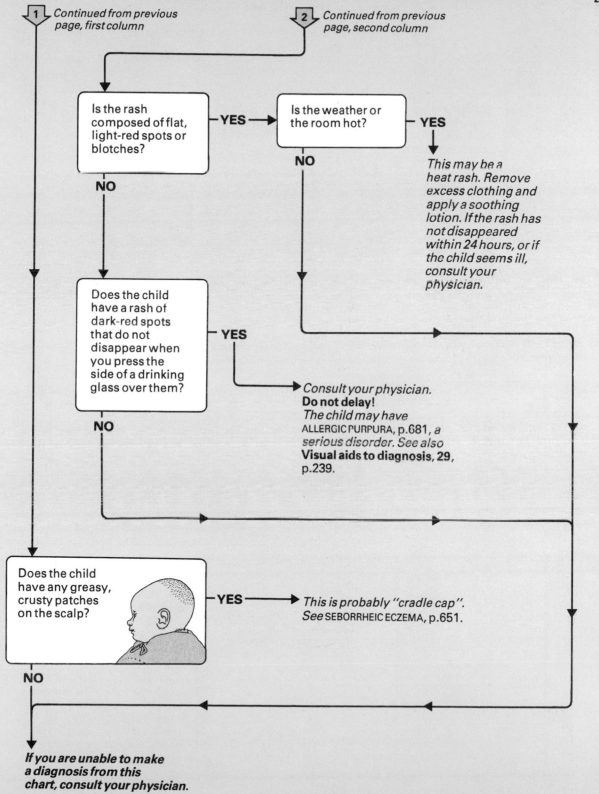

1 Continued from previous page, first column

2 Continued from previous page, second column

Is the rash composed of flat, light-red spots or blotches? — **YES** →

Is the weather or the room hot? — **YES** →

This may be a heat rash. Remove excess clothing and apply a soothing lotion. If the rash has not disappeared within 24 hours, or if the child seems ill, consult your physician.

NO (from first box)

NO (from weather box)

Does the child have a rash of dark-red spots that do not disappear when you press the side of a drinking glass over them? — **YES** →

Consult your physician. **Do not delay!** *The child may have* ALLERGIC PURPURA, p.681, *a serious disorder. See also* **Visual aids to diagnosis, 29**, p.239.

NO

Does the child have any greasy, crusty patches on the scalp? — **YES** →

This is probably "cradle cap". See SEBORRHEIC ECZEMA, p.651.

NO

If you are unable to make a diagnosis from this chart, consult your physician.

90
CHILDREN
0–5 years

Slow weight gain
Failure to gain weight or grow at the expected rate (see the box below and the growth charts on p.645).

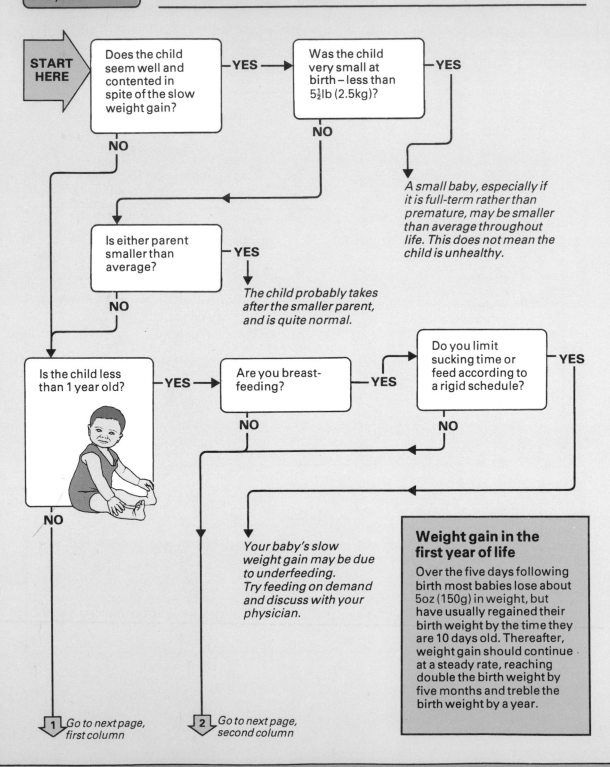

START HERE

Does the child seem well and contented in spite of the slow weight gain?

YES → Was the child very small at birth – less than 5½lb (2.5kg)?

YES →

A small baby, especially if it is full-term rather than premature, may be smaller than average throughout life. This does not mean the child is unhealthy.

NO (from first box)

NO (from second box)

Is either parent smaller than average?

YES

The child probably takes after the smaller parent, and is quite normal.

NO

Is the child less than 1 year old?

YES → Are you breast-feeding?

YES → Do you limit sucking time or feed according to a rigid schedule?

YES

NO (breast-feeding)

NO (rigid schedule)

Your baby's slow weight gain may be due to underfeeding. Try feeding on demand and discuss with your physician.

NO (less than 1 year old)

1 Go to next page, first column

2 Go to next page, second column

Weight gain in the first year of life

Over the five days following birth most babies lose about 5oz (150g) in weight, but have usually regained their birth weight by the time they are 10 days old. Thereafter, weight gain should continue at a steady rate, reaching double the birth weight by five months and treble the birth weight by a year.

1 Continued from previous page, first column

2 Continued from previous page, second column

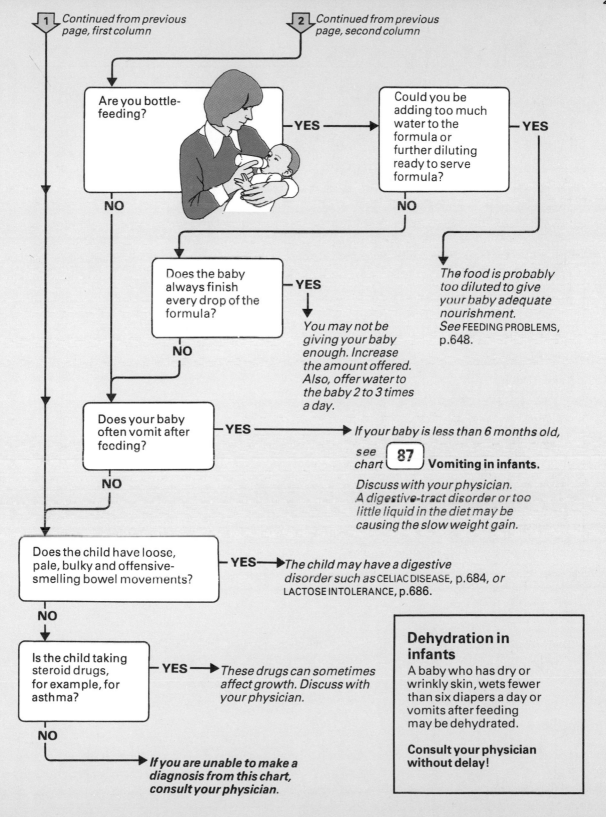

Are you bottle-feeding?

— **YES** → **Could you be adding too much water to the formula or further diluting ready to serve formula?**

— **YES** ↓

The food is probably too diluted to give your baby adequate nourishment. See FEEDING PROBLEMS, p.648.

NO (bottle-feeding) ↓

NO (water) ↓

Does the baby always finish every drop of the formula?

— **YES** ↓

You may not be giving your baby enough. Increase the amount offered. Also, offer water to the baby 2 to 3 times a day.

NO ↓

Does your baby often vomit after feeding?

— **YES** →

If your baby is less than 6 months old,

see chart **87** **Vomiting in infants.**

Discuss with your physician. A digestive-tract disorder or too little liquid in the diet may be causing the slow weight gain.

NO ↓

Does the child have loose, pale, bulky and offensive-smelling bowel movements?

— **YES** → *The child may have a digestive disorder such as* CELIAC DISEASE, p.684, *or* LACTOSE INTOLERANCE, p.686.

NO ↓

Is the child taking steroid drugs, for example, for asthma?

— **YES** → *These drugs can sometimes affect growth. Discuss with your physician.*

NO ↓

If you are unable to make a diagnosis from this chart, consult your physician.

Dehydration in infants

A baby who has dry or wrinkly skin, wets fewer than six diapers a day or vomits after feeding may be dehydrated.

Consult your physician without delay!

91

CHILDREN
0–2 years

Fever in infants

Temperature of 100°F (38°C) or above, which may make a baby flushed and irritable.

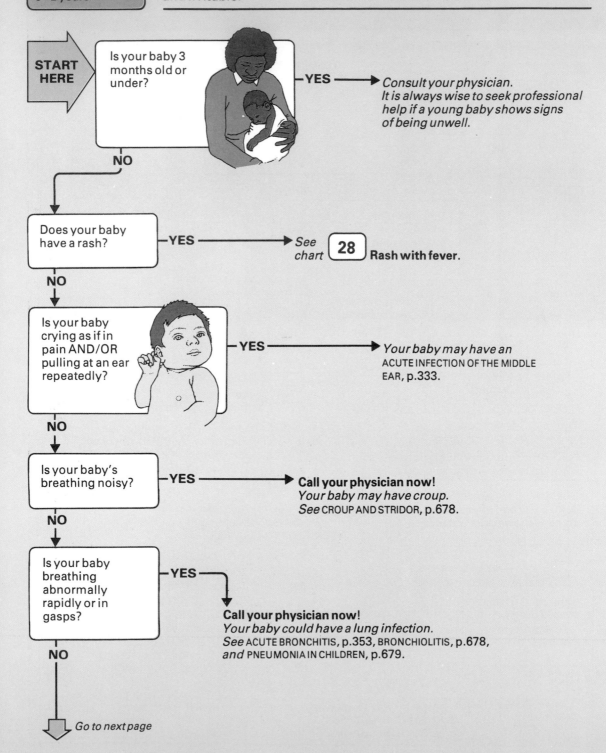

START HERE

Is your baby 3 months old or under? — **YES** → *Consult your physician. It is always wise to seek professional help if a young baby shows signs of being unwell.*

NO

Does your baby have a rash? — **YES** → *See chart* **28** **Rash with fever.**

NO

Is your baby crying as if in pain AND/OR pulling at an ear repeatedly? — **YES** → *Your baby may have an* ACUTE INFECTION OF THE MIDDLE EAR, p.333.

NO

Is your baby's breathing noisy? — **YES** → **Call your physician now!** *Your baby may have croup.* *See* CROUP AND STRIDOR, p.678.

NO

Is your baby breathing abnormally rapidly or in gasps? — **YES** → **Call your physician now!** *Your baby could have a lung infection.* *See* ACUTE BRONCHITIS, p.353, BRONCHIOLITIS, p.678, *and* PNEUMONIA IN CHILDREN, p.679.

NO

Go to next page

Continued from previous page

Does your baby have diarrhea? — **YES** →

Consult your physician.
Do not delay!
This may be an infection of the digestive tract.
See GASTROENTERITIS, p.459.
If your baby is less than 1 year old,
see GASTROENTERITIS IN INFANTS, p.649.

NO

Does your baby have a runny nose? — **YES** →

Has the baby been in contact with a contagious disease, such as measles, in the past 2 weeks? — **YES** →

Your baby may be developing that disease. See CHILDHOOD INFECTIOUS DISEASES, p.698.

NO

Your baby probably has a cold with a fever. See COLDS, p.342.

NO

Is the weather or the room hot AND Is your baby warmly dressed? — **YES**

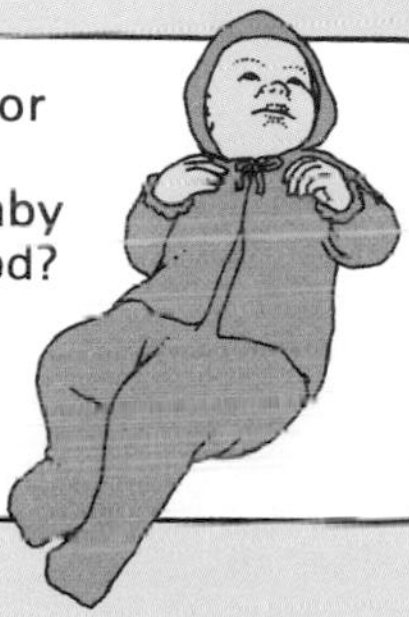

NO

The fever is probably the result of overheating. Try removing some of your baby's clothing and giving a drink of water.

If you are unable to make a diagnosis from this chart, consult your physician. Do not delay if your baby seems very ill or has a temperature of 102°F (39°C) or above.

Convulsions

Sometimes a high temperature in an infant can cause convulsions. (See CONVULSIONS IN CHILDREN, p.667.) If this happens, or if your baby's temperature reaches 102°F (39°C) or above, call your physician immediately.

While waiting for the doctor, see p.698 for advice on dealing with a fever.

92

Fever in children

A temperature of 100°F (38°C) or above, which may make the child flushed, irritable, or sleepy.

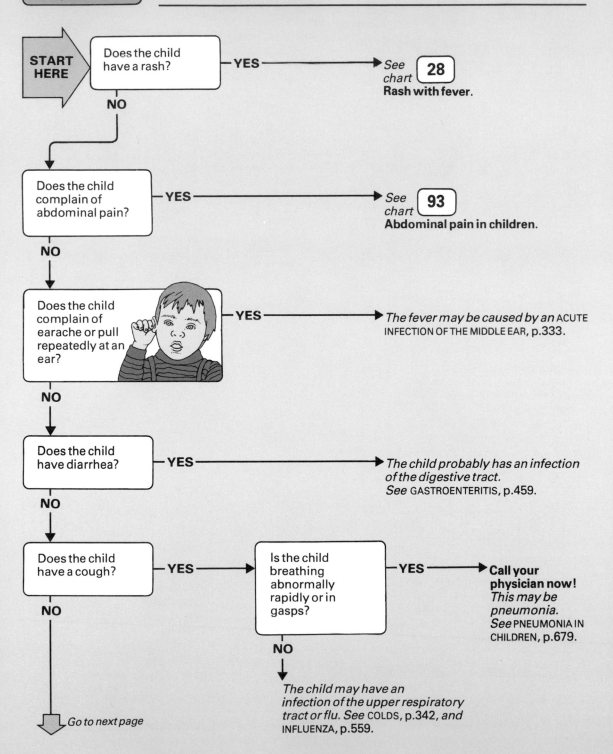

START HERE → Does the child have a rash? — YES → *See chart* **28** **Rash with fever**.

NO

Does the child complain of abdominal pain? — YES → *See chart* **93** **Abdominal pain in children**.

NO

Does the child complain of earache or pull repeatedly at an ear? — YES → *The fever may be caused by an* ACUTE INFECTION OF THE MIDDLE EAR, p.333.

NO

Does the child have diarrhea? — YES → *The child probably has an infection of the digestive tract.* *See* GASTROENTERITIS, p.459.

NO

Does the child have a cough? — YES → Is the child breathing abnormally rapidly or in gasps? — YES → **Call your physician now!** *This may be pneumonia. See* PNEUMONIA IN CHILDREN, p.679.

NO

The child may have an infection of the upper respiratory tract or flu. See COLDS, p.342, *and* INFLUENZA, p.559.

NO

Go to next page

Continued from previous page

Does the child complain of a sore throat, AND/OR is his or her voice faint or hoarse? —— YES —→ *The child may have an infection of the upper respiratory tract.* See TONSILLITIS IN CHILDREN, p.676, PHARYNGITIS, p.350, *and* LARYNGITIS, p.351.

NO
↓

Does the child have a runny nose? —— YES —→ **Has the child been in contact with anyone with a contagious disease such as measles?** —— YES —→ *The child may be in the early stages of an illness such as* MEASLES, p.699.

NO
↓

This is probably a feverish COLD, p.342.

NO
↓

Is there any swelling between the ear and the angle of the jaw, AND/OR is that area painful and tender? —— YES —→ *The child may have* MUMPS, p.700.

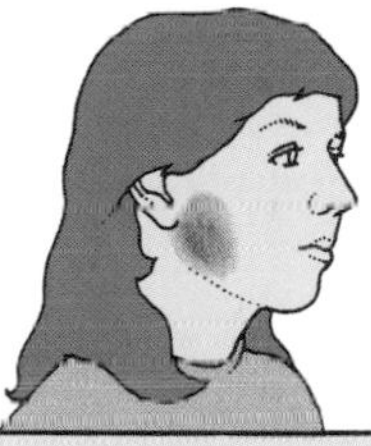

NO
↓

Does the child seem very ill and have two or more of the following symptoms?
☐ vomiting
☐ headache
☐ dislike of strong light
☐ stiff neck, or pain when trying to bend the head forward

—— YES ↓

Call your physician now! *These symptoms suggest the possibility of meningitis.* See MENINGITIS IN BABIES AND CHILDREN, p.668.

NO
↓

If you are unable to make a diagnosis from this chart and the child's temperature remains raised for more than 6 hours, consult your physician.

Convulsions and fever

A high temperature in a child under age 5 may bring on convulsions (see CONVULSIONS IN CHILDREN, p.667). If this happens, call your physician immediately. While waiting for the doctor, see p.698 for advice on dealing with a fever.

Temperature over 102°F

If a child of any age has a temperature of 102°F (39°C) or above call your physician immediately. While waiting for the doctor, see p.698 for advice on dealing with a fever.

93

Abdominal pain in children

Pain between the bottom of the ribcage and the groin, which may vary from a mild stomach ache to severe pain.

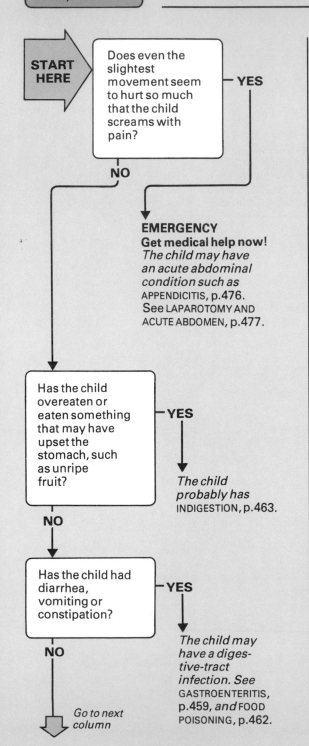

START HERE

Does even the slightest movement seem to hurt so much that the child screams with pain? — **YES**

NO

**EMERGENCY
Get medical help now!**
The child may have an acute abdominal condition such as APPENDICITIS, p.476. *See* LAPAROTOMY AND ACUTE ABDOMEN, p.477.

Has the child overeaten or eaten something that may have upset the stomach, such as unripe fruit? — **YES**

NO

The child probably has INDIGESTION, p.463.

Has the child had diarrhea, vomiting or constipation? — **YES**

NO

The child may have a diges-tive-tract infection. See GASTROENTERITIS, p.459, *and* FOOD POISONING, p.462.

Go to next column

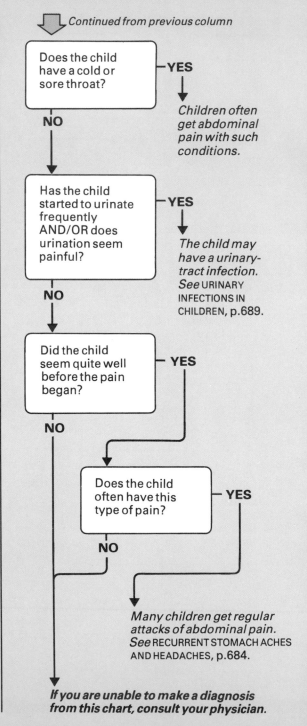

Continued from previous column

Does the child have a cold or sore throat? — **YES**

NO

Children often get abdominal pain with such conditions.

Has the child started to urinate frequently AND/OR does urination seem painful? — **YES**

NO

The child may have a urinary-tract infection. See URINARY INFECTIONS IN CHILDREN, p.689.

Did the child seem quite well before the pain began? — **YES**

NO

Does the child often have this type of pain? — **YES**

NO

Many children get regular attacks of abdominal pain. See RECURRENT STOMACH ACHES AND HEADACHES, p.684.

If you are unable to make a diagnosis from this chart, consult your physician.

94

CHILDREN
2–14 years

Itching in children

Generalized or local irritation of the skin, which makes the child want to scratch.

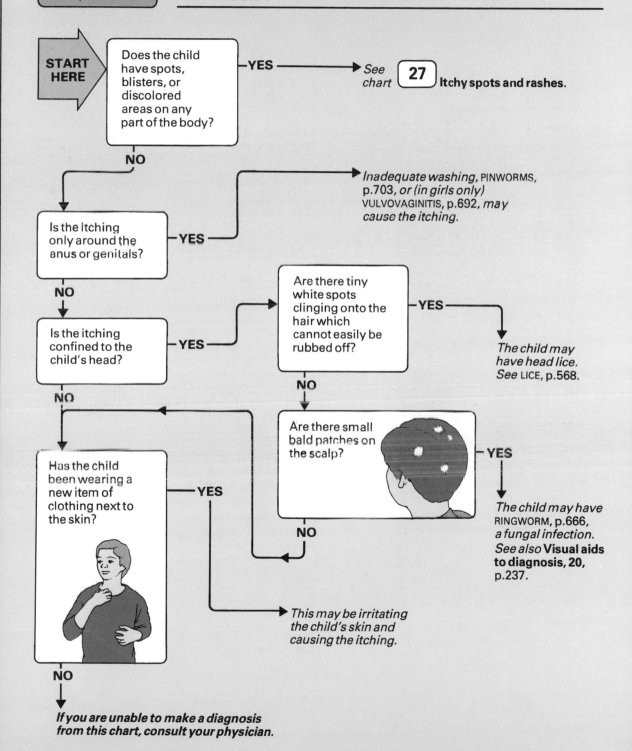

START HERE → Does the child have spots, blisters, or discolored areas on any part of the body?

—**YES** → See chart **27** **Itchy spots and rashes.**

NO ↓

Is the itching only around the anus or genitals?

—**YES** → *Inadequate washing*, PINWORMS, p.703, *or (in girls only)* VULVOVAGINITIS, p.692, *may cause the itching.*

NO ↓

Is the itching confined to the child's head?

—**YES** → Are there tiny white spots clinging onto the hair which cannot easily be rubbed off?

—**YES** → *The child may have head lice. See* LICE, p.568.

NO ↓

Are there small bald patches on the scalp?

—**YES** → *The child may have* RINGWORM, p.666, *a fungal infection. See also* **Visual aids to diagnosis, 20,** p.237.

NO ↓

Has the child been wearing a new item of clothing next to the skin?

—**YES** → *This may be irritating the child's skin and causing the itching.*

NO ↓

If you are unable to make a diagnosis from this chart, consult your physician.

Coughing in children
Noisy expulsion of air from the lungs.

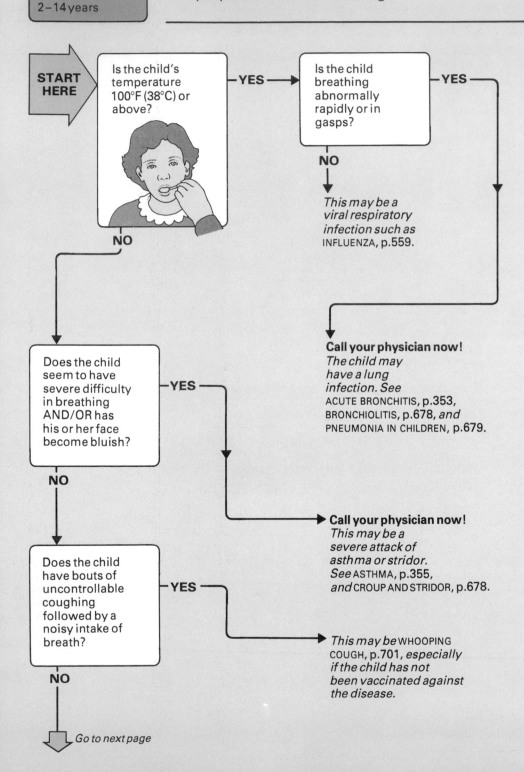

START HERE → Is the child's temperature 100°F (38°C) or above?

— **YES** → Is the child breathing abnormally rapidly or in gasps?

— **YES** → **Call your physician now!** *The child may have a lung infection. See* ACUTE BRONCHITIS, p.353, BRONCHIOLITIS, p.678, *and* PNEUMONIA IN CHILDREN, p.679.

NO ↓

This may be a viral respiratory infection such as INFLUENZA, p.559.

NO ↓ (from temperature question)

Does the child seem to have severe difficulty in breathing AND/OR has his or her face become bluish?

— **YES** → **Call your physician now!** *This may be a severe attack of asthma or stridor. See* ASTHMA, p.355, *and* CROUP AND STRIDOR, p.678.

NO ↓

Does the child have bouts of uncontrollable coughing followed by a noisy intake of breath?

— **YES** → *This may be* WHOOPING COUGH, p.701, *especially if the child has not been vaccinated against the disease.*

NO ↓

Go to next page

⬇ *Continued from previous page*

Is the child's breathing noisy or wheezy? ——**YES**——→ **Could the child have choked on or inhaled a small foreign object, such as a peanut, within the past few days?** ——**YES**——→ *This may be causing the coughing.* See INHALED FOREIGN OBJECT, p.678.

NO ↓

NO ↓

→ *The child may have asthma or croup. See* CROUP AND STRIDOR, p.678, *and* ASTHMA, p.355.

Does the child have a runny or blocked nose?

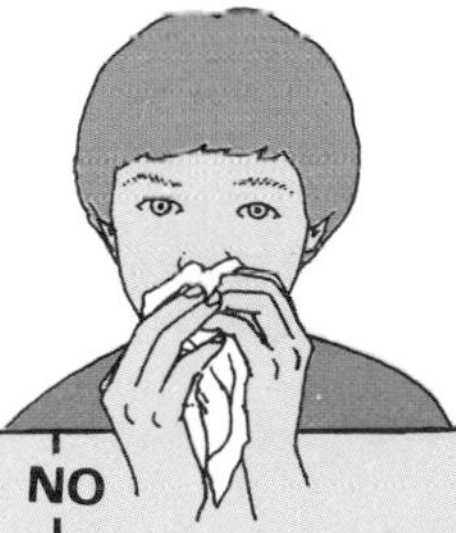

——**YES**——→ *Discharge from the back of the nose may be irritating the throat, causing the child to cough.* See RECURRENT COUGHS AND COLDS, p.680, *and* ADENOIDS, p.677.

NO ↓

Has the child had whooping cough within the last 3 months? ——**YES**——→ *Persistent coughing often follows* WHOOPING COUGH, p.701.

NO ↓

Does anyone in the house smoke heavily OR could the child be smoking? ——**YES**——→ *Smoking, or even living in a smoky environment, can cause coughing in a child. Giving up smoking will benefit your own and the child's health.*

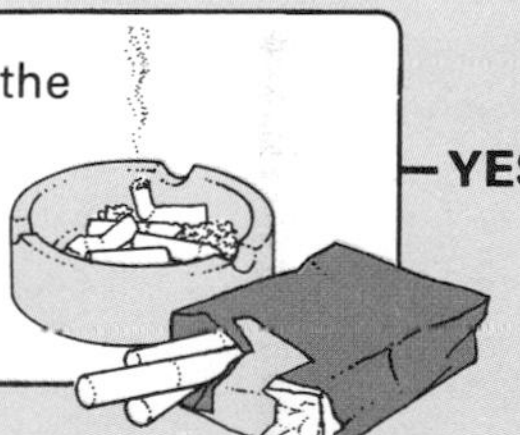

NO ↓

If you are unable to make a diagnosis from this chart, and the cough persists for more than 2 weeks, consult your physician.

96

Swellings in children

Any swellings or lumps in the neck or armpits, which may be tender or painful.

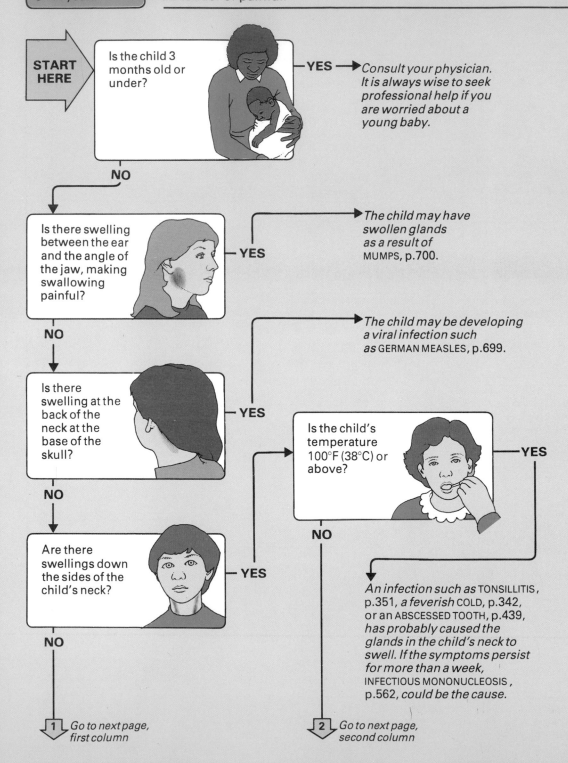

START HERE → Is the child 3 months old or under? — **YES** → *Consult your physician. It is always wise to seek professional help if you are worried about a young baby.*

NO ↓

Is there swelling between the ear and the angle of the jaw, making swallowing painful? — **YES** → *The child may have swollen glands as a result of* MUMPS, p.700.

NO ↓

Is there swelling at the back of the neck at the base of the skull? — **YES** → *The child may be developing a viral infection such as* GERMAN MEASLES, p.699.

NO ↓

Are there swellings down the sides of the child's neck? — **YES** → Is the child's temperature 100°F (38°C) or above? — **YES** →

NO ↓   **NO** ↓

An infection such as TONSILLITIS, p.351, *a feverish* COLD, p.342, or an ABSCESSED TOOTH, p.439, *has probably caused the glands in the child's neck to swell. If the symptoms persist for more than a week,* INFECTIOUS MONONUCLEOSIS, p.562, *could be the cause.*

1 *Go to next page, first column*

2 *Go to next page, second column*

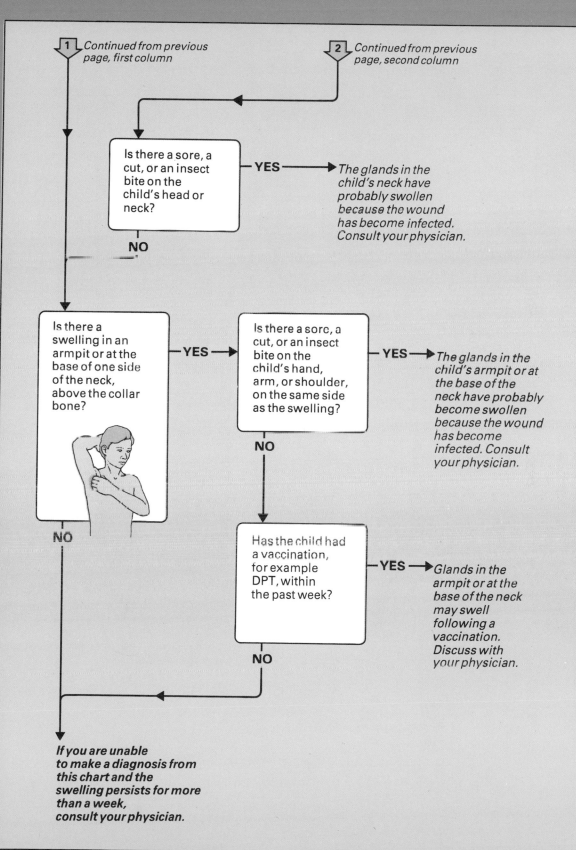

1 Continued from previous page, first column

2 Continued from previous page, second column

Is there a sore, a cut, or an insect bite on the child's head or neck?

YES → *The glands in the child's neck have probably swollen because the wound has become infected. Consult your physician.*

NO

Is there a swelling in an armpit or at the base of one side of the neck, above the collar bone?

YES →

Is there a sore, a cut, or an insect bite on the child's hand, arm, or shoulder, on the same side as the swelling?

YES → *The glands in the child's armpit or at the base of the neck have probably become swollen because the wound has become infected. Consult your physician.*

NO

Has the child had a vaccination, for example DPT, within the past week?

YES → *Glands in the armpit or at the base of the neck may swell following a vaccination. Discuss with your physician.*

NO

NO

If you are unable to make a diagnosis from this chart and the swelling persists for more than a week, consult your physician.

97

CHILDREN
2–14 years

Limping in children

A limp may be accompanied by pain in the affected hip, leg, or foot, and in a young child may result in a reluctance to walk.

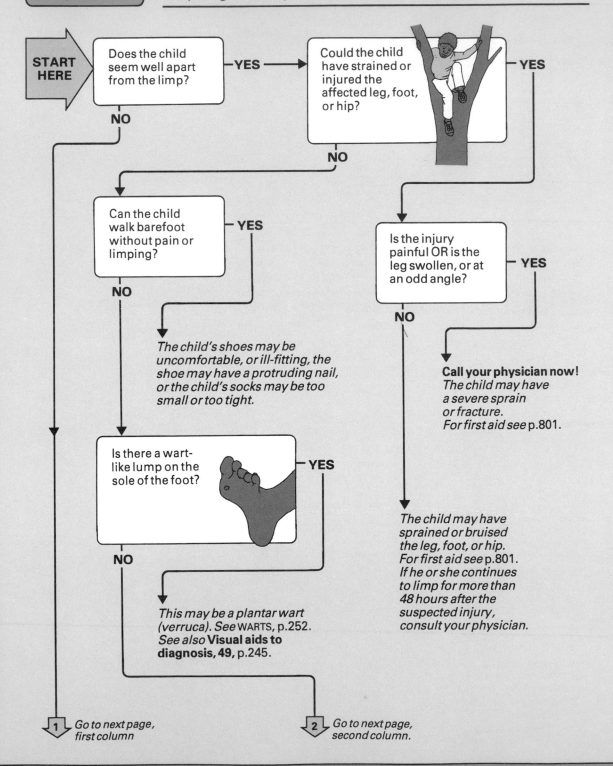

START HERE

Does the child seem well apart from the limp? — **YES** →

Could the child have strained or injured the affected leg, foot, or hip? — **YES** →

NO ↓

NO ↓

Can the child walk barefoot without pain or limping? — **YES**

Is the injury painful OR is the leg swollen, or at an odd angle? — **YES**

NO ↓

NO ↓

The child's shoes may be uncomfortable, or ill-fitting, the shoe may have a protruding nail, or the child's socks may be too small or too tight.

Call your physician now! *The child may have a severe sprain or fracture. For first aid see p.801.*

Is there a wart-like lump on the sole of the foot? — **YES**

NO ↓

The child may have sprained or bruised the leg, foot, or hip. For first aid see p.801. If he or she continues to limp for more than 48 hours after the suspected injury, consult your physician.

This may be a plantar wart (verruca). See WARTS, *p.252. See also* **Visual aids to diagnosis, 49,** *p.245.*

1 *Go to next page, first column*

2 *Go to next page, second column.*

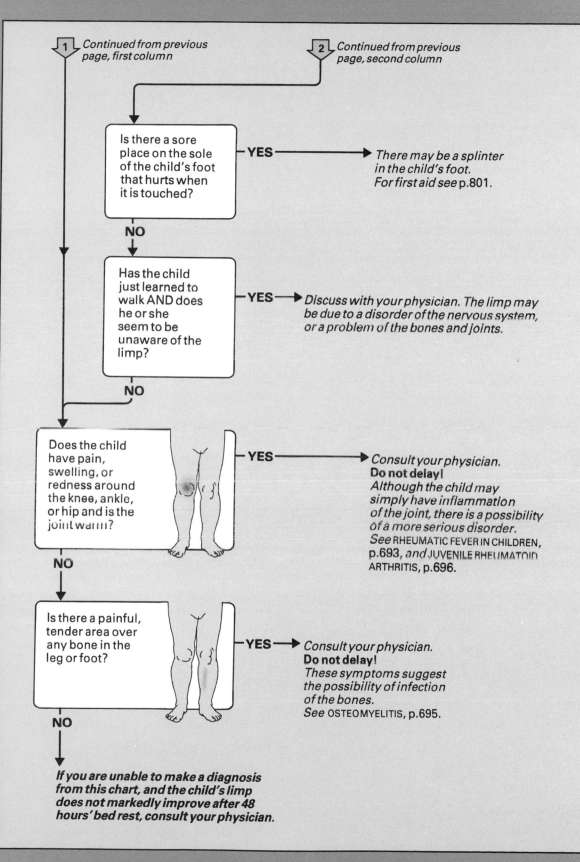

1 Continued from previous page, first column

2 Continued from previous page, second column

Is there a sore place on the sole of the child's foot that hurts when it is touched?

YES → There may be a splinter in the child's foot. For first aid see p.801.

NO

Has the child just learned to walk AND does he or she seem to be unaware of the limp?

YES → Discuss with your physician. The limp may be due to a disorder of the nervous system, or a problem of the bones and joints.

NO

Does the child have pain, swelling, or redness around the knee, ankle, or hip and is the joint warm?

YES → Consult your physician. **Do not delay!** Although the child may simply have inflammation of the joint, there is a possibility of a more serious disorder. See RHEUMATIC FEVER IN CHILDREN, p.693, and JUVENILE RHEUMATOID ARTHRITIS, p.696.

NO

Is there a painful, tender area over any bone in the leg or foot?

YES → Consult your physician. **Do not delay!** These symptoms suggest the possibility of infection of the bones. See OSTEOMYELITIS, p.695.

NO

If you are unable to make a diagnosis from this chart, and the child's limp does not markedly improve after 48 hours' bed rest, consult your physician.

98

ELDERLY
over 65 years

Incontinence in the elderly

Involuntary urination that may vary from a small leakage to complete emptying of the bladder.

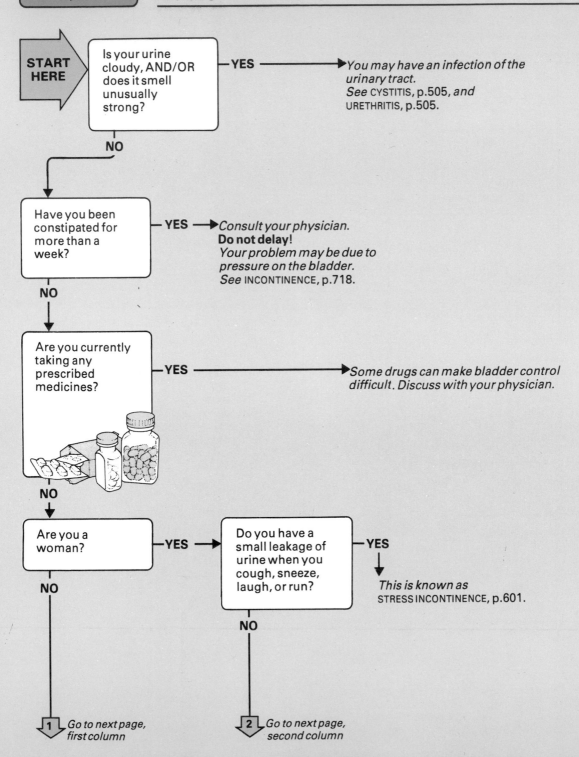

START HERE

Is your urine cloudy, AND/OR does it smell unusually strong? — **YES** → *You may have an infection of the urinary tract.
See* CYSTITIS, *p.505, and* URETHRITIS, *p.505.*

NO

Have you been constipated for more than a week? — **YES** → *Consult your physician.* **Do not delay!** *Your problem may be due to pressure on the bladder. See* INCONTINENCE, *p.718.*

NO

Are you currently taking any prescribed medicines? — **YES** → *Some drugs can make bladder control difficult. Discuss with your physician.*

NO

Are you a woman? — **YES** → **Do you have a small leakage of urine when you cough, sneeze, laugh, or run?** — **YES** ↓ *This is known as* STRESS INCONTINENCE, *p.601.*

NO (woman) | **NO** (leakage)

1 ↓ *Go to next page, first column*

2 ↓ *Go to next page, second column*

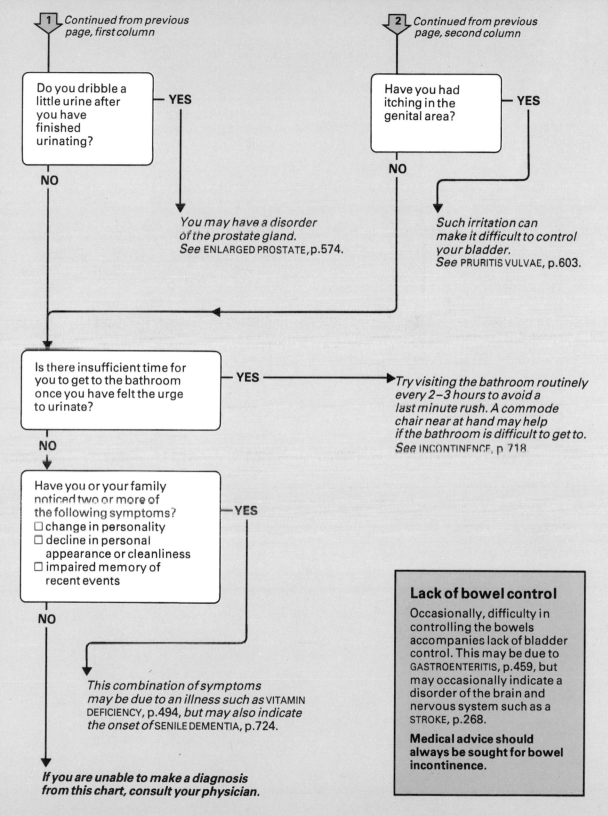

1 Continued from previous page, first column

2 Continued from previous page, second column

Do you dribble a little urine after you have finished urinating?

YES

NO

You may have a disorder of the prostate gland. See ENLARGED PROSTATE, p.574.

Have you had itching in the genital area?

YES

NO

Such irritation can make it difficult to control your bladder. See PRURITIS VULVAE, p.603.

Is there insufficient time for you to get to the bathroom once you have felt the urge to urinate?

YES

NO

Try visiting the bathroom routinely every 2–3 hours to avoid a last minute rush. A commode chair near at hand may help if the bathroom is difficult to get to. See INCONTINENCE, p.718

Have you or your family noticed two or more of the following symptoms?
☐ change in personality
☐ decline in personal appearance or cleanliness
☐ impaired memory of recent events

YES

NO

This combination of symptoms may be due to an illness such as VITAMIN DEFICIENCY, p.494, *but may also indicate the onset of* SENILE DEMENTIA, p.724.

If you are unable to make a diagnosis from this chart, consult your physician.

Lack of bowel control

Occasionally, difficulty in controlling the bowels accompanies lack of bladder control. This may be due to GASTROENTERITIS, p.459, but may occasionally indicate a disorder of the brain and nervous system such as a STROKE, p.268.

Medical advice should always be sought for bowel incontinence.

Confusion in the elderly

Any disorientation of times, places, and events, or loss of contact with reality. Use this chart only after consulting chart 15, **Confusion.**

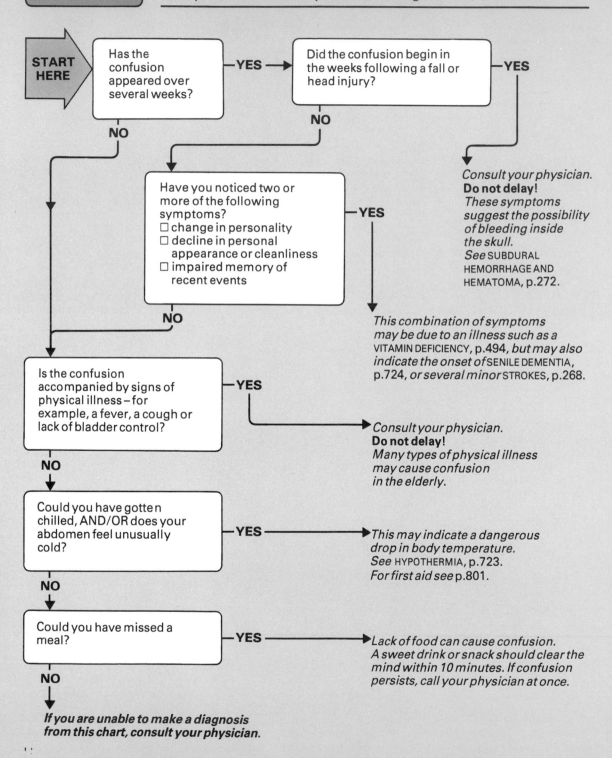

START HERE

Has the confusion appeared over several weeks? — **YES** → Did the confusion begin in the weeks following a fall or head injury? — **YES**

NO

NO

Consult your physician.
Do not delay!
These symptoms suggest the possibility of bleeding inside the skull.
See SUBDURAL HEMORRHAGE AND HEMATOMA, p.272.

Have you noticed two or more of the following symptoms?
☐ change in personality
☐ decline in personal appearance or cleanliness
☐ impaired memory of recent events
— **YES**

NO

This combination of symptoms may be due to an illness such as a VITAMIN DEFICIENCY, p.494, *but may also indicate the onset of* SENILE DEMENTIA, p.724, *or several minor* STROKES, p.268.

Is the confusion accompanied by signs of physical illness – for example, a fever, a cough or lack of bladder control? — **YES**

NO

Consult your physician.
Do not delay!
Many types of physical illness may cause confusion in the elderly.

Could you have gotten chilled, AND/OR does your abdomen feel unusually cold? — **YES**

NO

This may indicate a dangerous drop in body temperature.
See HYPOTHERMIA, p.723.
For first aid see p.801.

Could you have missed a meal? — **YES**

NO

Lack of food can cause confusion. A sweet drink or snack should clear the mind within 10 minutes. If confusion persists, call your physician at once.

If you are unable to make a diagnosis from this chart, consult your physician.

Visual aids to diagnosis

The purpose of this section of the book is to help you identify visual signs of illness. The pictures in the following pages show symptoms that appear on the skin in some disorders, the symptoms of skin disorders themselves, and also certain nail and eye problems. The best way to use these pictures is to adopt the following procedure. If you are concerned about any symptom, whether it is visible or not, begin by consulting the appropriate self diagnosis symptom chart (see p.66). The chart may then refer you not only to an article, but also to one of the visual aid illustrations in this section. Many kinds of skin problems look similar, and you might more easily be misled if you examine a picture *before* you study the chart, so do not use these illustrations as the only step, or even the first step, in the process of self-diagnosis. One additional word of warning: if the picture you have referred to does not really look like your own symptom, it is best to consult a physician. There can be a great deal of variation in the appearance of symptoms from case to case, and only a limited number of examples can be given here. Your physician is familiar, in most cases, with the full range of appearances of a disorder's visual symptoms.

If you are upset by medical illustrations showing sores, rashes, tumors and the like, you should probably not look at this section. The same is true if you are offended by pictures of any portions of the human body.

Birthmarks

An area of discolored skin present from birth (or soon after) may be called a birthmark. There are two main types: a concentration of tiny blood vessels in the skin (a blood vessel nevus), and a patch of discolored skin (a pigmented spot or pigmented nevus). Birthmarks usually are harmless, but they are often unattractive (see Birthmarks, p.652).

2 Port wine stain

A port wine stain is another type of nevus. It usually consists of a flat or pebbled patch of purplish-red skin. Generally this type of birthmark covers quite a large area and occurs singly, most commonly on the face or limbs. Port wine stains usually remain the same throughout life, though occasionally they may fade a little. If such a stain is considered disfiguring, makeup is one remedy or, in rare instances, plastic surgery may be helpful in solving the problem.

3 Pigmented spot

There are several types of pigmented spots. One, called a "cafe au lait" spot, is a flat patch of regularly darkened skin. It is harmless, but if several are present they should be examined by a physician for a hereditary disorder that may accompany this type of birthmark. Pigmented spots are usually small and occur singly. They tend to remain unchanged throughout your life. Makeup can be used to cover them if necessary. In rare cases, especially if a pigmented spot is present at birth and changes later, it may need to be removed surgically.

1 Strawberry nevus

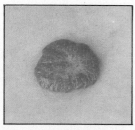

A strawberry nevus is a raised, bright-red patch of skin that grows in the first few months of life. After about six months the mark begins to shrink and fade. Most of these birthmarks disappear by the time the child reaches nine years of age.

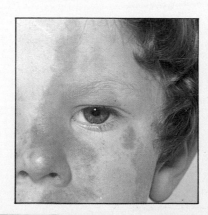

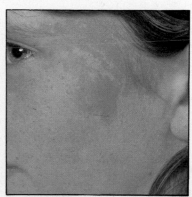

4 Diaper rash

Many babies have this redness around the thighs, buttocks and genitals at some time. The rash varies in severity from slight redness to severe, bright-red inflammation. Urine, wetness and bowel movements irritate the skin. The skin also becomes sore and moist. For mild diaper rash, frequent changing of diapers is often sufficient treatment. Wash the baby's buttocks gently without scrubbing. Also, exposing the baby's buttocks to warm air for a few hours each day, and applying a zinc oxide cream that also contains talcum and vaseline may be helpful (see Diaper rash, p.650).

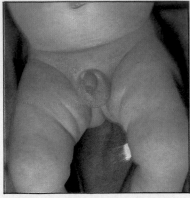

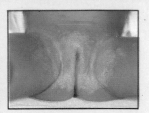

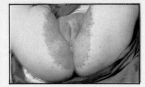

Severe diaper rash (above) may be treated with antibiotic ointment or mild steroid ointment for a while. In a boy, the foreskin may be inflamed, and urination may be difficult.

The photographs above show how the inflamed area is limited to the area of skin covered by the diaper.

Eczema in children

There are many different types of eczema (also known as dermatitis). All types are basically skin inflammations that usually itch. Babies with a tendency to have eczema are very sensitive to irritants. (See the articles on Eczema and dermatitis, p.253, Seborrheic eczema, p.651, and Infantile eczema, p.666.)

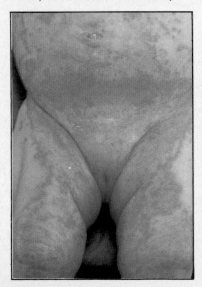

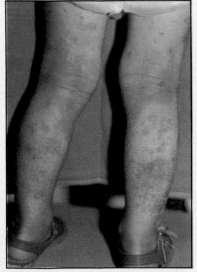

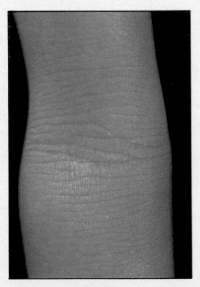

5 Seborrheic eczema in infants

This type of eczema usually takes the form of a red, scaly rash on the face and/or body (as shown above). It may also appear as yellowish, greasy-looking scales on the scalp, where it is known as "cradle cap." Seborrheic eczema usually appears during the first three months of life. Mild cases tend to clear up of their own accord, but occasionally a physician may prescribe a special cream to loosen the scales.

6 Infantile eczema

This red, itchy skin condition (shown in the photograph above) usually appears as a widespread rash in the first year of life, and improves as the child gets older. A mild case requires no specific treatment except regular applications of soothing creams or steroid ointments. Hot water should not be used, but bathing the area with bath oil should do no harm. This type of eczema may persist.

7 Skin changes in recurrent eczema

When eczema becomes a persistent problem, the skin in the affected areas may become dry, leathery, creased-looking and either darker or lighter than the surrounding skin, as a result of recurrent inflammation and repeated rubbing. In the photograph above, the changes occurred on the inside of the elbow, a common site for eczema. Such long-term skin changes can occur in adults as well as children.

Eczema in adults

There are several types of eczema and dermatitis that occur in adults. Some of them are pictured here. See the article on Eczema and dermatitis, p.253, for further information and descriptions.

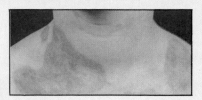

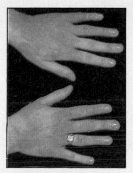

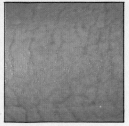

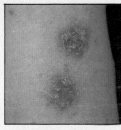

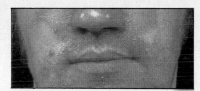

11 Seborrheic eczema on the body

In an adult, seborrheic eczema often occurs in the form of a red, flaky, itchy rash. It commonly appears on the scalp or the chest (above).

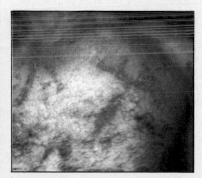

8 Housewife's hand eczema

This type of eczema is common to adults who have sensitive skin and constantly handle irritant chemicals.

9 Eczema in the elderly

Many elderly people have dry skin, particularly on the legs, that may crack and itch. Applying moisturizing ointment or cream, avoiding hot water, and bathing with bath oil may help.

10 Discoid eczema

In discoid eczema, round, red, flaky patches form. The photograph above shows the crusting produced when fluid from the patches oozes and dries. It is relatively rare and may spread.

12 Seborrheic eczema on the face

When seborrheic eczema affects the face (above) it is usually worst in the folds behind the nose, on the forehead, and in the eyebrows.

Contact (allergic) dermatitis

Some types of eczema or dermatitis are caused by certain substances coming into contact with the skin. Touching the substance produces an itchy, flaky rash that is usually limited to the area of contact. Contact dermatitis may be accompanied by allergies to other substances (see Allergies, p.705). A substance that affects one person may not cause a reaction in someone else.

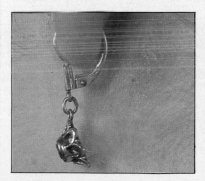

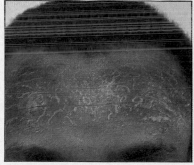

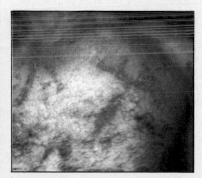

13 Metal contact

Some metals used to make items such as earrings, bracelets, watchbands and rings cause contact dermatitis. Pure gold or silver rarely causes a reaction, but other metals may be mixed in. Nickel often causes dermatitis.

14 Hatband contact

Some substances in fabric can occasionally produce contact eczema. The rash shown above was caused by material in the lining of a hat. The lining in gloves has also been known to cause contact eczema.

15 Plant contact

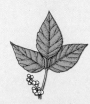

Touching certain plants such as poison ivy, poison oak and poison sumac may cause severe cases of contact dermatitis. The rash may spread to other parts of the body (above).

Allergic reactions

Many people have allergic reactions to external factors. Food, drugs, hair dyes, heat and cold are all known causes. Itchy lumps appear on the skin. They can occur anywhere on the body, and sometimes combine to cover large, patchy areas. Allergic reactions can be very uncomfortable but are usually harmless. However, in a severe reaction to hair dye or a sting in the head region, the scalp, face and throat may swell dramatically and endanger breathing.

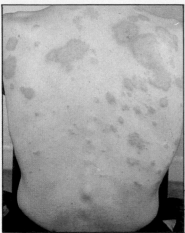

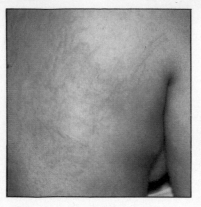

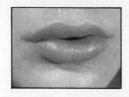

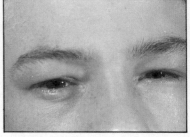

16 Hives

Hives (see p.255) is the most common form of allergic skin reaction. The rash usually takes the form of one or more raised, light-red patches called wheals (above). The wheals have clearly defined edges and are itchy. They can occur anywhere on the body and usually disappear within a few hours. Sometimes, however, they recur for longer periods. If the wheals cause persistent discomfort, a physician may prescribe antihistamine drugs.

17 Dermographism

Dermographism is a particular form of hives usually caused by scratching the skin. It consists of long, raised, narrow wheals (above) that exactly follow the lines where scratching or rubbing has occurred. It is relatively easy to confirm the cause of this type of allergic reaction, even though sometimes the wheals do not appear on the skin until several hours after the irritation that caused them.

18 Angioneurotic edema

When hives affect the face, considerable swelling may result, especially around the eyes (above) and lips (top). In these circumstances there is a risk that the tissues on the inside of the throat may also swell up and cause the person to suffocate. (For further information see the article on Hives, p.255.)

19 Pityriasis rosea

The patches that make up the pityriasis rosea rash have a slightly scaly surface. They look orangy-red in white skin, and dark brown in black skin. The condition is usually itchy and may persist for up to two to three months. It generally disappears by itself, though cream may be prescribed to relieve itching (see Pityriasis rosea, p.262).

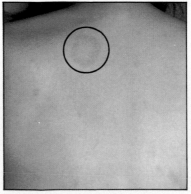

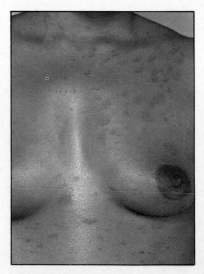

Pityriasis rosea starts as a single, oval patch, known as a herald patch, on the chest or back. (In the picture above the herald patch is circled.) Over the next few weeks several similar, but usually smaller, patches appear on the trunk (as shown on the right), the upper arms, and the thighs.

Bacterial and fungal infections

The skin is susceptible to several types of infection. Two of the most common are shown here: ringworm, which is caused by a fungus, not a worm; and impetigo, a fast-spreading bacterial infection. Most similar skin infections do not clear up, or clear up very slowly, unless you use a prescribed medication. It may be difficult to identify these infections, so if you seem to have one of them, consult your physician.

20 Ringworm

This fungal infection often appears as a red, itchy rash in the shape of a ring. It usually occurs on warm, moist areas such as the groin or between the breasts (below). Within two weeks of the appearance of the first ring, other rings appear close to the first one. Ringworm is rarely a serious condition, but it will heal more rapidly with professional help (see Ringworm, p.666).

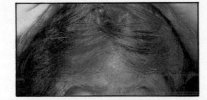

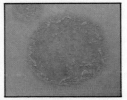

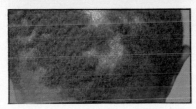

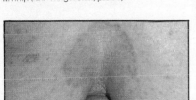

Ringworm on the scalp (above and top) can lead to temporary bald patches.

21 Animal ringworm

Some types of ringworm fungus that usually live on pets or wild animals can live on human skin. The ring (above) may appear on any part of the body and is likely to be more red or inflamed than the rings caused by human ringworm. It is treated in the same way, however. An infected pet should be treated by a veterinarian.

22 Impetigo

This bacterial infection most commonly affects the area around the nose and mouth. The appearance of groups of small blisters is the first sign of the condition. The blisters then burst to form a yellowish-brown crust. The infected area gradually spreads, and the condition usually has to be treated with antibiotic tablets.

Pictured at right is a case of impetigo at an early stage of the infection. Far right, the condition is shown at an advanced stage, after the yellowish-brown crust has formed (see Impetigo, p.257).

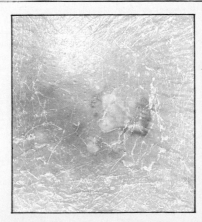

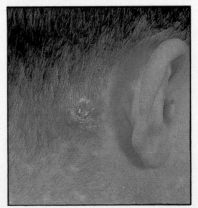

23 Boils

A boil is the result of several hair follicles becoming infected and inflamed. It starts as a red, usually painful, lump that gradually becomes swollen with pus. A head forms and the pain generally increases, until eventually the boil bursts. Boils may occur anywhere on the body (see Boils and carbuncles, p.251.)

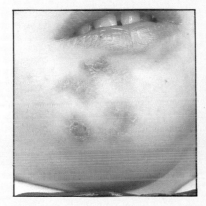

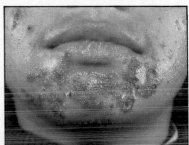

24 Cold sores

Cold sores are small blisters that are often found on the face, around the lips and nose. The blisters contain small areas of infection caused by a virus, herpes simplex. The infection occurs in two stages, as shown in the photo-graphs below. These blisters tend to appear when you are feeling tired and run down, when you have some other infection such as a cold (hence their name), or when you are exposed to wind or sunshine (see Cold sores, p.451).

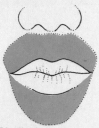

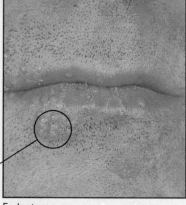

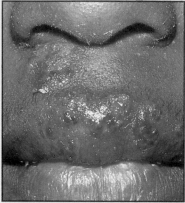

Distribution
Cold sores most commonly develop either around or on the lips.

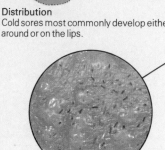

Early stages
In the early stages of cold sores, a group of tiny blisters appears (the inset photograph at left shows the blisters in more detail). Around the blisters is an area of red, in-flamed skin. The early stage may produce little or no discomfort in a child; adults tend to have burning, itching and pain.

Late stage
Within a few days of their appearance the blisters (shown above left) enlarge, burst and dry out. The yellowish crust that forms (above) is similar in appearance to the crust that forms in impetigo (see p.237). If the blisters persist or recur, you should be sure that you see your physician.

25 Shingles

Like cold sores (above), shingles is caused by a virus – in this case, herpes zoster, the same virus that causes chickenpox (see opposite page). Be-fore the rash appears, there is a burn-ing or stabbing pain in the affected area (see Shingles, p.562).

Distribution
Shingles usually develops along a long, thin area on only one side of the body. The trunk and the face are the most common sites. On the trunk, the rash often affects front and back.

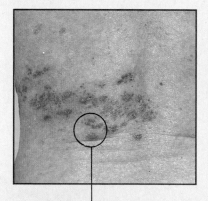

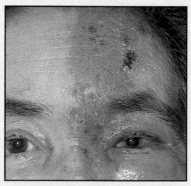

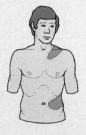

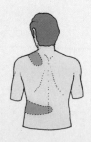

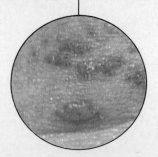

The shingles rash
The rash of shingles consists of numerous small blisters, shown in detail in the photo-graph at left. Within a week the blisters become dry and scab over. Then they slow-ly fade away. If the rash occurs near an eye (as shown above), it may cause severe pain, redness and watering in the eye. If this occurs, see your physician without delay. When the rash affects the body (above left) it tends to occur in a long, narrow strip along a rib. If you have shingles more than once, see your physician.

Common childhood infections

Several infectious diseases are usually caught in childhood. Three common examples – measles, German measles, and chickenpox – are shown below. These three infections each produce a characteristic skin rash that aids identifica-

tion. These diseases can have serious complications. Be sure to consult your physician if you or your child appears to have one of them. See also Childhood infectious diseases, p.698.

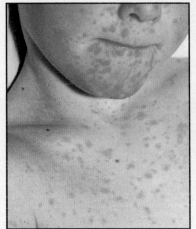

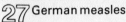

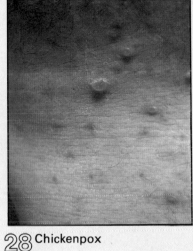

26 Measles

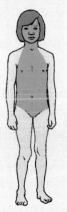

The rash of measles is flat, dark-pink spots that often join to form larger blotches (above). At first, the rash mainly affects the face, usually starting on the forehead and behind the ears. The rash spreads to cover the trunk (left) but it rarely appears on the limbs (see Measles, p.099).

27 German measles

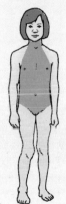

The rash of German measles (above) tends to be less severe than the measles rash (above left). German measles produces tiny, light-red spots that merge to form an evenly colored patch. The rash usually covers the neck and trunk (left). It usually lasts only a few days (see German measles, p.699).

28 Chickenpox

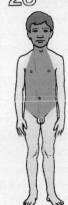

This infection is caused by the same virus that is responsible for shingles (opposite page). The photograph above shows the characteristic small, fluid-filled blisters. The rash covers mainly the face and trunk (left). It can also affect the scalp and the inside of the mouth (see Chickenpox, p.700).

Development of chickenpox

There are three typical stages in the development of the chickenpox rash. In the first, tiny red spots appear. Then the spots enlarge and fill with fluid to form raised blisters. In the third stage the blisters burst, dry out and crust over. They are very itchy.

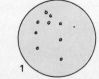

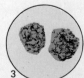

1 Small red spots
2 Fluid-filled blisters
3 Crusted scabs

29 Purpura

A "purpuric" rash may be produced by any of a number of disorders in which blood leaks through the walls of small blood vessels and into the skin. The rash consists of many flat, dark-red or

purplish spots or blotches. See Thrombocytopenia, p.425, Allergic purpura, p.681, and Skin problems of the elderly, p.722.

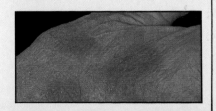

30 Acne

In acne, there is persistent, recurrent development of various types of spots on the skin. The condition is extremely common during adolescence – slightly more so in young men – and in most cases, but not all, it fades away during the late teens or early twenties (for further information see Acne, p.708).

Distribution
Acne pimples commonly appear on the face, mainly around the mouth, and often on the chest, shoulders, neck and the upper (and occasionally lower) portion of the back.

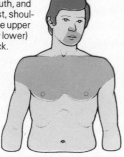

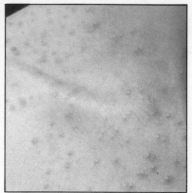

A pimple develops

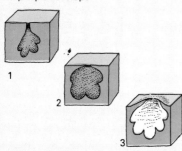

1
2
3

The opening of a sebaceous, or oil-producing, gland near the surface of the skin becomes blocked (1). There is a build-up of oily sebum within the gland (2). This accumulation leads to localized inflammation (redness and swelling) (3).

Blackheads
One type of pimple that appears in acne is the blackhead (photograph above). The black area for which it is named is a tiny plug of dark material stuck in a skin pore. Some experts believe the plug is a mixture of keratin and sebum and the color is melanin (the skin pigment). The "black" of the blackhead is therefore not dirt. Blackheads rarely become inflamed unless they are picked at or squeezed.

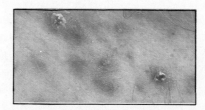

Pimples
The typical pimples that occur in acne (photograph above) may develop from blackheads (above left). Others develop from whiteheads. If picked or scratched, the pimples may become infected and pus-filled. Some acne pimples are just small red lumps, others have white tops. They tend to develop and then fade over several weeks.

Severe acne
The most severe form of acne produces painful, fluid-filled lumps called cysts under the skin (photograph left). The cysts may be up to 2 cm (about ¾ in) across, often persist for many weeks, and may leave pitted, scarred areas of skin.

31 Rosacea

Rosacea, sometimes called acne rosacea, occurs mainly in adults. The skin on the face, principally the cheeks and the nose, becomes abnormally red and flushed. After a time, pus-filled raised spots also appear in the affected skin. Why this occurs is not known. The rash tends to spread or become more prominent after eating hot or spicy food, or drinking alcohol. Rosacea is most common in women over 30 years of age (see Acne vulgaris and acne rosacea, p.255).

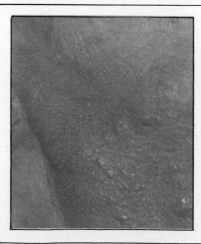

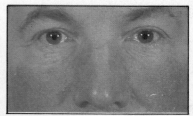

Distribution
Most people who get rosacea have the rash on their cheeks (right). The sides of the nose may also be affected (photograph above).

Abnormal skin formation

A number of skin conditions, some of which are shown below, are characterized by a fault in the normal maintenance of skin tissue. Though not always harmful to physical health, these conditions can cause embarrassment because they are unattractive. This often leads to considerable mental stress.

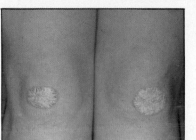

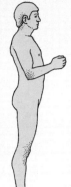

Distribution
Common sites for psoriasis are the knees, elbows and scalp.

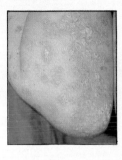

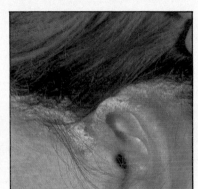

32 Psoriasis

Psoriasis consists of patches of thickened, silvery-white, scaly skin (photograph above). The patches often have a red rim. Skin affected by psoriasis generally causes little itching, but in a few cases it may be sore (see Psoriasis, p.254, for further information).

Severe psoriasis
In more severe cases of psoriasis (photograph above) the characteristic small patches join together to produce a more extensive area of affected skin. The fingernails and toenails (see p.245) become stippled, thickened and roughened.

Psoriasis of the scalp
When psoriasis occurs on the scalp, scaly, sometimes lumpy patches appear. In most cases the hair of the scalp remains unaffected, but sometimes temporary hair loss occurs. It is rare for psoriasis to spread from the scalp to the face.

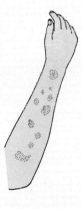

33 Lichen planus

This skin condition is extremely variable in appearance. In one typical example (photograph above), a rash of numerous, tiny, purplish-red lumps appears. The lumps are not scaly, but you may be able to see small white marks on the surface of the skin. The cause of the condition is not known (for further information see Lichen planus, p.261).

Distribution
Lichen planus may occur anywhere on your body, but the usual sites are the arms, wrists (above) and legs. It often also appears on the lining of the mouth (see Oral lichen planus, p.452).

Scar tissue

Whenever the skin is damaged, it is repaired by scar tissue. Scar tissue is formed by special cells called fibroblasts that manufacture collagen and other protein substances. The material they produce is stronger and tougher than ordinary skin, but tends to shrink slightly with age.

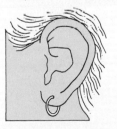

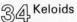

34 Keloids

A keloid is formed because of an abnormality in the mechanism for producing scar tissue. The scar tissue does not stop growing. Keloids can develop after an operation, a vaccination, or an injury. Even an ear lobe pierced for an earring (above left) may form a keloid (above right). The growths are more common in blacks than whites (see Keloid, p.261).

Warts and moles

Warts and moles are not related conditions, but they are sometimes thought to be because they look alike. Warts are small areas of long-standing viral infection. Moles are areas of skin that are heavily pigmented with melanin, the substance responsible for general skin coloring. Warts vary in appearance. Some common types are shown below. Warts are harmless, but may be a nuisance. A mole that is present from birth may develop into a malignant melanoma (opposite page). If this occurs it should be removed by a physician.

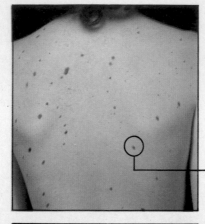

35 Moles

Moles can occur anywhere on the body. They are small, roughly circular areas of skin that are much darker than the surrounding skin. Large moles may have coarse hairs growing out of them. Some moles are present from birth. In some people a few develop during childhood.

Appearance
The dark patch that constitutes a mole may be flat or raised above the surrounding skin (inset photograph left).

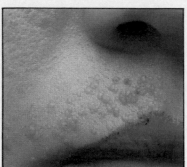

36 Plane warts

Plane warts are flat-topped, brownish spots that usually have a smooth surface. They often appear in groups, and may develop on the face or the back of the hand along the line of a scratch. This type of wart is most common in children and young adults. Plane warts (photograph above) commonly occur on the skin near the upper lip (see Warts, p.252).

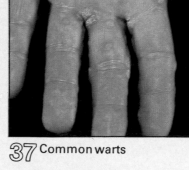

37 Common warts

This type of wart usually grows on the hands (photograph above) or on the feet (where they are known as verrucas – see p.245). The typical common wart is a hard lump with a roughened, cauliflower-like surface. Tiny black flecks may be visible in the body of the wart.

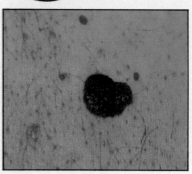

38 Seborrheic warts

These warts (above) are dark, sometimes rough-surfaced lumps that often appear on the skin in large numbers in later life. Like all warts, they are harmless, but because of their similarity to a malignant melanoma (opposite page) their appearance should always be reported to your physician. Seborrheic warts are not true warts (see Abnormal skin pigmentation, p.262).

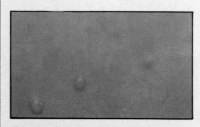

39 Molluscum contagiosum

These tiny, pale lumps are filled with cheesy material. They are not true warts, but like warts, they are caused by a viral infection. They appear in groups usually in children, especially those with eczema.

40 Sebaceous cysts

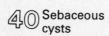

These cysts (right) are sometimes mistaken for warts, although they are not related. A sebaceous cyst typically appears as a soft, smooth, yellowish lump just under the surface of the skin. Sometimes a tiny dark dot can be seen in the skin over the center of the cyst. The scalp is a common site for these harmless growths (see Sebaceous cysts, p.261).

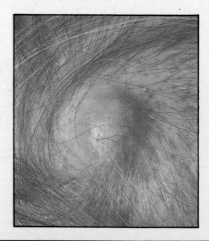

Skin cancers

There are three main types of *malignant*, or life-threatening, skin growths. These are basal cell carcinoma, squamous cell carcinoma and malignant melanoma. Skin cancers tend to be somewhat variable in appearance. As with most other malignant growths, early recognition and removal give a good chance of cure. For this reason, always report any suspicious lump, sore, or ulcer on the skin to your physician if it persists for more than a week.

41 Basal cell carcinoma

This type of skin cancer tends to grow very slowly, and rarely, if ever, spreads. It is variable in appearance. One common version (right) is the ulcerated (open-sore) form (see Basal cell carcinoma, p.258).

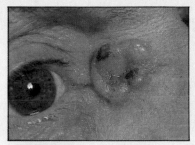

Common sites
Basal cell carcinomas usually appear on the face (left), near an eye or next to the nose.

Encrusted type
A basal cell ulcer can form a scab (round photograph right). When the scab detaches, the ulcer will show again.

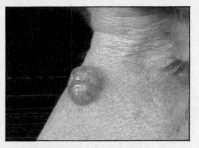

Cystic type
A cystic type of basal cell carcinoma growing on the bridge of the nose appears as a relatively smooth, skin-colored lump (photograph above). It gradually enlarges and may have blood vessels visible on the surface.

42 Squamous cell carcinoma

Common sites
Squamous cell growths typically appear on the face, especially on the lips (left) or near the ears, and on the hands (see Squamous cell carcinoma, p.259).

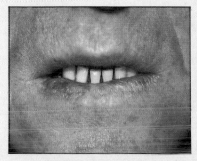

Ulcerated type
A typical ulcerated type of squamous cell carcinoma (above) is a persistent open sore that gradually enlarges.

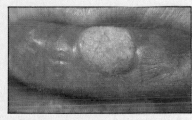

Warty type
Squamous cell carcinoma sometimes appears as a small, hard nodule that gradually enlarges into a wart-like lump (above). Like the ulcerated type (above left), the warty type of carcinoma is not usually painful.

43 Malignant melanoma

There are four kinds of malignant melanoma, but only one is shown here (right). The three that are not shown are: a large brown fleck on the face, which occurs in the elderly and takes 15 to 20 years to become malignant; a blue, brown or black lump that bleeds easily; and a dark area that enlarges near the tip of a finger.

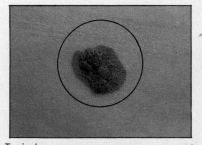

Typical appearance
A malignant melanoma usually takes the form of a dark, slightly raised lump (photograph above). Such a malignant growth may also occur in an existing mole, and cause it to enlarge and perhaps bleed.

IMPORTANT

The two photographs above show two harmless skin conditions: a seborrheic wart (above left) and a raised mole (above right). The third photograph in this box is of malignant melanoma, a very similar condition that is life-threatening if it is not treated in its very early stages. Always report a new pigmented spot to your physician (see Abnormal skin pigmentation, p.262).

Abnormal skin coloration

In these conditions, there is an abnormality in the natural coloring of the skin. The conditions are not harmful to general health but may, particularly in the case of vitiligo, cause mental or emotional stress because of their appearance (see Abnormal skin pigmentation, p.262).

44 Vitiligo

In vitiligo, irregularly shaped patches of skin on certain parts of the body (drawing right) lose their normal color and become much paler than the surrounding skin (photographs right). The nature of the skin surface and its texture do not alter. The cause of the condition is not clearly understood, but it may be an *autoimmune* problem; that is, a disorder of the body's natural defense system. If the appearance of the patches is embarrassing, you can learn to apply a special make-up to hide them.

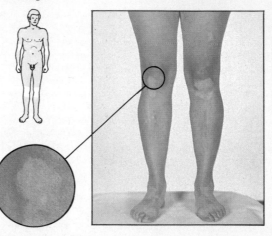

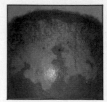

Vitiligo of the scalp
When vitiligo occurs on the scalp (above) it sometimes causes hairs in the affected areas to turn white.

45 Perfume pigmentation

Some perfumes, colognes and aftershaves contain chemicals that, when exposed to sunlight, temporarily increase pigmentation in the skin where they are applied. The skin returns to normal once the use of the chemical is discontinued. The neck (right) may be particularly susceptible. Some individuals are more susceptible to this condition than others.

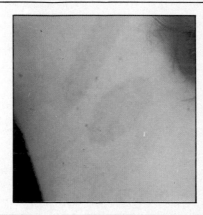

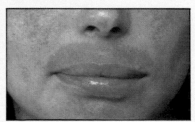

46 Chloasma

This condition may be due to hormonal changes such as those caused by oral contraceptives, pregnancy, or cirrhosis of the liver. Patches of skin become darker.

47 Jaundice

Skin color
Jaundice is not a disease, but a sign of one of several underlying diseases (see Jaundice, p.485). It is due to a build-up in the blood of bilirubin, a yellowish-brown substance that is normally extracted from the bloodstream by the liver and excreted in bile. In jaundice, the skin takes on a yellowish or greenish tinge (photograph right). The whites of the eyes also turn yellow (far right). The development of jaundice always requires the attention of a physician.

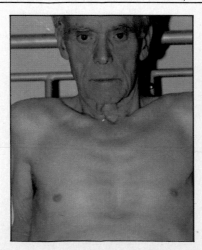

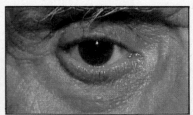

Eye color
Besides yellowing of the skin (left), jaundice also causes the whites of the eyes to take on a yellowish color (above). The change in eye coloration is usually a more reliable sign of jaundice than yellowing of the skin.

Common foot disorders

Athlete's foot and verrucas are common and harmless but irritating. Most other foot problems are also minor, but older people and those with diseases that may affect circulation (for example, diabetes) should not neglect sores, cuts and other foot conditions, because they may become serious without attention.

48 Athlete's foot

Athlete's foot (right) is a fungal infection in which the skin of the foot becomes damp, inflamed and itchy. The infection particularly affects the skin between and underneath the toes. The skin may peel and crack, sometimes producing sore areas. In severe cases (far right) the nails are also infected and look thickened and discolored (see Athlete's foot, p.256).

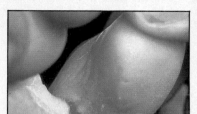

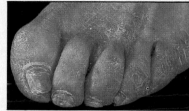

An example of severe athlete's foot that has affected the toenails.

49 Verruca

A verruca (right) is a name for the common wart (or plantar wart) on the sole of the foot (see Warts, p.202, and Warts and moles, p.242). Unlike other warts, the verruca does not usually grow as a raised lump. It is a flat area of hard, tough skin. Despite its flatness, walking on a verruca often feels like walking with a stone in your shoe.

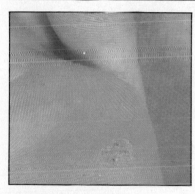

How a verruca develops

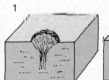

When a verruca first grows, it may be a raised lump like a common wart elsewhere on the body (1). It soon becomes pushed into the surface of the skin (2), which makes it more difficult to treat than a common wart elsewhere

Common nail disorders

Some disorders, such as psoriasis, may affect the nails as well as the skin. In other cases, such as paronychia, it is only the nails, and perhaps the cuticles and nail beds, that are involved (see Deformed and discolored nails, p.265).

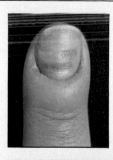

51 Paronychia

In this nail disorder the cuticles and nail fold become swollen and inflamed as a result of infection by bacteria or fungi. If the problem (left) persists, the nail itself may become darkened and deformed (see Paronychia, p.264).

50 Deformed nails

Deformed nails (right) are usually the result of generalized illness, when healthy nail growth is disrupted, or of injury to the nail bed at the base of the nail. Once the cause is removed the nails should grow healthily again, though it may take some months for the deformed portions to grow out completely (see Deformed and discolored nails, p.265).

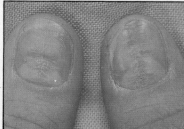

52 Psoriasis of the nails

Psoriasis may cause the nails to become pitted and roughened (above). In other cases, the nails become thickened. Only rarely are the nails alone affected by psoriasis (see p.254 and p.241). Sometimes the nail becomes completely detached.

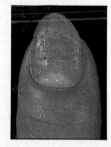

Common eye disorders

The common eye disorders shown below are all treatable. Sties and conjunctivitis are due to infection of the eye. Corneal ulcers may be caused by either infection or physical injury. Several other eye conditions, among them glaucoma (see p.320), do not produce obvious changes in the appearance of the eye, but do affect vision. Do not ignore unexplained or sudden changes in vision.

53 Sty

A sty (right) is an infected eyelash follicle (see Sty, p.314). A sty resembles a boil (see p.251) in that the follicle (the pit in the skin where the eyelash is formed) becomes inflamed and pus-filled due to a bacterial infection. Sties are uncomfortable and may be quite painful, but they usually clear up within a week if you apply warm, wet compresses and an antibacterial eye ointment.

54 Corneal ulcer

An ulcer on the cornea causes pain and discomfort in the eye, and may make the white of the eye turn pink or red. In addition, you may be able to see the ulcer as a whitish patch (right) and your vision in that eye may be misted over or otherwise impaired (see Corneal ulcers and infections, p.316). This condition needs immediate medical attention.

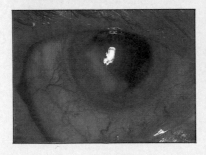

55 Conjunctivitis

In conjunctivitis, the surface of the eye and the inside lining of the eyelids, all of which are covered with a membrane called the conjunctiva, become inflamed and sore. The eye looks red and bloodshot, and there may be a discharge that makes it feel sticky and "gummed up." If the lower eyelid is pulled down (below) the redness of the lower eyelid lining is clearly visible (see Conjunctivitis, p.317).

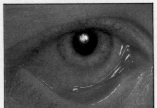

56 Foreign body on the cornea

A speck of grit or other small particle that enters the eye is usually moved to the edge of the eye by blinking, and you can remove it yourself (see within Accidents and emergencies, p.801). A corneal foreign body (below) needs expert medical care.

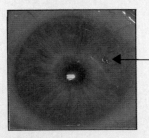

A foreign body stuck in the cornea, the dome-shaped front of the eye (see diagram right and photograph above) is a serious problem if mishandled. DO NOT attempt to move a particle embedded in the cornea. Get a physician to do it for you.

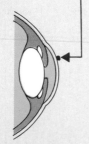

57 Chalazion

A chalazion (also called a meibomian cyst) is a painless swelling on the edge of the eyelid. Chalazions vary in size. Some are so small that they are barely noticeable, but others grow to be as large as a pea. Some become red and swollen (right), probably due to infection. Sometimes a chalazion will disappear by itself. In other cases, they have to be removed surgically (see Lumps on the eyelid, p.315).

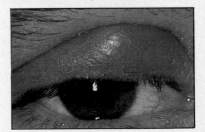

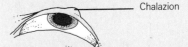

Chalazion

58 Xanthelasma

These are small patches of yellow material that grow in the skin around the eyes, particularly near the nose (right). In most cases they are harmless, but they can signify an underlying disease, so they should always receive medical attention. The patches are painless (see Lumps on the eyelid, p.315).

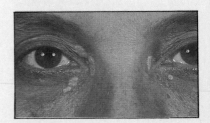

Eye problems in old age

The eye problems covered below occur mainly, but not exclusively, in older people. Entropion and ectropion are unlikely to pass unnoticed as they usually cause irritation and discomfort. Cataracts are much more difficult to detect at first.

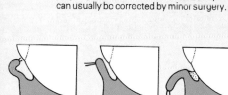

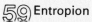 59 Entropion

In entropion the eyelid turns inwards ("in-turned eyelash"), so that the eyelashes rub on the surface of the eyeball. This irritates and inflames the eye (below) and may cause much pain and discomfort. Entropion can usually be corrected by minor surgery.

60 Ectropion

In ectropion (see p.315) the lower eyelid becomes slack and hangs away from the eyeball. This gives the appearance of "out-turned eyelashes" (above). The lining of the lid and the eye itself dry out and become sore. Also, tear fluid cannot drain away properly and runs down the face. Ectropion can usually be corrected by minor surgery.

61 Cataract

A cataract is an opaque area in the normally clear tissue of a healthy lens. In an advanced cataract (below and bottom) a misty circular area within the normally black-looking pupil is large and clearly visible. The upper eyelid has been pulled up slightly to give a clearer view of the cataract (see Cataracts, p.319).

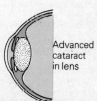

Lens

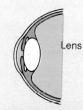

Advanced cataract in lens

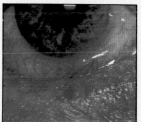

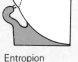

Entropion   Normal   Ectropion

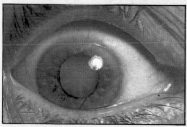

Other eye problems

62 Exophthalmos

Exophthalmos is the technical term for eyeballs that appear to bulge, stare, or protrude (right). Although the eyes appear to be enlarged, the eyeballs themselves are usually unchanged in size. Exophthalmos is due to a build-up of tissue behind the eyeball that pushes it forward within its bony socket (far right). An abnormally large amount of the whites of the eyes becomes visible, and it may be difficult to close the eyelids. Exophthalmos is a sign of any one of several underlying disorders (see Exophthalmos, p.326), and needs medical attention.

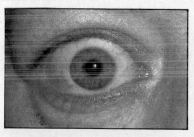

Normal

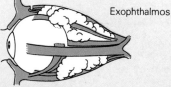

Exophthalmos

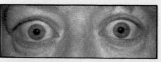

63 Ptosis

In ptosis (right), the upper eyelid starts to droop so that the eye will not completely close. Occasionally ptosis affects both eyes. The condition may be present from birth or may develop later. It may signify an underlying disorder (see Ptosis, p.314).

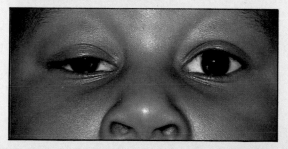

Mouth disorders

Three disorders that affect the lining of the mouth and the tongue and lips are mouth ulcers, geographical tongue, and black hairy tongue. None of these is serious but some ulcer-like growths in the mouth or on the tongue are *malignant*, or life-threatening. Early detection of any malignant growth is vital, so any lump or raw area that persists for more than about three weeks should be seen by a physician (see Mouth and tongue, p.450).

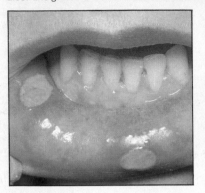

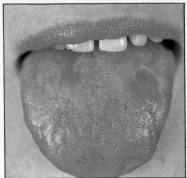

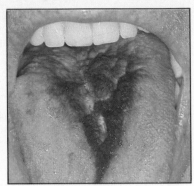

64 Mouth ulcers

These (above) are small, raw, painful areas inside the mouth or on the tongue or lips (see Mouth ulcers, p.450). They may occur as a result of injury (by a toothbrush, for instance) or illness. They usually heal within seven to ten days.

65 Geographical tongue

In this completely harmless condition (above), patches of the tongue's upper surface loose their pinkish, roughened covering. The smooth, dark-red muscular body of the tongue is exposed beneath. The tongue may be sore or uncomfortable when eating certain foods (see Tongue problems, p.455).

66 Black hairy tongue

Black hairy tongue (above) is a rare, harmless condition in which the hairlike papillae covering the upper surface of the tongue become elongated and stained a dark brown color. The cause of the condition is not known.

Parasites

There are a number of small animals that live on or in human skin and produce characteristic marks there. Some of the more common ones are shown here.

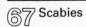

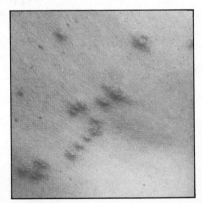

Scabies mite
This tiny, insectlike creature (right) is responsible for the rash of scabies (right center).

Nits
Nits are the eggs of lice (see p.568). They adhere tenaciously to human hair (right).

Bedbug
This small bloodsucking insect feeds mainly at night, while you sleep.

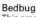

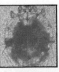

67 Scabies

A typical infestation of scabies shows various marks (above). Sometimes the burrows of the scabies mite can be seen as tiny white lines in the skin, and red lumps may also appear in this area. In most cases there is also a widespread, intensely itchy rash on the trunk. Common sites for this infestation are the hands, wrists and genitals (see Scabies, p.568).

68 Insect bites

Many small insects, including gnats, fleas, mosquitos, bedbugs and lice, produce small, inflamed, itchy spots where they bite the skin. Sensitivity to such bites varies; some individuals get large, puffy, red wheals that persist for several days, while others hardly notice a bite from the same insect. Often several bites (above) appear together (see Lice, p.568, Fleas, p.569 and Chiggers, p.569).

Part III

Diseases, disorders and other problems

Skin, hair and nail disorders
Disorders of the brain and nervous system
Mental and emotional problems
Eye disorders
Disorders of the ear
Disorders of the respiratory system
Disorders of the heart and circulation
Blood disorders
Disorders of digestion and nutrition
Disorders of the urinary tract
Hormonal disorders
Disorders of the muscles, bones and joints
General infections and infestations
Special problems of men
Special problems of women
Special problems of couples
Pregnancy and childbirth
Special problems of infants and children
Special problems of adolescents
Special problems of the elderly

Skin, hair and nail disorders

Introduction

Your skin is one of your largest organs. It is a supple, elastic tissue that conserves moisture and heat. In addition, it provides you with information about your surroundings. Buried in your skin are millions of tiny nerve endings called receptors, which sense touch, pressure, heat, cold and pain. Also embedded in your skin are many minute glands. There are sebaceous glands, which produce a waxy substance that helps to keep your skin surface supple and perhaps prevents it from drying out. There are also sweat glands, which produce a watery liquid called perspiration to cool you when you are too hot. It is the evaporation of the perspiration from your skin that cools you. To help with this temperature regulation, the small blood vessels in your skin dilate in hot weather to lose heat. This may make you look flushed. The same vessels constrict in cold weather to conserve heat.

There are thousands of hair follicles in your skin. These are pits of actively dividing cells that continuously make hairs. There are large hairs on your scalp and in your pubic region. In addition, there are smaller hairs all over your body, some that can barely be seen by the unaided eye. Your fingernails and toenails are also continuously produced by actively dividing cells. These cells, which are similar to those in hair follicles, are situated under the fold of skin at the cuticle, or the base of each of your nails.

Because your skin, hair and nails are on the outside of your body, you quickly notice any change in their appearance. In fact, most of the problems included here relate mainly to changes in appearance. There may be symptoms such as itching, swelling, or, occasionally, pain. Diseases of the skin, hair and nails can be irritating and uncomfortable. They can also be embarrassing because of their appearance. In rare cases, serious diseases of the skin such as cancer or severe blistering can occur. However, most skin diseases only cause self-consciousness and discomfort. This is not to minimize their effects, however, since they can be quite bothersome.

Go to your physician if you are worried about a skin, hair, or nail problem. Get medical advice before you try one of the many non-prescription preparations that are readily available at the local drugstore.

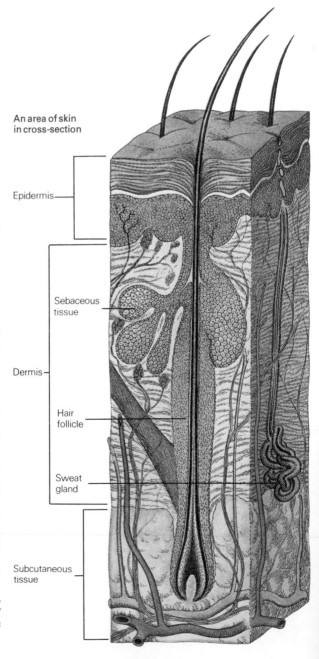

An area of skin in cross-section

Epidermis

Sebaceous tissue

Dermis

Hair follicle

Sweat gland

Subcutaneous tissue

Skin

Skin is composed of two layers. The surface layer that you see is a thin covering called the epidermis. Below the epidermis is a thicker layer, the dermis. The dermis contains many specialized structures such as hair follicles and sweat glands (see previous page). Below the dermis is a layer of fat that is called subcutaneous fat.

The surface skin layer, the epidermis, is a very active layer of cells. Cells at its base are continuously dividing to produce new cells, which gradually die as they fill up with a hard substance, keratin. As they die, they move up to the skin surface, to be shed or worn away by rubbing from your clothes, washing, or handling things. In fact, virtually any move-

ment that causes friction also causes some skin cells to be rubbed away. The continuous production of cells at the base of the epidermis keeps up with the continuous loss of cells from its surface. It takes an average of one month for any single epidermal cell to complete the journey from base to surface. On parts of the body where pressure and friction are greatest, the epidermis is thicker, and the journey takes longer. A number of skin problems are caused by a fault in the constant turnover of skin cells. In psoriasis, for example, there is an abnormal build-up of surface cells because there are increased numbers of cells being produced and pushed up from the base of the epidermis.

Skin renewal
The skin consists of two layers: the epidermis, a semi-transparent layer of cells, and the dermis, a permanent foundation of fat, supportive tissue and blood vessels. The cells at the surface constantly are being shed and rubbed off. Those at the base of the epidermis are dividing constantly to produce new cells, which after about a month, reach the surface to replace those being lost.

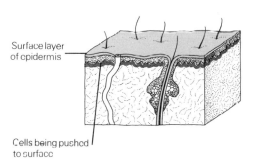

Surface layer of epidermis

Cells being pushed to surface

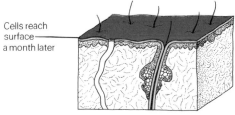

Cells reach surface a month later

Boils and carbuncles

See p.237,
Visual aids to diagnosis, 23.

A boil is an infection of a hair follicle (a tiny pit in the skin from which a hair grows) by certain bacteria, usually *Staphylococcus*. The follicle becomes inflamed and painful. White blood cells, which form part of the body's defense system against bacteria, collect at the site to combat the infection. White blood cells, bacteria, and dead skin cells form thick white or yellow pus within the inflamed area.

A carbuncle is either an unusually large, severe boil or a group of boils joined together by small tunnels in the skin.

Boils and carbuncles are localized infections and usually heal quickly. In a few cases, they are the result of poor resistance to infection or poor hygiene. Boils should not be confused with acne (see p.708) or with any other skin problems.

What are the symptoms?
A boil starts as a red, tender lump, which may throb. Over the next day or two, it becomes larger and more painful. As pus collects, it

develops a white or yellow head, or center. The pus is under pressure, which increases the pain and tenderness. Eventually, it either bursts through the skin or, less commonly, disperses inside. In either case, the pain is relieved and the boil heals.

Boils are extremely common. They affect virtually everybody at some time. Carbuncles are much rarer. Both may recur, because the bacteria that cause the boil or carbuncle may remain on the skin and produce more boils later. There is a risk that if the bacteria find their way from the boil or skin into warm food, they can multiply and produce *toxins* that cause food poisoning (see p.462). So if you have a boil you should wash your hands thoroughly before preparing food. If you have recurring boils, you should discuss the problem with your physician.

What should be done?
Most boils burst or disperse of their own accord within two weeks. If you have a boil

for longer than this, or if you have recurrent boils, see your physician. The doctor may take a sample of your blood and/or urine to rule out the unlikely possibility that an underlying disease such as diabetes mellitus (see p.519) is responsible for the boils. Successful treatment for any underlying disease should stop the boils from recurring.

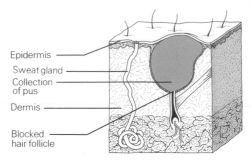

Epidermis
Sweat gland
Collection of pus
Dermis
Blocked hair follicle

What is the treatment?
Self-help: If you want to get rid of the boil as quickly as possible, apply a hot compress made of cotton cloth soaked in hot water to the boil every few hours. This will help relieve discomfort and hasten bursting.
Professional help: If the boil is about to burst, your physician may make a small cut in the center to allow the pus to drain away. In addition, or perhaps as an alternative, the doctor may prescribe an *antibiotic* to kill the bacteria. The treatment for recurrent boils is usually antibiotics and/or an *antiseptic* soap. This treatment may need to be carried out for several weeks to eradicate the bacteria that are causing the boils. If you have boils, it is best to take showers instead of baths and thus reduce the chances of spreading the infection to other parts of your body.

Warts
(*including verrucas*)

See p.242,
Visual aids to diagnosis 36, 37 and 39, and p.245, **visual aids 49.**

A wart is a lump on the skin produced when a virus invades skin cells and causes them to multiply rapidly. Some people have a low resistance to the various viruses that can cause warts and are therefore more likely to have them. Wart viruses spread by touch or by contact with the skin shed from a wart.

Warts are common in teenagers, less so in children, and even less so in adults. There are no serious health risks associated with warts, but they can cause embarrassment because of their appearance.

What are the symptoms?
There are several different types of warts, each produced by a specific virus. The common wart, also called a verruca or a plantar wart, is a small, hard, horny, white or pink lump with a cauliflower-like surface. Inside are small, clotted blood vessels that resemble black splinters. The common wart can grow anywhere on your body but is most likely to develop on your hands. On the bottoms of your feet and palms of your hands, a common wart tends to become pushed in so that its surface is level with the rest of the skin. Several warts may appear next to one another on your foot, forming a mosaic-like area 25 mm (1 in) or more across.

Common warts on most parts of the body are usually painless. However, a wart on the underside of your foot can make you feel quite uncomfortable, as though you are walking with a stone in your shoe.

Among the other types of warts are plane warts, which are small, brown, smooth warts that occur most often on children's faces.

Another type of wart is called molluscum contagiosum. These are tiny, white, pearly lumps, each with a central depression. These are also most common in children. Penile warts (see p.577) and vulval warts (see p.603) also occur.

What should be done?
Most warts disappear naturally, often within a few months but sometimes over several years. You may prefer to wait for this to happen. But if you have any warts that you consider unsightly or annoying, carry out the self-help described below to remove them.

However, there are two cases in which you should consult a physician. One is if you have penile or vulval warts. The other is if you develop any sort of wart and you are over the age of 45. In older people, what looks like a wart may be a more serious skin condition, such as skin cancer (see Basal cell carcinoma, p.258, Squamous cell carcinoma, p.259, and Malignant melanoma, p.259).

What is the treatment?
Self-help: There are many folk remedies for removing warts, but their apparent effectiveness is simply due to the fact that most warts eventually disappear of their own accord. The best way to treat unsightly warts is to apply a wart remedy in the form of paint, cream or plaster. These are available without a prescription at most drugstores. These preparations contain chemicals that destroy the abnormal skin cells. However, these chemicals will also damage surrounding healthy cells, so the preparations should always

be applied carefully to minimize soreness.

Do *not* treat warts on your face or genitals with a wart remedy, because the skin on these areas is very sensitive. And never allow these preparations to get into your eyes.

If you have an unsightly or annoying wart that does not respond to this treatment, see your physician.

Professional help: Your physician may prescribe a more effective kind of wart preparation. If this fails, the doctor can remove the wart by freezing it with liquid nitrogen or burning it off with electricity. A few days after this rather painful treatment, the wart will probably fall off. If it does not, repeated treatment should remove it. As an alternative to freezing or burning, a wart can be scraped off (*curettage*) after first being numbed by a local anesthetic. Occasionally a wart seems to be resistant to all forms of treatment.

Corns and calluses

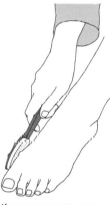

If you are prone to corns or calluses, it may be helpful to use a file or pumice stone to rub away the top layers and ease the discomfort.

Corns and calluses are areas of skin that have thickened because of constant pressure. This pressure causes tenderness in the tissues beneath the thickened skin. Corns are small (less than 5 mm or 1/5 in) and develop on the toes. Calluses are larger (up to 30 mm, or about 1 in) and commonly develop on the ball of the foot or over a bunion (see p.554). Both usually occur after you have been wearing a new or poorly fitted pair of shoes. A callus can also form if you wear high heels, since this type of shoe causes increased pressure on the ball of the foot. Some people seem to have less cushioning tissue than normal between the bones and skin of their feet, and so develop calluses and corns very easily. Calluses may develop on your palms, especially if you do heavy manual work.

What are the risks?

Corns and calluses are extremely common. Nearly everyone gets them at some time. But it is unusual for them to become so painful that you have to consult a physician.

If you have poor sensation and/or poor circulation in your feet due to some disease of the nerves (see Peripheral neuropathy, p.283), which sometimes is caused by diabetes mellitus, (see p.519), callus formation can be followed by deep *ulceration* of the area, which takes a long time to heal.

What is the treatment?

Self-help: Wear shoes that fit comfortably. After several weeks, the corn or callus should disappear. In the meantime, to ease any discomfort, regularly soften your feet with a bland ointment. You may also want to rub away the dead skin with a pumice stone. Calluses on the hands can be softened and trimmed in the same way. To prevent direct pressure on corns, put small spongy rings available at your pharmacy around them. If these self-help measures do not work, consult your physician who may decide to trim the corn or callus either surgically or chemically

---

Eczema and dermatitis

See p.234, **Visual aids to diagnosis 7** and p.235, **Visual aids 8–15.**

The word dermatitis means inflammation of the skin. Eczema is a specific form of dermatitis. Some physicians use the word eczema to describe internally-provoked inflammation of the skin, usually due to allergies, which may affect some people more than others. Dermatitis, on the other hand, also includes conditions that are caused by external factors and affect everybody in the same way, such as sunburn (see p.257). The distinction between eczema and dermatitis is not important for their treatment, so the terms are used interchangeably here.

In addition to inflammation of the skin, eczema is characterized by redness and flaking and/or blistering. Eventually, the skin in the affected area becomes thickened and changes color.

There are many types of eczema. Several of the more common varieties that adults get follow (see also Infantile eczema, p.666).

Contact dermatitis: This condition is caused by an allergy to certain substances that may touch the skin. If you are highly allergic, for example to poison ivy, the dermatitis develops within 48 hours after contact. The skin becomes red and itchy, even beyond the point of contact, and tiny blisters develop. These may join to form large blisters, which then break and crust over. If minute traces of chemicals from the plant are accidentally transferred from one part of the body to another, contact dermatitis may develop on the second part also.

Some forms of contact dermatitis are much less pronounced. For example, allergy to contact with nickel (on the underside of a wrist watch or earrings, for example), produces a red, flaky, itchy patch of skin, which may take weeks or even months to develop.

If an irritant remains in constant contact with your skin, the dermatitis will spread.

Seborrheic eczema: This type of eczema affects adults and young infants in different ways (for seborrheic eczema in infants, see p.651). In adults, the creases from the sides of the nose to the corners of the mouth may become red, flaky and itchy. In men, this inflammation may extend to the beard area and the hairy parts of the chest and back. The condition may also affect other skin creases such as the groin, armpits, and under the breasts. If it is found in a fold of skin and is moist, it is also known as intertrigo. Seborrheic eczema in a mild form also causes dandruff (see p.263).

The cause of seborrheic eczema is not known. It tends to run in families, and usually comes and goes over several years.

Housewife's hand eczema: People who are constantly using dishwashing liquids, detergents, household cleaners, and shampoos often damage the skin on their hands. The skin becomes dry, rough and reddened, particularly over the knuckles. It may thicken, crack, flake and itch. A similar type of eczema occurs among people whose hands are exposed to irritant chemicals on their jobs.

Irritant eczema: The skin of an elderly person tends to be dry, particularly on the legs. This can lead to mild redness, flaking and irritation. If you take hot showers, you may get this type of eczema.

Dyshidrosis: In this type of eczema, itchy blisters erupt on the palms of the hands and the soles of the feet. Some of the blisters may burst and weep, and the surrounding areas may become inflamed and tender. Other blisters do not burst, but die down to form a flat brown spot under the skin. An attack of this type of eczema usually lasts two to four weeks and then clears up of its own accord, though attacks tend to recur. At its worst, this type of eczema can be incapacitating.

Discoid eczema: Discs of red, flaking, weeping, itching skin appear, most commonly on the arms and legs. The condition lasts for several months, then usually clears up on its own, permanently. Its cause is not known.

What are the risks?
Seborrheic eczema, housewife's hand eczema, and irritant eczema seem to be more common than contact dermatitis, which is more common than discoid eczema and dyshidrosis. Eczema and dermatitis are not dangerous to your health, but they can be a nuisance. However, if blisters burst or if you scratch them, they may become infected by bacteria and look very unattractive.

What should be done?
If you have housewife's hand eczema, contact dermatitis of which you know the cause, or a mild form of any other eczema, try the self-help measures that follow. If they fail, or if your eczema is severe, see your physician.

What is the treatment?
Self-help: Eczema on the hand will improve if you wear rubber gloves over white cotton gloves when in contact with any irritants such as dish water. Dry your hands thoroughly after washing them, and apply an unscented hand cream several times a day.

If you avoid whatever is causing contact dermatitis, the condition should disappear within a few weeks. You may speed up the process by using a steroid cream that contains 0.5 per cent hydrocortisone. Such creams are available without a prescription.

Professional help: For any of the types of eczema described, your physician may prescribe a steroid cream or ointment of a different strength or substance. These preparations involve some slight risks (see Box, this page).

Severe itching may be slightly relieved by *antihistamine* tablets. However, these cause drowsiness and impair driving ability, so your physician may advise you to take them only at bedtime. Eczema worsened by a bacterial infection may be treated with *antibiotics*.

If your physician suspects you have a contact dermatitis, he or she will discuss the possible causes with you. Then *patch tests* (applying suspected irritants to the skin) can be used to try to identify the specific cause.

Psoriasis

See p.241, **Visual aids to diagnosis, 32** and p.245, **visual aids 52.**

As your skin is worn away, it is replaced by cells produced beneath the surface. In psoriasis, the normal rate of cell production is speeded up in some areas, and skin cells pile up faster than they can be shed. The result is an unsightly thickening of the skin, called psoriasis. An outbreak of psoriasis is often triggered by (among other things) emotional stress, damage to the skin, or a period of generally poor health.

What are the symptoms?
Deep pink, raised patches, covered by white scales, appear on your skin. They usually cause no discomfort, but they may be slightly itchy or sore. You may have anything from a single small patch to many large ones. The most common sites are the knees, elbows and scalp. Less commonly, patches appear under the armpits and breasts, on the genitals, and around the anus. When psoriasis occurs on

your hands and feet, it is usually in the form of raised areas with painful cracks or little blisters filled with white fluid. In some cases, your nails become thickened, pitted, and separated from the skin beneath.

Occasionally, psoriasis is associated with a mild form of arthritis, one that resembles rheumatoid arthritis (see p.552).

What are the risks?
Psoriasis appears most commonly between the ages of 10 and 30, and tends to run in families. In most cases, it does not affect general health. In the elderly and the very young, however, psoriasis may cause serious illness if the condition is severe and widely spread on the body, and if it is neglected.

What should be done?
Many people learn to live with mild forms of psoriasis. In time, you can become familiar with your particular form of the disorder, and you may be able to avoid the factors that trigger an outbreak. But if you have a severe case, or if it is causing serious discomfort or distress, consult your physician.

What is the treatment?
Self-help: Sunbathing or using an ultraviolet lamp helps to clear up psoriasis, but a sunburn can make the condition worse.

Professional help: Your physician will probably prescribe one of several ointments, creams or pastes to apply to the affected areas. Among them are *steroid* preparations, which are effective but, if used over a long period, may damage the skin (see Box, previous page). Some drugs used to treat psoriasis must be applied very carefully because they burn unaffected skin and may also stain your bedding and clothing.

In many cases, skin medications clear up most of the psoriasis. If they have little effect, the doctor may arrange for you to receive intensive ultraviolet treatment. You may have to be hospitalized for this treatment; intensive therapy should be carried out under medical supervision.

If intensive ultraviolet treatment fails, you may be advised to enter the hospital for one or two weeks to receive intensive applications of a skin preparation, or a treatment involving very low doses of a *cytotoxic* drug that slows down cell division. This treatment is not used widely because the drug may affect certain other cells in the body.

For most people who have it, psoriasis is a long-term condition, and there is no permanent cure. The condition usually reappears throughout life with varying degrees of severity, though treatment is usually successful in clearing up each outbreak.

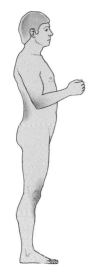
Common sites of psoriasis

Acne vulgaris and acne rosacea

See p.240,
Visual aids to diagnosis, 30–31.

Acne vulgaris, often called simply acne, is a condition in which spots of various types appear on the skin. As many adolescents know, it nearly always develops during puberty. For this reason it is discussed under Special problems of adolescents (see p.706).

Acne rosacea is a condition in which the tiny blood vessels under the skin of the cheeks, nose, and forehead enlarge over a period of weeks or months. Why this happens is not known. The blood vessels can be seen as red streaks on the face. In some cases, the skin becomes completely reddened. Eating hot spicy food, or drinking alcohol or strong tea or coffee, makes you flush brightly. In

some cases, pus-filled spots appear. About half of people with acne rosacea also get sore eyes, due to a type of conjunctivitis that develops (see p.317).

Acne rosacea is harmless. It affects adults and tends to persist for years, usually coming and going of its own accord in that time.

What should be done?
See your physician, who may prescribe an *antibiotic* drug. This is likely to improve the condition within a few weeks. However, after the antibiotic is discontinued, the condition may well recur and require antibiotic treatment again.

Hives
(urticaria)

See p.236,
Visual aids to diagnosis, 16–18.

In this very common disorder, red, itchy lumps, known as hives or wheals, develop on the skin. They sometimes have a white center of variable size, and they often join together to form large, irregular patches. The wheals may occur anywhere on the body.

Hives are sometimes triggered by an allergic reaction to a food such as shellfish, straw-

berries, nuts or food additives; or to a drug such as penicillin. Handling certain plants, particularly nettles, can also bring on the condition. In other people, wheals are raised simply when the skin is scratched or exposed to heat, cold, or sunlight. But in many cases it is impossible to discover what triggers the condition. Whatever the cause is, known or unknown, tension and stress of any kind usually make hives worse.

Usually, the condition clears up within a few hours and does not cause any other problems, but occasionally it may persist for days or months, even if it is treated.

Some people have a more distressing form of the disorder, called angioneurotic edema. In this condition, the tissues underlying the wheals swell, particularly on the face. In severe cases, the lips and skin around the eyes swell enormously. If the swelling spreads to the neck, breathing can become obstructed. Such cases are rare but serious, because it is possible to suffocate under these conditions. Very rarely, hives are part of a more serious disease, for example, systematic lupus erythematosus (see p.556). In most cases, however, hives are irritating but harmless.

What should be done?

If your urticaria is due to a food allergy, you will probably be able to identify the food responsible, because wheals will appear within a few minutes of eating that food. Identification of plants or drugs responsible for the disorder is also simple. Wheals will appear when you start to take the drugs and clear up when you finish. But you may not be able to identify the triggering factor and prevent outbreaks of hives. In that case, if the disorder is troublesome, consult your physician. If your lips and the skin around your eyes start to swell, see a doctor immediately.

To control troublesome hives, the physician may prescribe *antihistamine* tablets. In severe angioneurotic edema, the doctor may inject *steroids* to reduce the swelling and eliminate risk of suffocation.

Athlete's foot

In this irritating but harmless condition, a fungus grows on the skin between and under the toes, especially the fourth and fifth toes. The skin becomes red, flaky and itchy and smells unpleasant. Sweat or water makes the top layer of skin white and soggy. Other parts of the foot may also be affected.

Athlete's foot is slightly *contagious.* It can be caught from others through contact with shed fragments of their affected skin. It is very common, but it is seldom troublesome enough to require professional treatment.

See p.245,
Visual aids to diagnosis, 48.

What should be done?

Soggy skin between the toes, without underlying inflammation and itching, does not always harbor athlete's foot, but may be due to sweaty feet. Either condition will benefit from the following self-help.

Self-help: After taking a bath or shower, or swimming, dry between your toes carefully. Apply an antifungal cream, spray or powder. These are available without a prescription. If the skin is soggy, use an antifungal powder. Wear absorbent socks made of natural fibers, such as cotton, rather than artificial fibers. Wear open sandals or shoes with porous soles and uppers. Change your socks daily, and air your shoes well when you are not wearing them. Once the skin is dry, an antifungal cream will usually stop athlete's foot from recurring. If these measures fail to clear up the problem, see your physician.

Professional help: The physician may prescribe a different antifungal preparation from the one you have been using. If this produces no improvement, the doctor may prescribe antifungal tablets for four to six weeks.

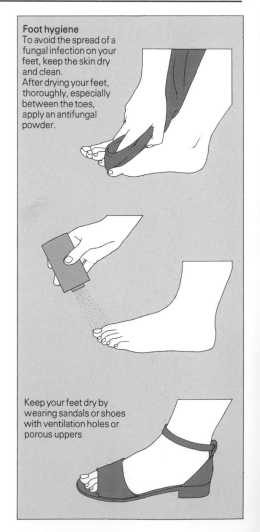

Foot hygiene
To avoid the spread of a fungal infection on your feet, keep the skin dry and clean.
After drying your feet, thoroughly, especially between the toes, apply an antifungal powder.

Keep your feet dry by wearing sandals or shoes with ventilation holes or porous uppers

Impetigo

See p.237,
Visual aids to diagnosis, 22.

Impetigo is a bacterial skin infection. It can occur almost anywhere, but usually appears in the area around your nose and mouth. It is *contagious* (catching), especially among children.

In impetigo, a small patch of tiny blisters appears, but you may not notice them since they soon break, exposing a patch of red, moist, weeping skin beneath. Gradually, the area becomes covered by a tan crust that looks like brown sugar. The infection then spreads at the edges, and newly infected areas may develop elsewhere.

Impetigo is common, and is more prevalent among children than adults. Usually, it is not a serious disease, but in a baby it can spread all over the skin and make the child very ill. Very rarely, if *Streptococcus* bacteria are the cause of the infection in a baby or child, acute glomerulonephritis (see p.690) can develop.

What should be done?
You should consult your physician. Left untreated, impetigo persists and spreads.

What is the treatment?
Self-help: Until you see your physician, gently wash away the crusts of impetigo with soap and water, so that the ointment your doctor may prescribe will be able to contact the affected area and hasten healing. Keep your own soap and towel away from others to avoid spreading the infection. Wash the surrounding skin twice a day to keep it free of bacteria. Children should stay out of school until the condition has healed.

Professional help: Your physician will probably prescribe *antibiotics*, to be taken by mouth or injected. An ointment may also be prescribed. This treatment should clear up the impetigo within seven to ten days.

Cellulitis
(*erysipelas*)

Cellulitis is a skin infection caused by *Streptococcus* bacteria that enter the skin tissue through a small cut or sore. The bacteria produce special chemicals called *enzymes* that break down the skin cells. Any part of the body can be infected but, for reasons that are not known, it is usually a cut or sore on your face or lower leg that becomes infected. A red, tender swelling develops and spreads gradually for a day or two. Red lines may appear on your skin, running from the infected area along lymph vessels to nearby lymph glands such as those in your groin. Your lymph glands may swell, your temperature rises, and you become feverish and ill.

What are the risks?
If the infection is not treated, the bacteria may get into the bloodstream and cause blood poisoning (see p.421). So consult your physician as soon as you become aware of the infection. The physician will probably prescribe an *antibiotic*, which should clear up the disorder.

Sunburn

Sunburn is inflammation of the skin and the tissues just beneath it caused by overexposure to the ultraviolet rays of the sun. The affected area becomes red, hot, tender and swollen, and in severe cases blisters may form. You are much more likely to become sunburned if you have light skin. In addition, a few people are extra-sensitive to the sun because they have a disease or they are taking a drug that makes them particularly sensitive to the sun.

You can become sunburned without sitting under the blazing sun. Ultraviolet rays will penetrate a hazy atmosphere in which you may feel quite comfortable. Also, if you are on the water or on sand, sun rays may reflect off those surfaces and burn parts of your skin that you think are protected.

Sunburn is a special problem throughout the year in the intense sunlight of the southeastern and southwestern United States. Vacationers are particularly susceptible, because they may unwisely try to acquire a tan too quickly.

Because cold temperatures do not block ultraviolet rays, and snow reflects them the same way that sand and water do, you can also get a sunburn on a skiing vacation.

What are the risks?
Repeated sunburn, or regular exposure to strong sun over many years, breaks down the elastic tissues in the skin and makes it look prematurely old and wrinkled. In addition, it can cause solar keratoses, which are roughened red patches of skin, to appear on exposed places, especially in fair-skinned people. Solar keratoses and/or long-term exposure to strong sun increase the risk of your getting skin cancer (see Squamous cell carcinoma, p.259).

What should be done?
Prevent sunburn by not sunbathing, or if you

must, sunbathe sensibly. On the first day spend only 20 to 30 minutes in the sun. Increase this by 30 minutes each day until you are beginning to tan, which usually takes four to five days. During this early period, use a sunscreen, or sunblock, lotion with an SPF (Sun Protection Factor) rating of 10 to 15. The rating should appear on the label. Try not to sunbathe between 11:00 am and 3:00 pm, when the sun is strongest. Once your tan is started, use plenty of suntan oil or lotion to soothe your skin.

If you do get a sunburn, adopt the following self-help measures. Protect sunburned skin, even while swimming, by wearing clothing or applying a sunscreen or sunblock lotion with an SPF rating of 15 or more, and use a soothing cream. You can take aspirin to relieve discomfort. Do not sunbathe again until all signs of sunburn have disappeared.

If the sunburn is very painful, consult a physician. A low dose, anti-inflammatory *steroid* cream may clear up the problem in a few days.

The sun's ultra-violet rays and your skin
The sun's ultra-violet rays can penetrate the semi-transparent epidermis and reach the underlying dermis.

Ultra-violet rays

The blood vessels under the epidermis dilate, allowing more blood to flow near the surface and causing the skin to look red. Or the redness may be caused simply by burned skin.

The ultra-violet rays eventually stimulate certain cells to produce more melanin, a skin pigment that protects the underlying tissues. The melanin moves toward the epidermis, darkening it.

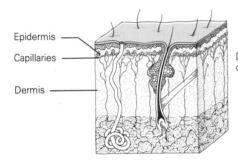

Epidermis
Capillaries
Dermis

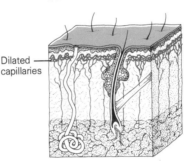

Dilated capillaries

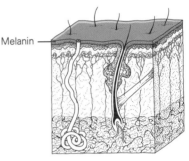

Melanin

Basal cell carcinoma

See p.243,
Visual aids to diagnosis, 41.

Basal cell carcinoma is the most common of the three types of skin cancer. The other two are squamous cell carcinoma (see next article), and malignant melanoma (see next page). In basal cell carcinoma, cells just below the surface of the skin become cancerous, and a tumor develops and becomes ulcerated. The cell damage usually seems to be caused by long-term exposure to strong sunlight, but it may be many years before skin cancer develops. The ulcer grows slowly as it destroys the tissue at its edges. Unlike many other *malignant* (life-threatening) growths, it does not *metastasize*, or spread to other parts of the body.

What are the symptoms?
A small, flesh-colored, or sometimes pearly-looking lump appears on the skin. A common site is the face, especially next to the eye or on the side of the nose. The lump grows steadily and within about six weeks becomes an ulcer with a hard border and a raw, moist center, which may bleed. Scabs may keep forming over the ulcer, but they come off and the ulcer does not heal. Sometimes basal cell car-

cinomas develop as flat sores on the back and chest that grow very slowly.

This type of skin cancer most commonly affects people with light skin who are middle-aged or elderly and have spent many years in a sunny environment.

What are the risks?
Because they grow slowly and do not metastasize, basal cell carcinomas cause only local destruction of tissue and disfigurement, and this only if they are neglected. A large, untreated ulcer will grow relentlessly and can destroy part of a nearby structure such as an eye or ear. Death resulting from this type of cancer is extremely rare. It occurs only when a large neglected ulcer eventually erodes some vital underlying structure of the body, such as an artery.

What should be done?
If you suspect you may have skin cancer, see your physician, who will probably make the diagnosis after a visual examination and a biopsy, in which a small sample of skin is removed for examination. A basal cell car-

cinoma can be removed in a number of ways. It may be cut out, frozen by *cryosurgery*, or destroyed by *radiation therapy*. All these methods have a high success rate, and any unsightly scar can be covered by a skin graft (see next page). Another method of removing these skin cancers is a combination of chemical destruction of the cancer and surgery, known as Moh's technique.

After treatment, your physician will probably want to see you regularly, because a small proportion of these cancers recur, usually within two years. If this happens, the ulcer will have to be treated again.

Squamous cell carcinoma

This is one of three types of skin cancer. The other two are basal cell carcinoma (see previous article) and malignant melanoma (see next article). In squamous cell carcinoma, underlying skin cells are damaged, and this leads to the development of a *malignant*, or life-threatening, tumor (lump). As with the other types of skin cancer, years of exposure to strong sunlight seem to be the main cause.

See p.243, **Visual aids to diagnosis, 42**.

What are the symptoms?
A firm, fleshy, hard-surfaced lump develops, and grows steadily. In some cases, it looks like a wart. In others it looks like an *ulcer*, but the ulceration never heals completely. A squamous cell tumor usually appears on a place that is constantly exposed to sunlight. The lower lip, the ears, and the hands are common sites.

What are the risks?
You are most at risk of having skin cancer if you have lived in a sunny area or worked outdoors for many years, have light skin, and are middle-aged or elderly. The disorder is very rare in people with dark skin.

If the cancer is allowed to reach an advanced stage, it may *metastasize*, or spread to other parts of the body. If this happens, the outlook is poor. Usually, if the problem is detected early, the treatment is effective.

What should be done?
Go to your physician without delay if you develop a lump that does not heal in two weeks. Your physician may want you to have a *biopsy*, in which a small sample of the suspected tumor is removed for analysis.

Most squamous cell tumors are removed by cutting them away. When the tumor is large, a skin graft (see next page) may be needed to cover the scar. Alternative treatments are *cryosurgery* (freezing), *chemosurgery* and *radiation therapy*. Most patients are completely cured, and regular checkups are advised over the next five years.

Malignant melanoma

Malignant melanoma is the most serious of the three types of skin cancer (see also Basal cell carcinoma, p.258, and Squamous cell carcinoma, previous article). This is because, unlike the other two, malignant melanoma often *metastasizes*, or spreads, throughout the body. Changes in the underlying skin cells that produce melanin, or skin-coloring pigment, cause a *malignant*, or life-threatening, tumor to develop. This cancerous lump sometimes develops from pigment cells in a mole present since birth, sometimes in a mole that developed later, and sometimes from pigment cells in what looks like ordinary skin. Many years of exposure to strong sunlight seem to play a part in the development of the disease.

See p.243, **Visual aids to diagnosis, 43**.

What are the symptoms?
The most common symptom is that a mole you have had since childhood changes in one of several ways. It may begin to spread, to become patchy, lighter or darker, to develop a black margin that spreads into the surrounding skin, to bleed spontaneously, or to itch. Later it develops a lump and becomes thicker. Another common symptom is the development of a new mole at any time after adolescence. These moles also develop a lump and thicken if the disease is present. Less commonly, a pale patch may develop.

What are the risks?
This form of skin cancer is not as common as the other two. Melanoma rarely occurs before adolescence. When it does it may occur in a mole present from birth. The tumors appear to be more prevalent among middle-aged or elderly people with light skin who have spent much of their lives in strong sunlight. Because the cancer may spread quickly, early recognition, diagnosis and treatment is essential. Otherwise the outlook is poor.

What should be done?
A change in a mole may not signal cancer, but may be due to some minor injury. In the same way, a change in the pigment of an area may

be caused by a harmless skin condition. However, if you develop any of the symptoms described, you should take no chances and should see a physician immediately. Even if the physician thinks the mole or paler skin is harmless, he or she may still recommend that you have it removed and examined under a microscope for signs of cancerous cells. If the diagnosis of malignant melanoma is confirmed, you will probably be hospitalized immediately for treatment. The melanoma is cut out along with a wide margin of nearby tissue. In addition, any nearby lymph glands may be removed, because the cancer can spread through them. A skin graft (see Box, this page) to cover the area is often done at the same time. In some cases, *cytotoxic*, or anticancer, drugs are also given.

Plastic surgery

Plastic surgery is done to repair or reconstruct a part of the body that has been injured, by a severe burn, for example, or that is malformed due to abnormal development (for instance, a cleft palate). It usually involves the technique of skin grafting and sometimes surgery on underlying tissues such as muscle and bone is also necessary. Plastic surgery may be done simply to improve a person's appearance; this is called cosmetic surgery.

Skin grafts
A wound caused by an accident, a severe burn, or an extensive operation may need a skin graft. Skin for grafting is taken from suitable areas of your own body. This skin will not then be attacked by your body's immune system as would the skin of a donor (see Transplants, p.402).

The most common skin grafting method, split-thickness grafts, involves shaving a thin layer of skin off of a large, healthy area, such as the thigh or back, and bandaging it in place over the wound for a week to ten days until it attaches itself to the underlying tissues. The area from which the skin has been taken usually heals in one to three weeks.

In a situation where such a graft is not likely to "take," a pedicle flap graft may be done. One type of pedicle flap graft involves loosening a strip of skin from a donor site near the area to be covered and pressing it over the damaged area. The grafted skin stays attached to the donor site by one of its edges, so that it is still supplied with blood. Depending on its size, the area from which the skin has been taken may be stitched together or may need a split-skin graft.

With recent advances in skin-culture techniques, it is now possible to take a small area of skin from a donor site and grow it under artificial conditions until it is large enough to cover a damaged site of virtually any size.

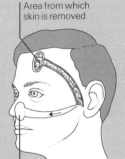
Area from which skin is removed

Area of skin graft

Cosmetic surgery
Although not usually a dangerous procedure, on rare occasions, cosmetic surgery may leave you worse off than before. Even less frequently there can be dangerous, even life-threatening, complications. Ask your doctor to recommend a plastic surgeon who is skilled at the procedure you are considering. Such a surgeon will tell you what you may realistically expect and whether you are a physically and psychologically sound candidate for cosmetic surgery.

Among the most common operations are nose reconstruction (rhinoplasty), facelift and breast enlargement (augmentation mammoplasty). Most involve only a few days' stay in the hospital and, with the exception of facelifts, are permanent and leave few noticeable scars. A facelift can last anywhere from two to ten years.

Varicose ulcers
(venous ulcers)

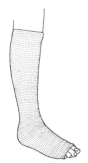

An elastic bandage can speed up sluggish blood flow.

If you have poor circulation in your legs, which becomes more likely as you grow older, the blood flow through the lower parts of your body, especially your calves and ankles, becomes sluggish. You may already have varicose veins (see p.409). In addition, any small injury or crack that appears in the skin is unlikely to heal because the tissues are filled with stagnant fluid and are not getting enough fresh blood. The injury or crack enlarges and gradually becomes a varicose *ulcer*. The condition is common in the elderly and in pregnant women.

What are the symptoms?
The ulcer is shallow, it weeps, and it may have pus in the center. Once it has formed, it may remain unchanged, or constantly keep healing and returning. The most common site for a varicose ulcer is the skin on the inside of the leg, just above the ankle. Quite often both legs are affected. The skin around the ulcer becomes red, flaky and itchy, and the ankles often swell. The ulcer may persist for months, or even years. If you think you have a varicose ulcer, see your physician and also adopt the self-help measures described below.

What is the treatment?
Self-help: Whenever you sit and relax at home, raise the affected ankle. Sleep with your feet higher than your chest. This can be done by raising the foot of your bed about 20 cm (8 in). Avoid standing for long periods of time, and exercise moderately by taking walks on a regular basis.

Professional help: Your physician may suggest that you wear a knee-high elastic bandage or thick elastic stocking during the day. If the ulcer is severe, the doctor or nurse may teach you to clean it with a mild antiseptic, and cover it with a dressing. This should be done frequently.

If the ulcer fails to heal, your physician may coat it with a white paste and then bandage it up. In some cases this still fails to clear up the problem, and you may be advised to go into the hospital for a few weeks. There you can rest in bed in the proper position, and your ulcer will be constantly observed and treated as necessary. To hasten healing, a skin graft (see Box, previous page) may be needed.

Sebaceous cysts

See p.242, **Visual aids to diagnosis, 40.**

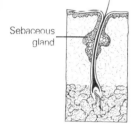

Sebaceous gland

A sebaceous gland is a tiny gland that lies just beneath the skin and produces an oily, waxy substance to keep the skin supple. A sebaceous cyst develops when the gland fills with a thick "cheesy" fluid that slowly accumulates. The cyst then grows slowly over many years. It can be seen as a pale lump beneath the skin. Such cysts are most often found in the scalp. In some cysts there is a narrow pore connecting the cyst and the skin surface. This pore is marked by a tiny, dark dot.

Sebaceous cysts usually occur singly. They are often painless and harmless, are quite common, and are often first noticed in young adults. The cause of these cysts is not known.

What are the risks?
If bacteria enter the pore, the cyst becomes infected. It then becomes enlarged, red, inflamed and tender. It may eventually burst and release foul-smelling pus. After this, the inflammation recedes but the cyst still remains and may become reinfected later. The cyst may also break beneath the skin. This causes a great deal of redness and pain. As the cyst heals, scar tissue may develop, and this may make it difficult to remove the cyst through surgery.

What should be done?
Most people with small cysts simply accept them. If a cyst becomes infected, or if you want one removed because it is unsightly, see your physician. *Antibiotics* are usually prescribed for an infected cyst. An obtrusive cyst can be removed by surgery in a simple outpatient operation, for which you may be given a local anesthetic. If, however, even a small part of the cyst is left behind, and this is sometimes unavoidable, it can recur.

Keloid

See p.241, **Visual aids to diagnosis, 34.**

A keloid is a scar that grows excessively. It can occur after an operation, a burn, a vaccination, severe acne (see p.708), or even the piercing of an ear lobe. At first the scar seems normal, but after several months it grows and becomes noticeably larger and thicker. Occasionally, for some reason, a keloid develops after a very minor scratch.

Keloids are harmless, but they can itch, and they sometimes cause deformity. They are quite common in people with black skin, but rare in those with light skin.

What should be done?
Some keloids stop growing, or even disappear, for no apparent reason. If you want one treated for cosmetic reasons, consult your physician, who will probably inject a steroid medication into it. This sometimes makes it smaller. An alternative is *X-ray* treatment. A keloid cannot simply be cut out. This would leave a scar that might turn into another keloid. Removing the keloid and treating the new scar with injections, X-rays, or both may result in only a small scar.

Lichen planus

See p.441, **Visual aids to diagnosis, 33.**

Lichen planus is an itchy skin rash of unknown origin. It is either small, shiny, reddish spots that appear suddenly, often on the wrists, or patches of thickened, discolored skin that gradually fade and leave a brown mark. Another type of lichen planus is a light, lacy pattern of slightly raised tissue in moist areas such as the vulva and also the inside of the mouth (see Oral lichen planus, p.452). Lichen planus can also make fingernails and toenails ridged.

Lichen planus is most common in middle-aged people. If you suspect you have it you should consult your physician, because there are many other skin conditions, some of them serious, that resemble lichen planus.

What is the treatment?
Most of the time, a dermatologist (skin specialist) can diagnose lichen planus on sight. If the diagnosis is in doubt, you may have to undergo a *biopsy*, in which a sample of skin is removed and examined. *Steroid* ointment usually relieves the irritation and reduces the rash. But the rash often returns and needs further treatment.

Pityriasis rosea

See p.236,
Visual aids to diagnosis, 19.

The cause of this skin rash is unknown, although some physicians suspect a virus is responsible. It starts as one or more large, red, scaly spots, generally on the trunk. Over the next few days the spots grow and spread to cover the trunk and upper arms (the same area that a T-shirt would cover) and perhaps the upper legs. The spots become oval patches of copper-colored skin with scaly surfaces. They often itch, and may persist for four to eight weeks. A slight sore throat may occur as the rash develops. The condition affects mainly children and young adults.

What should be done?
Pityriasis rosea is not dangerous, but you should visit your physician to be sure that you do not have some other similar, but more serious, skin disorder. Your physician may advise you to wait for the rash to disappear naturally. You can relieve any minor itching by applying cold cream to the rash. If the rash is very bad, the doctor may prescribe a *steroid* cream, and severe itching can be treated with *antihistamine* tablets. During the worst weeks of the condition, you should avoid hot baths or showers.

Ichthyosis

Ichthyosis is an inherited skin condition. In infancy or early childhood the skin is extremely dry, especially on the hands, and is broken up into diamond-shaped plates that resemble fish scales. Often the skin is darker than normal. Some types of ichthyosis improve considerably during adolescence.

What should be done?
There are various ointments, creams and special soaps your physician can recommend to make the skin less dry. Cold weather makes the condition worse, so make sure your child wears warm clothes and, in particular, good protective gloves.

Abnormal skin pigmentation

See p.242,
Visual aids to diagnosis, 35 and 38 and p.244,
visual aids 44–46.

Normal skin contains special cells called melanocytes that produce the brown skin-coloring pigment melanin. There are several conditions in which melanocytes are either abnormal or abnormally distributed. Sometimes they are fewer in number or less active than usual; this results in a pale area of skin that does not tan from the sun. Alternatively, the melanocytes may be more numerous or more active than usual. This results in a darker area of skin that tans very readily.

Albinism: This is a rare inherited condition. The melanocytes are unable to make melanin, so an albino is very pale-skinned and has white hair and pink or pale blue eyes. Albinos are advised to wear dark glasses and to avoid sunlight, because sun hurts their eyes and burns their skin easily.

Abnormal suntan: Certain diseases (see Addison's disease, p.524), and some drugs can provoke a "suntan" without exposure to sun. If this happens to you, see your physician.

Vitiligo: In vitiligo, pale irregular patches of skin appear, often symmetrically placed on either side of the body. The patches may grow, shrink, or stay the same size.

Pityriasis or tinea versicolor: This uncommon fungal infection causes patches of paler or darker skin to develop on the trunk. In addition, the affected skin may flake.

Chloasma: Hormonal changes during pregnancy or while taking oral contraceptives cause some women to develop patches of darker skin on the face, particularly over the cheeks. The condition disappears after childbirth or when the pill is stopped.

Moles: These are small dark areas of skin composed of dense collections of melanocytes. Some moles are hairy. Very occasionally, one may become *malignant* (see Malignant melanoma, p.259). If you have a mole that changes in size or shape, you should see your physician.

Seborrheic warts: These are not true warts (see p.252), but round or oval patches of dark skin 1 to 3 cm (up to about 1 in) across. They are common and often develop after middle-age. They have a crusty, greasy surface.

What should be done?
Most of these conditions are harmless, but if you are concerned, especially about a mole, consult your physician.

Self-help: You can find a number of non-prescription depigmenting creams available for lightening skin, but follow the instructions carefully and do not use one for more than a few weeks at a time. The darker your skin is, the more care you should take in using these preparations. Covering the discoloration with ordinary cosmetics may help.

Professional help: There are specific treatments available for some of these conditions. Vitiligo may be improved by ultraviolet-lamp treatment combined with drug therapy. Pityriasis can be cured by an *antifungal* ointment. Moles may be cut out. Special cosmetics can cover various skin blemishes.

Hair and nails

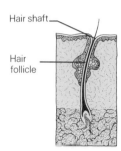

Hair shaft

Hair follicle

Hair and nails are dead, hardened structures that are very similar to the surface layer of your skin. Hairs grow from follicles, which are pits of actively-dividing cells that occur in varying numbers in your skin. Nails grow from folds under your skin. The substance that gives both hair and nails their hardness is the protein *keratin*, which is found in smaller amounts in the skin itself.

Because hair has little real function in human beings, diseases that affect it generally cause cosmetic and psychological problems rather than medical problems. Similarly, nail disorders can be unsightly and irritating but are not harmful to your physical health. Nevertheless, because appearance is usually of some importance to a feeling of well-being, hair and nail problems should be dealt with.

Dandruff

Dandruff comes from small flakes of dead skin on the scalp, which appear whenever the skin cells of the scalp grow unusually fast. The two main causes of this are a mild form of seborrheic eczema (see p.651), or, less commonly, psoriasis (see p.254) of the scalp. The hairs are not affected. Dandruff does not endanger health. It is simply unattractive.

What is the treatment?

Self-help: Use an anti-dandruff shampoo, preferably one that contains tar. Follow the instructions on the container. Massage the shampoo well into the scalp, and rinse at least three times with clean water. This should clear up the dandruff within two weeks, but the condition often recurs.

Professional help: If the shampoo does not work, your physician may prescribe a lotion containing a *steroid*, to suppress the underlying cause of the dandruff. Use the lotion as directed, and you should have less dandruff.

If the scaling is thick and sticks to your scalp, your physician may prescribe a lotion containing salicylic acid or tar. The lotion loosens the dead skin and allows an anti-dandruff shampoo to work more effectively on removing it from the area.

Hair care

To keep your hair in good condition, handle it gently and carefully. Brushing, combing and drying should not be done roughly or excessively. Excessive brushing (100 strokes each night for example) simply pulls hair out at the roots. Long hair may look unhealthy and have "split ends" simply because the free ends of long hair are older than the free ends of short hair. Also, hair that grows while you are ill is likely to be of poor quality. When you recover, the condition of the new hair should improve.

Moderate use of cosmetic hair styling will usually not damage your hair unacceptably. However, tight pony-tails, frequent brushing, cornrowing, permanent curling or straightening procedures, dyeing and bleaching all damage the hair to some extent.

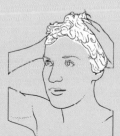

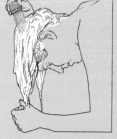

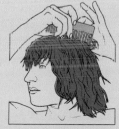

Washing your hair
One application of shampoo should be enough. You can use a mild shampoo designed for your type of hair (oily, dry etc.) and can usually dilute the shampoo by half. Use warm rather than hot water, wet your hair completely, apply the shampoo, and massage gently but thoroughly. If your hair is very oily, do not massage too much, as this encourages oil production. Rinse with cool, clean water. If you wish, use a special rinse or con-

ditioner at this stage. Wrap your dripping hair in a towel, then wait a few minutes and remove the towel and comb your hair out gently with a wide toothed comb.

Drying your hair
Hand-held or hood dryers are unlikely to damage hair if they are used properly, but heated rollers or curling irons should not be used too hot or too frequently. The best way to dry your hair is to let it dry on its own.

Removing unwanted hair
Many women (and some men) regularly remove hair from certain areas. Hair is usually removed if it is considered unsightly. Whether hair is unsightly or not is a matter of personal preference. Removal of unwanted hair is unlikely to improve hygiene or health.

Most methods of removing unwanted hair do not remove it permanently. Those most commonly used are described in the next column.

Shaving: suitable for most parts of the body, but may irritate and coarsen the skin if used on the face. Contrary to popular belief, the hair does not grow thicker as a result of shaving.

Depilatory creams and sprays: suitable for all parts of the body, but may irritate skin.

Abrasives: suitable for most areas but may cause soreness if used on the face.

Plucking: normally used for small areas such as eyebrows, often individual hairs. Has long-lasting results.

Waxing: suitable for most areas; has long-lasting results. Often done for customers by beauty salons.

Electrolysis: Usually permanent. Should only be done by an expert, generally on small areas (especially of the face).

Baldness

*(including
alopecia areata)*

In the vast majority of cases, baldness is a natural process. In men it tends to run in the family on the mother's side. The usual pattern is for the front hairline to recede while hair thins at the top of the head. In some men these balding areas eventually meet, and continued thinning may eventually occur over the whole scalp.

In most women, there is a gradual but slight loss of hair throughout life. Again, this is a normal process, although it may be distressing. Occasionally a woman's hair thins about three months after she has a baby. This is a fairly common occurrence and the hair grows back over the following weeks or months.

Rarely, baldness is due to some underlying disorder. It can occur after a severe, sudden illness. Many hairs stop growing during the illness and then fall out about three months later. Again, they will grow back. In certain severe or prolonged illnesses, such as thyroid diseases (see p.525) and iron-deficiency anemia (see p.419), hair is not only lost but also becomes fine and lusterless, giving the appearance of extensive loss. Usually, effective treatment of the underlying disease will restore hair to normal. Certain diseases that affect the skin, such as scleroderma (see p.557), may destroy the hair follicles. If such conditions are not treated early, patches of permanent baldness may result. And some

forms of treatment, in particular, *radiation therapy* and *cytotoxic* drugs used against cancer, can cause thinning or loss of hair. The hair usually grows back after the treatment.

Finally, there is a specific disease that can cause complete hair loss, though it usually causes only patchy loss. It is called alopecia areata. Round, bald patches appear suddenly where the hair follicles are temporarily damaged. The exposed scalp, which has normal skin, may contain a few fine, white hairs and/or "exclamation mark" hairs, which are narrower at the base than at the tip. In addition, the fingernails may become pitted. A more severe, but rare, form of alopecia causes permanent hair loss all over the body, including the armpits, pubic area, eyebrows and eyelashes.

What should be done?

Some people think of their balding as an acceptable part of the aging process. If you do not, there are two main options. The first is to obtain a toupee, or wig. The second is hair transplantation. Although it is not always successful, hair transplantation is the most effective treatment known for the type of hair loss normally found in men. The treatment is less successful for hair loss from other causes. There can be complications to hair transplant surgery, so be sure to discuss the advantages and disadvantages with your physician.

Baldness caused by alopecia areata often stops within a few months. Your physician may advise you to wait for this natural recovery or may attempt to hasten it by injecting steroids into the scalp. The effectiveness of this treatment is variable, and alopecia areata has a tendency to recur.

Baldness that occurs naturally in men generally runs in families. The front hairline may recede first and often meets a balding patch at the crown.

Paronychia

(including whitlow)

A paronychia is an infection of the skin adjacent to a nail; either the cuticle at the base of the nail, or the fold at the side of the nail. It occurs particularly in people who spend a lot of time with their hands in water. The infection may be caused by bacteria or fungi. Bacteria usually cause acute (sudden and severe) infections. Fungi, particularly *Candida*, which also causes thrush (see p.451), are usually responsible for chronic infections that develop slowly and are less painful, but may be very persistent.

What are the symptoms?

In acute paronychia, your cuticle or nail fold becomes swollen, red and painful. The cuticle may lift away from the base of your nail, and if you press on it pus may come out from

beneath it. When the nail fold is affected, a blister of pus (often called a whitlow) develops alongside the nail. Chronic infections produce similar, but less marked, symptoms. Often the skin around several nails is affected. The nail roots are no longer protected by the cuticles, and they are damaged. This causes deformed or discolored nails (see next article). Occasionally, the nails themselves are attacked by the fungi and become thick, whitish and powdery.

What should be done?

You can prevent paronychia by protecting your hands when they are immersed in water. Wear rubber gloves with white cotton gloves or a dusting of talcum powder inside. If you go to your physician with an acute bacterial

See p.245,
**Visual aids to
diagnosis, 51.**

infection in the early stages, *antibiotics* may clear up the problem. If pus has collected, the doctor may pierce the blister, which will allow pus to drain and relieve the pain.

If the infection is chronic, your physician will probably prescribe an *antifungal* cream or paint to apply to the affected nail(s) after you wash your hands. Do not force the medi-

cation under your nails. After several months of treatment, swelling usually subsides and any raised cuticles return to normal. In some cases, however, the treatment does not cure the condition and your physician may prescribe tablets of an antifungal drug for as long as it takes the infected areas to grow out and be replaced by normal nails.

Deformed and discolored nails

(*including ingrown toenails*)

See p.245,
Visual aids to diagnosis, 50.

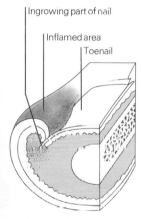

An ingrowing toenail curves into the sides of the toe and can be very painful.

Nails usually become deformed and/or discolored by injury or illness. Injury to the nail-forming area beneath the cuticle, which is sometimes caused by continuous pressure from poorly fitted shoes or by a decrease in the circulation due to arteriosclerosis (see p.404), can lead to thickening of the whole nail. Many disorders can produce nail deformities. Psoriasis (see p.254), lichen planus (see p.261), and chronic paronychia (see previous article) can cause the trimmed end of the nail to separate from the underlying skin. Bacteria entering this space may make the nail turn blackish-green. Iron-deficiency anemia (see p.419) can make nails spoon-shaped. Lung cancer (see p.366) and congenital heart disease (see p.656) can cause clubbing, or knobby enlarged ends of the fingers and toes, and the nails may grow around these ends. After any illness, temporary poor nail growth may cause a crosswise groove to appear in your nails. This gradually grows out and disappears.

Discoloration of a nail is caused by various illnesses. The nail bed appears pale in anemia (see p.419), and white in chronic liver disease. Small, black, splinterlike areas appear under the nails in infections of the heart valves (see p.392), in systemic lupus erythematosus (see p.556), and in dermatomyositis (see p.557).

An injury to the nail, or very rarely a vitamin or mineral deficiency, can cause one or more small white patches to appear in the nail and move out with the nail as it grows. Finally, the nail of the big toe sometimes curves under at the sides, catches in the flesh there and digs in, causing pain as the nail grows. This is an ingrown toenail. It is believed that the nail causes an injury to the skin that does not heal

What should be done?

Deformities and discoloration caused by an underlying illness grow out after the illness is over. Nails badly damaged by injury usually grow again naturally in about nine months. A nail that persistently grows in a deformed manner should be seen by your physician. He or she may be able to correct the problem.

If you have an ingrown toenail, try the following self-help measures. Wear loose-fitting shoes, keep the area clean and dry, and cut the nail straight across the top. If the pain increases or persists see your physician.

Occasionally, your physician may recommend a minor operation to remove the ingrowing edge of the nail and the toe's nail fold next to it. After the operation, your discomfort will be relieved, but you should follow the self-help treatment described, so that the condition does not recur.

Nail care
For healthy nails, observe the following guidelines.
1 Protect your hands from prolonged immersion in water, especially soapy water.
2 Keep nails short to prevent them from getting splits, which tend to trap dirt.
3 Trim your nails regularly with scissors, special nail clippers or a diamond chip file.
4 Either leave cuticles alone, or push them down with a cuticle stick or the thumbnail of the opposite hand.
5 If you use nail polish, touch up any chips in it rather than remove it with nail-polish remover. Nail polish remover makes nails weak and brittle. Do not use it more than once a week.

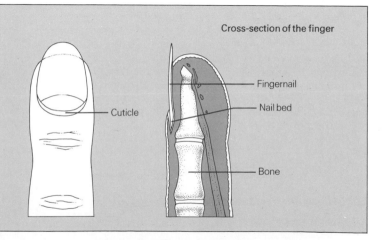

Cross-section of the finger

Cuticle

Fingernail

Nail bed

Bone

Disorders of the brain and nervous system

Introduction

Imagine the most complex and sophisticated electronic computer yet built. Your own brain is far more complex and sophisticated. Your entire nervous system is even more complex. It has two parts: a central system and a peripheral system. The central system is your brain and your spinal cord, both containing nerve fibers. The vast network of nerves throughout the rest of your body is your peripheral system. The peripheral nerves connect with the spinal cord at different levels, and it is through the spinal cord that information flows from these nerves to the brain and back again. This system controls all your conscious activities and profoundly affects even unconscious processes such as heartbeat rate and bowel functions.

Like the rest of the body, the nervous system is vulnerable to various problems. Defects in the part of the circulatory system that supplies the brain with blood (vascular disorders) can damage brain cells. The brain can also be damaged by injuries, infections, degeneration, structural defects and tumors. Because of their complexity, damage to the brain, spine or peripheral nervous system can cause extremely varied symptoms. Among them, for example, are headache, dizziness, loss of balance or coordination, weakness, numbness, tremors, memory loss, difficulty thinking of or understanding words, seizures and loss of consciousness.

Each of the following groupings of types of nervous system disorders covers a broad area of related possible problems. You may find it confusing that many of the same symptoms occur in different combinations for different individual disorders within the types. It *is* confusing. This is the reason that medical school students find the portion of their studies that pertains to the nervous system one of the most difficult to master.

When consulted about symptoms suggesting a nervous-system disorder, your physician or a neurologist, a physician who specializes in the nervous system, will search for answers to a number of questions including: What precisely is wrong? What is causing it? Where is the exact site of the problem? What treatment will be most effective? You can help by answering any questions as clearly and as accurately as possible.

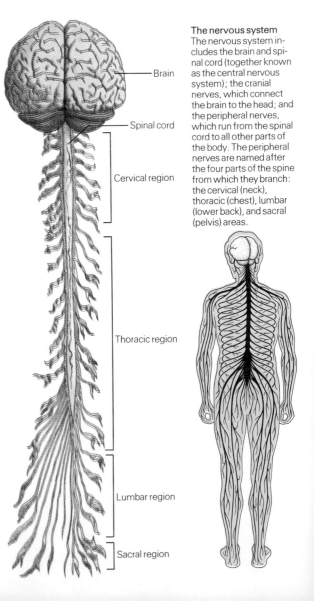

Brain

Spinal cord

Cervical region

Thoracic region

Lumbar region

Sacral region

The nervous system
The nervous system includes the brain and spinal cord (together known as the central nervous system); the cranial nerves, which connect the brain to the head; and the peripheral nerves, which run from the spinal cord to all other parts of the body. The peripheral nerves are named after the four parts of the spine from which they branch: the cervical (neck), thoracic (chest), lumbar (lower back), and sacral (pelvis) areas.

The brain

The brain lies well protected within the rigid, bony case of the skull. It has three main parts: the paired cerebral hemispheres; the cerebellum; and the brain stem. The cerebral hemispheres are responsible for controlling such "higher functions" as speech, memory, and intelligence. Some of these functions are controlled by specific areas; for example, the speech center controls speech. If the speech center is damaged by a stroke, the ability to translate thoughts into words is affected. Other functions such as memory cannot be localized, and seem to be controlled by the cerebral hemispheres generally.

The cerebellum is located under the cerebral hemispheres. It controls certain subconscious activities, especially coordinating movement and keeping your balance. The brain stem merges into the top of the spinal cord and maintains the vital functions of the body, such as breathing and circulation. Nerve signals travel up and down the spinal cord, which links the brain to the rest of the body.

The diagram (right) shows some of the better-defined areas of the brain and their functions.

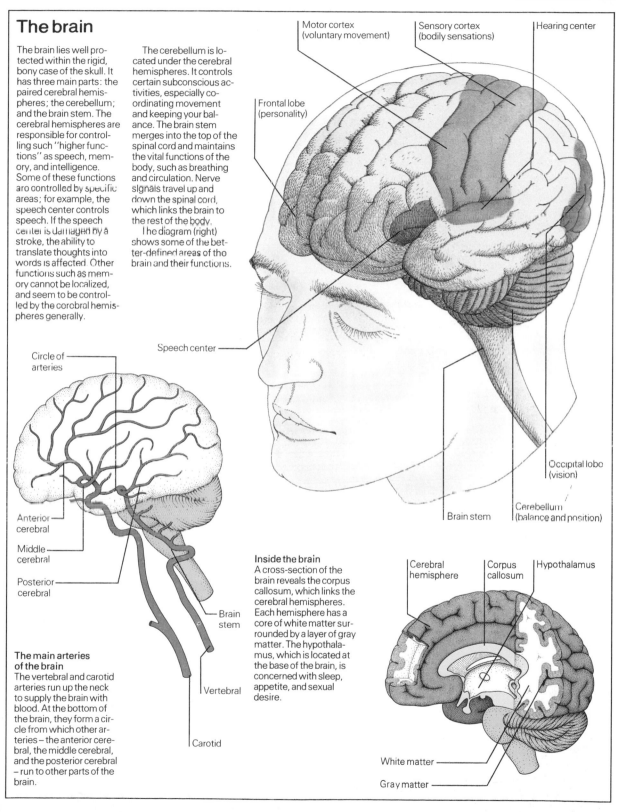

Motor cortex (voluntary movement)

Sensory cortex (bodily sensations)

Hearing center

Frontal lobe (personality)

Speech center

Circle of arteries

Anterior cerebral

Middle cerebral

Posterior cerebral

Brain stem

Vertebral

Carotid

Occipital lobe (vision)

Cerebellum (balance and position)

Brain stem

The main arteries of the brain
The vertebral and carotid arteries run up the neck to supply the brain with blood. At the bottom of the brain, they form a circle from which other arteries – the anterior cerebral, the middle cerebral, and the posterior cerebral – run to other parts of the brain.

Inside the brain
A cross-section of the brain reveals the corpus callosum, which links the cerebral hemispheres. Each hemisphere has a core of white matter surrounded by a layer of gray matter. The hypothalamus, which is located at the base of the brain, is concerned with sleep, appetite, and sexual desire.

Cerebral hemisphere

Corpus callosum

Hypothalamus

White matter

Gray matter

Vascular disorders

Four major blood vessels supply your brain with blood to provide it with essential nutrients and oxygen. There are the two carotid arteries in the front of your neck and the two vertebral arteries running up protective bony canals in the neck section of your spine. These major arteries join to form the brain's vascular system, a roughly circular arrangement at the base of your brain. Branches from the circle supply blood to all its parts. Areas that depend on only a single branch are especially vulnerable to any disturbance in the flow of blood.

The following articles deal with the principal ways in which the brain can be affected by defects in this system. These disorders, such as stroke, which are caused by inadequate blood supply or by bleeding in the brain tissue from diseased arteries, are serious ailments often marked by dramatic life-threatening attacks. Professional care is urgently needed for anyone who has an attack of this kind.

Stroke

A stroke occurs when part of the brain is damaged because its blood supply is disturbed. As a result, the physical or mental functions controlled by the injured area deteriorate. The disturbance may be due to one of three types of vascular disorders: cerebral *thrombosis*, cerebral *embolism*, or cerebral *hemorrhage*.

The first of these, cerebral thrombosis, can happen if an artery that supplies blood to the brain is narrowed down, usually due to atherosclerosis (see p.372). A *plaque*, or large deposit of fatty tissue, at the narrowed and roughened portion of the artery may break open and make a place where the blood can coagulate, and form a *thrombus*, or clot.

This thrombus may grow until it partially or completely blocks the artery.

A cerebral embolism is also a block, but it is caused by a type of foreign object, or *embolus*. The embolus may be a bit of arterial wall or a small blood clot from a roughened artery or a diseased heart. It is carried in the bloodstream until it becomes wedged in a place where it obstructs the flow of blood that goes to the brain.

In a cerebral hemorrhage the artery is not blocked; it bursts. Blood seeps from the rupture into surrounding brain tissue and continues to do so until the seepage is prevented by a pressure build-up as the blood "backs up" outside the rupture, and by the blood's clotting. The initial effects of a hemorrhage may be more severe than those of a thrombosis or embolism, but the long-term effects of all three types of stroke are similar. The results of a stroke, whatever the cause, depend on which part and how much of the brain is affected.

What are the symptoms?

Many of the symptoms of stroke are extremely frightening. You may wake up and find you cannot speak or move part of your body. Or you may, while conscious, feel an arm or leg become heavy, numb, or uncontrollable.

Sometimes a stroke begins with sudden loss of consciousness. Among the many other possible symptoms of a stroke are headache, numbness, blurred or double vision, confusion and dizziness. Often it is the functions of only one side of the body that are affected. This is because damage is usually limited to one side of the brain, and each side of the brain controls only one side of the body.

On the surface of the brain there are specific areas that control definite parts of the

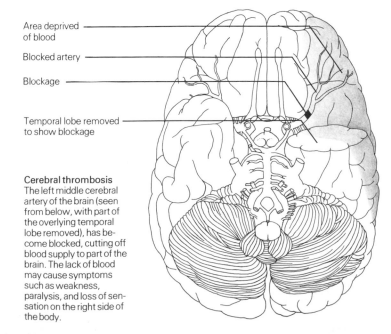

Area deprived
of blood

Blocked artery

Blockage

Temporal lobe removed
to show blockage

Cerebral thrombosis
The left middle cerebral artery of the brain (seen from below, with part of the overlying temporal lobe removed), has become blocked, cutting off blood supply to part of the brain. The lack of blood may cause symptoms such as weakness, paralysis, and loss of sensation on the right side of the body.

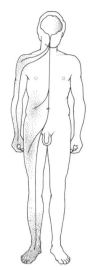

Each side of the body is controlled by the opposite side of the brain. This means that damage to the left side of the brain may result in paralysis and loss of sensation in the right side of the body.

body, or functions such as vision, memory and speech. Thus there is a characteristic pattern of symptoms that indicate which cerebral artery is malfunctioning. For example, you may have just weakness or numbness in your arm or hand, or on one side of your face. If a crucial control center such as the brain stem (which connects the brain and spinal cord) is involved, there may be a complex combination of symptoms or total physical collapse. In any event, the symptoms of a stroke, unlike those of a transient ischemic attack (see next article), persist for at least 24 hours, and usually much longer.

What are the risks?

Strokes and coronary artery disease (see p.374) are two of the most common causes of death in North America. Both problems are often the result of atherosclerosis (see p.372) and high blood pressure (see p.382).

Most people who have strokes are over 65 (more often men than women), have blood vessels that are narrowed by atherosclerosis and have high blood pressure. Abnormally high blood pressure at any age can cause a stroke by weakening arterial walls.

Whether or not your blood pressure is dangerously high, you are more likely than others to suffer a stroke if you smoke heavily. Strokes also seem to be more prevalent among diabetics and people with a high level of cholesterol in their blood.

About one in three strokes is fatal, one in three causes permanent damage or disability, and one in three has no lasting ill effects. If you survive a stroke, you may be partially paralyzed for many weeks before improvement becomes apparent. Even a mild stroke is a danger signal; it may be the first of a succession of increasingly severe attacks.

What should be done?

If you develop symptoms that suggest you may have had a stroke, get medical help immediately. Unless you have a very mild stroke, and weakness, numbness, or dizziness lasts for only a day or two, you will probably need to be admitted to a hospital. To assess the situation fully, your physician will probably require an *electrocardiogram* (*ECG*) and skull and chest *X-rays*. Although general treatment of all three forms of stroke is essentially the same, different types of investigation may be needed in order to determine the cause and location of the disturbance. If there is reason to believe that the stroke has been caused by an embolism, your physician may want you to have special X-rays of the neck arteries called *carotid arteriograms*. This is

because surgery to prevent further strokes is sometimes possible if the source of the embolus is tracked down to a carotid artery. For a more complete discussion of diagnostic tests for embolism, read the article on transient ischemic attack (see next article).

If someone loses consciousness in your presence, it may be because of a stroke. Whatever the cause, call for expert medical assistance and carry out first-aid measures (see within Accidents and emergencies, p.801) while you wait for help to arrive.

Remember that in cases of stroke an apparently unconscious person often senses what is going on around him or her. So do not panic, but try to speak words of comfort; they may be helpful.

What is the treatment?

Self-help: You can do nothing once you have had a stroke, but you can do much to guard against strokes or prevent them from recurring. Have your blood pressure checked regularly. If it is high, be sure to take the drugs your physician prescribes. Do not smoke or eat too much fatty food, and exercise moderately and regularly.

Professional help: The physician's first priority is to assess the severity of the attack and carry out necessary life-saving procedures to maintain breathing and circulation. But most people admitted to a hospital after a stroke are not unconscious, and their main requirement is rehabilitation including general medical care, physical therapy to restore function to affected areas of the body, and occupational therapy. People who have had a stroke often need patience and support, both physical and moral, from the people around them, to help them relearn old skills.

The nerves of a severely damaged portion of the brain cannot be regenerated. An undamaged area, however, can often be taught to take over the control of a function lost because of a stroke, and this is the goal of most rehabilitation programs. If a stroke weakens one of your legs, for example, you may be given exercises that slowly progress from using parallel bars to walking with a walker, crutch or cane to walking freely without help. Your relatives and friends should be involved in the relearning process, which is likely to continue long after you leave the hospital. Similarly, if your speech is impaired, a speech therapist will try to retrain you in skills of vocalization and pronunciation that were once as natural to you as breathing.

All this can, of course, be hard work. It will be easier if you can approach it with a positive attitude and a determination to succeed.

Prevention of further strokes is of prime importance. You will probably be warned not to smoke and will probably need to have regular doses of drugs such as a *diuretic* to keep your blood pressure down. If your stroke was caused by an embolism, surgical removal of the artery-blocking material may be advisable and recommended.

One frequent source of emboli is the roughened surface of part of a carotid artery that has been narrowed down by atherosclerosis. It is often possible to locate, clean out, and open up that section of the artery.

This operation, which is done under a general anesthetic, is usually successful, and later strokes from the same source are unlikely to occur. If surgery is not feasible, your physician may prescribe *anticoagulant* drugs for the rest of your life. These drugs are the so-called "blood thinners." They help prevent clots from forming around irregularities in your arterial walls.

Recovery from a stroke is more likely in people who are not only determined to get well, but who also have support and encouragement from friends and family.

Transient ischemic attack

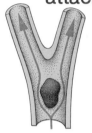

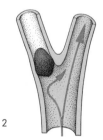

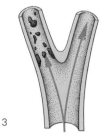

1
2
3

A transient ischemic attack often is caused by blood cells (1) blocking off a small artery in the brain (2). The attack is only temporary, because the blood cells are soon broken up and swept away (3), restoring blood flow.

In ischemia, tissues do not get enough oxygen because bloodflow through vessels that supply those tissues is impeded. An ischemic attack in the brain resembles a stroke due to cerebral embolism (see previous article), but a transient ischemic attack differs in that the symptoms last for only a short time. A sudden onset of weakness and numbness down one side of the body, for example, may last a few minutes or hours and then disappear, whereas the symptoms of a stroke last for more than 24 hours. It is important to understand this difference. But transient ischemic attacks are often signals of an impending stroke. Therefore, they should be treated to attempt to avoid a stroke that may occur later and cause more serious damage.

The narrowing or obstruction of arteries to the brain can be caused by several factors. Most often, however, an ischemic attack occurs because a small clot or a piece of *plaque* (see Atherosclerosis, p.372) breaks away from the wall of an artery or heart valve and is carried into the brain. As the fragment of clot or plaque (called an *embolus*) passes through blood vessels in the brain, it temporarily impedes the flow to an area of brain tissue, and causes stroke-like symptoms. The exact symptoms will vary, depending primarily on the portion of the brain affected. Circulation may soon be restored, however, and the temporarily deprived tissues soon recover. The block is therefore transient, or short lived. But the problem is likely to recur.

What are the symptoms?
The symptoms are like those of a stroke, but they do not last long. They may include headaches, dizziness, tingling, numbness, blurred or double vision, confusion, or loss of the use of part of one side of the body. If the embolus makes its way into an artery that supplies an eye, there may be temporary blindness in that eye.

What are the risks?
Recurring transient ischemic attacks often warn of an impending stroke. Nearly half of those who have transient ischemic attacks are apt to have a stroke within five years after they have their first attack.

What should be done?
If you have had stroke-like symptoms or sudden loss of vision in one eye, do not delay in consulting your physician, who may, after examining you, refer you to a neurologist. The first diagnostic step will be to try to identify the source of a possible embolus. A likely source of emboli is one of the two carotid arteries in your neck. To search for signs of narrowing of the carotid arteries, your physician may listen with a stethoscope to various places in your neck. The stethoscope may also be placed on your chest to pick up any sounds of an abnormal heart valve or irregularity in heartbeat rhythm. You may then need to have an *electrocardiogram* (*ECG*), a chest *X-ray*, other scanning tests, and special X-rays, called *arteriograms*, of those blood vessels that may be the source of the problem.

What is the treatment?
The purpose of treatment is to try to prevent a stroke. What preventive measures are used depend mainly on your age and general state of health. Medical treatment may consist simply of two aspirin tablets once a day for the rest of your life. Aspirin is a good weapon against recurrence of attacks, since it acts as an *anticoagulant*, reducing the likelihood of blood-clot formation. More powerful anticoagulant drugs may also be prescribed. In some cases surgery is advisable. If the precise location of the narrowing of an artery has been identified, the *atheroma*, or fatty deposit causing the narrowing, may be removed to improve the blood flow.

Subarachnoid hemorrhage

As with cerebral hemorrhages (see Stroke, p.268), the cause of a subarachnoid hemorrhage is a ruptured blood vessel. The disorder differs from a cerebral hemorrhage because the blood escapes over the surface of the brain instead of seeping into the brain tissue.

The surface of the brain is covered by three thin, membranous layers called the *meninges.* The outside membrane, the dura mater, adheres to the skull; the innermost one, the pia mater, adheres to the brain; and the middle one, the arachnoid, is much closer to the dura mater than to the pia mater. Thus there is a space between the arachnoid and the pia mater. This space is called the sub-arachnoid space and it is normally filled with a liquid called cerebrospinal fluid. A subarachnoid hemorrhage occurs when blood leaks into the subarachnoid space. This is usually caused by a burst aneurysm (see p.407) in a cerebral artery wall. The blood either remains in the fluid or seeps its way through the pia mater and into the brain tissue.

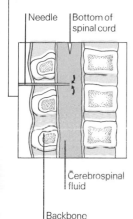

Site of lumbar puncture

Needle | Bottom of spinal cord

Cerebrospinal fluid

Backbone

Close-up of lumbar puncture

What are the symptoms?
The main symptom is a sudden headache, which is likely to be far more painful than an ordinary headache (see p.284) or even a migraine (see p.285). A stiff neck and virtual inability to endure bright light (photophobia) often follow, and there may also be faintness, dizziness, confusion, drowsiness, nausea and vomiting. A major attack can cause sudden loss of consciousness.

What are the risks?
Subarachnoid hemorrhage usually occurs in people aged 40 to 60 and is slightly more common in women. Anyone with high blood pressure (see p.382) or diabetes mellitus (see p.519) may be more susceptible.

Up to 45 per cent of major attacks (those that cause unconsciousness) are fatal, and one in three people who survive a first attack have additional attacks. There is a risk of permanent brain damage due to the pressure of blood on the brain surface. In many cases, either blood spreads into the brain tissue, causing stroke-like symptoms, or the blood vessels constrict, causing similar problems.

What should be done?
If you get a sudden severe headache, especially if it is accompanied by a stiff neck and sensitivity to light, call a physician without delay. If someone in your presence complains of a sudden headache and then lapses into unconsciousness, two possible causes are stroke and subarachnoid hemorrhage. In either case, while waiting for a physician, follow the first-aid instructions given in Accidents and emergencies (see p.801).

With an unconscious person the physician's first step is to initiate life-saving procedures to restore circulation and breathing. Once the patient is out of danger, the next step is to determine the cause of the problem. If an examination suggests a subarachnoid hemorrhage, the best way to confirm the diagnosis is to do a *lumbar puncture,* a test that involves taking a specimen of cerebrospinal fluid. (The fluid in the subarachnoid space of both the brain and the spinal cord is the same.) The easiest place to take the specimen and check it for blood is in the lumbar region, at the base of the spine.

What is the treatment?
If blood is found in your cerebrospinal fluid, your physician's main concern will be to prevent further bleeding. No drug treatment can heal a burst artery, but if you survive the first few days after a subarachnoid hemorrhage, the rupture that caused the problem has probably been sealed (at least temporarily) by natural clotting of blood, and healing is under way. The basic treatment then is several weeks of bed rest, usually in the hospital. One purpose of this rest is to prepare you for surgery, if it is necessary. (In some cases, surgery is done almost immediately.) During this period of rest, the doctor may prescribe a painkiller to relieve headaches. If your blood pressure is high, you will also have to take medication to reduce it.

Within three days of the attack, you will probably have special X-rays of the major arteries that supply your brain. These are called *arteriograms.* They are done to locate the site of an aneurysm or any other defective spots in arterial walls. If the arteriograms indicate a danger of later attacks, surgery to prevent more leakages may be advisable. The surgery involves sealing off an aneurysm by means of a tiny metal clip.

What are the long-term prospects?
If you regain consciousness after a major attack and survive for six months without further problems, you are probably out of danger. Chances of full recovery from surgery, if it is advised, are also good. Residual damage from an attack varies according to what areas of the brain are affected. Partial paralysis, weakness, or numbness may linger or even be permanent, as may sight and speech difficulties (for further information, see Stroke, p.268). You should have your blood pressure checked regularly, and high blood pressure controlled if possible.

Subdural hemorrhage and hematoma

In subdural hemorrhage blood leaks from vessels in the dura mater, the outermost of the three *meninges*, or membranous layers that cover the brain. It differs from extradural hemorrhage (see next article) in that the ruptured blood vessels are on the underside, rather than the outside, of the dura mater. Because these inner vessels are smaller than the outer ones, less blood is likely to leak out. The blood tends to seep quite slowly into the space between the dura mater and the arachnoid (the middle of the three meninges), and causes a *hematoma*, or collection of blood.

Among eventual symptoms of subdural hemorrhage are drowsiness, confusion, weakness or numbness down one side of the body, and persistent or recurrent headaches and nausea. During a period of days or weeks such symptoms may come and go, but they will gradually become worse.

Subdural hemorrhage occurs as a result of a head injury (see Brain injury, p.276). It occurs most often in elderly people who have fallen. These people have sometimes forgotten about the accident by the time symptoms develop.

What should be done?

Consult your physician without delay if you develop the symptoms described above. Because they are similar to those of a minor stroke (see p.268), be sure to tell the physician that you have recently injured your head, even if only slightly, if you remember any such incident. If any member of your family shows signs of mental deterioration and abnormal drowsiness, be sure that they see a physician. The affected person will probably be admitted to the hospital for diagnostic tests such as *X-rays*, *arteriography*, a *radioisotope scan*, and possibly a brain scan (known as *CAT scan*) to determine the cause of the symptoms. If the problem is diagnosed as subdural hemorrhage, treatment and chances for full recovery are similar to those of extradural hemorrhage (see next article).

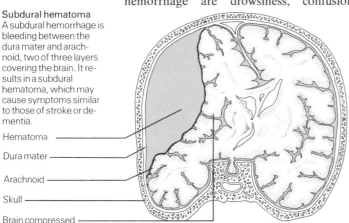

Subdural hematoma
A subdural hemorrhage is bleeding between the dura mater and arachnoid, two of three layers covering the brain. It results in a subdural hematoma, which may cause symptoms similar to those of stroke or dementia.

Hematoma —————
Dura mater —————
Arachnoid —————
Skull —————
Brain compressed —————

Extradural hemorrhage

Extradural hemorrhage occurs when blood vessels in the dura mater, the outermost of the three *meninges*, or membranous layers that cover the brain, rupture. Blood then flows outwards over the surface of the brain, between the dura mater and the skull. The problem usually results from a head injury that causes some of the blood vessels in the outer surface of the dura mater to burst (see Brain injury, p.276). Because these vessels are large, a substantial amount of blood leaks into the space between the dura mater and the skull. The symptoms of an extradural hemorrhage are likely to appear within 24 hours of the injury (see also Subdural hemorrhage and hematoma, previous article). Even if the original injury seemed trivial when it happened, the symptoms are not. They include a sudden severe headache; nausea, which often culminates in vomiting; and increasing drowsiness, all of which ultimately may lead to unconsciousness and death.

What are the risks?

Head injuries are very common, but only about ten per cent of them require hospital admission, and only one to two per cent cause extradural hemorrhage as a complication. This disorder creates an emergency situation, however, because pressure on the brain mounts as more and more blood floods into the narrow space between brain and skull.

What should be done?

If you or anyone in your presence shows symptoms of an extradural hemorrhage, get medical help fast, especially if there has been a blow to the head within the past several hours or the last day. Unless the person is treated promptly, there is a danger of permanent brain damage or even death. The person will be admitted to the hospital immediately for diagnostic tests and general treatment for head injury (see Brain injury, p.276). If tests indicate the presence of extradural hemorrhage, surgery will be necessary to stop the bleeding. The operation involves removing a portion of skull bone to release leaked blood and permit the surgeon to repair ruptured blood vessels. When the operation is done promptly, it usually results in complete recovery from all problems.

Infections

Infections of the nervous system are less frequent than infections of other systems such as the respiratory system, because the brain and spinal cord have no contact with the outside. Those infections that do occur gain entry through the bloodstream, the air spaces in the ears or sinuses, or through fractures caused by head injuries. Most nervous-system infections cause obvious, serious illness. Early diagnosis is important, since prompt treatment can save a life and prevent long-term damage to the brain, the spinal cord or the nerves. You should familiarize yourself with the symptoms of this type of infection so that you can act quickly and decisively if anyone in your family gets one.

Meningitis

Meningitis is an inflammation of the *meninges*, which are membranous coverings of the brain and spinal cord. There are three meninges. First, there is the outside membrane, the dura mater, which adheres to your skull. Next is the middle layer, the arachnoid. Finally, there is the innermost membrane, the pia mater, which adheres to the brain. The cause of infection of these membranes is usually an invasion by either bacteria or viruses. There are a number of ways that infection can reach the meninges. For example, infectious agents may spread through the bloodstream from some other part of the body, such as the lungs, where there is an infection. They can also spread to the brain from an infected ear or infected sinuses, through the cavities in the bones of the skull. Or if you have a head injury involving a fractured skull, this provides an easy entry for infection.

The brain and spinal cord are surrounded by cerebrospinal fluid, contained between two of three sheets of fibrous tissue called the meninges.

Meningitis occurs when the cerebrospinal fluid becomes infected, causing inflammation of the meninges

There are many forms and degrees of meningitis. Much depends on the type of bacterium or virus that causes the disease.

What are the symptoms?

Fever, headache, nausea and vomiting, a stiff neck, and *photophobia* (inability to tolerate bright light) usually develop over the course of a few hours. An occasional additional symptom is a deep red or purplish skin rash. If the infection continues to proceed unchecked, you become drowsy and you may eventually lose consciousness.

The symptoms of meningitis may be less obvious in infants and young children. For a full discussion on the differences, read the article on meningitis in babies and children (see p.668).

What are the risks?

Meningitis is an uncommon illness in this country. The most common form, a viral infection, spreads from person to person through the air. It therefore tends to occur in epidemics, as do many viral illnesses, often in winter when people are in close contact indoors. Bacterial meningitis may also occur in epidemics, but sporadic cases of this form are more commonly seen.

The sooner treatment of bacterial meningitis is started, the better the results. Untreated bacterial meningitis may well be fatal. With appropriate treatment, most people recover completely, but a few are left with permanent damage including deafness, blindness, and/or mental deterioration. Babies and elderly people are most in danger of either failing to recover or of being left with lasting residual damage. The reason for this may be that these people have relatively weak powers of resistance.

Viral meningitis tends to be a less severe illness than the bacterial type. In most cases there is full recovery with no after-effects.

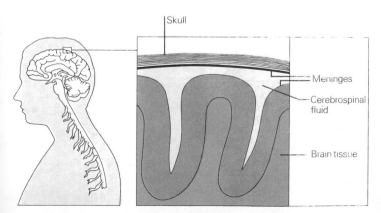

Skull

Meninges

Cerebrospinal fluid

Brain tissue

What should be done?

If you or anyone in your family develops symptoms of meningitis, particularly a combination of severe headache, stiff neck, and photophobia, consult your physician without delay. A tentative diagnosis of meningitis can be confirmed by an examination of a sample of cerebrospinal fluid, the liquid that bathes your central nervous system. This sample will be taken in a hospital. If the sample, which is obtained by a *lumbar puncture* (see illustration on page 271), looks cloudy and contains pus cells, the meninges are probably infected. Further tests of the liquid sample should be able to identify the infectious agent, and this will help your physician to plan treatment aimed at combating the particular organism involved.

What is the treatment?

You will have to remain in the hospital until the meningeal infection has cleared up. If the infection is bacterial, you will be given large doses of *antibiotics*, which may be dripped through a tube directly into a vein. This may be necessary for as long as two weeks. Since most viruses are not harmed by antibiotics, these drugs are not generally used for a case of viral meningitis. You can expect to be fully recovered in two to three weeks, depending on the severity of the attack.

While you are in the hospital, you will be made as comfortable as possible. Bed rest in a darkened room, plenty of liquids, and possibly drugs to lower your temperature and ease the pain of headaches will help your body overcome the infection.

Encephalitis
(*including Reyes disease*)

Encephalitis is inflammation of brain cells. It is usually caused by a viral infection. In a few cases, the virus is one that has caused an infectious disease such as mumps (see p.700), measles (see p.699), or infectious mononucleosis (see p.562) or from herpes simplex virus (see Cold sores, p.451). There are a few kinds of brain infection that are not caused by viruses. For example, one called African sleeping sickness is caused by a single-celled animal that is transmitted by the tsetse fly. But such diseases are virtually unknown in the United States.

In addition, there is Reyes disease, a disease of the brain and some abdominal organs such as the liver that affects children and adolescents primarily. The cause of Reyes disease is unknown, but typically it follows a viral illness. Some population studies have linked the disease with the use of aspirin, but the cause and effect relationship is unclear. The symptoms of Reyes disease are similar to those of encephalitis.

What are the symptoms?

The severity of encephalitis varies enormously. In mild cases the symptoms are those of any viral infection: fever, headache, and loss of energy and appetite. In more severe cases brain function is obviously affected, causing irritability, restlessness and drowsiness. In the most severe cases there may be loss of muscular power in the arms or legs, double vision, and impairment of speech and hearing. Also, in some cases, the drowsiness may deepen into a coma.

What are the risks?

Mild encephalitis is quite common and may not even be noticed. About 1 in 1,000 cases of measles causes mild encephalitis. Severe attacks are extremely rare. The risks vary with age and the kind of infectious agent that causes the disease. Encephalitis in babies and the elderly can be fatal, but people in the other age groups are likely to recover completely, sometimes after serious and prolonged illness. Although there is a risk of permanent brain damage, only a small percentage of cases have serious consequences.

What should be done?

If you develop the symptoms described, consult your physician, who will probably order various diagnostic tests, including blood tests, a skull *X-ray*, and an *electroencephalogram* (*EEG*). An essential test for diagnosis of infection of the nervous system is an examination of cerebrospinal fluid taken by a procedure called a *lumbar puncture* (see illustration on page 271), in which a tap, or sample, of cerebrospinal fluid is taken from the lumbar or low back region of the spine.

What is the treatment?

Since viruses do not usually respond to *antibiotic* drugs, the basic treatment consists of measures to ease symptoms and allow the body's natural defense system to overcome the infection. In most cases, you are simply kept comfortable and well nourished. Sometimes *steroid* drugs can help suppress inflammation. If you are unconscious, you will be fed through a *nasogastric* tube, and your breathing may have to be mechanically assisted by a *respirator*.

Recovery from a severe attack may be slow, and you may need the help of physical therapists, occupational therapists, or speech therapists to relearn fundamental skills such as clear speech, using a knife and fork, or sometimes even walking safely. You may be dependent on medical and family aid for up to a year after a severe attack of encephalitis.

Polio
(poliomyelitis)

Polio, or poliomyelitis, is a viral infection that attacks muscle-controlling nerves. It used to be universally feared, with parents dreading the "polio season," which occurred in summer. This is because in a small proportion of cases the disease caused permanent paralysis. But with modern preventive techniques the disease has been almost eliminated in the Western world. There is only an occasional case in the United States, because children are routinely given doses of anti-polio vaccine from early infancy onwards (see Immunization procedures, p.701). If you or members of your family are about to travel abroad, ask your physician about extra preventive doses of the vaccine.

Where polio exists, it is spread by personal contact or by eating or drinking contaminated foods or liquids. Its early symptoms are headache, sore throat and fever. These are followed by pain in the neck and back muscles. In severe cases, muscular weakness may then lead to paralysis.

With anti-polio vaccine readily available, everyone should be protected against polio. Children are routinely immunized in stages. If you or a member of your family have not been immunized, consult your physician. Travel to the tropics poses special risks as do rare epidemics of the disease.

Epidural abscess

An epidural *abscess* is a collection of pus in the space between the skull or spinal bones and the dura mater, which is the outermost of the three *meninges*, or membranes that cover the brain and spinal cord. The pus is usually due to a bacterial infection. As the pus collects it exerts pressure on the nerve tissue. In rare cases, *toxins*, or harmful chemicals that are produced by bacteria, may cause damage to the dura mater.

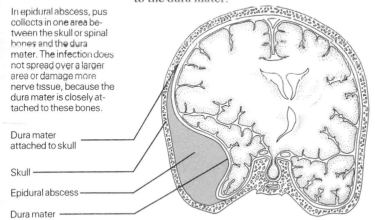

In epidural abscess, pus collects in one area between the skull or spinal bones and the dura mater. The infection does not spread over a larger area or damage more nerve tissue, because the dura mater is closely attached to these bones.

Dura mater attached to skull

Skull

Epidural abscess

Dura mater

What are the symptoms?
An abscess on the spinal cord can cause loss of muscular power in the legs and numbness of the entire lower part of the body. An abscess in the brain may have the same symptoms as a stroke (see p.268), causing weakness down one side of the body or difficulty with speech. The onset of stroke-like symptoms is seldom rapid; they usually appear gradually over several hours. In addition, you will probably have general symptoms caused by the infection, such as fever, confusion, and perhaps delirium or convulsions.

What are the risks?
Epidural abscesses are extremely rare, because the infections that used to cause them can now be treated with *antibiotics*. Such infections include acute infection of the middle ear (see p.333) and sinusitis (see p.347).

What should be done?
If you suspect that you have an abscess, consult your physician, who will probably consider the history of previous infection, and may order diagnostic tests. Among them may be blood tests to identify the invading bacteria, a skull *X-ray*, and perhaps an *electroencephalogram* (*EEG*). *Arteriography*, a *CAT scan* of the brain, and an examination of the spinal cord (*myelography*) may also be required for a diagnosis.

What is the treatment?
To combat infection, your physician will probably prescribe an antibiotic. In some cases, however, this will not solve the problem, and surgery will be necessary. The surgeon makes an opening in the skull or in the vertebral bone through which pus can be removed. After such an operation, antibiotic treatment is continued. If the original cause of infection is also dealt with, you have a good chance of full recovery.

Structural disorders

A structural disorder of the nervous system is one in which a portion of the system is in some way physically distorted or damaged. The cause may be an injury, a tumor, or a disorder of the nerves themselves or the bones and coverings that surround the system. While the skull protects the brain from external damage, the brain may also be damaged because of the inflexibility of the protective bones that make up the skull. For example, a small tumor on the brain cannot expand outward because of the skull, and so it may compress the brain and cause any of a number of severe problems.

Like many other maladies of the nervous system, structural disorders can often cause symptoms in areas far removed from the actual problem. This is because the nervous system is a far reaching, interlinked network that connects various parts of the body. Spinal cord injury, for example, may paralyze your arms, cause loss of bowel control, or trigger a number of other problems depending on what part of the cord is injured.

Brain injury

A substantial blow to the head will sometimes damage the brain, jolting and bruising it even though the skull is not fractured. As a result, the brain tissues may swell, and this will produce symptoms as pressure on the brain increases because outward expansion is obstructed by the rigid confines of the skull. If the skull is fractured, brain damage is even more likely. In either case, the extent of the damage and whether any loss of function will be temporary or permanent depend on the type and force of the injury.

What are the symptoms?
The symptoms depend on the strength of the blow and exactly what part of the head is damaged. Generally, however, a minor injury is followed almost immediately by a headache. A simple headache that clears up within a day or two usually signals minimal damage, rapid repair of brain tissues and, in all but rare cases, complete recovery. A more severe injury usually causes immediate unconsciousness, which may last only a few seconds or persist for weeks. When unconsciousness persists, you are commonly said to be "in a coma."

A person who has been temporarily knocked out is dazed and confused upon regaining consciousness. There may also be *amnesia*, or loss of memory. In addition, in some cases, there may be more headaches, mental lapses, and muscular weakness or paralysis (including difficulty with speech). Such symptoms tend to disappear gradually as healing progresses, but in extreme cases there may be residual damage that leads to lasting physical or psychological problems such as paralysis, abnormal irritability, depression, or decreased mental alertness.

What are the risks?
In only a small percentage of head injuries is the damage severe enough to cause permanent mental and physical disability. These injuries are most often caused by traffic accidents (especially those that injure people on motorcycles), industrial accidents, falls, fights, and explosions or gunshot wounds.

Because of the alarming number of head injuries that occur in motorcycle accidents, many states have enacted mandatory helmet laws for motorcyclists. Those who drive or ride as passengers on motorcycles, even in states that do not require helmets, should always wear a helmet to help avoid possible head and brain injury.

A severe head injury may rupture one or more blood vessels, which will cause a subarachnoid, subdural, or extradural hemorrhage (see p.271 and p.272). The symptoms of hemorrhage resulting from an injury may not appear until hours, days, or even weeks after the injury occurs. If the skull is fractured, there is a serious additional danger. Infectious agents may be able to enter through the fracture and infect brain tissues, causing meningitis (see p.273).

Finally, there is a possibility that lasting brain damage from a serious injury may cause occasional seizures or convulsions (see Epilepsy, p.287). This happens in about five percent of head injuries, excluding gunshot wounds. About 33 percent of those who survive gunshot head injuries have seizures or convulsions.

What should be done?
If you are present when someone loses consciousness because of an injury, follow the first-aid instructions in the Accidents and

The CAT scan

The CAT (computerized axial tomography) scanner takes a special type of X-ray of parts of the body, such as the brain, that do not form clear images on conventional X-rays.

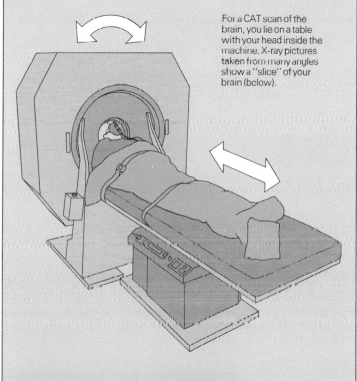

For a CAT scan of the brain, you lie on a table with your head inside the machine. X-ray pictures taken from many angles show a "slice" of your brain (below).

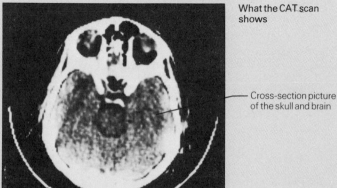

What the CAT scan shows

Cross-section picture of the skull and brain

emergencies section (see p.801) and summon medical help *at once.* An injured person who does not lose consciousness but has other symptoms of brain injury should see a physician as soon as possible.

If you were in an accident and you do not remember precisely what happened, it will help if someone who saw the incident can go with you in order to describe it to the physician who will treat you.

If you develop a headache for no apparent reason and begin to feel weak or mentally confused, think back over the past few days. Have you recently banged your head or had a slight accident? In any case, you should consult your physician. Depending on the severity of the symptoms and the results of your doctor's observations, you may need some in-hospital diagnostic tests to discover the extent of the damage. The first of these will be one or more skull *X-rays* to detect a possible fracture. Then, especially if symptoms persist, you may be required to have a brain scan (known as a *CAT scan*) and perhaps *arteriography* to look for evidence of a ruptured blood vessel.

What is the treatment?
Self-help: Medications should never be taken by someone who has been knocked unconscious unless a physician has been consulted and has recommended them. If you have had a fairly hard blow, your doctor may want you to spend a night or two in the hospital for observation, to check for complications. Two or three days of rest after a slight accident should be sufficient treatment. Most minor damage is self-healing.

Professional help: An unconscious person should be in the hospital, because intensive professional care is of paramount importance. A *steroid* drug may be administered directly into a vein to reduce brain swelling. In some cases of skull fracture, surgery that is performed to relocate bone fragments formed by the injury may be necessary.

What are the long-term prospects?
Recovery from severe brain injury usually takes many weeks, but chances for recovery of lost functions are fair. A few people are left with memory and thinking disorders, personality changes, slurred speech, or muscular weakness in an arm or leg. Encouragement and support from family and friends are an important part of the recovery process for these people, many of whom will also need occupational and physical therapy to overcome paralysis, muscle weakness, or poor coordination.

Spinal cord injury

The vertebrae, the bones that protect your spinal cord, are separated from each other by discs of flexible cartilage. The discs permit a certain amount of bending and twisting of your back. Injuries that primarily affect the bones or cartilage are discussed in another section of this book (see Backaches, p.546). In this article our concern is only with the spinal cord itself.

The nerve pathways that make up the spinal cord transmit nerve impulses between your brain and body. This allows you to control your movements and detect sensations such as touch or heat. If the spinal cord is damaged by an accident, part or parts of the body below the point of injury may be affected. The damage may be only temporary, but it usually leads to some degree of permanent disability, as these nerve pathways help control many body actions and functions. Prompt medical care by experts is a key factor in reducing the likelihood of damage and disability in spinal cord injury.

What are the symptoms?

The area of the body affected depends on the location of the damage to the spinal cord. There may be numbness and weakness, or paralysis of all muscles below the level of the injury, including those that control your bowels and bladder. Sometimes muscles on only one side of the body are affected. Pain is not always a symptom of injury to the spinal cord, but accompanying injury to nearby nerves sometimes causes severe pain, as, for example, in sciatica (see p.547).

Unlike the symptoms of certain types of brain injury (see previous article), which may become apparent only after some time has passed, symptoms of spinal cord damage almost always appear immediately after the injury that causes them.

What are the risks?

Spinal cord injuries are all too common today. Most spinal cord injuries are due to traffic accidents, falls, sports injuries such as diving accidents, and gunshot wounds.

Injury to the spinal cord in the neck can be fatal if it damages the nerves there that control breathing, or it can result in total paralysis of both arms and legs, as well as general numbness from the neck down. Injuries to other parts of the spinal cord are not

The spine and its nerves

Nerve signals from the brain go to the spinal cord and pass to the peripheral nerves. These nerves emerge from the spinal cord as two roots (the posterior and the anterior roots) in the gap between each vertebra, then join together to relay nerve signals to and from specific parts of the body. The peripheral nerves that emerge in the cervical region of the spine serve the neck and the arms; those that emerge in the thoracic region serve the ribcage and the abdominal wall; and those from the lumbar region serve the legs. The nerves that emerge from the sacral region control the bowels and the bladder.

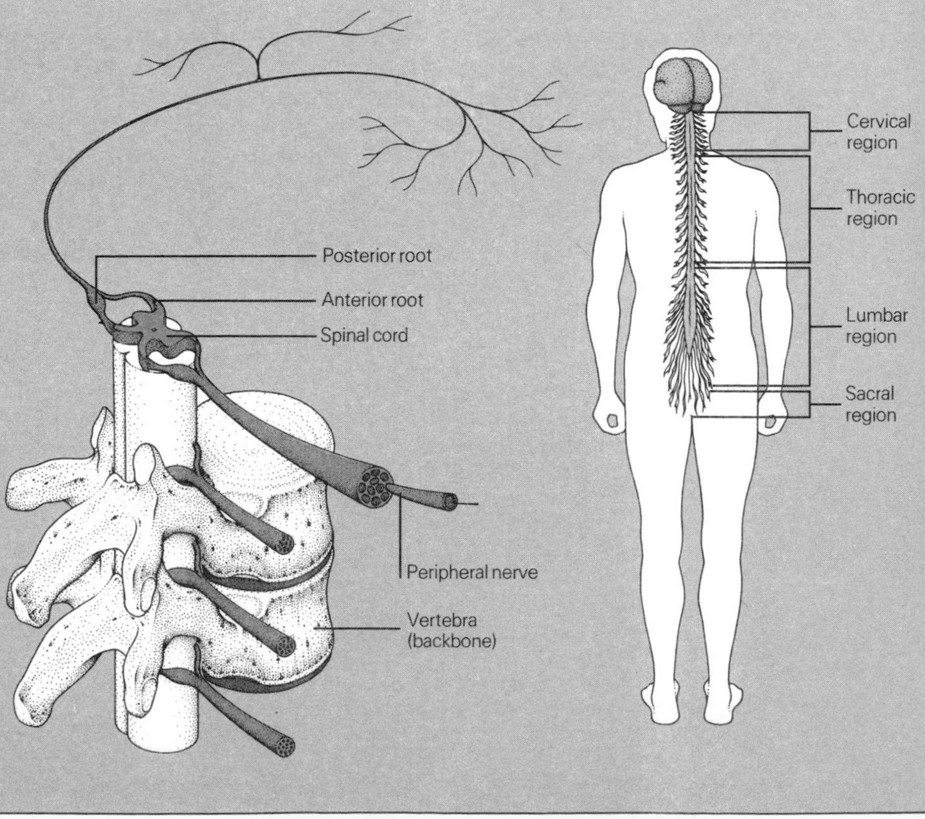

Posterior root
Anterior root
Spinal cord
Peripheral nerve
Vertebra (backbone)

Cervical region
Thoracic region
Lumbar region
Sacral region

usually fatal but may be permanent and cause severe disability. Bladder paralysis often leads to recurrent urinary tract infections (see p.502). Numb parts of the body are especially susceptible to various kinds of injury.

What should be done?

Serious injury to the spinal cord requires immediate hospitalization. If a person who has had an accident is unable to move the legs or complains of numbness, get professional help immediately. Do not try to move the injured person. The wrong kind of movement can do further damage to nerve pathways. Ambulances are equipped with special stretchers for carrying the injured, and the most helpful thing you can do is have someone get assistance, while you stay with the injured person, and let him or her know that help is on the way (see Accidents and emergencies, p.801 for further information).

Remember that many of the symptoms of this kind of injury are extremely frightening. For this reason you can help the injured person a great deal by staying calm and offering as much reassurance as you possibly can.

As soon as possible, the spine will be *X-rayed* in order to discover the site and extent of damage. The lower parts of the body will be tested for numbness.

In some cases a test called a *myelogram* will be done, to find out if pressure on the spinal cord can be relieved by surgery. In a myelogram, a dye that can be seen on an X-ray is injected into the fluid that encompasses the spinal cord and then the cord is X-rayed. Defects, breaks and obstructions can then usually be seen.

What is the treatment?

Self-help: The best treatment is prevention. Never dive into water head first until you are sure it is deep enough. Let yourself down into the water feet first. If you must jump in, do so feet first. It is still possible to break your back, but you should not damage your neck in this manner. Other tips are to always wear seat belts while driving, drive within the speed limit, and do not drink and drive. Hold onto railings while using stairs, and be careful on slippery surfaces, on ladders, and during sports activities.

Spinal cord injury with lasting effects will inevitably force a drastic change in your life style. If you have had such an injury, you will have to stay in the hospital for a long time; several months is not uncommon. With the aid of various medical professionals, you will learn new ways to move around and to cope with daily life.

Some modifications may be necessary in your home. For instance, you may not be able to walk up and down stairs. Of course, you should do everything possible to resume your former working routine. If this is not possible, ask your physician or a social worker for information about programs for vocational rehabilitation.

Professional help: The treatment of suspected spinal damage starts from the time of the injury. If there is severe damage to vertebrae, surgery is sometimes advisable, but bed rest will also be advised to promote healing. A severely damaged spinal cord, however, does not heal of its own accord and cannot be medically or surgically cured completely. At first you will be kept fairly immobile and under constant observation to see if your symptoms improve. While under observation, you will need intensive nursing care. You will have to be fed, turned regularly to prevent pressure sores, and helped with relieving your bladder and bowels.

This stage may last several weeks, after which, if you remain disabled, a team of physicians, nurses, physical therapists, and occupational therapists will start the process of rehabilitation. Their goal will be to help you make good use of the strength left in your muscles. Various mechanical and electrical aids are available to help develop physical skills and increase independence. The goals and manner of any such treatment depend in a large part on your motivation and, of course, on the precise location and the degree of injury. Counseling and guidance will probably be available to you for coping with a variety of problems, including sexual problems. It is expected that you will need considerable help in learning to deal with your disability. Your motivation to live as normal a life as possible is extremely important. Therefore, it is important that you try not to lose patience with yourself. If you are not willing to help yourself and work at rehabilitation, no one can help you.

It may be three or four months before the degree of disability and possibilities for future recovery can be fully assessed. Courage, determination, and good will during this difficult period can play a large part in your recovery as will the understanding, patience and aid of family and friends.

In recent years, increasing attention has been given to the rights of the handicapped. Curbs are being lowered, bathrooms and buildings made more accessible, and barriers removed. This is good for everyone, since most people either now have or someday will have some degree of disability.

Bell's palsy

Bell's palsy is a condition, usually only temporary, in which the muscles on one side of the face become paralyzed because of a disorder of the nerve that controls them. There are two facial nerves, one on each side, that run out from the brain through a small hole in the skull, just behind the ear. Bell's palsy occurs when one of those nerves becomes swollen and is pinched near the point where it leaves the skull. It is not yet known what causes the swellings or why only one of the two facial nerves is usually affected.

What are the symptoms?
The characteristic symptom of the disorder is weakness of one side of the face. The corner of the mouth droops, it may become impossible to close one eye, and facial expressions such as smiles or frowns are distorted since there is virtually no movement of the muscle from forehead to mouth on the paralyzed side. The attack usually comes on quite suddenly, often overnight, and it is sometimes accompanied by pain either in the ear or on the affected side of the face.

What are the risks?
Bell's palsy can occur in people of any age, and it is fairly common. A middle ear infection (see Acute infection of the middle ear, p.333) sometimes seems to bring it on.

Though it is disfiguring, Bell's palsy is not a dangerous condition. The main physical risk is of irritation of or injury to the eye. The eye does not close properly, so it is exposed to dust, and it may become abnormally dry. The eye may also develop ulcers if it is left unprotected (see Corneal ulcers, p.316).

Embarrassment over looking strange can cause troublesome psychological effects. The family and friends of a person with Bell's palsy should understand if he or she is reluctant to go out in public or has even stronger adverse reactions to the problem.

What should be done?
If you have symptoms of Bell's palsy, consult your physician, who will probably be able to recognize this disorder by simply looking at you. You may begin to recover within two to three weeks, and if this occurs your recovery will probably be complete. However, the first signs of returning muscle function may not appear for two months or longer. In such cases, recovery will not be complete, but may be satisfactory for most people.

Until you have fully recovered, you may need to wear a protective eye patch and apply moisturizing drops to the affected eye at regular intervals. Sometimes a *steroid* medication is prescribed. In the rare cases in which facial disfigurement persists, an operation may help to improve facial appearance and relieve the physical disability. Such an operation may be especially helpful in cases involving severe emotional distress.

Cervical spondylosis

Cervical spondylosis is a disorder that affects some of the cervical vertebrae, which are the seven vertebrae of the neck. It also affects the flexible discs of cartilage that are sandwiched between these vertebrae. Bony outgrowths develop on the vertebrae, frequently accompanied by a misalignment and/or hardening of the plate-like discs. As a result, the neck becomes stiff and the nerve pathways in the upper part of the spinal cord, especially those that run between the cord and the arms and hands, are subjected to an abnormal amount of pressure (see Neuralgia, p.290). The cause of this disorder is unknown. It is particularly prevalent among middle-aged and elderly people, perhaps simply because some bones tend to become knobby and irregular as the body ages. Men and women are equally susceptible to the malady.

What are the symptoms?
The main symptom of cervical spondylosis is a stiff neck. Pressure on the nerves that lead from the affected area to your hands and arms may cause such symptoms as tingling, "pins and needles," numbness, and, occasionally, pains in the shoulders or arms.

Pressure within the neck may in time affect other portions of the spinal cord. Thus, if cervical spondylosis becomes increasingly severe, there may be a gradual weakening of the legs, and perhaps problems with bladder control. Sometimes, too, blood vessels that run through the neck vertebrae to the brain can become constricted because of this disorder, and this can cause symptoms such as headache, dizziness, unsteadiness, or double vision, especially if you try to bend your neck.

What are the risks?
Cervical spondylosis is a common disorder. Minor symptoms of the disease cause discomfort but present no serious problems. Many people who have it do not need to see a physician about it. In most cases the symptoms do not worsen. If they do, and if lower parts of the spinal cord become affected, there is a risk of serious and irreversible

damage. In very severe cases the lower half of the body may become paralyzed.

What should be done?

If minor symptoms persist and seem to be getting worse, consult your physician, who, after examining you, may arrange for an *X-ray* to be taken of your neck. If your legs appear to be weakening, you may also have a test called *myelography* to determine the extent of pressure on the spinal cord.

What is the treatment?

The treatment for troublesome symptoms of cervical spondylosis is use of a supportive collar. During the day you will probably need to wear a rigid plastic collar. A more comfortable, soft collar is substituted at night. The collar prevents extreme movements of the head and supports it in a position that minimizes pressure on the cervical nerves and blood vessels. The collar is usually worn for about three months, and in some cases there are no further problems. While you are wearing the collar, you may be advised to take *analgesics*, or painkillers, such as aspirin. Your physician may also prescribe a tranquilizer to relax you and keep your neck muscles from tightening up and causing still more discomfort.

If the symptoms persist, or if new ones develop, you may have to be hospitalized for *traction* or for an operation. Surgery involves an enlargement of the constricted bony spinal canal, a fusing together of some of the cervical vertebrae, or both. Either or both of these procedures usually gives some relief from the symptoms, but you will be left with a reduced ability to turn or bend your neck.

Carpal tunnel syndrome

At certain points in the body, nerves run through confined spaces where they are apt to become severely pinched if surrounding tissues become swollen. A major nerve particularly subject to this kind of damage is one that carries signals between the brain and the hand. As it travels through the wrist, this nerve passes through a tunnel formed by the wrist bones (known as the carpals) and a tough membrane on the underside of the wrist that binds the bones together. The tunnel is rigid, so if tissues within it swell for some reason, they press on and pinch the nerve. This leads to the painful condition called carpal tunnel syndrome.

Carpal tunnel syndrome is a fairly common disorder, especially among women approaching middle age. There is some evidence that a change in the balance of female sex hormones may lead to an accumulation of fluid and consequent swelling in the wrists at the time of menopause.

What are the symptoms?

The symptoms of carpal tunnel syndrome are tingling and intermittent numbness of part of the hand, often accompanied by pains that shoot up the arm from the wrist. The pains are generally worse at night and may be severe enough to wake you from a deep sleep. If you hang your hand over the side of the bed and rub or shake it, the pain may lessen. If the condition is very severe it can result in permanent numbness and weakness of the thumb and one or more fingers. One or both hands may be affected.

What is the treatment?

In some cases the condition clears up of its own accord. In others a splint worn on the affected wrist at night seems to help. To reduce the amount of fluid in the swollen tissues, your physician may prescribe a *diuretic* drug. An injection of a *steroid* drug at the wrist can help combat inflammation. But if you are in pain and the condition persists, the best treatment is an operation. The surgeon frees the pinched nerve by cutting through the tough membrane, creating more space. This is usually a successful procedure that gives immediate relief, requires only a brief hospital stay, and leaves a barely noticeable scar on the inside of the wrist.

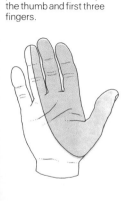

Pressure of swollen tissue on the median nerve where it passes through the carpal tunnel can result in loss of sensation in part of the hand, mainly in the thumb and first three fingers.

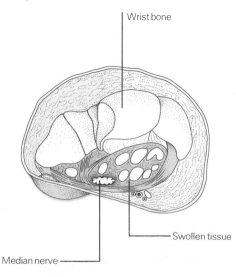

Cross-section through the wrist

Wrist bone

Swollen tissue

Median nerve

Brain tumor

An abnormal growth, or tumor, in the brain is a serious matter, whether the growth is *benign* (unlikely to spread) or *malignant* (likely to spread and threaten life). This is because the protective bones of the skull make it impossible for any type of tumor to expand outward, and so the soft brain tissue becomes dangerously compressed as the growth develops. So, since both are very dangerous, the distinction between benign and malignant tumors that develop in the brain is somewhat less clear-cut than it is in other body parts.

What are the symptoms?

As a tumor enlarges, it causes increased pressure within the skull. The result is frequent headaches, which are often most painful when you are lying down. The headaches are later accompanied by nausea and vomiting. Sometimes vomiting caused by a brain tumor seems to occur suddenly, without even a warning spell of nausea. Because the build-up of pressure can affect the nerves at the back of the eye, there may also be blurred or double vision. Other symptoms depend on the location of the growth in the brain. They include weakness down one side of the body, general unsteadiness, loss of the sense of smell, loss of memory, or even a major personality change. The presence of a brain tumor may also cause epileptic seizures (see Epilepsy, p.287).

What are the risks?

Tumors that originate in the brain are much less common than those that originate in the breast, lungs, or intestinal tract. However, spread of other cancers to the brain, creating secondary tumors, is relatively common. Such secondary tumors (those that have *metastasized*, or spread, from elsewhere in the body) are more common in later life, when most cancers are most likely to occur. Tumors of the brain will, if untreated, lead to permanent damage of the brain and can metastasize or spread to other tissues. Some types of brain tumors are fatal, especially if they are not treated. If a benign growth is discovered and treated early, however, there is often an excellent chance for full recovery.

What should be done?

If you have any of the characteristic symptoms, especially a headache that worsens when you lie down and is accompanied by vomiting, convulsions or progressive loss of vision, hearing, or use of your extremities, consult your physician. Your doctor may refer you to a neurologist for diagnostic tests. The tests may include *X-rays* (including X-rays of the chest, since secondary brain tumors frequently arise from cells from malignant tumors of the lung), a computerized brain scan (*CAT scan*), *angiography*, and possibly a *radioisotope scan* of brain tissues and *electroencephalogram (EEG)*.

What is the treatment?

Surgery to remove a benign tumor is often possible, and may well be completely successful. Even when the tumor involves a crucial part of the brain, it is sometimes possible to remove a portion of the growth to reduce pressure and relieve symptoms. Surgery, whether for full or partial removal of the tumor, is sometimes followed by *radiation therapy* to kill any remaining tumor cells.

Surgical treatment may not be as successful in the case of malignant brain tumors, but even in such cases there are ways of relieving your symptoms and making you more comfortable. *Steroid* drugs may help diminish the swelling of brain tissue, and thus the pressure, around the growth. *Anticonvulsant* drugs can be prescribed to control epileptic seizures related to the growth. There are also various *analgesics* available that reduce the pain of severe headaches.

Spinal cord tumor

Tumors of the spinal cord are similar to brain tumors (see previous article), but they produce different symptoms. Persistent back pain is the most characteristic symptom. Sometimes sensations of numbness or coldness and muscle weakness in one or more limbs may develop, and you may have difficulty in urinating or moving your bowels. The precise symptoms you have depend on what part of the spinal cord and which nerves are damaged by the tumor.

Spinal cord tumors are even rarer than brain tumors. If you have symptoms suggesting the possibility of a growth on your spinal cord, your physician will probably refer you to a neurologist for an examination, and for a *myelogram* (a special *X-ray* of the spine), and perhaps other diagnostic tests. If a tumor is found, an operation to chip away the surrounding vertebrae may be necessary. By relieving the pressure on spinal nerves and their pathways, such operations generally relieve pain immediately, and may also relieve other symptoms. As with brain tumors, further treatment depends on factors such as the type, size and site of the growth.

Peripheral neuropathy

Damage to peripheral nerves, which are nerves other than those in the brain and spinal cord, is called peripheral neuropathy. The damage sometimes occurs as a complication of a long-term disorder such as diabetes mellitus (see p.519), alcoholism (see p.304), certain vitamin deficiencies (see p.494, and also B_{12} deficiency anemia, p.420), or tumors in certain parts of the body. There are many other possible causes of peripheral nerve damage, including taking certain drugs for too long (see Box, p.513) and over-exposure to certain chemicals (especially arsenic, mercury, lead, and the organophosphates found in many insecticides). Avoiding toxic chemicals, injuries, and excessive intake of alcohol, along with observing good nutritional and exercise habits, can help you prevent neuropathy.

What are the symptoms?
In most forms of peripheral neuropathy, symptoms begin gradually, over many months. A dramatic exception is Guillain-Barre syndrome (see next article). The standard pattern is a tingling sensation that begins in the hands and feet and spreads slowly along all four limbs to the trunk. Then, in the same way, numbness may develop. Often the skin becomes very sensitive, and you may have neuralgic pain (see p.290). In some cases, there is a gradual weakening of muscle power throughout the body.

What are the risks?
Peripheral neuropathy is relatively common among alcoholics and diabetics. Cases caused by a build-up of *toxic*, or harmful, chemicals are rare in the general population, but occur more often among farm workers and people who work in other jobs where there is exposure to chemicals.

One of the risks associated with peripheral neuropathy is that if a numbed part of your body is injured, you may be unaware of the injury until infection or *ulceration* occurs. Numbness in the fingers can reduce dexterity, and make you more susceptible to accidents and injuries. A gradual wasting away of the muscles can accompany the weakness which can even become paralysis.

What should be done?
Because slow damage to the nerves either improves very gradually or is irreversible, early diagnosis is important. If your hands and feet are tingling, and especially if any of the factors that can cause this condition are applicable to you, see your physician, who will probably refer you to a neurologist for tests. The neurologist will take your medical and personal history and will examine you for signs of numbness, muscle weakness and changes in your reflexes. Special tests will depend on what the neurologist thinks may be causing the symptoms.

What is the treatment?
No direct medical or surgical treatment is possible. But if the cause of nerve damage is found to be diabetes or some other chronic disorder, stricter treatment of the underlying problem should slow or halt the progress of peripheral neuropathy. If toxic chemicals have caused the problem, you will be advised to stop your exposure to that substance. This may require a change of occupation.

In severe cases where muscles have been badly weakened, aids to mobility and independence, such as physical therapy, walking with a cane or other support, and bath rails may be prescribed. You will also be warned to remain actively aware of the possibility of unnoticed wounds on your numb limbs and to consult your physician without delay whenever you have a severe bruise or an open sore. Be sure to take good care of your feet and toe nails and wear shoes that fit well.

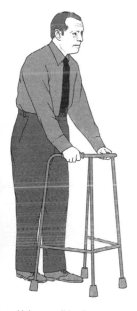

Using a walking frame

Guillain-Barre syndrome

This is an uncommon and acute form of peripheral neuropathy (see previous article), which can follow virtually any sort of viral infection or even an immunization. Why it occurs is not clear. Some physicians think it may be caused by an unpredictable allergic reaction to the virus that caused the illness or to the vaccine used in the immunization. The symptoms appear a few days after the causative illness has cleared up or the immunization has been given, and they are often severe. Within hours, a sensation of tingling, then numbness, then weakness or even paralysis may spread from your hands and feet to the rest of your body. Often, the paralysis is so extensive that it affects your breathing, and intensive hospital care becomes necessary.

Unlike other, longer-term forms of peripheral neuropathy, the nerve damage of Guillain-Barre syndrome is usually only temporary. With appropriate hospital care, full recovery from severe attacks is probable, but you may require physical and occupational therapy and it may take many months for you to return to normal health.

Functional disorders

The following disorders have one feature in common: They are generally caused not by a structural problem in the central nervous system, but by something wrong in the way it works. Typical symptoms of such functional faults are mainly localized in the head. They include dizziness and the pain of certain kinds of headache. But malfunction of the brain can also cause disturbing reactions in the whole body, such as blackouts or convulsions.

The physical reasons for such functional disorders as migraine and epilepsy, and even the common headache, remain largely unknown in spite of intensive research. This is why the conditions themselves are usually identified by their characteristic symptoms rather than by the processes that produce them. One achievement of modern medical research, however, has been the discovery of effective ways to relieve the symptoms of many of these disorders even though actual cure is not yet possible. As a result, most people who have conditions such as epilepsy now lead virtually normal lives.

There is reason to hope for even greater advances in the relatively near future. Scientists have focused much research on the chemistry and electrical nature of the nervous system. The result has been a gradually growing understanding of how this complex portion of our bodies works. From this understanding will spring new drugs and methods of dealing with functional disorders of the nervous system.

Headache

Headaches are sometimes a symptom of an underlying disorder. In fact, about a quarter of the disorders discussed in this book include headache as a possible symptom. However, if you get headaches, the strong probability is that they occur independent of any other disorder, develop gradually (often without apparent cause), clear up in a few hours, and leave no after-effects. In other words, most headaches do not indicate that there is anything seriously wrong with you. Your headaches, however painful, are likely only temporary, and brought on by tension that puts a strain on muscular tissues or blood vessels in the head, the neck, or both.

Brain tissues themselves never ache. They are insensitive to pain, since the brain itself does not contain *sensory* nerves. Sensitivity in this area exists only in the *meninges* (the membranes that cover the surface of the brain), the skin and muscles that cover the skull, and the many nerves that run from the brain to the head and face.

There are some types of headaches that are neither symptoms of underlying disorders nor insignificant and fleeting, but that can be considered as a specific disease. One of these is cluster headaches. These usually occur at night, and awaken you from sleep because the pain is intense. They are called cluster headaches because they occur every night for several weeks or even months, and then do not recur for a long time, sometimes several years. Another example of severe headache is migraine (see next article).

The headaches discussed in the following paragraphs are not of that kind. They are the simple, ordinary headaches that are almost universal. There are many factors that, either alone or in combination, can give you headaches. A few are stress, too little or too much sleep, over-eating or drinking, a noisy or stuffy environment, and heavy work indoors or outdoors.

You may not be able to figure out what has caused a particular headache. From a physiological standpoint, however, there are only two actual causes of headache pain. The first is strain on facial, neck, and scalp muscles, usually caused by tension. The second is swelling of blood vessels in the head area that results in strain within their walls. These two types are called tension headaches and vascular headaches respectively. If you have been under emotional stress, for example, you may think that worry or grief has given you a headache. This is true, but only indirectly. In fact, the strain has in some way affected your posture, creating a physical tension that results in pain. Similarly, if you have spent several hours concentrating on paperwork, the resultant headache probably comes from a hunched-over studying position, or perhaps eyestrain, not from the mental effort.

The typical morning-after, or hangover, headache that follows over-indulgence in alcohol is possibly due to a widening of the blood vessels in the brain. Alcohol is a *vasodilator*, which acts to dilate (widen) blood vessels in the body. In addition, a tension headache may develop because vascular pain leads to a straining of head and neck muscles.

What should be done?

If you have had headaches from time to time for several years, you probably know already whether they are migraines (see next article). If they have begun recently, however, your first priority is to find out what might be causing them. As a starting point, consult the Self-diagnosis symptom chart on Headache (see p.90). This is especially important if you have other symptoms in addition to headache. If you have recently had a head injury and you feel drowsy or nauseated, you could have an extradural hemorrhage (see p.272) or a subdural hemorrhage (see Sub-dural hemorrhage and hematoma, p.272). If it is painful to bend your head forward and you have been nauseated or been vomiting, you could have a subarachnoid hemorrhage (see p.271). In any of these cases, you should go to a hospital emergency room immediately. If you have a fever, light hurts your eyes, and it is painful to bend your head forward, you could have meningitis (see p.273), or migraine. You should see a physician as soon as possible, especially if you have a fever.

A headache that occurs alone and disappears overnight is probably no cause for concern. But if you have headaches that last for more than 24 hours or that recur as often as two or three times a week, you should consult your physician. After examining you, the doctor may refer you to a neurologist, a nervous system specialist, for diagnostic tests to make sure you do not have an underlying disorder of the central nervous system.

What is the treatment?

Self-help: One or more of the following measures should ease a simple tension or vascular headache. First, try to relax. Stretch and massage the muscles of your shoulders, neck, jaws and scalp. Take a hot bath, lie down, and place a warm, dry cloth or, if it feels better, a cold, wet one, over the aching area. Drink plenty of fruit juices or other non-alcoholic liquids, and take a mild painkiller such as aspirin. A nap or a good night's sleep is often the best treatment.

Professional help: If your physician finds that your headaches do not indicate an underlying disease, there may be little to do but recommend that you follow the above self-help measures, and possibly prescribe another type of painkiller.

Relieving a headache
Relaxation is often one cure for a tension headache. Take a leisurely, warm bath or lie down blindfolded or in a dark room and let all of your muscles relax.

Migraine

If you have migraine, you have periodic headaches, generally along with other symptoms such as nausea and disturbed vision, that almost completely incapacitate you for as long as they last. In spite of intensive medical research, it is not known why some people are subject to such attacks or what triggers them. Certain factors do appear to be involved in many cases. For instance, susceptibility to migraine headaches tends to run in families, leading to the strong suspicion that there is an inherited, or genetic, aspect of the disorder. In some cases, certain foods, including cheese, chocolate and red wine, have been found to provoke attacks. Often there is a relationship between the recurrent headaches and menstruation, stress, or even the anticipation of relaxation *after* stress. They can also be related to psychological illness. But your own migraines may seem to be unrelated to any of these factors.

The biological cause of an attack is probably the way the arteries leading to the brain react to the triggering factors, whatever they are. For some reason the arteries first become narrowed, then become swollen. This causes a disturbance in blood flow. In vascular headaches, which are less severe than migraine headaches, the arteries only swell (see previous article).

What are the symptoms?

In migraine, severe headaches are both preceded by and accompanied by other symptoms. The nature of each attack varies from person to person, but there is usually a warning period during which you feel abnormally tired and out of sorts. This is followed by nausea, vomiting, and sometimes diarrhea. You may find bright lights unbearable (a condition called *photophobia*). You may also have some sort of visual disturbance, usually worse in one eye, such as a misting over or a zig-zag distortion. Early warning symptoms can last for varying amounts of time, several minutes or several hours.

When the headache comes, the warning symptoms tend to fade away. You are likely to have intense, gripping pain, which starts at one side of your forehead but gradually spreads. The pain probably then begins to throb, and your entire head begins to ache. While you have the migraine headache, your eyes may be bloodshot and you will look pale and sick. In some cases the pain is centered between the nose and eye, and both the nose and eye tend to run.

The length of each migraine and the timing of headaches and headache-free periods are unpredictable, but you can learn to predict the nature and duration of each of your own attacks, based on your previous experience with the disorder.

Other less common symptoms experienced by some people are numbness or tingling in one arm or down one side of the body, dizziness, ringing in the ears, and temporary mental confusion.

What are the risks?

Migraine is a common complaint. Migraine headaches rarely start before puberty, but the unexplained recurrent abdominal pains of some children (see p.684) are sometimes an indication that they will have migraine headaches in later life. Only rarely does a first attack occur after the age of about 40. In fact, some people stop having attacks after reaching middle age. You are most likely to have migraine if it runs in your family and if you are female; migraines are slightly more common in women.

Although migraine headaches cause considerable suffering, they are not dangerous. It is unsafe, however, to attempt to drive or operate machinery while in enough pain to be distracted. In a few people some numbness, weakness, or visual disturbance has been known to become permanent. This is an extremely rare occurrence, however.

What should be done?

If you have recurrent severe headaches that you cannot control with simple painkilling drugs such as aspirin, consult your physician. There are no diagnostic tests for determining whether headaches are due to migraine or some other problem, but the doctor will probably be able to make a diagnosis based on your description of your symptoms.

What is the treatment?

Self-help: Try to make an objective study of your condition. After each attack, give some thought to what you were doing, thinking, feeling, eating, or drinking before the symptoms began. You may discover that you usually have indulged a special fondness for cheese, chocolate, or some other particular food before each attack. If this is the case, you may be able to prevent further attacks by avoiding that food in the future. Or you may find that you tend to have attacks just after periods of extra hard work or stress. In that case try to pace yourself differently. Avoid a crowded schedule, and leave yourself time for relaxation.

For some women, oral contraceptives appear to be the trigger factor. If you began to have migraine headaches about the same time you "went on" the pill, discuss the matter with your physician. Changing the type of drug or your contraceptive method (see Infertility and contraception, p.607) may eliminate the headaches.

As you come to recognize the early warning signs of an attack, you may be able to prevent it. The moment you suspect that a migraine headache is coming, splash your face with cold water, take two aspirin tablets, lie down in a darkened room, and stay there for two or three hours. Do not worry about the migraine during those hours. Simply relax, listen to a favorite record, take a nap, or meditate. Do not read at this time, even if reading normally relaxes you.

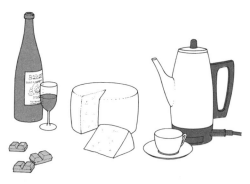

Foods can cause migraine
Many foods, notably cheese, chocolate, red wine, or coffee, may trigger migraine attacks in some people.

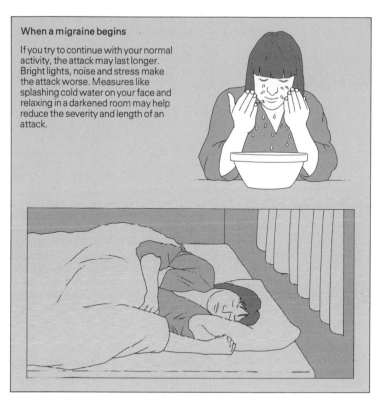

When a migraine begins

If you try to continue with your normal activity, the attack may last longer. Bright lights, noise and stress make the attack worse. Measures like splashing cold water on your face and relaxing in a darkened room may help reduce the severity and length of an attack.

Professional help: Although migraine cannot be cured, it can be relieved by drugs. There are two basic types of treatment. After a discussion of the illness as it affects you, your physician will suggest the treatment that is likely to be most helpful. If your migraines are not too severe and not too frequent, your physician may prescribe drugs that ease an attack after it has begun. These may be in the form of tablets, suppositories (drugs in a form that is inserted into the rectum), or injections and include one or more of the following drug types: *vasoconstrictors*, which act to narrow blood vessels; *antihistamines*, which expand the blood vessels; and *anti-emetics*, which control vomiting. You must take the drugs only when necessary, and exactly as prescribed, because an overdose can have unpleasant side-effects, including headaches as bad as or worse than the ones you are trying to avoid.

The second type of treatment is preventive. It is designed for people whose migraine headaches are so severe and frequent that they considerably disrupt ordinary functioning. This treatment consists of a type of relaxation therapy called *biofeedback*, and/or the use, on a continuing basis, of some of the same medications mentioned earlier.

Epilepsy

There are many forms of epilepsy, each with its own characteristic symptoms. Whatever its form, the disease is caused by a problem in communication between the brain's nerve cells. Normally, such cells communicate with one another by sending tiny electrical signals back and forth. In someone with epilepsy, the signals from one group of nerve cells occasionally become too strong; so strong that they overwhelm neighboring parts of the brain. It is this sudden, excessive electrical discharge that causes the basic symptom of epilepsy, which is called an epileptic seizure, fit, or convulsion.

It is not yet known what causes the brain's communication system to misfire in this fashion, or why such events recur in some people. Exhaustive research, including the testing of great numbers of epileptics, has shown that roughly two out of three epileptics have no identifiable structural abnormality in the brain, that is, there is nothing that is visibly wrong. The epilepsy of the remaining one-third can generally be traced back to an underlying problem such as brain damage at birth, severe head injury, or brain-tissue infection. Occasionally the condition may be caused by a brain tumor (see p.282). This is especially likely when the epilepsy appears for the first time in adulthood.

What are the symptoms?

The basic symptom of epilepsy is a brief, abnormal phase of behavior commonly known as a seizure, fit, or convulsion. It is important to realize that a single such episode does not indicate that you have epilepsy. By definition, epileptic seizures recur. There are many forms of the disease, but two major types are petit mal and grand mal.

Petit mal epilepsy is a disease of childhood that does not usually persist past late adolescence. A child may have this form of epilepsy if, from time to time, he or she suddenly stops whatever activity is going on and stares blankly around for a few seconds (sometimes up to half a minute). During the blank interval, known as a petit mal seizure, the child is unaware of what is happening. There may be a slight jerking movement of the head or an arm, but petit mal seizures do not generally involve falling to the ground. When the seizure ends, the child often does not realize that the brief blank spell has occurred. Such children are sometimes thought simply to be "day dreamers."

The most characteristic symptom of grand mal epilepsy is a much more dramatic seizure. The person falls to the ground unconscious. Then the entire body stiffens. Next it twitches or jerks uncontrollably. This may last for several minutes and is usually followed by a period of deep sleep or mental confusion. During a seizure some people lose bladder control and pass urine freely. In many cases the person gets a warning of an impending seizure by having certain strange sensations before losing consciousness. Any such warning is known as an aura, and an aura can occur just prior to the occurrence of the seizure or as much as several hours before it strikes. It may consist of nothing but a sense of tension or some other ill-defined feeling, but some epileptics have quite specific auras such as an impression of smelling unpleasant odors or hearing peculiar sounds, distorted vision, or an odd bodily sensation, particularly in the stomach. Many epileptics learn to recognize their special aura, and this may give them time to avoid accidents when they become unconscious.

Other types of epilepsy are much less common than petit and grand mal. Two additional types are called focal epilepsy and temporal lobe epilepsy. A person with focal epilepsy does not necessarily lose consciousness; the seizure begins with uncontrollable twitching of a small part of the body, and the twitch gradually spreads. The thumb of one hand, for instance, may start to jerk, followed by a jerking of the entire arm and then of the rest of that side of the body, after which there may be a more generalized seizure of the entire body. A person with temporal lobe epilepsy is likely to have an aura lasting only a few seconds. Then, without being aware of it, he or she does something entirely out of character, such as becoming suddenly angry, laugh-

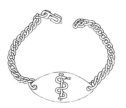

If you suffer from epilepsy, it is a good idea to wear a bracelet engraved with information about it If you have a seizure, those around you will know what is wrong and be able to get appropriate help

ing for no apparent reason, or interrupting normal activity with some sort of bizarre behavior. Strange, chewing movements of the mouth are apt to occur throughout any such episode.

What are the risks?
Between one and two per cent of the popula-

tion of the United States has some form of epilepsy. The disease may occur at a higher rate than this in some families. Both sexes are equally susceptible. Petit mal epilepsy occurs mainly in children, and epilepsy generally is more common in children than in adults. This is partly because petit mal epilepsy usually disappears before adulthood.

It should be emphasized that isolated, non-recurring convulsions, which are quite common in children, are often the result of the high fevers most often caused by infectious diseases (see Convulsions in children, p.667). A child who gets such convulsions and no others is not an epileptic. If you have any doubts about the nature of convulsions of a child, speak with your physician.

Modern drug treatment can control most forms of epilepsy, and epileptics can generally lead virtually normal lives. If occasional seizures do occur, however, there is a danger that they may happen in the wrong place at the wrong time. If your condition is not successfully controlled, you risk your life, and perhaps the lives of others, if you climb ladders, work with machinery, or drive a car. For this reason you should not drive at all unless your seizures are well controlled. Consult your physician about when it is safe for you to drive, and find out about possible legal restrictions on driving from the agency in your state that issues drivers' licenses.

Even in a relatively safe place, accidents can happen to you while you are having a seizure. When you clench your jaw, for instance, you may accidentally bite your tongue badly. Also, sharp objects are a danger when you fall and move about during your seizure. Bumping your head or another part of your body is also possible.

Recurrent uncontrolled convulsions have been known to cause permanent brain damage, but this is rare.

What should be done?
If you think someone in your family may have epilepsy, consult your physician, who will want a full description of the seizures from both the observer and the affected person, who may be a young child. The physician will also want to know how often the seizures occur. If there has been no recent illness or injury that might cause convulsions, the doctor can probably diagnose the condition as epilepsy based on the given facts. An *electroencephalogram* (*EEG*) test will probably be carried out to help confirm the diagnosis. And if there is a possibility that some identifiable brain damage or infection is causing the seizures, there may also be a skull *X-ray*,

blood tests, and perhaps a *CAT scan* of the brain. Some of the testing may have to be done in the hospital, and/or under the direction of a neurologist.

What is the treatment?

Self-help: If anyone in your family has epilepsy and is taking medicine for it, be sure that the drugs are taken exactly as prescribed. If pills are vomited up for any reason, another dose should be taken. However, if a dose is missed, you should not decide to compensate for it by taking more the next time. In such instances, contact your physician. He or she will know what is the best course of action.

Once the diagnosis of epilepsy is confirmed, ask your physician about how to obtain a card or tag that will tell strangers that you have epilepsy if you should ever have an unexpected attack and lose consciousness or act strangely. Some cards or tags include a telephone number or advice on what action any observer should take to help and protect you during a seizure. Carry your card at all times.

Professional help: Except in the relatively rare cases of epilepsy caused by curable brain damage, tumors, or infection, epilepsy cannot be cured. Anti-convulsant drugs taken as directed, however, effectively prevent most epileptics from having seizures. There are many such drugs, and your physician will prescribe one or more for you. You will need to take medication at regular intervals, and perhaps for the rest of your life if you have persistent attacks. As pointed out above, a child with petit mal epilepsy may grow out of it in time, and if this occurs your physician will let you know when the drugs are no longer necessary. Consult your physician if you have any questions.

Anti-convulsants occasionally have unpleasant side-effects, especially if they are taken in large amounts. So you should see your physician from time to time for check-ups and possibly blood tests to see if the dosage of the prescribed drug needs to be adjusted. If the drug is not completely effective, the doctor may increase the dose or may decide to try a different type of anti convulsant. If your condition is due to an underlying disorder, that disorder will also require treatment. Then, as the disorder improves, you should have fewer convulsions.

How to help someone who has a seizure

As explained in this article, some epileptic seizures are merely momentary blackouts, and the posture of the body remains virtually unaffected. If someone, probably a child with petit mal epilepsy, has such an attack in your presence, it is generally wise to ignore it. Just guide the person gently towards a safe place if any such minor convulsion occurs in a potentially dangerous situation – while crossing the street, for example. This advice applies equally in cases of temporal lobe epilepsy where the person may simply act strangely in some way. Just remember that no matter how active he or she may seem to be, the epileptic person is actually unaware of what he or she is doing, and should be gently guided away from danger, not forcibly restrained or scolded.

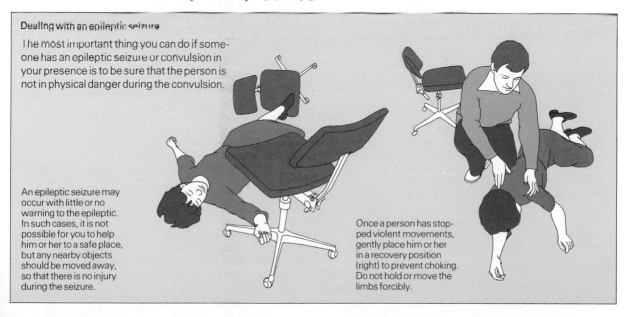

Dealing with an epileptic seizure

The most important thing you can do if someone has an epileptic seizure or convulsion in your presence is to be sure that the person is not in physical danger during the convulsion.

An epileptic seizure may occur with little or no warning to the epileptic. In such cases, it is not possible for you to help him or her to a safe place, but any nearby objects should be moved away, so that there is no injury during the seizure.

Once a person has stopped violent movements, gently place him or her in a recovery position (right) to prevent choking. Do not hold or move the limbs forcibly.

Someone who has a grand mal epileptic seizure will start to twitch or jerk, and may fall to the ground. If this happens, take the following steps:

1. Guide or push the person to a safe place *only* if he or she is in immediate danger – on a ladder, for example. Otherwise, do *not* attempt to move the person.

2. Move nearby objects so that they cannot cause injury. Do not hold down or restrain the person.

3. Loosen the person's collar and try to pull the jaw forward and extend the neck so he or she can breathe easily. During the active phase of a seizure, breathing may be much reduced, but artificial respiration is virtually impossible, and the epileptic will breathe normally as soon as the muscles relax again at the end of the seizure.

4. Most seizures last only a minute or two. If a seizure continues for more than about three minutes, or if another seizure starts a few minutes after the first, summon medical help immediately. The person may be carrying a card or tag that gives emergency information.

5. Many epileptics fall asleep after a seizure. If this happens, place him or her in a recovery position (see illustration, previous page) and allow the person to wake naturally. If possible, move him or her to a quiet place to allow undisturbed sleep, and check from time to time to be sure that everything is all right.

6. If the person does not have a card or tag, or if he or she is not known to be an epileptic, take the person to a physician or emergency room when the seizure has passed.

There is a common belief that the main thing you should do for convulsive epileptics is to force something between their teeth to keep them from biting or swallowing the tongue. This is poor advice. Any such attempt can actually damage the person's mouth.

Dizziness
(*vertigo*)

Dizziness, which is sometimes called vertigo, is a sensation of either spinning around yourself or of being stationary while everything that is around you spins. It is not a disease. It is a symptom of a disturbance in the brain and/or the organs of balance in your inner ears (see How you keep your balance, p.329). The disturbance may be caused by any of several underlying disorders.

Dizziness may be infrequent and mild, or you may have it very often and be so severely affected that you feel nauseated, vomit, lose your balance and fall down, or even faint.

The term vertigo is often incorrectly used to mean fear of heights. The correct term for fear of heights is acrophobia.

Dizziness is sometimes caused by a specific disease such as labyrinthitis (see p.338) or Meniere's disease (see p.337). More often, however, the functional disorder that causes it is minor and only temporary, and the dizziness is also only minor and temporary. It is frequently impossible to discover the cause of the problem. Dizziness is especially likely to occur in the elderly (see Aging and the senses, p.721).

What should be done?

If you have severe, prolonged, or repeated attacks of dizziness, consult your physician, who may arrange for special diagnostic tests to determine whether anything is seriously wrong. The best way to deal with dizziness is to lie down until it (and nausea, if any) goes away. If there is no identifiable underlying cause of persistent attacks, your physician may prescribe a drug that helps to stabilize the balancing mechanism in your inner ears.

Neuralgia

Neuralgia is pain from a damaged nerve. Several possible kinds of damage can lead to this disorder. The trouble may be temporary and mild, or it can be chronic and severe, as in sciatica (see p.547), peripheral neuropathy (see p.283), low back pain (see p.547), and trigeminal neuralgia (see p.722), a facial pain that mainly affects the elderly. The pain of neuralgia tends to be sharp and hard to bear. You feel it shooting along the affected nerve. It usually lasts only a few seconds, but several attacks may occur in quick succession.

Treatment of neuralgia depends on the location of the damaged nerve or nerves and on the cause of the damage. If you have occasional attacks that are only mildly painful, you can probably relieve the pain with *analgesics* such as aspirin. But if the pain becomes intolerable, consult your physician, who may prescribe a stronger painkiller. Your physician may also refer you to a neurologist, a doctor who specializes in problems of the brain and nervous system, for diagnostic tests and further treatment. In certain severe cases of neuralgia in the face, an operation to destroy the damaged nerve may be advisable. Also, drugs that change nerve conduction may be prescribed.

Degenerations

Grouped under this heading are a number of diseases in which nerve cells degenerate and die, usually quite slowly, taking months or years. The symptoms of the various diseases differ widely, depending on the area of the brain or spinal cord in which the degeneration of the nerve cells occurs. The results are distressing and sometimes even tragic. But there is hope because scientific research into causes and possible treatments is gradually increasing our understanding of these disorders. With this new understanding it is reasonable to hope for more and increasingly effective treatments.

Parkinson's disease

(paralysis agitans, shaking palsy)

Parkinson's disease is caused by gradual deterioration in certain nerve centers inside the brain. The centers are those that control movement, particularly semi-automatic movements such as swinging your arms while walking. Deterioration of these nerve centers upsets the delicate balance between two body chemicals, dopamine and acetylcholine, which are essential for controlling the transmission of nerve impulses within this part of the nervous system. The resultant lack of control produces the symptoms of Parkinson's disease.

Nobody knows what causes the more common forms of the illness. In rare cases the nerve degeneration results from such factors as carbon-monoxide poisoning or high levels of certain metals in body tissues. Sometimes Parkinson's disease is the result of an earlier infection of the brain, such as encephalitis (see p.274). High doses of certain drugs used in treating psychiatric conditions such as schizophrenia (see p.295) sometimes produce the symptoms of Parkinson's disease.

What are the symptoms?
One characteristic symptom is a type of *tremor* (sometimes incorrectly spoken of as "palsy," which actually means paralysis). There is an involuntary, rhythmic shaking of the hands, the head, or both, often accompanied by a continuous rubbing together of thumb and forefinger. Such tremors are most severe when the affected part of the body is not consciously in use. Once you begin to consciously move the involved body part the tremor disappears or diminishes. If the disorder worsens, there is a gradual loss of most automatic physical movements such as the natural swinging of the arms that makes walking smooth, or the ability to write legibly or move your mouth and tongue so as to speak clearly. It becomes increasingly difficult to initiate new movements, or to change from one position to another. There is no pain, numbness, or tingling, simply a decreasing ability to move. Falls may be frequent because it is difficult to retain balance while walking. Simple activities such as rising from a chair can become hard to manage. Further symptoms include excessive salivation, abdominal cramps, and sometimes in the later stages of the disease, deterioration of memory and thought processes.

What are the risks?
Most people who have Parkinson's disease are elderly or in late middle age. Men are slightly more susceptible than women, and there is some evidence that Parkinson's disease runs in families. Because the disease does not affect nerves that supply the heart or other vital organs, it is not directly life-threatening. A slowly progressing disability, however, can lead to mental depression.

What should be done?
There is no immediate cause for concern if, after age 50, you develop a mild tremor. Many people do so as they grow older. Consult your physician, however, if you have other symptoms of Parkinson's disease, or if the tremor worsens. Special diagnostic tests are not always necessary. Your doctor may be able to make a diagnosis based on a general physical examination.

What is the treatment?
Self-help: Encouragement and support from family and friends can be very helpful. Practical changes in the house, for example, bath-rail supports, special banisters along regular routes, and chairs with high arms will help you get around more easily and be more comfortable. Try to exercise regularly, and keep your spirits up by remaining or becoming as engaged in activities as possible.
Professional help: Modern drug treatment can do much to relieve the symptoms of Parkinson's disease, particularly stiffness and

immobility. In mild cases drugs are not usually prescribed, because they may have some troublesome side-effects. But your physician will probably want to see you about every six months to observe the progress of your condition. If drug treatment becomes necessary, medications that re-establish the balance of dopamine and acetylcholine within the affected area of the brain are usually prescribed. Some of these drugs tend to make the mouth unpleasantly dry, but that may seem more like a benefit than a side-effect if excessive salivation is a symptom of the disease in your case. New drugs are constantly being developed, but none has yet proved to be completely effective against the tremor that occurs in the disease. If tremors become a serious problem, it is sometimes possible to operate on the portion of the brain that is responsible for the problem, especially in younger people.

What are the long-term prospects?
As yet no treatment has been found that slows down the progression of Parkinson's disease, but the relief from symptoms that the various treatments give has kept many people with this disease in reasonable health.

Multiple sclerosis

Many nerve tracts, or pathways, in the brain and spinal cord are sheathed in a protective covering called myelin. The myelin sheath feeds nutrients to the nerves within it and also speeds up the passage of electrical impulses along the nerves. If a sheath becomes inflamed and swollen, and if this affects a number of nerve tracts in different parts of your central nervous system, you have the disease known as multiple sclerosis. Any part of the brain or spinal cord that contains myelin-covered nerves can be affected. There is some evidence that the damage may be due to a virus, or that the cause may be a deficiency or abnormality of the fatty substance that makes up myelin.

What are the symptoms?
Myelin is so widespread in the nervous system and the nervous system so widespread in the body, that multiple sclerosis can show up in many different ways. Most commonly, it begins with a vague, brief symptom that clears up completely within a few days or weeks. For example, you may get a feeling of tingling and numbness or weakness that may affect only one spot, one limb, or one side of the body. Temporary weakness of a limb may cause you to fumble, drop things or drag a foot. This type of symptom may be especially apparent after a hot bath or exercise.

Other possible indications of multiple sclerosis include *ataxia* (general physical unsteadiness), temporary blurring of vision, slurred speech, and either difficulty or lack of control in urinating. All symptoms disappear after the first episode in most cases, and sometimes there are no further problems.

But for some people there are repeated attacks. In these instances recovery is less complete after each attack, and permanent disability with progressive weakness of limbs or loss of vision develops. The periods between attacks are called remissions, and during remissions some people who have the disease continue to function in their usual activities for 20 to 30 years.

What are the risks?
Multiple sclerosis is not hereditary. In two-thirds of all cases, the first attack occurs between the ages of 20 and 40. The disease virtually never begins in children or in people over 60. Multiple sclerosis occurs slightly more often in women than in men.

Repeated attacks of multiple sclerosis can cause severe disability, but this does not occur in every case. If one of your symptoms is urinary incontinence (loss of bladder control), there is a risk of infection of the urinary tract (see p.502).

What should be done?
If you have symptoms of multiple sclerosis, your physician will probably refer you to a neurologist, or nerve specialist. There is no specific diagnostic test for the disease, but certain tests such as *ophthalmoscopy*, examination of spinal fluid, and special electrical brain wave tests can aid in diagnosis. Other tests will help rule out other possible reasons for your symptoms.

What is the treatment?
Self-help: The best thing anyone with severe multiple sclerosis can do is to try to accept the presence of the disease and its restrictions. Those who approach the problem optimistically and constructively succeed best at making whatever changes are required to continue to live as full a life as possible.
Professional help: Some cases are considerably relieved by *steroid* injections or tablets. These drugs may provide only limited help to other patients. Many drugs have been tried in the treatment of multiple sclerosis, but none

has proved to be particularly helpful. Some physicians may give vitamin supplements to make sure you do not have a vitamin B deficiency that might be contributing to the nerve damage.

Muscle-relaxant drugs sometimes relieve muscular stiffness or pain, and surgery for relief of spasms is advised in some cases. With particularly troublesome urinary incontinence it is sometimes necessary to have a *catheter*, or tube, introduced into the bladder. Urine drains through the catheter and into a bag, which you empty and clean daily. Final-ly, your physician may advise physical therapy to strengthen your muscles, and occupational therapy to help you remain active and able.

Only a limited number of people are crippled by multiple sclerosis. Many people have transient symptoms that pass without leaving ill-effects and may not return for many years. Many others are left with minor disabilities but lead almost normal lives. About 70 per cent of multiple sclerosis patients will still be actively engaged in their normal activities five years after the diagnosis.

Motor neuron disease
(*amyotrophic lateral sclerosis*)

This rare condition occurs when certain nerve cells die. These are the motor neurons that run from the brain to the muscles and control the muscles' movements. The affected muscles cannot be stimulated and used, and they gradually waste away. The affected part of the body becomes increasingly weak. The disease can cause difficulty in swallowing, breathing, walking, or any other muscle-powered activity. Thus it can interfere with virtually any of the body's physical functions.

Motor neuron disease occurs most often in people over 40. Little is known about its cause, and it cannot be cured. Treatment is directed at easing symptoms and helping you to remain relatively mobile and independent. In most cases death occurs within two to ten years of the onset of the disease.

Huntington's chorea

Huntington's chorea is a very rare degenerative nerve disease that starts in early middle age. Uncontrollable body movements, called chorea, gradually develop and are followed by mental deterioration. Sometimes mental deterioration occurs first. No treatment has yet been discovered to halt the progress of the disease or control its symptoms. The word "chorea" literally means "dance." The term is a rough description of the swift, jerky movements that occur in people who have this disease.

Huntington's chorea is an inherited disorder that seldom produces symptoms before marriage and childbearing. Therefore, a person with this disease may not know it until after having a child. If you know of anyone in any branch of your family who has had the disease, consult your physician about possible risks for yourself and your children.

Friedreich's ataxia

This is an exceedingly rare inherited disease in which certain groups of nerve fibers gradually deteriorate. The main symptom is *ataxia*, or loss of coordination of movement and balance, especially when walking. Gradually it also becomes difficult for the affected person to stand still, to speak, and to use the arms. The arms may begin to shake just when he or she intends to move them. This is called an intention tremor. Symptoms usually become apparent between the ages of 5 and 15. There is now no treatment for this disease. Friedreich's ataxia runs in families, so if you have relatives with the disease you should seek advice from your physician or a genetic counselor before starting a family.

Pre-senile dementia

Senile dementia (see p.724) is primarily a disorder of the elderly. Pre-senile dementia, or Alzheimer's disease, is either the same or a similar disorder that occurs in someone under 60. It may be due to an underlying disorder such as hypothyroidism (see p.526) or a brain tumor (see p.282), and in such cases it can sometimes be successfully treated if the cause is discovered in time. If this is not the case, it may be due to a progressive loss of brain cells, the cause of which is not known. Reasoning powers, memory, and other thought processes tend to deteriorate more quickly than they do in senile dementia, and the disease in a comparatively young person can be fatal within about five years.

Mental and emotional problems

Introduction

Mental illness is difficult to classify into clearly defined diseases. It is the symptoms of mental illness that distinguish one type of disorder from another, but those symptoms often vary much more widely in both kind and degree than the symptoms of physical illness. Because of this it is sometimes difficult to tell whether or not a person is actually mentally ill or, if illness is obvious, to determine the probable cause and work out a possible cure.

In general, if you are able to keep your mental balance during periods of emotional stress, you can call yourself mentally healthy. If you lose that balance you are ill, at least to some extent. The articles in this section are designed to help you recognize some of the warning signs of common forms of mental illness, not only in yourself but also in others. The arrangement of articles is based on two groupings. First, there are illnesses that arise primarily from internal influences, such as schizophrenia, depression and compulsions. The actual causes of such disorders are not known, but personality factors and slight variations in the amount and type of chemicals in the brain may be the cause. Second, there are addictions, or illnesses triggered off by external influences such as alcohol or other drugs. Certain personality types appear to be especially susceptible to these disorders.

Some people are overwhelmed by trivial crises such as minor marital quarrels. Others retain their balance in daunting circumstances such as the break-up of a once-happy home. Such mental health is not necessarily inborn. You can cultivate it in yourself and thus stand a better chance of coping well with the problems of living.

Psychiatric terms

There is a special vocabulary that relates to psychological problems and their treatment. Many general terms used in these pages have clearly defined meanings for medical people, but laymen sometimes find it difficult to distinguish among them. Here are definitions of eight such terms:

Psychiatrist: A psychiatrist is a medically qualified physician who can diagnose and prescribe drugs for any illness. As a psychiatrist, he or she specializes in mental illness.
Psychologist: A psychologist has been trained in human psychology, but not in medicine. Psychologists concentrate on psychotherapy (see below). They are not licensed to prescribe drugs.
Psychoanalyst: The term psychoanalyst refers to a person who treats mental disorders by probing into and analyzing the unconscious, as well as the conscious, contents of the minds of his or her patients.
Psychotherapy: Psychotherapy is a general term for the treatment of mental disorders by intellectual and verbal means, including suggestion, analysis and persuasion.

Such treatment may be supplemented by other forms of treatment such as drugs.
Neurotic: Neurotic people are particularly susceptible to symptoms of mental or emotional stress. They may sometimes weep uncontrollably for some apparently inappropriate cause, for example, or have an irrational fear of flying. But their "hang-ups" do not become so overpowering that they lose contact with the realities of daily life.
Psychotic: A person who is psychotic has lost contact with reality and is either occasionally or constantly incapable of rational behavior.
Psychosomatic: A psychosomatic disorder, sometimes called a psychogenic disorder, is a physical illness caused by a mental or emotional problem. A psychosomatic illness is real, *not* imaginary, but it can often be cured by treatment of an underlying psychological problem.
Psychopathic: Psychopathic people may seem on the surface to be normal. But they are mentally or emotionally irresponsible, and their behavior is chronically, and often dangerously, antisocial.

Mental illnesses

The chemistry of the brain probably plays an important part in causing mental illness. That is why drugs may be used along with *psychotherapy* in treating the disorders discussed below. But most cases of mental illnesses such as manic depression, anxiety, or hypochondriasis are thought to be largely the result of personality factors. Some people, for example, are by nature *neurotic*. They irritate easily, are over-sensitive, and may lack energy. When under stress, such people sometimes become depressed or anxious. Many others are *cyclothymic*. This means they have swings in mood from elation and energy to lethargy and withdrawal. Under stress, such people may become manic-depressive. Most people, however, overcome the drawbacks of inherited personality traits and manage to cope with emotional problems without treatment. If you have a neurotic or cyclothymic personality, you are not necessarily on the verge of a mental illness.

It is estimated that three to four per cent of most physicians' patients consult the doctor mainly because of an emotional problem. The physical disorders of many others are related to psychological stress. Many people who consult a physician are either neurotic and temporarily in need of help or have what can be *psychosomatic* symptoms such as palpitations or indigestion (for definitions of terms, see previous page).

When a doctor feels that your problems are mainly mental ones, you may be referred to a psychiatrist. But it is sometimes difficult to determine whether physical symptoms are the result of emotional or other causes. For this reason, if you or a family member have symptoms that you suspect might be totally or even just partly caused by emotional difficulties, be sure to tell your physician.

It is only when people lose touch with reality and behave in bizarre and perhaps life-threatening ways that they can be considered *psychotic* rather than neurotic. It is usually best to treat such patients in a hospital, where they are less likely to do harm to themselves or to others.

Schizophrenia

Schizophrenia (literally "split mind") is often thought of as a split or dual personality. However, this disease is best defined as a disorganization of normal thought and feeling. It is probably caused by the malfunctioning of the cells through which information flows within the brain. Symptoms usually appear in late adolescence or early adulthood, and extreme mental stress almost always triggers them. The illness is lifelong, but acute attacks tend to come and go, and usually occur at times of emotional upheaval or personal loss.

What are the symptoms?
Some popular novels, plays and movies have encouraged us to think of schizophrenia in extremely narrow and dramatic terms. Schizophrenia has been presented quite often in terms of the split personality, two seemingly individual and separate people living within the same body.

For most people with schizophrenia, an attack begins with a gradual, or occasionally sudden, withdrawal from day-to-day activities. The person's speech may become increasingly vague, and he or she may seem to be unable to follow a simple conversation. An acute attack happens unexpectedly. Often the onset is so gradual that it is difficult to know when *psychotic* symptoms appear. Among such symptoms are apparently disconnected remarks, along with blank looks, that are followed by sudden statements that seem to spring into the speaker's mind.

Schizophrenics often believe that others hear and "steal" their thoughts. Sometimes they fear they have lost control of bodily movement as well as thought, as if they were puppets. They frequently believe they hear voices, often hostile ones. Less commonly, they have hallucinations of odd physical sensations, of being given poison, or otherwise being attacked by others. In time many schizophrenics build up a set of beliefs in a fantasy world. They may express exaggerated feelings of happiness, bewilderment, or despair. They may laugh at a sad moment or cry without cause. Or they may seem devoid of feeling, so that it becomes almost impossible to make emotional contact with them.

There are several types of schizophrenia that are characterized by the predominant symptoms, but the only practical distinction that most doctors now make is between the *paranoid* and other types. The main symptom of a person with paranoid schizophrenia is constant suspicion and resentment, accompanied by fear that people are hostile or even plotting to destroy him or her.

What are the risks?

Most young and middle-aged patients in mental hospitals are there because they are schizophrenic. About 1 person in 1000 has been treated for the disorder. Men and women are equally susceptible. Paranoid schizophrenia is most common in early adulthood (late 20's through 30's).

The abnormality of brain chemistry that underlies schizophrenia can be inherited, but if it runs in your family, you will not necessarily have schizophrenic attacks. You may, however, have either a "schizoid personality" (a tendency towards extreme shyness and withdrawal) or a "paranoid personality" (a tendency towards over-sensitivity and distrustfulness).

People who have attacks of schizophrenia in its most severe forms may physically harm themselves or others, or may try to commit suicide (see p.298).

What should be done?

If you suspect that someone in your family is schizophrenic, try to get them to see a physician. It may not be easy. People who are becoming mentally ill often refuse to admit it. Even those who realize that something is wrong have a fear of being "put away." But medical care is vital. Do not leave a person who seems extremely disturbed alone. The presence of a relative or friend to reassure them, or even keep them from hurting themselves until help arrives, may be essential. People with symptoms similar to those of schizophrenia are usually admitted to a hospital for a preliminary period of observation. During this time tests are carried out to make sure these symptoms are not due to a physical illness such as a brain tumor (see p.282).

What is the treatment?

Severe cases must be treated in a hospital. Treatment usually involves the use of drugs, *psychotherapy* and rehabilitation.

The most effective drugs are regular doses of special tranquilizers designed to modify abnormal brain chemistry. As symptoms gradually disappear, doses are reduced, and all medication may be discontinued when the acute attack ends. Some people, however, need long-term medication. They may either take pills regularly or be given an injection every two to four weeks. Occasionally *antidepressant* drugs are also prescribed (see Depression, next article). In rare cases *electroshock therapy (EST)* may be recommended.

Techniques of psychotherapy vary, but the goal is the same: to help the patient understand the stresses that contributed to the current attack. This can help the person learn how to prevent future stresses from leading to further illness.

The final stage of treatment is rehabilitation, which helps people who are recovering from attacks to regain normal skills and behavior patterns. In the early stages of hospital treatment schizophrenics are generally given occupational therapy. As their condition improves, they are given increasingly complex tasks and pressures, and these eventually approximate the tasks and pressures of the world outside. Once the acute phase of the illness is over, the schizophrenic prepares for a return to the outside world by making periodic visits from hospital to home or to a half-way house.

What are the long-term prospects?

Many people recover from an attack of schizophrenia well enough to return to a relatively normal life. But they may have further attacks. In some people the condition becomes *chronic*. Such a person will always be withdrawn and emotionally unresponsive, but they generally avoid severe attacks of the disorder with the aid of constant medication.

What is a nervous breakdown?

The term "nervous breakdown" is often used by the public as a general term to say that a person has had an attack of a serious mental illness. In other words, a person who has a nervous breakdown becomes unable to deal with ordinary life because of mental or emotional problems. Usually temporary hospitalization is implied.

"Nervous breakdown" is not a medical term, and would not be used by a physician to describe the diagnosis of a patient who has a mental illness. Terms such as schizophrenia, depression, or anxiety are more useful.

Unfortunately, people who are known to have some form of mental illness are often feared and avoided by others in the community and sometimes by friends and family. But mental illness is not really very different from physical illness and is not catching or contagious. Just as in any other illness, help, concern and support will benefit the patient, society and yourself. Ignorance and prejudice can only be harmful.

Depression

Most people feel depressed occasionally. There is no question of their being mentally ill, though, if they continue with a daily routine and gradually recover. The difference between "feeling depressed" and having the mental illness known as depression is that people who are actually ill cannot lift themselves out of their misery. Their depression persists, deepens, and eventually interferes with their ability to lead normal lives. If you or others in your family have occasional periods of low spirits that disappear after a few days or weeks, you have no cause for concern. The symptoms of true depressive illness are described below (see also Manic depression, next article).

There are two main types of depressive illness. One type is caused by an extreme reaction to a specific emotional blow such as the death of someone you loved, the end of a marriage or love affair, or a financial loss. *Neurotic* people sometimes over-react to such misfortunes, and the result may be a depressive illness. The other type of depression usually occurs without apparent cause. It may result from hormonal changes after childbirth (see Postnatal depression, p.642) or may be associated with schizophrenia (see previous article).

There are periods of particular susceptibility to depressive illness in almost everyone's lifetime. Late adolescence, middle age, and the years after retirement are such periods. Many people find the transition from adolescence to adulthood difficult, especially when there are intense family conflicts or educational or work pressures. Loss of fertility or virility in middle age may seem like loss of sexuality, a loss that would trigger depression in many people. A person in late middle age may brood over the realization that he or she can advance no further in a career.

Depressive illness among elderly people is extremely common. This may be related to many factors, including the death of friends, the physical limitations of old age, and the realization that death is now in the foreseeable future.

Every severe depression is probably accompanied by a chemical change that affects the way the brain functions.

What are the symptoms?
Symptoms of depressive illness include not only overriding melancholy but also physical changes. It is common for the depressed person to become unconcerned or apathetic about the outside world. He or she may also lose interest in or have trouble with eating, sleeping and sex. Sometimes indigestion, constipation and headaches appear. Some depressed people have severe psychological symptoms. They may lose touch with reality, may feel guilty and worthless without cause, may believe that they are being persecuted or that their bodies are rotting away, and may have hallucinations. Sometimes acute anxiety (see p.300) accompanies the depression, and the resultant restlessness and agitation may mask the more expected symptoms.

Intensity of symptoms often varies with the time of day. Typically, a depressed person wakes up early in a sad mood that brightens as the day progresses. But some people have the worst symptoms at night. As the illness progresses, depression may deepen until it never lifts. The person then becomes totally withdrawn, and may spend most of the time huddled in bed.

What are the risks?
About 15 per cent of the population is likely to experience at least one period of depression severe enough to require medical help, though the symptoms may not be specifically identified as a depressive illness. Some types of depression tend to run in families.

The gravest risk of depression is suicide, the last resort of someone who finds life unbearable (see Box, next page). In rare cases the illness can unbalance a person's mind so much that they feel forced to kill others as well as themselves, to spare them the agony of being alive. Although they are too common in all age groups including the young, depression and suicide are particular problems of the elderly, and sometimes depression can resemble and be confused with senility (see Senile dementia, p.724). This confusion is particularly unfortunate since depression is often reversible. Thus a depressed elderly person may be thought to have senile dementia and get no treatment for his or her depression.

What should be done?
If you recognize the symptoms of increasing depressive illness (not just a passing sadness) in yourself, see a physician now. Do not be ashamed to tell him or her about your fears. If you recognize the symptoms in other people, try to persuade them to accept medical help.

What is the treatment?
Self-help: If you think a mild form of depression is lasting too long or beginning to deepen, a vacation, active sports, or a hobby may help you pull out of it. It may not be possible to do this, however, if you have a depressive illness, so if these measures fail,

see your physician. If a member of your family seems to be severely depressed, try gentle but firm persuasion to get him or her to a doctor. Threats of suicide should be considered an emergency.

Professional help: Treatment depends on the type and severity of symptoms. If you go to your family physician with symptoms of depression, he or she may refer you to a specialist for treatment. Treatment may consist of medications, *psychotherapy*, or a combination of both. *Antidepressants*, which are often used in treatment of depression, can usually begin to relieve a mild case within two to three weeks. In severe cases, especially when there is a risk of suicide, the physician may advise hospitalization, because in a hospital your symptoms can be monitored, you can be prevented from harming yourself, and drug treatment and psychotherapy can be closely supervised. In rare cases of persistent illness, *electroshock therapy* (*EST*) may be recommended.

If you are treated in a mental hospital, the goal of treatment is not only to cure your depression but also to prepare you for a return to normal life.

What are the long-term prospects?
People who have a depressive illness almost always respond well to treatment. Unfortunately, some types of depression tend to recur. Yet many people who have repeated attacks of depressive illness manage to function by getting treatment in the early stages of each attack.

Manic depression
(including mania)

A normal person has moods that shift from moderate liveliness to moderate lethargy, depending largely on circumstances. A person who has the disorder called manic depression has extreme moods that are not related to external events. Manic-depressive illness tends to be cyclical, with periods of elated over-activity (mania) irregularly alternating with deep depression (see previous article). Periods of normality, sandwiched between the extremes, may last a short time or years.

Extreme stress may trigger off a sudden attack of mania or depression, particularly in people who seldom have acute attacks. Often, however, there is no direct cause, and phases of the illness begin gradually. Very rarely manic depression is caused by a severe infection, a stroke (see p.268), or a brain injury (see p.276).

What are the symptoms?
Close associates of a person with this disorder are likely to be first to recognize the beginning of the manic phase, which starts gradually with hypomania, a moderate degree of mania. People in this phase begin to wake up earlier and earlier in the morning, until they find themselves leaping out of bed before sunrise. At the same time, their work output often falls because they are easily distracted and increasingly restless. They may be promiscuous sexually, go on spending sprees, and enthusiastically start (but rarely finish) new projects. They are often irritable, and may have sudden attacks of rage.

Hypomania seldom reaches a fully manic stage. If it does, total elation may result in wilder speech, full of rhyming, punning, and illogical word associations. Some people sing and dance or laugh uproariously for no reason. At times an underlying sadness may break through in fleeting moments of withdrawal. Because they lack concentration, manic people often forget to eat, so they tend to lose weight and become exhausted. Eventually, they may have delusions of grandeur or intense anger at their inability to carry out wild schemes.

The depressive phase is like depression (see previous article), but the symptoms are often more severe. The onset is gradual. The person becomes increasingly withdrawn. Sleep is frequently disturbed. Although there may be early-morning wakefulness, late rising becomes habitual. Sex drive decreases,

---

Suicide

Each year about 200,000 people in the United States try to kill themselves. About 22,000 succeed. Those who fail often want to fail; an unsuccessful attempt at suicide may be a lonely, frustrated, or ill person's way to attract attention. You can never be certain, however, that someone who tries to commit suicide and fails will not succeed some day. So if anyone you know seems emotionally disturbed and threatens to commit suicide, try to get him or her to see a physician. If quick action seems necessary, call your physician, a local crisis "hot line," or a hospital for help. While waiting for help, encourage the suicidal person to talk, and listen patiently without passing judgement. Do not leave such a person alone; wait with them at least until professional help arrives.

If you find someone who is unconscious or semi-conscious, whatever the cause, call an ambulance or take the person to a hospital emergency room. Disturbed individuals often seek death by taking an over-dose of sleeping pills. If you find tablets or a medicine container anywhere near the person, be sure to give them to the hospital staff or the ambulance crew. Meanwhile apply first aid (see Accidents and emergencies, p.801).

speech and movement slow down, and imagined problems multiply. Some manic depressives become unable to face the world, and simply stay in their rooms.

What are the risks?

Manic-depressive illness is rarer than depression. It is thought to occur in about three per cent of the population. It tends to run in families, and men and women are equally susceptible to it.

Although someone with this disorder may threaten suicide during depressions, he or she usually lacks the energy to carry it through. The danger increases with emergence from deep depression, when renewed energy may accompany a continuing death-wish. In the manic phase, outrageous behavior may ruin social and professional relationships, and lack of judgement can become serious enough to lead to financial disaster.

What should be done?

If you suspect someone you are close to is manic-depressive, persuade him or her to see a physician. If necessary, ask your own doctor for advice. If you think that you yourself may be becoming manic depressive, see your physician without delay. The illness is easier to treat effectively in its early stages.

What is the treatment?

After a diagnosis is made, in mild cases it is often possible for medications to be taken at home. Your physician may also refer you to a specialist for *psychotherapy*. In severe cases, especially when there is a risk of suicide or if irrational behavior gets out of hand, treatment in a hospital is usually necessary.

Drugs that alter brain chemistry are now generally used for manic-depressives. Because of possible side-effects, however, the person must have blood, kidney and thyroid-gland tests before some of these drugs can be prescribed. *Electroshock therapy* (*EST*) may also be recommended.

As the treatment in the hospital begins to show results, occupational therapy is added to the treatment to prepare the person for a return to normal life. If somebody in your family has been in the hospital for this disorder, you will probably be told both how to recognize signs of an impending attack and how to reduce the strains on the patient and lessen the risk of further attacks. After release from the hospital, many manic-depressives must continue to take drugs. They may need to have monthly checkups to guard against potentially harmful side effects of this drug regime.

What are the long-term prospects?

Not long ago most people who had one episode of manic-depressive illness could expect to have further attacks, which might become increasingly severe. However, this gloomy outlook can now often be brightened by long-term drug treatment.

Psychoanalysis

Psychoanalysis is the original technique on which all psychotherapy is based. It was developed by a Viennese neurologist, Sigmund Freud, in the late nineteenth century. The technique is based on Freud's theory that adult behavior is largely determined by early childhood conflicts. There are many variations on Freud's basic theory and technique, but all have the same goal: to help the patient recall memories buried deep in the subconscious mind. Once the root causes of a problem are recollected and understood, the patient may be able to change long-standing but unhealthy patterns of thought and behavior.

Treatment of this sort requires many meetings with the analyst, during which such matters as present and past dreams, recollections, thoughts and feelings are discussed, analyzed, and interpreted. Because full treatment involves several hour-long sessions per week for at least two or three years, often double this amount of time or more, psychoanalysis is not generally feasible except for people who have the money and time to invest in it. Moreover, the original technique has proved to be less effective than its early practitioners hoped. Many doctors now believe that the main value of Freud's work is that it provided a framework for modern psychiatry in emphasizing the vital influence of early experience on patterns of adult behavior.

Psychotherapy

Psychotherapy is treatment by verbal means. The original verbal technique for treating mentally disturbed people was psychoanalysis. Modern techniques have developed partly because of the need to develop less time-consuming methods. These vary widely but usually involve a number of counseling sessions, during which the patient discusses his or her special problems with the therapist, who offers clarification, understanding and challenges to possible new approaches for the patient without necessarily making a detailed investigation of childhood experiences. Sometimes people are treated in groups. The advantage of group psychotherapy is that members of the group learn from each other, and pressure each other to adopt a healthier attitude toward daily stresses. This type of therapy is particularly helpful for people who are not mentally ill but who have personality problems.

Anxiety

For most people, anxiety is a temporary reaction to stress. It becomes an illness only when it persists, and prevents you from leading a normal life. Some anxiety states are caused by severe stress, but in anxiety-prone people only slight stress, or none at all, may be involved. People who have "free-floating" anxiety live in a constant state of apparently causeless anxiety.

If you have an attack of anxiety, you will probably feel apprehensive and tense, and be unable to concentrate, to think clearly, or to sleep well. You may have frightening dreams and occasional symptoms of fear such as a pounding heart, sweating palms, trembling, or diarrhea. Some people in a state of anxiety find it hard to breathe, as if their lungs are under constant pressure. And they may become convinced that they have heart or stomach trouble when in fact they are physically healthy (see Hypochrondriasis, p.302). A man may have trouble maintaining an erection or may have premature ejaculation (see p.614). In so-called "anxiety attacks," which can occur apparently without cause at any time, the physical symptoms of fear intensify alarmingly.

What are the risks?
Anxiety is a very common form of psychological disorder. It is slightly more common in women than men, and adolescents and the elderly are especially susceptible. If severe anxiety is not treated, you may sink into *psychotic* depression (see p.297).

What should be done?
If your anxiety is caused by a specific stress, try to remove it. For example, consider changing jobs if your current work makes you anxious. If there is no way to deal with the stress, or if severe anxiety persists, consult your physician, who will examine you to determine whether your symptoms may be due to a physical condition such as an over-active thyroid gland (see Hyperthyroidism, p.525) or a vascular disorder of the brain (see p.268). If no physical cause for your symptoms is found, you may be referred to a specialist. The first time you have an anxiety attack, you may think you are having a heart attack. To be on the safe side, call your physician. If he or she is not available, call an ambulance to take you to a hospital.

What is the treatment?
Self-help: Various methods of relaxation can lessen the severity of symptoms. Whenever you feel tense and troubled, try doing relaxation exercises or some physical activity such as swimming, jogging, or brisk walking.
Professional help: Your physician may suggest exercises to relax tense muscles. In addition, or alternatively, your doctor may prescribe an anti-anxiety drug or recommend *psychotherapy*. Severe cases may also require a period of hospitalization.

What are the long-term prospects?
If your disorder is due to a stress that can be dealt with, you have a good chance of permanent cure. But if you are anxiety-prone or have free-floating anxiety, recurrent attacks are likely. You may be able to avoid them, or at least minimize symptoms, by continuing to do relaxation exercises even when you are not actively anxious. Ask your doctor if there is a drug that you can take as soon as you feel that an attack is beginning.

Phobias

A phobia is an irrational fear of a specific object or situation. For instance, you may dread the sight or touch of a spider, or you may have a morbid fear of heights (acrophobia). Such fears do not usually prevent you from leading a normal life; you simply avoid spiders or high places. Fear of confined spaces (claustrophobia) is more of a problem, since it may make you unable to use cars, trains and elevators, but most claustrophobic people manage to overcome their fears. Some phobias, however, may make normal life virtually impossible. A common example is agoraphobia, which is generally defined as fear of open spaces. For agoraphobic people an open space may be not just a park or field but anywhere outside their own home. The phobia may also involve extreme shyness – a fear of society that is closely associated with the withdrawal symptoms of depression (see p.297). If you suffer from agoraphobia or any other phobia, the need to face whatever you fear can bring on the symptoms of anxiety (see previous article), including anxiety attacks.

What is the treatment?
Self-help: To combat a relatively mild phobia, try to force yourself to come to grips with it gradually. This process is called "desensitization." If you abhor spiders, for example, start by looking at pictures of them. Next, make yourself stay in a room with one. Then look at one closely. Finally, let one run

over your hand. Or, if agoraphobia makes you dread shopping, begin by going to small shops and gradually increase store size until large stores no longer terrify you.

Professional help: If your symptoms are those of a general anxiety state, treatment is similar to treatment for anxiety. For agoraphobia associated with depression, many physicians prescribe *antidepressant* drugs. The most common type of *psychotherapy* for this disorder is *behavior therapy*, given either in or out of a hospital. There are two kinds of behavior therapy. The first, desensitization, has been described above. If you are unable to desensitize yourself, professional guidance may help.

The second technique is called "flooding."

It is not recommended as a self-help measure because it is very drastic. Whereas desensitization is like entering a cold sea gingerly, flooding is like the shock of a quick plunge. You are suddenly confronted with the feared object or placed in the feared situation, with no chance of escape. Thus, having experienced your phobia at its fullest intensity, you come to realize that the dreaded thing is not truly dangerous. As you can imagine, flooding is risky. Only a competent and experienced therapist should subject a phobic person to it.

Another technique for treating phobias is biofeedback training, in which relaxation techniques are used. Sometimes hypnotism is used by qualified professionals.

Psychosomatic illness

Almost every physical disorder has some connection with emotional factors. Even accidental injuries such as broken bones seem to happen more often to children with disturbed home backgrounds than to others. A psychosomatic disease, sometimes called a psychogenic disease, is one in which emotional factors are not merely present, but are dominant. This appears to be the case, for example, in many skin disorders, migraine, some types of asthma, and some gastrointestinal disorders.

The term "psychosomatic" should not be used in a derogatory sense, with the suggestion that psychosomatic illnesses are imaginary. They are not. They are real physical conditions. Imaginary physical disorders that are caused entirely by mental illness are called hysteria (see p.303).

You know from experience that your state of mind affects your body. For instance, your heart beats faster when you are excited or frightened, a stomach-ache often follows an emotional scene, fear can make you sweat, and so on. These are simple examples of the interaction of the body with the mind under stress. There are far more complex links known, such as one between chronic anxiety

and duodenal ulcers, though the mechanism of the linkage is not clearly understood.

There is much to be learned about psychosomatic illnesses. It may be that emotional stress is a final factor or "last straw" in precipitating health problems in people who have some genetic susceptibility to a disease already. Significantly, a tendency to develop disorders such as asthma, eczema, irritable colon, or migraine under stress seems to run in families.

What is the treatment?

If you develop an illness that is known to have a psychosomatic element, your physician may ask questions about your lifestyle. If straightforward medical treatment does not relieve your symptoms, he or she may begin to concentrate on helping you to handle the stresses of your day-to-day life. The knowledge that you can probably avoid or lessen certain symptoms by avoiding certain emotional strains may be helpful. For example, relaxation exercises, together with a change or two in your daily routine, can be particularly helpful in treating vascular, or circulatory, disorders such as some types of high blood pressure.

Compulsions and obsessions

A compulsion is an unreasonable need to behave in a certain way. An obsession is an idea or thought that lodges in the mind and cannot be forgotten. Obsessional mental activity often leads to compulsive behavior.

At one time or another most people have minor obsessions and compulsions. On a certain day, for example, you cannot get a popular tune out of your head. You are obsessed

with it. Or you may irrationally feel compelled to walk to work every day on the same side of the street. Obsessions and compulsive actions become disorders only when they are so intense and persistent that they interfere with normal life.

What are the symptoms?

Obsessions take hold gradually. You may

become interested in something such as politics, religion, or hygiene. Next you find yourself brooding about it. Eventually you can think of little else. At that point, the obsession may begin to affect your behavior. If, for instance, you have become obsessed with the idea that housebreaking is rampant, you may feel a compulsion to test your front door again after you have already locked it securely. This is a comparatively harmless compulsion. Some people, however, might carry it beyond the limits of normality by getting out of bed repeatedly during the night in order to test the door over and over again.

Compulsive disorders often center on irrational fears. Some women, for example, are so obsessed with fear of pregnancy that they will not use a bathtub previously used by a man. Other people become obsessed with fear of "germs," and wash their hands endlessly. Such a person may realize his or her behavior is irrational, but attempts to resist an overwhelming compulsion cause intense anxiety, which can be relieved only by giving in to the compulsion.

What should be done?
If you feel that any of your ideas or actions are slipping out of control, for example, if you cannot bring yourself to go to work because your customary route has been closed, consult your physician, who will probably refer you to a specialist for *psychotherapy*. Treatment for mild cases of this disorder is usually based on an effort to reassure you while trying gradually to discover what lies behind your compulsive behavior. Compulsions can sometimes be cured by a type of therapy that is known as "desensitization" (see Phobias, p.300).

Medical opinion is divided on the effectiveness of drugs for serious obsessional or compulsive disorders. Antidepressant and tranquilizer medications, however, help to reduce depression and anxiety, which are symptoms that commonly accompany these disorders.

Hypo-chondriasis

Most healthy people are scarcely conscious of the internal workings of their bodies. If you have hypochondriasis, which is commonly called hypochondria, you are excessively aware of them. You concentrate on them so much that they seem constantly troublesome. Mild cases of hypochondria are common. Concern about health becomes a form of mental illness, however, if it causes you to lose interest in virtually everything but your imagined ailments. The disorder usually occurs as a complication of an underlying mental condition such as anxiety (see p.300).

What are the symptoms?
The hypochondriac usually buys and uses great quantities of non-prescription medicines, repeatedly visits physicians, and may try various types of unproven medicine. If hypochondriasis is due to an underlying anxiety state, the person tends to interpret the physical symptoms of anxiety such as rapid heartbeat, trembling and breathlessness as signs of severe physical illness. People whose hypochondriasis is associated with depressive illness are often convinced that their bodies are degenerating – that, for instance, they have rotting brains and blocked bowels.

What should be done?
If you are constantly worried that you have a serious illness, and you are not convinced by your physician's repeated reassurances, try to accept that you may have a psychological problem. If you can at least admit the possibility and discuss it with your physician, you have made an important step towards resolving the problem. If your hypochrondriasis is due to an underlying mental illness such as depression, successful treatment of that disorder will usually cure the hypochondriasis. When hypochondriasis is the only problem, however, it is extremely difficult to treat. Mild tranquilizers are sometimes prescribed to combat hypochondriasis, and in some cases *psychotherapy* helps.

Organic psychosis

Psychosis is mental illness so severe that it causes loss of contact with reality. It is not known what causes psychosis in most cases. Sometimes, however, a psychosis may be caused by some physical factor such as a brain illness, an infection such as syphilis (see p.612), or a reaction to a drug. In such cases the psychosis is said to be "organic."

Organic psychoses cause obvious signs of illness such as a dazed expression and confused speech. Visual hallucinations (seeing imaginary objects or events) are common. The only satisfactory treatment is to deal with the underlying physical problem. If this is impossible, conventional drugs such as tranquilizers may give some temporary relief.

Hysteria

Hysteria is a *neurotic* over-reaction to an experience or situation. You are not hysterical in the medical sense of the word if you normally react to moments of stress by weeping uncontrollably or shrieking. Many people tend to over-dramatize their feelings, and they are not mentally ill because of this tendency. The illness known as hysteria, sometimes called a conversion reaction, occurs when someone (who may or may not be normally "highstrung") reacts to severe stress by developing physical symptoms that cannot be traced to physical factors. Such people do not realize that their symptoms are caused by hysteria. They, and usually their families and friends, simply assume they have been afflicted with a genuine physical disorder. The problem is often of a kind that helps the person with hysteria to escape from a stressful situation. For example, if you see a terrible accident where you work, you may develop a weakness of the legs that prevents you from leaving home the next day or even for much longer. Or a total loss of memory (*amnesia*) may follow an accident that you yearn to forget.

Do not confuse hysteria with psychosomatic illness (see p.301). Psychosomatic illnesses, though they are affected by stress, are actual physical disorders. Hysteria is purely imaginary illness.

What are the symptoms?

The hysterical reaction may be fairly mild (for instance, vague pains, weakness, or dizziness) or extremely severe (paralysis of the limbs, or sudden blindness). Less commonly, there may be loss of memory. Symptoms associated with hysteria are difficult to diagnose, especially since the ill person will deny that there is an emotional problem.

What should be done?

If you suspect that the disability of someone in your family is due to a neurotic reaction to some experience or situation, consult your physician. Whether or not your suspicion is correct, never accuse anyone of faking symptoms. Hysterical people are ill and often overly sensitive. Because hysteria is extremely difficult to diagnose, your doctor will probably want to arrange for in-hospital tests to rule out the possibility of a physical cause of the symptoms. If the cause appears to be hysteria, the person will probably be referred to a specialist.

What is the treatment?

The goal of treatment is to discover the underlying problem and help the person solve it. No medical treatment can cure symptoms of hysteria, so everything depends on sympathetic, patient *psychotherapy*. The only drug that may be prescribed for hysteria is a tranquilizer to help the person relax while the underlying problem is being uncovered and the symptoms gradually eliminated. In rare cases a treatment known as "abreaction," which does involve drugs, may be advised. It works best for people whose hysteria is due to a single, severe emotional shock.

A person undergoing abreaction must lie down in a quiet, darkened room. To overcome resistance to discussing a painful subject, the person is put into a hypnotic state either by breathing ether or being injected with a special drug. Then, when fully relaxed, he or she is asked to recall in detail the incident that triggered the hysterical reaction. Just reliving a suppressed experience in this way often removes symptoms of hysteria. Nobody knows why this happens, although there are a number of interesting theories.

Psychopathy
(*antisocial personality*)

A psychopathic person is by nature incapable of accepting the restraints that are normally imposed by the outside world. Psychopaths tend to be irresponsible, unable to hold down jobs, and incapable of having satisfactory relationships. Psychopathy might be described as a long-term mental illness that may or may not become a problem for the person and/or society. Some psychopaths achieve material or creative success in spite of their personality disorder. Most, however, are inadequate people who merely drift along through all or virtually all aspects of life and are almost constantly unhappy. A fair number of psychopaths become violent when they are frustrated, or habitually break the rules that create and maintain social order. Such psychopaths spend much of their lives in prison or under state care.

As yet, no way of altering the psychopath's personality has been discovered. It is possible to treat the disorders to which psychopaths are susceptible, such as extreme depression, alcoholism and drug addiction. But the basic personality remains the same. Some people who are extremely antisocial when young, however, become more emotionally mature in middle age. If you think the behavior of someone in your family may reflect a psychopathic personality, do not hesitate to consult your physician, who can help you to seek further guidance.

Addictions

Addictions are, or can become, mental illnesses in that an addict's craving for a drug or pleasurable activity is uncontrollable. The necessity to have whatever it is that the addict craves prevents him or her from living a normal life. An addiction often leads to lack of mental balance even when it does not cause any apparent physical damage. Three of the many possible types of addiction are singled out for discussion in the following pages: drugs, alcohol and gambling.

Alcohol is itself a drug, but it is discussed separately because, although addiction to alcohol has some features in common with addiction to other drugs, alcoholism is a particularly common disorder.

Abuse of and addiction to drugs is a growing problem in modern society. There are many dangerous drugs available both legally and illegally in the United States.

Smoking, the most widespread of all addictions, is not included in this group of articles because it is discussed elsewhere. For a general discussion of smoking, along with some ideas on how to give it up, see p.38. Read also the section on disorders of the respiratory system (see p.340) and disorders of the heart and circulation (see p.370).

Alcoholism

People who become addicted to alcohol usually begin to drink heavily to relieve personal, business, and/or social stress. Since they generally find the relief they are looking for, even though only temporarily and at the cost of occasional hangovers, they gradually begin to drink whenever they feel tense. The more they drink, the less tension they can tolerate without alcohol. You can consider yourself an alcoholic, or in danger of becoming one, if you have reached a point where you need to drink not only to relieve tension but also to make yourself feel "normal." The illness and resulting disability are severe and require immediate treatment if uncontrollable drinking has begun to affect your health and interfere with your personal and work life.

Some people can drink more, and more often, than others before reaching this stage. This difference depends in part on your physical tolerance for alcohol. The shift from social drinking to alcoholism can happen almost imperceptibly over many years, or it can occur with dramatic rapidity. Drinking habits, too, vary widely. Some alcoholics are "binge" drinkers, who go on one to several day sprees with "dry" or non-drinking, periods in between. Others drink constantly and are never quite sober. Some drink only wine, or gin, or beer, while others will drink anything alcoholic.

It is virtually impossible to generalize about what causes addiction to alcohol and how alcoholism develops. It is usually true, however, that people in the early stages of alcoholism can tolerate greater amounts of alcohol without showing symptoms of the disorder than they can in the later stages.

What are the symptoms?

Even relatives and close friends of people who are becoming alcoholics seldom notice the early symptoms. It usually seems like just a tendency to drink too much, and this appears to be confined to social occasions. Sometimes, however, such drinkers will admit that they have black-outs, which means they wake up in the morning with no memory of what happened the night before. If this happens to you or to someone in your family, recognize it as a sign of trouble. Before long the drinking will probably start earlier in the day and last longer.

In later stages an alcoholic may become secretive about drinking. Glasses of fruit juice may be surreptitiously spiked with alcohol. Bottles may be hidden around the house. Alcoholics often feel guilty about their addiction, and may become irritable and aggressive. Another symptom is repeated assertions that they are giving up drink altogether, alternating with denials that they have a drinking problem. They may become depressed, jealous, resentful, even *paranoid*, which means the person has unreasonable fears that other people are hostile or plotting to destroy him or her. Eventually there is likely to be a loss of memory and concentration, along with an inability to meet the demands of a steady job. Physically, an increasing dependence on alcohol may cause a flushed and veiny face, bruises on body and limbs, a husky voice, trembling hands, and chronic gastritis (see p.464).

What are the risks?

The disorder is more common in men than in

women. In the United States it is estimated that about ten per cent of adult males and about three per cent of adult females are alcoholics. People with alcoholic parents seem to be particularly susceptible, probably because of environmental rather than genetic factors. Some people have symptoms of alcoholism in adolescence or even earlier, but most alcoholics are between 35 and 55.

Alcoholism can affect every system of the body. Although exact figures are not known, it is thought that at least one in five long-term heavy drinkers develops cirrhosis of the liver (see p.487). Heavy drinking makes the liver particularly susceptible to infection and may cause serious diseases of the stomach, heart and brain. Because alcoholics seldom eat adequately, they are likely to have vitamin deficiencies, particularly vitamin B deficiency (see p.494). And a pregnant woman who drinks alcohol, whether she is an alcoholic or not, increases the chances of having a mentally retarded or physically deformed baby.

Another danger associated with alcoholism and heavy drinking is traffic accidents. Many injuries and deaths occur on the roads because the judgment of drivers is impaired by alcohol. Alcoholics also are difficult to live with because they are often irritable, and sometimes violent. As a result, the alcoholic risks breaking up his or her family. The same problems of irritability and impaired judgment that affect the alcoholic's home life and driving skill can also affect job performance, and may result in the loss of a job.

What should be done?
If you detect signs of an early stage of alcoholism in yourself, cut down on the amount and frequency of your social drinking for your family's sake as well as your own. If you find that this is impossible to do, seek help without further delay. Get in touch with a physician or the nearest branch of Alcoholics Anonymous, a world-wide organization that has been helpful to many people with drinking problems. If someone close to you shows symptoms of alcoholism but denies that he or she is drinking too much (as alcoholics often do), consult a physician about the problem. You cannot force someone to seek help, but persuasion by a physician, social worker or other professional is sometimes effective.

What is the treatment?
For treatment to be successful, the alcoholic must recognize the existence of the problem and be determined to grapple with it. The most satisfactory solution, of course, is simply to control your drinking. Unfortunately, total abstinence from alcohol is the only effective solution for many addicts. For people in later stages of alcoholism, an in-hospital "drying-out" process is usually necessary. This treatment involves complete abstinence, which often leads to withdrawal symptoms such as hallucinations, seizures, and *delirium tremens* (commonly known as the DTs). To help you through the most uncomfortable period at the beginning of this process, tranquilizers may be prescribed. You may also be given vitamins if you have a vitamin deficiency.

Psychotherapy is one way of continuing treatment after the initial drying-out period. Probably the most successful treatment is through Alcoholics Anonymous. There are local chapters throughout the country, made up of all kinds of people. In some cases a medication may be prescribed. The alcoholic takes this drug each morning, and this discourages drinking because the combination of alcohol with the drug produces nausea, vomiting and sweating. No such treatment will work, however, unless the alcoholic genuinely wants it to and never "forgets" to take a daily dose.

What are the long-term prospects?
The general outlook for alcoholics depends to a large extent on themselves. If you drink too much, it may be because of nearly unbearable social and business pressures. But if you are determined to give up alcohol, you can.

Drug addiction

People originally take drugs for one of two reasons. Either the drugs are prescribed by a physician to treat some physical or mental disorder, or they provide a pleasurable effect such as the warm, carefree drowsiness induced by heroin, or even the mild alertness produced by the caffeine in coffee, tea or cola. Whether or not a given drug is addictive varies considerably, not only from drug to drug, but also from person to person. Mildly addictive drugs such as codeine, together with such drugs as cannabis (marijuana) or cocaine are commonly known as "soft." "Hard" drugs are drugs that can lead to severe addiction; they are covered here.

Anyone who is addicted to a hard drug must take it in gradually increasing doses both to maintain the pleasurable effects of the drug and to keep from breaking down physically and emotionally. This is called

Drugs and their effects

A drug can be defined as any non-nutritional chemical substance that can be absorbed into the body. The word "drug" is commonly used to mean either a medicine or something taken (usually voluntarily) to produce a temporary (usually pleasurable) effect. Sometimes, the two categories overlap. Morphine may be prescribed as a medical treatment for relief of pain. Self-administered by an otherwise healthy person, it gives a temporary sense of well-being. Some drugs, including morphine and nicotine, are strongly addictive and harmful. Such apparently innocent substances as tea and coffee may be addictive (or more accurately the caffeine that they provide may be addictive) and also capable of harming some people.

The following list of drugs commonly used by addicts does not include caffeine, alcohol, nicotine, or tranquilizers, which are discussed elsewhere.

Type of drug	What it does	Outward signs of use	Some long-term effects
Amphetamines, often called pep pills, uppers, or diet pills.	Speeds up physical and mental processes, produces extreme energy and unusual excitement.	Weight loss, dilated pupils, insomnia, diarrhea, trembling.	Paranoia and violent behavior. Possible death from overdose.
Barbiturates, often called downers.	Produces extreme lethargy and drowsiness.	Blurred and confused speech, lack of coordination and balance.	Disruption of normal sleeping pattern; dangerously double vision; possible death from overdose, especially in conjunction with alcohol. Often ulcers at injection site.
Cannabis, including marijuana and hashish, often called pot, grass and hash.	Relaxes the mind and body, heightens perception, and causes mood swings.	Red eyes, dilated pupils, lack of physical coordination, lethargy, sometimes obvious nausea.	Long-term physical effects include brain, heart, lung and reproductive system damage. Decreased motivation.
Cocaine, often called coke or snow.	Stimulates nervous system and produces heightened sensations and sometimes hallucinations.	Dilated pupils, trembling, apparent intoxication.	Ulceration of nasal passages if drug is "sniffed;" generalized itching, which can produce open sores.
Opiates, including opium, morphine, heroin and methadone.	Relieves physical and mental pain, and produces temporary euphoria.	Weight loss, lethargy, mood swings, sweating, slurred speech, sore eyes.	Loss of appetite leading to malnutrition; extreme susceptibility to infection; absence of periods in women; possible death from overdose.
Psychedelic drugs, including Lysergic acid (LSD) and mescaline.	Unpredictable. Usually produces hallucinations, which may be pleasant or frightening.	Dilated pupils, sweating, trembling, sometimes fever and chills.	Possible irresponsible behavior; although apparently not addictive, a single drug-taking episode may cause long-term psychological upset.
Volatile substances such as inhaled fumes of glue, cleaning fluids, etc.	Produces hallucinations, giddiness, temporary euphoria, and sometimes unconsciousness.	Obvious confusion, dilated pupils, flushed face.	Risk of brain, liver, or kidney damage; possible suffocation from inhalation.

building up tolerance to the drug. If the addict's need for the drug is not satisfied, unpleasant physical and psychological effects called withdrawal symptoms will result. In some cases the withdrawal symptoms can be harmful, or even fatal, and withdrawal from the drug should be medically supervised.

What are the symptoms?
Every type of drug produces its own kind of mental and physical symptoms (see Table, previous page). In general, any addiction is likely to cause a gradual deterioration of the addict's standards of work, personal relationships, or both. The behavior of addicts is often erratic and their moods may be changeable, with periods of restlessness and irritability alternating with extreme drowsiness. There is often a loss of appetite, and unreasonable fatigue and surliness. If someone close to you has some of these symptoms, they do not necessarily indicate drug addiction. But if he or she also spends increasing amounts of time away from home and seems to be always out of money for no apparent reason, you have cause for suspicion.

What are the risks?
There are no reliable statistics available on the total number of drug addicts in the United States, partly because many addicts never receive treatment, and obtain drugs illegally. Estimates of the number of heroin users in this country range from about 400,000 to almost four million, and about seven million people are reported to use sleeping pills once a week or more. It is not known how many people are actually addicted to these drugs.

Hard drugs taken habitually violently upset the body's chemical system. In extreme cases the result can be serious physical or mental illness, or even death. With some drugs, an addict can build up a tolerance for the drug that is dangerously close to the dosage at which the drug can kill you. Also, when drugs are obtained illegally, there are no controls over the strength or purity of the drug. It is very possible to take a fatal dose by mistake.

What should be done?
Anyone who is addicted to a drug needs help, but addicts are unlikely to seek help unless desperate. If you are concerned about drug abuse in yourself or anyone else, consult your physician or a drug counseling center.

What is the treatment?
Self-help: No self-help is possible for severe addiction. If you seem to be dependent on regular doses of some prescribed drug such as a tranquilizer, do not hesitate to speak to your physician about the problem. The doctor will probably either allay your fear of possible addiction or recommend appropriate measures to break the habit.
Professional help: Hospital treatment, preferably in a special drug unit, is essential. The addictive drug is withheld either immediately or gradually, depending on the severity of withdrawal symptoms for that particular drug or combination of drugs. Once the withdrawal process is over, the second stage of treatment begins. It consists of an attempt to prevent renewed addiction by means of *psychotherapy* and vocational therapy. It is not easy to "kick" a drug habit permanently. Before they are discharged from the hospital, "cured" addicts may be offered temporary housing in a new environment and are usually advised to avoid their drug-taking friends and form new relationships.

Addictive gambling

Obsessive gambling is an addiction, not a compulsion. Gambling gives pleasure to the gambler, whereas a need for pleasure is usually not an important element in most compulsive activities. Obsessive gamblers are people who cannot resist the pleasurable excitement of a card game, the craps table, betting on horse races or other kinds of sports events, and similar games of chance. Unlike many people who enjoy an occasional fling, addicts no longer play primarily in order to win. Their gambling is an addiction because they cannot resist the constant repetition of periods of exciting tension that gambling provides, whether or not they are likely to gain anything from taking the risk. As a result, many obsessive gamblers gamble so recklessly that they gamble away all their own and their families' resources.

This addiction is more common than is generally recognized. It may affect more than a million people in the United States, and some estimates are as high as three million. It seems to affect about five times as many men as women.

What should be done?
If you have an obsessive gambler in your family, try to get him or her to seek help from a physician or Gamblers Anonymous. If your addicted relative refuses to get help, you should consult your physician for advice.

Eye disorders

Introduction

Sight is the most important of the five main senses. Your eyes tell you much more than your other senses do, and the part of the brain that deals with sight is far larger than the parts that deal with the other senses.

The eye is a complex, intricate, and fairly delicate structure (see the illustration opposite). Each eyeball is a sphere about 25 mm (1 in) in diameter. Three concentric layers of tissue cover the eyeball. The tough outermost layer is the sclera, which is visible as the white of the eye. Its exposed surface at the front of the eye has a transparent covering, the conjunctiva, which also lines the inner surface of the eyelids. At the front of the eye, the sclera and conjunctiva join the cornea, a dome-shaped structure sometimes called the "window" of the eye.

Beneath the sclera is the choroid, a layer rich in blood vessels that supply the eye tissues with oxygen and nutrients. Toward the front of the eye, this layer thickens to form the ciliary body. From the front of the ciliary body extends a circular area of fibers, the iris, which varies in color from person to person and determines eye-color. In the center of the iris is an opening, the pupil, which looks like a black disc. Through this opening, light enters the eye. The amount of light is controlled by the contraction or dilation (widening) of the pupil. This adjustment is regulated by the muscles of the iris.

Immediately behind the iris and pupil is a transparent elastic body, the crystalline lens, which is attached to the ciliary body. Muscles thicken or narrow the lens, enabling the eye to focus on objects at varying distances. The space between the cornea and the lens is filled with a watery substance called aqueous humor. Behind the lens is a jelly-like substance called the vitreous humor, which makes up the bulk of the eyeball.

The innermost layer, the retina, lines the rear three-quarters of the eyeball. The retina includes a layer of light-sensitive nerve cells that are called the *rods* and *cones* because of their shapes. Light passes through the pupil and lens to the retina in such a way as to form an upside-down image of whatever you are looking at. The rods are very sensitive to light intensity and enable you to see in dim light. The cones detect color and fine detail.

There are 125 million rods and 7 million cones in each eye. Between them, the rods and cones transform the sensations of color, form and light intensity that they receive into nerve impulses. These impulses are then transmitted along retinal nerve fibers to the optic nerve, a stalk-like collection of nerves that connect the rear of the retina to the brain. The brain interprets the impulses received from each eye, reverses the images, and integrates them into one three-dimensional image.

The eye disorders covered in this section are dealt with in four groups. The first consists of errors of refraction such as problems of nearsightedness and farsightedness. The second group is concerned with disorders of those parts of the eye that you can see, mainly the eyelids, eyelashes, sclera, iris and lens. The third group deals with two forms of glaucoma, a disease that arises from a problem with drainage of aqueous humor. The final group is concerned with disorders that affect the structures in the inner layer of the eye, including the retina and its blood supply. The muscles and other tissues that surround the eyeball in its bony socket, which is known as the orbit, are also covered in this section.

Drugs and the eye

Drugs used to treat existing eye conditions can have side-effects that also affect the eye. Although most such side-effects are inconvenient rather than dangerous, some can be serious and may occasionally cause cataracts (see p.319), glaucoma (see p.320) or blindness. For this reason, drugs used to treat eye conditions should only be administered by a physician.

The eyes can also be affected by some drugs that are used to treat general disorders. For example, *steroids* can cause cataracts, while tranquilizers taken by the elderly may cause acute glaucoma. Such side-effects do not occur in all cases, but you should suspect them if you are taking drugs for some other disorder and are beginning to have eye problems.

The eye

The main parts of your eye are many and complex. The bony socket, which provides support and protection, is not shown.

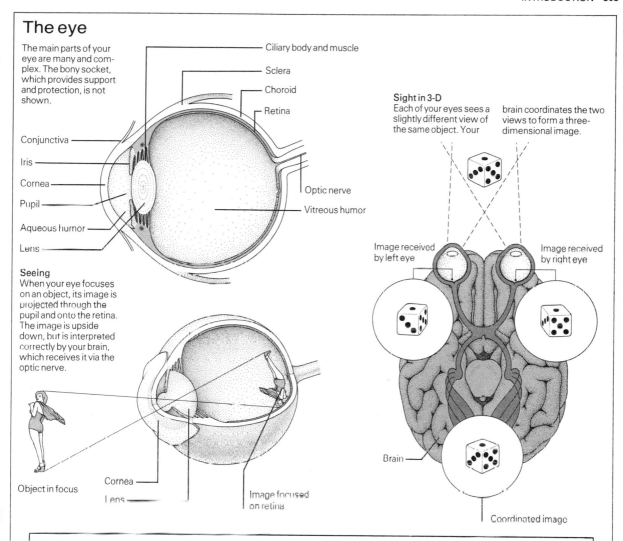

Ciliary body and muscle

Sclera

Choroid

Retina

Conjunctiva

Iris

Cornea

Pupil

Aqueous humor

Lens

Optic nerve

Vitreous humor

Seeing
When your eye focuses on an object, its image is projected through the pupil and onto the retina. The image is upside down, but is interpreted correctly by your brain, which receives it via the optic nerve.

Object in focus

Cornea

Lens

Image focused on retina

Sight in 3-D
Each of your eyes sees a slightly different view of the same object. Your brain coordinates the two views to form a three-dimensional image.

Image received by left eye

Image received by right eye

Brain

Coordinated image

Color blindness
Color blindness is the popular (and incorrect) term for the very common condition of being unable to distinguish between certain colors. Literal color blindness, or seeing everything in shades of gray, is extremely rare.

All the colors are made up of combinations of the three colors red, green and blue in the light rays that enter the eyes. Cells in the retina called *cones* each contain a light-sensitive substance that responds to one of these colors. But if you have a defect of color vision, you have either a partial or complete lack of one or more of the light-sensitive substances in the cones.

The most common form of color blindness is an inability to distinguish in dim light between reds and greens. In adequate light the colors are seen normally.

The second most common form is to have the same inability even in adequate light. If you have this condition, you will almost certainly be aware of it.

Defects of color vision affect men far more often than women. The defects are almost always hereditary and present from birth. They are passed on through the mother (see Genetics, p.704). They can be caused by an eye disease later in life, but this is rare.

There is no cure for color blindness, but it usually does not seriously interfere with day-to-day life. A colored filter on eyeglasses or a colored contact lens can be used to enhance your ability to see contrasts, but does not actually affect your ability to differentiate between colors. The device is usually worn over only one eye, though this may distort space perception. The device should not be worn while driving at night.

Errors of refraction

Refraction and sight
The cornea and the lens act as convex lenses to refract, or bend, light rays from an object and focus them on the retina. It is these focused rays that form the image you see.

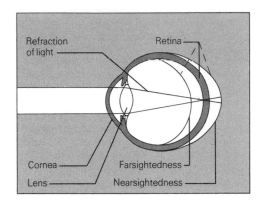

The way that light from objects is focused through the eye into an image on the retina is called *refraction*. In a normal eye, the point where the light focuses is exactly at the retina, and it is this precise focusing that assures that a clear image is seen. In some eyes, however, the eye focuses the light either behind or in front of the retina, so that the image is blurred.

The four most common disorders of refraction are nearsightedness (myopia), farsightedness (hypermetropia), astigmatism and presbyopia. Any of these disorders can be present in one or both eyes.

Nearsightedness
(*myopia*)

Correcting nearsightedness
In nearsightedness, the cornea and lens focus the light rays from a viewed object short of the retina, producing a blurred image. A concave lens held in front of the eye corrects the problem.

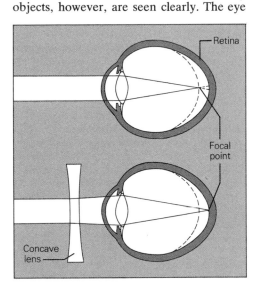

In nearsightedness the eye is too long from front to back, or, less often, the focusing power of the cornea and lens is too great. As a result, images of distant objects are focused in front of the retina and are blurred. Nearby objects, however, are seen clearly. The eye cannot counteract blurring as it sometimes can in farsightedness (see next article).

Nearsightedness is very common; about one person in five needs glasses for this problem. It usually develops at about the age of 12 and may worsen until about 20. It tends to run in families.

What should be done?
If you think you are nearsighted, consult an ophthalmologist (see p.312). If vision tests confirm your suspicion, glasses or contact lenses with concave (inwardly curved) lenses will be prescribed. These will move images of distant objects backward onto the retina and bring them into clear focus.

Once you have reached the age of about 30, your nearsightedness is unlikely to get any worse, but you should still visit your ophthalmologist every few years to check for subsequent errors of refraction.

There is a surgical procedure called radial keratotomy that has been tried to correct nearsightedness. It is still in experimental stages, however, and the long-term results are not known.

Farsightedness
(*hypermetropia*)

In farsightedness the eye is too short from front to back or, less often, there is a weakness in the focusing ability of the cornea and lens. In either case, the eye focuses images of objects at a distance behind the retina, and they appear to be blurred. If the defect is not too severe, the young eye can overcome it naturally by what is called *accommodation*. The ciliary muscles thicken and contract the lens, which brings the point of focus forward onto the retina and produces a clear image.

Farsightedness is generally present from birth and is usually diagnosed during childhood. It tends to run in families.

What are the symptoms?
Many people with mild farsightedness have no symptoms. Others have eyestrain (aching

Correcting farsighted-ness
In farsightedness, the cornea and lens focus the light rays from a viewed object beyond the retina, producing a blurred image. A convex lens held in front of the eye corrects the problem.

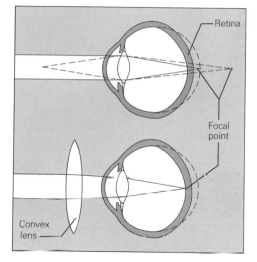

or discomfort in the eye), because they constantly have to use the ciliary muscles to see clearly. People with moderate to severe farsightedness have continuously blurred vision and may also have eyestrain. Neither symptom permanently damages vision.

What should be done?

If you have blurred vision and/or eyestrain, visit an ophthalmologist (see next page). If an examination establishes that you are farsighted, he or she will prescribe glasses or contact lenses with convex (outwardly curved) lenses. These reinforce the focusing power of the cornea and lens of your eye so that you can see more clearly.

With increasing age, the ciliary muscle may weaken. Therefore, you may need stronger glasses every few years.

Presbyopia

At rest, a normal eye is focused for distance vision. To enable the eye to focus on closer objects, the ciliary muscles of the eye thicken and contract the lens, a process that is known as *accommodation*. With age, the lens of the eye hardens and its ability to change shape to focus on close objects is reduced. This de-

terioration in the elasticity of the lens is called presbyopia.

Most people first notice the condition when they are in their mid-40s. It gradually becomes increasingly pronounced. If it is not corrected, you can read printed matter only by holding it further and further away from your eyes, until eventually you cannot see to read even at arm's length. If you are nearsighted (see previous page), you may need to take off your glasses to read print at a normal distance.

Correcting presbyopia
Presbyopia in people whose eyesight was formerly normal is corrected the same way as is farsightedness. A convex lens adjusts the focal point.

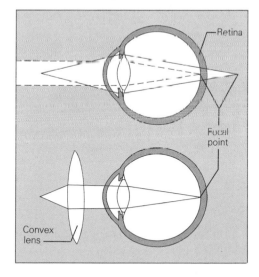

What should be done?

If you find that close objects are beginning to appear slightly blurred unless you hold them away from you, you should consult an ophthalmologist (see next page). If you have presbyopia, you will need glasses or, rarely, contact lenses, with convex (outwardly curved) lenses. These will reinforce the power of the lens of the eye and enable you to see close objects clearly.

You will need slightly stronger glasses every few years, to compensate for the decreasing power of your own lenses. This will continue until you are about 65. At this time the power of accommodation by the eyes virtually ceases.

If you are also nearsighted (see previous page), farsighted (see previous article), or astigmatic (see p.313), and are already wearing glasses for distance vision, you can avoid the need for two pairs of glasses by getting bifocals. In this type of glasses, the upper part of each lens is for distance viewing and the lower part for close vision. Some people have trouble adjusting to bifocals.

Bifocals
A bifocal lens is a combination of two lenses. The lower one is for reading and other close work. The upper lens helps you see distant objects.

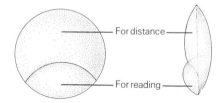

Going to the ophthalmologist

Why should you go?

Even if there is nothing apparently wrong with your eyes, you should have regular vision tests. Ideally, you should do this once every few years. If you are over 40, your eyes should be tested more often, preferably every two years. This is because some serious eye diseases, such as certain types of glaucoma (which can cause blindness), have no symptoms in the early stages and can be detected only by an eye examination. If they are detected early, these diseases usually can be treated.

Any sudden serious changes that occur in your eyesight should be reported immediately to your physician.

Three kinds of professionals with different training and skills can be involved in testing the eyes and correcting vision. Ophthalmologists are physicians who specialize in the treatment of eye disorders and in eye surgery. They can prescribe glasses, contact lenses and drugs. Optometrists are trained and licensed to test vision, and can prescribe glasses or contacts. However, an optometrist is not a physician, and usually cannot prescribe drugs. Opticians are trained only to fit glasses and contact lenses as they are prescribed by either an ophthalmologist or an optometrist.

What happens?

An ophthalmologist can test your eyes in various ways. He or she will test the *acuity*, or sharpness, of your vision by asking you to read the rows of letters on an eye chart. The letters vary in size from row to row. The top row has one large letter; the next row, smaller letters; the next, still smaller and so on.

The result is given as two figures, for example, 20/40. The first refers to the distance at which you read the letters – usually 20 feet. The second is related to the distance at which a person with normal vision can read the smallest letters that you were able to read correctly at 20 feet. The result 20/40 means that you were able to read letters at 20 feet that a person with normal vision would be able to read at 40 feet. The results may be different for each eye. Poor reading of the chart indicates a disorder of refraction, usually nearsightedness (see p.310) or farsightedness (see p.310). It could also mean a serious eye disease such as glaucoma (see p.320).

The doctor also looks at each eye through an instrument called an *ophthalmoscope*. With this, the backs of the eyes can be examined to see if you have any internal eye disorder such as retinal detachment (see p.324), or whether there are

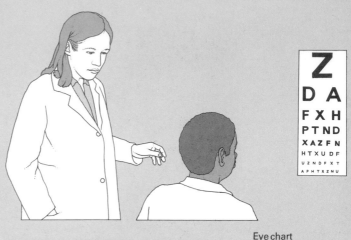

signs of any general disorder, such as anemia, high blood pressure, or diabetes.

The examiner will probably also test the balance of the muscles that control the movements of the eyes, to detect crossed eyes.

If the examiner discovers a disorder of refraction, glasses or contact lenses may be prescribed for you.

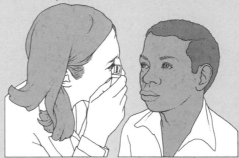

How do you obtain glasses?

If your test shows that you need glasses, you will be given a prescription. Take the prescription to an optician. Your ophthalmologist may recommend one. The optician can take the necessary head measurements, and you choose the type of lenses (glass or plastic) and the frame you want. Plastic lenses are lighter than glass, and they are safer because they break less easily. However, they also scratch more easily and, so must be more carefully cleaned and cared for.

Glasses usually take about two to three weeks to be made up. Any necessary adjustments to the frame can usually be made when you pick them up. Wear the glasses for a trial period, and if you find the lenses are not satisfactory, you should return to your ophthalmologist.

Eye chart
The letters on an eye chart are a standard size and should be read from a distance of 6 meters (20 ft).

Examining your eye
The physician examines the back of your eye by shining the light from an ophthalmoscope through your pupil and lens.

Astigmatism

Astigmatism is distorted vision caused by an uneven curvature of the cornea, the outside front portion of your eye. Vertical but not horizontal lines are in focus, or vice versa. Diagonal lines may also be out of focus. Astigmatism sometimes occurs in conjunction with farsightedness (see p.310) or nearsightedness (see p.310). It is usually present from birth and does not grow worse with age.

What should be done?

If you suspect that your vision is distorted in the way that is described here, visit an ophthalmologist (see previous page). If tests establish that you have astigmatism, glasses or hard contact lenses shaped to the curvature required to correct the unevenness of the cornea will be prescribed. These will enable you to see normally.

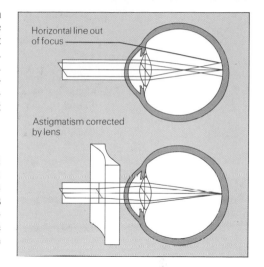

Horizontal line out of focus

Astigmatism corrected by lens

Contact lenses

Contact lenses are an alternative to glasses. They have become very popular in recent years.

Each contact lens is a circular plastic lens that fits closely over the front of the eye, to help correct errors of refraction. There are two types of contact lens: the hard lens, which is made of a plastic that is tough and hard-wearing, but that tends to irritate the sensitive eye; and the soft lens, which is more gentle to the eye, but which becomes scratched and worn more easily.

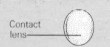

Contact lens

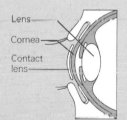

Lens
Cornea
Contact lens

Contact lenses go directly over the cornea, and work the same way glasses do.

How do you obtain contact lenses?

First, you go to an ophthalmologist for a thorough eye examination. The ophthalmologist will look for two things: first, whether your eyes are suitable for contact lenses (if you have hay fever, for example, you may not be able to wear them); and then, if they are suitable, whether you should wear hard lenses or soft ones. Once you are wearing contact lenses permanently, you will probably be advised to have your eyes checked once a year.

Inserting contact lenses
With clean hands, rinse your contact lenses thoroughly when you take them out of their storage solution. Place a lens you have lubricated with wetting agent cup side up on the tip of your forefinger.

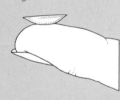

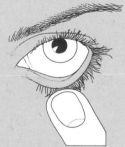

Hold your lids well apart with your other hand.

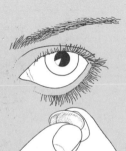

Look straight ahead or at the contact lens as you bring it up to your eye.

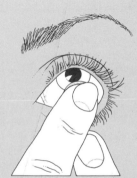

Place the lens gently over the center of your eye. Look downwards and release your lids.

Eyelids and the front of the eye

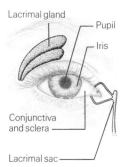

Lacrimal gland
Pupil
Iris
Conjunctiva and sclera
Lacrimal sac

The visible eye represents only about one-tenth of the surface area of the entire eyeball. The eyelids act as protective covers for this segment of the eye. Muscles in the lids open and close them, and act with fibrous tissue in the lids to keep them taut against the eyeball. The lid margins and the eyelashes are lubricated by a row of small glands, called the meibomian glands, on each lid margin.

The exposed surface of the eye (except for the cornea, which covers the iris and pupil) and the inner surface of each lid are lined with a sensitive transparent mucous membrane called the conjunctiva. They are also covered with a thin film of watery fluid called "tears," which is produced by the lacrimal glands above each eyeball. Apart from their use in expressing emotion, tears have two main functions: to lubricate the eye so that the lid can move over it smoothly as you blink; and to wash away foreign bodies. Tears drain away from each eye along two channels called the lacrimal tear ducts. A tiny hole at the inner edge of each lid marks the opening of the ducts. The ducts lead to the lacrimal sac at the side of the nose, and from there the tear fluid passes down into the nose, where it helps keep nasal tissues moist.

Ptosis

See p.247,
Visual aids to diagnosis, 63.

Consult your physician if a previously normal upper eyelid starts to droop and partially cover the eye. This may be a symptom of a muscular disorder such as myasthenia gravis.

Ptosis is permanent drooping of the upper eyelid so that it partially or completely covers the eye. The condition is caused by weakness of the muscle that raises the lid. Ptosis may be present from birth, in which case it usually affects only one eye and does not grow worse with age. It often runs in families. It can also occur at any age, after the nerve that controls the lid muscle or the muscle itself has been damaged. The nerve can be affected by injury; by one of several diseases, including diabetes mellitus (see p.519); or by a brain tumor (see p.282), in which case the ptosis is often accompanied by double vision. Muscle weakness can be caused by muscular dystrophy (see p.694) or myasthenia gravis (see p.542).

Ptosis may affect one or both eyes and may vary in severity during the course of the day. The condition may also occur as old age weakens the muscles of the upper eyelids.

Ptosis can be unattractive, and if it is severe it will block the vision of the affected eye or eyes. If it affects your vision, you should consult your physician. Successful treatment of any underlying disease will help to improve the ptosis. In other cases, either an operation to strengthen the muscle can be carried out or the lid can be kept raised by a support incorporated into eyeglasses.

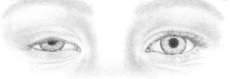

Sty

See p.246,
Visual aids to diagnosis, 53.

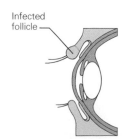

Infected follicle

Like all hairs, eyelashes grow from follicles, or depressions in the skin. It is quite common for one of these to become infected. When that happens a red, painful swelling like a boil (see p.251) develops on the lid margin, around the base of the eyelash. A white head of pus appears on the swelling, which is known as a sty.

A sty can be very painful, particularly if it is touched. Within a few days of a sty's formation, it bursts, which relieves the pain and causes the loss of the eyelash.

The sty subsides about seven days after it first appears, and the eyelid returns to normal. However, styes often recur within a short period, and sometimes several develop on the lids at the same time. In either case, this is probably because the bacteria that caused the initial sty have spread and infected other eyelash follicles.

What should be done?
You can hasten the relief of pain by making the sty burst early. As soon as the inflammation appears, apply hot compresses to it frequently. When these applications draw the pus to a head, do not squeeze the sty, but pull out the eyelash. The pus will be released. Wash the eyelid carefully to remove all pus.

If styes keep recurring, see your physician, who may prescribe an *antibiotic* to clear up the infection.

Lumps on the eyelid

See p.246,
Visual aids to diagnosis, 57–58.

The most common kinds of lump that can develop on the eyelid are styes (see previous article), chalazions, papillomas and xanthelasma.

A chalazion is a painless swelling on the lid margin. It is caused by the blockage of one of the meibomian glands, which lubricate the lid margin. Small chalazions usually disappear naturally within a month or two. You can speed up the process and get rid of them sooner yourself. You do this by gently massaging the lid towards the margin, which helps to release blocked-up fluid from the gland. Larger chalazions, which may grow to the size of a small pea, do not disappear spontaneously and are treated surgically. An incision is made in the eyelid and the contents of the chalazion are removed. This operation is not terribly complicated and, so, can be done in a physician's office or a hospital out-patient department, and requires only a local anesthetic. A chalazion can become infected, in which case it will become more

swollen, red and painful. In this event, you will want to get professional help as quickly as possible. Treatment, again, consists of an incision in the eyelid, in this case to allow the pus to drain away.

A papilloma is a harmless outgrowth of skin, ranging in color from pink to black, anywhere on the eyelid or lid margin. It may increase in size very slowly. If it is unattractive, it can be removed surgically using a local anesthetic. If it is small and inconspicuous and you do not want to have it removed, there is no reason to do so.

In xanthelasma, yellow patches of fatty material, for no certain reason, accumulate beneath the outer skin of the lids, especially near the nose. If the patches are unattractive they can be removed, but even then they may recur later.

Other less common lumps that may occur on the lid include a form of birthmark called an angioma, and a tumor growth known as a basal cell carcinoma (see p.258).

Entropion

(inturned eyelashes)

See p.247,
Visual aids to diagnosis, 59.

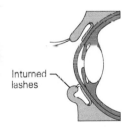

Inturned lashes

This is a condition in which the lid margin of either eyelid, most often the lower lid, turns inward so that the lashes rub on the surface of the eyeball—the conjunctiva and the cornea. This continuous rubbing causes irritation and may cause conjunctivitis (see p.317) and/or corneal ulcers (see next page). Persistent entropion can also damage the cornea and cause problems with vision.

The condition usually affects older people. As you grow older the fibrous tissue on the lower lids may become lax, which allows the muscle in the lid margin to contract excessively. It is this excessive contraction that can pull the margin of the lid in toward the eye. Occasionally, entropion occurs for a different reason. Such causes are all related to constant

irritation of the eye such as that which occurs in conjunctivitis, that causes the lids to become excessively scarred.

What should be done?
If your eye is already irritated when the condition occurs, see your physician to have it treated. Otherwise, turn the lid outward and keep it in this position by attaching one end of a piece of adhesive tape to the skin beneath your lower lashes and the other end to your cheek. After a few days, remove the tape and see if the condition clears up of its own accord. If it does not, consult your physician, who may arrange for you to have a minor operation on the eyelid (usually under a local anesthetic) to clear up the problem.

Ectropion

(outturned eyelashes)

See p.247,
Visual aids to diagnosis, 60.

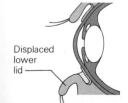

Displaced lower lid

In ectropion the lower lid of your eye hangs away from the eyeball, so that the lower half of the exposed surface of the eyeball and the lining of the lower lid become dry and sore. Also, the tears that normally lubricate the lining of of your eyelids and the front of the eye may be prevented from entering the tear duct in the lower lid. If this happens, the tears will run down your cheek.

What are the risks?
Ectropion usually occurs in older people because the muscle in the lower lid that keeps the lid taut against the eyeball may become

weak. The condition can also be caused at any age by a scar on the lower lid or cheek that has contracted and pulls down the lid. If ectropion is not treated, corneal ulcers (see next page) may develop on the exposed cornea and damage it permanently.

What should be done?
The condition rarely disappears of its own accord, so you should see your physician, who will arrange for you to have an operation on the tissues beneath the eye. This is a minor procedure that requires only a local anesthetic and should clear up the problem.

Blepharitis

Blepharitis is an inflammation of the lid margins that causes a persistent and unattractive redness and scaliness of the skin on and around the margins. The disorder is usually a form of sebhorrheic eczema (see p.651) and is sometimes accompanied by another form of eczema, dandruff (see p.263). In some cases bacteria infect the area and make the condition worse.

In severe cases, small ulcers may develop on the lid margins, and eyelashes may fall out. Often flakes from the lid enter the eye and cause conjunctivitis (see next page).

What should be done?
Try to treat the condition by washing away the scales, morning and night, with warm salt water, a warm solution of sodium bicarbonate, or a warm "soapless" shampoo. If this treatment does not improve the condition within two weeks, consult your physician, who may prescribe an ointment for you to rub into the lid margins after washing. This should clear the condition.

Blepharitis is a disorder that often recurs and needs repeated treatment. It is not, however, a threat to general health.

Dry eye

This condition is due to a deficiency of tear production by the lacrimal glands. The white of the eye becomes red and swollen, and the eye feels hot and gritty. Usually both eyes are affected. Dry eye often occurs in people who have rheumatoid arthritis (see p.552). In some cases it is caused by an allergy to an eye ointment or drops used for some other condition, but in many instances it occurs for no known reason.

The condition is most common in middle age and affects women more than men. There is usually no threat to sight, but you may also have a dry mouth, dry joints, and not enough digestive juices in your stomach.

To relieve the discomfort, your physician will probably prescribe artificial tear drops that you can apply to your eye as often as necessary. You may have to use the drops for the rest of your life.

Watering eye

Continuous watering of the eye may be caused by inward-growing eyelashes, which is called entropion (see previous page), or by a blockage in the lacrimal or nasolacrimal tear ducts that drain tears from the eye into the nose. Sometimes blockage follows an injury to the bone at the side of the nose. Sometimes it occurs in long-standing sinusitis (see p.347). But often the cause is unknown. Usually only one eye waters in this condition.

Blockage of the tear duct can lead to infection of the lacrimal sac. This causes a red and painful swelling in the skin beside the nose. In some babies the tear duct fails to open after birth, which causes tearing and a discharge from the eye.

Watering of the eye due to blockage is an uncommon problem. It usually occurs in middle age or later.

What should be done?
If your eye keeps watering, see your ophthalmologist, who will test your eyes to discover the cause of the problem.

In an infant, if the lacrimal duct or sac is blocked and the condition is in an early stage, the duct or sac can be cleared. This is accomplished by inserting a probe or by irrigating the eye while the child is either sedated or under a general anesthetic.

If blockage of the duct or sac is at too advanced a stage for these procedures, as is usually the case in adults, you may need an operation. The operation that is performed creates an artificial duct that by-passes the blockage. If the lacrimal sac is infected, you may have to take *antibiotics* (as tablets or eyedrops) to clear up the infection before further treatment is attempted.

Corneal ulcers and infections

See p.246,
Visual aids to diagnosis, 54.

The cornea is a transparent section of the eye's outer covering at the very front of the eye. Because of its position, it is the part of the eyeball that is most susceptible to injury and infection.

When an *ulcer* (an open sore) occurs on the cornea, infection can follow, and the reverse is also true. When an ulcer forms first, which is more common, it is usually the result of a foreign body striking or scratching the cornea. The ulcer then becomes infected by bacteria, viruses, or fungi. When an infection of the cornea occurs, it is almost always a virus that is responsible – usually *Herpes simplex*, the virus that also produces cold sores (see p.451) around the mouth. If you have a cold sore, never put your fingers to your eyes after touching your mouth.

What are the symptoms?

You will feel discomfort or pain in the eye, and the sharpness of your vision will be impaired to some degree. The effect on your vision is determined by the size of the ulcer. The white part of the eye will be reddened. In cases of infections other than those caused by *Herpes simplex*, the ulcer is sometimes readily visible, if you look closely, as a whitish patch. *Herpes simplex* infections produce what is called a dendritic ulcer, which has a branching pattern and is invisible to the unassisted eye. The symptoms are much more pronounced in bacterial infections than in viral or fungal infections.

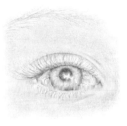

A corneal ulcer caused by bacteria may be visible as a white patch on the cornea.

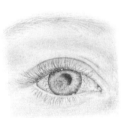

A dendritic ulcer of the cornea is normally invisible to the naked eye. But it can be made visible with a special stain.

What are the risks?

The majority of those affected by corneal ulcers are people who work at a job where their eyes are exposed to a spray of flying bodies, such as wood shavings or grit from car engines. If an ulcer is not treated promptly, a scar can form on the cornea and sometimes reduce vision. A neglected ulcer may perforate the cornea, cause pain and loss of vision, and allow infection to enter the eyeball, which can cause permanent loss of sight.

What should be done?

Because of the serious risks involved, as soon as you suspect you have a corneal ulcer or infection see your physician. If the doctor suspects a *Herpes simplex* infection, he or she may apply drops to the eye that stain and reveal any dendritic ulcer present, which can confirm the diagnosis.

Ulcers caused by injury to the cornea and the bacterial infections that follow them are treated with *antibiotics*, given as drops, ointment, tablets, or injections. For viral infections and the ulcers they produce, other drops and ointments are prescribed. Fungal ulcers are more difficult to treat. Dendritic ulcers tend to recur.

If scars from ulceration drastically reduce vision, you may need a corneal transplant – an operation to graft a new cornea onto the eye (see Transplants, p.402). If an ulcer has perforated the cornea, immediate surgery will be required to seal off the hole.

Conjunctivitis

See p.246,
**Visual aids to
diagnosis, 55.**

Conjunctivitis is inflammation of the conjunctiva, a transparent membrane that lines the eyelids and outer eye up to the edge of the cornea. The disorder can be caused by an infection or an allergy, or, in babies more than a week old, by incompletely opened tear drainage ducts.

An infection often comes from contaminated fingers, towels, handkerchiefs, or wash cloths touching the eye. In babies up to about three days old it is sometimes caught from the mother's birth canal. This condition, known as ophthalmia neonatorum, may be serious.

In all cases of infectious conjunctivitis, the white part of the eye turns red and feels gritty. There is then a discharge of yellow pus from the eye. Overnight this forms a crust. Bacterial infection usually occurs in both eyes and produces a marked discharge, whereas viral infection is usually limited to one eye and causes only a slight discharge.

Allergic conjunctivitis is caused by an allergy to pollen, cosmetics, or other substances. There is usually a longstanding redness and itchiness of the white of the eye, without any discharge of pus. The form that occurs in children and young adults all year round, but more severely in the pollen season, is a form of hay fever (see Allergic rhinitis, p.344). Less commonly, there is a sudden white puffiness of the conjunctiva, usually during the pollen season, that disappears after a few hours.

Conjunctivitis is very common. It is a troublesome disorder but, except in rare instances of opthalmia neonatorum, it is not usually serious.

What should be done?

If you suspect you or your child has conjunctivitis, see your physician immediately. If the symptoms are those of infectious conjunctivitis, avoid spreading the disease. Wash your hands after they have touched your eyes, and have your own separate washcloth and towel.

In cases of infectious conjunctivitis caused by bacteria, your physician may prescribe *antibiotic* drops or ointment to apply to your eyes after you have bathed away any discharge from the lids with warm water. One or two weeks of this treatment should clear up the condition. Viral infections will usually disappear of their own accord. Cases of ophthalmia neonatorum will be treated with antibiotic drops.

If you can identify the cause of allergic conjunctivitis, it may be possible to avoid the disorder. Consult your physician about using antihistamine medications or other non-prescription drugs that can relieve the inflammation of this form of the disorder.

Episcleritis

A transparent tissue called the episclera surrounds the eyeball. At the front of the eye, it lies between the sclera (the white of the eye) and the conjunctiva (a transparent mucous membrane overlying the sclera). In some young adults the tiny blood vessels in the episclera become inflamed for no known reason. One or both eyes may be affected.

The symptoms of episcleritis are a diffused or patchy redness over the white of the eye and a feeling of slight discomfort in the eye.

The condition is not serious and usually disappears by itself after a week or two, though it may recur from time to time. Natural healing of the inflammation can be hastened by anti-inflammatory drugs such as *steroids* which may be prescribed by your physician either as eye drops or ointment.

Scleritis

Scleritis is inflammation of the sclera, the outermost layer of tissue that covers the eyeball and that you can see as the white of the eye. The inflammation often accompanies rheumatoid arthritis (see p.552) or certain disorders of the digestive system, including Crohn's disease (see p.473). It can affect one or both eyes.

The symptoms are a dull pain in the eye and one or more areas of intense redness on the white of the eye. The inflammation can occur at the back of the eye, in which case there may be some loss of vision.

Scleritis is a rare disorder that occurs mainly in people between about 30 and 60. If the condition is not treated, there is a risk that wherever the sclera is inflamed the tissue will open. It is therefore essential that you see your physician right away if you suspect you have scleritis.

What is the treatment?
In mild or moderate cases, the inflammation can usually be cleared up with anti-inflammatory drugs such as *steroids*, either in tablet form or applied to the eye as drops. In severe cases, *immunosuppressive* drugs may be prescribed. If the sclera has become perforated, or opened, an operation will be needed to repair the damage.

Iritis

Iritis is inflammation of the iris (the part of the eye that determines eye color) and sometimes also of the ciliary body, which is behind the iris. In this disorder, microscopic white cells from the inflamed area and excess protein that leaks from the small blood vessels inside the eye float in the aqueous humor, the fluid between the iris and the cornea. If there are a lot of floating cells, they may become attached to the back of the cornea or they may settle to the bottom of the aqueous humor. The cause of iritis is not known. One or both eyes may be affected.

What are the symptoms?
There is a feeling of discomfort or pain in the eye, which becomes reddened. This is accompanied by a slight reduction in vision. Any cells that are stuck to the back of the cornea may be barely visible if you look in a mirror. Symptoms are often mild.

What are the risks?
Iritis is a fairly rare disorder. It can occur at any age, but is most common in young adults.

If it is treated early, iritis is not a serious problem. However, if you do not consult a physician because your symptoms are mild, complications will develop. So many white cells may accumulate in the aqueous humor that they block the opening through which the liquid drains out of the eye. This can cause acute glaucoma (see p.320). This complication may also develop if the back of the inflamed iris sticks to the front of the lens and aqueous humor is trapped behind the iris. Long-standing iritis can also cause cataracts (see next article).

What should be done?

At any sign of unexplainable redness or discomfort or any loss of vision in an eye, however slight, see your ophthalmologist. If you have iritis, the earlier treatment is started the easier it is to clear up an attack and the less likely it is that complications will occur.

What is the treatment?

Eye drops or ointment are given to reduce the inflammation. In severe cases, a drug may be injected into the outer layer of the eye after the use of a local anesthetic. You may also be given eye drops to prevent the back of the inflamed iris from sticking to the front of the lens. Any rise in pressure in the eye endangers the sensitive tissues of the eye and is controlled by medication.

Even when it is treated early, iritis often recurs. In most cases, however, it eventually disappears completely and with it goes any slight impairment of vision.

Cataracts

See p.247,
Visual aids to diagnosis, 61.

A cataract is an opaque (cloudy) area that occurs in the normally clear lens of the eye. Over a period of years, the cataract blocks or distorts light that is entering the eye and progressively reduces vision. In some cases the loss of vision is only slight and never becomes severe enough to warrant treatment. Cataracts usually occur in both eyes, but in most cases, one of the eyes is more severely affected than the other.

The most common cause of a cataract is deterioration of the lens in old age. Other causes include iritis (see previous article), injury to the eyeball (in which case only the injured eye will be affected), and diabetes mellitus (see p.519). The disorder tends to run in families, and in some cases it is present at birth or shortly after birth.

What are the symptoms?

The main symptom is a deterioration of vision in the affected eye. In some cases, vision is also blurred. In others, it is worse in bright sunlight. Except in some advanced cases, cataracts cannot easily be seen by an observer. In advanced cases, the lens may become white, opaque and quite readily visible through the pupil. A very advanced cataract may produce painful inflammation and pressure within the eye.

What are the risks?

Cataracts are fairly common, and you are more likely to have them as you get older.

The disorder may lead to severe deterioration of vision, but this can be rectified at any time by surgery.

What should be done?

If your vision deteriorates or becomes distorted, see an ophthalmologist. The physician may diagnose a cataract if glasses fail to improve your vision.

What is the treatment?

The only treatment possible for a cataract is an operation to remove the affected lens. This is the most common of all operations on the eye. If your vision is not too badly affected, your ophthalmologist will do nothing except make sure that you get glasses that give you the maximum benefit.

With a cataract that is causing inflammation and pressure in the eye, removal of the lens is essential. This is also necessary for a baby or young child with a cataract that is reducing vision severely. Usually an ophthalmologist will also recommend an operation for an adult if both eyes are affected and vision worsens to the extent that performing everyday activities becomes difficult, or if only one eye is affected but you need good vision in both eyes for your job.

Either a general or a local anesthetic is given for the operation. Usually the entire lens is taken out, but in some cases only the substance within the lens is removed, using a small needle, and the transparent capsule of the lens is left in the eye.

Removal of the lens from an eye makes the eye markedly farsighted (see p.310). This is corrected by eyeglasses, a contact lens, or a plastic lens placed in the eye at the time of the operation (an experimental procedure). If vision is then not as good as was anticipated, this is usually due to a defect in the retina at the back of the eye, which was obscured before the operation by the opacity of the lens. The most common retinal defect is macular degeneration (see p.323).

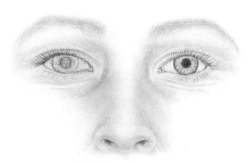

The pupil of the eye appears to be white in cases of severe cataract.

Glaucoma

Glaucoma is one of the most common and severe eye disorders in people over 60. Early treatment is vital, or the condition can ultimately lead to blindness.

The ciliary body in the eye constantly produces a fluid called aqueous humor, which circulates from behind the iris, through the pupil, and into the chamber between the iris and the cornea. In a healthy eye the fluid drains out of the eye through a network of tissue between the iris and the cornea, which is called the drainage angle. From there it flows into a channel that leads to a network of small veins on the outside of the eye. In some eyes the drainage angle does not work properly. As a result, the aqueous humor either flows away more slowly than it is produced or fails to flow away at all, and pressure builds up in the eye. Part of the extra pressure is exerted, via the lens, onto the vitreous humor, the jelly-like fluid that fills the eyeball behind the lens.

The pressure of the vitreous humor on the retina causes the collapse of tiny blood vessels that nourish the light-sensitive cells of the retina and the fibers of the optic nerve, both of which play a vital part in vision. Since they are deprived of the blood that provides them with essential nutrients and oxygen, the cells and nerve fibers begin to die, and vision begins to fade.

The cause, extent and type of glaucoma can vary considerably. Certain drugs can hasten the onset of the condition. The two most common types of the disease, both of which are described here, are acute glaucoma (also known as angle closure glaucoma) and chronic glaucoma (also known as open angle glaucoma).

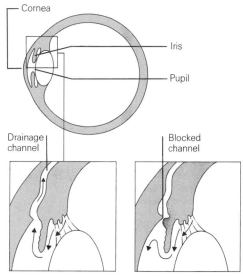

Normally, liquid circulates constantly through the pupil, between the iris and cornea, and is drained through a channel into veins. In glaucoma, the entrance to the drainage channel is blocked and the liquid builds up.

Acute glaucoma

(angle closure glaucoma)

Glaucoma is a disorder in which the circulation of aqueous humor, a fluid in the eye that is produced by the ciliary body, is blocked. The blockage occurs in a network of tissue between the iris and the cornea that is called the drainage angle. Pressure builds up in the eye because the aqueous humor cannot flow away, and this affects the functioning of both the retina and the optic nerve, which are essential to vision. For more about glaucoma in general, read above.

In acute glaucoma, the drainage angle becomes blocked suddenly. This type of glaucoma occurs mainly in farsighted elderly people. In farsightedness the distance between the cornea and the iris is shorter than normal, so the drainage angle is narrower. With age, the lens of the eye gradually enlarges and pushes the iris forward, and this narrows the angle further. In some cases where the drainage angle is extremely narrow, blockage can occur at any time. The outer edge of the iris blocks the drainage angle when the iris contracts to enlarge the pupil. This occurs naturally when you need to see in dim light or as part of your body's reaction to emotion. Aqueous humor, which is produced in the chamber behind the iris, cannot then drain away, and pressure builds up in the eyeball. The iris may recede from the drainage angle after the light has changed or the emotion has passed. If the liquid fails to drain and is caught in the drainage angle, the pressure in the eyeball continues to build, which causes acute glaucoma.

Usually, only one eye is affected, but the other eye is highly susceptible to an attack of glaucoma at a later date.

What are the symptoms?

In some cases there are short preliminary attacks months or weeks before a fully developed attack of acute glaucoma occurs. The attacks usually occur in the evening, when the light is dim, and last for as long as the iris blocks the drainage angle. Your vision becomes blurred, you may see halos around lights, the cornea begins to look hazy (as pressure in the eyeball forces aqueous humor into it), and often there is some pain and redness in the eye. No permanent damage to the vision usually occurs at this time.

In a fully developed attack, the same symptoms occur but they persist and become worse. Pain, often severe, may be felt in the head as well as in the eye. The pain is often accompanied by vomiting and even prostration. The cornea appears increasingly hazy and sometimes it even looks gray and granular. In addition, the eyeball may be painful and hard to the touch.

What are the risks?

Acute glaucoma is not a common condition. In the 40 to 65 age group, 1 person in 1000 has it. In the over-65 age group, 1 person in 500 may have the condition. Men and women are equally susceptible. About half of those who have the disease seek medical attention because of the warning symptoms that occur before a fully developed attack.

Acute glaucoma tends to run in families, partly because its predisposing factors, such as farsightedness, also run in families. If you are over 40, farsighted, and have two or more blood relatives who have (or have had) the disease, you should be especially aware of the possible symptoms.

If a fully developed attack of acute glaucoma is treated early, vision in the eye will return almost to normal. But once an attack is well under way, the fibers of the optic nerve at the back of the eye are often damaged, which causes some permanent loss of vision. If an attack is neglected altogether, the eye may become totally blind.

What should be done?

Because of the risks to sight, early treatment is essential. Most people seek treatment anyway, because of the extreme discomfort of the symptoms. At the first signs of an attack see your physician at once. If the attack occurs out of office hours, contact a physician on call or go to the emergency room of a nearby hospital. The physician will probably arrange for you to be admitted to the hospital under the care of an ophthalmologist.

What is the treatment?

In the hospital you may be given eye drops to encourage the iris to withdraw from the drainage angle. To reduce the production of aqueous humor, you may receive an injection of a drug and possibly also be given a dehydrating or drying agent, in the form of tablets or in an *intravenous drip*.

Usually, this treatment brings down the pressure in the eye within hours. A day or two later, a simple operation called an iridectomy may be performed to prevent any further attack (see Box, left). The operation can be done with a laser beam. A tiny artificial channel for the drainage of aqueous humor is made through the iris and directly into the drainage angle. The channel goes through the outer edge of the iris and beneath the upper eyelid, so that it does not show. Since your

---

OPERATION: **Iridectomy**

Because glaucoma usually affects both eyes, the operation will probably be done on both eyes, though symptoms may have occurred in only one. The eyes are done at separate times rather than both at once.

During the operation You are given either a local or general anesthetic. The surgeon makes an incision at the border of the conjunctiva and the cornea. A piece of iris is gently pulled through the incision and snipped off. This allows the aqueous humor to drain away, and relieves the symptom-producing pressure in the eye. The incision is then closed up. The operation usually takes about 30 minutes.

After the operation You will be given eye drops to suppress inflammation and will wear a patch over the eye for a few days. You will probably have to stay in the hospital for about five days.

Convalescence You should soon be able to resume normal activities, but you will probably be advised not to bend down or lift any heavy weights for a month.

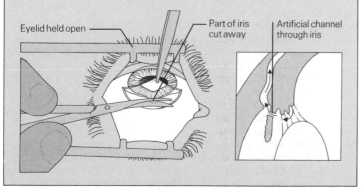

Eyelid held open — Part of iris cut away | Artificial channel through iris

other eye may be affected by glaucoma later, you will probably be advised to have an iridectomy performed later on that eye. Iridectomy usually prevents further attacks of glaucoma.

If you do not obtain immediate treatment, the iris may become stuck to the drainage angle and cause a permanent obstruction. If this occurs, you will need a more complex operation, possibly a trabeculectomy. In this procedure, aqueous humor is allowed to drain directly to small veins on the outside of the eye. Either a general or a local anesthetic is used. This operation also has a high success rate. In a few cases when it is only partially successful, it is sometimes possible to perform a second operation. If not, lifelong drug treatment, together with the partial drainage achieved by the operation, should keep the pressure under control.

Chronic glaucoma

(*open angle glaucoma*)

Medical myths

Watching too much television or working for a long time in poor light can harm the eyes.

Wrong. Extensive use of the eyes does not damage them any more than extensive walking damages your legs. However, your eyes can get tired, and you should read in adequate light.

In chronic glaucoma, the circulation of a fluid called aqueous humor, which is produced constantly by the ciliary body in the eye, is blocked gradually over a period of years. Aqueous humor builds up in the eye, and eventually creates an internal pressure that affects the blood supply to the retina and the optic nerve, both of which are essential to vision. The aqueous humor normally drains out of the eye through a network of tissue between the iris and the cornea. This network is called the drainage angle, and it is there that the blockage occurs.

As the disorder progresses, it becomes increasingly more difficult for the aqueous humor (which normally flows from behind the iris, through the pupil, and into the chamber between the iris and the cornea) to drain out of the eye through the drainage angle. The blockage causes a slow and steady build-up of internal pressure on the rest of the eyeball. For a more detailed description of how glaucoma occurs, read the introduction to this section (see p.320).

Unlike acute glaucoma (see previous article), chronic glaucoma often is not detected without an eye examination. This is because the blockage occurs and the pressure builds up so slowly. In most cases of chronic glaucoma, both eyes are affected by the disorder, one soon after the other.

What are the symptoms?
The development of the disorder is so gradual that the only symptom that occurs in the early stages is too slight to be noticeable. This is the loss of small areas of peripheral vision in one eye, on the side near the nose, caused by pressure in the eyeball that damages the fibers of the optic nerve. The loss passes unnoticed because the peripheral vision of the other eye compensates for it. Gradually, other areas of peripheral vision are lost, the areas lost increase in size, and the disorder affects the other eye. At some point in this process, you will become aware of the loss of part of your vision.

What are the risks?
Chronic glaucoma is more common than acute glaucoma (see previous article). It may affect one to two per cent of the population over the age of 40. The risk increases from middle age onwards. The disease tends to run in families, so you are more likely to get it if you have relatives who have it.

If the disease is allowed to continue unchecked, all your peripheral vision in both eyes is lost. Then the ability of the eye to see straight ahead gradually diminishes until it disappears altogether and both eyes become totally blind.

What should be done?
Since any vision that is lost through the disease cannot be regained, the sooner you receive treatment the better. In the early stages of this type of glaucoma, it is impossible to tell that you have it unless you are tested for it. For this and other good reasons, you should have regular eye examinations by a qualified physician. Be sure to go to an ophthalmologist for a checkup every two to three years after you reach the age of 40.

What is the treatment?
The treatment for chronic glaucoma is to try to bring down the pressure in the eyeball as quickly as possible. You will probably be given eye drops that partially unblock the drainage angles and/or drops or tablets to reduce the production of aqueous humor. All these drops and tablets generally have to be taken for life, and you will also need to have regular checkups by your physician to be certain that all is going well. Taking the drugs soon becomes part of your daily routine, and if you continue to take them you should not have any further loss of vision.

If drugs fail to reduce the pressure in the eye sufficiently, the ophthalmologist will probably recommend that you have an operation in which the surgeon creates an artificial drainage channel. This procedure has a high rate of success.

Back of the eye and eye orbit

The function of the back of the eye is to receive the light that is focused by the front of the eye and transform it into nerve impulses. These impulses then pass along the optic nerve, which leads from the back of the retina to the brain. The impulses are in a "code" that was determined by the specifics of what the eye saw. The brain "decodes" this message and you see what the eye saw an instant before.

The eye structure that receives the light is the retina, a layer of light-sensitive nerve cells that lines the back three-quarters of the eyeball. The nerve cells consist of *rods* and *cones*. They are particularly well adapted for detecting light.

The cones detect fine detail and color. They are most highly concentrated in the macula, which is an area in the center of the retina at the very back of the eye. This is why you have to look straight at an object to see it clearly. Most of the rods are located around the edges of the macula. They detect much less detail and no color, but are sensitive to the intensity of the light entering the eye. You can often see an object more clearly if it is in dim light by looking at it indirectly and slightly to one side.

The bony socket in which each eyeball lies is called the orbit. The eyeball swivels in the orbit by means of muscles attached to the outside of the eyeball and the inside of the orbit. Either an imbalance between these muscles or a defect in the nerves that control them causes the disorder known as crossed eyes. When this problem develops in an adult, it usually has a different cause from crossed eyes that appear in a child. Only the adult form of the disorder is covered in this section (see also p.674).

Macular degeneration

The macula, the area of the retina near the optic nerve at the back of the eye, is the part of the eye that distinguishes fine detail at the center of the field of vision. In some elderly people, the small blood vessels of the eye become constricted or narrowed and hardened. As a result, the macula does not get enough blood, and it requires a plentiful supply. This blood deficiency causes degeneration of the macula, and blurring of the central vision follows. In nearly all cases, both eyes are affected, either simultaneously or one after the other.

Macular degeneration usually develops gradually and is painless. For these reasons, you may not notice it coming on, particularly in its early stages. When both eyes are affected, reading and other activities that require sharp vision are not possible. Eventually, central vision disappears altogether, but the peripheral vision in each eye remains.

Most cases of the disease are untreatable, but if you notice the symptoms you should still see an ophthalmologist right away. Vision can sometimes be improved by eyeglasses with powerful magnifying lenses.

Diabetic retinopathy

In some people who have diabetes mellitus (see p.519), many of the small blood vessels of the retina, the layer of light-sensitive cells in the back of the eyeball, become constricted and die. The disorder usually occurs in both eyes. In a few cases, the remaining vessels may then leak blood into the retina and cause a permanent reduction in sharpness of vision. In addition, fragile new blood vessels may grow on the retina and in many cases they leak blood into the vitreous humor, the jelly-like bulk of the eyeball. This dims or obliterates vision temporarily. In both kinds of blood leakage, the blood is usually reabsorbed by the retina, but scar tissue then forms on the retina, and this may cause permanent, partial loss of vision. The disorder occurs more often in those diabetics who do not control their level of blood glucose properly, but all diabetics are susceptible and should have their eyes checked regularly.

Treatment usually is effective in controlling retinopathy. The vessels that leak blood can often be plugged by a *laser beam*, and any bleeding into the vitreous humor that has not cleared up within a year can be treated by draining the eye of vitreous humor with special instruments and replacing it with an artificial substitute.

The disorder tends to recur, but with repeated treatment your vision can usually be maintained.

Retinal detachment

The retina is a delicate layer of light-sensitive cells that lines the rear three-quarters of the eyeball. Beneath the retina is a layer of blood vessels called the choroid, which provides the retina with nutrients and oxygen.

Retinal detachment occurs when the retina lifts away from the choroid. A hole in the retina causes the detachment in most cases. The hole forms either because of degeneration of the retina or because the vitreous humor (the jelly-like bulk of the eyeball) has shrunk away from the retina and torn it. The hole usually forms near the front edge of the retina. Vitreous humor seeps through the hole and starts to detach the retina from the choroid. If the condition is not treated, this process continues, and more and more retina is lifted away. Eventually the retina is attached only at the front of the eye, to the ciliary body (an extension of the choroid), and at the rear of the eye, to the end of the optic nerve.

Both eyes may be affected, but rarely at the same time.

What are the symptoms?
The only symptoms are abnormalities of vision in the affected eye. Since the other eye is almost always normal, it may compensate for the affected eye, so that early symptoms may not be noticed. The first signs of a detached retina may be flashes of light, which often occur shortly before a hole is formed in the retina. Floating, black, often cobweb-like shapes may be seen when the hole is actually formed. Once detachment starts you may notice the loss of part of your peripheral vision in the affected eye. This often appears as a narrow black "curtain" coming from the top, the bottom, or one side of the eye. If

detachment continues unchecked, the loss of vision spreads. What vision remains becomes progressively blurred.

What are the risks?
Retinal detachment is rare. It occurs mainly from middle age onwards, and men and women are equally susceptible. You are particularly at risk if you are nearsighted (see p.310), because your retina is likely to be stretched due to the shape of your eyeball. If your eye is injured, or if you have the lens of your eye removed because of a cataract (see p.319), you are also at risk. If the disorder is neglected, there is a risk of permanent blindness in the affected eye.

What should be done?
If you experience any of the symptoms described, see your physician without delay. An ophthalmologist will be able to detect retinal detachment by looking into your eye through an instrument called an *ophthalmoscope.*

What is the treatment?
If a hole in the retina is discovered before detachment has started, you may need to have an operation to seal the hole permanently. This is done by freezing or by a *laser beam* after a local anesthetic has been given. If retinal detachment has begun, a different operation done under a local or general anesthetic may be necessary. In this procedure, the vitreous humor between the retina and the choroid is drained away, which allows the retina to sink back against the choroid and regain its blood supply. Then, the hole in the retina is sealed.

If the operation is carried out before detachment has started or when it has occurred only around the front edge of the retina, your vision will probably return to normal. If the detachment is more extensive and your central vision has been impaired, although the full field of vision will probably be restored, central vision will be permanently blurred to some extent. In five per cent of cases of complete detachment, the retina fails to sink back against the choroid after the operation, and the eye remains blind. After surgery, retinal detachment recurs in only a small minority of cases.

Following retinal detachment in one eye, there is a considerable risk that the condition will develop in the other eye. After the operation, you should see your ophthalmologist regularly to have the other eye examined. Any weak areas in the retina that are likely to develop into a hole can be detected and may be treated surgically.

Liquid can seep through one or more holes in the retina, causing it to become detached from the underlying choroid (right). To treat a detached retina, the surgeon pushes the choroid against the retina (below right) and seals them together with a freezing probe. Small portions left unsealed seal themselves later.

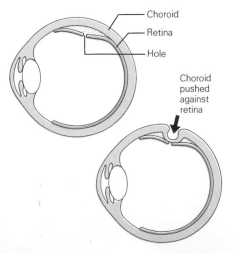

Choroid

Retina

Hole

Choroid pushed against retina

Retinal artery occlusion

The blood required by the light-sensitive cells of the retina in the back of the eyeball is supplied by the central retinal artery, a tiny vessel that enters the back of the eye near the optic nerve. Sometimes, usually in middle-aged or elderly people, the artery or one of its branches becomes blocked, either by a blood clot resulting from *thrombosis* or by an *embolus*, a tiny piece of a blood clot or of a fatty deposit that has traveled from a diseased blood vessel elsewhere in the body (see Arterial embolism, p.415). The clot or embolus cuts off all or part of the retina's blood supply. If the artery is blocked, there is immediate blindness in the eye that is involved. If a branch of the artery is blocked, only part of the vision, usually the upper or lower half, of that eye blacks out.

If you suddenly lose all or part of the vision of one eye, you should see your ophthalmologist or go to a hospital emergency room *immediately*. If the blockage can be treated within a few hours, it may be possible to restore some of the sight in the eye. This is done by giving you certain drugs that "thin" the blood and cause the clot or embolus to move further along the blood vessel to a position where less of the retina is affected. If the drugs do not work, there is an alternative treatment. This treatment is an emergency operation on the eye.

Whatever happens to the eye, your physician may arrange an *electrocardiogram* (*ECG*), an *arteriogram*, and other tests for you. These tests are done to find out what caused the blockage, so that the problem can be treated to prevent the same thing from happening to the other eye.

Retinal vein occlusion

The central retinal vein carries blood away from the retina and, therefore, plays a key role in supporting the mechanism of sight. In rare cases, mainly from middle age onward, the vein or one of its branches can become blocked by a blood clot. When this happens, blood leaks out of the blocked vessel and causes blurred vision. The blurring occurs gradually, but in most cases it becomes apparent to you quite suddenly.

The disorder may occur in the early stages of chronic glaucoma (see p.322) or it may be triggered by high blood pressure (see p.382). It can also be caused by a blood disease in which the blood tends to clot more readily than normal, such as polycythemia (see p.429), but this is rare.

The younger you are, the more likely it is that your vision will improve naturally because the leaked blood will be reabsorbed through the wall of the retina. If reabsorption does not occur, the blurring will be permanent, since there is no treatment available for the disorder.

Sometimes new blood vessels form and create complications. Any vessels that grow on the retina itself are fragile and tend to leak blood, which causes further blurred vision. This may also improve spontaneously, especially in younger people. If vessels grow on the surface of the iris, they can cause a painful form of glaucoma (see p.320) that may, in some cases, lead to complete loss of vision in the affected eye.

The early signs of retinal vein occlusion can sometimes be detected by examining the eye with an *ophthalmoscope*. This examination is carried out during a routine eye examination, which is one good reason for having such a test regularly (see Going to the ophthalmologist, p.312). Effective control of any underlying problem such as high blood pressure may then prevent the disorder from getting worse.

Choroiditis

Choroiditis is inflammation of the choroid, a layer of blood vessels beneath the retina, in the back of the eyeball. The retina and many cells in the vitreous humor, the jelly-like filling of the eyeball, also become inflamed. When the inflammation subsides, the choroid is left scarred. Usually the exact cause of the disorder cannot be determined, but in a few children who have it, it is due to infectious agents that enter the system from extremely close contact with a pet, often a dog. The inflammation causes blurred vision, and, sometimes, reddening of the eye and discomfort.

If you or your child have these symptoms, be sure to see your ophthalmologist without any delay. The ophthalmologist will probably arrange blood tests and *X-rays* to look for an underlying cause of the problem. *Steroid* drugs may be prescribed in a attempt to clear up the inflammation and the blurred vision.

If the outer edge of the choroid near the front of the eye is scarred, there will be some loss of peripheral vision, which you may not even notice. If the central choroid at the rear of the eye is affected, there will be some loss of clear central vision.

Tumors of the eye

Tumors are abnormal growths of tissue. They may be *malignant* (likely to spread and threaten life) or *benign* (unlikely to spread). Tumors of the eye are rare. They are usually malignant and painless.

Malignant melanoma

This is a type of eye tumor similar to a form of skin cancer (see Malignant melanoma, p.259). It occurs mainly in the choroid (the layer of blood vessels beneath the retina) or the ciliary body (an extension of the choroid in the front of the eye). Such tumors occasionally grow in the iris. Only one eye is affected, and the problem occurs mainly in the elderly. More than half of these tumors are discovered during a routine examination by an ophthalmologist. The rest are discovered because of a gradual loss of some vision in the affected eye. The ophthalmologist may arrange for you to have *fluorescein angiography*, *echography* and other tests, to show the nature of the tumor. The usual treatment for a young adult is to remove the affected eye to prevent the tumor from spreading to other parts of the body. In an elderly person, if the tumor is growing very slowly and is not causing any loss of vision, the eye may be watched for any major changes.

Secondary tumors

In some cancers, tumors *metastasize*, or spread, through either the bloodstream or the lymphatic system from the primary growth, and grow in other parts of the body. Such secondary tumors in the eye develop during the late stages of the primary cancer. If these tumors grow behind the eyeball, they may cause bulging of the eye (see Exophthalmos, below). Their effect on vision varies according to exactly where they are located in the eye, their rate of growth, and whether one or both eyes are involved. A secondary tumor in the eye can be destroyed, or at least controlled through the use of *radiation therapy*, but it may already have caused some permanent loss of vision. The primary tumor must be dealt with separately.

Retinoblastoma

A retinoblastoma is a malignant tumor of the retina that occurs in one or both eyes, usually in a child under the age of five. The child will not have any symptoms. If the central vision of only one eye is affected, the child may have crossed eyes, which is one reason why crossed eyes should be examined by a physician (see p.674). If the tumor is not discovered during its early growth, it may become visible through the pupil as a white area in the interior of the eye. The disease is often inherited. If you know that it runs in your family, it is sensible, before having children, to seek genetic counseling (see p.619). If you already have a child, tell your physician about the family history of retinoblastoma so that the youngster can have regular eye examinations. If this type of tumor is detected early, treatment with *radiation therapy*, a *laser beam*, or freezing is usually very effective. If the tumor is advanced, however, the eye will have to be removed to prevent secondary tumors from spreading to other parts of the body and endangering the child's life.

Optic neuritis

In some people between the ages of 20 and 40, the optic nerve in one eye becomes inflamed. The inflammation causes a gradual or sudden blurring of vision in the eye. In severe cases, the blurring progresses within a few days to temporary blindness. Often the eye is painful when you move it. If, in addition to the symptoms described, your fingers tingle or you have difficulty in urinating, this may mean that the condition is a symptom of multiple sclerosis (see p.292).

If your physician suspects you have multiple sclerosis, he or she may send you to a hospital for special tests or to another physician for a consultation, or second opinion. The treatment for optic neuritis is *steroid* medication, which hastens the spontaneous recovery that usually takes place. The problem may recur, however, in either eye. If it does recur, the disease usually does not respond to treatment, and it may cause progressive loss of vision.

Exophthalmos

See p.247,
Visual aids to diagnosis, 62.

Exophthalmos is bulging of one or both eyeballs. It is caused by a swelling of the soft tissue that lines the bony orbit in which the eyeball lies. The eyeball is pressed forward, which exposes an abnormally large amount of the front of the eye. The eye then tends to become dry and feel gritty. Eye movement is restricted, which can cause double vision. In severe cases, the eye is pressed forward so much that its blood supply is restricted and vision becomes seriously blurred. The lids may be prevented from closing.

The most common cause of the swelling is an abnormality in the production of thyroid hormones (see Hyperthyroidism, p.525). Other cases are caused by a tumor behind the eyeball (see Tumors of the eye, previous page) or inflammation of the tissue there (see Orbital cellulitis, next article).

Blood tests, *X-rays, echography, CAT scans* and an examination of the eye with an *ophthalmoscope* are carried out to find out what is causing the disorder.

What is the treatment?
If the thyroid gland is causing the condition, that disorder will be treated. Such treatment may not control the exophthalmos, however, and *steroid* drugs may be given, or part of the lids may be stitched together to prevent corneal ulcers (see p.316). In severe cases, an operation may be needed to relieve the pressure behind the eyeball. In this form of the disorder, early treatment nearly always returns normal vision.

Orbital cellulitis

The bony orbit in which the eyeball lies is lined with soft tissue. In rare cases, bacteria enter the tissue, usually from infected sinuses in the nose (see Sinusitis, p.347), or from a boil near the eye, and cause an inflammation. This is called orbital cellulitis.

The pressure of the swollen tissue pushes the eyeball forward, giving your eye a staring appearance (see Exophthalmos, previous article). Other symptoms are severe pain and redness in the eye, swollen eyelids that you may not be able to close, and usually a fever.

In rare cases the eye exudes pus. The condition often resembles conjunctivitis (see p.317). If there is pressure on the blood vessels that supply the eye, you may temporarily lose some vision. There is also a slight risk that the infection may spread to the brain and cause meningitis (see p.273).

Treatment consists of high doses of *antibiotics*, given as tablets or by injection. If infected sinuses are the source of the problem, you may need an operation to have them drained to prevent cellulitis from recurring.

Crossed eyes in adults

Normal eyes move together, so that both look at the same object at the same time. This is essential for good, clear vision. Crossed eyes occur when this co-ordination is absent. One eye looks at the object, and the other looks elsewhere.

Crossed eyes usually develop in infancy or early childhood (see p.674), usually as the result of another eye disorder that weakens the eye muscles. After childhood, crossed eyes almost always occur for a different reason and have a different effect. In almost all cases, crossed eyes that develop after childhood are caused by a disorder elsewhere in the body that affects either the nerves between the brain and the eye muscles or, less commonly, the muscles themselves. These disorders include diabetes mellitus (see p.519), high blood pressure (see p.382), temporal arteritis (see p.414), brain injury (see p.276) and muscular dystrophy (see p.694).

What are the symptoms?
In almost all cases, double vision occurs and you will also have the symptoms of some underlying disorder.

What should be done?
If you start to see double and have never had crossed eyes, see your physician. As a temporary measure to prevent double vision, cover one eye with a patch, which you can buy at a drug store. To discover the underlying cause of the problem, the physician will probably take your blood pressure, ask you to provide urine and blood samples for testing, and arrange for you to have various *X-rays.*

In most cases, good response to treatment of the underlying disorder corrects the double vision gradually within a few months. If the problem remains to some extent, this can usually be corrected by eyeglasses. Otherwise, an operation may be necessary.

Each eye is controlled by six muscles. An underlying illness affecting the control of these muscles can cause crossed eyes.

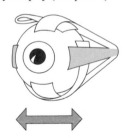
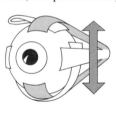
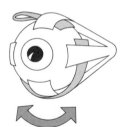

Disorders of the ear

Introduction

The ear is the organ of balance as well as hearing. It has three parts, the outer, middle and inner ear. The outer ear includes both the ear that we see – folds of skin and cartilage known as the pinna – and the outer ear canal, a passage about 20 mm ($\frac{3}{4}$ in) long that leads from the pinna to the eardrum. The opening of the canal is surrounded by cartilage. This cartilage is covered with skin that contains wax-producing glands and hairs. The deeper part of the canal is lined by a thin membrane and surrounded by bone. The eardrum is a thin membrane stretched across the end of the outer ear canal. It separates the outer ear from the middle ear.

The middle ear is a small cavity between the eardrum and the inner ear. It is bridged by three small, connected bones. These bones are named the hammer, anvil and stirrup because of their shapes. The hammer is attached to the inner lining of the eardrum. The stirrup is attached by a ligament to the oval window, an opening that leads to the inner ear. The anvil lies between the hammer and the stirrup, and is attached to both of them.

There are various openings in the middle ear. One of these leads into the air spaces in the mastoid region of the temporal bone (the bone that contains all of the internal regions of the ear). Two others lead into the inner ear. One opening, known as the eustachian or auditory tube, leads to the cavity at the back of the nose. The eustachian tube permits equalization of the air pressure on the inside of the eardrum with pressure on the outside. Sometimes the tube becomes blocked during a cold. When it becomes clear again, the sudden equalization of pressure makes you feel as if the ear has "popped."

The inner ear consists of two structures that contain membrane-lined chambers filled with fluid, the labyrinth and the cochlea. The labyrinth is the part of the ear used for balance. It consists of the semicircular canals, three connected tubes bent into half circles. The cochlea, which plays a role in hearing, starts on the inner side of the oval window and curls around like a snail's shell. The auditory nerve attaches to the labyrinth and the cochlea, and connects the hearing and balance functions of the inner ear to the appropriate parts of the brain.

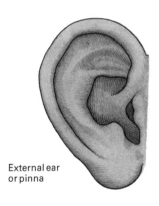

The structure of the ear
The outer ear collects sound waves and funnels them into the middle ear, which passes them on to the inner ear. The inner ear converts the waves into nerve impulses and transmits them to the brain. The inner ear also contains the mechanism for keeping your balance.

External ear or pinna

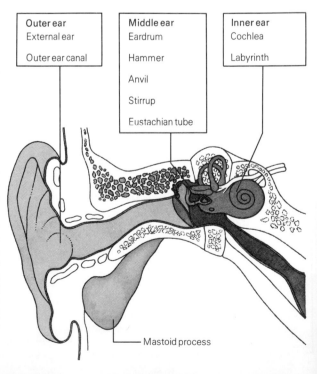

Outer ear	Middle ear	Inner ear
External ear	Eardrum	Cochlea
Outer ear canal	Hammer	Labyrinth
	Anvil	
	Stirrup	
	Eustachian tube	

Mastoid process

How the ear works

How you hear

A sound starts as a disturbance of the air, which produces sound waves. The visible ear helps to channel these waves down the outer ear canal, so that they hit the eardrum and make it vibrate. The vibrations pass through the hammer, anvil, stirrup and oval window into the fluid in the cochlea. Tiny hairs that line the cochlea change the vibrations in the fluid into nerve impulses, which are transmitted to the brain along the auditory nerve.

Most sounds reach you through this route, but this kind of hearing is supplemented by vibrations conducted through the bones of the skull to the inner ear. You hear your own voice mainly through this secondary kind of hearing.

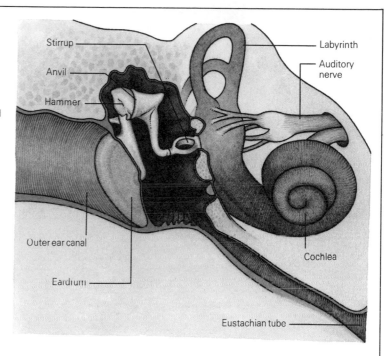

How you keep your balance

Your brain constantly monitors positions and movements of your head and body so that you are able to keep your balance. In each inner ear is a structure called the labyrinth, which monitors the positions and movements of the head by means of three semicircular canals. Each canal is at right angles to the other two, so whichever way you move your head – nod it (A), shake it (B) or tilt it (C) – one or more of the semicircular canals (below right) detects the movement, and relays the information to the brain. The brain coordinates this data with more information from your eyes, and from the muscles in your body and limbs, to assess your exact position and the movements you need to make to keep your balance.

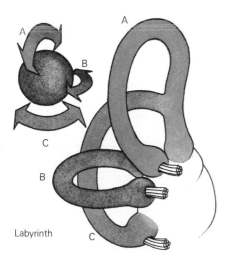

Each semicircular canal in the labyrinth detects movement in one of the three directions shown above left.

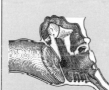

Conductive hearing loss
In conductive hearing loss, sounds do not reach the inner ear because of a mechanical defect in the middle ear.

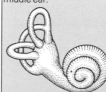

Sensorineural hearing loss
In sensorineural hearing loss, sounds reach the inner ear, but are not passed on to the brain.

Hearing loss and vertigo

There are two kinds of hearing loss, conductive and sensorineural. Conductive hearing loss is caused by a mechanical failure that keeps sounds from reaching the inner ear. This happens, for example, because of wax blockage in the outer ear (see next page). Sensorineural hearing loss is caused by nerve failure. Although sounds reach the inner ear, they are not perceived because the appropriate nerve impulses do not reach the brain. The usual cause of sensorineural hearing loss is damage to the cochlea or the auditory nerve. This sometimes happens in old age (see Aging and the senses, p.721). However, loud music, machinery noise, or rare side effects from medications can cause such damage at any age.

Vertigo is a false sense that you or your surroundings are spinning around. Vertigo often causes loss of balance. It is usually a symptom of disorders of the inner ear, the part of the ear that senses movement and maintains balance.

The outer ear

The lining of the outer ear canal is an extension of the skin of the visible ear, so most disorders of the outer ear are skin disorders. While the symptoms may be very troublesome, these disorders are generally not as serious as middle and inner ear diseases, since they do not affect the delicate mechanisms of hearing and balance.

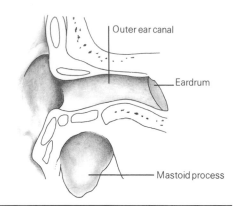

Outer ear canal

Eardrum

Mastoid process

Wax blockage

Glands in the outer ear canal produce wax to protect the canal. The amount produced varies from person to person. Some people produce so little wax that it never accumulates in the canal. Others produce enough to block the canal every few months.

The symptoms of wax blockage are a feeling that the ear is plugged, partial hearing loss, ringing in the ear, and sometimes earache. No serious risks are involved.

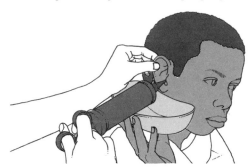

Syringing wax out
Warm water directed into the ear flows along the outer ear canal, bounces off the eardrum and flows back along the bottom of the canal, helping clean any blocking wax out. This wax-removing procedure is done by a physician.

What is the treatment?
Self-help: The best self-help for wax blockage is prevention. If you work in very dusty conditions, which can trigger wax blockage, consider wearing ear plugs.

Do not try to remove the wax with a stick or swab. It is all too easy to pack ear wax against the eardrum and cause damage.

Professional help: After examining your ear, your physician may soften the wax with eardrops before removing it. When wax is very difficult to remove, the doctor may dislodge it with a probe or electric suction apparatus.

Protruding ears

Most people's ears lie almost flat against the side of their heads, but in some people they protrude to some degree. In extreme cases, the ears may stick straight out. Protruding ears are not a risk to your physical health, but occasionally they can be the source of psychological distress. For some people this distress may become more acute than other people might imagine.

If you have protruding ears and are bothered by it, you can discuss it with your physician. The popular belief that the protrusion can be countered by simply strapping or taping your ears to the sides of your head at night is, unfortunately, not true. Mild protrusion may be concealed easily either by letting your hair grow longer or by changing your hair style so that it covers your ears. In extreme cases, the doctor may recommend an operation. The surgical procedure for cor-

The simple surgery
The ear is drawn back after a strip of skin has been removed from behind it. This surgery is not usually advised for children under five, since their ears are not yet fully developed.

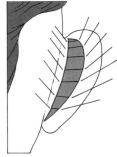

recting protruding ears is relatively simple. An incision is made near the crease of skin behind your ear, the ear is pulled back flat against your head, and the incision is sewn up. The scars from the operation are behind the ear, and they usually do not show. You will probably have to stay in the hospital for one or two days.

Infections of the outer-ear canal

(otitis externa)

Infections of the outer ear canal may take one of two forms: a localized infection such as a boil or *abscess*, or a generalized infection that affects the whole lining of the canal. Ear infections can occur after swimming. Persistent, excessive moisture in the ear canal can make the canal more susceptible to infection. Polluted water from lakes and rivers can cause infection by direct contact. Another cause of both localized and generalized infections is scratching inside the ear to relieve itching or while attempting to remove wax.

The first symptom of infection may be itching in your ear, usually followed by pain. Sometimes yellowish-green pus seeps from the ear, and this may relieve the pain. If the pus blocks your outer ear canal, you may lose some hearing. When you have this kind of ear infection, any movement of the head may cause pain in your ear.

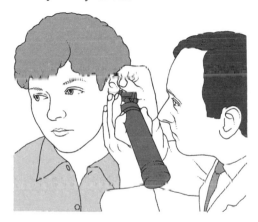

Inspecting the outer ear canal
A physician examines the ear through an otoscope. Pulling the top of the ear up and back gives a clearer view of the whole canal.

Infections of the outer ear are most common in young adults. If you do not get treatment for such an infection, it may spread and affect underlying cartilage and bone.

What is the treatment?

Self-help: Take aspirin and place a warm, clean cotton pad or an electric heating pad over your ear to help relieve pain until you see your physician.

Professional help: The physician will probably look into your ear with an *otoscope*, and may take a sample of any pus. The sample will be sent to a laboratory to see what has caused the infection. Then the doctor will probably clean your ear with a suction device or a cotton-tipped probe. This usually relieves irritation and pain. Your physician may prescribe any number of drugs in the form of pills, capsules, ear drops or cream. A combination of gentle daily cleaning of the ear and the use of the prescribed drugs should clear up the condition.

Usually, if the condition is not improved by this treatment within three to four days, your physician will take further action. Armed with the results of the laboratory tests, the physician may prescribe an *antibiotic* that is especially effective against the particular organisms, usually bacteria, causing the infection. If the pain is severe, the doctor may also prescribe a painkiller.

You must keep the infected ear dry. This means no swimming, and wearing ear plugs or a shower cap in the bath or shower.

The infection may recur and need treatment for many months if the microbes causing the infection are fungi, or if you develop an allergy (see p.705) to them. If this happens, your physician will probably prescribe a *steroid* cream or ear drops.

Tumors of the outer ear

Ear tumors
Tumors on the visible ear can be removed by surgery.

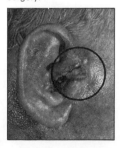

Like all tumors, those of the outer ear may be either *benign* (unlikely to spread) or *malignant* (likely to spread and threaten life).

On the visible ear, a benign tumor occurs as a painless wart. In the canal itself, it occurs as a hard growth of underlying bone tissue called an *osteoma*. With an osteoma, there may be no symptoms at all, or an accumulation of wax, discomfort, and hearing loss.

Malignant tumors on the visible ear occur as warty growths, like benign tumors, or as ulcers or bleeding sores that fail to heal. Malignant tumors are like skin cancer. The cells multiply uncontrollably. They may bleed, and eventually become painful. Malignant tumors in the outer ear canal cause intense earache and bloody drainage.

The dangers of a malignant tumor are the same as those of any malignant growth. If you notice any of the symptoms described, see your physician.

What is the treatment?

Benign tumors can be removed in a minor surgical procedure. Malignant tumors located on the visible ear require either surgery or *radiation therapy*. During surgery, the tumor and all or part of the visible ear are removed. The operation is sometimes followed by further radiation therapy. Tumors in the canal may require an operation known as a mastoidectomy or temporal bone resection (see p.336). This operation is followed by radiation therapy.

The middle ear

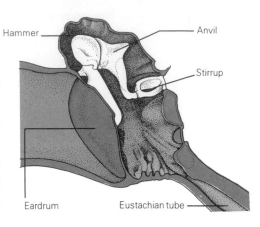

The most common disorders of the middle ear are infections and damage to the eardrum. Infections are commonly caused by bacteria or viruses, which enter the middle ear either through a perforated eardrum or along the eustachian, or auditory, tube from the back of the nasal cavity. The delicate bones that conduct sound to the inner ear are vulnerable to damage, so some conductive hearing loss (see p.329) is a common symptom in many middle ear disorders.

Otosclerosis

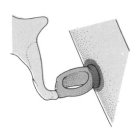

In otosclerosis, an abnormal growth prevents the stirrup from moving. This causes conductive hearing loss.

An abnormal growth of spongy bone can occur at the entrance to the inner ear and immobilize the base of the stirrup, a tiny bone through which sound waves pass into the inner ear. As a result, the stirrup cannot transmit some or all of the sound waves that enter the ear. This causes conductive hearing loss (see p.329) in that ear. In about 80 per cent of all cases of otosclerosis, both of the ears are affected, either the two at the same time or one after the other.

What are the symptoms?
Without treatment, otosclerosis usually leads to a slow loss of hearing, eventually ending with total deafness in both ears within 10 to 15 years. In a few cases, usually in children, the hearing loss progresses much faster. In some other cases the hearing loss stops well short of deafness. For example, someone with the disorder may be able to hear loud speech and other loud sounds.

At first, the affected person's voice sounds normal, unlike the abnormally loud voices of people with other types of hearing loss. As the disease progresses, some sensorineural hearing loss (see p.329) may occur. If this happens, it may cause noises in the ear and louder speech.

A woman with otosclerosis who becomes pregnant may find that the rate of hearing loss accelerates. Usually the change is not significant enough to cause added concern.

What are the risks?
The risks are the dangers associated with deafness and the emotional effects of the social isolation that this sometimes produces.

What should be done?
If your hearing deteriorates or you hear ringing in your ears, see your physician, who will examine your ears and probably give you some simple hearing tests. If otosclerosis is suspected, and particularly if you have a blood relative who has the disease, you will probably have to take several special hearing tests (see p.335).

What is the treatment?
The only treatment that will halt or cure otosclerosis is an operation called a *stapedectomy*. A stapedectomy improves hearing significantly in 90 per cent of cases. However, about two to five per cent of these operations result in total deafness in the affected ear. You and your physician should consider this risk as you decide whether you should undergo the procedure. If you have rapidly progressive otosclerosis in both ears, you will probably be advised to have the procedure done immediately to prevent quick onset of total deafness. Usually only one ear is operated on at a time, so that if the operation fails, there is a possibility of a successful operation on the other ear. If the procedure was successful, the second ear may be operated on a year after the first one.

In a stapedectomy, a surgeon folds the eardrum out of the way, removes the diseased stirrup, and replaces it with a tiny metal substitute. The patient usually feels dizzy for a short time after the operation, but can leave the hospital after one or two days. The eardrum heals naturally in one to two weeks. In another two to three weeks, the patient can usually return to normal activities.

In some cases, there is no immediate improvement in hearing after a stapedectomy because a blood clot is left in the middle ear and blocks sound conduction. The clot usually disappears in time and hearing improves.

Barotrauma

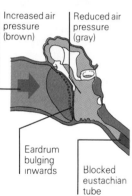

Increased air pressure (brown)

Reduced air pressure (gray)

Eardrum bulging inwards

Blocked eustachian tube

Normally, because of air passing along the eustachian, or auditory, tube, the air pressure in the middle ear is the same as the pressure in the outer ear. If a severe imbalance occurs, the eardrum can be damaged by the resulting pressure. This is called barotrauma.

Barotrauma often occurs when someone who has a nose or throat infection travels in an airplane. Before takeoff, the airplane is depressurized, which lowers the air pressure in the cabin. Air pressure in the ear also falls.

Before the airplane lands, the cabin is repressurized. The resulting raised air pressure in the outer ear canal would normally be balanced by air moving back along the eustachian tube to the middle ear, but if the tube is badly blocked because of an infection air cannot get through. This creates greater pressure on the outer surface of the eardrum than there is on its inner surface, and the eardrum is pushed inwards.

This is barotrauma, and its symptoms are moderate to severe pain in the ear, a plugged feeling, and some degree of hearing loss. You may also hear noises and feel a little dizzy. All of these symptoms usually clear up in three to five hours.

If you have a nose or throat infection and you must travel by air, use a decongestant spray or tablets. Suck candy or chew gum to encourage frequent swallowing. These measures will usually keep the eustachian tube open. You can also breathe in, hold your nose, and then try to force air up your eustachian tube by gently blowing out while keeping your mouth closed.

If you think you have barotrauma, see a physician. To equalize the air pressure within the ear, the physician may perforate your eardrum and remove any fluid from the middle ear. The eardrum will heal itself naturally in one to two weeks.

Ruptured eardrum

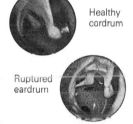

Healthy eardrum

Ruptured eardrum

A healthy eardrum is not quite transparent. But, when it ruptures, you may see the middle ear bones.

There are four common causes for ruptured eardrums: a sharp object put into the ear to relieve itching; an explosion; a severe middle ear infection; and a blow to the ear. A less frequent cause is a fractured skull.

What are the symptoms?
Some possible symptoms of a ruptured eardrum are pain in the ear (usually slight), partial loss of hearing, and slight discharge or bleeding from the ear. The symptoms usually last only a few hours.

What are the risks?
There is a risk that infection may enter the middle ear through the rupture. If you suspect that you have a ruptured eardrum, see your physician as soon as possible.

What is the treatment?
Self-help: To relieve pain, cover the affected area with an electric heating pad on a low setting and take aspirin.
Professional help: Your physician may prescribe an *antibiotic* and keep checking the ear until it heals naturally. This usually takes one to two weeks. The physician may also place a temporary plastic patch over the eardrum. If your eardrum has not healed within three months, your doctor may suggest that you have a minor operation in which a surgeon will graft a tiny piece of tissue, possibly from a vein, on to the eardrum. This simple procedure usually solves the problem. Once a ruptured eardrum has healed, it usually leaves no problems, and hearing loss is minimal.

Acute infection of he middle ear

(acute otitis media)

Acute otitis media is an infection, usually caused by a virus, but sometimes caused by bacteria, which inflames the cells lining the middle ear cavity. The disorder often develops when viruses from an infection of the nose and throat, such as a cold or measles, travel along the eustachian, or auditory, tube to the middle ear. Infection may also enter through a ruptured eardrum (see previous article). The disorder is often associated with nasal allergy (see Allergic rhinitis, p.344).

Middle ear infections occur often in children. At least half of them have an infected middle ear at some time, and often, repeated attacks of the problem occur.

What are the symptoms?
There is usually a feeling of fullness in the ear, followed by severe stabbing pain. This pain may prevent sleep and many other normal activities if it is severe and persistent enough. Other symptoms are fever, and hearing loss in the affected ear. If the infection is caused by bacteria and is not treated, the pressure of pus within the middle ear may eventually burst the eardrum. This produces a pus discharge that is accompanied by sudden relief from the pain. If the infection is caused by a virus, the symptoms are similar, but the problem will usually clear up by itself without bursting the eardrum.

What are the risks?

If the infection is viral, the risks are minimal. If the infection is bacterial, and if treatment is delayed too long, there is a danger that the problem may become chronic (see next article), or that the infection may spread to a portion of the bone behind the ear called the mastoid process. If it does spread to the mastoid process, an operation that is known as a mastoidectomy (see p.336) may become necessary. In this relatively simple operation, an incision is made behind the ear and the infected bone is removed.

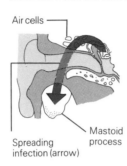

Air cells

The spread of infection Infections of the middle ear can spread to the mastoid process. If antibiotic treatment is unsuccessful, the only other treatment is surgery.

Spreading infection (arrow)

Mastoid process

What should be done?

You should see your physician for treatment as soon as possible.

What is the treatment?

Self-help: To provide some relief from pain, take aspirin and place an electric heating pad on the low temperature setting against the ear. Do not sleep with the heating pad under you. Carefully clean any pus off the pad after use to avoid reinfection.

Professional help: Your physician may prescribe drugs to help unblock the eustachian tube and clear up the infection.

If your eardrum is bulging, the physician may make a small cut, or *myringotomy*, in it to relieve the pressure and the pain. If the patient is a child, this may be done in a hospital, with a general anesthetic. The eardrum heals naturally in one to two weeks. Be sure to consult your physician before you stop any treatment. It may take as long as six weeks for the infection to clear up completely.

If a child has repeated middle ear infections, the adenoids (see p.677) may be acting as a reservoir of infection. In such cases, the doctor may suggest that the adenoids be removed. Persistent sinusitis (see p.347) also often leads to middle ear infection.

Your doctor will be able to determine if the middle ear infection has spread to the mastoid process, perhaps requiring a mastoidectomy operation.

Chronic infection of the middle ear

(chronic otitis media)

A chronic infection of the middle ear is far more serious than an acute infection. An acute infection flares up suddenly and often painfully, but usually causes little damage. A chronic infection is slow, relentless, and can cause permanent damage. Chronic infection of the middle ear is often the result of an untreated ear infection in childhood. The infection either never completely clears up, so that some of the organisms that caused it remain in the ear, or it eventually clears up but leaves a site that is particularly susceptible to subsequent infection. Pus produced continually from the chronic infection eventually causes a hole to form in the eardrum, and often damages or destroys the small bones of the middle ear.

Cholesteatoma (see next article) is another form of the disorder. It is potentially more dangerous, because it can lead to paralysis of the face or even to fatal brain infection in the worst cases.

What are the symptoms?

Grayish or yellowish pus will seep from the ear periodically. You may have some amount of hearing loss, depending on how long the infection has been present.

What are the risks?

If the infection reaches an advanced stage, it may spread to a portion of the bone behind the ear called the mastoid process. If this occurs, you may need to have an operation called a mastoidectomy (see p.336). In the rare cases of unsuccessful treatment, the bones of the ear may become damaged. This can cause permanent deafness.

What should be done?

See your physician, who will probably examine your ears with an *otoscope* and arrange for *X-rays* of your head to find out if the infection has spread to the mastoid area. Only then can the doctor determine if you need a mastoidectomy.

What is the treatment?

Self-help: Keep the ear dry and clean. Wipe away any discharge with a cotton swab.

Professional help: The physician will probably clean the ear and may prescribe an *antibiotic* in tablet form and ear drops containing an antibiotic. This treatment is aimed at eliminating the infection, drying up the ear, and preventing any discharge for a period of three months.

Hearing loss and hearing aids

Are you becoming hard of hearing?

Hearing loss is not in itself a disease. It is a symptom of some underlying disorder. Some hearing loss is common as you get older (see Aging and the senses, p.721), but if you are under 50 and becoming hard of hearing, you should see your physician without delay. The doctor will probably examine your ears and may give you some simple hearing tests in the office. If the tests indicate that your hearing is seriously impaired, you may need to take specialized hearing tests.

Audiometry

Audiometry takes place in a soundproof room. The first part of the test measures how well you hear sounds conducted through the air. You listen through earphones, with one ear at a time, to sound frequencies that range from deep, low tones to thin, high ones. For each frequency, the sound starts at an inaudible level, then increases in loudness until you can just hear it. That level is known as your threshold for that frequency.

The second part of the test measures how well you can hear sounds conducted through the bones of your head. The procedure is the same as in the first part of the test, but this time you wear special earphones that vibrate against your head. Your thresholds in both tests are recorded on a graph called an audiogram. In general, the first part of the test detects conductive hearing loss, while the second part detects sensorineural hearing loss (see p.329).

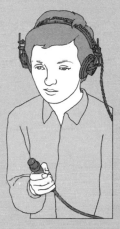

Impedance testing

In a healthy ear, the air pressure is the same inside and outside the eardrum. This allows the eardrum to vibrate freely when sound waves hit it. The vibrations pass through the ear, so that we hear, and also reflect back into the air. Too much or too little pressure on the inner side of the eardrum makes the eardrum too stiff to conduct, and reflect, sounds properly. This is one of the things that happens when you have a middle ear disorder and the auditory tube becomes blocked.

Impedance testing measures the ability of your eardrum to reflect sound waves. This will indicate how well your eardrum passes the sound waves into the ear. The tester puts a probe covered with a soundproof material such as cork into your outer ear canal, and seals up the entrance to the ear. A transmitter in the probe aims sounds at the eardrum. A receiver in the probe measures the reflections while air pumped through the probe changes the pressure in the canal rapidly from high to low. By looking at the measurements of the efficiency of sound reflection at various pressures, the doctor can deduce what is wrong with your ear and what stage the problem has reached.

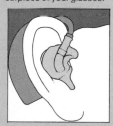

Hearing aids

Most modern hearing aids increase the volume of sound electrically, through an apparatus that usually fits unobtrusively behind the ear. The apparatus contains a tiny microphone that collects sounds and transforms them into electrical signals, an amplifier that increases the strength of the signals, and an earphone that turns the signals into louder sounds. A battery provides electrical power. The battery lasts a few months.

It is important to choose both the right kind of aid, and one that fits you properly. If you need a hearing aid, your physician will probably refer you to an audiologist for a hearing aid evaluation. In this test, you will try different kinds of aids. You should tell your physician or ear specialist immediately if you notice any change in your hearing between your regular check-ups, even after you get a hearing aid.

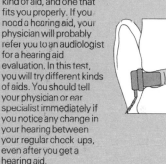

Behind-the-ear aid

The microphone, amplifier, and tiny battery are contained in a small, light, plastic case worn behind the ear. The earphone fits into your outer ear canal and seals it up so that no amplified sound is lost. The earphone is connected to the rest of the apparatus by a short plastic tube. This aid can be attached inside the earpiece of your glasses.

Bone-conduction aid

In cases of marked conductive hearing loss (see p.329), for example, when the middle ear bones are damaged (see Otosclerosis, p.332), sound is transmitted from the apparatus not through an earphone but through a vibrating pad that touches the bony mastoid process behind the ear. The vibrations pass through the bone to the inner ear.

Body-worn aid

In some more powerful hearing aids, the amplifier and battery are housed in a larger plastic case worn on the body. They are connected to the earphone by a thin plastic wire.

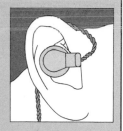

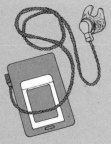

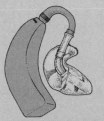

Your physician may then recommend an operation to remove the remaining infection and restore any lost hearing. In this operation, the surgeon removes any reservoir of infected tissue in the middle ear and mastoid area, and either mends the tiny bones in the middle ear or replaces them with metal substitutes if they are badly damaged. Then the eroded eardrum, which probably cannot heal naturally because of the scar tissue built up by incessant damage, is repaired by a tiny tissue graft. In 70 per cent of cases, damaged areas of the middle ear can be rebuilt and at least some hearing can be restored.

Cholesteatoma

In cholesteatoma the eustachian tube, which leads from the middle ear cavity to the nose and throat, either failed to open properly in infancy or has become blocked due to repeated middle ear infections. As a result, the air in the middle ear cavity becomes isolated. The air is gradually absorbed by the cells that line the cavity, and the air pressure in the cavity drops. The higher air pressure in the outer ear pushes the weakest part of the eardrum inwards. This forms a pocket in the eardrum. In that pocket, skin cells routinely shed by the eardrum collect into a ball called a cholesteatoma. The ball becomes infected, and produces pus. This erodes the bone that lines the cavity, and damages the delicate bones in the middle ear.

What are the symptoms?
Mild to moderately severe hearing loss is a common symptom. Sometimes pus will seep from the ear. Headache, earache, weakness of facial muscles and dizziness are also symptoms of cholesteatoma.

What are the risks?
If the cholesteatoma is not treated effectively, it can eat away the roof of the middle ear cavity. This sometimes causes epidural abcess (see p.275) or meningitis (see p.273). An abcess can also form behind the ear.

What should be done?
If you have any of the symptoms described, especially if you had a history of ear trouble as a child, see your physician. If your doctor suspects that you have a cholesteatoma, you will probably be referred to an ear, nose and throat specialist for an examination and perhaps a hearing test (see previous page).

If the cholesteatoma is small, or in an early stage, it may be possible to remove it and clean out the middle ear cavity thoroughly in a minor operation.

If the cholesteatoma is large or in a later stage, damage to the middle ear may be extensive. Then, removing the cholesteatoma becomes more complicated, involving an operation to rebuild the hearing structures and mend the broken eardrum.

In about 20 per cent of cases of cholesteatoma, the infection recurs. These infections are only dangerous if they are not treated right away. Your physician will probably check your ears at least once a year to make sure they are free of infection.

If your hearing is damaged badly, a hearing aid may help (see previous page).

OPERATION: **Mastoid removal**
Mastoidectomy

This is a short operation to remove infected tissue from the mastoid process, a honeycombed area of bone behind the ear. It is usually done when an infection of the middle ear has spread to the mastoid process and cannot be cured by antibiotic drugs.

During the operation The hair behind your ear is shaved off before you are taken to the operating room. You are given a general anesthetic. The ear surgeon makes an incision behind the flap of the ear, and delicately pares away the infected bone. The incision is then closed with stitches or clips. The operation usually takes one to two hours.

After the operation For a few days a drain draws excess fluid from the site of the operation. You will probably stay in the hospital for three to seven days.

Convalescence You should not work for two or three weeks, and must avoid water in your ear for two months or more. Your hair gradually grows over the scar.

Mastoid process

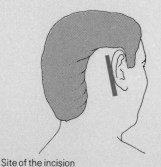

Site of the incision

The inner ear

Disorders of the inner ear affect two extremely sensitive structures: the cochlea, which transforms sound vibrations into electrical signals for transmission to the brain along the auditory nerve; and the labyrinth, which controls balance. If either of these structures is damaged, repair is impossible, because they are far too delicate for surgery. One result is often sensorineural hearing loss, which is caused by damage to either the cochlea or the auditory nerve. This type of hearing loss is usually permanent, because it can seldom be treated or cured.

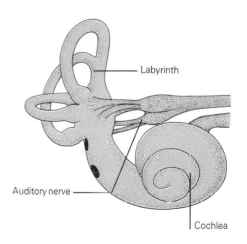

Labyrinth

Auditory nerve

Cochlea

Meniere's disease

In Meniere's disease there is an increase in the amount of fluid in the labyrinth, the part of the ear that controls balance. This increases pressure in the inner ear, which distorts, and sometimes ruptures, the membrane of the labyrinth wall. This disturbs your sense of balance. For a detailed description of how the labyrinth maintains your balance, read How the ear works (see p.329). The cochlea, which is adjacent to the labyrinth, may also be damaged by the pressure. If it is, the damage may impair your hearing.

The disease attacks one ear, then, about half of the time, it also affects the other ear. The cause of Meniere's disease is unknown, and the disorder is rare.

What are the symptoms?
Symptoms may be absent or mild most of the time, but they flare up periodically as attacks. These attacks vary in frequency from every few weeks to every few years. An attack may last from a few hours to several days. The main symptom of an attack is vertigo, or dizziness. This is often accompanied by noises in the ear and by muffled or distorted hearing, especially of low tones. Sometimes you feel pressure in the affected ear before or during an attack. In persistent cases the attacks usually become less severe, but some hearing loss and noises in the ear may persist between the attacks. Finally, it is possible for the severe attacks to return, and if they do they may become increasingly serious.

What are the risks?
In most people, the disorder is mild and clears up spontaneously. However, in a few particularly bad cases complete deafness occurs either in one or in both ears. These severe cases may be accompanied by anxiety (see p.300) and migraine headaches (see p.285).

What should be done?
If you have the symptoms described, see your physician, or an ear, nose and throat specialist, without delay. The physician will probably evaluate the problem by giving you several special tests.

The first test may be audiometry (see Hearing loss and hearing aids, p.335). If the result is unclear, the test may be repeated after you have dehydrated yourself by not drinking any liquids or by taking a *diuretic* drug, which increases your urination. Either method is thought to reduce pressure in the labyrinth by reducing the amount of fluid in it. If the second test shows that your hearing has improved by a specific amount, you may have Meniere's disease.

If the results are still not clear from the second test, or if your physician needs more information, you may need to have a different test. In this one, the ear is flooded with water at different temperatures. After each flooding, you experience a whirling sensation that makes your eyes flicker. How your eyes flicker is an indication of whether or not the labyrinth is diseased.

In rare cases, an additional test, called *electrocochleography*, may be necessary. This test requires a general anesthetic. The doctor inserts a needle-like probe through the eardrum of the affected ear. The probe registers information about the electrical activity in the cochlea. Certain kinds of distortions in this activity indicate to your physician that you have Meniere's disease.

What is the treatment?

Self-help: Lie still when you are having an attack. This should considerably ease the symptoms. Cut down generally on your intake of fluids and salt. This should reduce the frequency and severity of attacks.

Professional help: In most cases, the physician will prescribe medication to control nausea and vomiting. Drugs to reduce excess body fluid may also be prescribed.

If, despite treatment, there is enough fluid in the labyrinth to damage it, or if you are incapacitated by the symptoms of the disorder, you may need surgery. In one possible operation, a surgeon drills a hole through the bone of your middle ear into the labyrinth to release the excess fluid. In about 70 per cent of cases such an operation cures the vertigo and prevents further loss of hearing in the affected ear. In some cases the operation improves hearing.

If the disease is severe enough to cause vertigo that becomes so severe that it is disabling, the labyrinth may have to be deliberately destroyed by surgery. Before recommending that you have such a drastic operation, your physician will take into account the condition of your other ear and your age.

Labyrinthitis

In labyrinthitis, the labyrinth, a group of fluid-filled chambers that controls balance, becomes infected. The infection is usually caused by a virus. It inflames the labyrinth and totally disrupts its function.

What are the symptoms?

The main symptom is extreme vertigo, or dizziness. You feel off balance, and everything seems to be spinning in a circle. Your eyes move slowly sideways, then flick back to their original position. If you move your head, even only slightly, the vertigo gets worse. In some cases, there is extreme nausea and vomiting.

What are the risks?

Although labyrinthitis can be very debilitating, it is not a dangerous condition when cared for properly. The symptoms are often so distressing that few people who have it do not seek help.

What should be done?

If you have severe vertigo, see your physician at the first opportunity. If you cannot travel, ask your physician to come to you. The doctor will try to determine whether the vertigo has some cause other than labyrinthitis. One possibility is an infection that has spread from the middle ear.

What is the treatment?

You will probably have to rest quietly in bed for several days. Your physician will probably prescribe a tranquilizer and a drug that is used to combat nausea. The symptoms of labyrinthitis can be frightening, but they will probably disappear. Most cases clear up completely, within one to three weeks.

Occupational hearing loss

Prolonged exposure to noise at or above 90 decibels (see Sound and noise levels, next page), especially if the noise is high-pitched, can damage the sensitive hair cells lining the cochlea, the innermost part of the ear. This may cause partial to severe hearing loss. Some occupations that are particularly hazardous to unprotected ears are heavy construction, driving a tractor, and working around very noisy equipment. Exposure to loud rock music over long periods of time also endangers your hearing.

What should be done?

Sensorineural hearing loss (see p.329) that is caused by damage to the cochlea is irreversible. Therefore, prevention is crucial. If you are exposed to dangerous levels of noise, you should wear suitable ear protectors. Ear muffs that are designed for the purpose are the most effective. They resemble earphones and almost totally insulate the ears from noise. If the wearer needs to communicate with colleagues, as on the flight deck of an airplane, a small microphone and earphones can be added to the muffs. The second most effective protectors are ear plugs made of foam, plastic, wax or rubber.

If you work in very noisy conditions, have your physician test your hearing at regular intervals. If you detect loss of hearing early, you can take steps to prevent further damage to your ears. If you think that the noise level where you work is too high, you can contact the person responsible for safety in your plant or your union representative. You can also contact the local office of the Occupational Safety and Health Administration (OSHA) or the local health department, and file a complaint. See also next page.

Sound and noise levels

What are sound and noise?
Sound is a series of air pressure waves, or alternate peaks of high pressure and troughs of low pressure, travelling through the atmosphere. Noise is a term people use to describe a mixture of loud sounds, usually of different pitch, or frequency, that they find unpleasant.

Loud sound and noise
The loudness of sound or noise is measured in units called decibels by a decibel meter. Sounds quieter than 10 decibels are very difficult for the human ear to hear, and sounds that are 120 decibels are usually painful. A sound loud enough to cause pain can damage your ears, probably permanently. You should quickly eliminate the sound or get away from it to prevent damage to your ears. Exposure to noise that is loud enough to cause prolonged ringing in your ears may cause lasting damage to the sensitive hearing structures. There are recommended time limits on levels of sound exposure (see diagram).

If you are habitually exposed to noise levels above about 90 decibels, you may be in danger of occupational hearing loss (see previous article).

MAXIMUM NOISE EXPOSURE ALLOWED ON JOB BY LAW, IN HOURS PER DAY	
Decibels	Hours
90	8
92	6
95	4
97	3
100	2
102	1½
105	1
110	¼
115	¼ or less

Note: Measurements on the decibel scale do not equate with our own perception of loudness. To us, a rock concert that registers 100 decibels on a decibel meter sounds much more than twice as loud as a rushing stream that registers 50 decibels. Sound pressure doubles with each increase of six decibels.

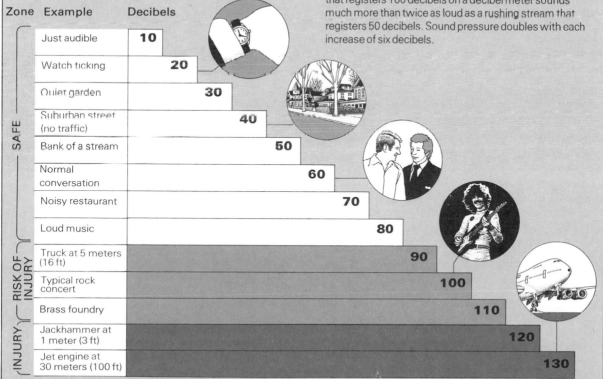

Zone	Example	Decibels
SAFE	Just audible	10
	Watch ticking	20
	Quiet garden	30
	Suburban street (no traffic)	40
	Bank of a stream	50
	Normal conversation	60
	Noisy restaurant	70
	Loud music	80
RISK OF INJURY	Truck at 5 meters (16 ft)	90
	Typical rock concert	100
	Brass foundry	110
INJURY	Jackhammer at 1 meter (3 ft)	120
	Jet engine at 30 meters (100 ft)	130

Disorders of the respiratory system

Introduction

You breathe to supply your body with oxygen and to get rid of carbon dioxide, a waste product of energy production. The lungs are the center of the respiratory system. In your lungs, the oxygen in the air you breathe is exchanged for carbon dioxide from the blood. The channel that the air follows in and out of your lungs is called the respiratory tract. It includes the nose, throat, and trachea, or windpipe. Deep in the chest the trachea divides into two main tubes, which are called bronchi. Each one goes into one lung, where it divides into increasingly smaller air passages called bronchioles. At the tip of each bronchiole there is a balloon-like cavity called an alveolus. There are about 300 million of these alveoli in each lung. The vital exchange of oxygen for carbon dioxide occurs through minute blood vessels in the thin walls of the alveoli.

You use several muscles to suck air into your lungs. The main one is the diaphragm. A dome-shaped muscular sheet attached to the lower ribs, the diaphragm divides the chest cavity from the abdomen. When the diaphragm contracts, along with other muscles between the ribs, a vacuum is created around your lungs. This causes them to expand, sucking air into the respiratory tract. When the muscles relax, the lungs contract, forcing the air back out. If this mechanism works well, you hardly notice that you are breathing. However, a number of things can go wrong, with the lungs themselves, with essential parts of the respiratory tract, or with the muscular action.

The articles in this section are arranged in three groups. Each group concentrates on disorders that affect one area of the respiratory system. The first group deals with problems that affect the nasal cavity and the sinuses, or air spaces behind the nose. The second group of articles deals with disorders of the throat. These include problems of both the larynx, or voice box, which is located at the top of the trachea, and the pharynx, the funnel that leads from the nasal cavity and the back of the mouth down to where the esophagus, which carries food and water to the stomach, separates from the trachea. The third group of articles deals with common diseases of the trachea, lungs and breathing mechanism.

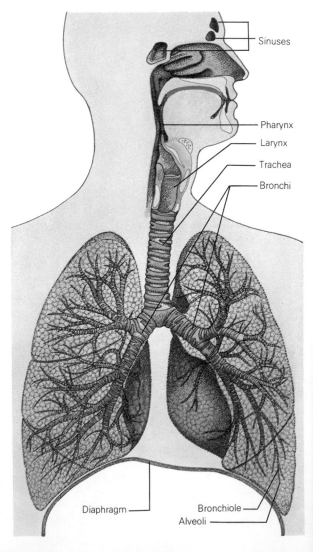

Sinuses
Pharynx
Larynx
Trachea
Bronchi
Diaphragm
Bronchiole
Alveoli

Details of the respiratory system

How you breathe

Air you breathe in through your nose is warmed and moistened by small blood vessels very close to the surface of the nasal cavity before it passes into the lungs. In addition, tiny hairs that line the nose provide a filtering system to keep foreign bodies such as dust particles from getting into your lungs.

When you breathe in, your diaphragm, which is dome shaped when relaxed, is pulled flat. At the same time, muscles between your ribs contract and pull your ribcage upwards and outwards. These movements increase the volume of your chest, which makes your lungs expand and suck air into them. The stronger the muscle action, the more air enters your lungs. Your rate of breathing in

and out is determined mainly by the amount of carbon dioxide that must be expelled from your bloodstream.

When you breathe out, your chest muscles and diaphragm relax. This makes your ribcage sink and your lungs, which are very elastic, contract and squeeze out air. The air that you breathe out still contains some oxygen. Otherwise, cardiopulmonary resuscitation (CPR) would not be effective in restoring breathing in an emergency.

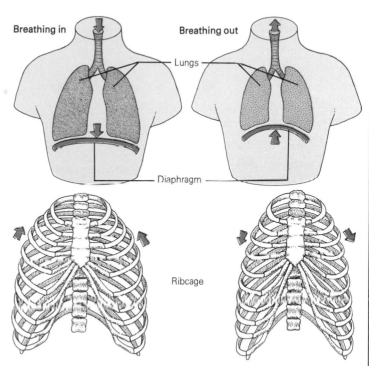

Breathing in   Breathing out

Lungs

Diaphragm

Ribcage

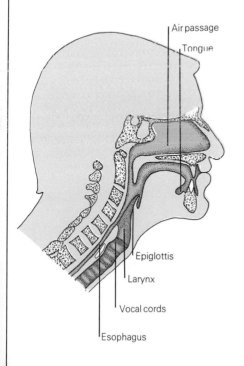

Air passage

Tongue

Epiglottis

Larynx

Vocal cords

Esophagus

The pleurae

Each lung is surrounded by a thin membranous covering called the pleura. This is folded back on itself to form a double layer all around each lung. There is a tiny space between the layers that

contains a small amount of fluid and forms a vacuum. The inner layer is attached to the lung and the outer layer is attached to the ribcage. The main function of the pleura is to lubricate the

lungs so that they can expand and contract smoothly and uniformly. When you breathe in and your ribcage lifts up and out, your lungs are pulled up and out at the same time.

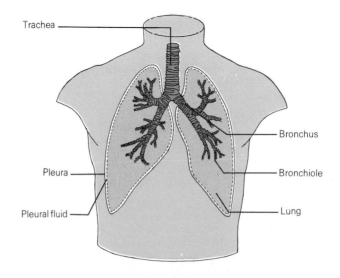

Trachea

Bronchus

Bronchiole

Pleura

Pleural fluid

Lung

The nose

The nose is the main entrance to your respiratory system. It is lined with a mucous membrane that contains many tiny blood vessels close to the surface. The front of the nose also has protective hairs. The nasal lining filters, moistens, and warms the air you breathe as it goes through the nasal passage toward your throat and lungs. The nasal passage runs along the top of the palate, or the shelf separating the nose from the mouth, and turns downward to join the passage from the mouth to the throat.

The nasal passage is not a simple tube. A series of baffles called turbinates make the passage winding rather than straight. Also, in several places, it branches into sinuses, which are pairs of air-filled cavities in the bones of the skull. Nasal infections, which are discussed in the following articles, sometimes spread into the sinuses as well as into the rest of the respiratory system.

The nose is also the organ of smell, and you may not be able to smell anything if a disorder "stuffs up" your nose. Permanent loss of smell is rare.

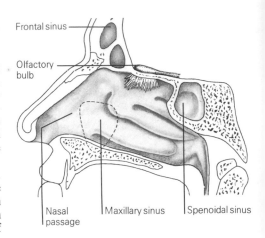

The nasal passage and sinuses
The nasal passage is linked to three pairs of sinuses or air-filled cavities in the skull. The sensitive hair-like endings of the olfactory nerves project into the nasal passage. They detect odors in the air and pass the information to the olfactory bulb in the brain.

Colds

The disease we call the common cold is really a group of minor illnesses that can be caused by any one of almost 200 different viruses. Usually a common, or head, cold is confined to the nose and throat, but the same viruses can also infect the larynx (see Laryngitis, p.351) and the lungs (see Acute bronchitis, p.353). These viral infections sometimes are followed by more serious bacterial infections of the throat, lungs, or ears.

All of us get colds. Most people have their first cold during their first year of life. Most children are extremely susceptible to nasal viral infection between the ages of one and three. Then they gradually become immune to many of the viruses that are common in their environment. The frequency of colds increases again during early school years, because the school environment contains new types of viruses. Most people acquire more immunity as they grow older, and catch fewer and less severe colds. (For more information about colds in babies, see recurrent colds in children, p.680.)

What are the symptoms?
To some extent the symptoms depend on

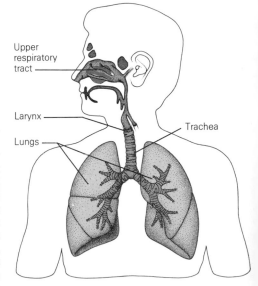

Where the common cold strikes
A cold can affect almost any part of the respiratory system. Sneezing and a runny nose mean that the upper-respiratory tract is affected. The infection may also irritate the trachea, and cause a cough, or the larynx, which makes your voice hoarse. Occasionally the lungs become infected, which can cause bronchitis.

what virus is responsible for the cold. Major symptoms include runny nose, sneezing, watering eyes, sore throat, hoarseness, and coughing. At first, the nasal discharge is usually rather watery. Then it becomes thick and greenish-yellow. You may also have a headache and a slight fever. This rise in temperature may cause shivering and chills. A very

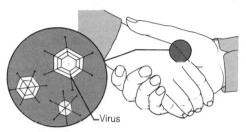

Spreading colds
Many people believe colds spread only through the air, but hand-to-hand contact is another possibility. If you have a cold, you may hold your hand in front of your mouth when you cough or sneeze and may then pass on the virus by hand.

—Virus

high temperature and general body pains, however, are more likely to be symptoms of influenza, or flu (see p.559).

Every person, regardless of age or sex, will get an occasional cold. Nobody is quite sure how colds are spread. One way seems to be through direct contact with other people who have colds. Also, coughs and sneezes spray the viruses into the air. Colds occur far less frequently in isolated communities, where everyone soon becomes immune to the viruses that are in circulation. An outbreak of colds is apt to follow the arrival of strangers.

What are the risks?
An ordinary cold often clears up in three to four days. Even with a bacterial infection, a head cold should not last longer than a week. But because the respiratory tract is a series of spaces connected by passages, an infection can spread from your nose and throat to your middle ear, sinuses, larynx, trachea, or lungs, and these secondary infections can lead to serious disorders of the respiratory tract.

What should be done?
Anyone with a cold should stay home in isolation if possible. This measure is mainly for the sake of other people, but it also gives you the chance to rest and recuperate. Consult your physician if the cold lasts more than ten days, if there are symptoms that suggest that the infection has spread beyond the nose and throat, or if you often get bronchitis or ear infections. Some symptoms should send you to your physician immediately. They in-

clude earache, pain in the face or forehead, a temperature above 102° F (39° C), and a combination of persistent hoarseness or sore throat, shortness of breath and wheeziness, and a dry, painful cough.

What is the treatment?
Self-help: There is no way to treat a common cold. There is only some advice that is worth following. Stay at home, in a warm (but not overheated) room, and increase the moisture in the air with some type of vaporizer or humidifier. Drink plenty of fluids, and take an aspirin or two at night to relieve any aches and pains and help you sleep. Over-the-counter cold tablets, cough syrups, and nasal sprays may also give you temporary relief, but you should use them only in moderation, and not expect them to cure your cold.
Professional help: There is little point in asking a physician to treat a normally healthy person who has a cold. Your doctor generally will not prescribe *antibiotics*, since viruses do not respond to them. An antibiotic might actually make matters worse by producing side-effects such as diarrhea.

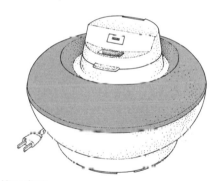

Vaporizers
Vaporizers moisturize the air in a room to help you recover from a cold or other respiratory infection. This commonly used type heats water to steam to add it to the dry air.

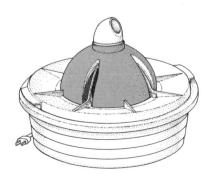

The cool vaporizer (above), a newer type, breaks water into tiny droplets and sprays them into the air of the room without using heat.

Self-help for a stuffy or runny nose

Many of the illnesses dealt with on these pages cause a nasal discharge. Although some of the illnesses – the common cold, for example – cannot be cured, the nasal discomfort they cause can be eased considerably by using the simple self-help advice on this page. In addition, always remember that the lining of the nasal passageways is fragile and has many tiny blood vessels just under its surface; be careful not to blow your nose too hard and cause a nosebleed.

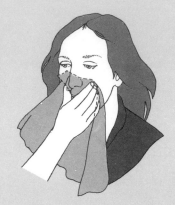

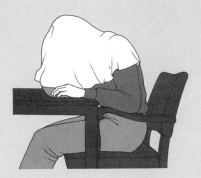

Blowing your nose
Blow into a disposable paper tissue or a clean handkerchief. Clear your nostrils one at a time, keeping the other one closed by pressing on that side of the nose. One common error is to press both nostrils almost closed as you blow. This not only prevents you from clearing your nose thoroughly, but also may encourage infection to spread to your ears. Also, if you blow too hard and the air cannot escape through the nose, it may travel along the eustachian tube to the middle ear, and it could possibly rupture or otherwise damage the eardrum.

Steam inhalation
There are several over-the-counter preparations available that are inhaled. They usually contain menthol or a similar substance. When dissolved in hot water and breathed into the nose they loosen mucus, which can then be cleared by blowing your nose thoroughly.

Nasal decongestants
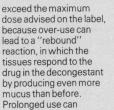
These over-the-counter preparations are intended to shrink and dry out the swollen, mucus-producing tissue inside the nose and sinuses, and liquify and free remaining mucus. They are available as tablets, sprays, or drops. Never exceed the maximum dose advised on the label, because over-use can lead to a "rebound" reaction, in which the tissues respond to the drug in the decongestant by producing even more mucus than before. Prolonged use can eventually damage and scar the nasal tissues, causing still other problems.

If you have recurrent attacks of bronchitis or frequent ear infections, however, you should see a physician at the first sign of a head cold. For you, a cold presents special problems. In your case, an antibiotic may be useful, since it will give you some protection against the bacteria-caused complications to which you are prone. Thus, in your case, the benefits of the drug will probably outweigh the possible drawbacks. Consult your physician who can explain your individual situation and recommend appropriate treatment.

Allergic rhinitis
(hay fever)

Allergic rhinitis, commonly called hay fever, is similar to asthma (see p.355) except in one respect. In asthma, an airborne substance causes an allergic, or hypersensitive, reaction in your lungs and chest. In allergic rhinitis, the reaction occurs in your eyes, nose, and throat. Exposure to an airborne irritant known as the *allergen* triggers the release of *histamine*, a body chemical. The release of this substance causes inflammation and fluid production in the fragile lining of the nasal passage, the sinuses, and the eyelids and surface layer of the eyes.

Nobody knows why some people are allergic to otherwise harmless pollen grains or other airborne particles. Presumably, there is a difference in some people's natural immune systems (see Allergies, p.705). Since allergy-based diseases such as asthma, contact dermatitis (see Eczema and dermatitis, p.253), and allergic rhinitis often run in families, the cause is probably partly genetic.

If you have allergic rhinitis, you react to specific allergens. For example, if you have hay fever, the most familiar variety of the disease, you may be sensitive to grass pollen, which is abundant in early summer, to tree pollen, which is in the air in spring, or to ragweed, which blooms in the fall.

In addition to pollen, almost any airborne substance derived from a living organism can cause allergic rhinitis, including bits of animal skin, hair, and feathers. You may also be allergic to house dust or, to be more precise, to the mites that infest the dust.

There are two types of allergic rhinitis, seasonal and perennial. Seasonal allergic rhinitis only bothers you part of the year because it is an allergy to a substance that is not in the air year round. Perennial allergic rhinitis occurs all year round because it is caused by exposure to airborne allergens that may be present at any time.

What are the symptoms?

If you have allergic rhinitis, you sneeze frequently, your nose runs, and your eyes are red, itchy, and watery. If you rub your eyes, it makes them worse. Itchy skin, dry throat, and wheezing can also occur. If you have hay fever, the symptoms are most severe when there is a lot of pollen in the air. Symptoms tend to be especially severe for 15 to 30 minute periods. These brief periods of acute symptoms are called allergy attacks.

Because airborne allergens are generally too small to see, it is difficult to predict when, or even why, you may have an attack. For example, if you are allergic to cat hair, you may start to sneeze on entering an empty room, because invisible bits of hair from a recent feline occupant are still in the air.

Allergic rhinitis is very common. Although there is a widespread belief that allergic rhinitis is a childhood disorder that you outgrow in your late teens or early twenties, this is not necessarily so. You can develop the disorder at any age, and later recover. You are particularly susceptible, however, if you are under 40 and have another allergic condition such as asthma or dermatitis, or if other members of your family have similar disorders. Many people react to more than one allergen, and some people have both seasonal and perennial bouts of allergic rhinitis.

What are the risks?

This disorder does not usually endanger your general health.

What should be done?

If you find that allergic rhinitis interferes with your daily routine, see your physician, who will probably first ask questions to find out how serious the problem is for you. The doctor may advise you against professional treatment, because the possible side-effects and the inconvenience of some kinds of treatment may cause more problems than the condition itself. If you do not know what causes your allergic rhinitis, your physician may suggest skin tests to find out which allergens make you react. The physician scratches the skin on your forearm and puts drops of liquid that contain a common allergen on the same spot. If the skin under any of the drops turns red and itchy, you are allergic to the allergen in that drop.

Substances that trigger off allergic rhinitis

Pollen
The pollen from any plant may trigger an allergy attack. Symptoms appear whenever the plant or plants to which you are allergic bloom and produce pollen.

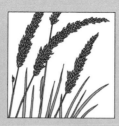

Animal hair
Those said to be allergic to animal hair, actually are not. They are affected by tiny skin flakes that the animal sheds and that often cling to the hairs.

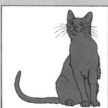

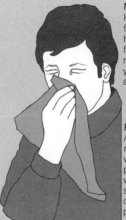

Mites in house dust
House-dust mites are found in almost every house. If anyone in your family is allergic to these mites, you should keep your house as free of dust as is possible.

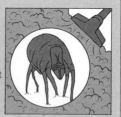

Feathers
An allergy to feathers is relatively easy to deal with. Simply avoid products that are stuffed with feathers or down, such as some jackets, coats, sleeping bags, and pillows.

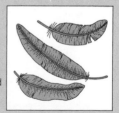

What is the treatment?

Self-help: If you get hay fever regularly, stay indoors as much as possible during the hay fever season, especially when the news media reports a high pollen count. You should avoid wearing contact lenses, because they can increase eye irritation. Resist the temptation to rub your eyes. If your allergic rhinitis is perennial rather than seasonal, try to find out what you are allergic to, and take steps to avoid it or minimize your exposure to it. Self-help recommendations for asthmatics (see p.356) also apply to those people who suffer from allergic rhinitis.

Whether your condition is seasonal or perennial, there are many drugs that ease the symptoms of allergic rhinitis. A large number of them are available without a prescription. The most commonly used drugs are *antihistamines*, which are generally effective for both preventing and stopping attacks. To be fully effective, antihistamines must be taken regularly, often for several days at a time. Some common side-effects from antihistamines are drowsiness, and dryness in the nose and throat. These may be more troublesome than the allergic rhinitis itself. Since antihistamines often make you sleepy, you should never take them if you intend to drive a motor vehicle or to operate machinery within the next few hours.

For quick relief from a stuffy nose, you can use decongestant nose drops or nasal sprays, which can ease symptoms within minutes. Do not use such medicines often or regularly, however. They eventually aggravate the very symptoms they are supposed to suppress.

Professional help: There are quite a few symptom-suppressing drugs that are available only with a prescription. If you do not get relief from any of the self-help measures suggested above, your physician may prescribe a type of antihistamine that works better for you than the non-prescription types. Another possible treatment for you is the use of a *steroid* spray.

All of these drug treatments merely suppress symptoms. They do not alter the basic allergic reaction. The only possible cure for allergic rhinitis is a series of injections designed to desensitize your system to the allergen or allergens that bother you. This is possible only if you have a skin test and successfully identify the substance or substances that bother you. In the treatment, your physician gives you a series of injections containing increasingly strong concentrations of your particular allergen in an attempt to stop your reactions.

This treatment is not always successful, and it takes a long time to complete the series of injections. Before you decide to have desensitization treatment, you should consider the possibility that it may not work for you and discuss the risks and benefits with your physician (see Allergies, p.705).

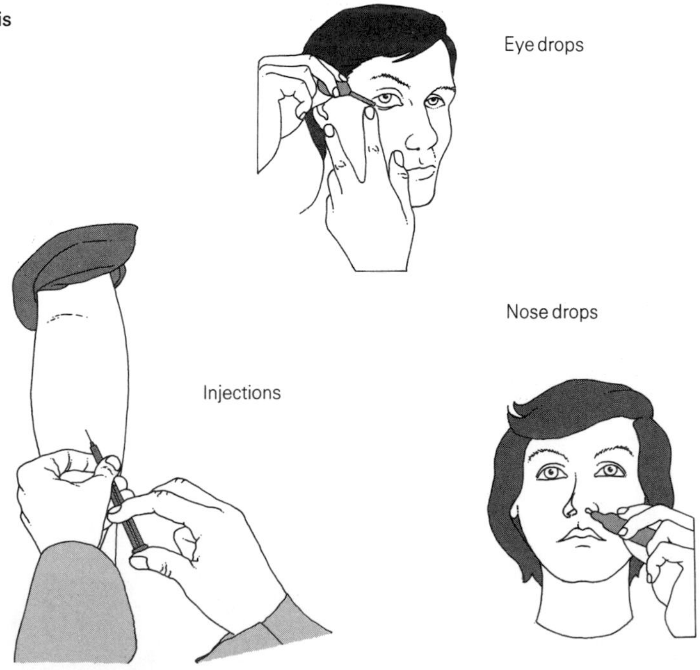

Treatment for allergic rhinitis
Sometimes an allergy may be cured by a series of desensitizing injections. Most treatments prescribed by your physician are designed to relieve the symptoms of the allergy rather than to cure the underlying cause. Irritation of the eyes and nose can be soothed by various antihistamine and decongestant drops and sprays.

Eye drops

Injections

Nose drops

Sinusitis

The sinuses are air spaces in the bones behind your nose. Sinusitis is an inflammation of the mucous membranes of the sinuses. It is caused by bacterial or viral infection. The frontal sinuses, which are in the forehead just above the eyes, and the maxillary sinuses, which are in the cheek-bones, are the ones that are most likely to be affected.

The organisms that cause sinusitis spread to the sinuses from the nose. This occurs easily because the mucous membranes of the main nasal cavity extend into and line the sinuses. Sinusitis usually occurs after a common cold, which is a viral infection (see p.342), is complicated by the occurrence of a secondary bacterial infection.

What are the symptoms?

After the first few days of a cold, when you would expect it to get better, the blockage in your nose may worsen and the greenish discharge may increase. Later, because the passages between the nose and the sinuses also become blocked, the discharge may stop. Your nose then becomes more stuffed up than ever. You have to breathe through your mouth, your speech becomes nasal, and you feel generally ill. If the frontal sinuses are affected, you may have a headache over one or both eyes. It is most painful when you wake up in the morning, or when you bend your head down and forward. The under-surface of your forehead just above the eyes may feel tender.

If the maxillary sinuses are affected, one or both cheeks may hurt. You may feel as if you have a toothache in your upper jaw. Occasionally, sinusitis may follow dental treatment, because infection can spread from the roots of your tooth into one of your sinuses (see Abscesses in teeth, p.439).

Sinusitis is common, but susceptibility varies. Some people never get it, while others get it every time they have a bad cold. Others may get sinusitis by jumping into water feet first without holding their noses. Damage to your nasal bones, or even a foreign body caught in your nostril, may make you more susceptible to infection and, thus, bring on an attack. A deformity of the nose, such as a deviated septum (see next page), may increase your susceptibility to sinusitis by obstructing the nasal airways.

What are the risks?

The risks of sinusitis are minimal if it is treated with *antibiotics*. Before the availability of antibiotics, the infection sometimes spread through the mucous membrane of the sinuses into the bones and even to the brain. Such serious complications of sinusitis almost never happen today.

What should be done?

Try the self-help measures recommended below. If the symptoms persist after three or four days, consult your physician, who may confirm the diagnosis of sinusitis by examining *X-rays* of your sinuses. The physician may also gently press the floor of the sinuses from inside your nose and mouth.

What is the treatment?

Self-help: Stay indoors, in a room with an

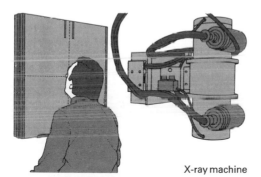

Frontal sinuses

Maxillary sinuses

Headache over one or both eyes indicates that your frontal sinuses are inflamed. Your cheeks may hurt if your maxillary sinuses are affected, but this is less common.

Examining the sinuses by X-ray
If you suffer from persistent sinusitis, your physician may arrange for you to have X-rays made of your sinuses, to examine them carefully before attempting to drain them. Several X-rays taken from different angles show the exact position of the sinuses. Healthy air-filled sinuses show up as dark patches surrounded by gray areas of bone. Any fluid in these sinuses can be seen on the X-rays as white areas filling what are normally black, air-filled spaces.

X-ray machine

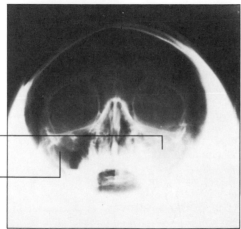

Blocked sinus

Unblocked sinus

X-ray picture

even temperature. Add moisture to the air with a vaporizer or humidifier. Blow your nose gently with tissues. To relieve the pain, inhale steam from a basin of hot water, or the spout of a kettle, *but be careful not to burn yourself; steam is very hot.*

Professional help: Your physician may prescribe a broad spectrum antibiotic and also suggest that you use decongestant tablets, nose drops, or a nasal spray. Decongestants shrink the swollen mucous membrane, which widens the airways, but for sinusitis they should be used only as prescribed by a doctor. If they are used incorrectly, decongestants can do more harm than good.

Further treatment should be unnecessary, but if the sinusitis persists, your physician may advise a minor operation under local anesthetic. In this procedure, the physician or surgeon pierces a bone between the nose and the sinuses to open an extra passageway, and washes the sinuses out with sterile water. This procedure relieves the obstruction. Material that is removed from the sinus can be analyzed to identify the cause of the infection and determine the best way to combat it. You may discover that you will need additional minor surgery to improve drainage if the infection becomes chronic, but this complication rarely happens.

Nasal polyps

If part of the mucous membrane that lines the nose becomes distended and protrudes into the nasal cavity, the growth that it forms is known as a nasal polyp. Polyps are caused by over-production of fluid in the cells of the membrane. This can be caused by a condition such as allergic rhinitis (see p.344). These polyps are harmless, but a big one or several little ones can obstruct your nasal passages, make breathing difficult, and impair your sense of smell. If the opening between the nasal cavity and one of the sinuses is blocked by a polyp, you may have headaches or pain in the muscles of your face.

What should be done?

If your nose is gradually becoming blocked, you may have nasal polyps. You may be able to see them in a mirror, by shining a light up your nostrils. They look like pearly gray lumps. However, polyps are often at the back of the nose, where you can only see them with a special instrument. If you suspect that you have nasal polyps, you should consult your

physician. The only way to treat nasal polyps is to remove them. If the diagnosis is confirmed, your doctor may refer you to a specialist for surgery. This minor operation is usually done under local anesthetic. Sometimes both the polyps and the lining of the sinuses where they originate must be removed. In these cases, more extensive surgery that is performed under a general anesthetic is required.

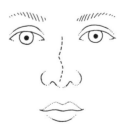

Examining the nose
To examine the inside of your nose, the physician may separate your nostrils with a special instrument, a nasal speculum, which looks like a pair of sugar tongs.

Deviated septum

If the nasal septum, or the wall between the nostrils, is very crooked, it makes the air passage on one side narrow. This obstruction can make breathing somewhat difficult, because the flow of air through the narrower passage may become blocked. Substantial deviation of the septum is not common. It usually happens because of an injury, and the nose can look straight. There are no significant symptoms other than the mild breathing problem and, rarely, an increased tendency to sinusitis (see previous page). The septum can be straightened by surgery if the deviation is troublesome. Most people who have a deviated septum simply live with it.

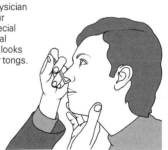
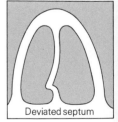

Deviated septum

Straightening a deviated septum
The operation used to straighten a deviated septum involves removing the bent or excess cartilage. It is usually done only if there are problems with breathing.

Anosmia

Anosmia is the technical term for a loss of the sense of smell and taste that persists even when there is no obvious cause such as a head cold. Most commonly, a chronic condition like allergic rhinitis (see p.344) or nasal polyps (see previous page) causes anosmia. It may be a symptom of a tumor of the brain (see p.282), but this is very rare. It may also occur because of a head injury. This is because such an injury sometimes damages the olfactory nerves. These are the nerves that carry smell sensations, as electrical impulses, from the nose to the brain.

What should be done?

If you notice that you have lost your sense of smell or taste, consult your physician. You will probably find that you have a nasal condition that your doctor can treat, and thus cure the anosmia. If there is no sign of abnormality in your nose, your physician may refer you to a neurologist for some diagnostic tests. It is unlikely that your olfactory nerves have been damaged.

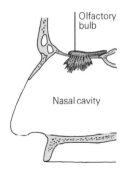

The position of the olfactory nerves
Olfactory nerves, fibers located at the top of the nose, below the olfactory bulb, convert smells into nerve impulses, which travel to the bulb and from there to other parts of the brain.

Nosebleed

When your nose begins to bleed, it is usually sudden and from only one nostril. This may occur quite often. In most cases of nosebleed, unless the nose has been injured, there is no apparent explanation for the bleeding. One relatively common cause is a cold or other infection, which causes crusting that damages the sensitive membrane that lines the nose. Nosebleeds are seldom cause for concern, since they are unlikely to be a symptom of any other disorder. A generalized bleeding disorder such as thrombocytopenia (see p.425) could cause nosebleeds, but in such cases there is usually a good deal of bleeding elsewhere in your body, such as from the gums or under the skin.

What is the treatment?

Self-help: Sit down and lean forward and breathe through your mouth. Close the lower part of your nose on the side that is bleeding by pressing it with the ball of your thumb. Keep pressing for five to ten minutes. This procedure stops most nosebleeds. Do not blow your nose for 12 hours. After that, blow gently so you will not dislodge the clot that has stopped the bleeding.

Professional help: If bleeding continues, consult your physician or, if necessary, go to an emergency room. Your physician will probably pack a strip of gauze into the bleeding nostril and tell you to leave it in for several hours. The purpose of the gauze packing is not simply to absorb the blood and stop its dripping from the nose. Rather, it is to apply pressure to the ruptured blood vessels. If the bleeding persists or keeps recurring, the bleeding area may have to be cauterized, or closed using heat. The doctor may take a specimen of your blood to make sure you have not become anemic (see p.419). This complication is unlikely, because generally, despite appearances, little blood is lost through nosebleeds.

Medical myth
Nosebleeds are often due to high blood pressure. They are nature's way of lowering it.

Wrong. A nosebleed comes from capillaries or small veins, while blood pressure is measured in a major artery. If a physician whom you consult about nosebleeds takes your blood pressure, it is partly to reassure you and partly because it is a good idea to test blood pressure.

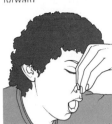

Sit with your head forward

Pinch the fleshy part of your nose

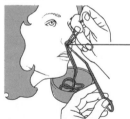

Physician packs the nostril with gauze

Stopping a nosebleed
If you have a nosebleed, sit down and lean over with your head forward. Close the lower part of your nose on the side that is bleeding by pressing it with your thumb, and breathe through your mouth. Hold it for about five minutes so that a blood clot forms and seals the damaged blood vessels. Do not blow your nose for 12 hours after the bleeding has stopped, so you will avoid dislodging the blood clot. If the bleeding has not stopped after about 20 minutes, go to your physician. The doctor will use a special instrument to pack strips of gauze into the affected nostril, and so apply constant pressure to the ruptured blood vessels.

The throat

The throat, also known as the pharynx, is part of a multi-purpose tube leading from the back of the nose and mouth down to the trachea, or windpipe, and to the esophagus, or gullet. When you breathe, air passes through your throat into the trachea on its way in and out of the lungs. When you swallow, chewed food lubricated with saliva moves down the throat into the esophagus on its way to the stomach.

When you speak, you use your larynx, or voice box, which is located in the throat at the top of the trachea. Air passing over the vocal cords, which are stretched flaps of tissue in the larynx, makes them vibrate and produce the relatively broad range of sounds that your mouth shapes into speech.

Like the rest of the respiratory system, the throat is mainly affected by infection, which often spreads upward, downward, or in both directions to involve the whole system. A sore throat is seldom a disorder in its own right. It usually indicates an infection somewhere else in the system.

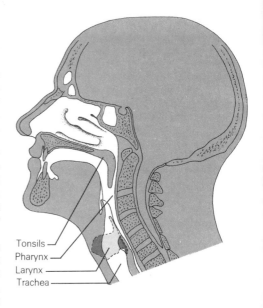

Tonsils
Pharynx
Larynx
Trachea

Pharyngitis

The pharynx is the part of the throat between the tonsils and the larynx, or voice box. Pharyngitis is acute inflammation of the pharynx. It is similar to acute inflammation of the tonsils, or tonsillitis (see next article). Both diseases are caused by the same bacteria and viruses, but pharyngitis tends to be less severe than tonsillitis. Some medical authorities simply refer to both conditions as acute sore throat. Persistent infection, or chronic pharyngitis, occurs when a chronic infection, usually a respiratory, sinus, or mouth disorder, spreads to the pharynx and remains. Pharyngitis can also be caused by irritation and inflammation of the pharynx without infection. Such irritation may be caused by cigarette smoke or alcohol.

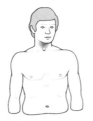

A sore throat
Although the sore throat of pharyngitis is rarely serious, it can make breathing, swallowing, and speaking painful and difficult.

Site of the pain

What are the symptoms?

If you have acute pharyngitis, your throat is sore, you have trouble swallowing, and you may feel feverish. As in tonsillitis, your throat is red and raw. If you have chronic pharyngitis, you also suffer from the symptoms associated with the infection that originally caused the pharyngitis.

What is the treatment?

Self-help: Whether your pharyngitis is acute or chronic, you should not smoke. Give your throat even more of a rest by switching to a mostly liquid diet for a short time. Nonprescription lozenges and mouthwashes should relieve the symptoms of acute pharyngitis. Gargling with salt water may also help. Aspirin or a substitute recommended by your physician may ease general aches and pains. If your sore throat persists for more then a few days, consult your physician.

Professional help: For an acute but particularly troublesome attack, your physician may prescribe an *antibiotic*, often in tablet form. For chronic pharyngitis your doctor will probably try to find and treat the primary source of infection. Your pharyngitis should then disappear.

Tonsillitis

Tonsillitis, or acute inflammation of the tonsils, is primarily a children's disease (see p.676). It occurs occasionally in adults, and the symptoms are very similar to those of influenza, or flu. If you feel ill, and have a sore throat, a headache, and chills and fever, examine your throat. If your tonsils are red and inflamed and seem larger than usual, you probably have tonsillitis. Another common symptom is swelling and tenderness of the glands surrounding the infected area. Check the glands in the neck and under the jaw.

What should be done?

Coddle yourself. Stay in bed for a day or two, take one or two aspirins every four hours, and drink plenty of liquids. Consult your physician if your sore throat and fever last for more than 48 hours.

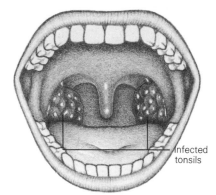

Infected tonsils

The tonsils
The tonsils are glandular swellings at either side of the throat that help to trap and destroy micro-organisms. If they become swollen and inflamed in the process, you have tonsillitis.

Laryngitis

Laryngitis is usually caused by bacterial or viral infection of the larynx, or voice box, which is at the top of the trachea, or windpipe. The infection causes general inflammation and swelling of the mucous membrane of the larynx, including the vocal cords. In young children, because the opening of the larynx is very narrow, the swollen membrane sometimes interferes with breathing (see Croup, p.678). Occasionally, laryngitis is caused simply by irritation and inflammation of the larynx without infection. This may be caused by tobacco smoke, alcohol, or excessive shouting, talking, or singing.

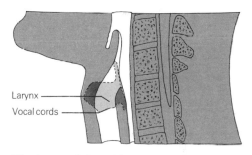

Larynx
Vocal cords

What happens in laryngitis
An infection of the upper-respiratory tract may affect the vocal cords, and they may become inflamed. When you speak, air passes over the swollen cords, and the sounds are distorted. This causes the hoarseness of laryngitis.

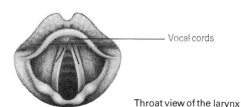

Vocal cords

Throat view of the larynx

The main symptom is hoarseness, which may lead to loss of voice in two or three days. Speaking may even become painful. There may be fever or other symptoms associated with influenza, or flu (see p.559). Most people recover in a few days.

What are the risks?

Uncomplicated attacks of laryngitis are not dangerous. The main risk is that a condition similar to laryngitis is one symptom of tumors in the larynx (see next article). Sometimes painful swallowing and earache associated with hoarseness are symptoms of tuberculosis (see p.563) that is spreading from the lungs. This is rare, but when it occurs the apparent laryngitis may be the first symptom.

What should be done?

If you think you have laryngitis and you are otherwise in good condition, stay home, rest your voice, and do not smoke or drink alcohol until the inflammation clears up and you can talk normally. This improvement should take no more than four or five days. If hoarseness persists for more than a week, you may have chronic laryngitis. Consult your physician, who may question you about your general health and examine your throat. If there is no inflammation, you do not have laryngitis, and you may need diagnostic tests.

If your physician finds that you have chronic bronchitis, sinusitis, or tuberculosis, treatment of the underlying condition should relieve the laryngitis-like symptoms.

Tumors of the larynx

A growth on the larynx may be either *benign* (unlikely to spread), or *malignant* (likely to spread and threaten life). There are two types of benign tumors of the larynx: papillomas, which usually appear several at a time; and polyps, which usually appear one at a time. Both types usually can be removed without permanent ill-effects. They seem to be caused by misuse or over-use of the vocal cords. Malignant tumors occur most often in people who smoke heavily.

What are the symptoms?

Hoarseness is usually the only symptom of a tumor in the larynx. There are no flu-like symptoms as in laryngitis (see previous article). If the tumor is malignant, its spread, which is cancer, may eventually make swallowing difficult, and you may have an increasingly obvious lump in your neck. In a child, because the airway through the larynx is narrow, a tumor of the larynx may give the voice a high-pitched crowing sound, known as stridor, because of the obstruction.

Hoarseness that is caused by benign growths is usually intermittent, but hoarseness due to cancer is continuous and gradually worsens. Since it is not painful and comes on slowly, you may scarcely notice it during its early stages.

Examining the larynx
To examine your larynx, the physician uses a system of mirrors. Light is reflected from a special eyepiece, which is basically a mirror with a hole in it for the doctor to look through. Another small mirror attached to a long handle is held at the back of your throat. It reflects the light into your larynx, and a view of the larynx back to the physician.

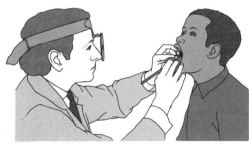

What are the risks?

Although neither type of tumor of the larynx is very common, benign tumors are slightly less common than malignant ones. The American Cancer Society estimates that there are about 11,000 new cases of cancer of the larynx each year, and that about 9,000 of those affected will be men.

The main risk is that if you ignore slowly increasing hoarseness, and if that hoarseness is caused by a malignant tumor, it may be too late to deal successfully with the cancer. Cancer of the larynx can almost always be cured if it is diagnosed early. If it is not discovered in time, it can either spread to

Speaking without your larynx
You may have surgery to create a breathing hole in your throat and to make a valve from your own esophageal tissue. This replaces your vocal cords. When you want to speak, you place a finger over the hole. Air from your lungs passes through the new valve, and makes it vibrate and produce sound.

Valve
Breathing hole
Esophagus
Trachea

other parts of the throat or get into the bloodstream and produce *metastases*, or secondary cancers, elsewhere in your body.

What should be done?

Do not ignore unexpected vocal changes. If you remain hoarse for more than a week, or if hoarseness keeps coming back, consult your physician. If your throat shows no signs of the inflammation that accompanies laryngitis, the physician may refer you to an ear, nose and throat specialist, who will examine your larynx by reflecting a light from a mirror held at the back of the throat. If there is swelling or any other sign of a growth, the specialist will probably do an *endoscopic* examination, and a *biopsy*, which determine whether you have a tumor and, if so, whether it is malignant.

What is the treatment?

Self-help: No self-help is possible.
Professional help: Benign growths, whether papillomas or polyps, can usually be removed in a minor operation done under local anesthetic. Malignant tumors discovered early are generally treated, and in most cases cured, by *radiation therapy*. If the cancer is more advanced, the larynx may have to be removed. Even then there is about an even chance of cure. To regain your voice, however, you will have to work with a speech therapist, who may teach you how to use the esophagus as a substitute for the larynx. An alternative technique involves implanting an artificial valve between the esophagus and the trachea. The valve permits air to move out of the lungs, through the valve, and up the esophagus, where you produce the sounds used in speech.

The lungs and chest

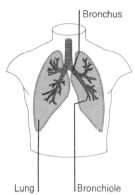

Bronchus

Lung | Bronchiole

Your body needs a constant supply of oxygen to stay alive. It also needs to dispose of carbon dioxide, a waste product of metabolism. In your lungs oxygen from the air you breathe is transferred to your blood and carbon dioxide is released from the blood. The blood transports the oxygen to all parts of your body. The carbon dioxide is exhaled. When the blood has less oxygen and lots of carbon dioxide in it, the heart pumps it back to the lungs through the pulmonary arteries.

The bronchus, or main airway that leads into each lung, divides into smaller and smaller airways called bronchioles. Each bron-

chiole ends in a cluster of tiny air-sacs called alveoli. Each alveolus contains several small capillaries. The walls of those capillaries are thin enough to allow oxygen and carbon dioxide to move between the air and the blood. There are millions of alveoli in each lung.

Your lungs are especially vulnerable to particles floating in the air. Bacteria that cause disorders like pneumonia (see p.359); irritants such as tobacco smoke, which can cause lung cancer (see p.366); and, in some people, airborne *allergens*, which cause asthma (see p.355), or farmer's lung (see p.365), can all interfere with lung functions.

Acute bronchitis

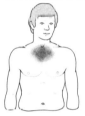

Site of the pain

Air pollution
Bronchitis occurs more often in areas with severe air pollution.

Inflammation of the mucous membrane that lines the bronchi, or main air passages of the lungs, is called bronchitis. If you have a respiratory infection, you may develop acute bronchitis, since the disorder is caused when the same viruses that cause colds (see p.342) and pharyngitis (see p.350) spread into the bronchi. If you have a healthy heart and healthy lungs, bronchitis usually clears up in a few days. In chronic bronchitis (see next article), prolonged, recurrent attacks cause gradual deterioration of the lungs.

What are the symptoms?
The main symptom of bronchitis is a deep cough that brings up grayish or yellowish phlegm, or sputum, from your lungs. Other

symptoms are breathlessness, wheezing and a fever. You may also have pain in the upper chest, which gets worse when you cough.

What are the risks?
Virtually everyone has an occasional attack of acute bronchitis. If you do not smoke cigarettes and you do not have chronic lung or heart trouble, you may have it once every few years. If you smoke, have a chest disorder such as asthma (see p.355) or bronchiectasis (see p.363), or live in an area where the air is very polluted, you are more likely to get the disease. If your lungs are congested because of heart failure (see p.381), you may also be particularly susceptible to acute bronchitis.

If you are a non-smoker who is generally healthy, there are few risks of complications from acute bronchitis. If you are particularly susceptible to bronchitis for any of the reasons mentioned above, you may have repeated attacks. These can damage the lining of the bronchi, impairing your ability to clear mucus from your air passages and leading to chronic bronchitis.

What should be done?
Do not ignore repeated attacks of acute bronchitis. Consult your physician to find out if there is an explanation. If you have not had bronchitis before, or if this is your first attack in several years, follow the self-help procedures suggested below.

What is the treatment?
Self-help: If you have a fever, take aspirin three or four times a day to bring it down. Take an over-the-counter cough medicine

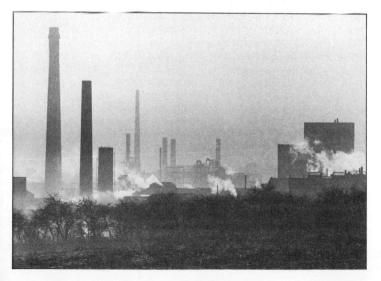

recommended by your physician, and follow the instructions on the label, to help soothe your cough. Stay home, not necessarily in bed but in a warm room. Use a vaporizer, a humidifier, or steam from hot water to moisten the air. This may help to clear your nasal passages and bronchi. This simple treatment is usually all that is needed. Call your physician if you become breathless, cough up blood, have a temperature above 101° F (38.5° C), or do not feel better in 48 hours.

If you have repeated attacks of bronchitis, remember that cold, damp living or working conditions can make you more susceptible to this disease. You may want to consider moving or changing your job.

Professional help: Because acute bronchitis is usually a viral infection, no specific treatment is possible. However, it is possible to relieve the symptoms. If your breathing is wheezy, your physician may prescribe a *bronchodilator* drug, which is usually taken by inhaling it. If your chest is sore from repeated attacks of coughing or if your cough is dry, your doctor may prescribe a cough suppressant. If your sputum becomes greenish-yellow, which indicates that you probably have a secondary bacterial infection, the physician may prescribe an *antibiotic*. Some physicians prescribe antibiotics in the early stages of the disease to try to prevent the occurrence of secondary bacterial infection.

Chronic bronchitis

Chronic bronchitis is similar to acute bronchitis (see previous article) but in chronic bronchitis the inflammation persists and gets worse. In its early stages, chronic bronchitis is difficult to detect. However, it is dangerous, because repeated infections of the bronchi and bronchioles thicken and distort the lining of these tubes. This causes them to narrow and become obstructed by the secretion of too much mucus and by excessive contraction of the muscles in their walls.

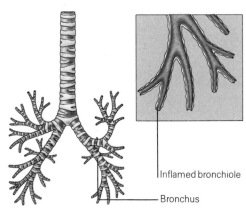

Inflamed bronchiole

Bronchus

Some risks of chronic bronchitis
Repeated infections of the bronchi and bronchioles damage the linings of these tubes, and leave the lungs susceptible to further infection. If the infection should spread to the alveoli (not shown), it could cause pneumonia or emphysema.

What are the symptoms?
The first symptom of chronic bronchitis is a morning cough that brings up phlegm, or sputum. Smokers may regard the cough, if they notice it at all, as a "normal" smoker's cough. Over the years the amount of phlegm gradually increases, and the coughing continues all day. Breathlessness and wheeziness become increasingly troublesome.

In the early stages of chronic bronchitis, only bad colds or influenza cause flare-ups. In the later stages, every minor head cold can bring on a severe attack. Many sufferers have several flare-ups every winter. One definition of chronic bronchitis is a recurrent cough with phlegm production that occurs on most days during at least three months a year, usually in winter, for at least two consecutive years.

In the last stages of the disease, coughing, breathlessness, and wheezing occur on a nearly continuous basis.

What are the risks?
If you smoke, you are more likely to get chronic bronchitis than if you are a non-smoker. Children of heavy smokers may be affected too. As infants they seem to be particularly susceptible to acute bronchitis and pneumonia (see p.359), and these disorders increase the risk of chronic bronchitis. The disease is more common in men than in women by three to one. Because air pollution can trigger it, it is also more common in industrialized countries and in urban areas than in developing countries and rural areas.

If you have chronic bronchitis and do not obtain treatment for it in its early stages, there are several risks, including death, involved. Usually, the disease has an established cyclical pattern of bronchial infection, which damages your lungs, and in turn leads to an increase in your vulnerability to further bronchial infection. If the infection eventually spreads into the alveoli, or air sacs at the ends of the bronchioles in the lungs, you may contract either pneumonia (see p.359) or emphysema (see p.358). Chronic bronchitis may also lead to pulmonary hypertension (see p.416) and right-sided heart failure (see p.381). Also, your entire respiratory system could fail, which is a medical emergency (see Accidents and emergencies section, p.801).

Some people who have chronic bronchitis gradually become blue around the lips and in the rest of the face because they are not getting enough oxygen. They may eventually experience respiratory failure because their lungs cannot supply their bodies with enough oxygen. Others develop lung cancer (see p.366), not because chronic bronchitis causes cancer, but because smoking is a cause of both diseases. If you have chronic bronchitis and you notice a marked increase in breathlessness and a change in the nature of your cough, these signs of deterioration in your condition may be the first signs of cancer.

What should be done?

If you have a morning cough with phlegm and if you smoke, you have even more reason to stop smoking. If the symptoms persist, consult your physician, who will probably consider such factors as your smoking habits and where you live and work before making any recommendations. If necessary, your doctor will recommend some diagnostic tests, which may include a chest *X-ray* and pulmonary function tests.

What is the treatment?

Self help: If you have chronic bronchitis, give up smoking and avoid smoke-filled rooms. Stay away from people who have colds. A cold, which is a minor illness to a person with healthy lungs, may cause an attack of bronchitis for you. If you work or live in a polluted atmosphere, you should consider changing jobs or moving. If you move, try to go to not only a cleaner, but also a warmer, drier environment. You are running a risk if you spend your winters in a cold, damp place.

Professional help: The treatment depends mainly on how far the disorder has progressed before you consult your physician. If you are already suffering from breathlessness, the doctor will probably prescribe an aerosol inhaler. Use it three or four times a day to relax the wall muscles of your bronchi. This will widen the airways in your lungs. If you are having a bad attack of infection and coughing up phlegm, your physician may prescribe an *antibiotic*. If you are having a particularly serious attack, your doctor may give you the antibiotic by injection, because that is by far the quickest way to get the drug to the source of the infection.

Your physician may prescribe small doses of an antibiotic for a period of several weeks or even months to prevent bacterial infection, or advise you to take a full dose only at the first sign of a flare-up of bronchitis. There is no consensus among physicians about the best way to treat chronic bronchitis. Although antibiotics are not effective against viral infection, they are often prescribed even when a virus rather than a bacterium causes an attack. This is because a viral infection may increase the chances of bacterial infection in the lungs.

Chronic bronchitis can adversely affect your heart. If there is any indication that this is happening or that you are likely to contract a second lung disease such as emphysema or cancer, treatment will be determined accordingly. Also, your physician may suggest that you undergo special lung and heart tests.

Asthma

Asthma is a chronic condition marked by periodic attacks of wheezing and difficulty in breathing. The cause of asthma attacks is partial obstruction of the bronchi and bronchioles due to contraction of the muscles in the bronchial walls. Whereas with bronchitis, you have constant wheeziness until you recover from the disease, with asthma, attacks come and go and there are wide variations in the degree of obstruction at different times. Asthma cannot be cured, but an attack can be relieved by treatment. If asthma attacks are not treated, they usually end naturally.

Most asthma is triggered by an allergy to such things as pollen, skin particles (dander) or hairs of cats or dogs, or miniscule mites in house dust. Some attacks start for no apparent reason. Attacks can also be caused by infections (especially of the respiratory tract), certain drugs, inhaled irritants, vigorous exercise, and psychological stress.

What are the symptoms?

The main symptoms of asthma are difficulty in breathing, a painless tightness in the chest, and varying amounts of wheezing. At times, the wheezing is audible only with a *stethoscope*, but sometimes it is loud enough to hear across a crowded room. In severe cases, breathing becomes so difficult that it may cause sweating, an increased pulse rate, and severe anxiety. In very severe attacks the face and lips may turn bluish because of the diminishing supply of oxygen in the body.

What are the risks?

Asthma is quite common in school age children. Most children outgrow the condition, and no more than two or three per cent of the adult population is asthmatic.

A succession of severe asthma attacks can be very disabling. Each year several thousand people die during an attack. However, most of these people are elderly and have other illnesses as well. Today, because of some recent medical discoveries, there is little risk of lasting disability or death for people who take their asthma seriously and consult a physician about it.

What should be done?

If you have asthma, there are some steps you can take to control asthma attacks. Study your own disease, take the self-help measures recommended below, and see your physician whenever you have a severe and persistent period of breathlessness. Asthma is an illness that you and your physician can work together to control. You can never be sure that the symptoms you have at home will be the same when your physician puts a stethoscope to your chest, so you must be able to give a clear description of what happened both before and during the attack.

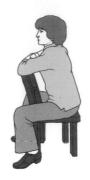

Self-help during an asthma attack
During an attack, it may help you to sit elbows up straddling a chair. This keeps your spine straight, stabilizes the top of your ribcage, and allows your chest muscles to move air efficiently.

What is the treatment?

Self-help: Because asthma is most often caused by an allergy, your first step in controlling the disease is to try to identify the *allergen*, or irritant, that bothers you. Your physician may be able to help by arranging skin tests (see p.345) with suspected allergens, but you can do much of the detective work yourself. Do you have your asthma attacks mainly at one time of the year, and do you also have hay fever? If so, your allergens are probably pollen grains. Do your attacks occur more often on certain days of the week than on others? This might suggest a link with dusts at work, such as flour in a bakery, or with something you are around only when you pursue a hobby, such as flowers in a greenhouse, or with some stressful situations, such as regular visits to a hospital. Is your asthma worse in one room of your house than another? You may be allergic to mites in house dust, especially in bedrooms, or to hair or feathers from a pet.

Another possibility is an allergy to a food or a drink. Shellfish, eggs, and chocolate are some common examples of foods that trigger asthma attacks in some people.

You can test your theory of what causes your asthma attacks by keeping a record of the frequency and severity of your attacks. Keep track of how often the attacks coincide with your exposure to the suspected allergen or allergens. One way to measure the severity of an attack is by means of a small *peak-flow meter*. Your physician may be able to lend you one if you cannot buy one. By measuring the maximum flow of air with the meter when you breathe out, you can keep precise records of how much the air passages in your lungs narrow during an attack.

Once you have identified an allergen, the best treatment for your asthma is to avoid exposure to that substance. This is fairly simple if the allergen is a particular food or a domestic animal. If it is something like grass pollen, you can only take precautions such as staying away from the countryside in mid-

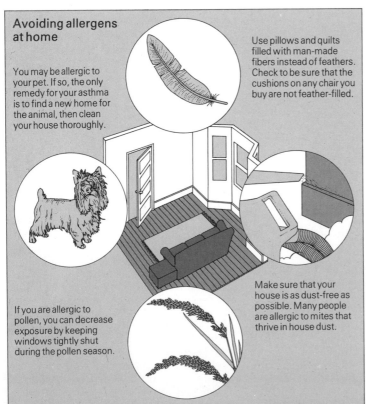

Avoiding allergens at home

You may be allergic to your pet. If so, the only remedy for your asthma is to find a new home for the animal, then clean your house thoroughly.

Use pillows and quilts filled with man-made fibers instead of feathers. Check to be sure that the cushions on any chair you buy are not feather-filled.

If you are allergic to pollen, you can decrease exposure by keeping windows tightly shut during the pollen season.

Make sure that your house is as dust-free as possible. Many people are allergic to mites that thrive in house dust.

summer. You will have to work in cooperation with your physician to try to control most of your symptoms.

Even if you cannot identify your allergen, you may have fewer attacks if you reduce the amount of dust in your house. Either replace feather pillows and fiber-filled mattresses with those filled with urethane foam, foam rubber or other non-allergic materials, or put airtight plastic covers on them. Use a vacuum cleaner to remove dust from crevices, and eliminate rugs or carpets or choose types that can be kept dust-free. Be aware, too, that other factors such as some forms of exercise or psychological stresses like tests in school can bring on attacks.

Professional help: Once the diagnosis is made, much can be done for you. The accuracy of your account of symptoms and probable allergens may help your physician make the diagnosis without allergy tests. In the past few years the treatment of asthma has been improved enormously with the introduction of new drugs, which can be taken as pills, liquid, or inhalants. These drugs fall into two categories. They are *prophylactics*, and *bronchodilators*. Prophylactics are taken regularly to prevent attacks. These are taken primarily by people who get very frequent attacks or who can predict when an attack is likely to occur. Bronchodilators, which are best for people who have only occasional asthma attacks, are taken only after an attack has started, to relieve the symptoms.

Some prophylactic drugs are inhaled four to six times a day to prevent attacks. These drugs relax the bronchial muscles and open obstructed airways. The best way to use these is to inhale them, since an inhalant goes directly to the site of the obstruction in the lungs. But they can be taken orally by anyone who finds inhalants difficult to use. If no pill, liquid, or inhalant succeeds in relieving a severe case of asthma, a bronchodilator drug may be injected into the bloodstream. This method almost always works. One group of drugs, *steroids*, is effective both in preventing asthma attacks and in relieving their symptoms once they are underway.

If your asthma attacks are clearly due to an allergen such as grass pollen, it may be possible to desensitize your lungs to that allergen with a series of injections (see p 346). But the drugs discussed above are effective enough that physicians seldom recommend such desensitization as a treatment for asthma.

Despite the success of drug treatment, an asthma attack is sometimes severe enough to require hospitalization. There are three things that can be done for you in the hospital

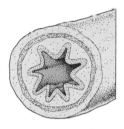

Cross-section of untreated bronchiole with blocked airway

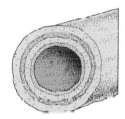

Cross-section of treated bronchiole with unobstructed airway

that you cannot do yourself at home. First, some drug treatments are most effective in the form of a fine mist which is given to the patient through a breathing apparatus. This apparatus requires professional maintenance. Second, if you are hospitalized, you can be given muscle-relaxant drugs and connected to a mechanical respirator. This treatment eliminates muscle spasms in the air passages inside the lungs. Your chest muscles can relax, also, since the work of breathing is done by the respirator. This gives your respiratory system a chance to recover from a severe attack. Third, the presence of nursing and medical staff 24 hours a day may relieve your anxiety about being unable to breathe.

What to do for an acute attack

A sudden, acute attack of asthma can be

The aerosol inhalant
Aerosol inhalants are prescribed to relieve symptoms of asthma attacks. You breathe out, and make an airtight seal with your mouth around the mouthpiece. Then, as you breathe in, you press the top down, so that a fine spray of the drug is released and inhaled into your lungs.

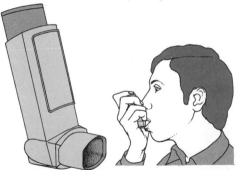

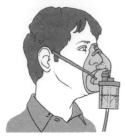
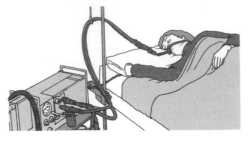

Hospital treatment for asthma
If your asthma attack is so severe that your normal dosage of drugs is ineffective, you may have to wear a specially designed oxygen mask (above left) that allows you to breathe in a fine mist of a drug combined with oxygen. If your condition still does not improve, you will be connected to an artificial respirator (above right), which forcibly pumps air in and out of your lungs. This treatment is usually given in combination with muscle-relaxant drugs and is rarely maintained for longer than 24 hours.

frightening for you and your family. In most cases the physician will have prescribed an inhalant of a bronchodilator or steroid drug. If one dose does not relieve your wheezing, you can repeat it in 30 minutes if this is suggested by your physician. However, you should not use the inhalant again if the second dose is ineffective. An overdose may be dangerous. Instead, call your physician. It is better to get in touch with a physician too soon than to wait until it is too late, since even with today's drugs severe asthma (*status asthmaticus*) may be difficult to treat.

Members of the family of an asthmatic are often alarmed by a severe attack, but feel helpless because they do not know what to do about it. Here is what to do:

1. Get the drugs and inhaling apparatus together on a table, and note the time the asthmatic takes the first dose of whatever medicine or medicines that the physician has prescribed for emergencies.

2. Help the asthmatic find the most comfortable position. Usually the best position is sitting up, leaning slightly forward, and resting on the elbows or arms. Plenty of fresh air is also important.

3. Don't stand around in a worried group. This only raises the asthmatic's level of anxiety. Someone calm and level-headed should stay with the patient. Everyone else should quietly go into another room.

4. Get the telephone number of the asthmatic's physician and be ready to call. If you call and the doctor is not in, be ready to take the asthmatic, quickly but calmly, to the nearest hospital emergency room.

Emphysema

In emphysema, the lungs become less and less efficient because of damage to some of the millions of alveoli, or air-sacs, at the ends of the bronchioles in the lungs. It is in the alveoli that oxygen and carbon dioxide exchange takes place. Healthy lungs have an elastic, spongy texture, so they contract and expand fully. If the alveoli become stretched or rupture, the elasticity of the lungs is gradually destroyed. This type of damage occurs when the alveoli are constantly subjected to higher pressure than normal. This happens to people who have a long-standing lung disease. Chronic bronchitis (see p.354) or asthma (see

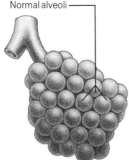

Normal alveoli

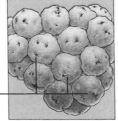

Damaged alveoli

What happens in emphysema
Damaged alveoli (air sacs in the lungs) may burst and merge to make fewer but larger alveoli. This causes a reduction in the lung's surface area. Less oxygen is able to travel through the walls of the alveoli and into the bloodstream.

previous article), for example, cause narrowing of the lung airways. The labored, forceful breathing that results strains, weakens and may ultimately damage the alveoli.

What are the symptoms?

The main symptom of emphysema is shortness of breath, which is likely to become gradually worse over a period of years. If you have emphysema, your chest is probably distended into a barrel-like shape. The name of the disease comes from the Greek word for inflation. If you also wheeze, cough, and bring up phlegm, these are symptoms of other kinds of lung trouble, not of emphysema.

What are the risks?

Emphysema usually occurs in people who have bronchitis or asthma. It is much more common in men than in women, and your chances of having it increase if you smoke and/or live in an area where the air is polluted. Some people are particularly susceptible to emphysema because of an inherited defect in the chemical make-up of their lungs. If your job requires exceptionally forceful use of lung power, you may also be highly susceptible. Some examples of such professions are glass-blowing and playing a wind musical instrument. If you have increasing shortness of breath, you risk death from eventual respiratory failure. Emphysema also makes you more susceptible to chest infections such as pneumonia that can be life-threatening.

Percussing the chest
Because emphysema patients have enlarged air sacs in their lungs, a physician can diagnose the condition by percussing the chest. The doctor places two fingers on the chest and taps them with the fingers of the other hand. The enlarged air sacs produce a hollower sound than normal ones.

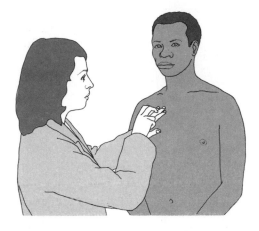

cuss, or finger-tap, your chest, and listen to it with a stethoscope. The doctor may also ask you to have a chest *X-ray*, and to blow hard into a *peak-flow meter*, a machine that measures your breathing capacity. Special breathing tests called pulmonary function tests may also be necessary. Because emphysema is usually associated with other lung disorders, it is not an easy disease to diagnose independently.

What is the treatment?
Self-help: If you smoke, stop. Avoid places with polluted air. Keep away from people who have coughs or colds. Exercise moderately but regularly in fresh, clean air.
Professional help: Physicians can relieve the symptoms and delay the progress of emphysema, but they cannot cure it. If you have bronchitis along with emphysema, you may be told to inhale *bronchodilator* drugs, which widen the airways and help prevent further damage to the alveoli. Since bronchitis and lung infections of any kind aggravate emphysema, the best way to help control the disease is to prevent respiratory infection. Thus your physician may prescribe *antibiotics* as a preventive measure.

There is also a risk of a pneumothorax (see p.362). In addition, since blood cannot flow freely through damaged alveoli, the resulting strain on the right side of the heart, which pumps blood to the lungs, can lead to heart failure (see p.381).

What should be done?
If you are troubled by breathlessness, you should consult your physician. In the initial examination, the physician will probably *per-*

Pneumonia

Pneumonia is not a specific disease. It is a general term for several kinds of inflammation of the lungs. Pneumonia is usually caused by a bacterial or viral infection, but it can also be caused by chemical damage to the lungs from inhaling a poisonous gas such as chlorine. The pneumonia, or lung inflammation, can be anything from a mild complication of an upper respiratory tract infection to a life-threatening illness.

The symptoms, the treatment, the impact, and the outcome of pneumonia depend on the cause, the general health of the person concerned, and on other factors. Viral pneumonia, for instance, does not respond to treatment with *antibiotics*. See the accom-

KINDS OF PNEUMONIA

Cause	Onset of symptoms	Temperature	Other possible symptoms
Influenza virus	Abrupt (within hours of infection)	104°F (40°C) or above	Bad cough, blood-stained sputum, blueness, dry cough
Other viruses	4 to 5 days after infection	About 101°F (38.3°C)	Dry cough
Mycoplasma (bacterium-like)	3 to 4 days after infection	About 101°F (38.3°C)	Dry troublesome cough, headache
Pneumococcus bacterium	Abrupt (within hours of infection)	Up to 104°F (40°C) or above	Chills, chest pain, blueness and, later, a cough with blood-stained sputum
Legionnaire's disease bacterium	2 to 10 days after infection	Up to 104°F (40°C) or above	Nausea, vomiting, chills, muscle aches, headache, blood-stained sputum, chest pain

panying table for a comparison of the causes and likely results of five of the most common types of pneumonia.

The variability of pneumonia has led to many popular and medical descriptive terms. If you are told that you have "double" pneumonia, it means that both your lungs are affected. If your attack is due to bacteria-like microbes called *Mycoplasma*, you may be said to have "atypical" pneumonia. "Bronchopneumonia" is patchy inflammation of one or both lungs, and "lobar" pneumonia affects the entire area of one or more lobes of the lung. When your physician determines what kind of pneumonia you have, you can ask for a description of that type.

What are the symptoms?

No single symptom is characteristic of all types of pneumonia. You should consider the possibility of pneumonia, however, if you already have a respiratory illness with symptoms such as a cough and fever, and you become short of breath while at rest and for no apparent reason. Additional symptoms to watch for besides coughing and a temperature are chills; sweating; chest pains; *cyanosis*, or a bluish tinge to the skin; blood in the phlegm; and, occasionally, mental confusion or delirium. The larger the lung area that is affected, the more severe the symptoms you experience will be.

How quickly the symptoms begin and which symptoms are most prominent varies with the cause of the infection. An especially virulent strain of the influenza virus can cause a pneumonia that can kill a feeble person within 24 hours. In a healthy young adult, pneumonia resulting from a mild respiratory infection might cause symptoms that are no worse than those of an ordinary cold.

What are the risks?

In the United States, about 15 people out of 1,000 have pneumonia each year. The disorder is often the final complication of some other debilitating disorder, and this is why many people who get pneumonia die. Anyone whose resistance is already low is very susceptible to pneumonia, so for people who are dying of heart failure, cancer, stroke or chronic bronchitis, the actual cause of death is often pneumonia. In anyone who is semiconscious or paralyzed, infection of the lungs is extremely likely. This is because under such conditions the normal coughing reflex that keeps the lungs clear of mucus and stagnant fluid is reduced, or even absent.

You are also more likely than other people to get pneumonia if you are very young (under 2) or very old (over 75), if you have a chronic chest disease such as asthma or some other chronic illness that reduces your body's resistance to infections, or if you are a heavy smoker or drinker. If you are under longterm treatment with *immunosuppressive* or anti-inflammatory drugs, especially *steroids*, you are also susceptible to pneumonia. These drugs decrease the body's normal defenses against infection.

Because pneumonia varies so much, no generalizations can be made about its outcome. In old, weak, or debilitated people, the main risk is death. Any type of pneumonia may lead to pleurisy (see next article), or empyema (see p.364). The most dangerous type of pneumonia is caused by viruses such as an influenza virus, because they do not respond to antibiotics. Compare the mortality rate for viral pneumonia in the accompanying table with that for a form of pneumonia caused by pneumococcus bacteria, which is similarly virulent but can be treated with antibiotic drugs. With increasing age or chronic illness, your chances of surviving even a mild case of pneumonia are reduced more and more with time.

What should be done?

Even if you have some of the symptoms usually associated with pneumonia, do not assume that you have it. Assume instead that you have a cold or some other infection of the respiratory tract, and take care of yourself accordingly. Consult your physician at once, however, if you become short of breath even when lying down, if your chest hurts when you breathe, or if you cough up blood-stained sputum. Your physician will probably listen to your chest through a *stethoscope, percuss,* or finger-tap, your chest, and ask you questions about the onset of symptoms and your smoking and drinking habits. It may be possible to make a firm diagnosis of pneumonia, and even of the type of pneumonia, based on such an examination. However, further tests such as a chest *X-ray* and laboratory examination of both blood and phlegm samples may also prove to be necessary.

What is the treatment?

Self-help: None is possible.

Professional help: Because pneumonia can unexpectedly become severe in a matter of hours, your physician may recommend hospitalization. The best treatment may be simply a combination of warmth, soothing cough medicines, and *antibiotics*. However, close professional supervision and observation are highly desirable during the early stages of pneumonia, especially if there is some doubt about the precise nature and extent of the inflammation.

Antibiotic drugs may be given orally or by injection. There is a wide variety of antibiotics, and the choice for your case will depend largely on the probable cause of your illness. Laboratory tests of your blood and sputum should indicate what is causing your infection. Your doctor will also need to find out if there are any antibiotics to which you are either allergic or particularly responsive.

Analgesics such as aspirin help to relieve chest pain. If you are very breathless and turning blue, you are probably in need of oxygen, which is generally supplied with a face mask or a tube in your nose. If your lungs remain troublesome in spite of all attempts at treatment, your physician may recommend further tests. For example, *bronchoscopy* may be done to exclude the possibility of lung cancer (see p.366).

A healthy young person should recover completely within two to three weeks. Even in cases of viral pneumonia, the chances of serious complications are minimal, since an-

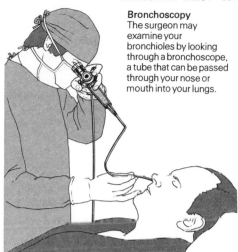

Bronchoscopy
The surgeon may examine your bronchioles by looking through a bronchoscope, a tube that can be passed through your nose or mouth into your lungs.

tibiotics can prevent secondary bacterial infection. Following recovery, you may still feel very tired for a long time after the infection is gone. A heavy cigarette smoker, or someone who is vulnerable in some other way, may take several months to recover from the illness or may die.

Pleurisy and pleural effusion

When you breathe normally, the lungs expand and contract easily and rhythmically inside your rib cage. Each lung is enclosed in a moist, smooth, two-layered membrane, which is called a pleura. The pleura lubricates the moving parts of the lungs and makes breathing easier. The outer layer of the pleura lines the rib cage. Between the two thin layers is a virtually imperceptible space,

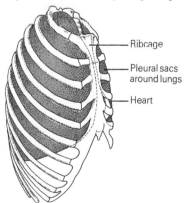

Ribcage

Pleural sacs around lungs

Heart

which is called the pleural space. It permits the layers to glide gently across each other. If either of your pleura becomes inflamed and roughened because of an infection, this seriously impedes the movement of the layers, and you have pleurisy.

Pleurisy is actually a symptom of an underlying disease rather than a disease in itself. The pleurae may become inflamed as a complication of a lung or chest infection such as pneumonia (see previous article) or tuberculosis (see p.563). The inflammation can be due to a slight pneumothorax (see next article), or a chest injury. Inflammation of the pleura sometimes creates a further complication by allowing fluid to seep into the pleural space. This causes a condition called pleural *effusion*. But pleurisy is not the only cause of pleural effusion; the condition may also be a complication of a generalized disease such as rheumatoid arthritis (see p.552), a liver or kidney disorder, or heart failure (see p.381). Cancer cells that are spreading from a tumor in the lungs, breast, or ovaries can also cause pleural effusion.

What are the symptoms?
If you have pleurisy, it hurts to breathe deeply or cough. You may also have severe, but one-sided, chest pain. These symptoms are accompanied by others that are associated with the underlying disorder. The pain will disappear if pleural effusion occurs as a result of pleurisy, because fluid will prevent the roughened or inflamed layers of the pleura from rubbing against each other. If this happens, you may become breathless.

What are the risks?

Pleurisy and pleural effusion due to infection have become rare disorders. This is because they now can be very effectively treated with antibiotics. Pleurisy is four times as common as pleural effusion.

In most cases the risks of pleurisy are the same as the risks associated with the underlying cause. Advanced pleural effusion can compress the lungs and cause severe breath-

Taking a sample of pleural effusion
A sample of fluid can be taken from the pleural space with a needle and a syringe. The needle is pushed between the ribs into the pleural space and fluid is drawn off.

lessness. Pleural effusion may also lead to empyema (see p.364).

What should be done?

Consult your physician if breathing becomes painful, you seem unusually short of breath, and either or both of these symptoms is accompanied by a fever, no matter how slight. After questioning you about symptoms and previous illness, the physician will probably listen to your chest with a stethoscope and will *percuss*, or finger-tap, your chest while listening for characteristic sounds made by irritated pleurae and pleural effusion. You may need a chest *X-ray* to help determine what disorder has caused the pleurisy. If you have pleural effusion, one way to diagnose the cause is to study the composition of the fluid, so a sample of fluid may be taken from the pleural space, with a needle and syringe.

What is the treatment?

Because pleurisy and pleural effusion are symptoms of other disorders, the only way to cure them is to treat the underlying disease. Meanwhile, to ease chest pains, the doctor may recommend that you use an *analgesic* such as aspirin.

Pneumo-thorax

As your healthy lungs expand and contract, each of the two layers of the pleura, a membrane that surrounds each lung, slips smoothly over the other. A pneumothorax occurs when air gets into the pleural space between

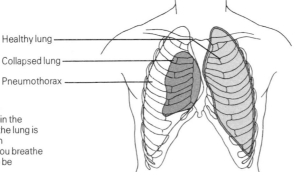

Healthy lung
Collapsed lung
Pneumothorax

Lung collapse
If air is present in the pleural space, the lung is prevented from expanding as you breathe in and is said to be collapsed.

the two layers, and separates them. Part of the lung, sometimes the whole lung, collapses, and is therefore emptied of air. A pneumothorax may be caused by a chest injury, or, more commonly, by air escaping into the pleura from the lung. A small pneumothorax will often simply disappear. But sometimes more air enters the pleural space, which can cause a larger and larger area of the lung to collapse.

What are the symptoms?

The major symptoms of a pneumothorax are breathlessness and chest pain, generally on the affected side, but sometimes at the bottom of the neck. The pain is usually sudden and sharp, though it may be hardly more than a sensation of discomfort. You may also have a feeling of tightness across your chest. The severity of the symptoms depends on the size of the damaged area and on your general health. If you are young and in good condition, you may have little pain and little difficulty in breathing, even if you have a large pneumothorax and a large portion of your lung collapses. If you are middle-aged and have chronic bronchitis, a small pneumothorax can be extremely painful and cause extreme difficulty in breathing.

What are the risks?

Pneumothorax is relatively rare. It occurs chiefly in otherwise healthy young men, for no apparent reason, and in middle-aged people, both men and women, whose lungs are already damaged by asthma, chronic bronchitis, or emphysema.

The seriousness of a pneumothorax depends on how air is getting into the pleura. Often a small pneumothorax is inconsequential and heals by itself. But if there is a hole that allows the pneumothorax to get larger, you will have increasing breathlessness and pain as more and more of the lung collapses. If the disorder remains untreated, death from *respiratory failure* can follow.

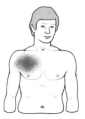

Site of the pain

What should be done?

If you suspect that you have this condition, consult your physician. An examination of your chest with a *stethoscope* should detect a large pneumothorax, but your doctor may need a chest *X-ray* to find a small one. In any

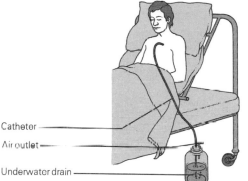

Catheter

Air outlet

Underwater drain

Treatment
To remove pleural air, a tube is inserted into the pleural space. As you breathe out and pleural volume decreases, air is squeezed out along the tube. An underwater drain ensures that the air travels only one way.

case, even if there is only a suspicion of a pneumothorax, you will probably be admitted to a hospital. There you will be carefully observed by your own doctor and others. Some tests may also be performed.

What is the treatment?

The treatment depends on the size of the pneumothorax and the condition of your lungs. Since the disorder may heal itself, you may need only a few days of X-ray observation and bed rest to make sure that the air in the pleural space is gone and that the collapsed portion of the lung has regained its elasticity and is full of air again. Treatment, if required, consists primarily of attempting to suck the air out of the pleural space with a tube known as a *catheter*, which is inserted between the ribs and into the pleural space. If this procedure does not improve the condition, your physician will need to get a clearer idea of the source of the problem. One possible approach is to inspect the inner side of each layer of the pleura, using an instrument called a *thoracoscope*. When a thoracoscope is inserted between the ribs and into the pleural space, it may be possible to find the hole through which air is seeping and seal it up.

Bronchi-ectasis

Bronchiectasis is the enlargement or distortion of one or more of the bronchi, or main air passages into the lungs, often as a result of frequent infections in childhood. The disorder takes years to develop. It leads to impaired drainage of the fluid that is normally secreted by bronchial cells, and this fluid may then remain in the lungs where it will then become stagnant. The stagnant fluid can lead to further infection.

What are the symptoms?

The main symptom of bronchiectasis is a frequent cough that brings up large quantities of green or yellow phlegm, or sputum, which sometimes is spotted with blood. The quantity of phlegm generally increases when you change position. This is especially true when you lie down.

If you have bronchiectasis, you are susceptible to repeated infections of the lung when you catch an ordinary cold. You may also have chronically bad breath.

What are the risks?

Bronchiectasis is rare because many childhood infections that caused the disorder, such as sinusitis and the chest infections that often followed measles or whooping cough, now

can be prevented by immunization or effectively treated with *antibiotics*. Similarly, tuberculosis, which also damages the lungs, has become extremely rare. Even people who have bronchiectasis can usually lead normal lives. They owe this to the effectiveness of antibiotics, which are usually given at the first sign of further infection.

If bronchiectasis is treated when the symptoms first appear, there is little danger.

What should be done?

If you repeatedly cough up large amounts of green or yellow phlegm, consult your physician, who will probably listen to your chest with a *stethoscope* and may also want you to have a chest *X-ray* and a *bronchoscopy*, a procedure in which an instrument called a bronchoscope is used to examine your bronchi. The results of these tests will help your physician to make a diagnosis.

What is the treatment?

Self-help: There is nothing you can do until bronchiectasis has been diagnosed. If you find that you have the condition, make a special effort to avoid getting colds and sore throats. Do not smoke, and stay out of smoke-filled rooms. If the lower part of your lung is infected, as it probably is if you have bronchiectasis, your physician probably will tell you about a self-help technique called postural drainage. This is a method of getting rid of bronchial secretions. In this technique, you place yourself so that the bronchus leading to the affected lobe of your lung is upside down. The fluid then drains out, and you can cough it up. Lying on a bed with your head and chest hanging over the edge for five to ten minutes twice a day can help keep your lungs fairly clear.

Professional help: At the first sign of bronchiectasis your physician will probably prescribe an antibiotic and instruct you to take the whole prescription even if the infection seems to clear up. If your condition is very localized, or if a lot of blood is mixed with the phlegm, your physician may advise you to have the affected part of the lung removed. Such surgery is seldom necessary for this condition, however. If it proves to be necessary in your case, your doctor will see that you are admitted to a hospital.

Lung abscess

An *abscess*, or a contained infectious area, in the lung is usually due to one of two conditions. It may be a complication of some type of pneumonia (see p.359), or it may be caused by inhaling material, such as food or a fragment of a tooth, while you are unconscious. You might inhale such a fragment while under an anesthetic, knocked out by a head injury, or drunk. Abscesses associated with pneumonia are very rare, because antibiotics usually prevent such complications. Lung abscesses occur most often among people who are suffering from malnutrition.

The main symptoms are alternating chills and fever. You may also have chest pain and a cough that brings up thick phlegm that contains pus and blood. If you have these symptoms, you must be admitted to a hospital for diagnostic tests. A chest *X-ray* will help your physician locate the site of the abscess, and tests of the phlegm will identify what has caused it. You should recover completely if you take the appropriate *antibiotics*.

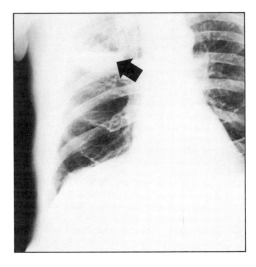

X-ray diagnosis of a lung abscess
An abscess in the lung is at least partially filled with fluid. The fluid-filled area shows up on an X-ray as a pale patch surrounded by a dark, air-filled area.

Empyema

Empyema means an accumulation of pus in any body cavity. The term is generally used to refer to an infected pleural effusion (see p.361). In pleural effusion, watery fluid seeps into the space between the two layers of the pleura, the membrane that surrounds each lung. In empyema, this fluid has thickened into pus. This may be a complication of a lung disease such as pneumonia (see p.359) or of an abdominal infection that spreads into the chest. There are no special symptoms of empyema, and the diagnosis is made based on an examination of a sample of the fluid in the pleural space. This fluid is taken from the pleura with a needle and syringe.

Empyema has become extremely rare since the advent of *antibiotics*. Most people who develop it are already under treatment for some underlying disorder. The treatment and prospects for full recovery depend on what the underlying disorder is.

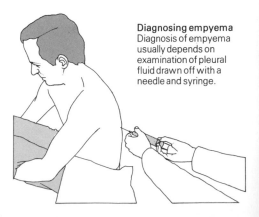

Diagnosing empyema
Diagnosis of empyema usually depends on examination of pleural fluid drawn off with a needle and syringe.

Pneumo-coniosis

(and other dust diseases)

Pneumoconiosis means dust in the lungs. The term refers to a number of occupational diseases that are caused by inhaling various kinds of dust particles. If you have been inhaling such particles continuously for many years, little patches of irritation may have formed in one or both of your lungs. If the scar tissue caused by the irritation has made your lungs less flexible and porous, you are suffering from some type of pneumoconiosis. A common form of the disorder in this country is appropriately named coal-miner's pneumoconiosis, or black lung disease. Silicosis is another form of pneumoconiosis. It affects workers in quarries, stone masons, metal grinders, and miners who drill rock. Others who may also be susceptible to pneumoconiosis are those who work with aluminum, asbestos, beryllium, iron, talc, cotton, sugar cane, and any of a number of synthetic fibers.

It usually takes at least ten years of continual daily exposure to contract a dust disease. However, some people who work with asbestos under poor conditions may succumb to asbestosis, a form of pneumoconiosis that is caused by asbestos dust, in much less time. Coal-miner's pneumoconiosis sometimes takes 25 years to develop.

What are the symptoms?
Breathlessness from exertion is the dominant symptom of pneumoconiosis. In silicosis the symptoms usually become progressively worse, and there may be other symptoms associated with tuberculosis of the lungs (see p.563). In all types of dust disease there is usually a cough with phlegm, or sputum, similar to the cough in chronic bronchitis (see p.354). The phlegm of coal-miners with pneumoconiosis is often black.

What should be done?
If you work where you are exposed to dust, find out what the dust is and if it carries some risk of pneumoconiosis. Check with your employee safety representative, management or your union. If the dust does cause lung damage, make sure you have a chest X-ray once a year, and consult your physician if you notice that you are increasingly short of breath. The physician will probably want to see a chest X-ray and results from pulmonary function tests to find out if you are severely affected. If you are, it may be advisable to change jobs, if possible. Even in a different job, you should continue to have periodic chest X-rays for the rest of your life, so that if you have later complications of your dust disease, you can discover them early.

If you smoke, give it up. There is a particularly good reason for not smoking if you have a potentially serious case of pneumoconiosis. Since only a small proportion of workers exposed to the dusts that cause the disorder actually become ill, we can assume that if you do, you are probably prone to lung diseases. Therefore, you may also be susceptible to other disorders that are caused by or intensified by tobacco smoke, including lung cancer (see next page).

What is the treatment?
Only a few of the pneumoconioses can be treated. Steroid drugs are usually used in these cases.

Farmer's lung

The disease known as farmer's lung is caused by frequent exposure to a fungus that grows in moldy hay or grain. It attacks only people who are allergic to the fungus. The allergy causes lung inflammation that narrows the air passages and thickens the alveoli walls. The effects of the disease are similar to those of pneumoconiosis (previous article), so it is sometimes called organic pneumoconiosis. A similar allergic reaction to certain kinds of fungus occurs among workers who deal with malt, mushrooms, and several other substances. Another similar disorder affects people who handle animals in laboratories, and pigeon breeders or others who have frequent contact with birds of various kinds.

The fungi that cause this disorder may be particularly numerous in the droppings of the animals involved.

What are the symptoms?
The main symptom of farmer's lung is breathlessness. This becomes troublesome a few hours after you have been exposed to the fungus. It generally goes away after another few hours. The breathlessness is usually accompanied by a dry cough. Since you may also have symptoms such as fever, chills and headache, you may mistake farmer's lung for persistent, recurring influenza or may even think that it is asthma.

What are the risks?
Farmer's lung and similar allergic reactions are rare, since only a small proportion of the people who are in constant contact with the fungi are susceptible to the disorder.

If you do get it, however, and do not discover the true cause of the constantly recurring symptoms, you may continue to be exposed to the fungus. Then your condition will probably get worse. When it is untreated over a long period, any inflammation of the lungs can destroy the elastic lung tissue, which is then replaced by stiff scar tissue. The result is a permanent, progressive breathlessness, which can lead to *respiratory failure* and heart failure (see p.381), both of which can be fatal.

What should be done?

Consult your physician if you have repeated attacks of breathlessness. If you are frequently exposed to any substance that can cause farmer's lung, be sure to tell your doctor. You will probably need to have a chest *X-ray* so that your physician can establish the nature and extent of the disease.

What is the treatment?

Self-help: Avoid further exposure to the fungus. Change your job if possible. Other-

wise, wear a protective mask over your nose and mouth whenever you may be exposed to the substance. In most cases no other treatment is necessary.

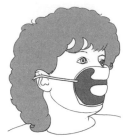

Avoiding farmer's lung
If you are often exposed to the types of fungus that cause farmer's lung, you should wear a protective face mask to filter out the tiny particles that may cause the damage.

Professional help: If you have had the condition for some time, it may be much more difficult to treat than it is in earlier stages. The most effective treatment may be *steroid* drugs, taken for several months.

Lung cancer
(bronchial carcinoma)

Although there are several kinds of lung cancer, only one, bronchial carcinoma, is common, and it is almost always caused by lung damage from smoking.

Inhaled tobacco smoke damages the cells that line the bronchi, and many scientists believe that the damaged cells themselves represent an early stage of cancer. Some of these cells may gradually form a wartlike tumor, which is the starting point of bronchial carcinoma. As the tumor grows, it spreads into the lungs from the bronchi. The cancer cells often get into the bloodstream and are carried to the brain, liver, bone, and skin where they establish *metastases*, or secondary cancers that also can be very dangerous.

What are the symptoms?

The first symptom of bronchial carcinoma is usually a cough, which is most often an increase in your smoker's cough. The disease is closely associated with chronic bronchitis (see p.354). More than half of the people who develop lung cancer have had bronchitis for years. Along with the cough there is generally some phlegm, which may be blood-stained. You may also be a little breathless. Often you will have chest pains. They are either sharp pains that become sharper when you take a deep breath, or dull and persistent pains. You may sometimes wheeze.

Sometimes the first symptoms of lung cancer occur in other organs to which the cancer has spread. Bronchial carcinoma spreads in about one out of eight cases, and it

is in those cases that the secondary cancer may alert your physician to the primary cancer of the lung. The symptoms of the secondary cancer depend on where the cancer cells have settled. If they are in your brain, you may have headaches, feel confused, or have an epileptic fit or a stroke. In the bones the symptoms are pain, swelling, or even fracture. If the cancer is in your skin, cystlike swellings appear. If it is in your liver the symptoms may be indigestion, dyspepsia, and eventually jaundice.

What are the risks?

Bronchial carcinoma is the most common form of cancer in the Western world. It affects more men than women, probably because lung cancer takes a long time to develop, and men smoked much more than women did 20 to 40 years ago. There has recently been a drop in the incidence of the disease among men and a rise in the incidence among women. This may be because men are smoking less than they did before, and many women only began to smoke heavily after World War II was over.

Your chances of getting the disease vary according to how much you smoke. If you have never smoked, you probably will not get bronchial carcinoma. Light smokers are ten times as susceptible as non-smokers, and heavy smokers are 25 times as susceptible. As soon as you stop smoking, the danger begins to decrease. After ten years of non-smoking, you have just about the same chance of es-

Medical myth

There is no point in giving up smoking if you have smoked for years. If you are going to get lung cancer, it can no longer be avoided.

Wrong. There is firm evidence that people who have smoked heavily for many years improve their chances of avoiding lung cancer by stopping.

caping coming down with bronchial cancer as do lifelong non-smokers.

If lung cancer is discovered early, either as soon as the symptoms develop, or by a routine chest *X-ray*, the affected portion of the lung can sometimes be removed surgically. Less than ten per cent of the people who get lung cancer are cured by surgery combined with *radiation therapy* and *chemotherapy*, however. Most people who have lung cancer do not seek help until the cancer has spread beyond the point where

surgery can be effective. Smokers increase their risk of contracting not only cancer, but also several other life-threatening diseases associated with smoking. These include coronary artery disease (see p.374), stroke (see p.268), and chronic bronchitis (see p.354).

What should be done?

To avoid bronchial carcinoma, stop smoking now, even if you do not have a smoker's cough (see How to stop smoking, p.40). A tumor takes years to develop, and if you remove the cause, the process may slow down or even stop. If you are experiencing symptoms such as increasingly severe smoker's cough, chest pains, and blood in the phlegm, see your physician, who will probably listen to your chest with a *stethoscope* and arrange for a chest X-ray. If the X-ray shows signs of possible cancer, you may be referred to a chest specialist, who may use a *bronchoscope* to look for cancerous growths in your bronchi. If there are such growths, their location can be more firmly established by bronchoscopy than by X-ray.

What is the treatment?

Self-help: No self-help is possible, except for giving up smoking.

Professional help: Surgical removal of the cancer is the best possible treatment for bronchial carcinoma, but in about two-thirds of the cases the cancer turns out to be too advanced for total removal when the chest is opened. Radiation therapy slows down the progress of the cancer and may relieve the symptoms for months or sometimes years.

Another possibility is treatment with *cytotoxic* drugs. These drugs kill cancer cells while doing little, or at least less, damage to normal cells. This treatment, also called chemotherapy, is similar to methods that have proved effective in cancers such as Hodgkin's disease (see p.433) and leukemia (see p.426). The treatment takes several months, and cytotoxic drugs have unpleasant side-effects, but the results are promising. Since this treatment is comparatively new, and different drugs are being tried, the results of long-term research trials are not yet available. However, it offers the best prospect for cure where surgery is not feasible.

The choice of which treatment is most suitable for you depends on the extent of the disease, what the *biopsy*, or laboratory examination of a piece of the tumor, shows and your general health. Discuss the possibilities with your physician. Although a diagnosis of lung cancer is serious, it is possible to treat it and sometimes to cure it.

Deaths caused by lung cancer

Lung cancer was a rare disease before cigarette smoking became a popular habit. Since records of deaths from lung cancer have been kept, the numbers rose steadily and steeply for men until only a few years ago. The number of women who died of lung cancer rose only slightly between 1900 and 1940 but in the last 40 years there has been a steady increase. This is because it has become more socially acceptable for women to smoke since World War II. Despite this, however, there are still approximately four times as many male as female fatalities from lung cancer in Western society.

OPERATION: ### lung removal
pneumonectomy or lobectomy

Pneumonectomy is an operation to remove a lung. If only part of the lung is removed, it is called a lobectomy. Either operation is done to treat cancer of the lung when the disease is diagnosed at an early stage, and occasionally for tuberculosis or bronchiectasis.

During the operation You are given a general anesthetic. The chest surgeon makes an incision from front to back on the affected side along the line of a lower rib. One rib is usually removed and the affected lung or part of the lung is removed through the gap. The operation usually takes between one and three hours.

After the operation You will spend a few days in the intensive-care unit. While there, some nutrients and drugs may be dripped into your arm and at least two drainage tubes will drain the incision. You may have to breathe through an oxygen mask. You can help yourself best by coughing frequently to bring up any secretions. The usual hospital stay is two to three weeks.

Convalescence You will need to convalesce for several months after you leave the hospital and will be advised to give up smoking for life.

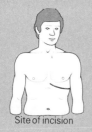
Site of incision

Interstitial fibrosis

Interstitial fibrosis is also called diffuse interstitial fibrosis or pulmonary alveolar fibrosis. In this disorder, the efficiency of the lungs is impaired by an accumulation of fibrous matter that obstructs the bronchioles, or air passages in the lungs, and thickens the walls of the alveoli. The alveoli are tiny air sacs at the ends of the bronchioles. It is at the walls of these tiny sacs that most of the oxygen we need to live is taken from breathed air by the blood. Here, too, the blood releases the waste gas carbon dioxide to the lung to be exhaled. Interstitial fibrosis is a rare, serious disorder. Its cause is unknown.

What are the symptoms?

Interstitial fibrosis may be either acute or chronic. In the acute form, the major symptom is increasingly severe shortness of breath, with coughing that may bring up blood-stained sputum. Another common symptom is chest pain. The progress of the disease is so rapid that most people who get it die within a year. The chronic form is more common. It starts in middle age, and the symptoms develop much more slowly. Another symptom that is found with chronic interstitial fibrosis is *clubbing*, a deformity of the fingertips that also occurs in a number of other chronic lung diseases.

What is the treatment?

Both acute and chronic forms of this condition end in *respiratory failure* and, ultimately, in death. Treatment with *steroid* drugs may relieve the symptoms and slow the progress of the disorder.

Fibrous tissue in the alveoli walls
Very rarely, fibrous tissue can develop in the walls of the alveoli, and reduce both their size and their potential for getting oxygen into the bloodstream. This tissue also affects the elasticity of the lungs, so that they expand and contract with less efficiency.

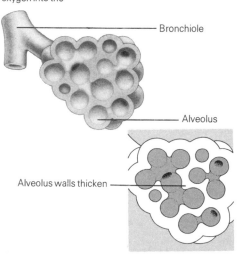

Bronchiole

Alveolus

Alveolus walls thicken

Clubbed fingers
Deformed fingers are a symptom of chronic lung disease. Your cuticles seem to disappear and your fingernails curve around the ends of your fingers. The tips of your fingers may also flatten out and become spatula-shaped. In particularly bad cases, the ends of your toes may be similarly affected. The reason for this strange deformity is not known.

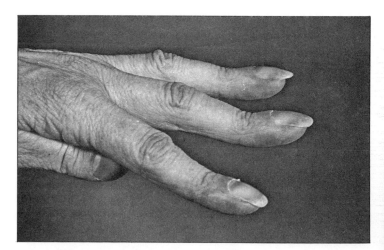

Pulmonary edema

Pulmonary edema is an acute, dramatic, and sometimes life-threatening symptom of heart failure (see p.381). The edema, or swollen tissue, results from inefficient pumping action of the left side of the heart. This causes the blood in the pulmonary veins, which bring oxygenated blood to the heart from the lungs, to become dammed up. This raises the pressure in these and other blood vessels in the lungs. As a result, fluid seeps from the blood vessels into the alveoli, the saclike parts of the lungs where oxygen and carbon dioxide are exchanged. An accumulation of fluid leads to swollen lungs. If you have this problem, and you suddenly become breathless, it is called an attack of pulmonary edema. This sometimes happens to someone who has heart failure and is not aware of it.

What are the symptoms?
An attack of pulmonary edema consists of breathlessness that becomes progressively worse over a few hours. This often occurs in the middle of the night. You may have a frightening sense of needing to fight for breath. The breathlessness is generally accompanied by a cough, which is dry and tickling in the early stages, but which may eventually bring up blood-stained, frothy phlegm, or sputum. In a severe attack you may also turn bluish because there is not enough oxygen in your blood.

What should be done?
If you have an attack of pulmonary edema, you may already be under treatment for heart failure. At the first sign of sudden severe breathlessness, contact your physician and call for an ambulance. This is an emergency that will respond to treatment, but delay may be fatal. Do not dispose of your sputum, since is will probably be tested to help your physician confirm that you have pulmonary edema, rather than some other malady with similar symptoms. Your blood pressure will probably be taken and your chest examined with a *stethoscope*. You will also probably be asked if you have chest pain. Pain in addition to breathlessness may indicate that you are also having a coronary thrombosis, or heart attack (see p.379).

What is the treatment?
Self-help: Try to keep calm. Sit up in a chair to make breathing easier. It will probably help you considerably if you straddle the chair, facing backwards, with your arms raised and resting on its back.
Professional help: The main objective is to relieve the breathlessness as quickly as possible. This is usually done best in a hospital, where you can be given oxygen. Your physician may prescribe one of several drugs, any of which can be injected directly into a vein to act swiftly. Morphine is used to slow and deepen breathing. A *diuretic* will help to drain fluid from your lungs, or open up blocked air spaces in the lungs. If you are not already taking digitalis, the doctor may also start you on it to strengthen the action of your heart. If the attack of pulmonary edema has been triggered by a chest infection, your physician may prescribe an *antibiotic* as well.

If pulmonary edema is treated rapidly and efficiently, and if your attack has not been brought on by a heart attack, your stay in the hospital may be no longer than a week or so. Your physician will probably continue to treat you for heart failure in order to prevent further complications.

Sarcoidosis

This is a rare disease in which multiple, tiny patches of inflammation suddenly appear in one or several parts of the body, frequently in the lungs. The word sarcoid should not be confused with *sarcoma*. A sarcoma is a type of tumor. The inflamed tissues of sarcoidosis are not a kind of tumor. They are also not due to an infection. Nobody knows just why sarcoidosis occurs, or why it clears up, as it usually does, of its own accord.

Often there are no symptoms. When there are, they depend entirely on what tissues or organs of your body are affected. If your lungs are affected, for example, you may have some shortness of breath, and scar tissue from the sarcoids may lead to bacterial infection or bronchiectasis (see p.363).

Other tissues and organs that may be affected include the skin, lungs, lymph glands, liver, spleen, eyes and the bones in the hands and the feet.

What should be done?
If your physician suspects you have sarcoidosis, a chest X-ray will nearly always confirm or disprove the diagnosis. Untreated sarcoidosis will generally disappear in two to three years. Your physician may prescribe a *steroid* drug, which seems to be the only effective medicine for sarcoidosis of the lungs.

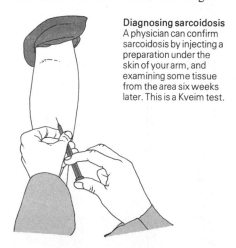

Diagnosing sarcoidosis
A physician can confirm sarcoidosis by injecting a preparation under the skin of your arm, and examining some tissue from the area six weeks later. This is a Kveim test.

Disorders of the heart and circulation

Introduction

Your blood is your body's transport system. Its main function is to carry both nutrients and oxygen, which provide raw materials and energy to the tissues of your body. The blood also carries waste away from the tissues and helps maintain body temperature. To do these things, your blood must circulate continuously.

Your heart is at the center of the circulatory system. Its steady beating pumps at least five quarts of blood through a full circuit of your body every minute. The heart consists of two pumps side by side. The pump on the right side moves blood to your lungs, where waste gases such as carbon dioxide are removed and oxygen is added. Freshly oxygenated blood returns to the pump on the left side, which moves it out into the rest of your body. Blood flows away from the heart, either to the lungs or to the rest of the body, through blood vessels called arteries. These branch many times, and the branches become smaller, forming blood vessels called arterioles. These, too, become smal-ler and smaller and branch repeatedly until they are tiny vessels called capillaries. Throughout the arteries and the smaller vessels that stem from them, your blood delivers nutrients and oxygen to the tissues and picks up wastes. This task is completed in the capillaries. As the blood moves on through the capillaries, the blood vessels gradually become larger, and eventually become veins. The veins carry the blood through organs such as the liver, which remove the wastes, and back to your heart. Then the cycle begins again.

Disorders of the heart and circulation are many and varied. Only the most common ones are covered in this chapter. Congenital, or inborn, heart disorders are covered elsewhere (see p.656). One disorder that has become especially common in this century is coronary artery disease, which is caused by atherosclerosis, a thickening of the internal lining of the blood vessels. The exact cause of this condition is uncertain, but the medical profession has found that certain factors are probably linked to it. These factors are heavy cigarette smoking, obesity, lack of exercise, and excessive fat in the diet.

If you are healthy, the two sides of your heart beat steadily. In some disorders the beats become uncoordinated or abnormally fast or slow. These disorders of rhythm, called *arrhythmias*, can usually be cured by drugs or by attaching a pacemaker (see p.391) to your heart to regulate your heartbeat.

Your heart contains one-way valves to ensure that the blood flows in one direction only. If these valves do not function properly, the result is called valvular heart disease. Fortunately, surgeons can repair or replace damaged valves. Finally, even if the heart is sound, damaged blood vessels elsewhere can cause disorders.

Treatment of heart and circulation disorders has improved significantly in the past 20 years, largely because of improved surgical techniques. In too many cases, however, the first symptom of serious trouble is permanent disability or even sudden death. Since several kinds of circulatory-system diseases probably can be prevented, physicians are increasing their emphasis on the importance of a healthy life style *before* problems begin.

How blood circulates
The heart pumps blood through the body. Deoxygenated, or "used" blood (gray) has made a full circuit of the body and is pumped from the right ventricle into the lungs. There it exchanges carbon dioxide for oxygen. The newly oxygenated blood (brown) enters the left side of the heart, and is then pumped out of the left ventricle to all body tissues.

The heart and blood vessels

The heart

The heart is basically a muscular bag made up of two pumps. Each pump is divided into two compartments linked by valves. The largest compartment is the left ventricle, which pumps blood, freshly oxygenated by the lungs, through the aorta to all parts of the body. The blood then returns to the heart, entering the right atrium through two large channels (the superior and inferior venae cavae). From the right atrium the blood passes through the tricuspid valve into the right ventricle. It is then pumped through the pulmonary artery into the lungs, where it receives oxygen. This oxygenated blood flows back to the left atrium of the heart via the pulmonary veins. From the left atrium it passes through the mitral valve into the left ventricle.

Blood vessels

Blood vessels that lead to and from the heart carry blood to all parts of the body. For a detailed illustration of how the blood circulates, see p.403.

Arteries

Arteries carry blood away from the heart. The walls of the arteries need to be strong, because blood is pumped along them under pressure from the heart. Arteries have four layers: a fibrous outer coating, strong muscle, a tough layer of elastic tissue, and a membranous inner lining.

Capillaries

Capillaries are tiny, very thin-walled projections of the smallest arteries. They carry blood to each cell of the body. Oxygen and other nutrients in the blood permeate the capillary walls (arrows) to reach body tissues, while waste matter is taken up to be carried to veins which take it to breakdown and disposal points.

Veins

Veins ultimately lead to the heart. Since the blood they carry is under much less pressure than that in the arteries, veins have thinner, less elastic, less muscular walls. Compression of the walls by ordinary muscle activity squeezes the blood along. Valves in the veins (bottom left) keep blood from flowing in the wrong direction. The veins have three layers: a fibrous outer coating, a thin layer of muscle and a membranous inner lining.

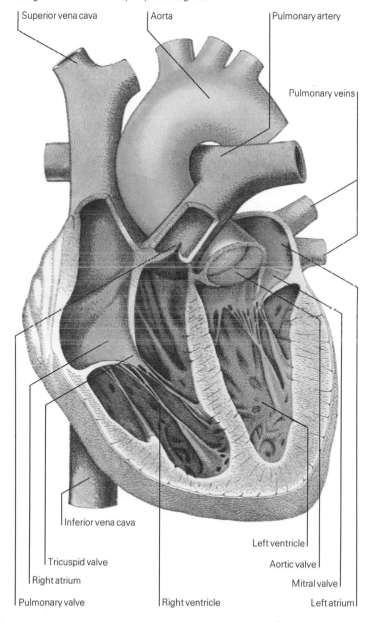

Superior vena cava

Aorta

Pulmonary artery

Pulmonary veins

Inferior vena cava

Tricuspid valve

Right atrium

Pulmonary valve

Right ventricle

Left ventricle

Aortic valve

Mitral valve

Left atrium

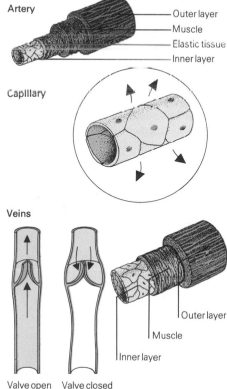

Artery

Outer layer
Muscle
Elastic tissue
Inner layer

Capillary

Veins

Valve open   Valve closed

Outer layer

Muscle

Inner layer

Major disorders

Heart disease accounts for almost one-third of all deaths in Western countries, and most of these deaths are due to coronary artery disease and hypertension, or high blood pressure. Coronary artery disease is caused by atherosclerosis, a thickening of the internal lining of the blood vessels seemingly linked with fatty substances, including *cholesterol*, in the blood. These disorders and their complications, including shock, heart failure, angina, and heart attack, are discussed in the opening pages of this chapter.

Athero-sclerosis

Your arteries are the vessels that carry blood from the heart to the rest of your body. If you are healthy, your arteries have walls that are muscular, smooth inside, and elastic enough to accommodate extreme variations in blood pressure, so that blood passes through freely. Sometimes, though, fatty streaks appear on the inner walls of arteries. These streaks may start at stress points, for example where an artery branches or where the wall is slightly damaged. As a fatty streak grows, it further damages the arterial wall. Eventually, the streak can become a hard mass of fatty tissue that erodes the wall, diminishes the elasticity of the artery, and narrows the passageway and interferes with the flow of blood. The fatty tissue is known as *atheroma*. A large mass of atheroma is called a *plaque*. The name of the disorder, atherosclerosis, means, literally, "hardening from atheroma." Atherosclerosis is an important contributory factor in arteriosclerosis (see Hardening of the arteries, p.404). It is also the cause of coronary artery disease (see next article).

Atherosclerosis is common in North America. Post-mortem examinations of bodies from fatal automobile accidents indicate that some degree of the disorder is almost universal, especially in men. Even children may be affected. A major reason for this is that atherosclerosis is associated with certains fats, including *cholesterol*, in the blood. Most people in the Western world eat large amounts of fatty and cholesterol-rich foods such as meat, butter, and eggs. Some research on the causes of atherosclerosis suggests that this kind of diet is a main cause of the frequency of the disorder.

Your chances of having the disease are highest if you have higher than normal levels of cholesterol in your blood, if you are a man of any age or a woman who is over 35, if you smoke, and if you have a condition such as diabetes (see p.519), kidney failure (see p.511), or high blood pressure (see p.382). (For further details on those who are at risk from atherosclerosis, see Coronary artery disease, next article.) The severity of atherosclerosis increases with age.

What are the symptoms?
There are rarely any symptoms of atherosclerosis until the damage it causes has become extensive. When you do develop symptoms, generally after several years, it is because a particular part of your body is being deprived of blood. Therefore, the symptoms depend on which part is affected. You may merely have cramps in your legs after exercise, or you may have a stroke (see p.268), kidney failure (see p.511), angina (see p.376), or a heart attack (see p.379).

What are the risks?
Severe atherosclerosis can exist without apparent ill-effects. Many parts of your body are supplied with blood not only by a particu-

Atheroma formation
An atheroma, or patch of fatty tissue that damages arterial walls, tends to form at the point at which an artery branches and the flow of blood is naturally disturbed. As atheroma increases, atherosclerosis develops.

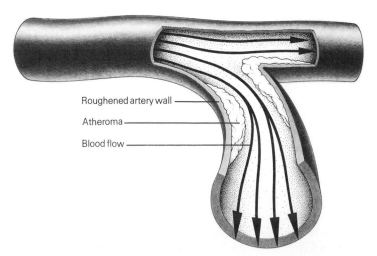

Roughened artery wall

Atheroma

Blood flow

lar artery and its branches, but also by minor branches of neighboring arteries. These may not be affected even though the major supply channel is badly damaged. As the supply of blood from the major artery decreases, other arteries can sometimes compensate by enlarging, which allows the total blood supply to that area of your body to remain almost constant. Even when the disorder affects body tissues that rely on a single artery for their blood supply, the channel can often be narrowed considerably without ill-effects. This is possible because the normal supply of blood to a tissue is usually more than it actually needs to remain healthy.

Thus, atherosclerosis may do you little or no harm for many years. It is more than likely, however, that as an artery becomes narrowed by fatty tissue, the part of your body that depends on that artery or one of its branches will eventually suffer from lack of blood. If this happens in the coronary arteries, which supply blood to the heart, you have coronary artery disease. If the cerebral arteries, which supply the brain, are affected, you may have a stroke (see p.268) or transient ischemic attack (see p.270). Other possible results of the disorder are dry gangrene in an arm or leg (see p.415) or kidney damage, which leads in many cases to chronic kidney failure (see p.512).

What should be done?

Do not wait for symptoms to develop before doing something about atherosclerosis. By the time symptoms appear, the disease will have produced troublesome consequences, and it will have been affecting your circulatory system for years. The time to begin taking the self-help measures recommended below is before symptoms develop. They may help you prevent or slow down the onset of atherosclerosis.

Research studies suggest that a fatty streak on the lining of an artery can be made to disappear, but that nothing can be done about an established *plaque*, or large, hard mass of fatty tissue. Vigorous treatment of atherosclerosis can reduce the likelihood of strokes, even in advanced stages of the disorder, but after a certain point, nothing seems to make a heart attack less likely. This is not to suggest that you should ask your physician for immediate tests to show whether you already have atherosclerosis and how advanced it is. Such tests are complicated and expensive, and self-help measures should be enough for almost everyone.

You should consult your physician, however, if you have two or three close relatives with heart or circulatory disorders, if you know that some of your close relatives have high levels of fatty substances in the blood, or if you have diabetes. Your doctor may suggest that you have a blood cholesterol test. Other possible tests include a blood-pressure check, a chest *X-ray*, an *electrocardiogram* (*ECG*) and ultimately, an *arteriogram*.

What is the treatment?

Self-help: Because the risk of developing severe atherosclerosis seems to be related to the level of fatty substances, including cholesterol, in your blood, you may want to reduce your intake of animal fats and other *saturated* (dairy) fats if your blood cholesterol level is high. There is some controversy about this in the scientific community, but as long as you continue to eat balanced meals (see p.26), you can avoid certain foods without harm and still derive pleasure and sustenance from your diet. In general, try to eat more poultry and fish and less pork, beef, and lamb. Remove fat from the meat that you do eat, and broil it instead of frying it. Restrict yourself to three eggs a week. Avoid cream. Use margarine high in *polyunsaturated* fats instead of butter. Eat more fruit and vegetables. Use cooking oils labelled "high in polyunsaturates," such as corn oil and sunflower oil, rather than oil labelled "vegetable oil" without further explanation. Try to reduce your total intake of fats.

People who are overweight, as well as heavy cigarette smokers, are known to be particularly susceptible to most of the disorders that can be caused by atherosclerosis. Heavy smokers, in particular, have a substantially higher frequency of heart attacks than do non-smokers. So give up cigarettes, and reduce if you are overweight. For a good reducing diet, see p.28.

Finally, follow a program of moderate physical exercise. Such activity may impede the development of atherosclerosis and increase your chances of living a long and healthy life. Do not overdo it, however. Get advice from your doctor if you have any reason to suspect that unaccustomed exercise may harm you.

Professional help: Your physician can help by keeping a watch on your blood pressure and treating you for hypertension if necessary. If you have an abnormally high blood-cholesterol level, the physician may prescribe a drug that will reduce it. As an alternative to drug treatment, your doctor may arrange for you to have several other types of blood tests and then counsel you on changes you can make in your diet.

Coronary artery disease

(coronary atherosclerosis, ischemic heart disease, coronary heart disease)

Your heart muscle requires a constant flow of oxygen- and nutrient-rich blood, just as all your other body organs do. This requirement is to keep the heart, itself, healthy and functioning and is only indirectly related to the blood required to fill the heart's chambers. Blood reaches your heart through two main coronary arteries, and a network of blood vessels over the surface of the heart muscle nourishes it.

Fatty deposits, or *atheroma*, can form in your arteries, and this narrowing of the passageways is part of a condition that is called atherosclerosis (see previous article). If your coronary arteries become narrowed, they can fail to provide your heart with enough oxygen. Also, the blood that flows through the arteries may form a clot, or *thrombus*, which can block an artery. When your heart beats faster in response to physical or psychological stress, and requires increased oxygen and nutrients, severely narrowed or blocked coronary arteries cannot cope. This strain causes angina, or heart pain (see next article). If the blood to part of your heart muscle is suddenly very severely reduced by a clot that becomes lodged in one of your coronary arteries, you will have a heart attack (see p.379).

What are the symptoms?

Often there are no symptoms of coronary artery disease, especially in the early stages. For recognizable symptoms that ultimately do occur, read the articles on angina (see next article) and heart attack (see p.379).

What are the risks?

Coronary artery disease is common in the Western world, where it accounts for 30 per cent of all deaths. More men than women are affected. The incidence of the disease is much lower in less affluent countries. Here are some additional facts that can help you determine whether you are especially likely to have coronary artery disease.

1. More young men than young women have coronary artery disease, but the risk to women increases after *menopause* and women over 60 are nearly as susceptible to the disorder as are men.

2. If you smoke cigarettes, you are at least twice as susceptible as a non-smoker. Deaths from the disorder in the 35 to 45 age group are five times more common in smokers.

3. There is an increased risk if you have high blood pressure or diabetes. Male diabetics are twice as susceptible as other men, and female diabetics are five times as susceptible as other women.

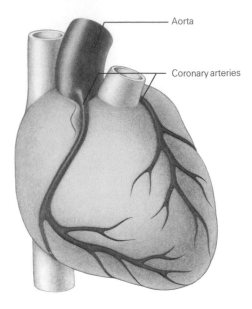

Aorta

Coronary arteries

The coronary arteries
Some of the freshly oxygenated blood that is pumped out of the aorta flows into two coronary arteries. These form a branching network over the surface of the heart and supply it with the nutrient-rich blood it needs to function.

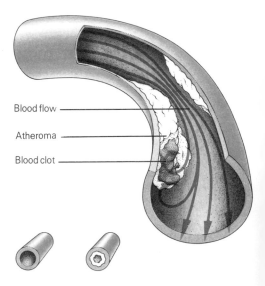

Blood flow

Atheroma

Blood clot

Normal   With atheroma

A blood clot forms in the arteries
An atheroma, or patch of fatty tissue, forms in a spot where the flow of blood is naturally disrupted. It roughens the arterial wall and causes increasing turbulence in blood flow. This can trigger the formation of a clot that may grow and block the artery.

4. Coronary artery disease seems to run in families. You are more at risk if several of your close relatives have had it.

5. If you are overweight, you are more at risk than a person of normal weight.

6. If you have a sedentary job you may be more susceptible than people whose work includes some hard physical labor.

7. If you are a woman over 35 who takes birth control pills, you are much more at risk of coronary artery disease than women who use other forms of contraception.

If you do have coronary artery disease, and the disease is not treated, your arteries may become increasingly blocked. Then the blood supply to your heart may be so reduced that there is a risk of a heart attack, which could be fatal. However, even after a major attack it may be possible to restore your heart to relative health. Sometimes, however, the heart muscle is damaged to such an extent that pumping action is weakened. This causes heart failure (see p.381).

Many people live for years with coronary artery disease and have no trouble. Others may be forced to restrict their activities because of recurrent attacks of angina. Many of these people can also lead relatively active lives as long as they keep the disease under control. Some must be much more careful, being certain not to put even slight strain on themselves. Yet, if they can adjust emotionally, even these people can be kept comfortable and happy.

What should be done?

For advice on what to do if you experience either of the main symptoms of coronary artery disease, read the articles on angina (see next article) and heart attack (see p.379). If you are worried that you may be susceptible, start taking preventive measures. Too often, sudden death is the first sign of the disease. The following recommendations for self-help are useful if you already have heart trouble, or if you want to improve your chances of avoiding it in the future.

If you want to check the state of your heart, see your physician, who, after examining you, may order some of the tests mentioned in the article on angina. You should also have your blood pressure checked from time to time (see High blood pressure, p.382).

What is the treatment?

Self-help: There is, as yet, no established way to dissolve *atheroma*, or fatty deposits, that have formed in the coronary arteries, but you can take steps to prevent or slow down further accumulations. If you smoke, give it

up, or at least switch from cigarettes to a form of smoking that does not involve inhaling the smoke, such as cigars or a pipe. If you are overweight, choose a moderate reducing diet (see p.28), and stick to it. Some studies indicate that there may be a link between the kinds of food eaten in a country and the incidence of coronary artery disease there. As a result, some heart specialists have drawn up certain dietary guidelines.

In the United States, as more of the population have seemed to adopt an "anti-coronary" diet, the number of deaths that occur from coronary artery disease has declined. The link between the changing American diet and the statistics on coronary artery disease cannot be proved at this time, but a more healthful lifestyle that includes no smoking, a proper change in diet and more exercise should do you no harm. Some suggestions on possible ingredients of an "anti-coronary life style" are:

1. Eat only small amounts of butter, cream, and fatty foods of all kinds.

2. Eat less meat than you are accustomed to, remove the fat from what you do eat, and broil the meat instead of frying it.

3. Eat no more than three eggs a week.

4. Eat plenty of fruit and vegetables but maintain a balanced diet.

5. Reduce your intake of salt. This advice is especially important if you have high blood pressure. A low salt diet may reduce both your blood pressure and the risk of coronary artery disease. If you are particularly fond of salt, do not despair. In time you will probably find that you will lose your craving.

6. Exercise regularly. There is some evidence that vigorous exercise two or more times a week diminishes the risk of heart disease. But, because sudden heavy exercise is dangerous, you must begin your exercise program gradually.

Professional help: If you have high blood pressure, your physician may prescribe drugs to lower it (see p.385). If you are a woman over 35 who takes birth control pills, and if you are also a heavy smoker, or have a family history of coronary heart disease, your physician will probably recommend a different form of contraception (see p.607).

If a blood test shows a high level of *cholesterol* or other fats in your blood, your physician may prescribe a drug to lower it. However, because such drugs may have unpleasant side-effects and must be taken constantly to be effective, most doctors prescribe them only if you have a very high cholesterol level or a high level that is combined with other predisposing factors.

A diseased coronary artery can sometimes be replaced by a length of vein from the patient's leg. This operation is called a coronary artery bypass (see p.378). The graft usually takes well because the surgeon uses your own tissue as opposed to tissue from a donor, which your body might reject . Such surgery may be recommended for active people who have been seriously disabled by painful angina. The graft may relieve the angina, but it does not control the underlying disease. And although the operation may be done on people of all ages, its success depends in part on your general health.

Angina

(angina pectoris)

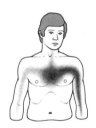

Site of the pain

Angina is not a disease in its own right. It is the name for pain that occurs when the muscular wall of the heart becomes temporarily short of oxygen. Normally, the coronary arteries that supply blood to the heart can cope with an increased demand, but this ability is restricted if you have coronary artery disease (see previous article) or high blood pressure (see p.382). Some other less common causes of angina are aortic stenosis (see p.398), anemia (see p.419) and hyperthyroidism (see p.525). If you have a condition that restricts the supply of oxygen to your heart, the supply may be adequate for some activities, but become inadequate when exercise, extremes of temperature, or strong emotion increase oxygen demand. When the oxygen requirement falls, the pain usually disappears.

What are the symptoms?

The main symptom of angina is pain in the center of your chest. The pain can spread to your throat and upper jaw, your back, and your arms (mainly the left one). Angina is a dull, heavy, constricting pain, which characteristically appears when you are active and fades when you stop activity and rest. Less commonly, the pain may occur only in your arms, wrists, or neck, but you can recognize it as angina if you know that it occurs whenever you are abnormally active or excited and disappears when you calm down. Additional symptoms that often accompany the pain are difficulty in breathing, sweating, nausea, and dizziness.

Angina is a common condition. In men it usually occurs after the age of 30 and it is nearly always caused by coronary artery disease. Angina tends to begin later in life for women. Although it is usually caused by coronary heart disease, some of the other causes of angina (anemia, for example) are more often found among women than they are among men.

What are the risks?

Since angina is a symptom rather than a disease, the risks are basically those of the condition that causes it. The heart may become so deprived of oxygen that there is a risk of heart attack (see next article). The angina may occur with less provocation as time goes by, and it may last longer. You may find that you have to become less and less active to avoid the pain.

What should be done?

If you think you are having attacks of angina, consult your physician. Some of the causes can be treated, and your physician can prescribe medication to help relieve the discomfort. *Consult your physician at once* if the pain of angina lasts longer than five minutes after you stop exercising, or if your attacks of chest pain are increasing rapidly in frequency, length, or severity. These are all signs that the condition is very severe and you are probably in great danger.

After examining you, the physician may take a blood specimen for tests to see if you have hyperthyroidism, anemia, or some other possible cause contributing to chest pain. You may need a separate blood test to determine the level of lipids, or fats, in your blood. For this test, the blood must be drawn in the morning before you have eaten. You may also need to have a urine test to determine if you have diabetes, since diabetics are particularly susceptible to heart disease. Diagnostic tests that may also be required include a chest *X-ray*, an *electrocardiogram* (*ECG*), a treadmill, or exercise tolerance, test and a coronary *angiogram* (sometimes called an arteriogram). The X-ray may show signs of heart strain such as an enlarged heart. The ECG will measure the electrical impulses arising in your heart and may confirm that the pain is indeed angina. Sometimes an ECG is done during or after exercise to see if the chest pain is related to exercise. The ECG will also help indicate how much of the heart muscle is affected by coronary artery disease. The angiogram, which involves injecting a dye into the bloodstream and then taking moving picture-type X-rays of the coronary arteries, can show exactly where the arteries are narrowed or blocked. Each spot will show up on the film as a constriction blocking the movement of the dye. Only after the results of all these tests are in can your physician determine the best course of treatment in your specific case.

What is the treatment?

Self-help: If you smoke, stop or cut down as much as you can. If you are overweight, go on a sensible diet (see p.28). Do not use your angina as an excuse to become inactive. You should certainly not reduce your physical activity unless your physician specifically advises you to do so.

Professional help: If and when the underlying cause of your angina is established, your physician will work toward relieving that condition. The angina will disappear or decrease if the treatment succeeds. Often, however, the underlying disorder is coronary artery disease, which cannot be "cured," and your physician will concentrate on preventing it from getting worse and on easing the discomfort and restrictions that are being caused by the angina itself.

Of the many drugs that effectively control or even prevent angina, the most commonly prescribed one is nitroglycerine, sometimes known as "nitro." What most people with angina find most surprising about this drug is the speed with which it usually works. In most cases it is literally only a matter of seconds between the time the tablet is put in the mouth and the relief of pain. If your physician prescribes this drug, make sure to keep your prescription up to date, because nitroglycerine tablets can lose their potency after only a few weeks, especially if the container is not sealed tightly. Your doctor will probably advise you to dissolve one tablet under your tongue the moment an anginal attack starts. Or if you know that some activity such as climbing the stairs at your office always brings on your angina, you can take a tablet shortly beforehand rather than waiting for the pain to occur. If you are under any psychological stress, you may also need to take a tranquilizer.

An unfortunate side-effect of the nitroglycerine is that it often causes temporary headaches. The headaches are usually mild, and not reason enough to discontinue the treatment. If you get severe headaches from

Medical myth

If you have angina, you must avoid exercise and lead the life of an invalid.

Wrong. Regular exercise is good for you, as long as you keep it within the limits imposed by the disorder. Experience and guidance from your physician will tell you how much you can do without pain. Do not be afraid, either, to participate in sexual intercourse if you desire to do so.

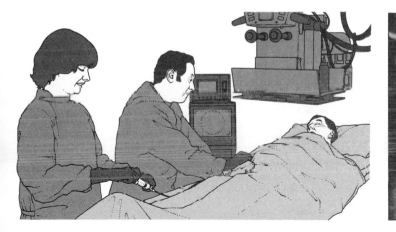

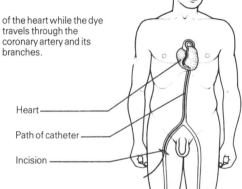

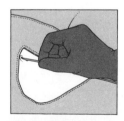

Coronary arteriography
A coronary arteriogram is done to discover where a coronary artery is narrowed or blocked. You will be sedated but conscious during the procedure. It involves injecting a dye, which shows up on an X-ray, into a coronary artery. A narrow tube (catheter) is inserted into an accessible artery, usually in the arm or groin, and then threaded up to the heart and into a coronary artery. To do this, the physician is guided by a picture on an X-ray screen. The special dye is then injected along the catheter. X-rays are taken of the heart while the dye travels through the coronary artery and its branches.

Inserting the catheter

Heart
Path of catheter
Incision

What the X-ray shows
The heart can be seen as a shadowy outline on the X-ray screen. The coronary artery and its branches show up as white lines while the dye flows through them. A narrowing of a line indicates the presence of plaque. Where a line stops abruptly, that part of the artery is completely blocked by atheroma or a clot.

taking a whole tablet, talk to your physician, who may suggest that you try reducing the dose by putting only part of a tablet under your tongue.

Among other drugs used for controlling angina, the most widely prescribed are a group known as the *beta-blockers*. Beta-blockers reduce the oxygen needs of the heart by reducing the heartbeat rate. One drawback of these drugs is that they must be taken exactly as prescribed, since an overdose can cause dizziness, fainting spells, and other unpleasant side-effects. Under certain circumstances, for example, if you have asthma, your doctor may not want to prescribe them.

Most patients with angina do not need, and might not benefit from, surgery. If, however, the angina is due to aortic stenosis, surgical valve replacement may be recommended. If your angina is caused by coronary artery disease, certain sections of your coronary network are blocked and your angina cannot be controlled by drugs, your physician may advise coronary artery bypass surgery. The operation can, in many cases, produce dramatic relief of symptoms.

What are the long-term prospects?

If you just found out that you have angina, and if you are otherwise in good health, you have a 50 per cent chance of living for another 10 to 12 years or more. The degree to which your life style will have to change depends on the cause and severity of the problem, your response to treatment and your normal degree of activity.

OPERATION: ## Coronary artery bypass

This operation is done to bypass a diseased coronary artery with a length of vein taken from the thigh. This relieves the pain associated with coronary artery disease but does not cure the underlying cause of the disease. The long-term effects of the operation are still being evaluated. **During the operation** You are under a general anesthetic, and for part of the time your circulation and breathing are taken over by a heart-lung machine. An incision is made down the length of your breastbone, and your ribcage is exposed to expose your heart. Meanwhile, a small incision is made in your leg, and a length of vein is removed. Wherever a blockage has been detected in the coronary arteries, a piece of this vein is grafted on to bypass the blockage. The usual operating time is four to five hours. **After the operation** You may spend a few days in an intensive-care unit, where your heartbeat will be constantly monitored. You will receive fluid and blood through intravenous drips. There will be surgical drains through tubes placed in your chest. You may need to breathe oxygen through a tube in your throat, and you may also need the help of a respirator. You will probably have to stay in the hospital for about two weeks. **Convalescence** You will need at least several weeks for convalescence, and as you recover, your physician will advise you on what activities you may participate in and when to start back to a regular routine.

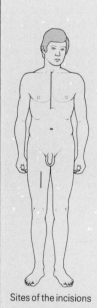

Sites of the incisions

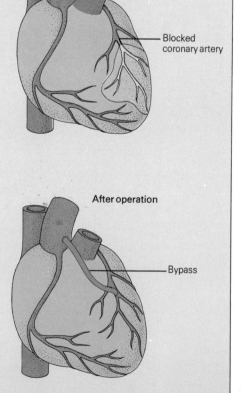

Before operation

Blocked coronary artery

After operation

Bypass

Heart attack

(coronary thrombosis, myocardial infarction)

The most common type of heart attack is caused by a thrombosis, or blockage, of one of the coronary arteries by a *thrombus*, or blood clot. This cuts off the blood supply to one region of the heart muscle. Lack of an adequate blood supply damages the deprived tissue. Heart attack generally occurs only if your coronary arteries are already narrowed by coronary artery disease (see p.374). If the size of the infarct, or damaged area of the heart, is small, and does not impair the electrical conducting system that regulates heartbeat, the attack should not be fatal and you will have a good chance of recovery.

In the United States there are more deaths from heart disease than from any other disorder. Heart attack is the most common cause of these deaths, but for every fatal heart attack there are at least two non-fatal ones. For most of this century the death rate from heart attack kept increasing in Western countries, but the rise stopped in the United States in the late 1960s and is now also slowing down in Europe. Some physicians attribute this improvement to greater awareness and adoption of the changes in life style that can prevent coronary disease.

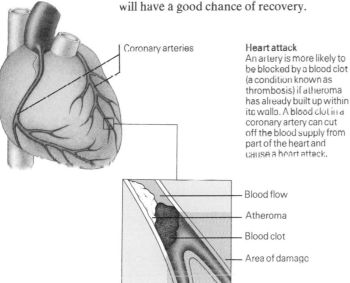

Coronary arteries

Heart attack
An artery is more likely to be blocked by a blood clot (a condition known as thrombosis) if atheroma has already built up within its wall. A blood clot in a coronary artery can cut off the blood supply from part of the heart and cause a heart attack.

Blood flow

Atheroma

Blood clot

Area of damage

What are the symptoms?

The main symptom of a heart attack is usually a crushing pain in the center of your chest. The pain may also appear in the neck, jaw, arms and stomach. A heart attack can come on gradually, preceded by a few weeks of angina (see previous article), but it can also happen without any warning. The pain may vary in degree from a feeling of tightness in the chest to an agonizing, bursting sensation. It may be continuous, or it may last for only a few minutes, then fade away, and then return. It may come on during exercise or emotional stress. Unlike the pain of angina, the pain that is brought on by a heart attack does not go away after the exercise or stress ceases.

Other possible symptoms of heart attack are dizziness, shortness of breath, sweating, chills, nausea and fainting. In a few instances, mainly in the elderly, there are few if any symptoms. This condition, which is known as a silent infarct, can be confirmed only by certain hospital tests.

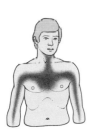

Site of the pain

What are the risks?

Two out of three people who have a heart attack recover, but the attack may be fatal if it interferes with the electrical impulses that regulate your heartbeat, or if it severely damages your heart muscle. Most deaths occur within two hours of the onset of symptoms. About ten per cent of patients admitted to hospitals with heart attacks go into shock (see p.386), which can also be fatal. Heart failure (see next article) may also develop.

After a heart attack, a thrombus, or clot, may form within one of the four chambers of the heart. If the thrombus becomes detached (it is then called an *embolus*) and is swept into the circulation, it can travel and cause damage elsewhere in the body. Fortunately, this rarely occurs, and even if it does, the embolus is usually too small to do much damage.

Damage caused by heart attack may weaken and stretch one of the walls of the heart chambers. The resultant aneurysms, or swellings, can lead to complications such as heart failure. There is the added risk that an enforced rest in bed may cause thrombosis in the veins, especially in the legs.

What should be done?

A heart attack is a medical emergency. Get professional help if you or anyone in your family seems to have the symptoms. Even if the discomfort is mild, do not try to travel to a physician. If your doctor is not immediately available, call an ambulance. While waiting for assistance, keep the person who is having the attack warm and calm. Do not leave him or her alone, because a comforting presence and reassurance are invaluable. If the affected person loses consciousness (see Cardiac arrest, p.388), do not give up. The problem may be only temporary. If someone with emergency training is present, the person's pulse should be taken, and if there is none, cardiopulmonary resuscitation, or CPR (see within Accidents and emergencies, p.801), should be given until help comes.

After a heart attack, most people are best off in a hospital. However, there is evidence that some patients do as well, or better, at home. A decision on what is best in your case will depend on your physician's assessment of the severity of the attack, how long you have had symptoms, and the facilities available both in and out of the hospital.

If you have had an attack, you may be put in an intensive-care or coronary-care unit of a hospital. There, or wherever you are, you will need to undergo a number of diagnostic tests, including an *electrocardiogram* (*ECG*). Several ECG recordings may be needed. In coronary-care units the ECG is continuously monitored. Blood specimens will also be taken at intervals to assess damage to your heart muscle. Your physician will also carry out other investigations to see whether drug treatment or a change in your way of life might help prevent another attack.

What is the treatment?

Self-help: None is possible.

Professional help: Your physician will probably try to control your pain with an analgesic drug, or painkiller. To reduce the risk of blood clots forming in the veins (see Deep-vein thrombosis, p.405), you may have to take a regular dose of an *anticoagulant* drug.

If your attack is a minor one, without complications, you may be allowed out of bed after 48 hours. Even if the attack is more serious, you will probably be permitted to use a bed-side commode or portable toilet almost as soon as treatment begins, since a certain amount of mobility is thought to reduce the risk of abnormal blood clotting.

What are the long-term prospects?

If you are reading this after having had a heart attack, the outlook is good. Mortality figures vary according to age and type of attack, but most deaths from heart attack occur within minutes or hours of the attack. This is why it is important to summon help immediately. If you show no sign of heart failure or disturbances of heart rhythm six hours after the pain disappears, you have an excellent chance of full recovery. If you are alive one month after even a severe attack, you have about an 85 per cent chance of surviving for at least a year and about a 70 per cent chance of surviving for five years.

After a heart attack you will naturally be concerned about your heart. It is important, though, not to be overly concerned. For comments about the best possible life style following a heart attack, see the accompanying box, After a heart attack.

After a heart attack

If you have just left the hospital after recovering from a heart attack, the most important thing to remember is that you are not an invalid. Damaged hearts heal, much as fractured bones do. Every month that passes improves your prospects for future health. Statistics show that ten years after a coronary thrombosis your life expectancy will be the same as if you had never had an attack.

You may find your activities limited by occasional pain in the chest (see Angina, p.376) or shortness of breath. If this is so, consult your physician, who can probably give you medication to relieve these symptoms. An operation is also a possibility (see p.378). If your physician has told you that you are well, it is more likely that you will find the only thing that is holding you back from your usual activities is your own anxiety. Whatever your job was before your heart attack, you will probably be able to return to it. Don't let well-meaning friends or colleagues persuade you to work part-time or take a less responsible job if your doctor says it is not necessary. There is no good evidence that such a move will help your health.

But how can you prevent another attack? Surely, you will say, there must have been something about your way of life that brought on the heart attack in the first place. If you

have a condition such as high blood pressure (see p.382) that may predispose you to circulatory-system disorders, cooperate with the treatment your physician recommends for it. For the most part, however, nobody knows why some people are affected and others are not. However, there are some guidelines for changes in behavior that most physicians believe will reduce your risk of further heart attacks.

1. Avoid sexual intercourse for four or five weeks after your attack, but do not be afraid to resume a full sex life thereafter, if you wish.
2. Do not smoke.
3. Keep your weight down to normal (see p.28), and eat less fat than usual.
4. Exercise regularly.

If you have not been accustomed to strenuous exercise, however, go gently. If you last played tennis 20 years ago, it would be unwise to take it up again. Start with something easier on you. Walking is ideal, but ultimately try to find a physical activity that you enjoy. You may be willing now to spend 20 minutes a day doing routine exercises before breakfast, but that enthusiasm is likely to fade. The "anti-coronary life style" can and should be enjoyable.

Heart failure

(and congestive heart failure)

In heart failure, the pumping action of your heart becomes inefficient, either because your heart muscle is weakened by disease or because there is a mechanical fault in the valves that control the flow of blood. Heart failure does not mean that your heart stops pumping, as in cardiac arrest, but that it is not working effectively.

Heart failure usually affects both sides of the heart, but sometimes affects only one side. When the entire heart is affected, the condition is known as *congestive* heart failure.

If your heart cannot pump out a normal volume, blood accumulates in the veins leading to it. In left-sided heart failure the blood accumulates in the veins that carry blood from the lungs. As a result, the lungs become swollen and congested with fluid. The fluid then passes from blood vessels into lung tissues (see Pulmonary edema, p.368). In right-sided heart failure blood accumulates in the veins that lead to the heart from other parts of the body. The affected parts, most obviously the legs, then become waterlogged.

Despite its name, heart failure is not an immediately life-threatening disease. The outcome depends on the seriousness of the underlying disorder and its treatment.

What are the symptoms?

Left-sided heart failure: The main symptom is breathlessness. At first you may feel breathless only after exercise, but the symptom becomes more and more apparent, especially in the evenings when you are tired. Because it may be hard to breathe when you lie down, you may need to sleep with several pillows under your head or even sitting up. Severe attacks of breathlessness can awaken you from sleep, and may become so bad that you want to lean out of a window to breathe fresh air. Difficult breathing is likely to be accompanied by wheezing. Bad attacks usually last no more than an hour, but the experience can be very disturbing.

Sometimes the lungs become so congested that you may hear a bubbling sound when you breathe. You may also have chest pain, and frothy, blood-flecked sputum, or phlegm. The fluid in your lungs decreases your resistance to infection; pneumonia (see p.359), for example, is a common complication of left-sided heart failure.

Right-sided heart failure: The most common symptom is fatigue, but this symptom is a sign of so many illnesses that on its own it is not a dependable indication of heart failure. A more reliable symptom is the swelling of the lowest part of your body from accummulation of fluid. If you are up and around, your ankles may swell. If you are bed-ridden, the swelling will be most noticeable in the lower part of your back. Internal organs such as the liver can also become swollen, and this can cause abdominal pain.

With congestive heart failure you are likely to have symptoms of both left-sided and right-sided heart failure. In addition, you may lose your appetite and experience mental confusion. As your blood supply fails, your arm and leg muscles will waste away, but this may not be apparent because of the swellings that accompany the condition.

What are the risks?

Untreated heart failure imposes a strain on your entire system that can be fatal. If heart failure is successfully treated, the main risks are those caused by the underlying disorder.

What should be done?

If you think you may have heart failure, see your physician, who will check your blood pressure and will probably have your blood and urine analyzed to find out whether your kidneys have been affected. Diagnostic tests may include a chest *X-ray* to look for lung problems and to check your heart size. An *electrocardiogram* (*ECG*) will help determine the type of heart problem, and there may be other tests that are appropriate for determining the underlying cause.

What is the treatment?

Self-help: Get plenty of rest to conserve energy. Although you should reduce your physical activities, do not let yourself become bedridden. A favorite armchair is better than a bed. An incident of heart failure does not mean you must lead a restricted life indefinitely. Treatment of heart failure and the underlying condition may eventually allow you to resume your normal activities.

Even while you are resting, keep your legs in motion by frequently shifting your position or relaxing and contracting your leg muscles. This helps because your circulation will be sluggish after you have heart failure, and your blood will tend to clot, especially in your legs and pelvis. The pumping action of your leg muscles helps move the blood along.

You should also cut down your daily intake of salt, because salt in your diet encourages fluid to stay in the body.

Professional help: Apart from treating the underlying cause, your physician can prescribe drugs that relieve your symptoms. Among these are *diuretics*, which cause you to pass more urine than usual and thus lower the fluid content of your body. It is usually

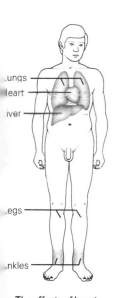

The effects of heart failure
Many parts of your body may be affected by heart failure. In left-sided failure, your lungs become congested. In right-sided failure, your liver, legs, ankles and a number of other parts of the body that accumulate fluid easily may be affected.

.ungs

.eart

iver

.egs

.nkles

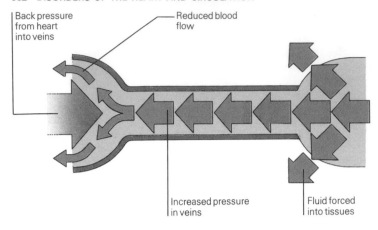

Back pressure from heart into veins

Reduced blood flow

Increased pressure in veins

Fluid forced into tissues

Heart failure forces fluid into tissues
When the heart fails, it is unable to maintain its normal output of blood. This, in turn, means that it can take in less blood from the vessels leading to it. These fill with a backlog of blood. The pressure then forces fluid into surrounding tissues.

best to take a diuretic in the morning, because most people find it more convenient to urinate frequently during the day than at night. Another drug commonly used in heart failure improves the strength of the heartbeat, especially if you have an irregularity of rhythm. Your physician will carefully control how much you take of the drug and when you take it, since too much of it can make you feel nauseous and cause other problems. It is important that you follow the doctor's instructions and do not discontinue the drugs until you are told to do so, even though you may feel you no longer need them.

If you must have a long period of bed rest, you may also need to take an *anticoagulant*, a drug that keeps blood from clotting. If your physician prescribes an anticoagulant, your blood must be tested at intervals to make sure the dose is correct. An overdose of such drugs

can cause bleeding into the intestines, skin, brain or other organs of the body.

Acute, or sudden, heart failure, with extremely severe breathlessness, is a medical emergency. If this occurs, you must go straight to a hospital, where oxygen can be administered and drugs given by injection to help relieve the symptoms quickly.

What are the long-term prospects?
With drug treatment your symptoms of breathlessness and swelling should subside. If you carefully follow a salt-free diet and take your medications regularly, you can probably expect many years of nearly normal life ahead of you. If heart failure reaches a point where it no longer responds to rest, diet and drugs, however, there is one other very rare form of treatment that offers some hope: heart transplantation. Replacing diseased hearts with healthy ones taken from accident victims has proved effective in certain cases, but the operation is still quite rare and experimental (see Transplants, p.402).

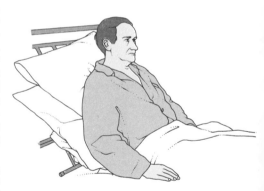

Coping with breathlessness
If you have left-sided heart failure, you may find it difficult to breathe when you lie down. To ease this, prop yourself up with several pillows.

High blood pressure
(hypertension)

As your heart pumps blood through your arteries, the force of the blood flow exerts pressure on the arterial walls, just as air pumped into a tire exerts pressure on its lining and surface. And just as too much air pressure is bad for the life of a tire, so too much blood pressure eventually damages your arteries. If your heart pumps blood through your circulatory system with a force that is much greater than necessary to maintain a steady flow, you have hypertension, or high blood pressure. This puts your whole circulatory system under a strain that may ultimately cause great problems.

Blood pressure varies from person to person and even in different parts of your body. For example, it is higher in your legs than in your arms. For the sake of convenience, it is usually measured in one of the large arteries of one or both arms (see p.384). Two types of pressure, *systolic* and *diastolic*, are measured. Systolic pressure is the peak pressure at the moment when your heart contracts in the process of pumping out blood. Diastolic pressure is the pressure at a moment when your heart relaxes to permit the inflow of blood. Thus the systolic figure, which represents the moment of greatest pressure, is always higher than the diastolic figure. If someone tells you that your blood pressure is 120 over 80, this means that your systolic pressure is 120, and your diastolic 80. Those figures are within the normal range for a healthy young adult. (See also Low blood pressure, p.417.)

Whether you have high blood pressure depends largely on medical judgment of your individual case. For instance, if you are over 65, and your blood pressure reading is 140/90, your physician may consider this to be normal pressure for you, since blood pressure tends to rise with age. But when you are in a relatively calm emotional and physical state and your blood pressure exceeds 150/100, there is probably cause for concern. Even if only one of the two figures is high, especially the diastolic figure, you may have high blood pressure.

There are actually two different types of high blood pressure, essential hypertension and secondary hypertension. In essential hypertension, you have raised blood pressure for no apparent reason. In secondary hypertension, the cause of the disorder has been identified by your physician. Some possible causes of hypertension are kidney disease, hormonal disorders such as Cushing's disease (see p.523) and aldosteronism (see p.524), and changes in the body produced by taking oral contraceptives (see p.607) or becoming pregnant (see p.624).

Essential hypertension is more common than secondary hypertension. A tendency toward essential hypertension seems to run in families. In other words, blood pressure appears to be influenced by heredity as well as by life style. It also seems likely that people who are overweight when they are young are more apt to have high blood pressure in middle age than their lean contemporaries, and that there is a link between high blood pressure and high salt intake. If you are hypertensive and overweight, you may be able to lower your blood pressure by reducing your weight and the amount of salt that you consume in your diet.

In most cases of hypertension, the blood pressure rises steadily over a number of years unless it is treated. Occasionally, however, an exceedingly high blood pressure develops very quickly. This dangerous condition, which can be either essential or secondary, is known as malignant hypertension. It is perhaps significant that malignant hypertension is most often found among smokers.

What are the symptoms?

High blood pressure is nearly always a symptomless disease. If you have hypertension,

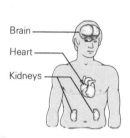

Organs affected by high blood pressure
High blood pressure, left untreated, can lead to heart failure or kidney failure. It can also affect vessels in the brain, causing a stroke.

Brain
Heart
Kidneys

you may feel fine, without the slightest indication of physical problems. Such symptoms as headaches, palpitations, and a general feeling of ill health usually occur only when your blood pressure is dangerously high. So it is risky to wait for treatment until symptoms develop. If you have malignant hypertension, you are more likely to have the symptoms described above.

You should always be aware that you may have high blood pressure, especially if you are over 40, if there is a history of hypertension in your family, and if you are overweight.

High blood pressure is extremely common, especially in North America. One study suggests that one in ten Americans is hypertensive. The incidence rises steeply with age and appears to be twice as high among black Americans as among whites. The study also indicates that women are only about one-half to three-quarters as likely to have high blood pressure as men. Above 95 per cent of all investigated cases, not including those resulting from pregnancy or the use of oral contraceptives, were cases of essential rather than secondary hypertension. Malignant hypertension is rare, but it does require rapid diagnosis and treatment.

What are the risks?

Even mild hypertension will lower your life expectancy to some degree if you do not get treatment for it. If you have untreated severe hypertension, the disorder may shorten your life considerably. In particular there are major risks to the heart and brain in such cases. Untreated malignant hypertension can be fatal within six months.

The reason high blood pressure is dangerous is that increased pressure in the circulatory system forces your heart to work harder to keep your blood moving. This extra work can damage the inner lining of your coronary arteries. Over a period of years fatty tissue called *atheroma* is likely to form where damage has occurred, and your coronary arteries may become narrowed or even close up completely. The result may be a heart attack (see p.379). Congestive heart failure (see previous article) is also a possible consequence. If you have hypertension, you are six times more likely to develop heart failure than someone who has normal blood pressure.

Moreover, if you have high blood pressure, your chances of having a stroke (see p.268) are four times greater than they would be if your blood pressure were normal. This is because increased blood pressure can lead to the formation of atheroma in the arteries that supply the brain with blood.

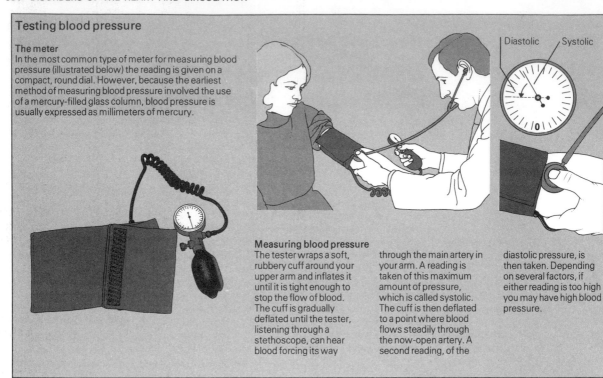

Testing blood pressure

The meter
In the most common type of meter for measuring blood pressure (illustrated below) the reading is given on a compact, round dial. However, because the earliest method of measuring blood pressure involved the use of a mercury-filled glass column, blood pressure is usually expressed as millimeters of mercury.

Diastolic   Systolic

Measuring blood pressure
The tester wraps a soft, rubbery cuff around your upper arm and inflates it until it is tight enough to stop the flow of blood. The cuff is gradually deflated until the tester, listening through a stethoscope, can hear blood forcing its way through the main artery in your arm. A reading is taken of this maximum amount of pressure, which is called systolic. The cuff is then deflated to a point where blood flows steadily through the now-open artery. A second reading, of the diastolic pressure, is then taken. Depending on several factors, if either reading is too high you may have high blood pressure.

Your kidneys may also be damaged, especially if you have malignant hypertension. Damage to your kidneys (see Chronic kidney failure, p.512) also leads to a further rise in blood pressure. The brain, eyes and other organs also can be affected by damage to the blood vessels that supply them with needed oxygen and nutrients.

High blood pressure during pregnancy (see p.624) should be treated. If it is allowed to persist, high blood pressure can decrease the efficiency of the *placenta*, which supplies the fetus, or unborn child, with nourishment.

What should be done?
Have your blood pressure checked once a year. However, if you are taking oral contraceptives or estrogen pills, or if you are pregnant, you should have your blood pressure checked more frequently. Some large department stores and drug stores now have do-it-yourself machines for testing blood pressure. Also, many health, community, and work organizations sponsor free blood pressure screening programs.

Even if you show signs of high blood pressure at a first examination, your physician may want to test your pressure again before treating you. Because exertion, excitement, or some other physical or psychological factor can result in a misleading reading at a given moment, it is preferable not to make an immediate diagnosis. In a second examination the physician will probably pay special attention to your chest and pulse rate. The physician may also spend a few minutes looking into your eyes with an *ophthalmoscope*, because the blood vessels on your retina are the only blood vessels that can be seen without elaborate equipment, and their condition often gives valuable information about the effects of abnormally high blood pressure.

Further investigation will depend on your age and whether your physician needs to check if your case is essential or secondary hypertension. You may be given a chest *X-ray* to determine whether your heart has become enlarged, an *electrocardiogram (ECG)* to check other aspects of your heart, and blood and urine tests to see if you have kidney trouble. If your doctor needs further information, you may also have an *intravenous pyelogram (IVP)*, a test in which dye is injected into your body and your kidneys are examined by X-ray.

What is the treatment?
Self-help: Secondary hypertension will generally be eliminated when and if the primary cause is treated successfully. If the primary cause cannot be dealt with, the treatment should be the same as it would be for essential

Assessing the condition of blood vessels
Blood vessels on your retina can be examined easily by a physician with an ophthalmoscope. Since these vessels are representative of the others in your body, they are used as a fast and easy check of general circulation.

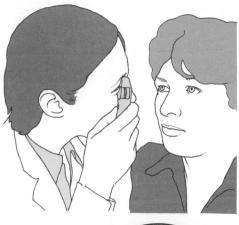

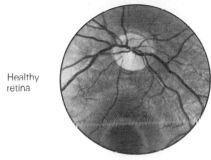

Healthy retina

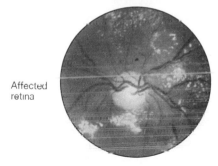

Affected retina

height, and then try to maintain that weight. Again, there is no firm evidence that hypertension is kept under control by weight reduction alone, but we do know that thin people are hypertensive less often than those who are overweight, and thin people are less likely to get certain serious diseases that are linked with hypertension.

3. Do not salt your food, and give up salt-rich foods such as salami and pickles, and salted foods such as potato chips and nuts.

4. Try to make your work schedule and recreation less demanding, and learn to side step crises. Some studies indicate that a person who is always pressing ahead to the next objective, talks rather than listens, and constantly looks at his watch is at greater risk of all heart and circulatory disease.

5. Drink alcohol in moderation. Some people maintain that small quantities of alcohol help lower blood pressure. There is no convincing evidence that this is so, but, in any case, small amounts of alcohol will probably do you no harm.

Professional help: If self-help does not lower your blood pressure to a normal range, you will need some form of drug treatment. The drugs used to treat hypertension must always be administered under the supervision of a physician. Continue your self-help measures, however, since all these drugs may have side-effects, and in general the lower the dose you need, the less chance you will have of experiencing the side-effects.

Since essential hypertension is usually a symptomless disease, you may be tempted to stop taking the drugs because you do not feel ill. Because high blood pressure cannot be cured, you will probably have to go on taking regular doses of medicine for the rest of your life. This may mean growing accustomed to some unpleasant side-effects of the medication. For instance, many of the drugs that are commonly prescribed for hypertension lessen the body's normal response to sudden changes in posture. Thus when you suddenly stand up from a sitting position, there may be a slight delay before the extra blood needed to adjust to the change is pumped to the brain. This may cause a temporary feeling of faintness or even an actual faint. Other side-effects may include a dry mouth, a stuffy nose, headaches or drowsiness.

For all these reasons your physician will not put you on drugs without being satisfied that you really need the treatment. Research has shown that it is best to prescribe a lifelong course of drugs for any comparatively young person with a diastolic blood pressure of 105 or more. In some cases, though, it may be

hypertension, which, although it cannot be cured, can be controlled.

In many cases, changes in your weight, diet and life style can lead to satisfactory lowering of the blood pressure without the use of drugs. Here are some suggestions of what you can do to accomplish this.

1. If you smoke, give it up, or at least cut down as much as possible. A link between cigarette smoking and hypertension has not yet been firmly established, but there *is* a link between smoking and coronary artery disease. Since we know that the chances of heart trouble are increased by both cigarettes and high blood pressure, by giving up smoking you can halve the risk instead of doubling it.

2. If you are overweight, choose a moderate reducing diet (see p.28), stick to it until you reach a suitable weight for your age, sex and

advisable to do so if the reading for diastolic pressure is only above 90.

Your doctor will base the decision on a number of considerations such as your age, general state of health, and sex (women appear to be less susceptible than men to the complications that result from hypertension). When the decision has been made, it is important that you both agree to the treatment, and that you follow your physician's instructions carefully and completely.

One group of drugs, the *diuretics*, are often used first in treating hypertension. A diuretic helps reduce your blood pressure by expelling fluid from your body, thus lowering the volume of the blood. Diuretics make you urinate frequently, so it is a good idea to take them in the morning rather than at bedtime. Some diuretics also cause you to lose potassium, which must be replaced by supplements or by eating foods that are rich in potassium, such as oranges, bananas or other fruits. If diuretic medications do not control your high blood pressure, your physician will probably prescribe other drugs that work in different ways to lower blood pressure. It is extremely important that you follow your physician's directions in taking these medications. High blood pressure is a serious disease that can be overcome by a working partnership between you and your doctor. If you develop any unpleasant side-effects or become tired of taking these medications, perhaps because there are no obvious results, discuss these problems with your physician.

What are the long-term prospects?

If you have had high blood pressure, but you control it carefully, you will avoid nearly all risk of heart failure and considerably reduce the likelihood of stroke. The effect of control on the chance of having a coronary thrombosis, or heart attack, is less clear-cut, probably because many other factors are involved, and the damage to the coronary circulation that is caused by high blood pressure is irreversible. Even so, it is logical to conclude that since your heart works under less strain when your blood pressure is lowered, you are less likely to suffer a heart attack than you were before treatment for the disorder brought it under control.

Generally, the outlook is good if you have hypertension but you are being treated for it successfully. Regular visits to your physician and careful attention to your physician's instructions are an important part of effective treatment for this disorder.

Shock

For medical purposes shock is defined as a condition in which the flow of blood throughout the body becomes suddenly inadequate, and vital parts, deprived of oxygen, cease to function, at least briefly. This usually happens for one of three reasons. One is that your heart fails to pump out a sufficient supply of blood. This is called cardiogenic shock. The second possible reason for shock is loss of blood or some other body fluid, to the point where there is not enough blood in your body to maintain pressure. This can be the result of an injury, some disorder such as a perforated ulcer (see p.468), a bad burn or prolonged diarrhea. This is called hypovolemic shock. The third possible cause of shock is that the diameter of your blood vessels may become so large that there is a relative shortage of blood, even though the actual quantity has not diminished. This may be the result of an intense allergic reaction or a severe infection; it is called anaphylactic, or septic, shock.

If shock develops, your body's condition enters a dangerous downward spiral. Lack of blood flowing to the brain deprives it of oxygen. As the brain becomes affected, the blood vessels become over-dilated and unresponsive because the nervous system cannot control blood vessel diameter as it normally does. The blood pressure then drops even further because your blood vessels are enlarged. Once in this downward spiral, your body cannot recover by itself.

What are the symptoms?

The symptoms of shock include sweating, faintness, nausea, panting, rapid pulse rate, and pale, cold, moist skin. Blood pressure plummets to levels far below what is needed (see Low blood pressure, p.417). As the blood supply to the brain falls, the person in shock becomes drowsy and confused, and may also lose consciousness.

What are the risks?

Apart from accident victims, the people most likely to go into shock are those with internal bleeding from any cause, severe blood poisoning (see p.421), heart or lung disorders that can lead to heart attack (see p.379), massive pericardial effusion (see Acute pericarditis, p.401) or a severe attack of asthma (see p.355).

Untreated shock leads to death because the body cannot recover on its own. Since the

Shock and circulation

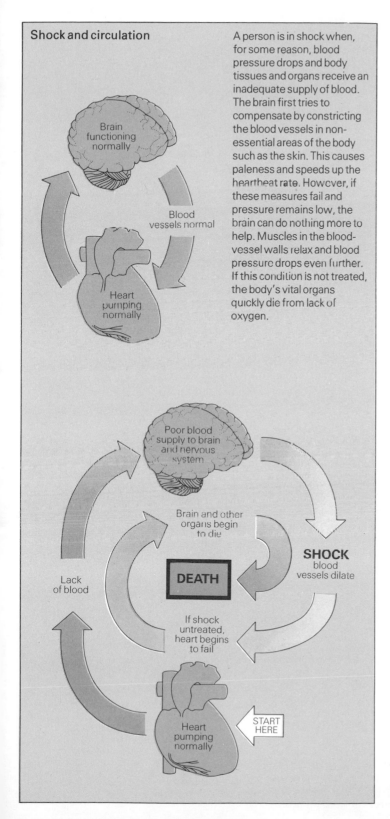

A person is in shock when, for some reason, blood pressure drops and body tissues and organs receive an inadequate supply of blood. The brain first tries to compensate by constricting the blood vessels in non-essential areas of the body such as the skin. This causes paleness and speeds up the heartbeat rate. However, if these measures fail and pressure remains low, the brain can do nothing more to help. Muscles in the blood-vessel walls relax and blood pressure drops even further. If this condition is not treated, the body's vital organs quickly die from lack of oxygen.

Brain functioning normally

Blood vessels normal

Heart pumping normally

Poor blood supply to brain and nervous system

Brain and other organs begin to die

SHOCK blood vessels dilate

Lack of blood

DEATH

If shock untreated, heart begins to fail

START HERE

Heart pumping normally

brain can function for only a few minutes without oxygen, prolonged shock can cause brain damage even if you otherwise recover physically. The kidneys are also affected quickly by lack of blood. Acute kidney failure (see p.511) can cause death even if recovery procedures begin within minutes. The chances for recovery from hypovolemic shock are fairly good if the underlying cause is dealt with immediately. But other types of shock are more likely to be fatal.

What should be done?

If someone is in shock, get professional medical aid right away. People who are in shock cannot do anything at all for themselves. For advice on what to do while awaiting help, read the article on shock within Accidents and emergencies (see p.801).

As soon as possible, the person in shock will be hospitalized, probably in an intensive care unit. Here the medical staff has special equipment available, such as a continuous blood-pressure recorder, which operates by a tube inserted into a vein, and a continuous *electrocardiogram* (*ECG*) recorder. Such equipment gives some immediate information on the patient's condition. The main tasks of the physician are, first, to stabilize the patient, second, to assess how severe the shock is, and third, to identify the cause.

What is the treatment?

In most cases the first goal of treatment is to restore blood pressure to normal, so that body organs get enough blood to stay alive. The physician inserts a fine tube into a vein, usually in the arm, and connects the tube to a container of plasma or blood that is matched to the patient's blood type (see p.428). This raises the volume of blood and, thus, the blood pressure. If the brain is not already damaged, it responds by regaining control of blood-vessel tone and diameter. In many cases, the kidneys receive particular attention to prevent the onset of kidney failure.

When emergency procedures have restored blood pressure to nearly normal levels, treatment for the underlying condition can begin. What that treatment is will depend on the severity and cause of the condition. For example, an operation may be carried out to repair a bleeding ulcer, or high doses of *antibiotics* may be injected into the bloodstream to combat severe infection. The prospects for a full recovery usually depend partly on the underlying cause and partly on the swiftness and effectiveness of whatever emergency treatment is given during the crucial minutes when the body is in shock.

Heart rate and rhythm

The muscles of the heart must contract in unison for the heart to function effectively as a pump. Your heart has four chambers: the left and right atria on the top; and the left and right ventricles on the bottom. Valves between these chambers keep the blood moving between them in the proper direction, but it is electrical impulses from a group of cells in the right atrium that help control the muscle contractions. These electrical impulses flow swiftly along nerve pathways that branch out in all directions to the muscles in all four chambers of the heart. If some portion of this complex conducting system goes wrong, the regular rhythmic pace of your heartbeats is disturbed, and one of the disorders that are described in the following group of articles may be the result.

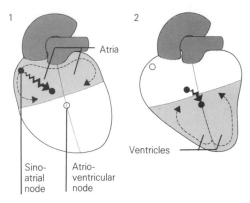

1

Atria

Sino-
atrial
node

Atrio-
ventricular
node

2

Ventricles

The electrical impulse that initiates a heartbeat originates at the sino-atrial node, passes through the atria walls to the atrioventricular node and is relayed to the ventricles.

Cardiac arrest
(and ventricular fibrillation)

In cardiac arrest, your heart stops beating. When your heart stops, your brain no longer gets the blood it needs to function, and you lose consciousness immediately. Cardiac arrest in someone who seems to be in good health is usually due to unsuspected coronary artery disease (see p.374). Cardiac arrest is sometimes caused by a disorder of rhythm known as ventricular fibrillation, which occurs if the muscles of the ventricles, or the two lower chambers of your heart, twitch without coordination and without effective pumping.

What should be done?
If cardiac arrest occurs when nobody else is present, it is fatal. However, it is possible to recover if the heartbeat and circulation can be restored by cardiac massage within a few minutes. For example, a person trained in cardiopulmonary rescuscitation (CPR) often can help to revive someone whose heart has stopped until he or she can be taken to the hospital. For information on this life-saving technique, read the section on Accidents and emergencies (see p.801) *before* an emergency of this kind occurs. Whether you are trained in CPR or not, have someone call for an ambulance immediately when a person around you suffers cardiac arrest.

The prospects for recovery from cardiac arrest are good if treatment is given promptly and the circulation is kept going until the victim reaches the hospital. If the cardiac arrest is caused by ventricular fibrillation, the heartbeat can often be restored with a defibrillator, an apparatus that briefly passes an electric current through the heart.

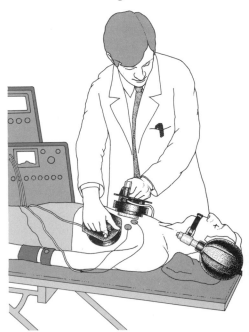

Using a defibrillator to restart the heart
A defibrillator sends an electrical shock to the heart via two metal plates placed on the chest wall. This method of restarting a stopped heart mimics the natural process in which impulses from the right atrium spread throughout the heart in the normal beating of the heart.

Atrial fibrillation and flutter

If you have atrial fibrillation, the muscles in the two atria, or upper chambers of the heart, contract at a rate of about 400 pulsations a minute. This is much too fast. The muscles in the ventricles, the two lower chambers of the heart, cannot contract faster than about 160 times a minute, and they are unable to keep pace with the atria. Atrial fibrillation reduces the efficiency of the heart as a pump, because the rapid atrial contractions push out too little blood. As a result, the ventricles have a shorter filling period, and the action of the upper and lower chambers of the heart is not coordinated.

Atrial flutter is the same as fibrillation, except that in atrial flutter the muscles contract more regularly and at a somewhat slower rate (up to about 300 beats a minute). Both fibrillation and flutter tend to come and go, with periods of normal heart function between attacks.

Atrial fibrillation and flutter usually occur as a consequence of coronary artery disease (see p.374) or heart disease brought on by rheumatic fever (see p.393). The fibrillation or flutter can also be caused by an over-active thyroid gland or a high fever. In about ten per cent of cases, especially among elderly persons, there is no obvious cause.

What are the symptoms?
Often there are no symptoms. The most common symptom is palpitations, or an enhanced awareness of your heartbeat. If you have atrial fibrillation, you may also experience dizziness, occasional attacks of angina (see p.376), and fainting spells. You may also develop some or all of the symptoms of heart failure (see p.381).

What are the risks?
One danger of atrial fibrillation or flutter is an increased risk of *embolism*. If a blood clot forms in either atrium, the clot may break into small pieces, which may travel through the circulatory system to a point where their size prevents them from going any further. This is called an embolism. It can block all flow of blood beyond that point. The damage caused by such an embolism depends on its size and location.

Another possible risk is heart failure. Normally, even though the atria are not functioning well, the ventricles alone can cope with the task of pumping blood. However, the ventricles are not pumping at maximum efficiency, so heart failure may develop with atrial fibrillation, especially if the ventricles are also diseased.

What should be done?
If you suffer from symptoms associated with either of these disorders, consult your physician, who will probably recommend an *electrocardiogram (ECG)*. Since atrial fibrillation is often intermittent, you may need to have a continuous ECG recording for 24 to 48 hours. This is done with lightweight, portable equipment, so that you can carry on normal activities while the recording is being made. Your physician may order other diagnostic tests for you if you show any signs of a possible underlying heart disorder.

What is the treatment?
Self-help: None is possible.

Professional help: Treatment largely depends on the cause of the disorder. A drug is usually prescribed to improve the efficiency of ventricular contractions, because your circulation will depend on efficient pumping by your ventricles if your atrial contractions are faulty. Drugs called *beta-blockers* are used to treat atrial flutter or fibrillation that is associated with thyroid disease. Your doctor may also prescribe an *anticoagulant* drug to prevent an embolism.

If your heart is basically healthy, or if the underlying cause of atrial fibrillation has been treated successfully and atrial flutter or fibrillation persists, your physician may consider a treatment sometimes called *electroversion*. This consists of an electric shock administered to your heart while you are under mild anesthesia. This treatment frequently restores normal heart rhythm.

Ectopic heartbeats

The word "ectopic" comes from a Greek word meaning "out of place." Ectopic heartbeats are simply small irregularities in an otherwise steady pulsation. If you feel that your heart has missed a beat, or gained an extra beat, you are experiencing this common and usually minor disorder. Do not worry about it. Usually, the condition is harmless, and does not require treatment.

If you find the occasional irregularities troublesome, though, your physician may prescribe a drug for the condition. Frequent ectopic heartbeats are often associated with excessive use of tobacco, alcohol or caffeine. If the condition bothers you, try cutting down on smoking and on drinking alcohol and coffee along with other caffeine-containing beverages such as cola soft drinks.

Heart block

Your heartbeat rate usually is controlled by a natural pacemaker, which consists of a group of specialized cells in the wall of the right atrium, or upper right chamber of the four heart chambers. This pacemaker transmits electrical impulses over the two atria, and ultimately to the ventricles. These impulses cause the rhythmic contractions of heart muscle that we call heartbeats. Heart block occurs when some abnormality in the system that conducts these impulses throughout the heart muscles causes the system to fail, either partially or completely. Then the beating of the atria, or the upper half of your heart, is not coordinated with the beating of the ventricles, or the lower half of your heart.

In first degree block the conduction of the heartbeat impulses is slower than normal, but it causes no symptoms. In second degree block some of the atrial impulses fail to get through to the ventricles, and your pulse becomes irregular. In the disorder known as third degree heart block, the impulses are not conducted at all, and the ventricles go on beating independently of the pacemaker and the atria. Normally your heartbeat rate, the pulse you can feel or hear in your arms or chest, quickens to cope with exertion or emotion. But during heart block this no longer happens. As a result, your heart pumps too little oxygenated blood to your brain and other parts of your body at times when a greater supply is needed.

Heart block can occur for no obvious reason, but it is often associated with coronary thrombosis, or heart attack (see p.379). An overdose of the drug digitalis can also cause heart block.

What are the symptoms?
There are often no symptoms of heart block. If you do not exercise much and do not experience emotional upsets, you may never know you have this disorder. On the other hand, complete, or third degree, heart block sometimes produces symptoms similar to those of heart failure (see p.381). The most severe symptoms are caused by what are called Stokes-Adams attacks. The main symptom of a Stokes-Adams type of heart block is sudden loss of consciousness, which is often accompanied by convulsions. Such attacks can occur if the ventricles are beating without any control from the pacemaker cells, and either slow down drastically or miss a few beats, not pumping enough blood to keep the brain functioning normally.

What are the risks?
There is very little risk that a minor degree of heart block will have serious consequences. Before the artificial pacemaker, an electrical device that can take over the job of your natural pacemaker, you would have had a 50 per cent chance of living for more than a year if you had third degree heart block. Today the odds are more favorable. The mortality rate for people who have Stokes-Adams attacks is still relatively high, but advances in the artificial pacemakers are constantly reducing these risks.

What should be done?
If you have attacks of extreme weakness and breathlessness, you may have heart block. If you have these symptoms, especially if you have episodes of unconsciousness, consult your physician without delay.

What is the treatment?
For many forms of heart block, no treatment is necessary. Even complete heart block may not require treatment if you do not have any symptoms. Heart block associated with coronary thrombosis, Stokes-Adams attacks or other serious problems is generally controlled with an artificial pacemaker. For more about pacemakers, see next page.

Paroxysmal tachycardia

If you are a healthy adult, your heart beats 50 to 100 times a minute, and rises to about 160 a minute during periods of exertion. If you have an attack, or paroxysm, of tachycardia, your heartbeat suddenly speeds up to a rate of 160 or more pulsations a minute. An attack of paroxysmal tachycardia can last for a minute or for several days.

What are the symptoms?
The main symptom of this disorder is palpitations, or enhanced awareness of your heartbeat. You suddenly become aware of your rapid heartbeats, and you may become anxious. Some people who have paroxysmal tachycardia say it is accompanied by a false premonition of impending death. Additional symptoms of the disorder may include breathlessness, fainting spells, chest pain, and abnormally frequent urination.

What are the risks?
Despite any anxiety or fright, paroxysmal tachycardia is not usually a serious disorder. There is a slight risk of congestive heart failure (see p.381) but there is usually no danger.

What should be done?

When you get the pounding feeling in the chest that characterizes paroxysmal tachycardia, you may be alarmed, especially if this is your first attack. Although there is little cause for concern, you should see your physician if the symptoms last for more than a few minutes. You may have an underlying disorder such as atrial fibrillation (see p.389), and it is easier to diagnose the basic trouble if the physician can examine you during an attack.

If you are young to middle-aged, with no background of heart trouble, tachycardia is unlikely to be serious. Try to relax, and practice the self-help measures suggested below. If, however, you get recurrent attacks, they may be worrisome and exhausting, and you probably should seek help. After examining you, the physician may order an *electrocardiogram (ECG)* to confirm the diagnosis and rule out other possible causes of palpitations.

What is the treatment?

Self-help: Heartbeat rate can be slowed down by certain nerve impulses, which can be induced in several ways. Try holding your breath for a while, or taking a slow drink of water, or bathing your face in cold water. If none of these measures works, it may help if you hold your nostrils closed and try to blow through your nose, which will make your eardrums "pop."

If you have had an attack of paroxysmal tachycardia, you may want to take some preventive measures against further attacks. Cigarettes, alcohol, tea and coffee may all increase your susceptibility. Try cutting down on whichever of these you usually use. There also seems to be a link between anxiety and tachycardia, but it is unclear whether anxiety causes tachycardia or vica versa.

Professional help: Your physician may massage an artery in your neck; a gentle pressure here will slow down the heart. If your attack warrants further treatment, your physician may give you an injection of a drug that combats rapid heartbeat. In extreme cases, your physician may advise you to have what is sometimes called *electroversion*, a procedure in which an electric shock is administered to your heart directly, while you are under a mild anesthetic.

As preventive medical treatment, your doctor may prescribe drugs that decrease the excitability of the heart muscle. These help keep your heart from speeding up.

Pacemakers

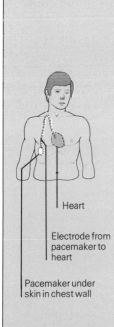

Heart

Electrode from pacemaker to heart

Pacemaker under skin in chest wall

A pacemaker is a device that provides an artificial, regular electrical impulse to replace an irregular or absent natural impulse in your heart. It is used to treat disorders such as heart block. An electrode is placed in contact with your heart wall, either directly or through a thin tube pushed into your circulatory system from a convenient vein. This electrode is connected to a small generating unit powered by a battery with a life span of up to 12 years, depending on what type of battery is used.

If a pacemaker is required for only a short time, such as when a heart attack temporarily disturbs your heart rhythm, you can wear the pacemaker's generating unit on a belt. Otherwise it is implanted under your skin, usually in the loose tissues of your chest wall. If you have a pacemaker, you should be examined at intervals by your physician to make sure the device is working well. Checks by telephone using special equipment are also possible. A battery that is low on power can be replaced quickly and easily.

Modern pacemakers are remarkably resistant to outside interference. If you have a pacemaker, however, you should stay away from powerful radio or radar transmitters, and avoid going through security devices at airports, shops and libraries. Some models can be influenced by electromagnetic impulses from microwave ovens, electric shavers, auto magnetos and the like. If you undergo surgery, your surgeon may also need to take certain precautions since some *diathermy* techniques for controlling bleeding can adversely affect the function of your pacemaker.

Positioning a pacemaker
The pacemaker wire is fed to your heart along a vein that runs close to your collar bone. If the pacemaker is permanent, the physician will insert it under the skin on your chest wall.

Heart valve diseases

The heart has four valves. The mitral valve controls the flow of blood from the left atrium (one of two chambers in the top of the heart) into the left ventricle (one of two chambers in the bottom of the heart). The tricuspid valve is the equivalent of the mitral valve on the right side. The pulmonary valve controls the exit from the right ventricle into the pulmonary artery, which carries blood into the lungs. The aortic valve controls the output of blood from the left ventricle into the aorta, the artery through which blood flows to the body. Inflammation of a valve can cause stenosis or incompetence. Stenosis is a thickening of the valve, which narrows the valve's opening. Incompetence is a distortion of the valve, which prevents it from closing fully.

The diseases described here involve stenosis or incompetence, except for rheumatic fever and bacterial endocarditis. They are included because they are common causes of heart valve disease.

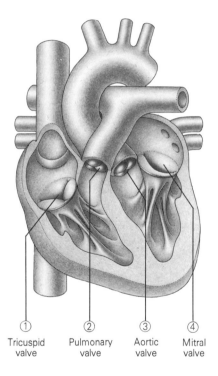

Tricuspid valve Pulmonary valve Aortic valve Mitral valve

How the valves work
With each heartbeat the ventricles contract and force the blood out of the heart. The aortic and pulmonary valves open to let the blood out.

Between heartbeats the ventricles relax and the aortic and pulmonary valves close. The mitral and tricuspid valves then open to allow blood to flow into the heart from the veins. The constant and regular repetition of this cycle keeps the blood flowing throughout your body.

Blood out

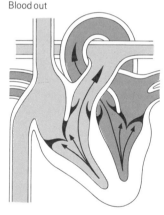

Valves ② and ③ open
Blood pumped out of heart to lungs and body tissues

Blood in

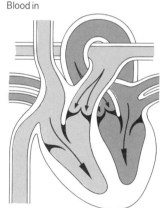

Valves ① and ④ open
Blood passes into the heart from the body tissues and the lungs

What can go wrong
When a valve does not open wide enough, the heart must generate more pressure to pump through an adequate supply of blood. When a valve does not close completely, some of the blood that has flowed through it leaks back into the heart, which must pump it out again. Both conditions increase the heart's work load and can lead to heart failure.

Normal opening

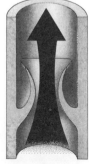

Inadequate opening (stenosis)

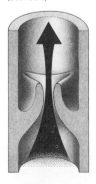

Normal closing

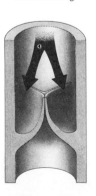

Inadequate closing (incompetence)

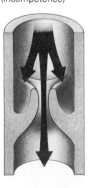

Rheumatic fever

Rheumatic fever is not technically a heart disorder since it affects many other parts of the body. It is included here because its most important consequence may be some type of valvular heart disease. Rheumatic fever begins with a throat infection that is caused by certain kinds of *Streptococcus* bacteria. The streptococcal infection is followed by general illness, the main symptoms of which are fever, aching and swollen joints, a characteristic rash, and often inflammation of and damage to various body tissues.

All heart tissues, including the pericardium, which is a membranous bag that encloses the heart, can be affected. But it is the heart's valves that are most often involved. In addition to the heart, the joints are likely to be inflamed and damaged by rheumatic fever. Heart problems used to be much more common than joint problems in rheumatic fever patients. Until recently, the heart was involved in the majority of cases. Today, however, the pattern is changing, perhaps because of the widespread use of *antibiotics*, and heart disease seems to have become less common than joint disease among people who have had rheumatic fever. Although rheumatic fever is not as widespread as it once was, children and adults under 30 are still fairly susceptible. Up to one per cent of teenagers show signs of heart disease associated with the disorder.

What are the symptoms?

Most commonly, rheumatic fever begins with a sore throat that seems to clear up quickly, but you begin to feel tired and feverish one to six weeks later. Thereafter your symptoms depend on which organ or organs are most affected. Inflammation of the heart rarely produces symptoms that you can identify. Inflamed joints are easier to recognize. The disorder usually affects the knees and ankles, but it may extend to the fingers, wrists and shoulders. Joints inflamed by rheumatic fever are apt to be swollen, tender, hot, red and extremely painful. More than one joint is usually involved, and the pain and swelling migrate from one to another.

In as many as ten per cent of rheumatic fever cases a complication known as chorea occurs about two to six months after the *Streptococcus* infection. Chorea affects the brain. Its main symptoms are involuntary jerky movements of the hands, arms and face. Speech may also be slurred temporarily. This condition does not cause permanent damage to the brain.

If you have rheumatic fever, you may also develop one or more red, ring-shaped rashes

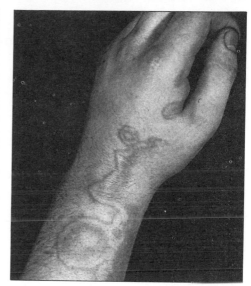

Swollen joints
Swollen joints are a common symptom of rheumatic fever. Usually only one or two joints swell at a time. An affected joint feels stiff and painful. After a few days the swelling subsides and another joint may begin to swell. This pattern can continue for several weeks.

with a white center. Such rashes usually appear on your torso. As one fades away, another may appear. Similarly, rheumatic nodules, or lumps, may appear on your knuckles, wrists, elbows or knees. The rashes do not itch, the lumps are painless, and they all disappear in time.

What are the risks?

If you have had rheumatic fever, the risk of further attacks is greater for you than for someone who has never had the disease. Before preventive treatment was possible, one in every four children aged 4 to 13 who had had rheumatic fever suffered a recurrence of the disease. With penicillin treatment the risk is much reduced. But about 60 per cent of rheumatic-fever cases still develop valvular heart disease. The severity of the heart trouble is often related to the number of attacks of rheumatic fever. There is also a slight risk of heart failure (see p.381) as the result of a very severe attack.

What should be done?

Always consult your physician if you or any member of your family has aching, swollen joints along with a feverish illness. The physician will suspect rheumatic fever and will pay special attention to the heart, listening with a *stethoscope* for any indication of trouble. Diagnostic tests may include analysis of blood specimens to determine changes, if any, that may have occurred from rheumatic fever; a chest *X-ray* to look for signs of heart enlargement; and an *electrocardiogram (ECG).* If a joint is swollen, it may be necessary to withdraw some fluid from it while you are under a local anesthetic, to establish the cause of the swelling.

What is the treatment?

Self-help: None is possible.

Professional help: If there are signs of heart involvement, your physician will keep you in

bed until your condition improves. Bed rest may also be prescribed if the disease has attacked your joints. While in bed, you will probably be given regular doses of aspirin to reduce inflammation and ease pain. *Steroid* drugs may be prescribed as an alternative.

Long-term treatment with an *antibiotic* is almost always prescribed for people who have had an attack of rheumatic fever. This treatment guards against streptococcal infections, and it has greatly reduced the recurrence rate for rheumatic fever. Only about four per cent of those who get the disease have more than one attack during the course of their lifetime. The antibiotic must be taken regularly for many years; a child who has had the disease must continue to take the drug even as an adult.

What are the long-term prospects?

Once an attack of rheumatic fever is over, there will be few, if any, symptoms. The joints and skin generally heal completely. The chance of damaged heart valves remains, especially in a person who has had more than one attack. Sometimes this heart damage may not become evident for many years. With modern treatment for valve disorders, however, the prospects are good even if your heart is affected.

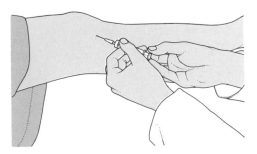

Removing fluid from an inflamed joint

If you seem to have rheumatic fever, your physician may draw fluid out of a swollen joint.

Some of the fluid is analyzed. Also, removing the fluid relieves some discomfort.

Bacterial endocarditis

The endocardium is the inner lining of the heart muscle. It also covers the heart valves. If the endocardium is damaged, as it might be, for example, in mitral incompetence (see p.396), bacteria (or occasionally fungi) may infect the damaged area. As the organisms multiply, they damage the area further, and some of them may move through the circulatory system to other parts of the body. They can form *emboli,* which can block small arteries and prevent blood from reaching tissues supplied by those arteries (see Arterial embolism, p.415). But it is the heart valves themselves that are primarily affected by bacterial endocarditis. As the valves are gradually destroyed by the multiplying bacteria, heart failure (see p.381) is apt to develop.

What are the symptoms?

No single symptom will tell you that you have this disease. There is usually some fever, but your temperature will rarely exceed 102°F (approximately 39°C). In addition, you may have sudden chills (especially when the bacteria form an embolus), headaches, aching joints, fatigue and loss of appetite. If the valves have been affected, eventually some or

all of the symptoms of heart failure may appear as well.

Other symptoms depend on the location of each embolus. You may have painful lumps in the tips of your fingers or small bruises behind your nails. It is fairly common for emboli to lodge in the brain, and this may cause weakness on one side of your body or loss of your vision (see Transient ischemic attacks, p.270). Emboli from bacterial endocarditis can lodge in any part of your body.

Although exact figures are not available, it is known that bacterial endocarditis is rare, especially among children and the elderly. Most cases of the disease occur in people between the ages of 15 and 55.

What are the risks?

Over 50 per cent of bacterial endocarditis cases are caused by heart trouble resulting from rheumatic fever (see previous article). Other possible, but much less common, causes are congenital heart disorders (see p.656), syphilitic heart disease (see p.612), and heart-valve replacement (see p.397). Bacteria can be introduced into the bloodstream during minor operations, dental extractions, and some diagnostic procedures, but this rarely causes endocarditis. More risk is associated with major heart surgery.

People who are susceptible to bacterial endocarditis, that is, chiefly those who already have heart trouble, are generally given a prescription for an *antibiotic* immediately before medical or dental surgery or when they develop boils or other skin infections. This precaution helps kill any bacteria that might otherwise get into the bloodstream and cause bacterial endocarditis.

If bacterial endocarditis is not discovered and treated within a few weeks of the initial infection, it can cause irreversible heart damage. Emboli may also do permanent damage to the brain and other parts of the body.

What should be done?

If you suspect that you may have this disease, consult your physician immediately. The symptoms can be confused with a wide variety of complaints, and it will help a physician who has not seen you recently if you point out that you have, or have had, any heart valve disease or heart murmur, or any of the symptoms commonly associated with endocarditis.

If a diagnosis of bacterial endocarditis seems likely, your doctor will probably admit you to a hospital. There you may undergo any of several tests. Samples of your blood will be tested to discover what kind of bacterium is causing your endocarditis.

Your bacterial endocarditis may also cause you to become anemic. If so, your doctor may have you take an iron supplement.

What is the treatment?

The treatment depends largely on what bacterium is responsible for causing the disorder. Your physician will choose a suitable antibiotic to combat that organism. If your case of bacterial endocarditis is diagnosed and effectively treated within six weeks of the initial infection, you have a 90 per cent chance of complete cure.

Mitral stenosis

Mitral stenosis occurs when the mitral valve, which is between the left atrium (one of the two upper heart chambers), and the left ventricle (one of the two lower heart chambers), becomes abnormally narrow. In order to force blood through the narrow opening, the atrium enlarges and pressure within the chamber gradually rises. This pressure is transmitted back through the pulmonary veins to the lungs, which makes them become congested. To keep blood flowing through the lungs at a normal rate, the right ventricle must also pump more and more vigorously, and it too becomes enlarged.

What are the symptoms?

The main symptom of mitral stenosis is breathlessness, which is caused by congestion in the lungs. It is most apparent after exercise, but it can occur at night or whenever you are lying down. You may also cough up small amounts of blood. You may become increasingly susceptible to attacks of bronchitis (see p.354), and you may even have chest pain similar to angina (see p.376).

As pressure builds up through the entire circulatory system, you may experience general fatigue, swollen ankles, and other symptoms that indicate right-sided heart failure (see p.381). If this happens, chest symptoms usually become less troublesome because the heart failure relieves pressure on the lungs.

About 60 per cent of people who have had rheumatic fever later develop some kind of heart disease. Almost 75 per cent of these people have some degree of mitral stenosis. But the number of cases of rheumatic fever has been declining in recent years, so mitral stenosis is less common than it used to be.

What are the risks?

Breathlessness and general weakness can be disabling, especially if you are pregnant or if you have a chest infection or an over-active thyroid gland (see Hyperthyroidism, p.525). But the main danger is of atrial fibrillation (see p.389), with its accompanying complications of heart failure or formation of an *embolus,* or blockage, in a blood vessel. Nearly half of those who have mitral stenosis eventually develop atrial fibrillation, and some of these will also develop emboli. Your chance of avoiding this complication is good, however, if you are under 45.

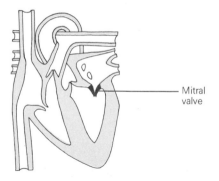

Mitral valve

What should be done?

Consult your physician if you have any of the symptoms mentioned above. Sometimes mitral stenosis is discovered by accident at a regular check-up. After examining you, with special attention to your heart and lungs, the physician may be able to diagnose mitral stenosis by listening for a heart murmur (see p.657). If additional testing is needed, your doctor may want to order a chest *X-ray*, an *electrocardiogram (ECG)*, and possibly an *echocardiogram.*

What is the treatment?

Self-help: None is possible. If you have no disabling symptoms, you can live a normal life without any treatment for mitral stenosis. However, if you have this condition, you should always ask your physician for an *antibiotic* treatment before you undergo dental or medical surgery to protect you from bacterial endocarditis (see previous article).

Professional help: If breathlessness is troubling you, your physician may prescribe a *diuretic* drug, which causes frequent urination. This treatment can help by draining fluid from your body. However, diuretics may also cause you to lose potassium. This mineral, an essential component of your body fluid and digestive juices, must be replaced. For this reason your doctor may prescribe supplementary potassium.

If you have developed atrial fibrillation, it can usually be controlled by certain heart drugs and you may be given *anticoagulants* to prevent the formation of emboli.

If your mitral stenosis is so severe that it restricts your daily activities, your physician may advise you to have surgery. It may also be necessary if you become pregnant and your symptoms worsen. The usual operation is called mitral *valvotomy*. It involves widening the narrowed valve. Such an operation involves some danger, but if your health is otherwise good, the mortality risk from the operation is only two per cent. In general the results are highly successful, and often the symptoms do not return for many years. If your symptoms do return, you may require a second valvotomy, or you may have to have your mitral valve replaced with an artificial one. About 80 per cent of those who have had the valve replacement operation have survived for at least five years. Read the following article, on mitral incompetence, for more about mitral-valve replacement.

Mitral incompetence

If your mitral valve does not close properly, blood may leak back into the left atrium (one of the two upper heart chambers) from the left ventricle (one of the two lower heart chambers). This is called mitral incompetence. If you have this disorder, your heart has to work harder than usual, and the muscular heart wall enlarges in an attempt to cope with the additional work load. Rheumatic fever (see p.393) is usually the cause of the disorder, but mitral incompetence may be present from birth (see Congenital heart disorders, p.656) or may arise in connection with some other type of heart disorder.

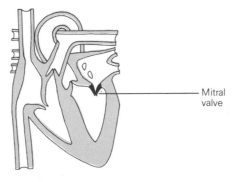

Mitral valve

What are the symptoms?

Often there are no symptoms, but mitral incompetence can lead to shortness of breath, fatigue, and other symptoms of congestive heart failure (see p.381). In later stages of the disorder, you may have some difficulty in swallowing if the enlarged wall of the left atrium presses on your esophagus.

Mitral incompetence can be permanent if the valve itself is damaged, or temporary, as in some cases of rheumatic fever. But because the number of cases of rheumatic fever has declined in recent years, mitral incompetence is less common than it used to be.

What are the risks?

The risks are similar to those of mitral stenosis. If you are among the relatively few people who have mitral incompetence without mitral stenosis, however, you are less susceptible to atrial fibrillation (see p.389) than those who have both disorders. Bacterial endocarditis (see p.394) is a more frequent consequence of mitral incompetence.

What should be done?

For precise advice read the previous article, on mitral stenosis. Diagnostic tests for the two disorders are similar.

OPERATION: Heart-valve replacement

Ball and cage

Tissue

Types of valves
A tissue valve is made from your own tendons. A ball and cage valve is made of plastic and metal.

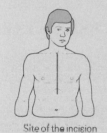

Site of the incision

This is an operation to replace damaged heart valves either with specially designed plastic and metal valves or with valves made from some of your own tendon tissues.

During the operation You are under a general anesthetic and your circulation and breathing are taken over by a heart-lung machine. An incision is made either along your breastbone or along the line of a lower rib on your left side. Your ribs are parted and your heart is opened up. Any damaged valves are cut out. The new valves are then sewn into place with stitches that will dissolve once you have healed. The operation takes from two to four hours.

After the operation You will spend the first few days in the intensive-care unit. One or two drainage tubes will be in place at the bottom of the incision. You will breathe oxygen through a tube leading into your throat, and may need the help of a respirator. Your bladder will be drained by a catheter. You will receive fluid and blood through intravenous drips and your heart will be monitored constantly by an ECG machine.

Convalescence Recovery may take several months. If you have had an artificial-valve replacement, you will have to take anticoagulant drugs for life. You may hear the artificial valves clicking in your chest; this is quite normal.

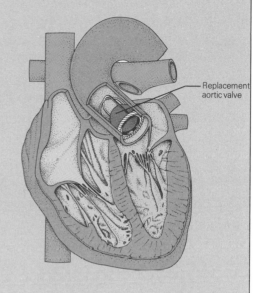

Replacement aortic valve

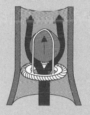 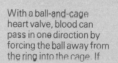

With a ball-and-cage heart valve, blood can pass in one direction by forcing the ball away from the ring into the cage. If

blood begins to flow in the opposite direction, it forces the ball firmly against the ring and closes the valve.

What is the treatment?

As with mitral stenosis, no treatment is likely to be required unless you have symptoms. If you have discovered that you have mitral incompetence, be sure to get *antibiotic* treatment before having teeth extracted or undergoing any kind of surgery. This is to protect you against the risk of bacterial endocarditis.

Medical treatment for mitral incompetence is much the same as for stenosis (see previous article). If the symptoms of mitral incompetence are extremely severe, your physician may advise you to have surgery in order to have the incompetent valve replaced with an artificial one.

There are two possible types of replacement, a mechanical valve or a valve formed from grafted tissue. Your surgeon must decide which of these is more appropriate for

your particular case. Mechanical replacements are efficient, but they cause clotting of blood five to ten per cent of the time. If you have a mechanical valve replacement, you will need to take an *anticoagulant* drug to guard against this complication. Anticoagulants are not suitable for anyone with a peptic ulcer that may bleed, or for anyone who lives far away from the laboratory facilities that are essential for monitoring this sort of treatment. Tissue-graft valves involve much less risk of clotting, but they may be less durable.

If, at any time after the operation, you suddenly become short of breath, faint, or dizzy, or if your urine looks abnormally dark or your chest begins to ache, see your physician as soon as possible. Any of these symptoms may indicate there is a mechanical failure of the replacement valve.

Aortic stenosis

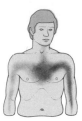

Site of the pain

Aortic stenosis occurs when your aortic valve, the valve between the aorta and the left ventricle, becomes abnormally narrow. The aorta is the artery through which the left ventricle, one of the two lower heart chambers, pumps blood into the body. Thus, the narrowing decreases the quantity of blood that the heart can pump throughout the body. In an effort to squeeze more blood through the valve, the left ventricle then develops a thickened muscular wall. This thicker, harder-working tissue requires more and more blood to supply it with the oxygen and nutrients it needs to work so hard.

What are the symptoms?

At first, aortic stenosis may produce no symptoms at all. As the condition worsens, you will begin to feel breathless after physical activity. You may then develop angina (see p.376), dizzy spells, or even faintness whenever you exert yourself. Eventually your symptoms may be those of left-sided heart failure (see p.381).

Rheumatic fever (see p.393), which is associated with other valve disorders, is often the cause of aortic stenosis. The aortic valve is affected in about 40 per cent of people who get heart-valve trouble after an attack of rheumatic fever. If you have this disorder alone, without first having rheumatic fever and without any other valve defects, you probably were born with it (see Congenital aortic stenosis, p.658). The chances of having the problem are three times greater for a man than for a woman. The reasons for this difference between the sexes is not known.

What are the risks?

A shortage of blood throughout your body means a shortage of blood, and therefore a shortage of oxygen, in the heart itself. This can cause ventricular fibrillation and cardiac arrest (see p.388).

What should be done?

As with mitral stenosis (see p.395), you may first learn that you have aortic stenosis because your physician discovers it in a routine medical examination. If you have any of the symptoms of aortic stenosis, do not delay in consulting your physician, who will examine you, listen to your heart, and probably order diagnostic tests without delay. A chest *X-ray* should show whether or not the heart is enlarged. An *electrocardiogram (ECG)* can help your physician to determine how much your heart is enlarged, if, indeed, it is. The diagnosis can then be confirmed or perhaps disproved, with *ultrasound*, an *echocardiogram*,

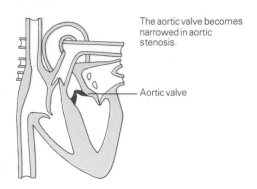

The aortic valve becomes narrowed in aortic stenosis.

— Aortic valve

cardiac catheterization, and *coronary arteriography.*

What is the treatment?

Self-help: If you know you have mild aortic stenosis, avoid strenuous activity. There is no reason, however, to treat yourself as an invalid. Moderate exercise is still possible and, in fact, desirable. For example, play golf and go for walks, but do not play squash or run for buses. Do not be afraid to have sexual intercourse, but take it at a relatively leisurely pace. Ask your physician to prescribe *antibiotics* for you before you have surgery or a dental extraction, to protect you from the risk of bacterial endocarditis (see p.394). And make sure that you have your heart examined yearly by your physician.

Professional help: The only treatment for severe aortic stenosis is surgery, and the most common form of surgery is valve replacement (see previous page). Decisions that must be made, the possible risks of the operation, and prospects for recovery are similar for all heart valve disorders. Your physician should be able to help clarify these matters for you.

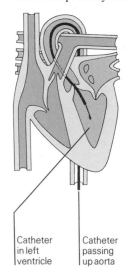

Cardiac catheterization
Aortic stenosis can be confirmed by cardiac catheterization. A catheter containing an electronic device to measure pressure is threaded along an artery to the heart. It measures the pressure in the left ventricle and in the aorta.

Catheter in left ventricle

Catheter passing up aorta

Aortic incompetence

If your aortic valve, the valve between your aorta and your left ventricle, does not close properly, you may develop aortic incompetence. The aorta is the artery through which the left ventricle, one of the two lower heart chambers, pumps blood into the body. But if the valve does not close right, blood may leak back to the left ventricle. The most likely cause of the disorder is rheumatic fever. The aortic valve can also be damaged by syphilis (see p.612), but this now causes only about one per cent of all aortic incompetence cases. If you have severe aortic incompetence, your left ventricle will enlarge and its walls will thicken. This is a response to the fact that the ventricle must work harder to pump blood through the aorta to the body. Sometimes, too, part of the valve ruptures because of damage to the tissues from bacterial endocarditis (see p.394).

What are the symptoms?
There are often no symptoms for years, but symptoms develop swiftly if the valve is ruptured. The main symptom is breathlessness. You may also have angina (see p.376) and all the symptoms of congestive heart failure (see p.381). If aortic incompetence is left untreated, the disorder can lead to heart failure (see p.381).

What should be done?
Consult your physician if you find that you have any of the symptoms of aortic incompetence. Examination and diagnostic tests are similar to those that are carried out for other heart-valve disorders. A common exception is that blood tests may be included to find out whether you have syphilis (see p.612). Treatment is the same as it is for aortic stenosis (see previous article).

Tricuspid stenosis and incompetence

Tricuspid stenosis and incompetence involve narrowing and leakage of the tricuspid valve of the heart. These disorders generally occur only in conjunction with other valvular disease that is caused by rheumatic fever, and account for less than five per cent of all valvular heart diseases.

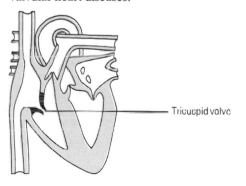

Tricuspid valve

What are the symptoms?
The symptoms of these tricuspid disorders are much like those of congestive heart failure (see p.381).

What are the risks?
The symptoms of heart failure may gradually get worse. Finally, you may become disabled by the disease. As is true with other heart-valve diseases, tricuspid stenosis and incompetence poses an additional risk that you will get bacterial endocarditis (p.394).

What is the treatment?
No treatment is required for mild cases. If treatment proves necessary, it is similar to that for mitral stenosis (see p.395), except that *valvotomy*, or widening of the valve, is rarely successful. A valve-replacement operation may be necessary.

Pulmonary stenosis and incompetence

Non-congenital pulmonary valve disorders, usually caused by rheumatic fever, are rare, comprising only about two per cent of all heart-valve disorders resulting from rheumatic fever. Symptoms and diagnostic tests are similar to those for other valve problems.

Pulmonary stenosis and incompetence may only be discovered during a routine examination. If the pulmonary valve is severely affected, your doctor may advise you to have a valve replacement operation (see Mitral stenosis, p.395).

Pulmonary stenosis may also occur as a congenital disease (see p.658).

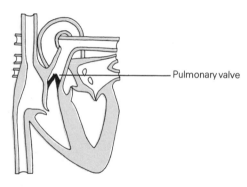

Pulmonary valve

Heart muscle and pericardium

The walls of your heart are made of muscle that contracts rhythmically about 100,000 times a day. If this muscle becomes diseased, the force of your heartbeat decreases and this affects the circulation of blood. There are several forms of a heart-muscle disorder known as cardiomyopathy. The tiny fibers of the muscle may be weakened by an internal chemical change. In some cases the disease is confined to the heart. In others, the heart is only one of the affected organs. Cardiomyopathies are generally less common than most other types of heart disease. The three most common kinds are covered in this section. In addition, two disorders of the pericardium, which is the membraneous bag that surrounds your heart, are discussed in the following articles.

Myocarditis

Myocarditis, or inflammation of the heart muscle, occurs as a rare complication of one of several diseases. In mild cases, the only symptom may be slight chest pain and shortness of breath. In more serious cases, such as those caused by diphtheria (see p.703), myocarditis can lead to heart failure (see p.381), and death.

If, while treating you for the underlying disease, your physician suspects you may have myocarditis, you may need to have a chest *X-ray* and an *electrocardiogram (ECG)* so that your physician can verify the diagnosis. Other possible diagnostic tests include an *ultrasound* scan and a *biopsy*. In a biopsy, a small amount of tissue is removed and examined in detail.

The primary aim of treatment for myocarditis is to eliminate the underlying infection. In addition, you will be advised to rest completely. In some forms of myocarditis, treatment with *steroids* speeds healing.

Nutritional cardio-myopathy

Like any muscle, the heart muscle can be damaged by a vitamin or mineral deficiency or by poisoning. The most important form of such nutritional cardiomyopathy in Western societies is found among alcoholics (see Alcoholism, p.304). Heart specialists attribute the damage either directly to the alcohol or to the lack of vitamin B_1 that may be characteristic of the alcoholic's diet. In non-alcoholics, nutritional cardiomyopathy can also occur because of vitamin B_1 deficiency. It can also be caused by a lack of potassium in the bloodstream. This is a potentially serious deficiency that occasionally develops in people who for some reason suffer from persistent diarrhea or who are under long-term treatment with *diuretic* drugs.

The symptoms of nutritional cardiomyopathy vary greatly. You may simply have palpitations, which is increased awareness of your heartbeat, and swollen hands and feet. Since the damage can cause disorders such as atrial fibrillation (see p.389) or even heart failure (see p.381), you also may have the symptoms of those ailments.

Treatment will probably consist of an attempt to correct the dietary deficiency. How this is done depends on the circumstances, but if your problem is alcoholism, only total abstinence can halt the disease.

Hypertrophic cardio-myopathy

If, for some reason, there are defective cells in your heart muscle, the walls of your heart may thicken in an effort to compensate for the weakness. In severe cases the swollen walls may impede the flow of blood into and out of your heart. The symptoms of this disorder, which is called hypertrophic cardiomyopathy, include fatigue, chest pain, shortness of breath, and palpitations, which is increased awareness of your heartbeat. If you have any of these symptoms, see your physician, who may order diagnostic tests such as a chest *X-ray*, an *electrocardiogram (ECG)*, and perhaps a *biopsy*.

There is no treatment for the disease, but the symptoms may be relieved by certain drugs that help regulate the heart, and *diuretics*, which help rid the body of excess fluid. A few people who have been in danger of fatal heart failure as a result of hypertrophic cardiomyopathy have had successful heart transplants (see p.402).

Acute pericarditis

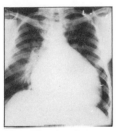

X-ray of pericardial effusion
The fluid that collects around the heart (pericardial effusion) is opaque to X-rays and makes the heart look much larger than normal.

Pericarditis is an inflammation of the pericardium, which is a membranous bag that surrounds your heart. When the pericardium becomes inflamed, fluid can collect in the space between it and the heart. This condition, which is called pericardial *effusion*, may cause further complications. In acute pericarditis, there is a severe attack of chest pain that comes on suddenly. The inflammation in acute pericarditis is usually caused by a viral infection, but it may also be caused by rheumatic fever (see p.393), diseases of the connective tissue such as systemic lupus erythematosus (see p.556), or chronic kidney failure (see p.512). Acute pericarditis can also follow either heart attack (see p.379) or a physical injury to the chest, but these causes of the disorder are rare.

Mild pericarditis is probably a common feature of viral illnesses. But pericarditis severe enough to cause acute pain is unusual.

What are the symptoms?
The main symptom of acute pericarditis is pain, which is usually in the center of your chest. The pain may radiate to your left shoulder. Unlike the pain of angina (see p.376), it becomes worse if you breathe deeply, cough, or twist your body. You may also be short of breath.

What are the risks?
There is a slight risk that a pericardial effusion will grow rapidly enough to cause dangerous pressure on the heart. Although pericarditis generally is not a serious disorder by itself, it can be associated with more severe and serious illness.

What should be done?
Chest pain, especially if it is associated with difficulty in breathing, can be a symptom of several serious illnesses, including pleurisy (see p.361), pneumonia (see p.359), pulmonary embolism (see p.406) and heart attack (see p.379). If the pain is severe and lasts for more than a few minutes, consult your physician. After examining you, your doctor will probably order diagnostic tests such as a chest X-ray, an *electrocardiogram (ECG)*, and blood tests. These will help determine whether you have pericarditis and, if so, what has caused the inflammation.

What is the treatment?
Pericarditis due to a viral infection usually clears up without treatment. The inflammation subsides within 10 to 14 days, and leaves no ill effects. In rare cases, when pericarditis is associated with a heart attack for example, your physician may prescribe a *steroid* drug to speed up healing. When acute pericarditis is due to a connective-tissue or metabolic disorder, the underlying disease must be treated. Your physician may insert a needle into your chest to remove some of the fluid either if a pericardial effusion endangers your heart, or for diagnostic purposes.

Constrictive pericarditis

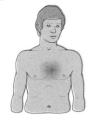

Site of the pain

When pericarditis, or inflammation of the membranous bag that surrounds the heart, is due to a chronic infection such as tuberculosis (see p.563), the course of the illness is very different from that of acute pericarditis (see previous article). Long-standing inflammation can thicken, scar, and contract the pericardium until it shrinks so much that the normal beating of the heart is restricted. This disorder is called constrictive pericarditis. Because tuberculosis is no longer widespread, constrictive pericarditis has become less of a problem than it used to be.

What are the symptoms?
The main symptom is that your legs and abdomen swell because fluid accumulates in those areas. Any or all of the other symptoms of heart failure (see p.381) may also develop from constrictive pericarditis.

In fact, without surgical treatment, heart failure is virtually inevitable, and becomes more and more severe.

What should be done?
Whatever the cause, you should consult your physician if you have any of the symptoms that indicate you might have heart failure. Recommended diagnostic tests will probably include a chest X-ray, an *electrocardiogram (ECG)*, and perhaps further studies. Your physician may also recommend that you have *cardiac catheterization*, which is a special X-ray of your heart, to get a detailed assessment of the condition of your heart.

Also, your sputum will probably be tested for indications of tuberculosis.

What is the treatment?
No self-help or treatment by drugs is possible. But constrictive pericarditis can be cured by an operation that is called a *pericardectomy*. In this procedure, the surgeon carefully removes the thickened pericardium from the surface of your heart. The prospects for full recovery from the disease after surgery are usually excellent.

Transplants

Surgery to replace some damaged body organs with healthy ones is now routine. Several thousand such operations are done every year around the world. Healthy replacements come either from people who have consented (or whose surviving relations consent) to the medical use of parts of the body after death, or from living donors who are usually related to the person who needs a transplant. Many state and national medical organizations will provide organ donor cards for those who are willing to donate their vital organs. It is sometimes difficult to get donated organs so donating your organs is a real service.

Quick action is of critical importance. For instance, a kidney must be removed within 30 minutes after the donor's death and can be kept in storage for no more than 24 hours before transplantation. With the help of cooperating medical organizations, physicians quickly locate suitable recipients for donated kidneys.

What are the difficulties?

With modern medical techniques the operation itself is straightforward. Yet kidney transplants are not commonly performed. This is due to the shortage of donated kidneys and to the fact that the body's defense system treats any transplanted organ as if it were an infecting organism and tries to destroy it through the action of white blood cells and *antibodies*. An ideal transplant would have tissues identical to those of the organ it replaces. Donated organs are matched to the patient by *tissue type*, but a perfect match is almost impossible. The body's fight to reject a new organ must be counterbalanced by treatment with *immunosuppressive* drugs. Such treatment carries very great risks and must be given with a precision that is difficult to achieve. Because this aspect of the treatment is so risky, it is impossible to predict the success of most transplants.

There are are two exceptions to this rule. First, an organ transplant between identical twins involves no risk of rejection, because the tissues of identical twins are a perfect match and do not provoke a response from the defense system. Of course, this can only be done with an organ the donating twin can survive without, such as a single kidney. The second exception is corneal transplants, which "take" easily because the cornea has no blood supply and therefore lacks the rejecting weapons of white blood cells and antibodies.

Rejection of a transplanted heart, liver, or lung may mean sudden death. Kidney transplants are far less risky, since rejection of the transplanted organ is not necessarily fatal. The patient can be kept alive with an artificial kidney machine, or *dialysis* (see Artificial Kidney aids, p.512), until another transplant becomes available. Because no comparable alternative exists for other vital organs such as the heart, surgeons tend to suggest transplantation only if the patient is near death from the failure of the organ to be replaced.

What are the long-term prospects?

Treatment with immunosuppressive drugs begins immediately after the transplant operation, and must continue for the rest of the patient's life. Unfortunately, such treatment reduces resistance to infection, may encourage the growth of malignant, or life-threatening, tumors and may damage bones as well as other body organs. The drug dosage must be meticulously calculated. Too little can lead to rejection of the transplant at any time, and too much can have fatal side-effects. In spite of the difficulties, however, some recipients of kidney transplants live for 15 years or more after the operation, and a few recipients of donated hearts, lungs, or livers are leading productive lives five years or more after the operation.

How a transplant is done

In many heart-transplant operations the surgeon does not remove the entire heart but cuts away only the two main pumping chambers (the ventricles), the main heart valves, and part of the two smaller chambers (the atria). Most of the connections to the major blood vessels are left intact, making it easier to connect up the donated heart tissues. This "partial" heart transplant is possible because it is usually only the main heart valves or the muscular walls of the ventricles that are damaged.

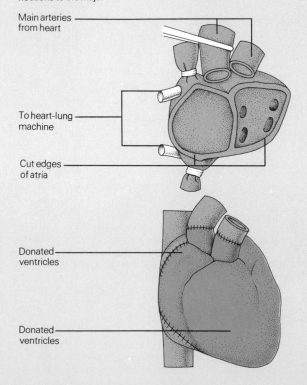

Main arteries from heart

To heart-lung machine

Cut edges of atria

Donated ventricles

Donated ventricles

Circulation

Your blood makes two separate circuits through your body, from and to its central pump, the heart. In the shorter of these two circuits, the pulmonary circulation, "used" blood is pumped to your lungs where it picks up oxygen and discards carbon dioxide. Then it returns to your heart. From there the oxygenated blood is pumped throughout your body. This is called the systemic circulation. Its purpose is to supply all your tissues with nutrients and pick up waste products before returning the blood to your heart to become reoxygenated in the pulmonary circulation.

The arteries that carry blood away from the heart have thick, muscular walls to restrain and absorb the peaks of blood pressure that occur each time your heart beats. The main artery, the aorta, has an internal diameter of about 30 mm ($1\frac{1}{4}$ in). It branches into smaller arteries, then into tiny arterioles, and finally into microscopic capillaries, whose thin, porous walls permit easy exchange of nutrients and oxygen for waste products between the blood and the tissues. Gradually the capillaries merge to form venules, and they merge to form soft-walled, flexible veins, which return oxygen-depleted blood to the heart.

Your blood does not flow at a constant rate to all parts of your body. The rate varies according to how much blood is needed by certain tissues at a given moment. For example, the uterus of a pregnant woman makes greater demands on the circulation than the uterus of a woman who is not pregnant. When you run, blood is diverted to your leg muscles at the expense of your abdominal organs. These organs, however, may need and get more blood at other times, such as to aid digestion after a large meal. When you feel cold, less blood flows in vessels near the chilled skin, and more flows in deeper vessels, to conserve heat. This pattern is reversed, and you flush, when you are overheated.

Your circulatory system is highly complex, and it can go awry not only if the central pump malfunctions, but also if problems arise within the blood vessels. There can be a weakness in an artery wall, or the hardening of an artery that makes it unable to absorb increased blood pressure. Blood clots that cause blockages can form, and a variety of other disorders, some severe and some merely annoying, can affect your circulation. The most common of these conditions are described in the following group of articles.

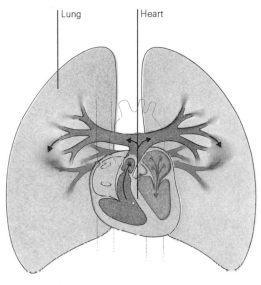

Lung   Heart

Pulmonary circulation "Used" blood is pumped from the right ventricle through the pulmonary artery into the lungs. Capillaries in the lungs surround tiny air sacs (alveoli, which are not shown here). There, the blood absorbs oxygen and expels carbon dioxide. The capillaries merge to become pulmonary veins. These carry the freshly oxygenated blood into the left side of the heart.

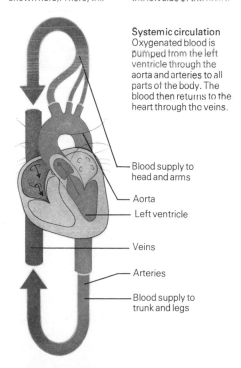

Systemic circulation Oxygenated blood is pumped from the left ventricle through the aorta and arteries to all parts of the body. The blood then returns to the heart through the veins.

Blood supply to head and arms

Aorta

Left ventricle

Veins

Arteries

Blood supply to trunk and legs

Hardening of the arteries

(arteriosclerosis)

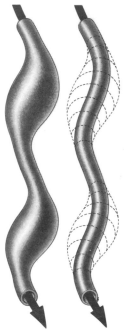

Normal   Hardened

How hardened arteries affect blood flow
Hardened arteries cannot dilate and constrict to regulate blood flow in the same way as normal arteries do. This rigidity encourages the formation of blood clots, which can further affect blood flow.

As people grow older, their arteries tend to harden, so most adults have some degree of arteriosclerosis. But although gradual loss of elasticity in arterial walls is inescapable, the seriousness of the condition is directly linked to how much you are affected by atherosclerosis, or fatty deposits in your blood vessels (see p.372). A combination of arterial aging and fatty deposits makes the arteries increasingly narrow, and also more brittle, that is, less and less able to expand. Both these effects decrease the amount of blood that can pass through the arteries.

Arteriosclerosis sometimes affects a major artery, but more often, the arteries in which the blood supply is seriously reduced are the smaller ones that carry blood to your brain and to your legs.

What are the symptoms?
Arteriosclerosis that impairs the flow of blood to your legs can cause pain, most often in your calves. You will probably feel pain only when your legs are active. The pain increases with activity and disappears with rest. Another possible symptom is pain in your toes, which persists even when you are resting. It tends to be worst at night; the best way to relieve it, at least in the early stages, is to dangle your legs over the edge of the bed. This causes more blood to flow into your toes, temporarily eliminating the problems.

If your brain is affected, you may get dizzy when you move your head in a certain way, or you may have attacks of temporary loss of vision (see Transient ischemic attacks, p.270). This is a particularly frightening symptom. Much more dangerous, *thrombosis*, the formation of a blood clot in a blood vessel, is more likely to cause a stroke (see p.268), if it occurs in a diseased artery. Although nearly everyone has arteriosclerosis to some extent, most people are not aware that they have it.

What are the risks?
As with atherosclerosis (see p.372), the risks associated with arteriosclerosis depend on what part of your body is affected. Among possible serious complications are stroke (see p.268), coronary artery disease (see p.374), dry gangrene (see p.415), and aneurysm formation (see p.407).

Cigarette smokers are particularly at risk. The older you are, the more likely you are to be severely affected. The disease seems to run in families, and its effects are likely to be more serious if you already have anemia (see p.419), diabetes mellitus (see p.519), or heart failure (see p.381).

What should be done?
Start now on self-help measures to slow down the development of atherosclerosis, even if you feel fine. If you think you have symptoms of arteriosclerosis, consult your physician, who, after examining you, may want you to have an *electrocardiogram* (*ECG*), since your coronary arteries may be affected by this disorder. A chest *X-ray* and tests on samples of blood and urine can also be helpful in diagnosing your condition.

What is the treatment?
Self-help: Recommendations in the article on atherosclerosis (see "What is the treatment?" p.373) are generally applicable to arteriosclerosis. It is particularly important that if you smoke cigarettes you stop. In addition, if your legs are affected, try to keep them as warm and dry as possible. When you cut your toenails, avoid cutting the flesh, since an open wound on the affected part of your body is highly susceptible to infection when you have arteriosclerosis.

Professional help: Your physician can help you by treating conditions such as anemia, diabetes, or heart failure that aggravate the effects of arteriosclerosis. Among medicines sometimes prescribed for arteriosclerosis patients are *vasodilator* drugs, which widen your blood vessels, and *anticoagulant* or *antithrombotic* drugs, which help prevent your blood from clotting as readily as it normally would. If your physician prescribes any such drugs, you will need to take them on a long-term basis.

If you are having problems with your feet, your physician may recommend that you see a podiatrist.

Surgery is a possible treatment if your case of arteriosclerosis is not extensive. The procedure usually involves replacing a narrowed stretch of artery with either an artificial tube or a section of vein taken from another part of your body. Even if this operation is successful, it cannot remove the factors that can cause further arteriosclerosis.

What are the long-term prospects?
Although arteriosclerosis is almost certain to become more severe as you grow older, symptoms such as the pain in your legs may become less troublesome. This occurs because your body compensates for the inadequate quantity of blood flowing through some arteries by expanding other, healthy arteries that supply the same area. If you eat sensibly, do not smoke, and exercise regularly and moderately, you will probably delay or even prevent complications.

Deep-vein thrombosis

Thrombosis is the formation of a *thrombus*, or blood clot, which may partially or completely block a blood vessel. Thrombosis in a vein near the surface of the skin causes thrombophlebitis (see p.407). But if blood clots form in a deeper vein, the result is called deep-vein thrombosis. There are many causes of deep-vein thrombosis. Although the condition occurs most frequently in the legs and lower abdomen, it can occur anywhere in your body.

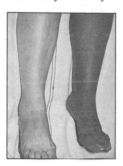

Thrombosis in the leg
The leg may become extremely red all over, It also swells and becomes painful at the site of the blood clot.

Deep-vein thrombosis is fairly rare, but if you are elderly or overweight, you are particularly susceptible. The disorder also may affect anyone with a blood disease such as polycythemia (see p.429), and women who are taking *estrogen*, either in the form of birth control pills or as post-menopausal therapy. The condition often develops after long periods of immobility, especially while you recover from an illness. This is because at such times your blood flow has a tendency to become quite sluggish.

What are the symptoms?
The area drained by the vein, usually your calf or thigh, becomes swollen and painful as the normal flow of blood is obstructed. This raises the pressure in your veins and capillaries. In your leg this causes edema, or cushion-like swellings that can remain indented if you press them with a finger. If the thrombosis is not in your leg, there may be no symptoms unless pieces of the clot break off, enter the blood, and cause an embolism (see Pulmonary embolism, next article).

What should be done?
If you think you may have a deep-vein thrombosis, see your physician, who will examine you, particularly your heart, lungs and circulation. To locate a deep-vein thrombosis in your leg, the doctor may require *venography*, or *X-rays* taken after a dye is injected into a vein in your foot. Among the tests that may be used in certain cases are *ultrasound* and *radioactive fibrinogen* tests.

What is the treatment?
Self-help: If you are a woman over 35 and you are taking oral contraceptives, ask your physician about alternative methods of birth control. The risks of thrombosis associated with birth control pills increase with age. Also, if you smoke, stop.

Professional help: If you are about to have surgery for another reason and your physician believes you are susceptible to deep-vein thrombosis, you may be given injections of an *anticoagulant* drug both before and after the operation. If you are bedridden, you will probably be encouraged to flex your leg muscles, wiggle your toes, and bend your ankles to keep your circulation active. If you are immobilized for a long time, your legs also may be mechanically elevated and put in plastic bags, which are alternately filled with air and deflated. The resultant pumping effect keeps your blood flowing normally.

If deep-vein thrombosis has already occurred, you may be given high doses of anticoagulant drugs, initially by injection and then in tablet form. Because these drugs can cause unwanted bleeding if you use them incorrectly, you must take them exactly as they are prescribed, usually for a period of several weeks. An analgesic prescribed by your physician will help relieve any pain that you may be suffering with.

Most clots are gradually reabsorbed into the bloodstream. In obstinate cases a *thrombolytic* drug is sometimes used to dissolve the clots, but such cases are rare. Sometimes, surgery is necessary to remove blood clots. The only lasting cure for deep-vein thrombosis, however, is to remove the factors that predispose you to thrombus formation.

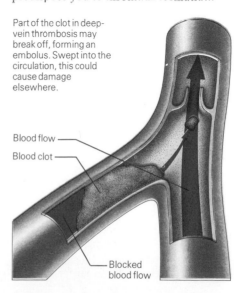

Part of the clot in deep-vein thrombosis may break off, forming an embolus. Swept into the circulation, this could cause damage elsewhere.

Blood flow

Blood clot

Blocked blood flow

Pulmonary embolism

Pulmonary embolism nearly always occurs as a complication of deep-vein thrombosis (see previous article). A blood clot detaches from the wall of a deep vein and moves into your bloodstream, through your heart, and along your pulmonary artery towards your lungs. If the loose clot, or *embolus*, is fairly large, it may become lodged in an artery inside your lungs, where it can block off some of the blood. This reduces the volume of freshly

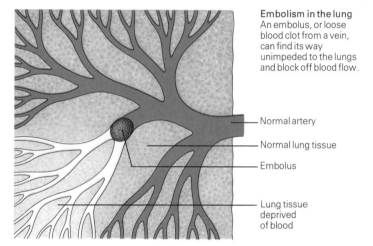

Embolism in the lung
An embolus, or loose blood clot from a vein, can find its way unimpeded to the lungs and block off blood flow.

— Normal artery

— Normal lung tissue

— Embolus

— Lung tissue deprived of blood

oxygenated blood that is returning to the left side of your heart. Any such pulmonary embolism is apt to be a serious matter.

In the United States, there are 630,000 cases of pulmonary embolism during an average year, and 1 out of every 380 cases results in death. Pulmonary embolism affects three women for every two men, and people who are in bed recovering from operations are particularly at risk from the disorder. Massive pulmonary embolism, an attack in which most of the blood flow in the lungs is blocked off, is very serious. Nearly one of every five cases results in death.

What are the symptoms?

The symptoms of pulmonary embolism depend on the size of the embolism and its location in your lungs. Because your heart and body tissues do not get all the oxygen they need, some degree of breathlessness is usually present. You may also feel faint and have chest pain. You may have a cough, bloody sputum and *cyanosis*, or blueness, around your mouth. In some cases, a massive pulmonary embolism can cause collapse and death within minutes.

What are the risks?

Any blockage of the flow of blood into your lungs can lead to right-sided heart failure (see

p.381). Your susceptibility to chest infection is increased by even a small pulmonary embolism, and if you have a massive pulmonary embolism, you can die from the collapse of your circulatory system.

What should be done?

Anything that predisposes you to deep vein thrombosis also increases your chances of having a pulmonary embolism. See your physician if you have symptoms of either disorder, especially if you have been confined to bed. The physician will examine your lungs and heart with a *stethoscope* and, if pulmonary embolism is suspected, will want a chest *X-ray* and an *electrocardiogram* (*ECG*) to see if your heart, especially the right side, is under strain. Then, to confirm the diagnosis, a pulmonary *arteriogram* might be advisable.

If you collapse with suspected massive pulmonary embolism, the physician's first task is to revive you by giving emergency treatment. But collapse from pulmonary embolism resembles collapse from heart attack (see p.379), so the physician will probably take a blood sample as quickly as possible in order to determine the cause of the collapse.

What is the treatment?

Self-help: To prevent pulmonary embolism, follow the self-help advice of the article on deep-vein thrombosis (see previous article). If the symptoms of an embolism occur, you must get professional help.

Professional help: You will probably have to be hospitalized. You may be given an injection of a *thrombolytic* drug to dissolve blood clots. Often, the treatment is an *anticoagulant* drug, given by mouth.

If the embolism is severe, emergency treatment may be required. This will probably involve a procedure called cardiac massage, and oxygen given with a face mask or tube. The blockage will then be removed surgically. This is a major operation done under general anesthetic.

What are the long-term prospects?

If you survive the critical first few days of massive pulmonary embolism, you stand a good chance of complete recovery. Chances are even better when the source of emboli, or blood clots that are moving through your bloodstream, is found and treated. A less severe embolism may damage part of the lung, but you will almost always make a satisfactory recovery if emboli are prevented from reforming. Your physician may prescribe an anticoagulant drug to help prevent further embolisms.

Thrombo-phlebitis

Phlebitis is inflammation of a vein, usually caused by infection or injury. When this happens, blood flow through the roughened, swollen vein may be disturbed. Then *thrombi*, or blood clots, may develop and adhere to the wall of the inflamed vein. The resultant disorder is called thrombophlebitis, and it generally occurs in veins of the legs.

Women are slightly more susceptible than men to the disorder. It is rarely a cause of death. You are more likely than others to get thrombophlebitis if you have varicose veins (see p.409), or if you are undergoing medical treatment that involves piercing your veins with tubes or needles. Though it is sometimes necessary, any such procedure can cause phlebitis simply through physical irritation, but this rarely occurs.

What are the symptoms?

The main symptoms of thrombophlebitis are pain, redness, tenderness, itching, and a hard, cord-like swelling along the length of the vein that is affected. If infection is present, you may also have a fever.

What are the risks?

If there is infection and it remains untreated, it can lead to blood poisoning (see p.421). There is also a slight chance that blood clots may be carried away in the circulation and become lodged in a more vulnerable spot, such as a deeper vein (see Deep-vein thrombosis, p.405), most likely in your leg or in your lower abdomen.

What should be done?

If you do not have a prolonged infection, thrombophlebitis usually clears up in a week or so. If it does not, consult your physician, who will probably be able to diagnose your ailment without special tests.

What is the treatment?

Self-help: To ease the pain of thrombophlebitis, you can take aspirin as directed on the container. Some sort of zinc ointment, which can be purchased without a prescription, should be effective in relieving any itching with which you are suffering.

Professional help: If there is infection, your physician may prescribe an *antibiotic* drug, and suggest that you rest in bed, elevate the affected leg, and apply hot compresses. Your physician may also advise you to wrap the affected area with an elastic bandage. This often hastens recovery by speeding up blood return in the vein, so that the blood carries away blood clots and prevents further clots from forming. With treatment, thrombophlebitis nearly always clears up completely in a couple of weeks.

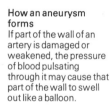

Thrombophlebitis usually affects the veins near the skin. It often occurs in the legs.

Aneurysms

An aneurysm is a permanent swelling of an artery due to a weakness in its wall. Aneurysms can form anywhere, but the most common and troublesome sites are the arteries of the brain, and the aorta, the large major artery through which the heart pumps blood to the rest of the body. There are, basically, three reasons why an aneurysm might develop in one of your arteries:

1. There are three layers of tissue in your arterial walls. The supportive strength of your arteries is supplied by the muscular middle layer, and this layer may be congenitally defective. The normal pressure of blood in the affected artery causes a balloon-like swelling, which is called a saccular aneurysm, to develop at that point. Aneurysms due to congenital defects are nearly always found in arteries at the base of the brain. Because of their shape and because several of them are often clustered together, they are known as "berry" aneurysms.

2. Inflammation, whatever the cause, may weaken an arterial wall. Most arterial inflammation is caused by disorders such as polyarteritis nodosa (see p.556), or bacterial endocarditis (see p.394).

3. A portion of the muscular middle layer of an arterial wall may slowly degenerate as the result of a chronic condition such as atherosclerosis (see p.372) or high blood pressure (see p.382). An aneurysm that is caused by atherosclerosis is likely to be a sausage-shaped swelling called a fusiform aneurysm that runs along a short length of the artery. A similar type of swelling may be caused by high blood pressure. Increased pressure of blood

How an aneurysm forms
If part of the wall of an artery is damaged or weakened, the pressure of blood pulsating through it may cause that part of the wall to swell out like a balloon.

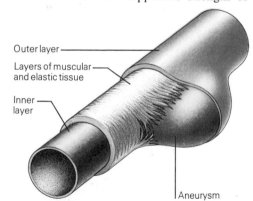

Outer layer

Layers of muscular and elastic tissue

Inner layer

Aneurysm

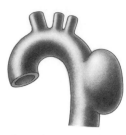

A saccular aneurysm develops when part of the muscular middle layer of the artery has been damaged.

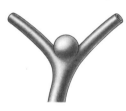

Berry aneurysms are found at the base of the brain, where an artery branches. A congenital defect causes them.

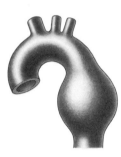

Fusiform aneurysms are formed when the arterial wall is weakened all the way around.

Dissecting aneurysms
High blood pressure may cause the inner and outer layers of an artery to split apart. Blood is then forced between the layers, and causes the outer wall to swell. The blood that is trapped between the layers tends to form a clot, which may eventually fill the aneurysm and seal it off.

in an artery, however, can stretch the wall in many different ways. It can even split the layers, and force blood between them. This is called a dissecting aneurysm.

Aneurysms can cause trouble in several ways. They can burst, which leads to a loss of blood supply for certain tissues, and to *hemorrhage*, or internal bleeding, at the site of the aneurysm. They can swell so much that they press on and damage neighboring organs, nerves, or other blood vessels. They also can disturb the flow of blood to such an extent that its eddying and whirlpooling cause dangerous clots to form.

What are the symptoms?

The symptoms of aneurysm vary according to the type, size, and location of the swelling. Berry aneurysms, or those at the base of the brain, usually cause no symptoms until they burst. A sudden severe headache at the back of your head, or even unconsciousness, may be the first sign of this type of aneurysm (see also Subarachnoid hemorrhage, p.271).

If you have an aneurysm of the aorta, your symptoms will depend on two factors: what section of the aorta is affected; and what type of aneurysm you have. The most common symptoms of a saccular or fusiform aneurysm in the thoracic aorta, or the portion of that artery that passes through your chest, are chest pain, hoarseness, difficulty in swallowing, and a persistent cough that is not helped by cough medicine. If you have a dissecting aneurysm in the same area of your aorta, you are likely to have pain that can easily be mistaken for a heart attack (see p.379). In either case, you will not be able to see or feel the swelling on the surface of your chest, because your thoracic aorta is confined within your rib cage.

A saccular or fusiform aneurysm in the abdominal portion of your aorta can usually be seen as a throbbing lump. Other symptoms

include loss of appetite and loss of weight. If the aneurysm is located towards your back, it may press on the bones of your spine, and cause severe backache. Dissecting aneurysms of the abdominal aorta are relatively rare. When they do occur, the main symptom is severe abdominal pain. Aneurysms in other parts of the body are rare and generally of little consequence.

What are the risks?

The major risk of an aneurysm is that it may burst, and cause a hemorrhage. A burst aneurysm allows blood to flow into the surrounding tissues, which causes serious local damage. Moreover, the entire circulatory system may collapse if the leak drastically reduces the volume of blood in the circulation. Unless expert medical help is available, a burst aneurysm in the aorta can be fatal. More than 40 per cent of all people who have a burst berry aneurysm die as a result.

Even when it does not burst, an aneurysm of the aorta causes turbulence in the flow of blood that can cause the formation of a *thrombus*, or clot, with all the associated dangers. *Emboli*, or parts of a blood clot that break away from the thrombus, can block smaller arteries such as those that supply the kidneys or other organs, and this can lead to many problems. Turbulence in the aorta also can stretch the aortic valve of the heart and cause aortic incompetence (see p.399).

Aneurysms sometimes occur in more peripheral arteries, such as those of the arms and legs, but in these locations they are generally less hazardous.

What should be done?

You can do nothing about berry aneurysms, since you probably will not know that you have one unless it bursts. If you have any of the symptoms of an aneurysm of the aorta or if you inexplicably develop a lump anywhere on your body, especially on your abdomen, and particularly if it throbs, consult your physician immediately. Many of the symptoms can be caused by other, often trivial conditions, so the physician will probably want to give you a full examination before making a definite diagnosis. To find out the size, type and location of an aneurysm, if you have one, you may need to have extensive *X-rays*, chiefly to verify and locate the atherosclerosis that probably caused it. You may have to have *arteriography* and *ultrasound* tests to help identify the aneurysm.

What is the treatment?

Self-help: The best ways to prevent aneur-

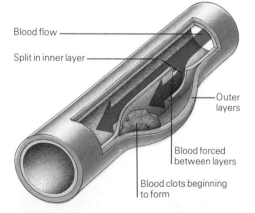

Blood flow

Split in inner layer

Outer layers

Blood forced between layers

Blood clots beginning to form

ysms are to take steps to prevent or slow down atherosclerosis (see recommendations on p.373), and to keep your high blood pressure under control (see p.382). If you have already developed an aneurysm, there is no effective self-help.

Professional help: Surgery is the usual treatment for an aneurysm, but the surgeon must consider the location and size of the aneurysm and the condition of the rest of your arteries before recommending the procedure. The operation is difficult and risky.

What are the long-term prospects?
About 30 per cent of people with ruptured berry aneurysms die instantly, and another 15 per cent die from further bleeding within a few weeks. The outlook for long-term survival is excellent if you have a successful operation and live for six months after the first hemorrhage occurs.

Surgery for aneurysms of the thoracic aorta is often impossible, and in such cases the long-term outlook is poor. With operable chest aneurysms there is an 80 to 90 per cent chance of survival. Abdominal aneurysms are frequently a much less serious problem. In general, they need to be removed only if they are very large or if they are found to be growing. With or without surgery, the outlook is good for most of these. The same is true for aneurysms in peripheral arteries.

Varicose veins

Varicose veins are veins that have become twisted and swollen. This disfiguring and sometimes painful condition usually occurs in the legs as a result of the strain imposed on leg veins by our upright posture. It is through the veins that blood is returned to the heart from the tissues of the legs. Since the heart is not strong enough to pump the blood up unaided, it must be helped by the pumping action of your leg muscles.

Normally, blood is collected from leg tissues in a network of superficial veins, or those on the surface of the muscles, which are connected to deep veins, or those embedded in the muscles, through what are called perforating veins. When a muscle relaxes, the deep veins and perforating veins expand and suck blood in from the superficial veins. All deep veins and perforating veins have one-way valves that prevent blood from flowing back into superficial veins. So when the muscle contracts, blood is pumped up the deep veins toward the heart.

If, for some reason, the valves of the perforating veins do not work efficiently, some blood may be pumped the wrong way, back into the superficial veins. They respond to the increased pressure by dilating and twisting. Thus, varicose veins are often visible because they lie just under the skin.

What are the symptoms?
The most common early symptom of varicose veins is the appearance of a prominent, bluish, swollen vein in your leg when you stand up. The most usual site is either at the back of the calf or up the inside of the leg anywhere between your ankle and your groin. Varicose veins can also occur around your anus (see Hemorrhoids, p.483) or in your vagina if you are pregnant (see p.623).

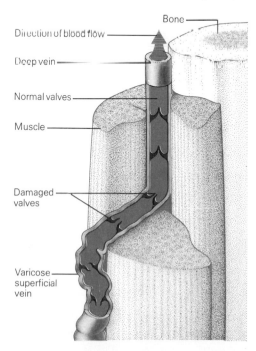

Bone

Direction of blood flow

Deep vein

Normal valves

Muscle

Damaged valves

Varicose superficial vein

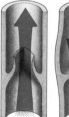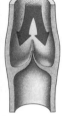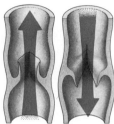

Normal vein

Varicose vein

Varicose veins occur when the valves in veins become damaged. This may occur because the veins are swollen due to extra pressure on them from standing or some other cause.

When valves in the veins become inefficient, blood is forced from the deep veins into the veins lying just under the skin. The increased pressure of fluid in these superficial veins makes them twist and bulge.

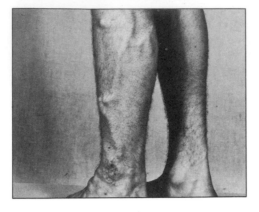

A swollen leg vein will probably grow increasingly prominent. The vein may become tender to the touch, and the skin above it or at your ankle may begin to itch. Your whole leg will ache, and you may find that your feet become swollen after a short period of standing and your shoes seem too tight by the end of the day. A shopping expedition, or waiting for a bus, may make both legs feel extremely sore and tired even when you only have varicose veins in one leg. Women usually find that all these symptoms are intensified for a few days before and during menstruation.

Your symptoms may not worsen beyond this stage. But some people with severe varicose veins find that the impaired circulation causes a brownish discoloration of the skin, especially near the ankles. Eczema (see p.253) of the skin near the veins is another possible symptom.

What are the risks?

Varicose veins are usually troublesome rather than disabling, but they occasionally have serious consequences. For example, a combination of the force of gravity and valve failure in perforating veins can give your tissues so little blood that the undernourished skin breaks down and an ulcer develops. Varicose ulcers (see p.260) will not heal as long as the veins associated with them remain under pressure.

Another risk, which is rare, is that bumping or cutting the skin over a varicose vein may release a torrential flow of blood from the swollen vein. This will need immediate medical attention. The greatest risk of varicose veins is inflammation of the wall of the vein. Blood tends to clot on the inflamed, roughened wall, and this can lead to thrombophlebitis (see p.407).

What should be done?

If you think you are susceptible to varicose

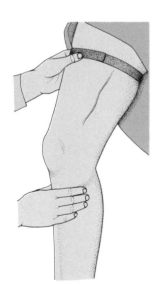

Finding the faulty valves
The physician applies a tourniquet to your leg while you are lying down. The tourniquet should stop the flow of blood through the vein. But if a valve is damaged at that point, some blood will leak through when you stand up, and the varicose vein stands out below the tourniquet. This is repeated at various points down your leg.

veins, especially if you are pregnant, guard against them by adopting the self-help measures recommended below. If you already have varicose veins, the self-help measures will ease your symptoms and slow down the progress of the condition, but they will not cure it, and your physician may advise you to have surgery. If your discomfort increases, consult your physician. The doctor probably will not need special tests to confirm the diagnosis. A simple procedure involving the use of elastic tourniquets on your leg will usually show which of your perforating veins have damaged valves.

If further investigation is required, the performance of your leg veins can be observed through *venography* or *thermography*. In venography, dye is injected into a varicose vein and its progress through the circulation is observed by taking *X-rays* of your leg. In thermography, the temperatures of various parts of your leg are recorded to produce a heat map. The aim of both techniques is to discover the precise location of weak valves.

What is the treatment?

Self-help: Try to keep off of your feet as much as possible. Whenever you can, sit with your legs raised. If your symptoms are very troublesome, lie down or sit down as often as you can, with your legs raised above the level of your chest. This ensures good drainage from your ankles and feet. Ask your physician if you need support stockings, and put them on before you get out of bed every day. Some people prefer elastic bandages, but you will need to have a nurse or doctor show you how to put them on properly. Also, they can be uncomfortable, especially in hot weather.

If you break your skin, and blood begins to flow from a varicose vein, lie down, raise the affected leg, and keep it raised. Do this no matter where you are, even in a public place. The bleeding will immediately slow down, and you can control it by moderate pressure with a clean handkerchief. You should then get professional medical help to clean and dress the wound.

Do not try to cope with varicose ulcers or eczema without professional advice. And never scratch an itch caused by varicose veins, because this can cause ulceration.

Professional help: Your physician can recommend support stockings or soothing dressings to relieve skin irritation, but the most satisfactory treatment for varicose veins is surgery. In the most common form of surgery, the affected veins are simply stripped from your leg. This procedure does not leave a noticeable scar, since a large section of vein can be removed through a tiny incision. The malfunctioning valves in the perforating veins are tied up with thread to close them permanently. The remaining small veins rapidly enlarge to take over the function of collecting blood and channeling it to the deep veins.

As an alternative to traditional surgery, varicose veins can sometimes be treated by injection. A small amount of a *sclerosant*

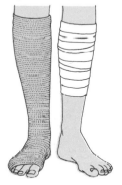

Simple self-help
If you have varicose veins, you should wear support stockings or elastic bandages. Also, try to sit with your feet propped up.

chemical is injected into the swollen veins. This makes the walls become inflamed and mat together, so that the veins stop carrying blood. If you have such treatment, it will

probably be as an out-patient and involve only two or three visits to your physician. There are several drawbacks to the injection treatment. For example, injection is unlikely to succeed if the varicose vein is in your thigh. Therefore, many physicians recommend stripping the veins first. If there are minor recurrences of the complaint later, they can usually be treated fairly easily by injection.

After either treatment, you will have to

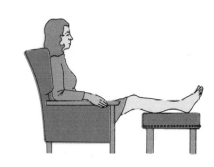

wear support stockings or elastic bandages for about six weeks. You should walk as much as possible, and avoid standing or sitting with your legs hanging down.

OPERATION: Varicose-vein removal

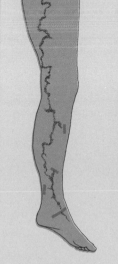

Sites of the incisions

Varicose veins can be removed by an operation. Their work will be taken over by other, nearby veins.

During the operation You are under a general anesthetic. Incisions about two inches long are made at the top of your inner thigh and at the ankle to reveal parts of the affected vein. Several very small cuts are also made down the leg where branches of the main vein go deeper into the leg. The branches are severed, then tied to stop them from bleeding. A flexible wire is passed from the ankle to the thigh along the main vein. A hook is attached to the wire at the upper end. As the wire is withdrawn, the hook pulls the vein from beneath the skin. At the same time the leg is bandaged tightly to prevent bleeding. The operation usually takes 30 minutes for each leg.

After the operation Your legs will remain bandaged for several weeks and you will later have to wear elastic bandages. You will probably leave the hospital within one week after the operation.

Convalescence Once you are at home you will probably be advised to walk up to several miles a

day and always relax with your feet up. Your physician will encourage you to gradually increase your activity and return to work as soon as you are ready.

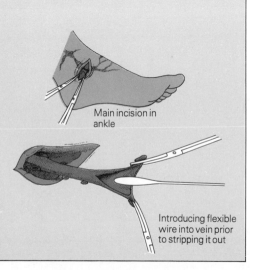

Main incision in ankle

Introducing flexible wire into vein prior to stripping it out

Raynaud's disease

(and Raynaud's phenomenon)

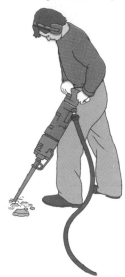

Regular use of high-vibration machinery such as pneumatic drills can damage the blood vessels and lead to Raynaud's disease.

This circulatory system disorder affects your fingers, and occasionally your toes. It occurs when the small arteries that supply them with blood become extra sensitive to cold and suddenly contract. This reduces the flow of blood to the affected area. At first the contraction is only a temporary *spasm* that can be eased by warmth, but it may eventually become permanent. Lack of oxygenated blood makes the affected area pale, often with a bluish tinge. When a temporary spasm ends, blood flows in, and the paleness disappears.

The disease may also occur as a secondary effect of conditions other than cold. It is sometimes an occupational disorder of people who work with chain saws, pneumatic drills and similar equipment. It can be caused by a disorder of the connective tissue such as scleroderma (see p.557), by pulmonary hypertension (see p.416), Buerger's disease (see next page), an emotional disturbance, or a nerve disorder. And it can be brought on by sensitivity to certain drugs that can affect the blood vessels. In all cases where it is secondary to another disorder, this condition is called Raynaud's phenomenon instead of Raynaud's disease. The condition is quite common, especially among women. It nearly always occurs first in young adulthood.

What are the symptoms?

Change of color in the fingers or other affected areas is the main symptom. Normally the color changes from white to bluish red at a rate that varies according to the temperature to which those areas are exposed. There is generally no pain, but there may be numbness or a feeling of "pins and needles" in the affected area.

Raynaud's disease worsens very gradually. Raynaud's phenomenon, on the other hand, may worsen quickly. In late stages of the disorder the affected flesh may shrink, and small ulcers may form as the tissues become damaged because the tissues do not receive an adequate blood supply.

What are the risks?

Prolonged contraction of the arteries may result in dry gangrene (see p.415), but this is rare. More often the poor blood supply eventually weakens your fingers and diminishes your sense of touch.

What should be done?

If self-help measures suggested below do not work, consult your physician, who may have to diagnose your condition on the strength of what you say, since your fingers or toes may look perfectly healthy by the time you reach the doctor's office.

What is the treatment?

Self-help: Keep your hands and feet warm and dry. Wear loose-fitting gloves and socks and comfortable, roomy shoes. If you smoke, give it up, because cigarette smoking further deteriorates inadequate circulation. A warm climate is probably the best solution for the problem, but it is a solution that not everyone can pursue. Try, at least, to stay indoors during very cold weather.

Professional help: Medical treatment of Raynaud's disease is based on attempts to encourage your small arteries to expand. Even when your arterial walls have been permanently damaged, *vasodilator* drugs sometimes improve circulation. Alcohol is a vasodilator, and your physician may suggest that you should have a drink now and then, because moderate quantities of alcohol seem to ease the symptoms of Raynaud's disease. However, the benefits may come mainly from the increased sense of well-being that alcohol often induces. Raynaud's disease is sometimes treated by an operation called a *sympathectomy*, in which the nerves that control contraction of the arteries are cut. Although this procedure often produces a dramatic improvement in the disorder, the nerves tend to grow back. If the condition has become permanent, there may not even be temporary improvement. For some reason, too, sympathectomy is more successful when the toes rather than the fingers are affected by the disorder.

Most people simply learn to live with Raynaud's disease. For Raynaud's phenomenon, the treatment depends on the underlying cause of the condition.

Frostbite

Frostbite is freezing of the skin and underlying body tissues. It occurs when part of your body is severely affected by temperatures well below freezing. The flow of blood to the affected area stops, and skin cells may be permanently damaged in severe cases. Any part of your body may be affected, but your hands, feet, nose and ears are most at risk. Frostbitten skin is hard, pale and cold, and has no feeling. When it has thawed out, it becomes red and painful. Anyone subjected to several hours of extreme cold, on a ski slope, for instance, may become frostbitten, but people who have atherosclerosis (see p.372) or who are taking *beta-blocker* drugs, which decrease the flow of blood to the skin, are particularly susceptible.

What should be done?

When you must go out in extreme cold, wear several layers of warm clothes under a waterproof, windproof outer garment. Make sure that your ears, hands and feet (and nose, if possible) are protected. Remember that fatigue, drinking alcohol, and lack of oxygen due to high elevations can affect your judgement, which can cause you to disregard the bodily discomfort that shows you have had enough cold and ought to go indoors.

Infants and children may lack the ability or knowledge to dress protectively enough to avoid frostbite. Parents should be sure their children are dressed adequately.

Frostbite must be treated promptly. Every minute of delay lessens your chances of recovery. So memorize the instructions for dealing with this problem (see within Accidents and emergencies, p.801) before you venture into the cold, especially if you will be in a place where professional medical help may not be available. If, after warming the frozen area, you do not fully recover, see your physician as soon as possible. There is a risk of dry gangrene (see p.415). If this occurs, you may need to have the affected part amputated, especially if it is a finger or toe. If frostbite is treated quickly, however, it may have no long-term ill-effects.

Medical myth

The best way to deal with frostbite is to rub the affected area with snow.

Wrong. Rapid rewarming is the right treatment. For complete instructions, see within Accidents and emergencies, p.801.

Acro-cyanosis

You have the condition known as acrocyanosis if your extremities, that is, your fingers, toes, wrists or ankles, sometimes look blue. The bluish tinge comes from the sudden contraction of tiny arteries that supply blood to your hands and feet. Because of such spasms, these parts get less blood than they need, and waste products build up in local veins. This gives the skin its abnormal color. Nobody knows why acrocyanosis develops. The condition is intensified by cold. It is present to an equal degree in both hands or both feet. It is not painful, but the affected parts nearly always feel cold and may be sweaty. Acrocyanosis does not cause ulceration or other skin problems.

What should be done?

Do not be too concerned if you have acrocyanosis. It is fairly common, especially among women. It is not a sign of a major disorder, and it does not need or respond to treatment. All you can do about it is protect your hands and feet from extreme cold.

Buerger's disease

(thromboangiitis obliterans)

Buerger's disease is caused by recurrent attacks of inflammation of the arteries, and sometimes the veins. These attacks eventually cause *thrombosis*, or the development of blood clots in blood vessels, and disruption of circulation. Thrombosis in an artery prevents oxygenated blood from reaching the tissues served by that artery, and the starved tissues may die as a consequence. Thrombosis in a vein prevents blood from returning to the heart, which causes swelling because the blood is not drained away from the tissues.

Any blood vessels may be affected by this disease, but Buerger's disease is most commonly found in the legs. The attacks of inflammation followed by thrombosis may be caused by a disorder of the connective tissue (see Collagen diseases, p.556), but the cause has not been definitely established. Some researchers think that the disease is not an entity in itself, but is a symptom of hardening of the arteries (see p.404).

What are the symptoms?

The symptoms depend on what areas are affected. Probably the most common symptoms are coldness and pain in your legs. The pain is felt after exercise and usually disappears with rest. Your legs may also tingle, and can become painfully hot and swollen if your veins are mainly affected. If your arteries are affected, there may be ulceration or even dry gangrene (see p.415). Other possible symptoms are those of Raynaud's phenomenon (see previous page), which is sometimes brought on by Buerger's disease.

What are the risks?

This disorder is rare. Those who get it are nearly always male cigarette-smokers between 25 and 40 years old. The major danger of Buerger's disease is that you may get gangrene of a leg or, occasionally, an arm, and have to have the limb amputated. Otherwise the risks are those of hardening of the arteries. If your veins are affected, you may develop thrombophlebitis (see p.407).

What should be done?

If you have any of the symptoms of this

disorder, consult your physician, who will probably examine you with Buerger's disease in mind, especially if you are a man under 45. You may have blood tests to determine, among other things, your blood-cholesterol level, which is usually normal or low with Buerger's disease, and can be high with arteriosclerosis. To identify the site and nature of the circulatory obstruction, your physician may also want you to undergo *angiography*.

What is the treatment?
Self-help: Since smoking increases the frequency and severity of attacks, do not smoke. The most positive step you can take is to give up cigarettes if you are still using them. Never expose your arms or legs to extreme cold. Your physician can give you advice about foot and hand care, and will warn you to be careful not to wound the flesh when you cut your toenails. The reason for this is to minimize the risk of infection and gangrene. Your physician may also recommend that a podiatrist or visiting nurse see you on a regular basis for foot and hand care.

Professional help: Your physician may prescribe *vasodilator* drugs for relief of pain, or a *sympathectomy*, a surgical procedure in which the nerves that are causing your blood vessels to constrict are severed. But neither of these measures is guaranteed to help. If gangrene sets in, amputation of the affected areas may be unavoidable. However, even if each flare-up of Buerger's disease leaves some residual disability, it is common for the attacks to stop occurring eventually.

Temporal arteritis

(cranial arteritis, giant-cell arteritis)

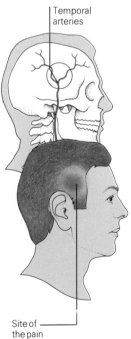

Temporal arteries

Site of the pain

If any of your arteries are chronically inflamed, and if the inflammation causes thickening of their lining and a reduction in the amount of blood that they can carry, you have the disease known as arteritis. Temporal arteritis gets its name because the arteries chiefly affected are the two that run behind the temples in your scalp. These temporal arteries are branches of the carotid arteries, which supply blood to your head and brain.

Temporal arteritis affects mainly people over 55. Women are twice as susceptible to the condition as are men.

What are the symptoms?
The most common symptom of temporal arteritis is a dull, throbbing headache on one or both sides of your forehead. The artery that is the source of the headache may be swollen, red, and painful if you touch it. Among other possible symptoms are mild fever, loss of weight, loss of appetite, and a generalized muscular ache. Such muscle aches, however, are more characteristic of a similar disease called polymyalgia rheumatica (see p.557).

What are the risks?
In severe cases, temporal arteritis can cause a stroke (see p.268). But the disease more commonly affects the eyes. Half of the people who have this disease have eye trouble, and this involvement can lead to some loss of vision. Before modern drugs were available, about 30 per cent of people with temporal arteritis became blind.

What should be done?
If you have persistent headaches from any cause, you should consult a physician. If your headaches are accompanied by some of the other symptoms of temporal arteritis, and if you are over 55, your physician will suspect that you may have this condition. A blood test will help indicate whether temporal arteritis is causing your symptoms. The doctor may also decide that a *biopsy*, in which a small piece of one of your temporal arteries is removed for microscopic examination, is needed to identify the disease. This procedure can be done while you are under a local anesthetic. More than one biopsy may be necessary. To confirm the diagnosis or help determine which piece of artery to remove for a biopsy, your physician may require an *arteriogram*, but this is rarely necessary.

What is the treatment?
Self-help: None is possible.

Professional help: Your physician will probably prescribe a *steroid* drug, which you may need to take for a long time. Regular blood tests will show whether the steriod is suppressing the disease by damping down the inflammation of the affected arteries. There are several possible side-effects of steriods, but most of them are unlikely to occur from the dose required to treat temporal arteritis. Once you start on the drug, however, you must continue to take it regularly until your physician says you may stop. You should continue to see your physician regularly.

What are the long-term prospects?
If you see your physician early enough, and if you cooperate with the steroid treatment, you have a 75 per cent chance of complete recovery. Successful treatment is less likely if the disease is not diagnosed in an early stage.

Arterial embolism

An *embolus* is a solid particle, usually a fragment of clotted blood or a piece of *plaque* (fatty deposit), that is carried along in your bloodstream. The embolus may be very small, but because arteries divide into successively smaller vessels – first arterioles, then capillaries – eventually the embolus can go no farther. At that point, it creates an *embolism*, or blockage, that prevents the tissues in the affected area from getting an adequate blood supply. The embolus may originate in your heart, because of a heart attack (see p.379) or some other heart disorder. It may be a fragment of bacterial growth resulting from bacterial endocarditis (see p.394). In rare cases, it may even be a tiny foreign object that entered an artery through a wound.

The severity of an arterial embolism depends on its size and location. The parts of the body that are most commonly affected are the brain and legs. But embolisms can occur anywhere in your body.

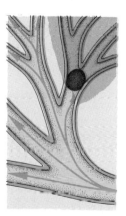

An embolus lodges
An embolus is carried along with the flow of blood in the arteries. It may lodge where the arteries branch or narrow. An area that depends on the blocked artery for blood supply will die if the problem is not treated.

What are the symptoms?
An embolism in an internal organ usually goes unnoticed unless it affects a large area. It may cause loss of function in part of the intestine, however, and cause the same symptoms as intestinal obstruction (see p.471). For the symptoms of cerebral embolisms, read the articles on stroke (see p.268) and transient ischemic attacks (see p.270). In other parts of the body, particularly the limbs, pain may be the earliest symptom. This is followed by a tingling or prickling sensation and the affected area eventually becomes numb, weak and cold. If the embolism is in an arm or leg, the skin is pale at first but later turns bluish from lack of oxygen. Both legs may be affected if a large embolus blocks the arteries at the bottom of your back, where the aorta (the main artery from your heart to your body) divides in two. Such embolisms, which are called saddle embolisms, can cause severe pain in your abdomen and in your back as well as in your legs.

What are the risks?
If one of your major arteries is blocked, the tissues it supplies will die within hours if the blockage is not treated; in other words, dry gangrene (see next article) will set in. In the brain the result of an embolism can be a fatal stroke. If you have blockage in your aorta (for example, a saddle embolism) you have only a 50 per cent chance of surviving.

The more extensive and severe the symptoms, the more quickly you should consult your physician, who will probably make a swift diagnosis without special tests. Your physician may want you to have diagnostic *arteriography*, however.

What is the treatment?
Self-help: If the symptoms are in an arm or leg, you should keep the affected limb cool and immobile until medical help arrives. This reduces the need for oxygen. No self-help is possible for embolisms in any part of the body other than the limbs.

Professional help: Minor embolisms are usually treated with *vasodilator* drugs or aspirin. If your case is severe, you may be given an analgesic to relieve the pain and injections of an *anticoagulant* drug to prevent further clotting. Additional treatment of the disorder depends on the location and the size of the embolism.

In most cases when an arterial embolism severely affects an arm or leg, immediate surgery is necessary to prevent gangrene (see next two articles). The operation, which is called an *embolectomy*, involves inserting a tube into the artery and mechanically sucking the embolus out through it. If this is done in time, complete recovery is possible.

Dry gangrene

Gangrene is dead flesh. Its characteristic black color is a sign that the skin, and often underlying muscle and bone, are dead. There are two basic types of gangrene: dry and wet (see next article). Dry gangrene does not involve bacterial infection. It occurs when the flow of blood to certain tissues is stopped or reduced. This may be the result of arterial embolism (see previous article), poor circulation due to diabetes (see p.519), or hardening of the arteries (see p.404). It is occasionally caused by prolonged frostbite (see p.412).

The oxygen-deprived area dies, but dry gangrene does not spread beyond that area.

As the flesh dies, it can be extremely painful. Once dead, it becomes numb and slowly turns black. A visible line separates the dead tissue from living tissue.

Because dead tissues lack resistance to infection, there is always a chance that the dry gangrene will lead to wet gangrene. There is also a risk of blood poisoning (see p.421).

What should be done?

If you have one of the disorders mentioned above, there are several ways to improve your chances of avoiding dry gangrene. Do not smoke. If you are a diabetic, make sure the disorder is kept under control by observing your diet and following your physician's instructions. Your doctor may recommend that you have a podiatrist or visiting nurse take care of your feet to prevent flesh wounds. You should wear comfortable, properly fitted shoes. If you think you may be getting dry gangrene, you should consult your physician immediately.

What is the treatment?

Your physician will try various measures to improve circulation to the affected part of your body before it is too late. *Anticoagulant* drugs or *vasodilators* may prove helpful, but surgery to unblock or bypass a clogged artery may also be advisable. If the gangrene appears to become infected, you will be given *antibiotics* to prevent wet gangrene. If the dry gangrene does not respond to treatment, amputation of the affected part, with some adjacent tissues, will be unavoidable.

Wet gangrene

Gangrene means dead flesh. Wet gangrene develops when either a wound or dry gangrene (see previous article) becomes infected by bacteria. Some of the invading bacteria produce poisons that break down the surrounding tissues, and so the gangrene spreads rapidly. A particularly virulent type of wet gangrene, which is called gas gangrene, is caused by certain strains of bacteria that not only spread rapidly but also produce a foul-smelling gas within the affected tissues. These bacteria flourish in dirty conditions. Wet gangrene, therefore, usually results from a major injury in which large, dirty wounds occur and are not thoroughly cleaned.

Mild forms of wet gangrene can complicate any case of dry gangrene. The more severe forms are now rare in countries where standards of medical care and hygiene are high.

What are the symptoms?

The dying tissues can be extremely painful. When they are dead, they are numb and blackened. There is a redness and swelling around the blackened area, and a thin pus oozes from it. There may also be an unpleasant smell. In severe cases there is fever as well, and gas bubbles may appear in the dead tissue, making the skin and muscles crackle and pop if you press them. If gas gangrene is not swiftly dealt with, it can cause shock (see p.386), which can be fatal.

What should be done?

If you are in danger of developing gangrene, see your physician or go to a hospital without delay. A dirty injury must be properly cleaned as quickly as possible. A physician can recognize wet gangrene almost instantly by sight, touch, and often by smell.

What is the treatment?

If you have wet gangrene, the entire affected area may have to be removed surgically. You will also be given high doses of *antibiotics.* Severe cases are also treated with a specially prepared *antiserum* to combat the invading bacteria. A modern technique that seems to improve the chances for preventing further spread of severe wet gangrene is known as *hyperbaric* oxygen treatment. After the dead tissue is removed, you may be placed inside a special chamber into which oxygen is pumped under high pressure. The oxygen permeates the flesh and the bacteria cannot survive, for they can live only in oxygen-free tissues.

Pulmonary hypertension
(cor pulmonale)

Pulmonary hypertension is raised blood pressure in the lungs. It is a disorder of the circulation that can be caused by any disease that blocks the flow of blood through the lungs. Among the common causes are bronchitis (see p.353, 354) and emphysema (see p.358). People who live for a long time at high altitudes are especially susceptible to pulmonary hypertension, but almost any lung disease can lead to this condition.

Whatever the cause, the main result is increased pressure within the pulmonary arteries, which carry blood from your heart to your lungs. In time this leads to thickening of the arteries, which further obstructs the flow of blood. In its effort to compensate for poor circulation, the right side of your heart becomes enlarged, and the extra work the heart must do can eventually cause right-sided heart failure (see p.381).

What are the symptoms?
There are often no symptoms of pulmonary hypertension until the condition is well advanced. Thereafter the main symptom is swollen ankles. The swelling is usually noticeable only when your chest ailment is particularly troublesome. If the pulmonary hypertension is caused by chronic bronchitis or emphysema, your skin may have a bluish tinge because it contains less oxygen and more waste products than it should. If you already suffer from breathlessness because of the underlying lung disease, pulmonary hypertension is likely to make you even more breathless. You may also have certain symptoms of right-sided heart failure.

The main risks are from the lung disease that causes pulmonary hypertension, but if the disorder itself leads to heart failure, there is an added risk of complications such as the failure of your digestive system or your kidneys and other organs.

What should be done?
If you notice that your ankles are swelling at times when your chest condition seems par

ticularly acute, tell your physician, who will examine you and take a specimen of urine to test the health of your kidneys, because they may be affected by prolonged heart failure. If there is evidence of possible heart failure, you may need to undergo further diagnostic tests to find out if it is present.

What is the treatment?
Self-help: If you are still smoking in spite of lung trouble, give it up now.
Professional help: Heart failure due to pulmonary hypertension can be relieved by bed rest and treatment with oxygen, which reduces spasm in your pulmonary arteries, and *diuretics,* which take excess fluid out of your system. Further attacks are likely, though, unless the underlying disorder is treated, and treatment depends on the disease. Prolonged treatment with oxygen sometimes helps to lower pulmonary blood pressure, and your physician may prescribe daily home treatment with oxygen.

If your pulmonary hypertension is due to chronic lung disease, long-term treatment will aim at halting further deterioration. Your physician may prescribe *antibiotics* and immunize you against influenza to help prevent acute chest infections.

Pulmonary hypertension is hard to reverse once it has developed. With careful treatment, however, the disease can be kept under control and its effects minimized.

Low blood pressure
(hypotension)

Chronic high blood pressure (see p.382) is a serious problem, but chronic lower-than-average blood pressure is not. The only type of low blood pressure that may cause problems is the kind that comes on abruptly and causes dizziness or faintness. The most common such condition is a phenomenon known as postural hypotension. When you stand up abruptly from a sitting or lying position, your blood vessels have to contract to maintain normal blood pressure in the new posture. This process occurs automatically by reflex action of your nervous system. If you have postural hypotension, however, the reflex action is defective in some way. As a result, your blood pressure falls and the flow of blood to your brain is temporarily reduced if you suddenly change your posture. This causes dizziness or can even cause a brief loss of consciousness.

Postural hypotension may be due to medications prescribed for *high* blood pressure. Such drugs have an effect on the nervous system, which can cause postural hypoten

sion if the dosage is too high. The simple treatment is to reduce the dose. Occasionally, too, postural hypotension may occur as a minor complication of pregnancy or certain other conditions such as diabetes (see p.519) or hardening of the arteries (see p.404).

Sometimes low blood pressure causes such a diminished flow of blood to your brain that you will faint. This can be due to illness or to a physical reaction to sudden emotion, undernourishment, or standing too long in the heat. Occasional fainting spells due to hypotension are seldom cause for concern.

What should be done?
If you have dizzy spells or feel faint when you stand up abruptly, make a habit of standing up slowly from a sitting or lying position. If you have frequent fainting spells, consult your physician, who will check your blood pressure and may need further diagnostic tests to determine the underlying cause of the trouble. No special treatment for chronic hypotension is likely to be necessary.

Blood disorders

Introduction

Your blood has two basic parts: blood cells, which are also called blood corpuscles; and plasma, the fluid in which the blood cells are suspended. The disorders of the blood that are discussed in this section are principally concerned with the blood cells.

Most of the blood cells in your body are red blood cells. Their main function is to carry oxygen from the lungs to all parts of the body. Red blood cells contain a protein called hemoglobin, which combines with oxygen in the lungs and releases it to the tissues as the blood circulates through your body. The red blood cells also carry the waste product carbon dioxide from the tissues to the lungs so that it can be exhaled.

Your body also contains white blood cells, which protect the body from infection. There are several different kinds of white blood cells. Most of them are neutrophils, which attack and engulf bacteria. Another kind, the lymphocyte, recognizes foreign cells, infectious agents, and other foreign substances and participates in the body's immune reaction against them. There are other varieties of white blood cells, but these two are the most numerous.

A third type of blood cell is the platelet. Platelets gather wherever a blood vessel is injured, to plug the hole. This is the first stage in the blood clotting process. Chemical substances in the plasma then assist in forming a clot that seals the wound.

Most blood cells are produced in the bone marrow. However, lymphocytes are made in the spleen or in the lymph glands, which are found in the neck, armpits, groin and many other parts of the body. The spleen and lymph glands, together with the channels and ducts connecting them, are called the lymphatic system. When red blood cells and platelets become old or defective they are filtered out of the bloodstream and broken down by the spleen, and also by the liver and lymph glands.

Disorders of the blood are grouped as follows: lack of hemoglobin, which causes anemia; disorders in clotting, which cause bleeding and bruising; cancerous changes in the white cells, which cause leukemia; disorders in the production of blood cells in the bone marrow; and disorders that affect the lymphatic system.

Basic parts of the blood

Blood can easily be separated into its different parts like cream from milk. Red blood cells are heavier than white blood cells and platelets, which are heavier than the plasma.

Plasma
Plasma is a yellowish fluid that contains salts, antibodies, and blood-clotting factors.

White blood cells
White blood cells protect the body against infection by destroying bacteria and producing antibodies.

Platelets
Platelets help plug damaged blood vessel walls and form the first stage of a blood clot.

Red blood cells
Red blood cells account for almost half of your blood, and contain a protein, hemoglobin, that carries oxygen throughout the body.

Plasma

White blood cells and platelets

Red blood cells

White blood cells
1. Neutrophil
2. Lymphocyte

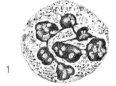

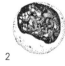

1

2

Platelets

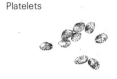

Red blood cells

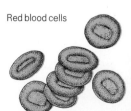

Anemia

The main component of red blood cells is the protein hemoglobin, which combines with oxygen in the lungs and carries it throughout your body, and releases it to those tissues that require it. Anemia is defined as a decrease in either hemoglobin or red blood cells to below the normal level.

Iron is an essential ingredient in hemoglobin. If you do not have enough iron in your body, you cannot make enough hemoglobin. This form of anemia is called iron-deficiency anemia. A severe shortage of vitamin B_{12} in your body also affects the production of red blood cells. This is called B_{12} deficiency anemia. Lack of folic acid in your body has the same effect, and this is called folic acid deficiency. If red blood cells are destroyed more quickly than they normally would be, the number of red blood cells in your body may fall well below normal, and cause hemolytic anemia. Inherited defects of the blood such as sickle-cell anemia cause your body to produce abnormal hemoglobin.

The characteristic symptoms of anemia include paleness, fatigue, weakness, fainting, breathlessness, and palpitations. Palpitations, or an increased awareness of your heartbeat, can occur when your heart tries to compensate for the anemia by pumping blood faster than is normal.

Iron-deficiency anemia

Iron is an essential component of hemoglobin, the protein in red blood cells. Insufficient iron in your body causes an inadequate production of hemoglobin, and therefore leads to iron deficiency anemia.

Normally, extra iron is stored in your body and then used to produce hemoglobin in newly developed red blood cells. Most of this iron is recovered as old red blood cells are destroyed. The small amount of iron lost from the body is replaced by iron absorbed from your diet. Some people, for a variety of reasons, have little or no iron stored in their bodies. If you are one of these people, you can stay healthy if you balance the iron you lose with iron absorbed from your diet. If you lose more iron than you are able to absorb, you may become anemic.

There are three general causes for a lack of iron reserves. The first is that there may not be enough iron in your diet to replace the amount that is lost each day. This problem occurs mainly in young children (see Iron deficiency anemia in children, p.681) and in people who, for one of several reasons, are living on restricted diets.

The second major reason for iron deficiency is that the digestive system is unable to absorb iron, even though there may be enough of the right forms of it in the diet. This occurs most often because part of the stomach has been removed surgically (see Stomach ulcer, p.465, and Cancer of the stomach, p.466).

The third reason for iron deficiency is that the iron reserves may become depleted through excessive loss of blood. This is the most common cause. If the blood loss is caused by a temporary problem, reserves of iron will rebuild in time. Many women have heavy menstrual periods, which can gradually deplete their iron reserves. In other cases, blood loss may occur in the intestinal tract. This type of blood loss, in sufficient quantity, can produce bloody or black stools. But, if it is limited in quantity, there may be no sign of the bleeding. Some of the common causes of intestinal blood loss are gastritis (see p.464), stomach ulcer (see p.465), duodenal ulcer (see p.468), cancer of the stomach (see p.466), cancer of the large intestine (see p.481), and hemorrhoids (see p.483).

What are the symptoms?

Symptoms are those characteristic of most forms of anemia. You may be weak, pale, tired, faint and/or breathless. You may also have palpitations, or an increased awareness of your heartbeat that occurs when your heart tries to compensate for the anemia by pumping blood faster than is normal.

What are the risks?

Iron deficiency anemia itself is very unlikely to lead to death. However, it does weaken your body's resistance to the effects of other illness or injury, especially if you lose large amounts of blood. It can also limit your productivity and your energy.

What should be done?

If you have anemia, see your physician. Do *not* attempt to treat the condition yourself. You may prevent your physician from diagnosing a serious but treatable disease that has produced the anemia. The doctor diagnoses anemia by taking a blood sample and having it tested. If the cause of the anemia is not obvious, further tests may be required. These may include measurements of the blood iron level, an examination of your bone marrow, and a look for blood in a bowel-movement sample. If bleeding is detected, other tests, such as an *upper gastro-intestinal (GI) series*, a *barium enema*, or *endoscopy* may be needed.

What is the treatment?

Iron deficiency anemia must be treated by dealing with the underlying disorder. It is very important that any correctable cause be appropriately treated. Usually the iron deficiency itself can be treated with iron tablets. These can cause indigestion or bowel upsets, but this should not happen if you take the tablets right after you eat and do not take more than your physician has prescribed. If you continue to have difficulty with the tablets, your physician may give you iron by injecting it into a vein, or into a muscle. Ordinarily the anemia disappears after several weeks of treatment. If the anemia is severe, or if it must be corrected fairly quickly, your physician can arrange for a blood transfusion.

When your anemia has cleared up, your physician will usually suggest that you continue to take iron for an additional six months, to build up your iron reserves. If the cause of the anemia was a poor diet, your physician can advise you on how you should change your diet in the future to prevent the problem from recurring.

The prospects for people with iron deficiency anemia are generally excellent. In many cases, treatment of the underlying disorder will permanently eliminate the iron deficiency. If it does not, you can prevent the anemia from recurring if you continue to take the iron tablets.

Anemia of chronic disease

This type of anemia frequently complicates other diseases. Disorders that often bring on this type of anemia include rheumatoid arthritis (see p.552), hepatitis (see p.486) and tuberculosis (see p.563). It can also occur in anyone who has an acute infection such as pneumonia (see p.359).

The symptoms of anemia of chronic disease are the same as those for other forms of anemia, combined with the symptoms of the underlying disease. It cannot be treated, except by transfusions, but it should improve when the disease that produces it improves in response to treatment.

B$_{12}$ deficiency anemia and folic acid deficiency

Red blood cell production takes place in the bone marrow, and depends substantially on two vitamins, vitamin B$_{12}$ and folic acid. Your body absorbs these vitamins from certain foods (see Vitamin guide, p.496). If you do not get enough of either vitamin, red blood cell production falls. Also, those red blood cells that are formed are defective. The result is one of these forms of anemia.

In North America, nearly everyone's diet contains sufficient quantities of B$_{12}$. A deficiency of the vitamin usually occurs because your body cannot absorb it. In a healthy person the liver contains reserves of vitamin B$_{12}$. If you develop an inability to absorb B$_{12}$, your body will eventually deplete these reserves and anemia will develop.

There are various reasons why some people cannot absorb B$_{12}$. Your body normally absorbs B$_{12}$ from the lower small intestine. But before this can occur the vitamin must combine in the stomach with a special substance known as intrinsic factor, which is secreted by the stomach lining. In some people, for reasons that are not fully understood, the stomach lining stops secreting enough intrinsic factor. Without it, sufficient quantities of vitamin B$_{12}$ cannot be absorbed. This is the most common type of B$_{12}$ deficiency, and it is called pernicious anemia.

If you have had some forms of digestive-tract surgery, your body's ability to absorb B$_{12}$ may be reduced, sometimes to the point where it cannot absorb any of the vitamin.

Folic acid deficiency is usually due to inadequate amounts of the vitamin in the diet. Folic acid is generally supplied by green vegetables. Your body cannot build large reserves of this vitamin, so any deficiency shows up within a few weeks as a form of anemia called folic acid deficiency. If you have celiac disease (see p.474), you are also susceptible to folic acid deficiency because you cannot absorb sufficient amounts of folic acid, even if it is plentiful in your diet. Finally, there are some people who have an increased requirement for folic acid, and they need more of the vitamin than an ordinary diet provides.

Both types of anemia produce the symptoms associated with anemia in general, but

B_{12} deficiency anemia is more serious, because B_{12} is vital to the maintenance of the nervous system as well as to the production of red blood cells. Deficiency of B_{12} therefore damages the brain and spinal cord, which causes additional symptoms.

What are the symptoms?
The main symptoms of B_{12} and folic acid deficiency anemia are those of other anemias. They include paleness, fatigue, shortness of breath, and palpitations, or heart fluttering, particularly if you exert yourself. In both disorders, your mouth and tongue may be sore, and your skin may become yellow in color. If the spinal cord is affected by B_{12} deficiency, you may not be able to walk or keep your balance properly, and you may feel continuous tingling in your hands and feet. You may also suffer some memory loss, confusion and depression.

Pernicious anemia, the most common type of B_{12} deficiency, is equally common in men and women, and rare before the age of 40. If you have a close relative who has pernicious anemia, you have a greater than average risk of contracting it. Folic acid deficiency is somewhat more common than B_{12} deficiency. It often occurs in elderly people, who may live on a poor diet. It also occurs in pregnant women, who need extra supplies of the vitamin for the developing baby. It is particularly common in cases of severe alcoholism, because alcoholics often do not eat properly.

What are the risks?
If you have B_{12} or folic acid deficiency anemia, and if it is treated promptly, you will probably recover completely. If you do not obtain prompt treatment for B_{12} deficiency anemia you risk permanent damage to your spinal cord and, to a lesser extent, irreversible intellectual impairment.

What should be done?
If you have symptoms of anemia, see your physician. If your movement, balance or memory are also affected, make the appointment without delay. Be sure to tell the physician if you have a close relative who has pernicious anemia. Tests on a blood sample can usually establish whether or not you have either of these vitamin deficiencies. But if you have one of them, the underlying cause usually can be determined only by examining the results of further tests.

What is the treatment?
Once your ability to absorb vitamin B_{12} through the digestive tract has been lost, it can never be regained. Treatment of pernicious anemia and other types of B_{12} deficiency consists of a life-long series of vitamin B_{12} injections. You may eventually be able to give them to yourself. It is important that you do not miss an injection; if you do, your symptoms will return. Problems with walking and balancing may take several months to improve. If these symptoms existed for a long time before treatment began, they may never disappear completely.

Folic acid deficiency that is caused by an inadequate diet can be cleared up completely. At first, your physician may prescribe folic acid tablets. After that, you will probably be told how to make sure that your diet contains adequate amounts of the vitamin (see p.496). If the deficiency is caused by a failure to absorb normal quantities of folic acid, or by an increased requirement for it, extra folic acid may be prescribed in tablet form for an indefinite period.

Blood poisoning
Blood poisoning, or septicemia, is not a single disease. It is a condition that is caused by the spread of bacterial infection in your blood. The "poison" is either the bacteria that is causing the infection, or poisonous substances called *toxins* that are made by the bacteria.

Even a minor infection such as a boil (see p.251) or a small contaminated wound releases a few bacteria into your bloodstream. Many routine dental procedures, such as extractions, also release bacteria into your blood. If you are healthy, your body destroys these automatically. If you contract a more severe infection such as pyelonephritis (see p.502), the level of bacteria or toxins in your blood may be higher than with most other diseases. This produces fever, chills, fatigue, loss of appetite, and a generally ill feeling. *Antibiotic* drugs can aid your body's natural defenses in combating such an infection. A blood test can identify the infecting organism and help your physician choose the proper antibiotic.

It is important that you consult your physician for treatment of urinary tract infections, wound infections and major burns, because bacteria tend to invade the bloodstream in these conditions. Large numbers of bacteria and/or toxins in your blood may cause septic shock (see p.386). You may have severe chills and become pale, cold, and clammy, accompanied by a serious drop in blood pressure. This usually, but not always, begins from an infection in some part of your body. This is a very serious condition, and you should get immediate medical help.

Sickle-cell anemia

In the inherited disease called sickle-cell anemia, the red blood cells contain an abnormal hemoglobin, called hemoglobin S. If you have this disease, you have no normal hemoglobin in your red blood cells, because you have inherited a sickle-cell gene from each of your parents. This condition must be distinguished from sickle-cell trait, in which you inherit only one sickle-cell gene from one parent. Then you have red cells that contain half normal hemoglobin and half hemoglobin S, and your health is not impaired. In addition to hemolysis, or premature destruction of red blood cells, hemoglobin S causes red cells of persons with sickle-cell anemia to become deformed in shape, or "sickled," especially in parts of the body where the amount of oxygen is relatively low. These abnormal blood cells do not flow smoothly through the capillaries, or smaller blood vessels. They may clog the vessels, and prevent blood from reaching the tissues. This blockage causes *anoxia*, or lack of oxygen, which makes the sickling worse. Attacks of this kind are called sickle-cell "crises." They can be very painful.

What are the symptoms?

If you have sickle-cell anemia, you will have all the symptoms of anemia (see p.419). In addition, you may have occasional sickle-cell crises, which produce attacks of pain in the bones and abdomen. You may also develop blood clots in the lungs, kidneys, brain, and most other organs.

How often crises occur varies a great deal from one person with the disease to another. Crises are more likely to occur during infections and after an accident or injury. They also occur with anesthesia and surgery if appropriate precautions are not taken.

Both the sickle-cell trait and sickle-cell anemia are virtually unknown except in people of African descent and in persons from parts of Italy, Greece, Arabia and India. About 1 in every 1000 black Americans has sickle-cell anemia.

What are the risks?

There is virtually no risk from sickle-cell trait, but a man and woman who both have the trait can produce a child with sickle-cell anemia. If you have sickle-cell anemia, you risk painful crises. Abnormalities of bone growth and severe infection from certain bacteria may also occur. Severe sickle-cell crises can damage most organs in your body by impairing blood flow, and this damage can lead to death from heart failure (see p.381), kidney failure (see p.511) or stroke (see p.268).

What should be done?

If you or your child displays any of the symptoms described, see your physician, who will consider the possibility of sickle-cell anemia, especially if the disease is known to run in your family. Analysis of a blood sample will disclose whether the disease is present.

If you are of African descent and you are considering getting married or having a child, it is wise for you to be tested for sickle-cell trait. Because the trait is relatively common in the black population, about 6 of every 1000 black couples will have the capability of producing a child with sickle-cell anemia.

What is the treatment?

There is now no cure for an inherited disease such as sickle-cell anemia, but the symptoms can be treated. Crises of acute pain are the most common problem. These are treated with painkillers, and you often have to be admitted to the hospital for them. It is extremely important that you do everything possible to maintain good health, and that you obtain prompt treatment for infections, injuries and other illnesses. Also, you should see a physician regularly who is thoroughly familiar with the disease. Special precautions are necessary before you have any surgery, including dental surgery. Also, you should not fly in an unpressurized airplane or be at altitudes above about 6000 feet, at least not without special precautions and instructions.

Thalass-emia

In this disorder an inherited defect prevents the formation of normal amounts of hemoglobin A, the type of hemoglobin that is found in the red blood cells after the first few months of life. As a partial compensation, the cells contain hemoglobin F, a type of hemoglobin that is usually found only in newborn babies. However, only a relatively small amount of hemoglobin F is made in adults who have thalassemia, so their red blood cells contain less hemoglobin than normal. In addition, the majority of the red blood cells produced in this condition are destroyed within the bone marrow, and those that remain can survive only a short time.

The full-blown form of the disorder, called thalassemia major, occurs only if you inherit the defect from both of your parents (see p.704). It produces severe anemia. When you inherit the defect from only one parent, the result is the thalassemia "trait." This rarely causes any symptoms or disability.

What are the symptoms?
The symptoms of thalassemia major are similar to those of hemolytic anemia (see next article). They include paleness, tiredness, weakness, breathlessness and palpitations, or increased awareness of your heartbeat. A child who has the disease will be relatively inactive and will also be unable to keep up with his or her playmates.

What are the risks?
Thalassemia trait is several times more common than thalassemia major. Both forms of the disorder are relatively common in persons from the Mediterranean area, the Middle East and the Far East.

If you have the trait, you are at little or no risk. If you have thalassemia major, repeated blood transfusions are needed to treat the anemia. This treatment eventually causes a build-up of iron in your body, which damages the liver and the heart. At one time, this led to death from liver or heart failure. There is now a treatment available that makes it possible to remove the iron.

What should be done?
If you or your child displays any of the symptoms described, see your physician, who will consider the possibility of thalassemia, especially if this disease is known to run in your family. Initially the doctor will arrange for a blood sample to be taken and tested to confirm or reject this possibility.

If you have any form of the disease in your family, even as the trait, and you are considering having a child, be sure to see your physician about the possibility of your child being affected by the disease.

What is the treatment?
The underlying genetic defect that causes thalassemia cannot now be cured. If you have the disease, regular blood transfusions throughout your life will relieve the symptoms of anemia, and it is now possible to use only young red cells in the transfusions. These survive longer, and therefore you can reduce the frequency of the transfusions. Also, you need a drug that causes your body to eliminate excess iron.

Hemolytic anemia

Hemolysis is a disorder in which your red blood cells are destroyed prematurely. When this occurs, your body attempts to compensate by producing new red cells at a faster rate. If destruction exceeds production, the resulting disorder is called hemolytic anemia.

Hemolytic anemia may be hereditary, in which case it is present at birth or soon afterwards, or you may acquire it later in life. In the hereditary hemolytic anemias, hemolysis occurs because a specific component of your red blood cells is abnormal. Certain drugs can damage red cells and so produce hemolysis and hemolytic anemia. This occurs if you have inherited a specific type of abnormality that triggers anemia when you take a certain type of drug or develop special infections. Then your red blood cells become less able to protect themselves against the chemical reactions caused by the drug or the infection, and they are destroyed.

One type of acquired hemolytic anemia occurs when your body produces *antibodies,* or substances that normally protect you from infections, that attack the body's own red blood cells. Hemolysis may also occur when your body produces antibodies against recently transfused red blood cells. Finally, red cells may also be destroyed after they are damaged by artificial heart valves, abnormal blood vessel walls, or *toxins.*

The disease is rarely fatal in any of its forms, though some forms of hemolytic anemia are difficult to treat.

What are the symptoms?
The main symptoms of hemolytic anemia are paleness, fatigue, breathlessness, and palpitations, or heart fluttering, especially with exertion. In addition, your skin may become yellow, and your urine may contain blood pigment and so be darker than normal. If your red blood cells continue to be destroyed prematurely for many years, gallstones (see p.489) often result.

What should be done?
If you have the symptoms described, see your physician. You will probably be questioned about your symptoms, and the physician will probably arrange for a blood test.

What is the treatment?
The principal treatment for one type of hemolytic anemia, hereditary spherocytosis, is a *splenectomy,* an operation to remove the spleen. Most red blood cells are destroyed by the spleen as they wear out. Removing the spleen can considerably improve hemolytic anemia, but does not cure it.

Hemolytic anemia that is caused by drugs is treated by discontinuing the drugs. If the disease is caused by antibodies, your physician may prescribe various drugs.

Bleeding and bruising

Bleeding occurs when a blood vessel is damaged. If the vessel is internal, blood seeps into surrounding tissue, and a bruise forms. Where delicate blood vessels are near the surface of tissue, as they are in the nose, for example, a very slight injury or irritation may cause bleeding.

For most people, minor bleeding causes no harm because the body soon stops it. It does

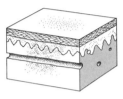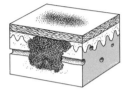

Bruises
Blood from an internal injury collects in surrounding tissue to form a bruise. Once the internal bleeding has stopped, white blood cells called monocytes help to break down the leaked red blood cells. A bruise is blue because red cells look blue when seen through the skin.

this by means of three main mechanisms that act together. The nearby blood vessels contract, and restrict the flow of blood to the area of the wound. The platelets in the blood gather where the blood vessels are damaged, and stick to the vessel walls and to each other to form a plug. In addition, interlacing strands of a material called *fibrin* form in the damaged area. Blood cells are then trapped in the fibrin mesh and form a clot that seals the break and stops the bleeding.

In diseases that cause abnormal bleeding, one or more of the mechanisms that halt blood loss does not work right. Bleeding from a cut, which would normally stop within five or ten minutes, may continue for hours, or even days. Minor injuries may cause extensive bruising. There may be internal bleeding, and bleeding in the joints may produce acute pain and eventually cause crippling damage. Two of the most common of such disorders, hemophilia and thrombocytopenia, are discussed here.

Hemophilia

Hemophilia is the best known of the bleeding diseases. Although it is the most common of these diseases, it is still rather rare. In this disorder, there is a marked reduction in the amount of a protein called anti-hemophilic globulin, or Factor VIII, in the blood. Factor VIII is vital to the clotting mechanism of the blood. Because of the way hemophilia is inherited, only males have the disease, but it is passed from generation to generation by female "carriers." In the United States about 1 male in 10,000 has hemophilia. In about 75 per cent of cases, there is a family history of the disease, but in the remaining cases, the hemophiliac is the first of his line, probably because of a mutation, or spontaneous change, in the genes of his mother.

What are the symptoms?
Symptoms usually appear in childhood, as soon as the affected male child becomes active. He gets bruises on his knees and elbows after he crawls, and cuts bleed for a long time. Internal bleeding caused by falls may cause large, deep bruises, which may make a limb swollen and painful for several days. Repeated bleeding into joints and accumulation of scarred tissue produce stiff joints that limit the child's movement. There is a great deal of variation in the amount of bleeding from one patient to another.

What are the risks?
Today the risks of being crippled or dying from hemophilia are greatly reduced because of effective treatment. However, a major injury is still particularly dangerous for anyone who has hemophilia. Also, if you are a hemophiliac, special precautions must be taken before you have any operation, even a tooth extraction.

What should be done?
Any member of a family with a history of hemophilia should seek genetic counseling before starting a family. Your physician or local public health organizations can tell you where to find such counseling. If you have a male child who shows any of the symptoms described, see your physician.

If you are an adult male and you notice that you bruise or bleed in a way that seems abnormal to you, you should also see your physician. After questioning you, the physician may refer you to a hematologist, or blood specialist. If you or your child have hemophilia, you may be given a card that describes the disease. The hemophiliac should carry the card at all times, so that if an accident occurs the appropriate treatment will be given.

What is the treatment?

Self-help: If you have hemophilia, unless it is a very mild case, your physician will advise against activities that could cause even minor injury. This means that you must avoid most physical contact sports. Solitary exercise such as running or gymnastics may be advised in moderation. Your physician will also advise that you not take aspirin or any drugs that contain it. This is because aspirin increases the chance of bleeding.

Professional help: If severe bleeding or bruising does occur, you should know who to contact, usually your own physician or a spe-cial hospital. Such bleeding is treated by in-fusing a concentrated form of Factor VIII, the missing clotting factor, into a vein. De-pending on the severity of the bleeding and its location in your body, it is often necessary to continue the infusions of Factor VIII regular-ly for five to ten days after a bleeding episode.

What are the long term prospects?

There is no question that hemophilia is, in many ways, a limiting disease. It is probably most difficult to deal with in childhood when much of normal play must be avoided. Adults with hemophilia generally work out satisfac-tory lives within the limitations that are im-posed by the disease. Those who are ex-tremely upset by feelings of restriction or vulnerability should seek psychiatric aid.

Thrombo-cytopenia

The blood cells known as platelets play a vital part in the mechanisms of the body that stop bleeding. If you have thrombocytopenia, your blood contains about one-third or less of the normal number of platelets. As a result, you will bleed longer than is normal if you are injured or if you begin to bleed internally or externally for any reason.

Thrombocytopenia is usually caused by the body forming *antibodies* (normally protective biochemicals) that attack its own platelets. Healthy platelets are damaged and then re-moved from the bloodstream at a high rate. This type of thrombocytopenia is known as acute ITP, which stands for immune throm-bocytopenic purpura. Its cause is unknown. Thrombocytopenia may also occur because of a drug you are taking for an unrelated purpose. It occurs relatively often in people who are receiving *radiation therapy* or *chemotherapy* for cancer.

Thrombocytopenia can occur as a symp-tom of other blood disorders such as leukemia (see next article). Also, your platelet count can be reduced when you are given many blood transfusions in a short period of time, during major surgery, for example, or when abnormal bleeding and clotting occur with another disorder.

What are the symptoms?

The main symptom of thrombocytopenia is a rash that consists of minute, bright red and dark red dots. These dots are actually tiny areas of bleeding in your skin. The rash can appear on any part of your body, but it often begins on the legs and wherever your skin has been irritated. Nose bleeds and a tendency to bruise are also very common symptoms. Bleeding from cuts is also prolonged, and major internal bleeding often occurs when your platelet count is low.

What should be done?

Consult your physician immediately if you notice the characteristic rash or any other abnormal bleeding. The physician will proba-bly review any drugs you may be taking for another disorder, and will take a blood sam-ple for laboratory analysis. The blood test will show the platelet level, and indicate whether the thrombocytopenia is a sign of another disease. Usually a bone marrow examination is required to determine if platelets are being made in the marrow.

What is the treatment?

Your physician will probably stop most or all drugs you may be taking, because virtually any drug can produce thrombocytopenia. If the cause appears to be an antibody, your physician may prescribe a *steroid* drug to decrease the destruction caused by an-tibodies. This will allow the level of platelets in your blood to rise. The disease often im-proves or disappears after a few weeks. If it does not, your physician may advise you to have a *splenectomy*, an operation in which your spleen is removed. The spleen normally destroys worn out red cells, but it can become enlarged and overactive. If this occurs, the spleen may also destroy platelets, and pre-vent you from recovering quickly.

If you have thrombocytopenia that is caused by underproduction of platelets by the bone marrow or by blood loss caused by bleeding or abnormal clotting, you may need transfusions of platelets.

Leukemia

Leukemia is a cancer of white blood cells. Normally the number of white blood cells that are produced equals the number that die off as part of the natural process of cell turnover in the body. This keeps the total number of white blood cells constant. In leukemia, white blood cells often multiply at an increased rate. It is also significant that the cancerous cells tend to live longer than normal white blood cells. Thus the number of abnormal cells increases, either gradually or rapidly, and this causes an over-accumulation of leukemic cells throughout the body. These cells often interfere with the functions of various organs. And, be-cause the cells are abnormal, they do not cope effectively with infectious agents that the normal white blood cells help to elimi-nate from the body.

There are two main types of leukemia, which affect different types of white blood cells. Lymphocytic leukemia is a malignan-cy of lymphocytes (see p.432) and/or the cells from which they originate. Myelogen-ous (or granulocytic) leukemia is a cancer of the cells from which granulocytes originate. Both of these leukemias may be acute or chronic. Acute lymphocytic leukemia main-ly affects children; it is discussed elsewhere (see p.682).

Acute myelogenous leukemia

This disease, which is also called acute granulocytic leukemia, is caused by a *malig-nant*, or life-threatening, change in cells that produce granulocytes, one of the types of white blood cells made in the bone marrow. The resulting leukemic granulocytes multiply and survive longer than normal cells. As their numbers increase, the leukemic cells invade the bone marrow. This invasion disrupts the production of normal granulocytes, red blood cells and platelets.

Then, the leukemic granulocytes begin to enter the bloodstream, and their numbers increase fairly rapidly. Next they invade or-gans and tissues, particularly the spleen and liver. These organs become enlarged.

What are the symptoms?

The common early symptoms of acute myelogenous leukemia are fatigue, infections (especially of the mouth and throat), fever, lip and mouth ulcers, and a tendency to bruise and bleed. You may also have the usual symptoms of anemia (see Iron deficiency anemia, p.419).

The disease often occurs suddenly, with the symptoms becoming pronounced over one or two weeks. But, sometimes, the symptoms appear gradually over two or three months. An elderly person may have what is called smoldering leukemia, in which the onset of the disease is very gradual. In such cases, treatment is usually postponed.

What are the risks?

There is no cure for acute myelogenous leukemia. If it is not treated, it can be fatal within a few days or weeks. Even with suc-cessful treatment the average survival time after the disease is identified is about one year. The main hazards of this form of leukemia are serious infection and bleeding (see Thrombocytopenia, previous page).

What should be done?

Anyone with the symptoms described should see a physician immediately. After examining you, the doctor will probably arrange for you to have blood tests and usually a bone mar-row *biopsy*. In a biopsy some of your bone marrow is removed and examined carefully under a microscope. If they are present, the cancer cells will be visible.

What is the treatment?

As soon as the diagnosis of this disease has been confirmed, you will probably be admit-ted to a hospital. Because the treatment is complicated and difficult, it should generally be done by a physician who treats acute leukemia regularly. You should probably be in a large medical center where physicians are available around the clock. In the hospital, you will get transfusions of red blood cells and platelets when you need them. An *an-tibiotic* is usually prescribed to reduce the chance of infection. If you develop a fever or other evidence of infection, the infectious agent will be identified and antibiotics that are effective against it will be given to you intravenously. Transfusions of granulocytes may also be necessary. Platelet transfusions are usually done to prevent bleeding due to thrombocytopenia (see previous page).

The treatment for the leukemia itself is the administration of strong *cytotoxic*, or anti-cancer, drugs. These drugs are given intravenously. Their purpose is to eliminate leukemic cells from the bone marrow, but they also destroy many of the normal blood cells that are in the bone marrow. This is, unfortunately, unavoidable.

Once the leukemic cells in the bone marrow are destroyed, which may take more than one series of treatments, it takes at least two weeks before significant numbers of healthy cells start to repopulate the marrow and enter the bloodstream. This period of very low blood cell count can be extremely dangerous. If necessary, you will be placed in a special care area of the hospital, and precautions will be taken to prevent any infection. You may also require further transfusions of red blood cells and platelets.

When the danger period is over, your condition should improve dramatically. If the treatment is successful, at some time from three weeks to three months after the beginning of treatment all signs of leukemia disappear. The bone marrow then produces normal cells, and the disease is said to have gone into remission. This means that the symptoms of the disease have disappeared or diminished, but only temporarily. The drug treatment produces a complete remission in 50 to 80 per cent of patients. You may need further drug treatment at four to six week intervals to try to prevent the disease from returning. Eventually, however, leukemia does return. Further intensive treatment may produce several more remissions, but the chances for a remission and the duration of each remission decrease with each repeated treatment. There is growing evidence that bone marrow transplantation that is carried out at the time of the first remission, both improves the long-term survival rate and produces some cures.

Chronic lymphocytic leukemia

The disease begins when one or more lymphocytes, a type of white blood cell, become *malignant*, or life-threatening. Instead of maturing and dying in the normal way, the leukemic cell multiplies and produces more of its kind. These also produce leukemic cells, and so on. After some time, perhaps several years, the leukemic cells gradually crowd out normal white blood cells in the lymph glands, and reduce the ability of the remaining healthy cells to fight infections. The leukemic cells also overflow from the lymph glands into the bloodstream, and from there into the spleen, the liver, the bone marrow and other parts of the body. As the number of leukemic cells in the marrow rises, they interfere increasingly with the ability of the marrow to produce other blood cells. This leads to a number of problems, including anemia, susceptibility to infections, and bleeding.

What are the symptoms?
The disease often produces no symptoms for awhile and is most often discovered by a blood test done for another purpose. In some cases, the first signs of the illness are enlarged lymph glands in the neck, armpits, or groin, or a feeling of fullness in the upper left portion of the abdomen, due to an enlarged spleen. In other cases of the disease, the first symptoms may be those that are caused by anemia (see p.419) or infection. In some cases, general ill health, loss of appetite and weight, fever, and sweating at night are the first indications of the disease.

What should be done?
Anyone who has some of the symptoms listed above should see a physician, who can arrange for a blood sample to be taken and tested. If you do have the disease, other tests can determine it extent.

What is the treatment?
When the disease is in an early stage, you do not require any treatment, and only periodic checkups are necessary. Treatment is required, however, when symptoms or signs of the disease appear, such as significant increases in the size of your lymph glands, spleen or liver; anemia; a low platelet count in your blood; or fever and weight loss.

The treatment your physician will probably use initially for chronic lymphocytic leukemia is an anticancer drug that is very well tolerated and is usually effective in eliminating or greatly reducing most symptoms of the disease. Your enlarged lymph glands and your spleen will probably decrease in size. Your blood count will improve, and your symptoms will go away. If this drug is ineffective, or if it stops working after a period of successful treatment, you will probably be treated with a combination of other anticancer drugs. These often produce improvement again.

The average lifespan after a diagnosis of chronic lymphocytic leukemia is three to four years. However, if you have this disease and you either do not need treatment or respond to it very well, you have a good chance of living much longer.

Chronic granulocytic leukemia

Chronic granulocytic leukemia begins in the same way as acute myelogenous leukemia (see p.426). A *malignant*, or life-threatening, change occurs in bone marrow cells that produce granulocytes, a type of white blood cell. As a result, the number of granulocytes in your blood rises excessively, often to between 20 and 40 times the normal level. When the disease is not treated, the multiplication of granulocytes may limit the production of red blood cells, so you may also become anemic. In addition, the accumulation of leukemic cells may cause enlargement of both your spleen and your liver.

What are the symptoms?

If you have chronic granulocytic leukemia, you feel generally ill, have little appetite, and lose weight. You may have a fever and sweat at night. In addition, your enlarged spleen may cause a sense of fullness in the left upper portion of the abdomen. You may also have symptoms of anemia (see p.419).

What are the risks?

If chronic granulocytic leukemia is not treated, it is likely to be fatal within weeks or months. The disease usually responds very well to initial treatment, which gives most patients at least two to three more years of fairly normal life. Eventually, the disease begins to resemble acute leukemia, and it no longer responds to treatment.

What should be done?

If you have any of the symptoms described, you should see your physician, who will probably examine you and arrange for blood tests. The blood tests will either rule out the disease, or indicate the need to take further blood tests. To establish a clear diagnosis, there may also be a bone marrow *biopsy*, in which a small sample of marrow is removed to be examined.

What is the treatment?

Most people who have the disease can be treated as out-patients. The basic treatment is tablets of anticancer drugs that usually restore bone marrow production to normal and clear up the symptoms. Some people need to continue to take the medication regularly, while others require it only intermittently. Your physician will watch your condition, and take blood tests every two to four weeks. This is important because the dose of medication often needs to be adjusted, and too much of the drug decreases your blood count to dangerous levels.

After some time, treatment with drugs will no longer control the disease. The average length of time before this occurs is three years, but it can be much shorter or much longer. Eventually the leukemia becomes much worse and you will probably be admitted to a hospital. At this stage of the disease, stronger anticancer drugs may help you for a short time, but often it is only a matter of weeks before the disease proves fatal.

Blood groups

What are blood groups?

The surface of each red blood cell is covered with molecules called *antigens*. There are various groups of antigens, including the ABO group, the Rh (or Rhesus) group, and many others, on each red blood cell. Your red blood cells contain specific antigens from each of these groups. For example, you might have type A antigens from the ABO group on all your red cells. This means you have blood type A. Your Rh type may be positive (Rh+) or negative (Rh−). Your blood type is determined by the genes you inherit from your parents (see p.704).

Why are they important?

If you have a transfusion of the wrong type of blood, the red blood cells may be destroyed by *antibodies*. This can cause shock (see p.386), acute kidney failure (see p.511), and death. If you need a blood transfusion, whoever is giving the transfusion must identify the major antigens on your blood cells and then select the correct, matched blood for the transfusion. Mismatched ABO and Rh types are the most likely to cause transfusion reactions, but other types are also important at times. Blood groups are also important in certain cases when a woman becomes pregnant (see Rhesus incompatibility, p.626).

If you are going to have an elective operation that will require a transfusion, such as a hip joint replacement, the best way to avoid any difficulty in matching blood is to "bank" several pints of your own blood during the months before surgery is scheduled. This also avoids the danger of contracting blood-transmitted hepatitis.

How common is my blood type?

The easiest way to find out your blood type is to donate blood at a blood donor center or hospital. Donating blood is harmless to healthy persons and is a fine way to contribute to the health of others. Many companies and community groups have annual blood drives.

You can find out how common your blood type is by looking at the table.

Major blood-type frequencies

| Types | White Americans | | Black Americans | |
	Rh+	Rh−	Rh+	Rh−
A	38.0%	7.0%	26.0%	2.0%
B	7.0	1.0	17.0	1.5
AB	3.0	0.6	4.0	0.4
O	37.0	6.0	45.0	4.0

Bone marrow

The marrow inside your bones is an active tissue with a rich blood supply. Your bone marrow produces most of your blood cells, including all of the red cells and platelets, and most of the white cells (see p.418).

The blood that flows through the marrow moves the blood cells that the marrow produces into the bloodstream. In an adult, active blood-forming marrow is only in the bones of the body's trunk. The limb bones contain fatty, non-active marrow, which can change to active, blood-forming marrow if the body needs to produce more blood cells. In a young child, all the bones have active blood-forming marrow.

This section includes diseases in which the bone marrow produces either too many or too few blood cells. These disorders may affect all types of blood cells, as in aplastic anemia and polycythemia, or may only affect one type of cell, as in multiple myeloma and agranulocytosis.

Poly-cythemia

Normally your body adjusts the production of blood cells in the bone marrow, so that the number of blood cells that are made equals the number that are destroyed. If you have polycythemia, the mechanism becomes faulty and your marrow produces far more blood cells than usual.

There are two main types of the disorder. The first, polycythemia vera, is an overproduction of red blood cells, granulocytes and platelets.

The second type of polycythemia is called secondary polycythemia. It occurs as a result of an underlying cause such as a severe lung disease, certain kinds of congenital heart disease (see p.656), cigarette and cigar smoking, and living at high altitudes. These conditions can prevent the red blood cells from obtaining enough oxygen to pass on to the body's tissues, and the bone marrow responds by producing many more red blood cells.

There is a third and less important type of the disorder, which is called stress polycythemia or pseudopolycythemia. In this condition, the number of red blood cells in a blood sample is high, but the cause is a decrease in the amount of plasma in the blood. This is usually due to smoking, but it can be caused by taking *diuretic* drugs or by becoming *dehydrated.*

Currently, secondary polycythemia and stress polycythemia are not treated directly. Rather, the problems that cause them are dealt with. Polycythemia vera is the most serious form of the disease, however, and it can be treated directly.

What are the symptoms?
The typical symptoms of polycythemia vera include recurrent headaches, dizziness, a feeling of fullness in the head, and a ruddy complexion. Sometimes there is severe itching, and hot baths make the itching worse. A physician who examines you may find that you have an enlarged spleen.

What are the risks?
Although polycythemia vera cannot be cured, it is almost always readily controlled by treatment. Many people who have the disease live for many years. Possible complications from the disease include heart attack (see p.379), deep-vein thrombosis (see p.405), stroke (see p.268), peripheral arterial thrombosis, bleeding, and gout (see p.498).

What should be done?
If you have the symptoms of polycythemia, you should see a physician. The physician will arrange for a blood test, which should show whether or not you have some form of the disease. If polycythemia is diagnosed, further tests are necessary to discover which type of the disorder you have. The tests may include additional blood tests, an *intravenous pyelogram*, or *X-rays* of the kidneys, and a measurement of blood volume. In this last test, for example, a small amount of radioactive albumin and a small quantity of your own red blood cells labelled with radioactive chromium are injected into a vein in one of your arms, and a blood sample is taken from your other arm about 30 minutes later. Then the volume of red blood cells and plasma in your bloodstream can be determined.

What is the treatment?
If you have polycythemia vera, you may be able to receive treatment as an out-patient. The first goal of treatment is to lower the number of red cells in your blood to reduce the risk of thrombosis, or blockage from a

clot. To do this, about a pint of blood is regularly taken from a vein in your arm. In some cases, this treatment is only needed once to clear up the condition.

Drugs are usually used to control the over-production of blood cells. Depending on what drug your physician prescribes, you may take it in tablet form for several weeks or it may be injected into a vein. Drug treatment may control the disease for up to several years. Treatment is repeated when the blood counts begin to increase again.

Multiple myeloma

The plasma cells are among the less common types of white blood cell in the bone marrow. They produce *antibodies* that help to destroy bacteria, viruses and other infectious agents and foreign cells. They also produce antibodies in response to vaccination or immunization. Normally, plasma cells make up only a small percentage of the cells in the marrow, but in multiple myeloma one plasma cell undergoes a *malignant*, or life-threatening, change and begins to multiply excessively. This has three serious effects. First, it disrupts the production of red blood cells, platelets and granulocytes (a type of white blood cell) in the marrow, which leads to anemia (see p.419), thrombocytopenia (see p.425) and a reduction of granulocytes in the blood. Second, the excess plasma cells cause destruction of bone. Third, the remaining normal plasma cells produce fewer antibodies and this reduces resistance to infection.

What are the symptoms?
Usually the first symptoms of myeloma are the symptoms associated with anemia (see Iron deficiency anemia, p.419). Increased susceptibility to infection may also appear early. The most characteristic symptom of the disease is pain in your bones, particularly in the vertebrae, or backbones.

What are the risks?
Myeloma is a rare disease, occurring in less than 4 of every 100,000 people in the United States. Myeloma affects mainly people over 50 and it is somewhat more common in men than it is in women.

Myeloma cannot be cured, but if you have the disease, treatment can give you several years of fairly normal life. Recurrent infection is a common problem with this disease, and it can be quite serious. There is a risk of chronic kidney failure (see p.512), and bleeding is another common problem.

What should be done?
If you are over 50 and you have developed bone pain, especially in your back, you should see a physician. If you have multiple myeloma, laboratory analysis of blood and urine samples and *X-rays* of the skeleton will usually detect it.

What is the treatment?
In the early stages of multiple myeloma, if there are no complications, the usual treatment that is currently used is an anticancer drug. The amount of the medication that is given must be carefully controlled, because too much of the drug can damage too many of the other cells in the bone marrow, and too little of it will not be able to halt the progress of the disease. Blood samples are taken during treatment to find an effective, safe dosage. Often *steroids* are also prescribed.

This treatment controls the disease in many but not all cases. Because your resistance to infection remains low during this treatment, *antibiotics* may be prescribed if you have any symptoms of an infection. Troublesome bone pain can usually be relieved by *radiation therapy*. If you respond to treatment at first, and then have a relapse, your physician may try different drugs.

If the disease is not in an advanced stage when it is diagnosed, and if you respond well to treatment, you will probably survive for about two years.

Aplastic anemia

If you have aplastic anemia, your bone marrow's production of blood cells decreases. This causes a reduction in the total number of cells in your bloodstream. This may occur gradually or suddenly. In most cases the cause of the problem cannot be identified. Sometimes the cause can be tentatively traced to exposure to a toxic substance such as benzene, certain substances used to dye hair, a drug taken for another disorder, or radiation. Most anticancer drugs produce similar changes in the bone marrow, but the condition usually improves when the drug is discontinued for awhile.

What are the symptoms?
There are three main groups of symptoms. The decrease in production of red blood cells

causes the symptoms of anemia (see p.419). The decrease in production of granulocytes, a type of white blood cell, makes you more susceptible to infection. Finally, the decrease in platelet production (see Thrombocytopenia, p.425) leads to spontaneous bruising, red dots on the skin, and bleeding from the nose, mouth and other sites.

What are the risks?

The main risks associated with aplastic anemia are infection and bleeding. Both of these may be severe enough to become life-threatening. You may improve spontaneously or with treatment, but progressive failure of the bone marrow, worsening your condition, may also occur.

What should be done?

If you develop any of the symptoms described, see your physician at once. This is especially important if you are taking a drug or working with chemicals or radioactive materials. The physician will probably arrange for a blood test. If the test results show that aplastic anemia may be present, you may need to have a bone marrow *biopsy*, in which a small amount of bone marrow is removed and examined under the microscope. This examination should allow your physician to make a definite diagnosis.

What is the treatment?

In cases where the disease is associated with a drug that is being taken for another problem, your physician will strongly consider stopping the drug and finding a suitable substitute. If there is any suspicion of continuing exposure to a *toxic* compound, you should remove yourself from contact with it.

Your physician will probably treat anemia and hemorrhage, or bleeding, with blood transfusions, and infections with *antibiotics*, which are usually given intravenously for best results. If you do not have an infection, but your granulocyte count is very low, you still may be given an antibiotic to reduce the chance of infection.

If the disease is severe or if it is growing worse, a bone marrow transplant offers the best hope of recovery. However, the bone marrow transplant has its own hazards. There is also a medication available, but it helps only a few patients.

Agranulo-cytosis

The white blood cells known as neutrophils act as the body's first defense against infections. Normally the neutrophils are produced in the bone marrow and are released into the bloodstream. In agranulocytosis, most or all of the neutrophils are destroyed, and there is a severe reduction in the number of neutrophils that are circulating in the blood. The result of this reduction in circulating neutrophils is decreased resistance to infection.

The disease is often caused by a drug that you are taking for some other disorder. It can also be caused by a viral infection or by an *antibody*, or normally protective biochemical in your blood, that you develop against your own white blood cells. The disease may be the first sign of leukemia (see p.426) or aplastic anemia (previous article).

What are the symptoms?

The characteristic symptom of the disease is susceptibility to infection. This is especially true in the mouth and throat, where ulcers often occur. Sometimes, if you have agranulocytosis, infections such as pneumonia (see p.359) progress unusually rapidly and are extremely severe, or even fatal.

What should be done?

If you have had one infection after another, see your physician, particularly if you are taking a prescription, or even a non-prescription drug. Some drugs are known to carry a particular risk of damaging bone marrow, and your physician will be alert to this possibility. The doctor will probably arrange for a blood test. If the results show that you may have agranulocytosis, a bone marrow *biopsy*, in which a small amount of bone marrow is removed and examined, will be necessary before your physician can make a definite diagnosis.

What is the treatment?

Your physician will probably instruct you to stop taking any drug in case it is the cause of the disorder. If the level of granulocytes in your blood is very low, you will probably be given an *antibiotic* drug to prevent infection. If you already have an infection, or if you have a fever, you will probably be given antibiotics intravenously right away.

In most cases, the outlook for complete recovery from agranulocytosis is very good. Either the drug or the infection causing the disease is eliminated and recovery begins. Cases caused by one of the types of leukemia or aplastic anemia are more complex and so are those in which a difficult-to-control infection develops.

Lymphatic system

The lymphatic system consists of lymph glands, or nodes, that are found throughout your body, the small vessels called lymphatics that link them, and the spleen.

The lymph glands produce the lymphocytes, a type of white blood cell. Lymphocytes recognize foreign cells, infectious agents, and other foreign substances, and participate in your body's immune reaction against them. The glands also act as barriers to the spread of infection through the lymphatics, because they trap infectious agents. This is why the lymph glands often become swollen when you have an infection.

The spleen is part of the lymphatic system. It is actually a large lymph gland and is located in the upper left part of the abdomen, behind the ribs.

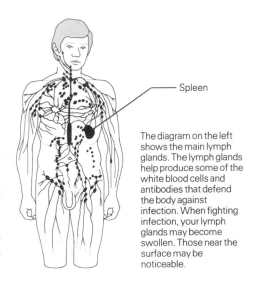

Spleen

The diagram on the left shows the main lymph glands. The lymph glands help produce some of the white blood cells and antibodies that defend the body against infection. When fighting infection, your lymph glands may become swollen. Those near the surface may be noticeable.

Lymphomas

A lymphoma is a *malignant*, or a life-threatening, tumor of the lymph glands. There are two general types of lymphomas. One is called Hodgkin's disease (see next page). The other is non-Hodgkin's lymphomas. These are discussed below.

What are the symptoms?
The first symptom of non-Hodgkin's lymphomas is usually a swollen gland. This can occur anywhere in your body, but the first ones commonly appear in your neck, armpit or groin. Other possible symptoms include feeling generally ill, losing your appetite, losing weight, fever and night sweats.

What are the risks?
Lymphomas are a very rare form of tumor. All types of lymphomas are ultimately fatal if they are not treated. Different types, however, respond very differently to treatment. The potential for cure also differs according to the type of lymphoma you have.

What should be done?
If you have a swelling or lump that persists for no obvious reason for more than two weeks, see your physician. If the swelling is an enlarged lymph gland, and there is no evidence that the swelling has been caused by an ordinary infection, the physician may take a blood sample and arrange for you to have the gland examined and probably removed. The blood test and an examination of the gland tissue will usually permit your physician to determine if you have a lymphoma and, if so, what type you have.

If a lymphoma is present, more tests are needed to determine the extent of the disease. A chest *X-ray* may reveal enlarged glands in the chest. A *lymphangiogram* may be performed to detect any enlarged glands in the abdomen. A bone marrow *biopsy*, the removal and examination of a small amount of marrow, may also be necessary to determine if lymphoma is present there. Other tests may be necessary as well.

What is the treatment?
If only the glands in a single part of your body, such as the neck, are affected, you may be treated with *radiation therapy*, or radiation therapy followed by *chemotherapy*. In chemotherapy, *cytotoxic*, or anticancer drugs are used. If the disease is more wide-spread, chemotherapy will probably be the main form of treatment. Most chemotherapy is given intravenously. Radiation therapy may be used to supplement chemotherapy.

Treatment usually requires that you stay in a hospital for a short time initially while you are given a combination of drugs. The treatment is repeated at intervals of a few weeks, in your physician's office. Your response will depend on two factors. The first and most important one is the type of lymphoma you have. The second factor is the extent to which the disease has spread in your body.

Hodgkin's disease

Hodgkin's disease produces swelling in the lymph glands, or nodes, and to that extent it is similar to non-Hodgkin's lymphomas (see previous article). However, non-Hodgkin's lymphomas are believed to be caused by *malignant*, or life-threatening, transformation of a lymphocyte, a type of white blood cell, while Hodgkin's disease is probably caused by malignant transformation of another type of cell (a macrophage). Another difference between the disorders is Hodgkin's disease is much easier to cure.

What are the symptoms?

The main symptom of Hodgkin's disease is persistent swollen glands, usually in the neck, armpit or groin. Other possible symptoms include fever, sweating, fatigue, weakness, weight loss and itching.

If Hodgkin's disease is treated early, the rate of cure is high. Therefore, it is vital that you report any unexplained swellings to your physician as soon as possible. The physician will probably arrange for samples of blood to be taken and a swollen gland to be removed, so that they can be examined and a diagnosis can be made.

If you have Hodgkin's disease, you will need to have tests in the hospital to determine the extent of the disease. You will have a bone marrow *biopsy*, in which a small amount of bone marrow is removed and examined, and a chest *X-ray*. There will also probably be a *lymphangiogram*, and a laparotomy (see p.477), to see if your abdomen shows signs of disease. The test results and the type of Hodgkin's disease you have will determine what treatment you need.

What is the treatment?

Radiation therapy is used to treat the disease if it is detected at a relatively early stage. Depending on the type of Hodgkin's disease you have, radiation therapy has an 80 to 90 per cent success rate in such cases. If the disease is at an advanced stage when it is discovered, you will be treated with one or more *cytotoxic*, or anticancer, drugs, sometimes in combination with radiation therapy. The treatment usually continues for about six months. About 40 per cent of patients with advanced Hodgkin's disease are cured by this intensive drug therapy.

Once treatment is completed, your progress is monitored by checkups every few months for about five years. If no signs of the disease have reappeared during that time, you have almost certainly been cured.

Immuno-deficiency

An immunodeficiency is a decrease in your body's immune defenses. There are two general types of immunodeficiency. In one, there is an inadequate production of *antibodies* (substances that protect your body from infectious diseases), in response to a previous infection or an immunization. This may affect only one type of antibody, or several at once. Because of this immunodeficiency, your resistance to some kinds of infection, especially bacterial, is decreased.

The second type of immunodeficiency results from disorders of, or decreased numbers of, the various kinds of lymphocytes. These are white blood cells from the bone marrow and the lymph glands. In this form of the disorder, the ability of the lymphocytes in your bloodstream to gather around and kill invading organisms is decreased. As a result, your resistance to infections caused by fungi, certain viruses, and the organisms that cause tuberculosis is impaired. It is possible to have both general types of immunodeficiency at the same time.

There are many types of inherited defects of the immune system. If you are born with one of these you are susceptible to certain types of infections. Many diseases also impair the functioning of the immune system. These diseases include the leukemias (see p.426), the lymphomas (see previous page, and Hodgkin's disease, see previous article), cancer in general, diabetes mellitus (see p.519) and uremia. Finally, some drugs that are used to treat many disorders, especially *steroids*, and *cytotoxic* (anticancer) drugs, and also *radiation therapy*, can significantly affect your immune system.

What is the treatment?

If you have an inherited deficiency of antibody production, injections of antibodies collected from other persons may be helpful. This treatment must be repeated every few weeks. If you have certain types of inherited deficiencies of lymphocytes, transplantation of tissue from the thymus, a small gland in the neck, offers some hope. This still highly experimental treatment is based on the thymus gland's influence on certain lymphocytes. Another possible treatment is long-term *antibiotic* therapy. For most people with an immunodeficiency, however, there is no specific treatment, and you must be careful to avoid infection and be sure to get immediate treatment if you do become ill.

Disorders of digestion and nutrition

Introduction

Your body needs a regular supply of nutrients to grow, to replace worn-out tissue, and to supply energy for the thousands of chemical reactions occurring in your body all the time. These nutrients are extracted from the food you eat as it passes through the digestive system. This system consists of the digestive tract, which is essentially a tube running from the mouth to the anus, and the digestive glands, including the liver and pancreas. The tract and glands work together as a system, to take in food and break it down so that the nutrients in it can be absorbed into the bloodstream.

The first part of the tract is the mouth, where the teeth tear and chew the food into small pieces and mix it with saliva. This functions as a lubricant, and also contains an *enzyme*, or digestive juice, that breaks down starch.

The tongue moves the food around the mouth as it is chewed, and then forms it into a ball called a *bolus* for swallowing. Few people appreciate the importance of the tongue in eating. Most people think of it only in its role in speech. If you are one of these people, imagine yourself trying to chew and swallow a mouthful of food without having the aid of your tongue.

The second section of the tract is the esophagus, or gullet. When you swallow, food slips down this muscular tube and through a ring of muscles that relaxes to let it through into the third section of the tract, the stomach. Muscles in the stomach wall pummel the food into a pulp as digestive juices, manufactured in the stomach wall, start to break the food chemically into yet smaller pieces. The half-digested food then passes through another ring of muscles and along a short tube, the duodenum, which is the first part of the small intestine. In the small intestine, further breakdown of food requires help from some other organs of the body.

Just beneath your liver lies the gallbladder, a pear-shaped sac about 9 cm (3½ in) long. Your gallbladder stores and concentrates an enzyme called bile, which is produced by the liver and trickles into the gallbladder, along with other substances, through a network of tiny tubes. Your gallbladder releases the bile, when it is needed, into your small intestine through an opening that

is called the bile duct. The bile helps digest fats. Your pancreas releases other digestive juices besides the bile, through a duct that joins the bile duct just before it enters your small intestine.

The food is pushed along the intestine by waves of contraction of the muscles in its wall. As this is happening, enzymes and other chemicals reduce the food to smaller and smaller pieces that can seep through the wall of the small intestine and be absorbed into the bloodstream.

Once in the blood, the nutrients are transported to all parts of the body. These nutrients ultimately end up afloat in the liquid that surrounds each cell in your body. The cells "eat" the nutrients as they need them, pulling them inside their cell membranes through a number of simple but effective mechanisms. Once inside the cell, the nutrients are sorted and broken down still further. Finally some nutrients are used to provide energy and others are used to make new tissues and other biological substances such as the enzymes.

The next-to-last section of the tract is the large intestine. Here, water is absorbed into your body from the undigested and indigestible remains of food. What is left becomes semi-solid waste. Finally, the waste is expelled as bowel movements at convenient intervals through the last part of the tract, the anus.

Most disorders of the digestive tract affect only one section. Such disorders are grouped together, along with a general description of what that particular part of the tract looks like and how it works. Some disorders affect two or more sections of the tract, and these are also grouped together. Finally there is a short group of articles describing disorders of nutrition. These are problems related to the amount or type of food you eat, or the ability of your digestive system to absorb certain chemicals in the food.

Some nutritional disorders are rare, inherited diseases that require that you eat a special diet for the rest of your life. Others can affect anybody and may be extremely widespread in the general population. Obesity is a particularly good example of such a disorder. It is covered at length in this section along with other problems related to nutrition and metabolism.

The digestive system

The digestive system is divided into a number of sections, each of which has its own part to play either in the breakdown and absorption of food, or in the expulsion of waste matter. Digestive enzymes (biological substances that speed up chemical reactions), assist in the process of breaking food down into pieces small enough to pass through the wall of the small intestine and into the bloodstream.

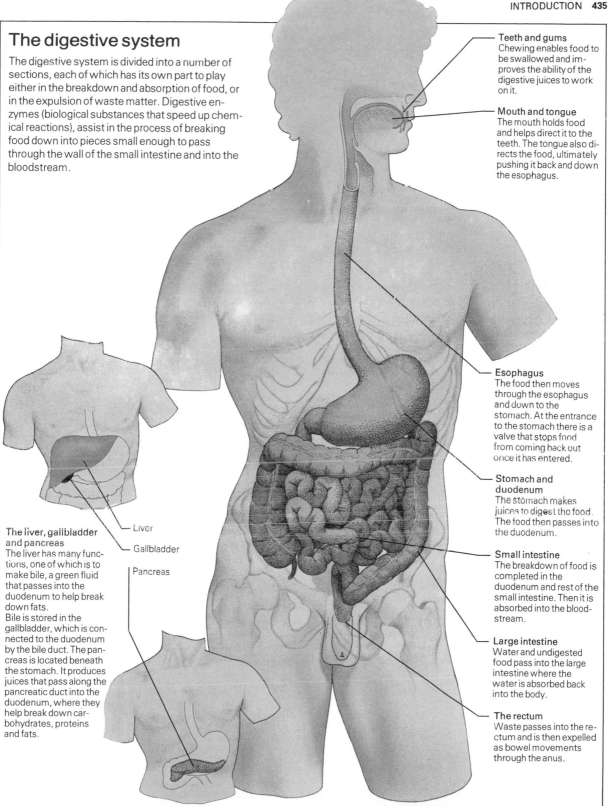

Teeth and gums
Chewing enables food to be swallowed and improves the ability of the digestive juices to work on it.

Mouth and tongue
The mouth holds food and helps direct it to the teeth. The tongue also directs the food, ultimately pushing it back and down the esophagus.

Esophagus
The food then moves through the esophagus and down to the stomach. At the entrance to the stomach there is a valve that stops food from coming back out once it has entered.

Stomach and duodenum
The stomach makes juices to digest the food. The food then passes into the duodenum.

Small intestine
The breakdown of food is completed in the duodenum and rest of the small intestine. Then it is absorbed into the bloodstream.

Large intestine
Water and undigested food pass into the large intestine where the water is absorbed back into the body.

The rectum
Waste passes into the rectum and is then expelled as bowel movements through the anus.

Liver

Gallbladder

Pancreas

The liver, gallbladder and pancreas
The liver has many functions, one of which is to make bile, a green fluid that passes into the duodenum to help break down fats.
Bile is stored in the gallbladder, which is connected to the duodenum by the bile duct. The pancreas is located beneath the stomach. It produces juices that pass along the pancreatic duct into the duodenum, where they help break down carbohydrates, proteins and fats.

Teeth and gums

Your teeth break the food you eat into pieces that can be easily swallowed and digested. Teeth are alive. The pulp at the heart of each tooth contains blood vessels and nerves that sense heat, cold, pressure and pain. A hard substance called dentin surrounds the pulp. On the crown, the part of the tooth above the gum, the dentin is covered by enamel. The root of the tooth, which is buried in the gum, is covered by a sensitive bone-like material called cementum. The gums fit tightly around the teeth, and the roots of the teeth fit into sockets in the jawbone. A shock-absorbent material, periodontal ligament, lines the socket of each tooth, to prevent the skull and jawbone from being jarred.

Enamel is the hardest substance in your body, but acids produced by the action of bacteria on sugar and other carbohydrates can erode the enamel and cause dental decay. If it is unchecked, decay progresses through the dentin and into the pulp, to kill the tooth or cause an abscess. Too much sugar in the diet is largely responsible for decay.

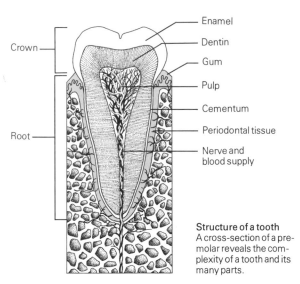

Crown
Root

Enamel
Dentin
Gum
Pulp
Cementum
Periodontal tissue
Nerve and blood supply

Structure of a tooth
A cross-section of a premolar reveals the complexity of a tooth and its many parts.

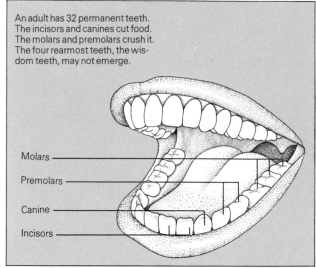

An adult has 32 permanent teeth. The incisors and canines cut food. The molars and premolars crush it. The four rearmost teeth, the wisdom teeth, may not emerge.

Molars
Premolars
Canine
Incisors

Dental decay
(caries)

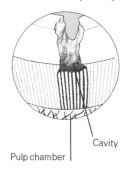

Pulp chamber
Cavity

If you pass the tip of your tongue over your teeth some hours after brushing them, you can feel patches of a slightly rough, sticky substance. This substance is called dental *plaque*. It consists of mucus, food particles, and bacteria, and forms mainly in two places: between the teeth and where the teeth meet the gums. The bacteria in the plaque break down the sugar in your food, and this process forms acid. The acid erodes the calcium in the tooth's enamel, and forms a minute cavity. This is the beginning of dental decay.

If the decay is not treated, the acid eats through the enamel and erodes the dentin beneath it. Dentin contains minute canals that lead to the pulp, and the bacteria eventually inflame the pulp. Your body responds by sending more white blood cells to the pulp to combat the bacteria. The blood vessels around the tooth enlarge to accommodate the extra blood and white cells. The enlarged vessels press on the nerves entering the tooth,

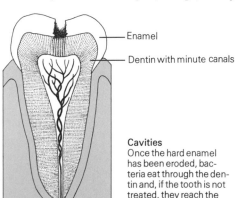

Enamel
Dentin with minute canals

Cavities
Once the hard enamel has been eroded, bacteria eat through the dentin and, if the tooth is not treated, they reach the pulp chamber.

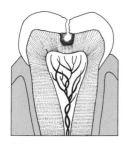

Acid starts decay

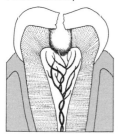

Acid eats into dentin

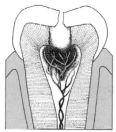

Pulp becomes inflamed

and this causes toothache. If a significant number of bacteria physically invade the pulp chambers the nerve of the tooth will probably die, even though the white blood cells are fighting the infection (see Dead teeth, next article). This will end the toothache, but may lead to an abscess (see p.439).

What are the symptoms?
In the early stages of decay the main symptom is a mild toothache when you eat something sweet, very hot, or very cold. If the decay continues, you may have an unpleasant taste in your mouth that comes from stagnant food and bacteria packed into the cavity.

In the final stage of decay, the pulp of the tooth becomes inflamed. If this occurs, you may suffer persistent pain after eating sweet, hot, or cold food. You may also have sharp, stabbing pains, sometimes in the jaw above or below the decayed tooth. It may be difficult to tell which tooth is painful.

What are the risks?
Tooth decay generally presents no serious danger to health if it is caught and treated early. But there is a risk for people who have heart diseases. If bacteria from an infected tooth enter the bloodstream, the disease may worsen (see Bacterial endocarditis, p.394). Also, if you have a bleeding disease such as hemophilia (see p.424), you should have a tooth extracted only after you have consulted your physician.

What should be done?
Keep dental decay to a minimum by taking good care of your teeth (see next page). Brush and floss them regularly, reduce your sugar intake, use a fluoride toothpaste, drink fluoridated water, and visit your dentist regularly to have your teeth cleaned and examined. Allow *X-rays* to be taken every year or two if your dentist recommends it. These will reveal any new small cavities and other problems you may have developed that may not be detectable by other means.

If you have young children, do not allow them to go to sleep with a bottle of juice as a pacifier. The sugary juice can bathe the tooth all night, promoting tooth decay. Also, children probably should have annual fluoride applications starting at about age three to four, even if your water supply is fluoridated.

What is the treatment?
Self-help: By the time the symptoms of dental decay cause distress, little self-help is possible. Pain-relieving tablets such as aspirin may help until you can get to your dentist.
Professional help: In the early stages of the disease, your dentist will usually fill the cavity immediately, if time permits. If the decay is advanced, the dentist may perform a *root canal* procedure, which involves removing the inflamed pulp tissues and filling the canals in the roots of the tooth (see illustration, below). In rare cases, the dentist may extract, or pull out, the tooth.

Dead teeth
(endodontics)

At the heart of every healthy tooth is the pulp, a living tissue that makes the tooth sensitive to heat, cold, pressure and pain. When the pulp dies, the tooth dies.

The pulp may die after dental decay (see previous article) has penetrated to it, or sometimes after a blow to the tooth. Occasionally, a tooth dies for no apparent reason. No symptoms signal the death of a tooth, except that a decayed tooth will no longer be painful. You may not know you have a dead tooth until your dentist tells you. Eventually, most dead teeth turn slightly gray.

Once a dead tooth has been detected, it almost always should be treated. There is a risk, especially after dental decay, that bacteria from the dead pulp will seep out through the end of the root and cause an abscess to form (see p.439).

What is the treatment?
A dead tooth can continue to function efficiently, so there is usually no reason for it to

be extracted unless it is badly decayed. The dentist usually cleans out the tooth, disinfects it, and fills the pulp chamber and root canal. Any cavities in the crown are filled in the usual way (see Going to the dentist, p.448). Sometimes discolored or broken dead teeth are crowned (see p.448).

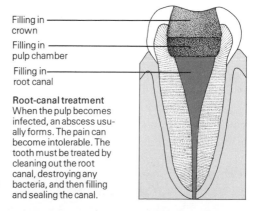

Filling in crown

Filling in pulp chamber

Filling in root canal

Root-canal treatment
When the pulp becomes infected, an abscess usually forms. The pain can become intolerable. The tooth must be treated by cleaning out the root canal, destroying any bacteria, and then filling and sealing the canal.

Keeping your teeth and gums healthy

Almost anyone who eats the usual diet of an advanced Western nation will find it virtually impossible to avoid tooth decay completely. However, you can cut it down to a minimum, and retain your own teeth in a healthy condition until old age, by taking four simple steps.

1. Brush your teeth thoroughly at least twice each day, in the morning, and before you go to bed. You should also use dental floss to dislodge food particles and *plaque* from places that you cannot reach with your brush.

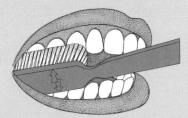

Your dentist or hygienist will show you how to use the floss properly, since incorrect use can damage your gums. To check the efficiency of your cleaning, chew a disclosing tablet occasionally. The dye in the tablet colors the plaque on your teeth.

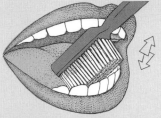

2. Reduce your sugar intake and eat a balanced diet. Candy, other sweet snacks, and sweet drinks between meals are especially harmful, because after you eat or drink them your teeth are attacked for up to one hour by acid. Try to eat sweet foods only during meals. Better still, cut them out altogether and finish your meals with fruit or cheese rather than with ice cream or cake. Cheese is particularly effective in neutralizing acid formation.

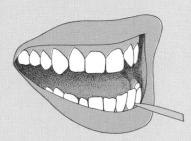

Using toothpicks
Toothpicks should not be used to remove plaque, since they can easily damage your gums.

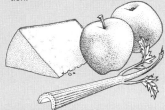

Using dental floss
Dental floss, either waxed or unwaxed, is thread that you draw between your teeth to remove plaque and food particles. Take about 45 cm (18 in) of dental floss and wind most of it around one of the fingers on each hand, with about 2½ cm (1 in) of floss between your fingers. Place the back of one finger into the mouth and then draw the floss between the teeth, and with a sawing action, rub the sides of each tooth.

3. Strengthen your tooth enamel with fluoride. The level of fluoride in the water should be between 0.7 and 1.2 parts per million, depending on the climate. Your dentist, local water authority, or public health department can tell you what the fluoride level is in your community's water supply. Also, children under 12 should have fluoride applied to their teeth every year, because their enamel is still forming. Your dentist will advise you on the use of fluoride mouthwash or tablets, and may apply a fluoride gel to your teeth. In addition, the family should use a fluoride toothpaste.

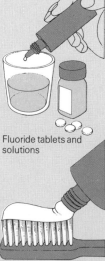

Fluoride tablets and solutions

4. See your dentist regularly. An examination and cleaning every six months should ensure that any new cavity is filled before decay can spread, and that any gum disease is treated before it can become serious.

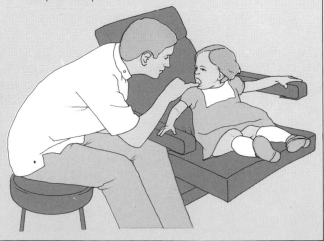

Disclosing tablets
These tablets contain a dye that stains plaque. Remove the plaque with floss and a toothbrush.

Fluoride toothpaste

Abscesses in teeth

A tooth abscess is a pus-filled sac in the tissue around the tip of the tooth's root, which is embedded in the jawbone. The abscess usually forms when a tooth is decaying (see p.436) or dead (see p.437), or when the gums have receded severely. A tooth's dead pulp, together with invading bacteria, can infect the surrounding tissue. Even when a dead tooth has been root-filled (see p.437), bacteria occasionally remain in the tissue around the base of the roots of the tooth and cause the formation of an abscess.

If the abscess is not treated, it may eat into the jawbone until it has eroded a small canal, or sinus, through the bone and its overlying gum. Just before the canal reaches the surface of the gum, it can form a swelling, or boil. The swelling may remain for weeks, but in some cases the boil bursts. In these cases, foul-tasting pus drains into the mouth and there is sudden relief of pain.

Anyone who does not visit the dentist regularly is likely to have a tooth abscess at some time. Untreated decayed teeth will die, and some dead teeth eventually cause abscesses.

What are the symptoms?
The abscessed tooth aches persistently or throbs, and usually is extremely painful when you bite or chew. The glands in your neck may swell and become tender, and if the abscess spreads, the side of your face may become swollen. Often you also have a fever and feel generally unwell.

What are the risks?
If the abscess is not treated by a dentist or physician, there is a slight risk that the spreading infection could cause generalized blood poisoning (see p.421) or affect the adjacent bones. If the dead pulp and bacteria in the tooth are not removed by a dentist, the infection will keep returning.

What should be done?
See a dentist as soon as possible; immediately if the swelling is spreading into the face or neck. If a dentist is not available, call your physician, who may prescribe an *antibiotic* to prevent the infection from spreading further. Then be sure that you visit your dentist at the first opportunity.

What is the treatment?
Self-help: Take aspirin to provide some relief from the pain. Rinse your mouth every hour with warm salt water. This will hasten the bursting of the boil, and the resulting relief of pain. When the boil has burst, wash away the pus with an extra rinse.

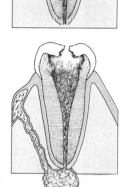

How a boil forms
If dental decay is not treated, the pulp may become infected. Pus may begin to form. Infected pus in the base of the tooth may develop into an abscess and seep out through the root of the tooth. The pus may then eat through the jawbone, and erode a channel called a sinus. It emerges in the gum and causes a painful swelling called a boil.

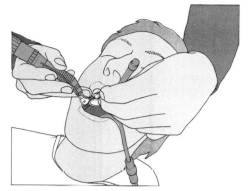

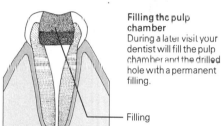

Treating an abscess
Your dentist may try to save an abscessed tooth by drilling a small hole through the crown to release the pus. The dentist can then clean out the pulp chamber, disinfect it, and put in a temporary filling. Later, he will put in a permanent filling.

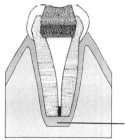

Filling the pulp chamber
During a later visit your dentist will fill the pulp chamber and the drilled hole with a permanent filling.

— Filling

Apicectomy
Occasionally a dentist will perform an apicectomy. This is an operation in which the infected tissue at the base of the tooth is removed.

— Infected tissue removed

Professional help: The dentist may extract a very badly infected back tooth or a baby tooth. To save a tooth, the dentist drills a small hole through the crown and into the pulp chamber. If the abscess has not yet burst, the drilled hole releases the pressurized pus, and this relieves the pain. The dentist cleans out and disinfects the pulp chamber. At a later visit, if the infection has cleared up, the dentist will put a permanent filling in the pulp chamber and the drilled hole. About six months later, the dentist will probably take *X-rays* of the area to make sure that new bone and tissue are growing into the cavity left by the abscess. If this is occurring, no further treatment is likely to be required.

In a few cases of abscessed teeth, the abscess does not clear up and a small affected area remains at the tip of the root. Antibiotics cannot clear up the infection permanently, and to treat persistent bacteria, your dentist may refer you to an oral surgeon for an operation called an *apicectomy*. After deadening the gum with a local anesthetic, the oral surgeon makes a small cut through it, drills away the bone that covers the tip of the root, removes the infected tissue, and fills the root canal (see Dead teeth, illustration, p.437). In rare cases this fails to clear up the trouble, and the tooth must be extracted (see Going to the dentist, p.449). If you wish, the tooth can be replaced with a bridge.

Discolored teeth

Teeth may become discolored, which is different from the slight yellowing that occurs with age, for a variety of reasons. Smoking can cause brown surface staining. The death of a tooth (see p.437) can turn it gray. Certain drugs, if they are taken in large doses during childhood, can cause faulty, discolored enamel to form. Severe attacks of certain childhood infections, such as whooping cough and measles, can produce patches of discoloration on the teeth. And extremely excessive amounts of natural fluoride in the water, as found in some parts of the world, can cause fluorosis, or white or brown markings in the teeth. This does not happen in areas where a controlled amount of fluoride is added to the water to reduce tooth decay.

tooth or by attaching a synthetic veneer. If a dead tooth is brittle, the crown may be ground down to gum level and replaced with a new artificial crown (see Going to the dentist, p.447).

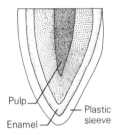

One possible treatment for a discolored tooth is to cover it with either a hard plastic sleeve or a porcelain crown. The covering material is closely matched for color with the neighboring teeth. The sleeve or crown is cemented permanently into position.

Pulp
Enamel
Plastic sleeve

What is the treatment?
If the discoloration is superficial, your dentist or dental hygienist will clean the tooth or teeth with a rotary polisher and polishing paste. Deeper discoloration, such as the gray of a dead tooth, can be treated by bonding a tough white porcelain or plastic crown to the

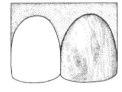
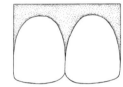

Orthodontia

In the ideal set of teeth, the teeth are straight, regularly spaced with neither overlap nor gaps, and exactly the right size for the jaws. The *occlusion*, or the relationship of the upper and lower teeth when the mouth is closed, is such that the upper teeth slightly overlap the lower teeth, and the points of the molars alternate.

Few people have perfect teeth, however. One reason for this is that you inherit different characteristics from each of your parents, and sometimes the two do not match. For example, your teeth may be too big for your jaws. If so, they can develop only by sloping backwards or forwards or by overlapping with their neighbors. If your teeth are too

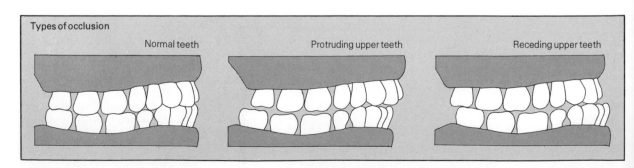

Types of occlusion

Normal teeth   Protruding upper teeth   Receding upper teeth small for your jaws, there will be some gaps between your teeth. If your lower jaw is smaller than your upper jaw and your lips are also small, the teeth in your upper jaw may protrude. This is called a faulty bite, or malocclusion. Another type of malocclusion occurs when the permanent upper front teeth bite just behind the lower teeth. This often develops in children of about seven or eight, and may change as the jaw grows.

Heredity is not the only cause of irregularity of teeth. Crowding is sometimes the result of loss of primary (baby) teeth through decay. For example, when primary molars are lost prematurely, the permanent molars move forward in the jaw to fill the gaps. Then, when the permanent premolars and canines appear, between the ages of 11 and 13, they are crowded out of the natural arch of the teeth. In some cases, they fail to appear at all (see Missing teeth, next article). Sometimes the crowding that takes place when the adult teeth appear is only temporary. This is particularly true with the lower front teeth.

In these mild cases of crowding, there is a slightly increased risk of dental decay and gum disease, because it is more difficult to keep crowded teeth clean. In rare cases, when the crowding is severe, it can cause difficulty in chewing food comfortably, and sometimes concern over the appearance of the teeth.

Many teenagers could benefit from treatment of crowded teeth. Such treatment could help them keep their teeth and gums clean.

What should be done?

If you are an adult with a minor problem such as a few crowded or twisted teeth, your dentist will probably tell you that the problem can be corrected by a specialist, if you are willing to spend the time and money. If the problem is severe, and may cause damage to or loss of your permanent teeth, you may have to have the problem corrected.

If your children are developing crowded or maloccluded teeth, ask your dentist when to begin to correct the condition. Orthodontic treatment usually is most effective during childhood and early adolescence, when the teeth and jaws are still growing and developing. Also, the texture of the bone facilitates tooth movement at this time.

What is the treatment?

If you are an adult and have a minor problem, your dentist will probably extract some teeth and/or fit you with braces, to correct the crowding or malocclusion. You may find the braces embarrassing, but they are usually temporary and eventually improve the func-

tion of your teeth and your appearance.

If, as an adult, you have severely crowded or maloccluded teeth, or if your jaw protrudes or recedes, it is possible to have corrective surgery. In this procedure, an oral surgeon repositions or removes pieces of the jawbone and some teeth. The operation usually requires hospitalization. Another possible treatment is to have crowns and bridges made (see p.448, 449).

In the case of children, your dentist may be able to treat minor crowding, but for major treatment the child is referred to an orthodontist, who specializes in correcting irregularly positioned teeth.

The orthodontist will use *X-rays* to check that all the adult teeth have formed and are likely to emerge. In most cases, the orthodontist will make plaster casts of the teeth and the jaw. If crowding seems likely, one possible treatment is to extract a neighboring tooth that has already appeared, to provide space. Generally, the treatment for irregularly positioned teeth is to use an appliance, or braces, over a period of months. This appliance is anchored by fitting it around several teeth, or by attaching wires to straps that are put around each tooth. The appliance often has springs that exert continuous force on a tooth to twist it, push it backwards or forwards, or move it sideways along the jawbone, depending on which way the tooth needs to be realigned.

Appliances are often used when a child's upper incisors protrude and the canines are prominent and crowded. Some premolars may be extracted first. Then an appliance can be fitted to move the canines into the correct position, and later refitted to pull back the upper incisors and prevent a gap between them and the canines. Such treatment starts around the age of 10 to 13 and lasts for 18 to 24 months. Visits are made to the orthodontist every month to adjust the appliance. The

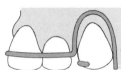

Retainer plate in position
This is a simple device without springs that holds the teeth in their new position.

final part of the treatment is to fit a retainer to hold all the teeth in their new positions for 6 to 18 months, while the surrounding tissue has a chance to stabilize.

An appliance can trap *plaque*, the sticky substance that forms on your teeth from food particles, mucus and bacteria. This material can cause tooth decay, so you must clean both teeth and appliance after every meal.

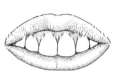

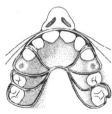

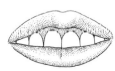

Crowding can produce front teeth that protrude so much that the mouth cannot be closed normally (top). A plate can pull back these teeth and premolars may be removed to make room (center). The result is not only cosmetically more desirable (bottom), but also allows normal movement of the teeth and jaw.

Missing teeth

Permanent teeth that are missing from a child's mouth after loss of the first teeth can cause dental trouble in later life unless steps are taken to prevent it.

Adult teeth may be missing for one of three reasons. The most common reason is that they may have been lost through early decay or an accident. Molars and premolars (see p.436) are most susceptible to early decay. Another reason is that the teeth may have failed to develop. This happens most commonly with the upper side, or lateral, incisors and the premolars (see p.436). Finally, they may be impacted, or prevented from erupting above the gum by the root of an adjacent tooth. This can cause a number of problems. Some of the teeth that most commonly are impacted are the upper canines, premolars and wisdom teeth (see next article).

Problems caused by a missing molar
The tooth above a missing molar descends to fill the gap and the teeth around the gap tilt. Chewing becomes difficult and, because cleaning is also difficult, decay is likely.

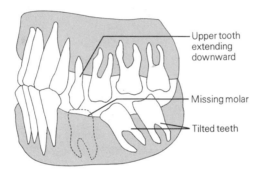

Upper tooth extending downward

Missing molar

Tilted teeth

Even if a child loses only a single molar through an accident or tooth decay, this can cause several problems in later life. One is that the molar in the jaw above or below the space has too much room to grow into. When you chew, your jaw moves from side to side as well as up and down, and if a molar fits into a space in the row of teeth above or below it, it interferes with the sideways motion of your jaw. The dentist will probably extract the molar or grind its points down, because this condition can prevent you from chewing your food properly.

Another common problem is that, because the teeth on either side of the missing molar do not receive the usual supporting pressure, they tilt and twist around in the gum.

Other teeth naturally tend to grow into the spaces left by missing teeth. To do so, they may emerge too much from the gum or grow at an angle. This can produce maloccluded teeth, or a faulty bite (see previous article). Then, when you bite or chew, your teeth do not close correctly, which puts stresses on the teeth and jaw. These stresses occasionally cause temporal mandibular joint (TMJ) disease, which involves pain in the joints of the jaw. Other problems caused by malocclusion include wear or loosening of some teeth, and difficulties with the muscles of the face.

A more common risk of teeth growing into gaps at an angle is that cleaning these areas may be difficult. Food may become wedged in hard-to-reach spaces. This can lead to dental decay (see p.436) and periodontal disease (see p.446).

What should be done?
If you think that your child has a missing primary (baby) or permanent tooth, take the child to the dentist. If you have had teeth missing since childhood yourself and you suffer from any of the problems described, you should also discuss it with your dentist.

What is the treatment?
Your dentist may choose to restore your occlusion by inserting a permanent prosthesis (false tooth) by bridgework, or by making a partial denture that you can remove, at night for example. (See Going to the dentist, p.449.) Your dentist may refer you to an orthodontist, a dentist who specializes in treating irregularly positioned teeth.

To treat pain in the jaw caused by malocclusion, your dentist may either fit a bite-plane over your upper teeth and gums, or file down the high spots in your teeth, in order to correct the bite.

Problems with wisdom teeth

The last teeth in the back of each group of molars are the wisdom teeth. In most people the four wisdom teeth appear between the ages of 17 and 21, but in some people one or more of them never emerge. This is nothing to worry about. In fact, it may well be an advantage, since wisdom teeth often cause problems as they emerge. Even when they form normally, wisdom teeth are difficult to clean, and therefore they decay more commonly than other teeth.

Sometimes a wisdom tooth emerges at an angle. The space between it and the next tooth traps food particles, and they can stagnate there. Often a wisdom tooth fails to emerge properly because it becomes impacted, or blocked, under the gum, sometimes by the tooth next to it. This can cause problems: The gum forms a pocket around an impacted tooth where food tends to be caught. Bacteria can produce an infection, called pericoronitis, around the tooth.

If one of your wisdom teeth simply fails to appear, you probably will not have any symptoms. If it erupts at an angle and forms a stagnation area for food particles, you may

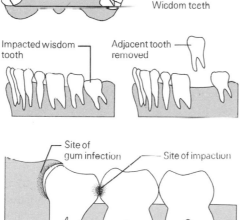

Position of wisdom teeth
The wisdom teeth are behind the first two molars in both upper and lower jaws.

— Molars

Wisdom teeth

Impacted wisdom tooth
An impacted wisdom tooth is one that is blocked when it grows at an angle against the adjacent tooth. The problem can be solved by removing either the adjacent tooth or the wisdom tooth itself.

Impacted wisdom tooth

Adjacent tooth removed

Gum infection
If an impacted wisdom tooth has partially emerged, food and bacteria can become trapped under the gum flap and cause decay and bad breath.

— Site of gum infection

— Site of impaction

have bad breath and possibly an unpleasant taste in your mouth.

The main symptoms of pericoronitis are pain when you bite on the tooth or the gum partially covering the tooth, and an unpleasant taste. You will probably also have redness and swelling of the gum around the tooth. If you have any of these symptoms, see your dentist or physician as soon as possible.

What is the treatment?
Self-help: You can obtain temporary relief from the pain by taking aspirin or rinsing the area around the tooth with warm salt water.
Professional help: Your dentist or physician may prescribe an *antibiotic* to clear up the infection, and will probably advise you to continue to use mouthwashes to keep the area clean, and relieve the pain. However, the antibiotic will usually give only temporary relief, and the long-term solution to the problem is to have the wisdom tooth extracted soon after the infection has subsided. Your dentist will take *X-rays* to determine the position of the tooth. If it lies at a difficult angle, or if the other wisdom teeth are similarly affected, you may need a general anesthetic for the extraction, and you may have to be hospitalized for the procedure. In many cases, however, one or more wisdom teeth may be removed by an oral surgeon or a dentist in the office. A local anesthetic is commonly used.

Denture problems

Most modern dentures, or false teeth, look natural and fit well, but no denture is as efficient and comfortable as your own teeth. With natural teeth, the stresses of biting and chewing are absorbed by the teeth, the roots of the teeth, and the special shock-absorbent material, called the periodontal ligament, that lines the tooth sockets in the jawbone. With dentures, the stresses are absorbed in unnatural ways. The most critical of these is the pressure that the baseplate, or false gums, places on the ridges of the natural gums, especially if the dentures are worn day and night. This pressure can cause inflammation of the gums and, eventually, mouth ulcers and degeneration of the jawbone underneath the gum tissue.

The base of a partial denture also puts an abnormal sideways load on the natural teeth around which the denture base fits. Partial dentures, especially poorly-fitted ones, have another disadvantage. They trap food particles, which can cause decay in the remaining teeth (see p.436) and may lead to gingivitis

(see next article) or even periodontal disease (see p.446). The fungus that causes oral thrush (see p.451) can also lead to a painful mouth condition, especially if you have been taking *antibiotic* drugs.

What are the symptoms?
The early symptoms of excessive pressure on the ridges of the gums are pain when the dentures are in place, especially when you are eating, and either white and patchy or red and inflamed gums. If the inflammation persists, the gums become deep red and soft, and bleed easily – after you scratch them with your toothbrush, for example. A mouth ulcer (see p.450) may form on any spot where your denture rubs your gums. After a denture has been worn for many years, hard, pale pads called dental granulomas form at the main pressure points, especially near the edges of the denture.

Further symptoms arise when the gums and jawbone shrink, which is bound to happen after a few years of continuous pressure

Biting and chewing with false teeth

With the loss of your teeth you lose periodontal tissue, a shock-absorbent material that lines the sockets of the jaw bones. Dentures can press against your gums, leading to soreness, inflammation and mouth ulcers. Regular visits to the dentist and proper denture care will minimize the problem.

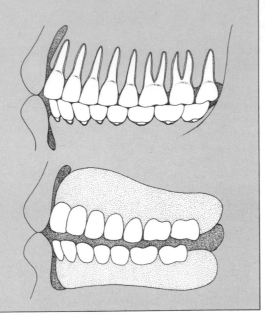

Caring for your dentures

Always remove your dentures at night and keep them in a glass of water mixed with a cleansing agent, so that they do not dry out and warp.

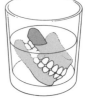

Clean your dentures daily and make sure that all food and plaque are removed. Your dentist will show you the best method.

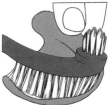

It is vital to clean any natural teeth thoroughly, especially where these teeth meet your gums.

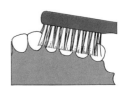

even if the denture has caused no other problems. When this happens, you have to close your mouth further to bite properly, and even further if your dentures are worn down. The common symptoms of gum and jawbone shrinkage are loose dentures, sunken cheeks, and a protruding lower jaw. Sometimes, there are pains in the jawbone joints from the extra movement needed to bite.

What are the risks?

A long-term risk of problems with dentures is that your jaw and mouth movement and appearance may change a great deal to cope with the slow shrinkage of your jawbone and gums. Also, chronic inflammation and pressure can lead to infection, or even cancerous changes in the gums.

What should be done?

If you have full dentures, have them checked by a dentist at least every two years. If you have a partial denture or a bridge (see Going to the dentist, p.449), go to the dentist at least once every six months to safeguard your natural teeth. If you have pain, sores, or bleeding in your mouth, consult your dentist within a few days.

What is the treatment?

Self-help: Always remove your dentures at night, to give your gum tissues a regular rest period. When they are not in your mouth, many dentures must be kept in a glass of

water or they warp when they dry out. Partial dentures often feel a little tight when you insert them in the morning, but this is quite normal and the feeling disappears after five minutes or so. Clean your dentures daily, according to your dentist's instructions, and clean your natural teeth and gums thoroughly, especially around the base of the teeth.

If you wear dentures, and have a sore mouth, be sure to keep your dentures scrupulously clean, and soak them overnight in a cleaning solution designed for this purpose. Also, you should clean and massage your gums with a finger, cloth, or brush.

Professional help: The useful life of dentures varies from six months to five years or more, depending on the condition of your gums and jawbone, the denture material, and how well the dentures fit. When your dentures become worn or your gums and jawbone shrink, your dentist will make new dentures, or if your dentures are not too worn, the dentist can sometimes adapt the existing baseplate to the new shape of your gums.

To clear up inflamed gums your dentist may prescribe an anti-fungal agent. In addition, it is likely that your dentist will encourage and teach you how to take better care of your gums and dentures to avoid future problems.

Some people have great problems coping with dentures, and never really adapt to them. It also may become difficult to adapt to new dentures as you grow older.

Gingivitis

Gingivitis is inflamed and swollen gums. It is most commonly caused by *plaque*, a sticky deposit of mucus, food particles and bacteria that forms at the base of the teeth. It may also be caused by a vitamin deficiency, by certain medications, and by some glandular disorders and blood diseases.

Some researchers think that irritation from plaque creates microscopic ulcers at the edge of the gums, which become infected and swollen. As the gum margin swells, a pocket forms between the gum and a tooth. This

Avoiding gingivitis
If plaque builds up, bacteria in its deeper layers die and then mineralize and harden into calculus. Proper tooth brushing and flossing and regular care by your dentist prevent calculus formation and the gingivitis it causes.

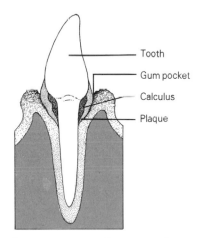

Tooth

Gum pocket

Calculus

Plaque

becomes a trap for more plaque, the gum swells even more, and the pocket deepens. If the condition is not treated, it may develop into periodontitis (see next article).

Gingivitis is very common in adults, usually in a mild form. Pregnant women and diabetics are particularly susceptible. The disorder is less common in healthy children.

What are the symptoms?

Healthy gums are pale pink and firm, and look speckled. In gingivitis, they become red, soft, and shiny, as well as swollen. They bleed easily, even from gentle brushing. Unless it is checked, gingivitis can eventually lead to destructive gum and bone disease (see Periodontitis, next article).

What should be done?

Only mild gingivitis is likely to develop if you keep your teeth and gums clean and have regular dental care. If you have not taken care of your teeth, and gingivitis has developed, see a dentist as soon as possible.

What is the treatment?

Self-help: Brush your teeth after meals and use dental floss at least once a day, to remove all plaque. To see how successfully you are doing this, use a disclosing tablet occasionally (see Keeping teeth and gums healthy, p.438).
Professional help: In serious cases, your dentist may prescribe an antibacterial mouthwash after removing any plaque and *calculus*, a hard, chalky deposit that traps plaque, from the base of your teeth. Calculus is removed with a scaler (see Going to the dentist, p.448). The dentist or dental hygienist will also show you the most effective way to use a toothbrush and dental floss. Some people develop calculus despite careful tooth care, and need to have their teeth cleaned professionally every few months.

Most cases of gingivitis respond to treatment, and the gums return to normal. It is then up to you to keep your teeth and gums clean to avoid recurrence of the disease.

Neglect and gum disease
Inadequate brushing allows plaque buildup, which promotes gum disease. The inflamed and sore gums will stay that way until the plaque is removed. If this is not done, teeth may have to be extracted.

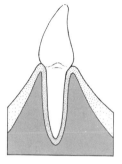 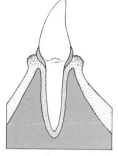 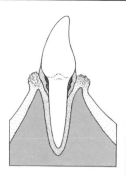

Healthy gums fit firmly around the neck of the tooth. They are pink and will not bleed easily. Plaque allowed to build up between the teeth and

the gums can cause painful inflammation. Unchecked plaque between tooth and gums finds its way to some of the bone and fibers that

anchor the tooth. Here, the bacteria that the plaque harbors can do severe damage.

Perio-dontitis

Periodontitis is the end result of gingivitis (see previous article) that has been treated too late or not at all. In gingivitis, *plaque*, a sticky deposit of mucus, food particles and bacteria, collects in pockets between swollen gums and the base of your teeth. Some dentists think that this protected plaque contains bacteria that, over a period of years, cause destruction of the bone that surrounds and supports your teeth. Eventually, the bony sockets can become so eroded that the teeth become loose and must be extracted.

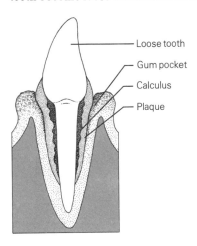

Damage caused by gum disease
The bacteria in unchecked plaque will eat into the bone and tissue that surround and anchor the tooth. They also form calculus, which can pry the gum away from the tooth. Both processes can loosen and ultimately make it necessary to pull the tooth.

Loose tooth
Gum pocket
Calculus
Plaque

What are the symptoms?

The pockets between gums and teeth gradually deepen and the plaque in the pockets causes an unpleasant taste and bad breath. As the disease progresses, the teeth loosen in their sockets. Tapping them produces a dull sound, instead of the sharp noise of firmly-set teeth. More and more cementum, the sensitive tissue that covers the root of the tooth, is exposed, and it aches when you eat very hot,

Treatment of periodontitis
Plaque and calculus building up between tooth and gum form a deep pocket between them. In treatment, the pocket is cut away so the area can be kept clean and new gum can grow.

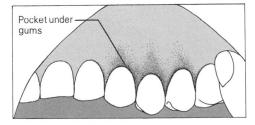

Pocket under gums

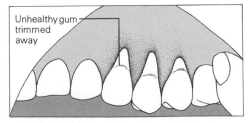

Unhealthy gum trimmed away

very cold or sweet food. Sometimes an abscess (see p.439) forms deep inside a pocket and eats away more bone.

What are the risks?

Adults lose more teeth from periodontal disease than from dental decay. The problem is common among young adults, and the likelihood of having it increases with age.

If you have periodontitis, you can lose all your teeth. They will have to be replaced with dentures, and you may then have denture problems (see p.443).

What should be done?

The disease often can be halted before it reaches an advanced stage. See a dentist as soon as you notice any of the symptoms described. To find out how advanced the disease is, the dentist usually measures the depth of the pockets and takes *X-rays* to determine the condition of the underlying bone. This is an important factor in how the dentist will decide to treat the problem.

What is the treatment?

Self-help: Follow the measures described in "Keeping your teeth and gums healthy" (see p.438), and pay special attention to cleaning your gums and the base of your teeth.

Professional help: If the disease is at an early stage, your dentist can help to keep it under control by treating any dental disorders that encourage plaque to form or allow it to persist, such as crowded or twisted teeth (see Orthodontia, p.440). Your cooperation in cleaning your teeth thoroughly is also very important to the treatment.

If the pockets have become very deep, periodontal surgery may be required. A *gingivectomy* is a minor operation performed in the office by a dental specialist, in which the gums are trimmed to reduce the depth of the pockets. If your bone has been damaged, it too will be trimmed. After the surgery, the gumline is covered with a protective coating called a periodontal pack, which should stay in place for one to two weeks until the gums heal. The coating should not prevent normal eating and drinking. If you have any problems with it, you should call your dentist or the specialist who did the surgery.

Cementum that has been worn away can be replaced by synthetic material bonded to the tooth. Particularly sensitive cementum can be protected with a layer of sodium fluoride, or your dentist may prescribe a toothpaste that also provides protection. Very loose teeth can be anchored. Ask your dentist about possible procedures for this.

Going to the dentist

When should you go?
You should visit a dentist about every six months. Regular examinations are necessary not only to minimize tooth decay, but also to check the health of your whole mouth. A neglected mouth, besides being vulnerable to the various disorders described in this section, can create the risk of infections entering the bloodstream, which can endanger your general health. Dentures, like natural teeth, need to be checked regularly, and all dentures eventually wear down and need to be replaced. If you have a full set of dentures and have no problems with them, you should visit a dentist about once every two years.

What happens at the examination?
The dentist first examines your mouth for signs of any diseases that are not confined to the teeth. Red, puffy gums indicate gingivitis (see p.445) or periodontitis (see previous page). A white discoloration of the inside of the mouth may signify oral thrush (see p.451), leukoplakia (see p.452), or oral lichen planus (see p.452).

The dentist then inspects your teeth with a mirror and a needle-shaped probe, looking for any color changes that indicate decay or any crack that indicates the beginning of a cavity. Existing fillings are examined to see if any parts have been chipped off or if any fresh cavities are developing around the edge of a filling.

If you have dentures, the dentist will check them for fit, and examine their effects on the gums and teeth.

Before the examination, the dentist or dental assistant usually will ask about your general health. This is very important. It may have a direct bearing on your treatment. If, for example, you have some types of heart condition and have a tooth extracted, or any other treatment that causes bleeding of the gums, you run the risk of contracting bacterial endocarditis (see p.394). Diabetics whose disease is not carefully controlled may become ill if they undergo stress in the dentist's chair. Also, if dental treatment of a person with diabetes requires a general anesthetic, it may have to be carried out in a hospital. People who have had some types of jaundice may be symptomless carriers of hepatitis (see p.486) and may need a blood test before the dentist can decide how to treat them. If you have an allergy, you may react dangerously to certain drugs, such as penicillin. If you are a pregnant woman, the dentist will examine your gums with particular care, looking for signs of gingivitis. And if you are taking any medication, the dentist must be careful to avoid possible harmful reactions between them and any drug the dentist may want to give you.

Why are X-rays taken?
Every year or two, "bite-wing" X-rays will be taken to check for dental faults that are not detected during a normal examination. X-rays are also taken of dead teeth (see p.437), if their roots have been filled, to make sure an abscess (see p.439) is not forming at the base. They may also be used to check the growth of your wisdom teeth (see p.443), or to show how much bone is supporting the teeth if you have periodontal disease (see Gingivitis, p.445 and Periodontitis, previous page).

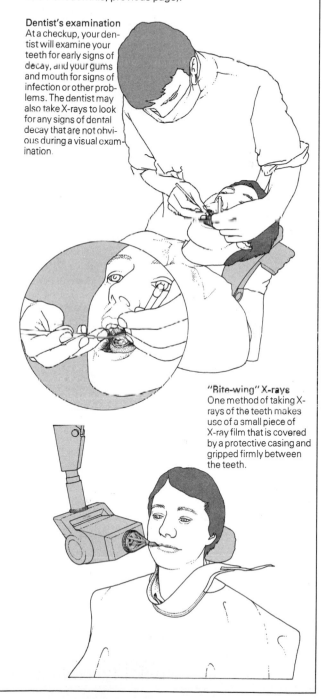

Dentist's examination
At a checkup, your dentist will examine your teeth for early signs of decay, and your gums and mouth for signs of infection or other problems. The dentist may also take X-rays to look for any signs of dental decay that are not obvious during a visual examination.

"Bite-wing" X-rays
One method of taking X-rays of the teeth makes use of a small piece of X-ray film that is covered by a protective casing and gripped firmly between the teeth.

What are the various kinds of treatment?

Cleaning and polishing If any of your teeth are covered by *calculus,* which is a chalky deposit that can cover plaque, it will be removed by probe-like instruments, ultrasonic units or other mechanical implements called scalers. Because they

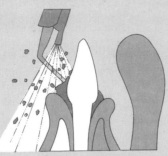

have to operate down to the base of the tooth, scalers may cause the gums to bleed slightly. After scaling, the teeth are polished, because a smooth surface slows down the deposit of calculus.

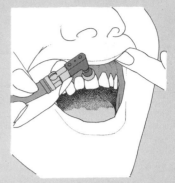

Filling When a tooth is partly decayed or chipped, the dentist replaces the damaged area with a filling. White fillings often are used on front teeth. Silver amalgam, a mixture of silver, tin and mercury, is generally used on back teeth. If the treatment is likely to cause pain, the dentist will inject your gum with a local anesthetic. The dentist removes any decayed area, and shapes the hole to retain the filling securely. If a front tooth is chipped, the dentist roughens the surface and bonds the filling to it. After having a local anesthetic you must be careful to avoid biting your lip or tongue while they are still numb, especially when you eat.

The dentist will fill a tooth if the enamel has been damaged. This is because bacteria can destroy the dentin within and, if not checked, will then attack the pulp.

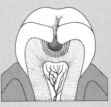

The dentist drills out a hole and removes all traces of decay. He shapes the hole so that the filling will not fall out.

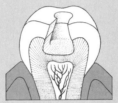

The hole is filled with a mixture of silver, tin and mercury. If a filling will be easily visible, the tooth is filled with a white filling made of quartz in a plastic resin.

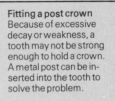

Fitting a post crown Because of excessive decay or weakness, a tooth may not be strong enough to hold a crown. A metal post can be inserted into the tooth to solve the problem.

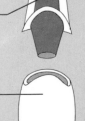

Tooth root (in gum) ——————

Damaged portion ——————

The tooth is trimmed down to the gum and the pulp is removed from the root canal, which is then filled with an antiseptic material. The post is then fitted into the root.

Cleaned out root canal ——————

Trimmed ——————

Crowns When a tooth is severely decayed, broken, discolored, or brittle, the dentist will usually make an artificial crown for it if the base of the tooth and the roots are sound. Generally, a white porcelain crown is fitted on a tooth that can be seen. On back teeth, gold or a less expensive alloy is used, because of the strength of these metals. The treatment usually requires two or three visits; the first one or two to prepare the tooth, and the last to put on the crown. Between visits a temporary plastic or aluminum crown may be worn.

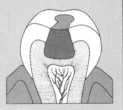

A broken, cracked, or heavily filled tooth can be repaired with a crown. The remaining part of the tooth is shaped to receive the crown.

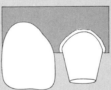

The crown, a hollow shell, is fitted over the old tooth and cemented on.

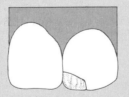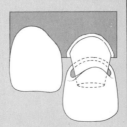

The post secure in the root, a crown is fitted over it.

Gold post in root canal ——————

Crown ——————

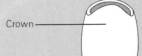
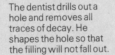

Bridges If you have a gap or gaps of up to about four teeth, flanked by sound natural teeth, you may need a bridge, an artificial tooth or teeth to bridge the gap. The dentist will prepare your natural teeth for crowning, then cement the bridge and the crowns, to which the bridge is attached, into place. There should be enough of a gap left between the base of the bridge and the gum ridge so that you can clean the area properly. Bridges at the front of the mouth are made of an alloy faced with porcelain. Those at the back are usually made of gold or other less expensive alloys. Putting in a bridge normally requires three or four visits to the dentist.

Extractions There are several reasons for pulling a tooth. It may be too decayed or badly broken to be saved by root canal therapy or crowning, or it may be causing crowding or malocclusion (see Orthodontia, p.440). It may be loose because of advanced gum disease, or it may be preventing another tooth from erupting above the gum. Before most extractions, the dentist will inject a local anesthetic to numb the tooth and gum. A general anesthetic may be used for a small child, to extract badly impacted wisdom teeth (see p.443), to extract several teeth at once, or for extremely apprehensive patients. After an extraction you must not do anything that might dislodge the clot that forms on the wound. If the socket bleeds persistently, bite on a clean, tightly folded handkerchief or a gauze pad, as a compress. Keep it in place for half an hour by clenching your teeth. A small amount of oozing may continue for several hours.

Dentures To replace many missing teeth, a partial denture is required. A full denture replaces all your natural teeth. Dentures are made of tough plastic or a combination of metal and plastic.

Full dentures stay in place by resting on the gum ridges and by suction in the case of upper dentures. On a partial denture, the baseplate (artificial gums) often has clasps that fit around natural teeth to help keep the denture in place.

Fitting a denture normally requires several visits to the dentist. The dentist takes impressions of the gums, and the relationship between the upper and lower jaws is recorded. The dentist also discusses with you the size and color of your false teeth. In most cases, the dentist makes a preliminary denture with the artificial teeth in a wax baseplate, and makes any necessary adjustments with this preliminary model of the denture. After the final denture is made, the dentist fits and adjusts it so that you bite evenly.

Replacing a missing tooth
If all of a tooth is missing, the gap can only be filled by building a bridge.

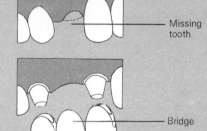

Missing tooth

The two teeth on either side of the gap will be shaped so that they can anchor the bridge.

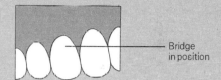

Bridge

The bridge is cemented to the two shaped teeth so that they hold the replacement in position.

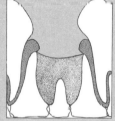

Bridge in position

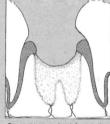 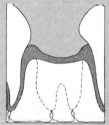

After a tooth extraction When a tooth is pulled, a blood clot will usually form in the socket.

Sometimes the blood clot breaks down. This leaves what is called a dry socket.

Eventually new bone will grow into the gap and gum will grow over the bone.

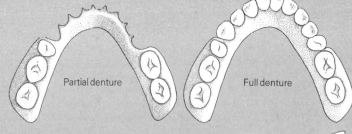

Partial denture

Full denture

The trays (right) are filled with a putty-like substance to take impressions of your gums. The one with a recess is used for the lower jaw, the other for the upper jaw.

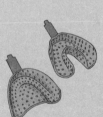 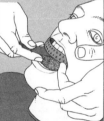

Mouth and tongue

The inside of your mouth is covered by a delicate lining of mucous membrane. It is kept moist and lubricated by saliva, which is produced in three pairs of salivary glands in your mouth. These are the sublingual glands, which are located under your tongue, the submandibular glands, which are in the floor of your mouth, and the parotid glands, which are found above the angle of your jaw.

Your tongue has a complex system of muscles that enables it to move food around as you chew, and then to mold chewed food into a ball for swallowing. The surface of your tongue is covered with hair-like projections called papillae, and groups of tastebuds are clustered around them.

The tastebuds can distinguish four main types of flavor: sweet, salt, sour and bitter. It is to these tastebuds that you are indebted for the pleasure of a fine meal. More important, it is often your tastebuds that warn you if you begin to eat food that has spoiled.

Changes in the shape of your mouth, tongue and lips enable you to form a variety of sounds, including those that are necessary for speech.

The majority of disorders that affect your mouth and tongue are not serious and are simple to treat. However, because it is possible for *malignant*, or life-threatening, tumors to form there, you should consult your physician or dentist about any condition of the mouth or tongue that persists for more than ten days.

If you have any reason to suspect that you have a tumor, read the articles on salivary gland tumors and tumors of the mouth and tongue in the following pages. If after that you still think you have or may have a tumor, you will want to see a physician as quickly as possible.

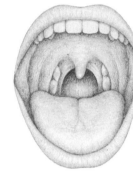

The mouth
The mouth is the first part of the digestive tract. The teeth crush the food so that enzymes can break it down, while saliva lubricates it, to make it easier to swallow.

Mouth ulcers
(*including canker sores*)

See p.248,
Visual aids to diagnosis, 64.

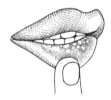

Mouth ulcers
One type of mouth ulcer may appear in clusters on the lower lip. These ulcers are white, and may be very painful.

A mouth ulcer is a break in the lining of the mouth that uncovers the sensitive tissue beneath. All mouth ulcers look very much the same, but they vary considerably in cause and seriousness. The two most common and painful types of ulcers are aphthous ulcers, which tend to occur when you are under stress, run down or ill, and traumatic ulcers, which result from an injury to the lining of your mouth. Such an injury may be caused by a toothbrush, a rough denture, or hot food.

Some mouth ulcers are caused by infection by a virus. A virus that commonly causes mouth ulcers is herpes simplex (see next article). This virus causes blisters that eventually turn into ulcers. Rarely, an ulcer may be the first sign of a tumor of the mouth (see p.454), or a more generalized disease such as anemia (see p.419) or leukemia (see p.426).

Mouth ulcers are very common; about ten per cent of people get them. Aphthous ulcers occur most often in adolescents and young adults, and more often in women (especially just before a menstrual period).

What are the symptoms?
You usually first become aware of an ulcer when you eat something spicy or acidic that makes it sting. All ulcers look much the same. You can usually see them in a mirror as pale yellow spots with red borders. Aphthous ulcers are small, measuring 2 to 3 mm ($\frac{1}{10}$ in) across. They usually appear in clusters on the sides of your mouth or gum, and last for three to four days. A traumatic ulcer is usually larger and lasts for a week or more. When a traumatic ulcer is caused by a rough tooth or denture, it will not heal until the cause is dealt with in some way.

What should be done?
The vast majority of mouth ulcers do not indicate any major health problem and usually heal by themselves. But if an ulcer fails to heal within ten days, or if ulcers keep recurring, then see your physician to find out if the ulcers are caused by a more serious underlying condition. Your physician may want you to have blood tests taken, and you may also

have to undergo a *biopsy* of the ulcer. In this procedure, part of the ulcer is removed under a local anesthetic, so that it can be examined. The results of these tests will show whether the ulcer signifies a serious disorder, which will then be dealt with as necessary.

If you suspect that a jagged tooth or rough denture is causing traumatic ulcers, consult your dentist about it.

What is the treatment?
Self-help: You can buy various non-prescription applications and lozenges that numb and protect the exposed tissue in an ulcer. These preparations relieve the pain and may help the ulcer to heal. Antiseptic mouthwashes or rinsing your mouth with warm, salt water may also help. To minimize discomfort, avoid eating spices (such as chili and pepper) or acidic foods (grapefruits and oranges, for example). The ulcer will also be sensitive to hot food or drinks.
Professional help: To deal with persistent aphthous ulcers, your physician may prescribe a mouth rinse or a cream containing a *steroid* drug.

Cold sores
(Herpes simplex)

See p.238,
Visual aids to diagnosis, 24.

Herpes simplex is a virus that causes blisters to form on your lips and on the inside of your mouth. These blisters, called cold sores, develop into painful ulcers. Your gums become swollen and deep red, and often the tongue is furred. You may have a fever and feel generally unwell. The older you are, the more severe the infection. In young children, the initial attack is usually so mild that it may pass unnoticed.

After the infection has cleared up, the virus lies dormant. Later, another infection (commonly a cold), or exposure to sunshine or wind, reactivates it. This causes a blister to form that bursts and forms an encrusted cold sore on the edge of your lip or somewhere else near your mouth.

Herpes simplex infection of the mouth is very common and seems to present no serious risks to your general health. The main danger involved is that, during the first infection, if you touch the ulcers and then your eye it could cause a herpetic corneal ulcer (see p.316) to form on that eye.

What is the treatment?
Mild cases of the first infection need no treatment. In severe cases your physician may advise you to rest, take aspirin if you have a fever, and use a mild mouthwash.

Cold sores generally clear up uneventfully. However, if the blisters are especially painful, your physician may prescribe a medication that you can apply to the sores to ease the pain as the sores heal.

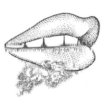

Most cold sores appear around the mouth. Tingling and numbness may precede or follow their appearance.

Oral thrush

Oral thrush is an outbreak of the fungus *Candida albicans*, one of the many microbes that are usually present in small numbers in your mouth. If your natural resistance to infection is low because of an illness, or if a course of *antibiotics* has upset the natural balance among the microbes in your mouth, this fungus may multiply out of control. As it does so, it produces sore patches in your mouth. Sometimes it can cause similar sore areas to form in your throat as well. The patches are creamy-yellow and slightly raised. If they are rubbed off when you eat or as you brush your teeth, they leave a painful raw area. The fungus can also cause denture problems (see p.443).

Many people have oral thrush at some time in their lives. It is most prevalent in very young children and elderly people. The same fungus can infect a woman's vagina and cause vaginal irritation and discharge (see Vaginal yeast infection, p.602).

If you have the symptoms described for oral thrush, you should see your physician within a day or two.

What is the treatment?
Your physician will examine you and may take a sample of a patch for laboratory analysis, or perhaps arrange for you to have blood tests to rule out the possibility of any serious underlying disease. One possible cause is iron deficiency anemia (see p.419). Meanwhile, the thrush may be treated with an antifungal agent, often taken as lozenges for seven to ten days. Oral thrush in itself is not serious and is quickly cleared up by this treatment, but it has a tendency to recur.

Leukoplakia

In leukoplakia, a part of the soft, delicate lining of your mouth or tongue thickens and hardens. This usually occurs to protect an area made sore by the repeated rubbing of a rough tooth or denture. It may also be caused by a protective reaction to the heat of inhaled tobacco smoke, in which case it is known as smoker's keratosis. The patch, which develops over a period of weeks, is white or gray and may be any size. At first it causes no discomfort, but later it feels rough and stiff and may be sensitive to hot or spicy foods.

Anyone can develop leukoplakia, but it is most common in the elderly. If you develop the symptoms described, see your dentist or your physician.

What is the treatment?
The treatment is to deal with the source of irritation that has caused the patch to form.

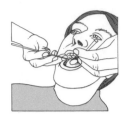

Taking a biopsy
Your dentist or your physician may remove a small piece of tissue from the affected area for analysis in a laboratory.

This means that a rough tooth or denture may have to be filed smooth, or, in the case of smoker's keratosis, you may be advised to give up smoking. This is usually all that is needed to make the patch disappear. If it has not gone away within two weeks, your doctor will arrange for a *biopsy* of the patch, in which a small sample of it is removed and examined. This is necessary because about three per cent of such patches are an early sign of a tumor of the mouth (see p.454).

Oral lichen planus

In oral lichen planus, changes occur in the lining of your mouth that often cause minor discomfort. Most commonly the disorder starts as a number of small, pale pimples that gradually join to form a fine, white, lacy network of slightly raised tissue. In other cases the disorder takes the form of shiny, red, slightly raised patches. The changes usually occur on the inside of your cheeks and the sides of your tongue.

The symptoms may include a sore mouth and a dry, metallic taste, or there may be no noticeable symptoms.

The cause of oral lichen planus is unclear. It can be brought on by emotional stress, by patches or irritation in the mouth such as those that are caused by ill-fitting dentures (see Denture problems, p.443), or by poor oral hygiene.

Oral lichen planus is rare. It can affect any adult but occurs most often in middle-aged and elderly women. Half of those who get oral lichen planus also have lichen planus on the skin (see p.261).

What should be done?
Any color or texture changes inside your mouth that do not clear up within ten days should be seen by your physician. The best way to prevent or treat the disorder is to keep your mouth healthy by brushing your teeth and gums thoroughly twice each day. If brushing is painful, try a very soft toothbrush, and use it gently. If you have dentures, ask your dentist to make sure that they fit properly and have no rough spots. These will be eliminated if present. If the condition is very irritating, your physician may prescribe a drug in tablet form, to be sucked every few hours. This treatment usually causes the patches to shrink and then they will disappear within a few days.

Trench mouth

Trench mouth, which is also sometimes called either acute ulcerative gingivitis or Vincent's disease, is a painful infection and ulceration of the gums, usually between the teeth. The infection is usually caused by bacteria, and results from a combination of factors that include failure to clean your teeth and gums properly, throat infections, and smoking. It often develops from gingivitis (see p.445). It may also occur along with some serious illness such as leukemia.

Trench mouth is rare. It usually occurs in young adults. Lack of rest, stress, and poor nutrition help bring on trench mouth. It is not thought to be contagious and is not a dangerous condition, but can cause considerable discomfort. This is particularly true when the throat is also infected.

What are the symptoms?
Your gums become red, swollen, and sometimes so painful that you cannot eat. After a while, ulcers appear on the gums, and they bleed. You may have a metallic taste in your mouth, and bad breath. Sometimes a fever develops. If you have these symptoms, it is

Gingivitis can trigger trench mouth. As trench mouth develops, ulcers appear in the mouth, especially on the already painful and inflamed gums.

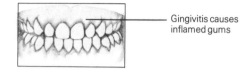

Gingivitis causes inflamed gums

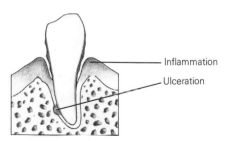

Inflammation

Ulceration

important that you see your dentist or physician as soon as possible.

What is the treatment?

Use of hydrogen peroxide mouthwash usually relieves the pain and inflammation of the gums. After a few days, your dentist can clean your teeth and gums with a scaler (see p.448). A prescription for an *antibiotic* may be given to clear up the infection. Regular follow-up visits about every two weeks, often to a dental hygienist, may be necessary.

When the disease has been eradicated, the dentist may advise minor surgery on your gums, to trim them to a smooth shape. This will make them easier to clean. It will also minimize the areas in your mouth in which another infection may develop.

Salivary gland infections

A salivary gland becomes infected and swollen most commonly as a result of mumps (see p.700). However, such an infection can also be caused by bacteria, especially if you are run down or if one of your glands has been damaged by salivary duct stones (see next article). When it is infected, the salivary gland becomes swollen and painful, and the lymph glands in your neck beneath the angle of your jaw may also feel enlarged and tender. Pus from the infected gland trickles into your mouth and tastes bitter. Sometimes an infection persists, and this may cause so much scarring in the gland that it may cease to function. If you have any swelling in your mouth, under your chin, or around your jaw, you should consult your physician.

What is the treatment?

Your physician will probably treat an infection of the salivary glands with an *antibiotic*, if the problem seems to be caused by bacteria. If the infection is persistent, you may be sent to a radiologist for a *sialogram*, a test to show whether the gland has been damaged. If it has, you will probably be advised to have it removed. Your other salivary glands will compensate for the one you have lost.

Salivary duct stones

A stone, or tiny hard particle, forms in the duct of a salivary gland when chemicals in the saliva encrust a minute bit of solid material in the duct. The stone partially blocks the duct and at mealtimes most of the large quantity of saliva produced cannot pass the stone, which causes the gland to swell. The submandibular salivary glands, in the floor of your mouth, are the most susceptible of your salivary glands to this uncommon disorder.

What should be done?

If you have any swelling under your chin or behind or under the angle of your jaw, particularly at mealtimes, consult your physician, who may arrange for you to have an *X-ray* taken of your mouth. If the cause of the swelling is not clear from this, you may also have a test called a *sialogram*.

What is the treatment?

If you have a salivary duct stone it can usually be removed under local anesthetic. If it recurs, a permanent opening can be cut along the duct so that saliva can drain into your mouth almost directly from the gland. Then the possibility of further stones and subsequent scarring of the duct is avoided.

The openings of the salivary ducts under the tongue are the ones most often affected by a stone.

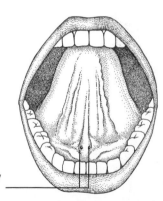

Openings of salivary ducts under tongue

Salivary gland tumors

Sometimes cells in a salivary gland may multiply to form a tumor. Why this happens is not known. Most such tumors form in one of the two parotid glands, which are located above the angle of your jaw. Most of them are *benign*, or unlikely to spread and threaten life. They generally develop slowly over several years, and gradually cause the gland to swell. It remains swollen, but there are no other symptoms. However, there is a very small risk that the growth may be, or may become, *malignant*, or likely to spread and threaten life.

If one of your salivary glands is swollen or if you have any pain or discomfort in your mouth, see your physician. You may have to go to a radiologist for a *sialogram*, a test that will help to disclose whether or not a tumor is causing the problem.

What is the treatment?
If you do have such a tumor, you will probably be advised to have it removed surgically. If the tumor is found to be malignant, *radiation therapy* will probably be advised.

In operations on the parotid gland, there is a risk of damage to an adjacent nerve that controls the movements of your lower face. However, surgery can usually repair such damage if it occurs.

Tumors of the mouth and tongue

Tumors can occur anywhere in or on your mouth, except on the teeth. There are two types of tumors, *benign* and *malignant*. The causes of both of these types are unknown. A benign tumor is usually a slow-growing lump that does not spread to surrounding areas and threaten life. A malignant tumor is a cancer. Its cells spread to the surrounding area, then further afield, and ultimately threaten life. This dangerous spread of cancer cells is called *metastasis*. Malignant tumors of the tongue may spread within a few months, while those in other parts of the mouth spread over several years. (See also Salivary gland tumors, previous article.)

What are the symptoms?
Benign tumors of the mouth usually occur singly. Such a tumor starts as a small, pale lump, which then grows slowly over several years. If it grows larger than 10 mm (about ⅓ in) across, it may cause fitting problems with dentures, and even slight distortion of the face. A benign tumor on your tongue may rupture and bleed extensively. Benign tumors are hardly ever painful.

A malignant tumor also begins as a single, small, pale lump, but then turns into an ulcer with a hard, raised rim and a fragile center that bleeds easily. The ulcer grows and erodes the surrounding area of your mouth. If the ulcer spreads over your tongue, the cancerous cells make the tongue muscles stiff and fixed, which causes difficulty in eating, swallowing and speaking. Malignant tumors are not usually painful until they grow and reach an advanced stage.

What are the risks?
Malignant tumors of the mouth are very rare generally, and they are extremely rare in people under 40. They are most common among those people who are over 60. Tumors of the tongue occur more frequently in men than they do in women. The opposite is true for tumors in the rest of the mouth. Benign tumors of the mouth seem to be about as rare as malignant tumors.

Benign tumors usually present no risk, but in rare cases they can become malignant. Malignant tumors carry the risk of spreading, or *metastasizing*, to other parts of your body. The later it is when a malignant tumor anywhere in your body is diagnosed and treated, the more likely it is that the cancer will become life-threatening.

What should be done?
Consult your physician at once if you have any lump, ulcer, or unexplained color change in your mouth that does not clear up within ten days, or if your dentures have begun to fit badly, or if your tongue has become stiff and difficult to control.

If the trouble is caused by a tumor, a small sample of the tissue will be removed for laboratory examination to find out whether it is benign or malignant. This is a *biopsy*, a procedure that is easily done in a few minutes, with local anesthesia. The results of this procedure will determine how your physician treats the tumor

What is the treatment?
Most benign tumors cause no problems. However, your physician will probably want to observe the growth of the lump or lumps at six-month or annual checkups, to insure that they have not become malignant during that time. Large benign tumors on the lips can be removed surgically, and your natural features can usually be restored by cosmetic surgery (see p.260). Special dentures or plates can restore the natural appearance of your gums.

The treatment for malignant tumors and the success of the treatment depend on the stage the disease has reached at the time the problem is diagnosed and the treatment is begun. If this is an early stage and the tumor has not spread, it is removed surgically. If the tumor has spread, *radiation therapy* is often used to destroy the cancerous cells. In some cases, both surgery and radiation therapy are used in the treatment. Cases that are diagnosed in an early stage are usually completely cured by these treatments.

Tongue problems

See p.248, **Visual aids to diagnosis, 65 and 66.**

The upper surface of the tongue is covered by papillae, or tiny hair-like projections of tissue. Groups of taste buds are clustered around them. Normally, the papillae are pink and velvety and are crossed by fissures, which expose the deep-red muscular body of the tongue beneath. But in some people various alterations take place in this normal color and texture. Most of these tongue problems are minor and need no professional treatment. If, however, you have any tongue problem that persists for more than ten days, you should consult your physician.

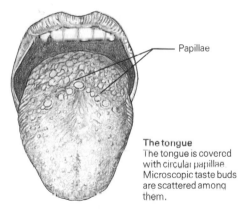

Papillae

The tongue
The tongue is covered with circular papillae. Microscopic taste buds are scattered among them.

Lumps or ulcers on the tongue
If a lump or ulcer forms on your tongue and fails to heal in ten days, see your physician without delay, even if the affected area is painless. The lump or ulcer could be harmless, but it could be a benign or malignant tumor (see Tumors of the mouth and tongue, previous article).

Glossitis and geographical tongue
Glossitis is a treatable inflammation of the tongue in which the papillae no longer form properly, and no longer cover the body of the tongue. Geographical tongue is a similar disorder, but it differs from glossitis in two ways. First, it occurs in patches that come and go, and second, there is no known cause or treatment for it. In either disorder, the exposed surface of your tongue becomes smooth and dark red, and often feels sore, especially if you eat spicy foods.

Glossitis can have many causes, including infection, injury and allergic reactions. It is often a symptom of a nutritional deficiency, such as iron deficiency anemia (see p.419) or B_{12} deficiency anemia (see p.420). If you have the symptoms described for glossitis, see your physician. If you have an underlying disorder, treatment of it will also clear up the glossitis. If there is no underlying cause, there is no need for concern. The glossitis will probably heal rapidly.

Your physician may prescribe an antiseptic mouthwash. Also, if you avoid hot or spicy foods, alcohol and tobacco, it may help relieve the soreness caused by either glossitis or geographical tongue.

Discolored and fissured tongue
Your tongue may become discolored for any of several reasons, but this is usually not a cause for concern. Some people have tongues that are fissured, or creased, more deeply or extensively than usual. Sometimes bacteria, which are present in everyone's mouth, accumulate in the fissures or on the papillae. This can make your tongue appear to be black or dark brown. The discoloration may also be caused by fungal infections such as oral thrush (see p.451), by smoking, or by taking *antibiotics*. Sometimes the papillae will become long and hair-like. Neither the fissures, the hair-like papillae, nor the discoloration need concern you. To restore your tongue to normal, you can brush it gently twice a day with a toothbrush if it does not hurt to do so. Dip the toothbrush in a diluted antiseptic, such as a mouthwash.

Another type of discoloration, called furred tongue, may occur when you are ill, especially with a fever. You may notice a whitish or yellowish furry coating on the surface of your tongue. This occurs because you may be talking and eating less than usual, and your tongue may be less active, which allows a film of bacteria, food particles, and excess cells to accumulate on it. Also, during illness your mouth is often dry, and there is not enough saliva to wash away this film. Your tongue will probably return to normal as soon as the illness clears up. No other treatment is needed for furred tongue.

Esophagus

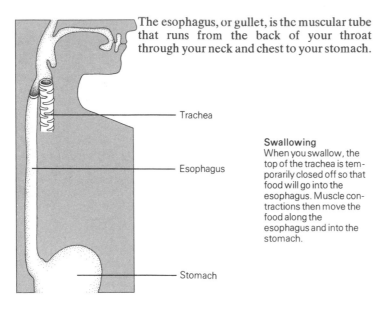

The esophagus, or gullet, is the muscular tube that runs from the back of your throat through your neck and chest to your stomach.

Trachea

Esophagus

Swallowing
When you swallow, the top of the trachea is temporarily closed off so that food will go into the esophagus. Muscle contractions then move the food along the esophagus and into the stomach.

Stomach

As you swallow, the back of your tongue pushes a ball of food into the esophagus. The soft palate closes off the passage to your nose, and the top of the windpipe closes so that food cannot get into your trachea, or lower windpipe, and then into your lungs. Rhythmic contractions of the esophageal muscles send the food down through the chest into the base of the esophagus, where a muscular valve at the entrance to your stomach relaxes to let the food pass through.

Difficult swallowing or pain while swallowing is called *dysphagia.* It is not a disease, but it is a symptom of nearly all diseases of the esophagus. And since it is the major symptom of a *malignant,* or life-threatening, growth in your esophagus, *always consult your physician immediately if you begin to have trouble swallowing.* Chances of a serious disorder are slight, but if you do have a serious condition, an early diagnosis is essential.

Heartburn and hiatus hernia

A domed sheet of muscle, the diaphragm, separates your chest from your abdomen. The esophagus has to pass through an opening, or *hiatus,* in the diaphragm to reach your stomach. A hiatus hernia occurs when the muscular tissue around the hiatus weakens and the abdominal portion of the esophagus, often along with part of the upper stomach, protrudes upwards through the hiatus into your chest. The protrusion, or hernia, forms a bell-shaped swelling at the base of the esophagus. Most people who have this type of hernia are not troubled by it. In some cases, however, it affects the efficiency of the muscular valve that maintains a one-way flow from the esophagus to the stomach. The result is that acid fluid from the stomach wells up into the lower esophagus. This process is

A hiatus hernia
The stomach is below the diaphragm. The esophagus passes through a hole in the diaphragm and enters the stomach. A hiatus hernia is when part of the stomach squeezes back through this hole into the chest.

called acid reflux, and it is more commonly known as heartburn.

What are the symptoms?
The main symptom, if you have any, is usually a painful burning sensation in your chest. Very rarely, the pain may extend into your neck and arms. If it is severe, you may mistake it for the pain of a heart attack (see p.379). If you bend forward or lie down, stomach acid can more easily flow into the esophagus, so heartburn is often particularly troublesome at night.

Another possible symptom is sudden regurgitation of acid fluid into your throat. Belching is often common.

What are the risks?
Hiatus hernia is quite common, especially among overweight, elderly people. But again, everyone with hiatus hernia does not experience heartburn. It is not in itself a severe or dangerous ailment. But persistent acid reflux, no matter what causes it, can lead to inflammation or even ulceration of the esophagus. Inflammation can lead in turn to stricture of the esophagus (see p.458). In rare cases, esophageal ulcers bleed, which may cause anemia (see p.419). Some degree of hiatus hernia often occurs during pregnancy (see Heartburn during pregnancy, p.622).

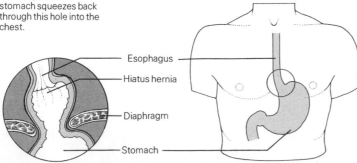

Esophagus

Hiatus hernia

Diaphragm

Stomach

What should be done?

If the symptoms are troublesome, adopt the self-help measures suggested below. If the symptoms persist, consult your physician. The physician may advise you to have diagnostic tests such as an *electrocardiogram (ECG)*, a *barium swallow X-ray*, and also perhaps *endoscopy*.

What is the treatment?

Self-help: If you are overweight, one of the most effective, self-help measures is to lose weight, as this sometimes helps relieve the symptoms of a hiatus hernia (see Obesity, p.492). Avoid stooping, particularly after a meal. Do not wear tight girdles or belts. Raise the head of your bed about four inches by standing the front legs on books or bricks, to reduce acid reflux at night. Avoid alcoholic drinks, which tend to aggravate the symptoms. And do not smoke, since smoking encourages the production of stomach acid. Try taking one of the antacids that is available without prescription. Be sure to follow the directions on the label. These preparations help relieve heartburn from acid reflux by neutralizing stomach acid, and some also may coat and protect the lining of the esophagus. As with a duodenal ulcer (see p.468), the symptoms of hiatus hernia can often be relieved by eating several small meals each day instead of two or three large ones.

Professional help: If non-prescription antacids are ineffective, your physician may prescribe another type of medication. To reduce the backflow of acid from the stomach to the esophagus, the doctor may also prescribe a medication that increases the speed with which food passes through the stomach and into the intestines.

The above measures usually prevent acid reflux, and relieve heartburn. If it persists and you do have a documented hiatus hernia, your physician may recommend that it be repaired surgically. The operation is relatively simple and results are usually good.

Cancer of the esophagus

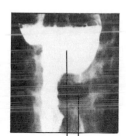

Esophagus

Tumor

An X-ray taken after a patient has swallowed a special dye reveals a cancerous growth narrowing the esophagus.

In this disorder, cells in the lining of the esophagus start to multiply rapidly and form a tumor. The tumor eventually causes narrowing and constriction of the passageway to your stomach. As with other types of cancer, the cause is unknown, though cancer of the esophagus has been linked with prolonged exposure to irritants such as tobacco smoke and alcohol.

What are the symptoms?

The main symptom is difficulty or pain when swallowing that worsens rapidly. At first only solids are hard to swallow, but then liquids also become troublesome. An additional symptom is rapid, progressive weight loss. Occasionally, you may belch up bloody mucus as well.

What are the risks?

Cancer of the esophagus is very rare. Men are about twice as susceptible as women, and the risk seems to be greatest for heavy smokers and drinkers who are 50 to 60 years old.

If the condition is detected in an early stage, chances for successful treatment are fair. Otherwise, it can spread swiftly, blocking the esophagus and spreading to vital neighboring organs. About ten per cent of those who have cancer of the esophagus survive for five or more years after the condition is discovered.

What should be done?

If food seems to stick in your throat when you try to swallow it, see your physician right away. Even though the chance of a cancerous tumor is slight, the doctor will probably order diagnostic tests, including a *barium swallow X-ray,* other *X-rays,* a thorough examination of the esophagus by *endoscopy,* and a *biopsy,* in which a sample of tissue is removed for careful examination.

If you have cancer of the esophagus, the usual treatment is to remove the affected part. *Radiation therapy* may then be used to attempt to destroy any remaining cancer cells. If an operation is not possible, radiation therapy will probably be used to slow down the progress of the disease.

Achalasia

When you swallow normally, food is guided down the esophagus by rhythmic contractions of the muscles in its wall. In the rare disorder known as achalasia, the nerves that control the muscles of the lower end of your esophagus become defective, and the contractions become irregular and uncoordinated. Why this happens is not known, but if it does, the lower part of your esophagus becomes constricted, distorted, and swollen with food that cannot move on into the rest of the digestive system.

What are the symptoms?

The main symptoms of achalasia are discomfort and pain on swallowing. There is also usually continuous discomfort or pain in your chest. Because food accumulates in the esophagus, you are likely to have a foul taste in your mouth and bad breath. Occasionally you may regurgitate food into your mouth. At first, only solids will be hard to swallow, but eventually you will have trouble with liquids as well.

As achalasia worsens, the esophagus is never properly emptied, and there is always a chance that you might inhale food particles while you sleep. These can cause chest infections such as pneumonia (see p.359). Because of the difficulty in eating, weight loss and signs of malnutrition may also occur.

What should be done?

If you suspect you may have achalasia, consult your physician, who, after examining you, will probably arrange a *barium swallow X-ray*. Visual examination of the esophagus by *endoscopy* may also be used to confirm the diagnosis. One form of treatment for achalasia involves passing a slender rubber bag down the esophagus and filling the bag with water or air, in order to stretch the muscles at the bottom. This procedure allows food to pass into your stomach more easily. But this only relieves the problem temporarily. The only permanently effective treatment is an operation called a cardiomyotomy, in which some of the muscles at the stomach entrance are cut in order to widen the passageway for food.

Pharyngeal pouch

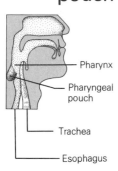

Pharynx

Pharyngeal pouch

Trachea

Esophagus

A pharyngeal pouch is a small bulge or sac that develops at the pharynx, which is in the back of the throat just at the top of the esophagus. This rare disorder occurs most often in elderly men. It usually happens because the muscles become uncoordinated during swallowing. Food enters the bulge during swallowing, and the bulge stretches downward to form a baglike pouch. Over the years the pouch gradually grows bigger, and it becomes increasingly difficult to swallow. The pouch itself may show up as a swelling in your neck, and it is most prominent after you drink. Another symptom of the disorder is regurgitation of fluid or undigested food from the pouch into your mouth, which generally occurs several hours after you eat. An irritating cough, and a metallic taste in your mouth may also occur.

The main risk of a pharyngeal pouch is that fluid from the pouch may enter your lungs while you sleep, and cause an infection.

What should be done?

Consult your physician if you have any difficulty in swallowing. The doctor will usually be able to diagnose pharyngeal pouch from a physical examination and a description of your symptoms. However, a *barium swallow X-ray* may be needed to confirm this. Often the disorder needs no treatment, but in some cases your physician will recommend removal of the pouch, which is a relatively,simple and safe operation.

Diffuse spasm of the esophagus

This is a rare condition for which there is no known cause. It consists of irregular, repeated spasms of the muscles of the esophageal wall, which can cause chest pains, difficulty in swallowing, and acid reflux (see Heartburn and hiatus hernia, p.456). The condition develops gradually, with intermittent attacks over a period of years. If you have this condition you will probably have to learn to live with it; there is no cure. To help relieve the spasms, an *antispasmodic* drug may be prescribed.

Stricture of the esophagus

This is a rare disorder that usually occurs in elderly people. It is the result of an accumulation of scar tissue in the esophagus, often caused by persistent acid reflux (see Heartburn and hiatus hernia, p.456). Because the scarred portions of the esophagus gradually become enlarged, the passageway for food becomes increasingly constricted. The result is difficulty in swallowing. You should always consult your physician as soon as possible if you have this symptom.

The usual treatment for stricture is to enlarge the passageway with either a water-filled rubber bag (see Achalasia, previous page), or a flexible metal rod called a "bougie." This procedure, which is done while you are under a general anesthetic, must be repeated every few weeks or so to be effective. Surgery to remove the scar tissue may be necessary.

Infections of the digestive tract

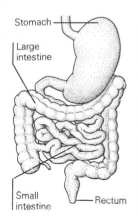

Stomach

Large intestine

Small intestine — Rectum

A digestive-tract, or gastrointestinal, infection occurs when certain infectious agents multiply rapidly in your stomach and intestines. This causes disorders of various kinds and varying severity.

The intestines normally contain many bacteria that are harmless. In fact, some of them are essential to the manufacture of some vitamins and are, therefore, desirable "intruders." The presence of such organisms is not considered an infection, for this term is generally used only to describe the presence of large numbers of dangerous organisms such as those that cause disease. The unchecked multiplication of such infectious agents will bring on a number of symptoms such as diarrhea and vomiting, along with more generalized illness if the organisms ultimately enter your bloodstream.

The gastrointestinal malady called gastroenteritis may have causes other than infection. Such causes include food allergies (see p.705), excessive use of alcohol, very spicy foods, certain medications, and toxic substances. In such cases the symptoms may be difficult to distinguish from those caused by minor infections. For this reason, gastroenteritis is included in this group of articles that deal primarily with infections that occur in the digestive tract.

Gastro-enteritis

Gastroenteritis is an irritation and inflammation of the digestive tract that produces the symptoms of an upset stomach. It is most commonly caused by a viral infection, which can easily be passed from one person to another without involving the consumption of food or drink. Such infections are the most common cause of the 24- or 36-hour attacks of vomiting and/or diarrhea that are often called intestinal or stomach flu.

Gastroenteritis can also be caused by eating or drinking contaminated food or water. A different kind of "food poisoning" can occur if you eat something that contains a *toxic* substance, for example, a non-edible mushroom or a rhubarb leaf. Also, some foods cause a similar reaction in individuals who are allergic to them. Tomatoes, berries, eggs, milk products and shellfish have been known to act in this way for some people, and there are many other possibilities. Such kinds of food poisoning are not caused by microbial infection, but they are capable of bringing on attacks of gastroenteritis that can be very serious (see Box, p.462).

Another possible cause of gastroenteritis is a change in the natural bacterial population of the digestive tract. If you have an illness that weakens you, or if you suddenly make drastic changes in your diet (for example, when you visit a foreign country), the balance may be disturbed so that certain bacterial strains become stronger at the expense of others, and this can cause an upset stomach. *Antibiotic* drugs often have a similar effect by acting selectively and disrupting the bacterial equilibrium in your intestines.

What are the symptoms?

The symptoms of gastroenteritis range from a mild attack of nausea followed by diarrhea, which happens to nearly everybody at some time, to a severe illness. You may have one or two bouts of vomiting and some soft bowel movements that hardly interfere with your routine. Or you may vomit repeatedly and have recurrent attacks of watery diarrhea with abdominal pains and cramps, fever and extreme weakness. Occasionally, an extreme case of gastroenteritis lasts so long that it disables you, but usually the symptoms go away within 24 to 48 hours.

What are the risks?

Gastroenteritis is a very common ailment, and most people get their first attack early in life (see Gastroenteritis in infants, p.649).

Risks depend on the type and number of infectious agents, the amount and virulence, or strength, of the poisonous food substances that you have eaten, and your age and general health. The danger of severe illness is greatest for newborn babies, infants less than about 18 months old, and chronically ill elderly people. Repeated attacks of diarrhea cause *dehydration* and loss of certain crucial body salts, which upsets body chemistry and, if unchecked, can lead to shock (see p.386). In a normally healthy person a few bouts of vomiting and diarrhea are no more significant than a common cold. But if there is also severe and persistent pain in the abdomen (not just an occasional cramp), the symptoms may be due to some other abdominal disorder such as appendicitis (see p.476).

What should be done?

If the self-help measures recommended below do not relieve, or at least greatly improve, the symptoms within two or, at most, three days, consult your physician. After examining you, your physician may decide to send a sample of your bowel movements to a laboratory for analysis. More probably, your answers to questions about what you have eaten and whether other family members or associates are ill, the doctor's observations of the state of your health, and any information your doctor may have about a local epidemic of this disorder will confirm the diagnosis. Analysis of bowel movements may be necessary, however, if diarrhea is prolonged, to make sure that your gastroenteritis is not due to a severe intestinal infection such as amebic dysentery (see next page).

What is the treatment?

Self-help: If you have an attack of gastroenteritis, stay at home, rest, and drink plenty of fluids until the attack subsides. To avoid dehydration because of diarrhea, you may need to drink at least an extra pint or so of fluid per day. Do not eat at all unless you are especially hungry, and drink only water or weak tea for the first 12 hours (a few sips every 15 minutes or so if you are having bad spells of vomiting). Then increase your intake of fluids to include unsweetened fruit juices, tea, clear broth or boullion, cooked cereal, and other bland, soft foods. Avoid sugar, because it can prolong diarrhea. The broth replaces the body salts lost because of the diarrhea. After about two days of this care you should be able to resume your normal diet.

Over-the-counter antidiarrhea medicines may help after the nausea and vomiting have subsided, but do not take aspirin or other painkillers. Such drugs are likely to aggravate the condition. Also, *antibiotics* tend to upset the equilibrium of intestinal bacteria, and make the diarrhea worse. Remember, too, that gastroenteritis is often caused by poor hygiene and is easily passed on to others. So be sure that you wash your hands thoroughly after you have a bowel movement and, also, before you touch food.

Professional help: There is no specific treatment for viral gastroenteritis. If the diagnosis is clear and your nausea and diarrhea are relatively mild and not due to some other disorder such as a generalized infection or appendicitis, your physician will probably advise you to continue the self-help measures recommended above. If your vomiting is severe, an *anti-emetic* drug may be prescribed in suppository form, or given to you by injection. Persistent diarrhea is sometimes treated with other medications such as narcotic-type drugs, which harden your bowel movements, *antispasmodic* drugs, and drugs that slow down bowel activity. Any such treatment is usually stopped as soon as the bowels begin to function normally.

If your vomiting and diarrhea are so severe that you become dehydrated, and especially if you also have a chronic disease such as diabetes mellitus (see p.519) or kidney problems (see p.511), your physician will probably admit you to the hospital so that fluid can be replaced *intravenously*, or through a tube into a vein and your blood chemistry can be restored to a proper balance.

Salmonellosis

Bacteria known as *Salmonella* are often present in the bodies of farm animals and poultry without making them appear to be sick. A human who eats *Salmonella*-infected meat, however, may get gastroenteritis (see previous article) and some additional unpleasant symptoms. *Salmonella* bacteria are not killed by freezing and even fresh, apparently safe meats can contain them. The bacteria are killed, however, by thorough cooking.

One cause of infection is failure to thaw food sufficiently before it is cooked, so that it does not cook all the way through. Also, sometimes meat is not frozen quickly enough after an animal is slaughtered. The delay permits a small number of bacteria to multiply, and the meat becomes infected.

Salmonellosis often occurs as an epidemic, if a number of people eat the same contaminated food, at a picnic or a party for example. But, you need not eat infected food to get salmonellosis. The bacteria can also spread from person to person on the fingers of anyone who handles infected foods or by the use of contaminated kitchen utensils. Finally, it is possible to carry the bacteria even after you recover from the infection. So it is important that you wash your hands carefully before you handle food.

What are the symptoms?

The main symptom is diarrhea. It is often accompanied by abdominal cramps, vomiting and fever. Occasionally there is blood in the bowel movements. The type and degree of diarrhea varies. You may have only one or two loose bowel movements a day, or you may have an acute attack of watery diarrhea

Food that can cause salmonellosis

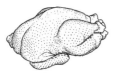

Insufficiently
thawed poultry

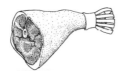

Improperly
cooked meat

Cooked meat
poorly reheated

every 10 to 15 minutes. If this continues for several hours, it can cause total prostration, or collapse. A relatively mild attack of salmonellosis can easily be taken for a simple attack of gastroenteritis.

What are the risks?

Children under the age of six are the most likely to get the disease. Apart from an occasional small epidemic, salmonellosis is not specifically identified, since the bowel movements of most people with upset stomachs are not sent to a laboratory for analysis. Nobody, therefore, knows how many cases of this disorder are diagnosed as gastroenteritis.

If the *Salmonella* bacteria spread from your digestive tract into your bloodstream, they may settle in other organs such as the liver, kidneys, gallbladder or heart, or in the joints, and cause inflammation or perhaps even a liver abscess. This seldom happens, however. Most *Salmonella* infections are mild and do not require treatment. In a severe attack, excessive loss of body liquid from repeated bouts of diarrhea can cause death from *dehydration*, if the disease is not treated.

What should be done?

If you have diarrhea that lasts for more than two or three days, or if you have a combination of fever, diarrhea, vomiting, and abdominal pain, consult your physician (see also Gastroenteritis, previous article).

What is the treatment?

If *Salmonella* infection spreads from the digestive tract, treatment will depend on the resultant disorder. Treatment for the disease itself will probably include an *antibiotic* medication. Complete recovery can be expected.

Very rarely, after the diarrhea has gone and you are completely recovered, a few live *Salmonella* organisms may remain in your digestive tract and may be excreted occasionally in bowel movements. Nothing can be done about this, and it seldom continues for more than three months. It is a problem, however, because it poses a continuing risk of spreading infection, or even a possibility of reinfecting yourself.

Bacillary dysentery

This is a fairly rare disease in developed countries, but epidemics of it may occur in densely populated areas with poor sanitation. It is possible to get it while traveling in such an area. It is caused by *Shigella bacillus*, a bacterium that invades the lining of the colon, and it is spread from person to person in unhygienic conditions. The main symptoms of bacillary dysentery, abdominal cramps, fever and diarrhea, are similar to those of gastroenteritis (see p.459), but the diarrhea may be bloody and contain pus.

Preventive measures and treatment are much the same as they are for most other gastrointestinal infections (see Salmonellosis, previous article). Sometimes, however, the symptoms may be extremely severe. In such cases *antibiotics* may have to be prescribed in combination with a variety of measures to restore body liquids.

Amebic dysentery

Amebic dysentery, which is caused by a microscopic single-celled animal, is rare in developed countries and more common in tropical climates where there is poor sanitation. The main symptom is bloody diarrhea, which may persist for a few weeks if not treated and then, after subsiding, may recur from time to time. Occasionally the organisms spread from the digestive tract into the bloodstream and settle in the liver, where they form *abscesses*, or pus-filled sacs.

This infection is usually caught abroad, most often in a tropical area. It is spread by unhygienic handlers of food.

What is the treatment?

If your physician suspects that you have amebic dysentery, samples of your bowel movements will probably be taken for analysis. Material for analysis may be obtained instead through a *proctoscope* examination. Treatment involves taking specific anti-amebic drugs, usually for one to three weeks. After diarrhea has ceased, bowel movement samples should be examined monthly until no infecting organisms are found. Meanwhile, be careful to wash your hands thoroughly after every bowel movement to avoid spreading the infection.

Typhoid fever

Typhoid fever is an infectious disease spread under unsanitary conditions either from person to person or through contaminated food, drink or water. Some people carry typhoid-causing bacteria in their bodies and infect others without getting the disease themselves. The symptoms of typhoid fever begin suddenly with headache, loss of appetite and vomiting. These are followed by persistent fever of around 104°F (40°C), increasing weakness, diarrhea (usually bloody), and often delirium. Early in the disease, you may have a pink abdominal rash, which then fades. Recovery takes two or three weeks if there are no complications. But typhoid fever can be a life-threatening disease because there may be very dangerous complications along with it such as extensive gastrointestinal bleeding or rupture of the intestines.

Typhoid fever is rare in Western countries. Nearly all cases can be traced back to recent travel or residence in an underdeveloped part of the world. If you are in such an area, or have been recently, and if you have developed the symptoms described above, see a physician without delay.

If typhoid fever is suspected, you will be admitted to an isolation unit in a hospital, for diagnosis and treatment. *Antibiotics* will probably be prescribed for about two weeks. It may take several more weeks before your digestive tract is entirely free of infectious bacteria, and you can leave the hospital without fear of passing on the infection.

Cholera

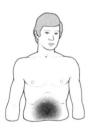

Site of the pain

Cholera is caused by bacteria that damage the intestinal lining and cause such severe diarrhea that up to 15 liters (about 4 gal) of liquid per day are lost. The bacteria spread through polluted water or raw fruits and vegetables in places where hygiene is poor. This disease almost never appears in developed nations, and when it does, it can be traced to visits to or residence in underdeveloped areas of the world. The symptoms of the disease are abdominal pain and severe diarrhea. Bowel movements of people with cholera resemble murky water and may be excreted almost continuously. You become extremely thirsty, have no fever, but vomit intermittently without feeling nauseous. You may also have muscle cramps. If cholera is not treated, *dehydration* can quickly lead to death.

If you are abroad or have been recently, and have extremely watery diarrhea that does not improve within a few hours, get medical help immediately. Drink as much non-alcoholic fluid as you can. If your illness is diagnosed as cholera, you will be hospitalized. The main treatment is to replenish body fluids directly into your veins. You may also be given an *antibiotic*. You will probably recover completely within two weeks.

Food poisoning

The term "food poisoning" has several meanings. It most commonly refers to illnesses that result from eating bacteria and/or bacterial products called toxins. The most significant types of food poisoning are listed below.

Staphylococcal food poisoning comes from eating food contaminated with the toxin of *Staphylococcus* bacteria. It can cause gastroenteritis (see p.459), an acute bout of vomiting, abdominal cramps, and sometimes diarrhea. The illness develops within one to six hours after eating contaminated food, and rarely lasts for 24 hours. If it is severe, your physician can prescribe a medication to prevent vomiting, but the disease subsides without treatment.

Since this bacteria is normally present on the hands of 50% of the population, staphylococcal food poisoning is common. Food is usually contaminated after cooking. While the food is cooling, the bacteria multiply and produce a toxin that survives reheating or boiling. Preventive measures include hand washing when handling food, cooling foods rapidly in the refrigerator, and immediate reheating.

Clostridial food poisoning, named for the clostridia bacteria, also causes gastroenteritis. The illness develops within 24 hours of eating contaminated meat, and symptoms subside in the next 24 hours. A syrup mixture to stop the diarrhea is the only treatment necessary.

Clostridia bacteria inhabit soil, insects, animals and raw meat. Food requires a temperature of 100°C (212°F) during cooking to kill the organisms. To prevent clostridial food poisoning, food should be served immediately after cooking, cooled rapidly, and preserved at safe temperatures.

Salmonella infections (other than typhoid) come from eating food contaminated with bacteria. For details, read the article on Salmonellosis (see p.460).

Botulism is a rare food poisoning caused by another Clostridia bacteria that produces a toxin in food that is smoked and preserved, but not cooked to 100°C (212°F). Home-preserved vegetables, and canned fruit and fish products have been sources of botulism outbreaks. Symptoms include abdominal pain, vomiting, blurring of vision, muscle weakness, and eventual paralysis, since the toxin prevents the nerves from conducting messages from the brain. Hospitalization is required. An injection of an antitoxin may reverse the muscle paralysis from the original toxin.

Stomach and duodenum

The stomach stores and processes food. In the stomach, the bulk of a chewed and swallowed meal is transformed into a slow trickle of pulp. Food enters the stomach through a muscular one-way valve, the esophageal sphincter. Inside the stomach, rhythmical contractions of powerful muscles in the stomach wall crush and pulverize the food, and the chemical action of acid and *enzymes*, made in the stomach lining, breaks it down further. All this activity continues while food remains in your stomach. In an empty stomach there is little muscular activity and virtually no release of acid or enzymes.

The processed matter trickles out of the stomach through another muscular valve, the pyloric sphincter, and into the duodenum, the upper section of the small intestine. In the duodenum, a tube about 25 cm (10 in) long, more enzymes are secreted and further digest the pulp before it passes into the rest of the small intestine. It takes three to five hours for the contents of a meal to reach the lower parts of the small intestine, and leave the stomach and duodenum empty. Because the chemicals of the stomach and duodenum are very strong, over-production or faulty production of them can damage the mucous membrane that lines these organs. Also, in some people this membrane is easily irritated by certain foods, drugs, or fluids. In most cases the irritation causes only the familiar symptoms of indigestion or gastritis. But sometimes the action of powerful stomach chemicals can lead to a more serious disorder such as an ulcer in either the stomach or the duodenum.

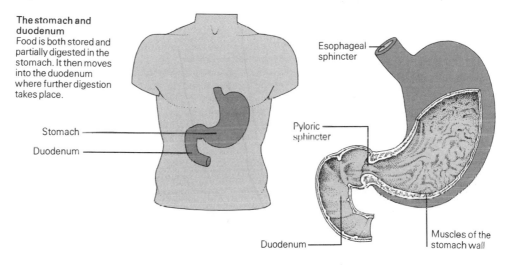

The stomach and duodenum
Food is both stored and partially digested in the stomach. It then moves into the duodenum where further digestion takes place.

Stomach

Duodenum

Esophageal sphincter

Pyloric sphincter

Duodenum

Muscles of the stomach wall

Indigestion
(dyspepsia)

Indigestion is a collection of symptoms that usually occur during or soon after eating or drinking. A variety of disorders, only a few of them serious, can cause indigestion, but often the cause is difficult to identify.

What are the symptoms?
Different people have different symptoms and tend to describe them in different terms. What one person calls heartburn another will call pain in the chest. What one person thinks of as a belch may be a hiccup to someone else. If you have indigestion, you may feel a general sense of discomfort or distension in your abdomen, or a sharp, dull, or gnawing pain in your chest. You may complain of heartburn, nausea, or the taste of acid fluid in your mouth. You may need to belch or pass gas frequently. You may have more than one of these symptoms. But most bouts of indigestion have one thing in common: They are related to food or drink. The one exception is that the same symptoms can be caused by swallowing air while eating, talking, or chewing gum. The discomfort of indigestion may be aggravated by wearing tight clothes.

What are the risks?
Indigestion is almost universal. Some people get one or more of the symptoms after eating

particular foods such as cabbage, beans, onions, or cucumbers, or after drinking wine or carbonated drinks. Others suffer if they eat too fast or have an especially rich or big meal. And others get indigestion whenever they are anxious, nervous, or depressed. Pregnant women are particularly susceptible to indigestion, as are heavy smokers, people who are constipated, and the obese.

Indigestion is troublesome and may even be painful, but it is not dangerous in itself. Many people have indigestion on and off throughout their lives without further complications. There is always a chance, however, that the symptoms may be caused by a severe illness. You probably know how your stomach behaves in given situations, and you either use self-prescribed remedies for indigestion whenever it occurs or try to prevent it by avoiding the things that cause it. Perhaps you take an occasional calculated risk by eating or drinking unwisely (for you) simply because the temporary pleasure outweighs the near-certainty of later discomfort. There are usually no serious risks in such behavior. What you should watch out for, however, is a change in the symptoms. If their character or timing is different, or if they become more frequent or severe, something other than your familiar indigestion may be causing them. You may have heartburn (see p.456), a gallbladder disorder (see Cholecystitis, p.490), a duodenal ulcer (see p.468), or even, very rarely, stomach cancer (see p.466).

What should be done?

Learn to recognize your particular symptoms, and deal with them by the self-help methods recommended below. If the pattern of symptoms changes, consult your physician right away. Some examples of changes are a feeling of nausea after eating that becomes actual vomiting, a significant increase in the frequency of attacks, or especially, loss of weight or appetite. If an underlying disease seems to be causing the new type of symptom, your physician will probably arrange for you to have diagnostic tests, usually including *X-rays* of the stomach and duodenum, for which you will need a *barium swallow*. Other possible tests may be an X-ray of the gallbladder, *endoscopy*, and a laboratory analysis of your blood, bowel movement samples, and sometimes also digestive juices from your stomach.

What is the treatment?

Self-help: If you can, avoid whatever causes your indigestion. Adjust your eating and drinking habits to your stomach's idiosyncrasies. Do not smoke. Try to avoid losing your temper or becoming over-excited during meals. Do not eat too quickly. Try to relax for half an hour after a meal. Some people find that commercially available antacid preparations help relieve the symptoms. If you take any such drug, be sure to follow the instructions on the label.

Professional help: Your physician's first task is to find out whether your indigestion is caused by an underlying disease. The more accurately you can describe your symptoms and their relationship to food and drink, the easier it will be for your doctor to discover the probable cause. Do not neglect to point out any recent developments that do not match the familiar pattern. In some cases, for instance, a long-term, gradual loss of appetite indicates cancer of the stomach; yet some people fail to mention this symptom to the doctor. If, after a physical examination and appropriate diagnostic tests, no serious disorder appears to be responsible for the symptoms, your physician will probably advise you along the lines suggested here as self-help. The doctor may also prescribe a stronger antacid than you will be able to purchase without a prescription.

Gastritis

Gastritis is inflammation of the mucous membrane that lines the stomach. It may sometimes be caused by a viral infection, or it may be a side-effect of certain drugs such as aspirin and other anti-arthritis medicines. But in most cases this disorder is the direct result of heavy drinking, smoking, or simply eating too much. Gastritis can also be caused by eating a food that "disagrees" with you, such as something that is either too spicy or too acidic. Finally, you can also develop a case of gastritis if you eat something to which you have an allergic reaction.

What are the symptoms?

The symptoms of viral gastritis are similar to those of gastroenteritis (see p.459). If the disorder is due to imprudent drinking, smoking, or eating, or to irritation from a drug, the symptoms will resemble those of indigestion (see previous article).

What are the risks?

Nearly everyone has an occasional, relatively mild attack of gastritis. Only rarely do pain and/or vomiting caused by gastritis alone persist for more than a day or two. You may be more susceptible if you smoke and/or drink large quantities of alcohol.

There is virtually no danger of lasting damage to health from occasional attacks of gastritis. If you have recurrent severe attacks in which vomiting and pain continue for more than 24 hours, you run the risk of developing gastric erosion (see p.467).

What should be done?

If you have gastritis often, it may be related to your life style. You probably smoke, eat or drink either too much or carelessly. Once you have found a likely cause, try to avoid further attacks. If you still have symptoms you should consult your physician.

To ease a current attack adopt the self-help measures suggested below, but see your physician without delay if you begin to vomit blood (see Box, p.469) or if the attack lasts longer than 48 hours. After considering the general state of your health and the possible side-effects of any drugs that you have been taking, the doctor may want you to have a series of diagnostic tests to make sure your trouble is simply gastritis. The tests will probably be those usually used to look for a suspected stomach ulcer (see next article).

What is the treatment?

Self-help: Eat nothing during the first full day of an attack. Instead, take frequent small amounts of non-alcoholic liquids, preferably milk or water. After 24 hours, begin to eat, but eat only foods that you know "agree" with you, and eat only a little at a time. If your abdominal pain is troublesome, take antacids but avoid aspirin. If you have repeated attacks of gastritis that seem to be related to your intake of alcoholic drinks or tobacco smoke, try to give up drinking or smoking for a month. If this works, the rest is up to you.

Professional help: If your disorder is clearly gastritis, your doctor will probably prescribe an antacid. For severe nausea and vomiting you may be given an injection of an *antiemetic* drug. If a drug seems to be causing the gastritis, your physician may advise a change of medication and talk with you about the best timing for taking regular doses.

Stomach ulcer

(gastric ulcer, peptic ulcer)

A stomach ulcer is a raw spot, often about 30 mm (more than one inch) wide, that develops in the lining of the stomach. The exact cause of such ulcers in not known. There is evidence, however, that irritation of the stomach lining from bile juices regurgitated into the stomach from the duodenum is sometimes a factor.

What are the symptoms?

The major symptom is a burning, gnawing pain, which is usually felt throughout the upper part of the abdomen but occasionally is confined to the lower chest. The pain lasts for from half an hour to three hours. Bouts of pain come and go, weeks of intermittent pain alternating with short painfree periods. Although there is certainly a relationship between pain and eating, the nature of the relationship is unclear. Your pain may begin right after you have eaten something, or it may not occur until hours afterward. Other possible symptoms are loss of appetite and weight, anemia (see p.419), and occasional vomiting of acid fluid that almost always relieves the pain.

What are the risks?

Probably one in five men and one in ten women in Western nations get either a stomach ulcer or a duodenal ulcer at some time. However, for no known reason, the number of such ulcers is declining. Stomach ulcers are about equally common in both sexes. Women seem more susceptible to this type than to duodenal ulcers. You are especially likely to develop a stomach ulcer if you smoke or drink heavily, if you consume large amounts of painkillers that contain aspirin, if you are elderly, or if you are a manual worker. Anyone whose job makes it impossible to have regular, unhurried meals is also more likely to develop an ulcer.

Bleeding from a stomach ulcer is not common but can be dangerous, particularly in the elderly. A sudden severe hemorrhage can cause shock (see p.386). Less severe bleeding, if it continues undetected for several months, may cause anemia (see p.419). Another risk, though only a slight one, is that the ulcer may erode through the wall of the stomach. This is called *perforation*. This complication is about 20 times more likely to arise if you have a duodenal ulcer (see p.468).

If a stomach ulcer remains untreated there may be serious loss of weight. Poor nutrition caused by reduced eating due to your pain, a lack of appetite, or both can predispose you to infections. There is a slight chance, too, that a recurrent stomach ulcer may cause pyloric stenosis (see p.468), or may undergo a *malignant*, or life-threatening, change and become a cancer (see Cancer of the stomach, next article).

What should be done?

If your symptoms suggest that you have a stomach ulcer, try following the self-help procedures below. If pain persists for more than two or three weeks, consult your physician. To determine if you have an ulcer and whether it is in the stomach or duodenum, your doctor will arrange for you to have *endoscopy* and/or a *barium swallow*. Other possible procedures include a blood test, a test of stomach fluid acidity, and laboratory analysis of a bowel movement to see if there is any internal bleeding.

What is the treatment?

Self-help: A stomach ulcer will often heal completely if you stay in bed for about two weeks, eat small, frequent meals, take antacid pills (which can be purchased without a prescription) to relieve pain, and avoid smoking and drinking alcohol. If your symptoms are not severe enough to justify two weeks in bed, try at least to eat little but often, to avoid alcohol, caffeine, and tobacco, and to sleep or rest as much as possible. If pain stops and does not recur, there are no grounds for concern. If it persists, even though antacids temporarily ease it, do not rely on self-treatment. See your physician.

Professional help: Your doctor may supplement the self-help measures recommended above by prescribing stronger antacids and a drug to try to speed up the normal healing process. Since about half of all peptic ulcers go away without treatment or with self-help measures alone, no further treatment may be required. But because another half of apparently cured ulcers recur within a few years, your physician will probably want to examine you again. If the ulcer does not heal after six to eight weeks of drug treatment, or if your recovery is only temporary, surgery may be advisable. Removal of a small portion of the stomach that contains the ulcer will generally eliminate the problem (see Box, next page).

What are the long-term prospects?

Prospects for a cure without surgery are improved if treatment is begun early, if drugs are used exactly as prescribed, if you continue to eat and drink moderately, and if you do not smoke. Surgery, whether for perforation, bleeding, or a stubbornly persistent ulcer, involves little risk unless you are over 70 years of age. Even then, only a small percentage of elderly patients do not survive surgery for this condition. In most cases the cure is both complete and permanent.

Cancer of the stomach

A stomach cancer usually starts as an ulcer in the lining of the stomach. This does not mean that if you have a stomach ulcer (see previous article) it will inevitably lead to cancer. The reason why a small proportion of ulcers become cancerous is not known.

As in all cancers, the *malignant,* or life-threatening, cells may spread to other parts of the body such as the lungs, the bones, or the liver. There are sometimes no symptoms at all until the disease has already spread too widely to be stopped.

What are the symptoms?

The first symptoms are easy to ignore. They are vague indigestion, with discomfort and occasional vomiting rather than pain after eating, combined with loss of appetite. Loss of appetite occurs far more often with stomach cancer than with peptic ulcers. Only fairly late in the disease do symptoms such as severe pain in the upper abdomen, loss of weight, and frequent vomiting develop. Indications of prolonged bleeding from the cancer such as anemia (see p.419), and bloody vomit and bowel movements, are also symptoms that appear in the later stages of stomach cancer.

What are the risks?

Cancer of the stomach is one of the leading causes of death in the United States, but it has become significantly less common over the past 30 years. It is twice as common in men as in women, and the chances of getting it increase with age. It is particularly common among low-income workers, and this suggests diet as a factor, but there is no evidence against any particular type of diet.

If, when a stomach cancer is discovered, it is too far advanced to be removed, treatment cannot cure it, but drugs may help alleviate the symptoms.

What should be done?

If you develop symptoms of indigestion (see p.463) for the first time in your life, or if your usual indigestion changes in character, consult your physician without delay. A long-standing stomach ulcer sometimes leads to stomach cancer. If you also have lost your appetite, and this persists for more than two or three days, be sure to tell the doctor, who will probably arrange for you to have a *barium swallow* and *endoscopy.* You may also have a *biopsy,* in which a small piece of tissue is removed for laboratory analysis.

OPERATION:
Stomach removal
Gastrectomy

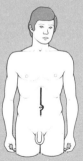

Site of incision

An operation to remove part of the stomach is called a partial gastrectomy. One that removes all of it is a total gastrectomy. They are performed when stomach ulcers fail to heal despite drug treatment or dietary changes, when an ulcer bleeds badly or perforates (breaks through the stomach wall), or for cancer of the stomach.

During the operation You are given a general anesthetic and your stomach is emptied by a tube passed into your nose and down your esophagus. The surgeon makes an incision in the upper abdomen and removes part or all of the stomach, then sews together the remaining cut edges to maintain a passageway for food. The operation usually takes about two hours.

After the operation You will be fed with an *intravenous drip,* and tubes will drain off excess fluid. After a few days your digestive tract will probably recover sufficiently for you to resume eating and drinking.

Convalescence Your physician may prescribe drugs to control side-effects such as nausea and diarrhea. Eating small, frequent meals is often advised. Most patients make a full recovery in one to two months.

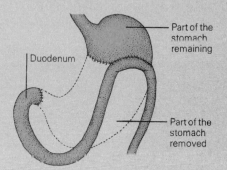

Duodenum

Part of the stomach remaining

Part of the stomach removed

In one form of partial gastrectomy (illustrated), the remaining part of the stomach is attached to the area of the small intestine between the duodenum and the ileum. In another method, the duodenum is re-attached to the stomach.

What is the treatment?
If the condition is discovered early, the cancer, along with part or all of the stomach surrounding it, will be removed surgically.

If surgery is not feasible, it is sometimes possible to slow down the development of cancer with *radiation therapy* or the use of *cytotoxic,* or anticancer, drugs

Gastric erosion

Gastric erosion is an area of inflammation in the mucous membrane that lines the stomach. It is usually caused by certain drugs that can irritate the membrane when taken in tablet form. Aspirin is the most familiar of these, and it is sometimes taken regularly in large doses by people who have rheumatoid arthritis (see p.552). Other anti-arthritis drugs, *steroids* used in treating severe asthma (see p.355), and conditions such as temporal arteritis (see p.414) and Addison's disease (see p.524) can also cause gastric erosion.

What are the symptoms?
This disorder is distinguished from gastritis (see p.464) in that the main, and often only, symptom is bleeding of the inflamed area. If you vomit, there may be blood in your vomit. The blood may be red but is more likely, because it is partly digested, to be black and to resemble coffee grounds. Blood will probably also appear in your bowel movements. If

bleeding begins gradually, you may not even be aware of it, but you will eventually show symptoms of anemia (see p.419).

What are the risks?
Gastric erosion is not common and cases severe enough to cause bloody vomit are rare. If you take large amounts of aspirin or other anti-arthritis drugs, however, you are particularly susceptible.

If persistent internal bleeding is not detected and treated, you will lose a large amount of blood, and anemia will result. There is a slight risk, too, of sudden severe bleeding, which will be vomited as red blood and/or passed as black bowel movements. To minimize the risks, many doctors recommend other drugs instead of aspirin to their arthritic patients. New anti-arthritis drugs are now being developed that may be even less irritating to the stomach lining than those currently prescribed. If you are taking a painkiller, including anti-arthritis drugs, regularly, consult your physician if you have any of the following symptoms: bloody vomit; feeling abnormally fatigued (which is often a symptom of anemia); persistent indigestion; or black bowel movements.

What is the treatment?
Self-help: No self-help is possible if you already have gastric erosion. To guard against the disorder, make a habit of swallowing any potentially causative drug during or immediately after a meal, and never take such drugs on an empty stomach.

Professional help: If you have been vomiting blood, you will probably be admitted to a hospital immediately, and given a blood transfusion if necessary. In less severe cases, your physician will probably take you off the causative drug, whatever it may be, and prescribe a less irritating one. You will also be treated for anemia if you have it (see Iron-deficiency anemia, p.419). An *endoscopy* may be done to observe the inside of your stomach. If there is no serious underlying disease, and if you avoid taking the drug that has irritated your stomach lining, gastric erosion should not recur.

Pyloric stenosis

Pyloric stenosis is a rare disorder that occurs when the outlet from the stomach to the duodenum, which is called the pylorus, becomes partly or completely blocked. This usually happens as a result of a stomach ulcer (see p.465) or duodenal ulcer (see next article), but occasionally it is caused by cancer of the stomach (see p.466). Whatever the underlying cause, your stomach cannot empty normally. This produces an uncomfortable, swollen abdomen, copious vomiting, and foul-smelling gas that you belch up.

If the pylorus becomes totally blocked, repeated vomiting may eventually result in loss of weight, *dehydration* (loss of body fluid), malnutrition, and a dangerous disturbance in the body's chemical balance. (For Congenital pyloric stenosis, a different disorder, see p.660.)

What should be done?
If you repeatedly belch foul-smelling gas and/or vomit recognizable bits of food, consult your physician. If pyloric stenosis is suspected, you may need to undergo *endoscopy*, to confirm the diagnosis and to determine the best course of treatment.

If an ulcer is causing the problem, it may respond to treatment with drugs. If this proves ineffective, or if the stenosis is a result of cancer, surgery will be necessary (see Stomach removal, previous page).

Duodenal ulcer
(peptic ulcer)

A duodenal ulcer is a raw area in the lining of the duodenum, which is a tube that leads from the stomach to the intestines. The ulcer is usually less than 15 mm (about ½ in) wide. It is caused by erosion of the surface of the duodenum by acid and digestive *enzymes* secreted by the stomach. The pain of a duodenal ulcer is due to the action of stomach acid on the exposed surface of the ulcer. Duodenal ulcers are one type of peptic ulcer. The other type is the stomach ulcer (see p.465), also called gastric ulcer.

What are the symptoms?
The main symptom of duodenal ulcer is recurrent bouts of gnawing abdominal pain that is usually localized in a small spot somewhere in your upper middle abdomen. Sometimes though, when the ulcerated area is on the back wall of the duodenum, you may feel it in your back. Typically, the pain, which resembles a "hunger pain," occurs several hours after a meal. It can generally be relieved by antacid tablets, a glass of milk, or a couple of crackers. You may have a bloated feeling after you eat, and you may also vomit.

What are the risks?
More than ten per cent of men develop a duodenal ulcer at some time. The disorder is much more common in men than in women and occurs most frequently in young and middle-aged adults.

Heavy smokers are particularly susceptible to duodenal ulcers, as are people who naturally produce particularly large quantities of stomach acid.

Although duodenal ulcers are painful, the risk of severe or permanent damage from complications is low, and the ulcers often disappear in time even if they are left untreated. Cancer does not develop from a duodenal ulcer.

A duodenal ulcer may bleed, and even slight bleeding can result in anemia (see p.419) if it persists. Sudden, heavy bleeding may cause you to vomit blood (see Box, next page) or have black, tarry bowel movements.

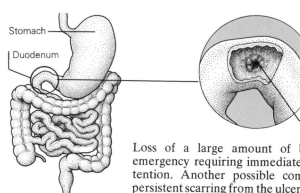

Stomach

Duodenum

Ulcer

The exact cause of a duodenal ulcer is not known. It may result from excess acid that flows from the stomach into duodenum. An additional factor may be an abnormality in the protective mucus lining of the duodenum.

Loss of a large amount of blood is an emergency requiring immediate medical attention. Another possible complication is persistent scarring from the ulcer that leads to obstruction of the entrance to the duodenum (see Pyloric stenosis, previous article).

In a few cases, perhaps one or two per cent of all duodenal ulcers, the ulcer erodes through the duodenal wall into the abdominal cavity. This will cause peritonitis (see next page) unless surgical treatment is carried out quickly. This *perforation* also causes sudden, intense pain, sometimes followed by shock (see p.386) and collapse. Any such emergency requires immediate hospitalization.

What should be done?

If you think you might have a duodenal ulcer, try the self-help measures recommended below. If the symptoms do not disappear within two weeks, see your physician, who may order the same diagnostic tests as for a stomach ulcer (see p.465).

What is the treatment?

Self-help: If you smoke, stop. Reduce your intake of alcoholic beverages. In general, you may eat whatever you like, but eat slowly and try to rest for half an hour after a meal. It is also wise to eat several small meals each day instead of two or three large ones. Food in your stomach tends to neutralize the stomach acid that causes pain. Missing meals or eating irregularly is likely to make your symptoms worse. Antacids taken regularly will also help. These simple measures may well be enough to cure your ulcer.

Professional help: At first your physician may simply prescribe an antacid other than the one you may be using. If antacids do not help, another drug, which reduces production of stomach acid, will probably be prescribed. It is important to follow the instructions exactly, because there is a risk that the ulcer will recur if you use the drug improperly or suddenly stop taking it.

Surgery is seldom necessary. An operation is usually performed only when an ulcer fails to respond to a long period of treatment or when complications occur. The type of operation varies, but the general goal is to reduce the acid-producing capacity of the stomach. This can be done either by cutting away a section of the stomach (see Box, p.467) or by cutting the nerves that control its acid production. This operation, called a vagotomy, is safe and usually successful, but occasionally there are troublesome aftereffects. These may include faintness, drowsiness, or trembling and sweating soon after eating; loss of weight and diarrhea; anemia; or vitamin D deficiency (see Vitamin deficiency, p.494). These aftereffects generally respond quickly to simple treatment.

Swallowed object (foreign body)

Normally, air goes down your windpipe into your lungs, and food goes down your esophagus into your stomach. If solid matter is accidentally "breathed in," it may get stuck in your throat (and is generally coughed up), or it may slip into your respiratory tract and cause choking. If this happens, prompt first aid is essential (see within Accidents and emergencies, p.801).

Most foreign bodies that go down the esophagus – even, amazingly enough, sharp and awkwardly shaped ones – are carried through the digestive tract and excreted without trouble. To be on the safe side, though, consult your physician if you have swallowed anything sharp (like a fish bone or needle) or bigger than about 10 mm ($\frac{1}{4}$in) in diameter.

If you find it difficult to swallow, or have abdominal pain or a fever, you may need to have your digestive tract *X-rayed*. This nearly always allows your doctor to locate and identify the foreign body, and it can usually be removed using an *endoscope* with a special attachment. Surgery is usually required only to remove an object that is large, firmly stuck and/or pointed.

Vomiting blood

Vomiting can be simply a sign of unwise eating or drinking. But you should never disregard blood in your vomit. It could indicate a serious disorder such as a bleeding stomach ulcer (see p.465).

Fresh blood is recognizable as such. It is bright red, and may occur as streaks in the vomit or may be virtually the only substance you bring up. On the other hand, blood that stays in the stomach for some hours turns black and may look like coffee grounds.

Consult your physician without delay if you suspect there is blood in your vomit, unless you are absolutely sure that it came from a recent nosebleed. If possible, take a sample of the vomit with you to aid diagnosis. If you have blood in your vomit and, in addition, your skin is cold, you are sweating, and you feel weak, get to a hospital now!

Generalized intestinal problems

The intestines are the section of the digestive tract from the beginning of the duodenum to the anus. They consist of a long, thin, coiled tube called the small intestine that leads to a shorter, wider tube, the colon. The colon leads into a final, short tube called the rectum. The colon and rectum together are often termed the large intestine.

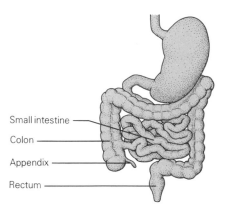

Small intestine

Colon

Appendix

Rectum

The intestines
The intestines are made up of the small intestine, the appendix, and the large intestine (colon and rectum). They form a long coil that fits into the abdomen. Nutrients from food pass through the walls of the small intestine and are absorbed into the bloodstream. Wastes move on through the large intestine and out of the body.

Food passes from the stomach into the duodenum and the rest of the small intestine, where it is further broken down by various digestive juices. As the food travels along the small intestine, propelled by rhythmic muscular contractions, nutrients are absorbed into the bloodstream through the thin intestinal walls. Most of the fluid is removed from the food as it passes through the colon. What remains is a mixture of undigested and undigestible food, largely vegetable fibers ("roughage"), along with bacteria, mucus and dead cells from the lining of the digestive tract. This material makes up the feces, which pass into the rectum and remain there until excreted through the anus as a bowel movement. In general, the entire digestive process from mouth to anus takes about 24 hours.

Problems that may occur anywhere within the intestinal tract rather than in one specific section are discussed in the following group of articles. Also included is peritonitis, a serious disease that affects the peritoneum, the thin membrane that lines the abdominal cavity and encloses many abdominal organs, including all the intestines.

Peritonitis

Peritonitis is inflammation of the peritoneum, a two-layered membrane that lines the abdominal cavity and also covers the stomach, intestines and other abdominal organs. This condition is almost always due to an underlying disease. It may occur as a complication of a disorder in which your digestive tract is irritated or ruptured, such as a duodenal ulcer (see p.468), diverticulitis (see p.479), or appendicitis (see p.476). It may also develop as a complication of certain problems of the fallopian tubes. These tubes are not enclosed within the peritoneum, but they touch its outside layer. Another possible cause of peritonitis is infection from an injury or wound that pierces the abdominal wall. Finally, peritonitis may occur as a complication of abdominal surgery, though this is an uncommon occurrence.

What are the symptoms?
The symptoms vary depending on the source of irritation or infection, but there is always severe abdominal pain. It is most severe near the site of the original problem. For example, it is worst in the right side of the abdomen if it

is caused by appendicitis. The pain increases when you move. If you press the most tender spot, it hurts. You may be nauseous and vomit, and you will probably have a fever. After two or three hours your abdomen may swell up as the pain becomes less severe and less localized. This decrease of pain does not indicate that you are getting better. In fact, it is just the opposite; it is a danger sign that signals an immediate need for emergency medical treatment.

What are the risks?
Peritonitis is rare in countries that have a high standard of medical care. However, if treatment for such abdominal problems as a duodenal ulcer, appendicitis, or an abdominal injury is delayed, peritonitis will almost inevitably develop. If peritonitis is neglected the risks are great. You can become *dehydrated*, or lose a dangerous amount of body fluid, from repeated vomiting. Decrease of severe pain indicates that your intestines have become paralyzed (see Ileus, p.472), and death will follow unless you quickly obtain emergency medical treatment.

What should be done?

Peritonitis is a serious disorder. Have someone call your physician or an ambulance immediately if you get severe abdominal pain that lasts for more than 10 to 20 minutes and is accompanied by any of the symptoms mentioned above. To establish the underlying cause of the attack, the doctor will question you and press on your abdomen in several places to pinpoint the inflamed area. If there

The examination
The doctor will palpate, or gently press, your abdomen, if peritonitis is suspected. The characteristic hardness and pain can often be detected during such an examination.

is time, you may also be given diagnostic tests such as blood tests and *X-rays* (see also Laparotomy and acute abdomen, p.477).

What is the treatment?

Prompt surgery to correct the underlying cause of peritoneal inflammation is generally the only possible treatment. After you reach the hospital, the contents of your stomach and intestines may be removed through a long tube passed down through your mouth. To treat the inflammation and strengthen you for the operation if you are weak and dehydrated, you may be given *antibiotics*, often along with nutrients and fluids, in an intravenous *drip*. Your abdomen will then be opened, and the organ that is causing the trouble will be either removed (as in appendicitis) or repaired (as in the case of a perforated ulcer). Prospects for full recovery are excellent. With the help of antibiotics, few people today die of peritonitis.

Intestinal obstruction

An intestinal obstruction is a partial or complete blockage of your intestines that makes it impossible for the digestive process to run its full course. Any one of several factors can cause an intestinal obstruction. The most common causes include a strangulated hernia (see p.537) or a blockage of the intestine by an *adhesion*, or a band of tissue, that is usually due to a prior inflammatory disease or an operation. However, the intestines can also be blocked by a growth such as cancer of the colon (see p.481). Sometimes part of a healthy intestine can become knotted or twisted, a condition known as volvulus. Rarely, the cause of intestinal obstruction is a nondigestible object such as a large coin that you have swallowed by accident (see Swallowed object, p.469).

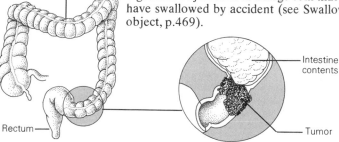

Blockage by a tumor
Part of the intestine has become completely blocked by a cancerous tumor, preventing the intestinal contents from passing down into the rectum.

What are the symptoms?

Symptoms depend on the location of the obstruction and on whether it is complete or partial. An obstruction in the small intestine causes intermittent cramp-like pains in the middle of your abdomen, along with increasingly frequent bouts of vomiting. But if the

blockage is in your large intestine you may vomit very little or not at all. Complete blockage anywhere in the digestive tract naturally causes constipation. If your large intestine is blocked, this may be so extreme that you cannot even pass gas. Partial obstruction is more likely to cause diarrhea than constipation, because only the liquid portion of a bowel movement can pass the obstruction. In an obstruction resulting from volvulus, the twisted portion of your intestine sometimes relaxes, which allows relief from pain and the passing of large amounts of gas and diarrhea. The relaxation of the obstruction is usually only temporary, however.

What are the risks?

Intestinal obstruction is fairly common. Fortunately, the underlying cause is usually discovered and dealt with before blockage becomes complete. Any disruption of the normal functioning of the intestines can lead to their paralysis (see Ileus, next article). Persistent vomiting can cause *dehydration* and, eventually, shock (see p.386). If the blockage is not relieved, there is also a danger that the intestine will rupture, and cause peritonitis (see previous article). If the obstruction is due to cancer, there is the additional risk that the disease may spread.

What should be done?

If you have a combination of symptoms that suggest intestinal obstruction, call your physician or an ambulance immediately. The doctor may suspect this disorder from a clear account of the symptoms and an examination of your abdomen. You will then be admitted to a hospital without delay so that the cause and exact site of the obstruction can be identified. *X-rays* will probably provide sufficient information for treatment to be started immediately, but an exploratory operation called a laparotomy (see p.477) is sometimes necessary to locate and remove the obstruction. You will probably be given fluids in an intravenous *drip* to prevent dehydration and shock, and the contents of your digestive tract will probably be removed by passing a long tube down through your mouth.

What is the treatment?

Surgery to relieve the blockage is virtually inevitable. It can usually be done at the same time as a laparotomy, if one is necessary. If the source of the trouble is a volvulus, the surgeon may be able to untwist the intestine in a way that will prevent the problem from recurring. Often, however, the preferred procedure is to remove the small part of the intestine that has become twisted, and rejoin the severed ends.

Prospects for full recovery from an intestinal obstruction are excellent after surgery unless the underlying disorder does not respond to treatment.

Ileus

Ileus is a serious disorder in which the intestines become paralyzed because of disruption of normal digestive processes. This can be caused by disorders such as intestinal obstruction (see previous article) or a perforated ulcer (see Duodenal ulcer, p.468), or by abdominal surgery. Bacteria stagnate in trapped, partly digested food, and produce gas that distends your intestines and abdomen. The swollen abdomen presses on your chest, and impairs breathing. In addition to being badly constipated, you may develop a fever and may repeatedly vomit foul-smelling liquid. In the beginning of an attack of ileus there is a dull, persistent pain in your abdomen. This may soon disappear, but relief from pain does not mean the condition has improved, and it may be fatal unless the underlying cause is successfully treated.

Some degree of ileus follows many abdominal operations and is routinely dealt with after surgery, so that you are unlikely to know you have had it. In other cases, treatment depends on the underlying disorder. For example, when the condition arises from a serious disorder such as a perforated ulcer, you are likely to be extremely ill and in need of urgent treatment.

Carcinoids
(and the carcinoid syndrome)

A carcinoid is a rare type of growth in the wall of the intestines. Although the growths are *malignant*, they develop so slowly that over half of the people who have them never know. If they are discovered at all, the growths are usually found during a diagnostic test or surgery for some other, unrelated disorder. The growths can become large enough, however, to cause intestinal obstruction (see previous page).

In about ten per cent of all cases, carcinoid cells spread through the bloodstream to the liver, where they multiply, and form hormone-producing tumors (see p.518) that have widespread effects on the body. The result is a characteristic group of symptoms called the carcinoid syndrome.

What are the symptoms?

The main symptom of the carcinoid syndrome is flushing of the skin on your head and neck, which is triggered off by some activity such as exercising or drinking alcohol. It looks like a blush, but it lasts up to several hours because it is caused by the abnormal secretion of a hormone that has this effect. Other probable symptoms include swollen and watery eyes; explosive diarrhea, often with abdominal cramps; wheezing and other symptoms of asthma (see p.355); and the symptoms of heart failure (see p.381), including breathlessness.

If you have these symptoms, your physician may arrange for you to have an abdominal *X-ray*, *endoscopy* to view the inside of your digestive tract, and a *biopsy* of any growth that is found. In a biopsy, a portion of the growth is removed and examined.

What is the treatment?

If carcinoids are discovered in their early stages, they can often be surgically removed, but surgery does not cure the carcinoid syndrome. Treatment is therefore aimed at easing symptoms. Appropriate drugs may be prescribed to help reduce the frequency and length of flushing attacks and to control diarrhea. Asthma is relieved by *bronchodilators*. A *cytotoxic* drug may be used to slow the progress of the disease.

Small intestine

The small intestine is a tube about 35 mm (1½ in) in diameter and about 5 m (16 ft) long. It runs from the stomach to the colon and is the main site where nutrients are absorbed into the bloodstream.

In the small intestine the process of breaking down food into small particles, already begun in the stomach, continues. This process is aided by the secretion of additional *enzymes*, or digestive juices, by the small-intestine wall. Once food particles are small enough, they pass through the thin lining of the intestine into the bloodstream. To make sure that as much food as possible is absorbed, the inside surface of the small-intestine wall is covered with tiny fingerlike projections called villi. These projections provide a large surface area for the material to pass through.

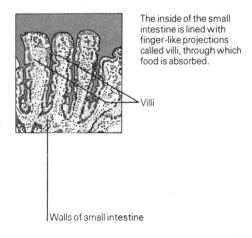

The inside of the small intestine is lined with finger-like projections called villi, through which food is absorbed.

Villi

Walls of small intestine

Crohn's disease

(regional ileitis)

Crohn's disease is a chronic, or long-term, inflammation of part of the digestive tract. The part most commonly affected is the final section of the small intestine, although patchy inflammation can occur anywhere in the intestines. The cause of the disease is not known, but it does not seem to be either hereditary or infectious. It begins with the development of patches of inflammation in the intestinal wall, which sometimes grow or spread from one part of the digestive system to another, and sometimes develop in only one place. Some of the spots heal, but they may leave scar tissue that thickens intestinal walls and narrows the passageways.

What are the symptoms?
Crohn's disease usually appears as periodic attacks of cramps, abdominal pain (especially after eating), diarrhea, and a general sense of feeling ill. You may also have a slight fever. Attacks tend to begin when you are in your twenties and to recur, sometimes every few months, sometimes every few years, for the rest of your life. In about one-quarter of cases, the symptoms only appear once or twice, and the disease does not recur.

What are the risks?
This has been a rare disorder in the Western world, but it is gradually becoming more common. There are about twice as many cases of it today as there were 20 years ago.

If Crohn's disease continues for years, it causes a gradual deterioration of bowel functioning. Sometimes the inflamed intestinal wall may leak, and cause peritonitis (see p.470). There is a risk of poor absorption of nutrients, with the associated loss of appetite and weight (see Malabsorption, p.475), or of intestinal obstruction (see p.471). Severe bleeding that causes iron-deficiency anemia (see p.419) can also occur. There is also a slight chance that Crohn's disease, if it is not treated, can increase your susceptibility to cancer of the intestine.

What should be done?
If your symptoms suggest the possibility of Crohn's disease, consult your physician, who, after examining you, will probably want *X-rays* of your digestive tract, for which you will need a *barium swallow* and perhaps a *barium enema.* You may also have to undergo *endoscopy* of the intestines in order to locate the inflamed areas. Blood and bowel movement samples may be required to see if you show signs of internal bleeding such as bloody bowel movements or anemia.

What is the treatment?
Self-help: Follow your physician's advice about diet and rest during an attack.
Professional help: In most cases treatment by drugs eases attacks of Crohn's disease. Among the drugs used are *analgesics,* an-

tidiarrhea tablets, vitamin supplements to ensure adequate nutrition, and a drug that reduces inflammation. Your physician may also recommend certain foods and warn against others, and may suggest that you modify your daily routine to relieve tension that may affect your nervous and digestive systems.

To guard against further attacks, long-term treatment with *steroids* may be prescribed. Another drug that helps, especially if your colon is affected, is an antibacterial medication. Initial high doses of such drugs may be decreased gradually. Such treatment should reduce the severity of the attacks.

If repeated attacks have scarred and narrowed your intestines so badly that the inflammation does not respond to drug treatment, you will probably need surgery to remove the section of intestine that is most affected. Occasionally an ileostomy (see Box, p.482) is necessary. Surgery cannot cure Crohn's disease, but it can provide dramatic improvement and postpone further progress of the disease for many years.

Celiac disease in adults

In celiac disease, the lining of your small intestine reacts adversely to gluten, a protein that is present in wheat and other grains. It is very rare for celiac disease to appear for the first time in adulthood; it nearly always shows up in infancy. For this reason it is discussed fully in the children's section (see p.684).

If celiac disease does appear for the first time in an adult, the symptoms are abdominal pain and swelling, diarrhea, weight loss, and a general lack of energy. If you develop these symptoms, see your physician. Diagnosis and treatment of the disease is basically the same for adults and children.

Tumors of the small intestine

Like those in other parts of the body, tumors of the small intestine can be *benign* (unlikely to spread) or *malignant* (likely to spread and threaten life). Most are benign and symptom-free, and these usually remain undetected unless they are found through tests or treatment for some other disorder. But in about one out of ten cases, the growths are malignant. Very rarely they are of a type known as carcinoids (see p.472).

What are the symptoms?
Malignant tumors in the small intestine may cause loss of weight, the symptoms of anemia (paleness, tiredness, and palpitations on exertion), and, occasionally, black or bloody bowel movements.

What are the risks?
Tumors of the small intestine are extremely rare, comprising fewer than five per cent of all digestive-tract tumors, even though the small intestine is the most extensive part of the tract. If you have Crohn's disease (see previous page) or celiac disease (see previous article), your chance of developing cancerous small-intestinal growths is probably slightly greater than normal.

There is the risk of intestinal obstruction (see p.471) from any large growth. A malignant tumor is life-threatening unless it is discovered and treated in an early stage, so the main risk is that the vague symptoms of cancerous small-intestine tumors may be ignored until it is too late for effective treatment.

What should be done?
If you lose weight for no clear reason, if you have abdominal pain, if you notice any

---

Constipation and diarrhea

There is no "normal" pattern for bowel movements. Most people have about one a day, but some have as many as three. At the other extreme there are people who regularly have only three bowel movements a week. In general, the more frequent the bowel actions the looser the movements. Consider yourself constipated only if your normal pattern changes and you begin to have irregular, unusually infrequent, and/or difficult movements. Similarly, you have diarrhea only if you have unusually frequent and particularly loose bowel movements.

Constipation and diarrhea usually are symptoms of disorders that may be serious but often are not. Some people are constipated largely because they worry so much about their bowels that they overuse laxatives, which may lead to bowel inactivity. Others lose their normal bowel activity because they tend to be "too busy" to take time out for a regular few minutes in the bathroom. Other possible causes include diet, especially a low-roughage diet; the use of certain medicines, especially cough mixtures; hemorrhoids or an anal fissure, which can inhibit bowel activity through fear of pain; or a disorder such as severe depression. Diarrhea can be brought on by stress, certain foods such as prunes or beans, over-consumption of alcohol, medicines such as antacids or antibiotics, specific food sensitivities, or similar factors.

If constipation persists for more than two weeks or diarrhea for more than 48 hours, or if you notice any other change in your bowel habits, always seek medical advice. The cause of your problem is unlikely to be serious, but have your physician evaluate it, to be safe.

change in your bowel habits, and/or if your bowel movements are dark, consult your physician, who will examine your abdomen and will probably arrange for diagnostic tests. A *barium swallow* and *X-rays* will help reveal tumors, if there are any. To determine whether they are benign or malignant, you may also have an *endoscopic* examination, and a *biopsy*, in which a portion of the growth is removed for examination.

What is the treatment?

Once they have been detected, small-intestine tumors are usually removed surgically even if they are benign. Sometimes malignant growths are either too numerous or too widespread for surgical treatment. In such cases *steroid* drugs, *chemotherapy*, and *radiation therapy*, either one at a time or in combination, are prescribed to help to keep them under control.

Meckel's diverticulum

In Meckel's diverticulum, a pouch forms near the lower end of the small intestine. The disorder is congenital, or present at birth. The pouch is like an appendix, in that it is significant only when it becomes inflamed. About 1 person in 50 has such a pouch, but most of these pouches do not cause any trouble. Symptoms of this disorder are severe bleeding from the rectum (the blood is maroon in color), sometimes preceded by pain, and usually combined with vomiting. More men than women get this disorder.

Inflammation of the diverticulum may be diagnosed as appendicitis (see next page), with or without peritonitis (see p.470), or even as a perforated duodenal ulcer (see p.468). But the initial treatment in all such conditions is to open up the abdomen surgically (see Laparotomy and acute abdomen, p.477). The surgeon then discovers that Meckel's diverticulum is causing the symptoms, and removes the pouch. This treatment, along with the treatment for peritonitis if necessary, cures the condition.

Malabsorption

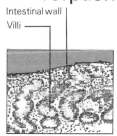

Intestinal wall
Villi

Flattened villi
Malabsorption may be caused by flattened villi. Such flattening reduces the amount of surface available for absorption.

If there is something wrong with the structure of your small intestine, or if the chemicals and *enzymes* within it are not properly assisting the digestive process, certain elements of your diet may not be fully absorbed. This is called malabsorption, and it can appear as a symptom of many diseases or conditions. For example, a physical change in the absorptive inner surface of the small intestine, such as the scars that result from Crohn's disease (see p.473), may not allow enough nutrients to pass through the intestinal wall. Similar damage to the intestine may be due to a reaction to one element in your diet such as gluten (see Celiac disease, previous page). In a rare inherited disease called lactase deficiency, one digestive enzyme (lactase) is missing, which causes an inability to digest and absorb lactose, the form of sugar present in milk (see Lactose intolerance, p.686).

Other causes of malabsorption include iron deficiency anemia (see p.419), B_{12} deficiency anemia (see p.420) and pancreatitis (see p.490). Malabsorption may also occur as a complication of diabetes mellitus (see p.519), cystic fibrosis (see p.685) and, in some cases, digestive-tract surgery.

What are the symptoms?

The usual symptoms are occasional abdominal discomfort, generally loose bowels, and yellowish-gray, greasy-looking bowel movements that have a peculiarly strong odor and tend to float because of a high fat content. Over months or years, unchecked malabsorption leads to loss of weight and energy, breathlessness, and the various symptoms of vitamin or mineral deficiency such as a sore tongue, prickling sensations and numbness in arms and legs, muscle cramps, and bone pain (see Vitamin deficiency, p.494).

What are the risks?

Severe, generalized malabsorption is extremely rare in the Western world. Prolonged malabsorption can cause emaciation and even death from starvation.

What should be done?

If you have reason to believe that you have malabsorption, and especially if you have grayish bowel movements that look greasy, soft and bulky, consult your physician. After giving you a full physical examination, the doctor will probably want several blood tests done to estimate the levels of various proteins, fats and minerals in your bloodstream. Laboratory analysis of bowel movement samples may also be done.

Once malabsorption is diagnosed, the physician's main task is to discover the underlying cause and treat that disorder. A high-protein, high-calorie diet with vitamin and mineral supplements may aid recovery.

Large intestine

The large intestine, a tube about 5 cm (2 in) in diameter and about 1.5 m (5 ft) long, consists of two main sections: the colon and the rectum. The small intestine opens into a pouch-like chamber called the cecum, which is the first part of the colon. The rest of the colon then runs up the right side of the abdomen, across under the rib cage, and down the left side, thus forming a frame for the highly convoluted small intestine. The rectum is a short tube about 12 cm (5 in) long that leads downwards from the end of the colon to the anus. Fluid and various mineral salts from the intestinal contents are absorbed into the bloodstream through the membranous wall of the colon, while indigestible solids are compacted and moved towards the rectum, where waste is stored until it is released through the anus as a bowel movement.

The large intestine can become troublesome for any one of several reasons. It is particularly subject to inflammation because of infection, and it is more susceptible than other sections of the digestive tract to tumors and polyps. Moreover, the large intestine, like the teeth, appears to be adversely affected by many of the kinds of food most Americans now eat. The evidence for this is that colonic and rectal disorders are far more common in the United States than they are in Africa and Asia.

The large intestine
Undigested food in liquid form flows from the small intestine into the large intestine, where most of the water content is absorbed back into the body. The semi-solid waste that remains moves down into the rectum, and is excreted in bowel movements.

Colon

Appendix

Rectum

Appendicitis

The appendix is a thin, worm-shaped pouch, around 9 cm (3½ in) long, that projects out from the first part of the colon. In some animals, such as rabbits, the appendix is relatively large and plays an important role in the digestive process. In humans, however, the appendix is small and seems to have no function. Its only known importance, unfortunately, is that it can become diseased.

In the condition known as appendicitis, for reasons that are not fully understood, the appendix becomes swollen and inflamed, and fills with pus.

What are the symptoms?
The principal symptom is severe abdominal pain that usually starts as vague discomfort around the navel, but becomes sharper and more localized during the course of a few hours. If you have appendicitis, you will probably feel pain and tenderness in a small spot in the lower right-hand part of your abdomen (the site of the inflamed appendix). Even slight pressure on the spot will increase the pain. You will also feel feverish and nauseated and may actually vomit. You will lose your appetite, and you may be constipated. A few individuals have diarrhea instead of constipation.

What are the risks?
Every year, about 1 person in 500 has an attack of appendicitis. Anyone may be affected, but the disease is rare among children under two years old.

If surgical treatment is delayed, there is a chance that the swollen appendix will *perforate*, or rupture. When this happens, the contents are released into the abdomen and this

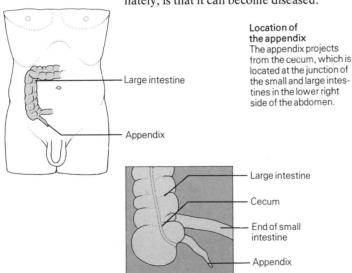

Large intestine

Appendix

Location of the appendix
The appendix projects from the cecum, which is located at the junction of the small and large intestines in the lower right side of the abdomen.

Large intestine

Cecum

End of small intestine

Appendix

OPERATION: **Appendix removal**
Appendectomy

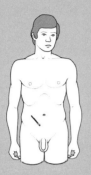

Site of incision

The appendix is usually removed for appendicitis, when the organ becomes inflamed and may burst. However, the surgeon may not be able to confirm the diagnosis of appendicitis until your abdomen has been opened up and examined, by a procedure called a laparotomy (see below).

During the operation The appendix is cut away and removed through an incision in the lower right side of your abdomen. If there are no further abdominal problems, the operation may take less than one hour.

After the operation You should be able to resume eating and drinking within 24 hours, and be ready to leave the hospital within one week of the operation.

Convalescence You will probably be back to normal two to three weeks after leaving the hospital. Lack of an appendix has no known effect on future health.

In its normal location (top right) the appendix is curved toward surrounding tissue. It is held away from the tissue (bottom right) during an appendectomy.

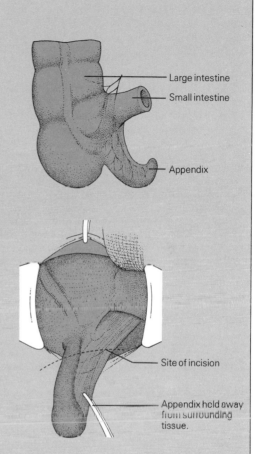

Large intestine

Small intestine

Appendix

Site of incision

Appendix held away from surrounding tissue.

Laparotomy and acute abdomen

If your intestines and the inner lining of your abdominal cavity become inflamed (see Peritonitis, p.470), the result will be pain, vomiting and fever. As the inflammation worsens, these symptoms become more marked, and the muscles of your abdominal wall will probably go into spasm, so that your abdomen feels hard and boardlike. The symptoms will be similar whether your inflammation is caused by a perforated duodenal ulcer (see p.468), an inflamed appendix (see previous page), Crohn's disease (see p.473), an inflamed diverticulum (see Diverticular disease, p.479), or bleeding from an abdominal injury, such as a severe blow. If you have the above symptoms, there is no time for delay. You should call your physician or get to a hospital immediately; this is an emergency.

When no certain diagnosis can be made immediately, your physician may use "acute abdomen" as a working diagnosis. After your physician examines you, the best course of action may then be for a surgeon to "take a look inside." That is, to do an operation called an exploratory laparotomy.

The term laparotomy refers to an operation in which the surgeon opens the abdomen and explores for an unknown source of infection or disease. The operation is not always performed as an emergency. For example, if you have a fever for several weeks that is undiagnosed even after extensive testing, or if you have Hodgkin's disease, you may need to have a laparotomy.

Once your abdomen is open, the surgeon will remove or repair the affected organ.

usually causes peritonitis (see p.470). But it is possible that the *omentum*, an apron of tissue that covers the intestines, will envelop the inflamed appendix, enclose the area, and prevent the spread of infection. When infection is localized in this way, the result is an *abscess* of the appendix.

What should be done?

If you have a pain in your abdomen along with any of the other symptoms of appendicitis, consult your physician without delay. *Do not take a laxative.* It can cause an inflamed appendix to burst. The doctor will question you about your symptoms and will carefully examine your abdomen to test for the location and severity of the pain.

If the physician decides that you probably have appendicitis, you will be admitted to a hospital as soon as possible. If there is some doubt about the diagnosis, and if your symptoms do not indicate an urgent need for surgery, you may undergo further diagnostic procedures such as blood tests and an abdominal *X-ray*. Alternatively, an exploratory operation called a laparotomy may be done immediately (see Laparotomy and acute abdomen, previous page).

What is the treatment?

The treatment for appendicitis is swift removal of the affected organ. The operation, known as an appendectomy, is straightforward and there are few risks associated with it. Usually, the appendectomy can be started as soon as a laparotomy has established the cause of the problem.

If diagnostic tests or a laparotomy show that your appendix is abscessed, then it is less likely that the appendix will be removed immediately. If the omentum is adhering to the inflamed organ the operation is more difficult. The abscess may be drained and you will probably receive large doses of *antibiotics* to reduce the infection. You may be allowed to go home after a few days, though the antibiotics may be continued for several weeks. Because appendicitis is likely to flare up again, you will later be readmitted to the hospital to have your appendix removed, but only when further tests show that the abscess has subsided.

Irritable colon

(spastic colon, mucous colitis, irritable bowel syndrome)

Normally, the contents of the intestine are propelled along by regular, coordinated waves of muscular contraction known as *peristalsis*. In a so-called irritable colon, the waves are irregular and uncoordinated, and this interferes with the progress of waste matter through the intestines. The cause of the disorder is not fully understood, but many people have it without ever seeking medical advice about it. Some physicians believe that the cause is mainly psychological, since the disorder appears to be most prevalent among people under stress.

This condition appears to be twice as common in women as in men. Many people simply learn to live with it. Although an irritable colon may cause discomfort over many years, there is no danger of further complications.

What are the symptoms?

The predominant symptoms may be either diarrhea or constipation; in other words, the bowel movements may either be too loose or too hard. Constipation with hard, dry, pellet-like bowel movements may alternate with diarrhea, which is usually worse in the morning. Pain when you move your bowels is common. The most consistent symptoms are cramp-like, spasmodic pains, usually on one side of the lower abdomen. These are usually relieved when you move your bowels.

If you have an irritable colon, you will occasionally feel mildly nauseated, bloated, and full of gas, and you may not have much interest in eating.

What should be done?

Because some of the symptoms are similar to those of cancer of the colon (see p.481), ulcerative colitis (see p.480), and Crohn's disease (see p.473), all of which are potentially dangerous, you should consult your physician about them. A series of tests such as *X-rays, sigmoidoscopy,* and examination of samples of bowel movements for traces of blood or infectious agents should enable your physician to diagnose your trouble.

What is the treatment?

Self-help: If you have an irritable colon, you can try to discover the factors that make the symptoms worse. Emotional stress may be important, in which case you will need to try to lead a calm, orderly life. If you discover that fried foods, raw vegetables or some other type of foods seem to aggravate your symptoms, try to avoid them. It may be helpful to cut out alcohol and tobacco. Often a dramatic improvement results from a high-fiber diet similar to that recommended for diverticular disease (see next article). Other people do better with a bland diet.

Professional help: If constipation is your predominant symptom, your physician may recommend either a mild, non-irritating laxative or a preparation that softens bowel movements. If, however, your main problem is diarrhea, your doctor may prescribe a drug for this if it is severe. If you have severe abdominal pain, the doctor may also prescribe an *antispasmodic* drug. If you are extremely tense and anxious or are under unusual stress, you may be given mild sedatives or tranquilizers for a while.

Such drugs can relieve the symptoms of an irritable colon. They cannot cure the disorder, however. In most cases, irritable colon will persist throughout life, with the symptoms alternately easing and worsening at irregular intervals.

Diverticular disease
(diverticulosis and diverticulitis)

Small, sac-like swellings known as diverticula (singular: diverticulum) sometimes develop in the walls of the lowest part of your colon. Many older people develop diverticula without ever knowing it. This symptom-free, or almost symptom-free, diverticular disease is diverticulosis. Occasionally, however, for no known reason, one or more of the diverticula becomes inflamed, and causes the diverticular disease known as diverticulitis.

There seems to be some connection between diverticular disease and the Western diet, which is low in fiber content. Diverticulitis rarely occurs in Africa and Asia, where more fiber is consumed.

What are the symptoms?
If you have diverticulosis, you may have no symptoms at all, or you may have cramping pains and sometimes tenderness in the left side of your abdomen. The symptoms may be temporarily relieved when you pass gas or move your bowels. Your bowel movements are often small and hard and you may have occasional attacks of diarrhea. Sometimes the diverticula will bleed, which will cause you to pass bright red blood in some of your bowel movements.

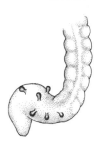

In diverticulosis, small pouches form in the wall of the colon and project into the abdominal cavity.

If you get diverticulitis, you will have severe abdominal pain, often spasmodic at first but becoming more constant, in the lower left side of your abdomen. You may also feel nauseous and have a fever. The abdominal pain is aggravated if you touch the sore spot. In some people diverticulitis flares up and then causes disabling pain within a few hours.

In other people with the disorder the symptoms may linger on in a mild form for several days before becoming severe.

What are the risks?
Fortunately, only a minority of those with diverticulosis ever develop the symptoms of diverticulitis but, left untreated, diverticulitis can lead to serious complications. One possibility is the formation of an *abscess* in the colon around an inflamed diverticulum. If the abscess *perforates* the intestinal wall, peritonitis (see p.470) can develop. If this happens, there is a risk of death unless you obtain treatment within an hour or so.

What should be done?
Always consult a physician if your bowels behave in an unusual manner for more than a week or two, or if you have a persistent pain in the lower part of your abdomen. After examining you, your physician may arrange for tests of your blood and samples of your bowel movements, a *sigmoidoscopy* of your lower bowel, and a *barium enema*, to make sure that cancer of the large intestine (see p.481), which has similar symptoms, is not causing your problem.

If your symptoms indicate that you may be having a severe attack of diverticulitis, get medical help without delay.

What is the treatment?
Self-help: It may be possible to prevent the formation of diverticula by modifying your diet. Eat whole grain breads, breakfast on oatmeal or bran cereals, and eat plenty of fibrous fresh fruits and vegetables. Many individuals with mild symptoms of diverticulosis have found that the symptoms disappear within 7 to 14 days of beginning such a diet. A high-fiber diet of this kind can, however, cause your abdomen to become distended, and you may pass a lot of gas. It may be necessary to adjust the amount of fiber in your diet until you find what suits you. Nonprescription preparations that soften your bowel movements may also be helpful. If

diverticulitis develops, no self-help measures are possible.

Professional help: If you have diverticulitis, you may be admitted to a hospital, where the contents of your stomach will be sucked out through a *nasogastric tube.* You may not be allowed to eat or drink at first, and may be given the fluids you need through an intravenous drip. This will free your diverticula of solid matter and allow them to recover. To clear up any infection, you may be given injections of *antibiotics* and, if necessary, of painkillers. After a few days, when your symptoms have subsided, you will gradually be able to eat and drink again.

If, however, your physician feels that diverticulitis is likely to recur, an operation may be advised to remove the affected section of your colon. Such surgery may require at least a week's stay in the hospital.

The prospects of full recovery from even a severe attack of diverticulitis are excellent if you consult your physician early enough about your symptoms.

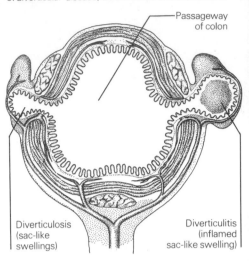

A cross section of the colon reveals the two forms of diverticular disease, diverticulosis and diverticulitis.

Passageway of colon

Diverticulosis (sac-like swellings)

Diverticulitis (inflamed sac-like swelling)

Adapted from an original painting by Frank H. Netter, M.D., from THE CIBA COLLECTION OF MEDICAL ILLUSTRATIONS, copyright by CIBA Pharmaceutical Company, Division of CIBA-GEIGY Corporation.

Ulcerative colitis

Ulcerative colitis is a long-term condition in which raw, inflamed areas called ulcers, and small *abscesses* develop in the lining of the large intestine. These may first appear in the rectum and may gradually spread upward into the lower colon. In many cases the entire large intestine may become involved. No one knows why some people are susceptible to this disorder or what causes it.

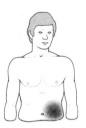

Site of the pain

What are the symptoms?

Symptoms usually recur over a period of years. You may have an attack of ulcerative colitis without any warning, or the disease may come on gradually. A characteristic early symptom is left-sided abdominal pain that is relieved by a bowel movement. But the act of moving the bowels is itself painful, and you will probably have diarrhea that contains blood and pus. In a severe attack, there may also be sweating, nausea, loss of appetite, and a fever of up to 104°F (40°C).

Ulcerative colitis is a relatively rare condition. It is more common in women and is most likely to occur in young adults.

What are the risks?

In a severe attack of the disease there is the danger that you may lose large amounts of blood, and that substances from the ulcerated area will cause blood poisoning (see p.421). This can be fatal. However, the attacks are usually intermittent and not so severe. If you

have had ulcerative colitis for ten years or longer, you are slightly more likely to get cancer of the large intestine (see next page) than someone who has never had the disease.

What should be done?

If you have an attack of painful diarrhea, with blood, pus and mucus in it, or if other symptoms suggest you may have ulcerative colitis, consult your physician. If laboratory analysis of samples of blood and bowel movements show no evidence of infection, the most usual cause of such symptoms, the next step is to arrange for hospital tests that will help the doctor make a firm diagnosis.

If you are in great pain or bleeding profusely, you will be hospitalized and these tests will be carried out right away. Your rectum and large intestine may be examined by *sigmoidoscopy,* and perhaps by *colonoscopy* as well. A *biopsy* from the intestinal wall will probably be taken during one of these tests. You may also need to have a *barium enema.*

What is the treatment?

Self-help: If your condition is diagnosed as ulcerative colitis, you will probably be under a physician's care for several weeks. During that period and thereafter, you can help prevent further attacks by changing your diet to one that is high in fiber. Some physicians suggest that you also cut down on your intake of milk and other dairy products.

This disease can be aggravated by certain *antibiotics* that often cause diarrhea as a side-effect. If you have had earlier attacks of ulcerative colitis, be sure to point this out to any physician who may not know your medical history and, so, might decide to prescribe an antibiotic medication for some other, unrelated, disorder.

Professional help: The usual treatment is a four- to six-week course of drugs aimed at healing the ulcers. The main drugs used are *steroids*, sometimes in combination with other drugs. These medications may be given as tablets, and steroids may also be given as enemas or rectal suppositories.

Treatment for a severe attack of ulcerative colitis is generally carried out, at least for the first two weeks, in the hospital. Nutrients and steroid drugs may be administered through an intravenous *drip*, or orally in concentrated liquid form. If you have lost a lot of blood, you may be given a transfusion. To try to prevent further attacks of ulcerative colitis, another drug may be prescribed in tablet form to be taken indefinitely.

If you have recurrent attacks of ulcerative colitis, your physician may advise you to have an operation to remove the colon. This would prevent further attacks of the disease, and also eliminate the risk of cancer of the colon.

Benign tumors of the large intestine
(including polyps)

Some tumors of the large intestines are *malignant*, or likely to spread and threaten life (see Cancer of the large intestine, next article). But *benign* growths, which are unlikely to spread, are more common in this part of your body. They occur singly or in groups, for no known reason. Most of them are small, grape-shaped growths known as *polyps*, though an occasional benign tumor can grow large enough to create an intestinal obstruction (see p.471). Since about 1 out of 100 benign tumors becomes malignant, polyps are removed if they are discovered.

Many people have symptom-free tumors without knowing it. Often they are discovered only as a result of *X-rays* done for another reason. Sometimes, however, benign tumors signal their presence by producing streaks of dark blood in bowel movements, or a mucous discharge from the anus that stains underclothing. They are frequently both diagnosed and removed by means of *colonoscopy*, *sigmoidoscopy*, or *proctoscopy*. If this is not feasible in your case, you may need a relatively simple laparotomy (see p.477) to remove the tumors.

Cancer of the large intestine
(cancer of the colon, cancer of the rectum)

Cancer of the large intestine, which is made up of the colon and rectum, occurs most often in the lowest part, in or near the rectum. As cancerous cells multiply, the smooth intestinal lining roughens, enlarges, and hardens, until it develops into an ulcerous area that bleeds easily or into a constriction that hinders bowel movement. If it is allowed to progress, the disease spreads along the intestinal wall and through it to adjacent abdominal organs. It may also enter the bloodstream and spread to other parts of the body. The cause of the disease is not known, but the higher rate of its occurrence in countries where a highly refined, low-roughage diet is common suggests that this type of diet is an important factor.

What are the symptoms?
There are several possible symptoms, depending on the site of the cancer and how far it has developed. One symptom that should not be ignored if it lasts for more than seven to ten days is a change in type of bowel movements. Persistent, inexplicable, abnormal constipation or diarrhea (see p.474) are

usually early warning signs. Bloody bowel movements, too, should always be reported to your physician. Never ignore this symptom or assume that it is merely caused by hemorrhoids (see p.483).

There may also be vague indications of indigestion (see p.463) and pain along with tenderness in the lower part of the abdomen. Sometimes the major symptom is simply a lump somewhere in the lower abdomen. And sometimes there are no symptoms at all until the cancer causes an intestinal obstruction (see p.471) or until the intestine ruptures and causes peritonitis (see p.470).

What are the risks?
Cancer of the large intestine is the third most common type of cancer. Only lung cancer and breast cancer are more common. Men and women are equally susceptible to cancer of the large intestine, which is most prevalent among people over 40, especially among those who are in their 60s and 70s. Also, about 1 out of every 20 people who have ulcerative colitis (see previous page) eventually develops cancer of the colon.

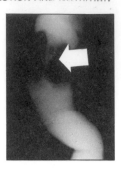

Cancer of the colon appears on an X-ray as a dark mass (arrow) on the inside wall of the colon.

Because most cancers of the large intestine develop and *metastasize*, or spread, slowly, you have a good chance of complete cure if the disease is diagnosed early. If the malignancy has already spread, to the liver for example, the outlook is much less favorable.

What should be done?

If you have any of the symptoms mentioned above, consult your physician, who will examine your abdomen carefully to see if you have developed a lump and will insert a rubber-gloved finger into your rectum to check for a rectal growth. Your physician may want you to have *proctoscopy*, and you may also need to provide bowel movement samples for laboratory tests. If the doctor suspects either cancer or a benign tumor of the large intestine (see previous article) you will need to undergo other diagnostic procedures such as a *barium enema*, *sigmoidoscopy* and possibly *colonoscopy*.

What is the treatment?

Surgery is the best treatment for this type of cancer if it has not progressed too far. If the cancer is in your colon, the growth is removed along with a section of the healthy colon around it. The two ends of the colon are then sewn together. If the cancer is in the rectum, a colostomy (see below) is usually necessary.

If the cancer has become too widespread for surgery, its progress can often be arrested by *radiation therapy* and/or *cytotoxic* (anti-cancer) drugs.

What are the long-term prospects?

Most people who have operations for cancer of the large intestine survive in good health for five years or longer. After five years, you can consider yourself cured. The success rate for treatment with only radiation therapy and drugs is lower, however.

OPERATION: ## Colostomy and ileostomy

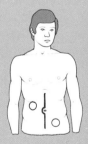

Colostomy incision (line) and possible stoma positions (circles).

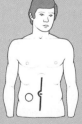

Incision site (line) and position of stoma (circle) in ileostomy.

In the treatment of certain digestive-tract diseases such as cancer of the large intestine, diverticulitis, and ulcerative colitis, it may be necessary to remove part of the tract (intestinal resection). If possible the two cut ends are sewn together to maintain a passageway for food. When this is not feasible, an opening called a "stoma" is made in the abdominal wall, through which undigested material can pass into a bag. This operation is called a colostomy when the colon opens through the stoma, and an ileostomy when the lower part of the small intestine (the ileum) opens through the stoma.

Before the operation you will probably be given laxatives, an enema, and perhaps drugs to reduce the natural population of bacteria and other organisms in your intestines.

During the operation You are given a general anesthetic, and the diseased part of the digestive tract is removed through an incision in the abdominal wall. The upper end of the tract is joined to the lower end if possible. Otherwise it is stitched into a second incision to form the stoma. The operation takes about two to three hours.

After the operation You will receive nutrients via an intravenous *drip*, and fluid will be drained from your abdomen. Within two or three days you will be given a special diet, and begin to pass waste materials and gases into the bag.

Convalescence You will need about two months to recover from the operation, and you should gradually become adept at emptying and cleaning the bag. People with colostomies can eventually return to an almost normal bowel routine, emptying their bag at regular intervals. Sometimes bowel control becomes so good that the wearer needs only a pad over the stoma for most of the day. Those with ileostomies usually need to keep the bag in place all the time.

The anus

The anus is a canal 4 cm (1½ in) long. It leads from the rectum, down through a ring of muscles called the anal sphincter, to the anal orifice, through which solid wastes are eliminated as bowel movements. If you are healthy and past early childhood, you normally control the anal sphincter, keeping the orifice closed or letting it open when it is appropriate. This part of the digestive tract is relatively simple in structure and function and the only common anal disorder is hemorrhoids.

One reason why so many people have hemorrhoids may be our highly refined diet. Waste products of such non-fibrous foods create small, hard bowel movements that can injure the sphincter walls as they pass through. And because they do not pass easily, nearly every bowel movement requires enough straining to potentially damage the anus. Another reason for the prevalence of hemorrhoids is that many people worry unnecessarily about their bowels and work too hard at forcing sphincter muscles to do what they do naturally if given enough time.

Hemor-rhoids
(piles)

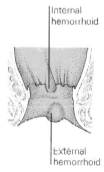

An internal hemorrhoid forms inside the lower part of the rectum and may not be visible from the outside. An external hemorrhoid forms at or just inside the anal orifice and may become visible if it prolapses (protrudes) through the anal orifice.

Hemorrhoids are varicose veins (see p.409) in your anus. The affected veins lie just under the mucous membrane that lines the lowest part of the rectum and the anus. They become swollen because of repeatedly raised pressure within them, usually as a result of persistent straining as you move your bowels. Hemorrhoids often appear during pregnancy and immediately after delivery (see Varicose veins during pregnancy, p.623). Many people who are obese (see p.492) also have them. If you have hemorrhoids, the swollen, twisted veins in your anus are thin-walled and easily ruptured by the passage of a bowel movement. An internal hemorrhoid is one near the beginning of the anal canal. If the bulging vein is farther down, virtually at the anal *orifice*, or opening, it is considered external.

External hemorrhoids sometimes *prolapse*, or protrude outside the orifice. This may happen only as you move your bowels, and then the prolapsed vein springs back into place. Thrombosis may also occur. In thrombosis, the blood in the hemorrhoid clots and this causes pain.

What are the symptoms?
Bleeding is the main, and in many people, the only, symptom. The blood is bright red and appears as streaks on toilet paper or on the bowel movement itself, or there may be a brief flow of blood. In addition, bowel movements may become increasingly uncomfortable and even painful. Prolapsed hemorrhoids often produce a mucous discharge and itching around the anal orifice. Moreover, severe hemorrhoids sometimes prolapse unexpectedly even when you are not attempting to move your bowels. If there is thrombosis, there may be severe pain.

What are the risks?
Hemorrhoids are very common; most people have occasional bleeding from them. Serious trouble is less common. Hemorrhoids themselves are not dangerous, though they can be annoying and uncomfortable. The risk is that bleeding thought to be from hemorrhoids may actually be caused by cancer of the rectum or colon (see Cancer of the large intestine, p.481), especially if you are over 40. That is why you should always see a physician at the first sign of anal bleeding. Also, too much loss of blood may cause iron deficiency anemia (see p.419).

What should be done?
Consult your physician if you detect signs of anal bleeding. He or she may examine your anus with a rubber-gloved finger and look at the area through a *proctoscope*. To exclude the possibility of cancer, you may also need a *barium enema* and *sigmoidoscopy*. If there is a diagnosis of hemorrhoids, treatment will depend on the details of the problem.

What is the treatment?
Self-help: To produce soft, easily passed bowel movements, eat plenty of fresh fruit, vegetables, and whole grain or bran cereals and bread. If you already have hemorrhoids, wash yourself thoroughly but gently after every bowel movement by using soft, moist paper and drying yourself carefully afterwards. A sensible diet and good hygiene will generally keep hemorrhoids under control and may even clear up a mild case. To assist the process you can buy astringents in the form of rectal suppositories (no prescription is needed) that will often help to shrink painful hemorrhoids.

OPERATION: ## Removing hemorrhoids
Hemorrhoidectomy and ligation

There are several different methods for removing painful or bleeding hemorrhoids. The traditional method is to cut them out. You may need to take painkillers for the first few bowel movements following the operation. Alternatively your anal opening may be manually stretched, or a small cut made in it. The idea behind these methods is to weaken the anus, and diminish the abdominal straining that often contributes to hemorrhoids. All of these methods require a general anesthetic.

Another method is to place a tight rubber band over the base of each hemorrhoid, which then withers painlessly over the next few days. This process, called ligation, can be done during a brief visit to an out-patient clinic and may not even require a local anesthetic.

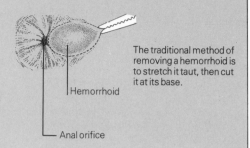

The traditional method of removing a hemorrhoid is to stretch it taut, then cut it at its base.

Hemorrhoid

Anal orifice

For a particularly painful attack, which is usually caused by a prolapsed and/or thrombosed vein, stay in bed for a full day. An ice compress may relieve the swelling enough for the exposed hemorrhoid to recede. Soaking in a warm bath may also help. If pain persists for more than 12 hours, see your physician.
Professional help: If a thrombosed hemorrhoid causes extreme pain, your physician may remove the clot. A local anesthetic may be used. A persistent prolapsed hemorrhoid may have to be manipulated manually through the sphincter. A physician usually treats chronic hemorrhoids by prescribing soothing or painkilling ointments or suppositories that contain *steroid* drugs. Some suppositories also contain a local anesthetic to numb the area and allow you to move your bowels with less discomfort. Additional measures, if constipation persists, include a combination of bulk-additives in the diet and a preparation to soften bowel movements.

If your hemorrhoids do not heal, a more active type of treatment may be necessary. Two possible procedures are to inject a special shrinking agent into an internal hemorrhoid or to destroy the hemorrhoids by a process called *cryosurgery*, which involves freezing the affected tissue. Occasionally, the swollen veins are removed surgically. This is called a hemorrhoidectomy. It is a relatively simple operation (see above).

Anal fissure

A fissure is an elongated ulcer that extends upward into the anal canal from the anal sphincter. When you have a bowel movement, irritation of the ulcer causes spasm of the sphincter, which causes severe pain and sometimes bleeding. This rare condition, which occurs most often in women, can sometimes be cured by adding roughage to the diet, and taking a preparation that softens your bowel movements. If the fissure is persistent or recurs, however, you may need to have a minor operation to stretch the anus and relax the sphincter muscles. This treatment stops spasms and relieves irritation, and the ulcer nearly always heals without further treatment within a few days.

Anal fistula

Erosion of tissues because of a spreading *abscess* within the anus causes the rare condition known as anal fistula. The fistula itself is a tiny tube that leads directly from the anal canal to a tiny hole in the skin near the anal *orifice*, or opening. The continual discharge of watery pus through this small hole irritates the skin and may cause discomfort and itching. Sometimes, too, the underlying abscess is painful. There is a very slight possibility that an anal fistula indicates the presence of Crohn's disease (see p.473), ulcerative colitis (see p.480), or cancer of the large intestine (see p.481). If you consult your physician about this complaint, you may need to have diagnostic *X-rays* of the intestines.

The usual treatment is a minor operation to remove the fistula and drain the abscess.

Liver, gallbladder and pancreas

The liver, gallbladder and pancreas, together with the digestive tract, make up the digestive system. The liver is the largest single internal organ. It fills the upper right-hand part of the abdomen behind the lower ribs. The liver has a crucial and complex role in regulating the composition of the blood, and also plays a large part in many other body processes. Many red blood cells, which contain the oxygen-carrying protein, hemoglobin, are broken down in the liver. The hemoglobin is converted into another substance, bilirubin. A fluid called bile that contains bilirubin and various other substances (among them cholesterol) trickles along tiny tubes to the gallbladder, a collecting bag that nestles within the lobes of the liver. When you eat a meal, the gallbladder empties its contents, the bile, along the bile duct into the duodenum, the first part of the small intestine. Bile is a waste product, but it plays an important role in digestion by helping to counteract stomach acid and by aiding in the digestion of fats.

The pancreas lies just behind the lower part of the stomach. It has two distinct functions, one of which is to make certain hormones, including insulin (see Diabetes mellitus, p.519). Its other function is to make *enzymes*, or digestive juices, that periodically flow down the pancreatic duct and into the duodenum, where they break food down into molecules that are small enough to be absorbed into the body.

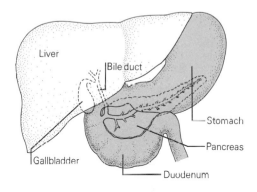

Liver and stomach (front view)

Liver
Bile duct
Stomach
Pancreas
Gallbladder
Duodenum

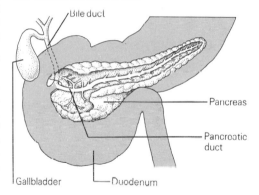

Liver omitted and closer view

Bile duct
Pancreas
Pancreatic duct
Gallbladder
Duodenum

Jaundice

See p.244,
Visual aids to diagnosis, 47.

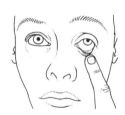

Looking at the whites of the eyes may help diagnose jaundice.

The term jaundice refers to a condition that discolors the skin and whites of the eyes with a yellow pigment. It is caused by an overabundance of bilirubin in the bloodstream. Bilirubin is a byproduct of the breaking down of aged red blood cells by the liver. The liver filters bilirubin from the bloodstream and excretes it into the bile ducts, which carry it to the gallbladder, and from there it eventually flows into the small intestine. Most of the bilirubin is then broken down by bacteria and it is finally eliminated from the body in bowel movements.

Jaundice most frequently results from liver diseases, including viral infections such as hepatitis (see next articles) and cirrhosis (see p.487). Drug reactions can also cause it. Another possible cause is obstruction of the bile ducts. This can prevent bilirubin from entering the intestines, which creates pressure in the liver. This can happen with gallstones (see p.489) and pancreatic tumors (see Cancer of the pancreas, p.491). Jaundice also occurs in hemolytic anemia (see p.423). In this blood disease, many red blood cells are destroyed, and an abundance of bilirubin is released into the bloodstream. In this case, the liver functions normally, but it is unable to remove bilirubin from the blood rapidly enough. This causes jaundice.

What should be done?
If you notice the symptoms described, you should consult your physician immediately. The treatment will depend on what underlying disorder is causing the jaundice. Once the underlying cause is treated and cured, the jaundice should disappear.

Acute hepatitis A

Acute hepatitis A is a viral infection of the liver. The liver becomes tender and swollen, and bilirubin, a substance produced when the liver breaks down aged red blood cells, accumulates in the bloodstream.

If you have this type of hepatitis, the virus will be present in your blood and bowel movements for two to three weeks before any symptoms develop, and for two to three weeks afterwards. During this time, the hepatitis A virus can infect anyone who handles anything contaminated by your blood or bowel movements.

What are the symptoms?
The symptoms of any kind of hepatitis include some or all of the following: jaundice (see previous article), weakness, loss of appetite, nausea, brownish or tea-colored urine, abdominal discomfort, and whitish bowel movements. How ill you feel and which symptoms you have may vary from case to case. Usually, after four to six weeks, the symptoms gradually disappear.

What should be done?
If you are jaundiced, or have several of the other symptoms described, consult your physician. A blood test will probably be necessary to diagnose hepatitis A. Additional blood tests will be done periodically to follow the course of the disease.

Your physician can inject all household contacts of the person with hepatitis A with a preparation to prevent infection. This is effective for up to two weeks after initial contact with the infected person. It is also useful when traveling to areas of the world where hepatitis A is relatively common.

What is the treatment?
Self-help: If someone in your household develops hepatitis A, certain precautions are necessary to prevent the spread of infection. Be careful not to touch contaminated bowel movements. Flush bowel movements directly down the toilet, and then wash your hands. The infected person can share toilet facilities and dishes with other family members. Clothing and bed linen require special handling only when they are visibly soiled, and then they should be laundered with a detergent that kills germs. Contaminated toilets and floors should be cleaned with a disinfectant.
Professional help: There is no specific medical treatment for hepatitis A, except bed rest and progressive activity as you feel better. You can eat your usual diet, but alcohol, which may put a strain on your liver, is prohibited during the first few weeks of the infection. After you recover, there are no restrictions on reasonable alcohol consumption. Ask your physician when it is safe for you to begin to drink again.

The chances of complete recovery from hepatitis A are excellent, and you will develop an immunity to the disease, so you will not have it again.

Acute hepatitis B

Acute hepatitis B is caused by a virus that infects the liver. If you have this disease, your blood, either fresh or dried, is highly contagious during the four to six weeks before the symptoms of the disease appear and for a short time afterwards, because particles of the hepatitis B virus are already circulating in your bloodstream.

The symptoms of hepatitis B are the same as those of hepatitis A (see previous article). Jaundice (see previous page) is the most obvious one, but it does not occur in every case. Others include weakness, loss of appetite, nausea, brownish urine, whitish bowel movements, and abdominal discomfort. One difference between the diseases is the severity and duration of the symptoms. In hepatitis B they are more severe and last longer.

What are the risks?
In the United States, ten per cent of all persons with hepatitis B develop some form of chronic liver disease. Some common sources of hepatitis B infection are needle punctures from acupuncture, tattooing and injections of drugs; blood transfusions; and sexual contact. The virus can spread through contact with saliva, nasal mucus, sperm and menstrual blood.

What should be done?
If your skin or the whites of your eyes turn yellow, or if you have any of the other symptoms of hepatitis, see your physician. If you have hepatitis B, a blood test can show liver damage, and also some tiny particles of the hepatitis B virus.

Your physician can inject members of your household with a special preparation to prevent hepatitis B. This is also effective if you come in contact with the blood of any infected person.

What is the treatment?
Self-help: Read the self-help in the article on hepatitis A (see previous article). The same

precautions apply with hepatitis B. You should clean any blood stains with a germ-killing detergent, do not share your toothbrush and razor blades with anyone with the disease, and avoid sexual contact with them. **Professional help:** Treatment for hepatitis B consists mainly of bed rest, proper nourish-

ment, restrictions on alcohol intake, and periodic blood tests to monitor the disease. If your symptoms are severe and you become *dehydrated*, or dried out, your physician may admit you to a hospital. There, steps can be taken to reverse dehydration under the watchful eyes of a professional staff.

Non-A, non-B hepatitis

This viral infection of the liver was not discovered until 1975. It was first found in hospitalized patients who had blood transfusions and developed hepatitis, but did not have either A or B hepatitis virus in their blood. This difficult-to-identify virus causes most of the hepatitis spread through blood transfusions, because it cannot be identified in donated blood. It often leads to chronic liver disease (see Chronic active hepatitis, next article, and Cirrhosis of the liver, below).

Researchers are still gathering information about this disease, but it appears that non-A, non-B hepatitis is spread through sexual activity and contact with infected blood. The symptoms are similar to those of hepatitis A (see previous page) and hepatitis B (see previous article), but they are often milder and may not include jaundice. The treatment is also similar, but your physician will probably check your blood more frequently for chronic liver disease.

Chronic active hepatitis

Chronic active hepatitis is an inflammation of cells in your liver that may continue for several years. No one is sure what causes the disorder, but some people who contract hepatitis B (see previous page) or non-A, non-B hepatitis (see previous article) will develop chronic active hepatitis. In some cases it occurs as a reaction to certain drugs.

Chronic active hepatitis is an *autoimmune* disease; that is, your body forms *antibodies*, or normally protective substances, that attack liver cells and cause the inflammation. Nobody knows why such self-destructive reactions take place.

The severity of the symptoms varies from case to case. Some people will have no symptoms for long periods of time, and occasionally experience episodes of the other forms of hepatitis, with jaundice (see p.485), joint pains, nausea, fever and loss of appetite.

Others will have no symptoms despite having mild liver inflammation for many years. For them, the disorder can only be detected by blood tests. Chronic active hepatitis can also progress rapidly, and lead to liver failure.

What should be done?
Your physician will suspect the disease when blood tests show your liver is inflamed and releasing substances into the bloodstream. A definite diagnosis can be made only with a liver *biopsy*, a procedure in which a small sample of tissue is removed for examination.

If you have symptoms, your physician will probably prescribe *steroid* drugs to reduce inflammation. Most people treated for chronic active hepatitis will recover within one to three years. The others usually develop cirrhosis of the liver (see next article), which eventually causes death.

Cirrhosis of the liver

Cirrhosis is a chronic disease that is the result of slow deterioration of the liver. In this disease, damage to the liver from one of many causes changes its structure gradually, and the liver becomes progressively less able to carry out its functions, which include regulating the content of the blood.

The most common cause of the disease in North America is alcoholism (see p.304). Malnutrition, hepatitis (see previous articles), parasites, toxic chemicals, and congestive heart failure (see p.381) are some other possible causes of the disease.

What are the symptoms?
In the very early stages, while there are still plenty of healthy liver cells, symptoms are mild. As the disease progresses, loss of appetite and weight, nausea, vomiting, general malaise and weakness, indigestion, and abdominal distention all become increasingly pronounced. There is a tendency to bleed and bruise easily that leads to nosebleeds. Small, red, spidery marks called spider nevi may appear on your face, arms and upper trunk.

In the later stages jaundice (see p.485) may occur. Men can lose interest in sex, their breasts enlarge, and they become impotent. Women usually stop having periods (see Absence of periods, p.583). Eventually, *liver failure* may develop. In this condition, fluid retention in the abdomen and ankles, irritability, and an inability to concentrate are the main symptoms. Memory is impaired and the hands tremble markedly. Confusion and drowsiness occur and increase as the condition worsens. Life-threatening bleeding from enlarged veins in the esophagus may also occur.

What are the risks?

Cirrhosis is relatively common, especially among heavy drinkers. The heavy drinker who does not eat properly is especially at risk. The disease progresses at different rates depending on the individual case. If the disease is detected at an early stage, you can slow its progress by following the treatment carefully. If you cannot give up alcohol, however, the disease may eventually cause liver failure. Cirrhosis of the liver also increases the risk of severe bleeding in the digestive tract. If this happens it is usually difficult to control and may cause liver failure. Very rarely, a tumor develops in the liver as a result of cirrhosis (see next article).

What should be done?

If you suspect that you have cirrhosis, and it is a distinct possibility if you drink heavily and regularly, you should consult your physician. A physical examination is often sufficient for a diagnosis, though you may have to have blood tests and a liver *biopsy*, in which a small portion of the liver is removed and examined, to assess the extent of the damage.

What is the treatment?

Self-help: Whatever the underlying cause of the cirrhosis, stop drinking alcohol immediately. If you continue to drink, the disease is certain to get worse. Your liver will remain particularly sensitive to alcohol, and amounts that would have no effect on a healthy person may kill you.

If you suspect, even slightly, that you may be an alcoholic, see your physician and discuss the matter frankly. There are several ways of treating alcoholism, but until you admit your suspicions and confirm them, nobody else can help. Inaction and denial can cost you your life.

Never take any drugs without your physician's approval. Try to follow a nutritious diet that contains plenty of protein, carbohydrates, and vitamins, but is low in fats and salt.

Professional help: Your physician can prescribe drugs to counteract the symptoms of cirrhosis. For example, *diuretics* reduce the fluid in your body, and *antacids* may relieve abdominal discomfort. To guard against malnutrition, you may also be given dietary and vitamin supplements. Depending on the cause of the cirrhosis *steroids* or other *immunosuppressive* drugs may also be prescribed. If you vomit blood (see p.469) you should get emergency medical help; you may need blood transfusions and surgery.

The prospects for a person with cirrhosis vary enormously. The heavy drinker who develops cirrhosis, but who then cuts out alcohol completely and eats a nutritious diet, should be able to lead an otherwise normal life. But the alcoholic who will not or cannot abstain will eventually develop liver failure. Hospital treatment with an intravenous *drip* that contains drugs and nutrients can usually bring about some improvement, but repeated episodes of liver failure make this treatment progressively less effective.

Tumors of the liver

Like tumors elsewhere in the body, liver tumors may be either *benign* (unlikely to spread) or *malignant* (likely to spread and threaten life). Benign tumors are extremely rare. If they are discovered at all, benign liver tumors can usually be removed surgically.

There are two types of malignant tumors. The majority are *metastases*, or cancers that have spread from other parts of the body through the bloodstream to the liver. About one third of all cancers spread to the liver in this way, and in some cases it is the symptoms of the secondary liver cancer that draw attention to a primary cancer elsewhere. Cancer may start in the liver (primary liver cancer) but, like benign liver tumors, this is very rare.

What are the symptoms?

The symptoms may initially be only those from the primary cancer, most often of the breast, lung or gastrointestinal tract. As secondary liver cancer develops, it causes further loss of weight and appetite, abdominal discomfort, and general ill-health. Jaundice (see p.485) may appear in the late stages.

What should be done?

Consult your physician if you have the symptoms described above, or if jaundice develops. The outlook is poor once cancer has spread to the liver. *Radiation therapy* and *chemotherapy* may not reduce the size of the tumor, and surgical removal is not possible.

Gallstones

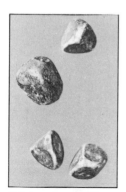

Gallstones form in different shapes and sizes. They may be large and smooth or small, sharp and crystalline.

Stones of varying composition sometimes form in the gallbladder, the reservoir where bile collects. Bile is a waste product that flows from the liver to the gallbladder. From there it is excreted into the intestines, where it combats stomach acid to some degree and aids in fat digestion.

Bile is rich in fatty substances, especially cholesterol, that are extracted from the blood by the liver. Bile also contains bilirubin, a substance formed by the breakdown of hemoglobin from old red blood cells. Sometimes if the balance of these substances is upset, a tiny solid particle forms in the gallbladder. The particle may grow as more material solidifies around it. Some people may have only one gallstone and others may have more than one.

What are the symptoms?

Between one third and one half of gallstones do not produce any symptoms. But some gallstones flow out with the bile, and may get stuck in the bile duct. If this happens the result is biliary colic, an intense pain either in the upper right side of your abdomen or sometimes between your shoulder blades. Over a period of a few hours the pain builds to a peak and then fades. It makes you feel sick, possibly causing you to vomit.

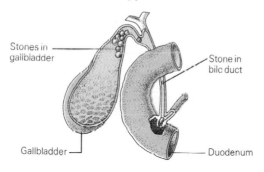

Stones in gallbladder

Stone in bile duct

Gallbladder

Duodenum

Gallstone sites
Gallstones may remain in the gallbladder or pass through the bile duct into the duodenum. In either case you will probably have no symptoms. Problems arise if the gallstones are trapped in the bile duct.

Biliary colic is a result of the gallbladder trying unsuccessfully to empty bile into the intestines. If the stone falls back into the gallbladder, or is forced along the bile duct into the intestines, the blockage that had been causing the problem is gone and the pain ceases.

What are the risks?

Some 20 million people in the United States have gallstones. About 1 million new cases of the malady develop each year. Autopsy studies show that 20 per cent of all women have gallstones when they die. The comparable figure for men in the United States is only eight per cent.

For reasons that are not yet understood, some groups may be more likely to have gallstones that are others. For example, among American Indian women, about 70 per cent of those who are over 30 years old have gallstones.

The older you are, the more likely you are to have gallstones. Up to one in five elderly people are estimated to have them. And as the autopsy studies indicate, for some unknown reason, women are far more likely than men to have them.

If a gallstone remains lodged in your bile duct for any length of time, it may block the exit for bile and cause obstructive jaundice (see Neonatal jaundice, p.647). Another risk is inflammation and perhaps infection of the gallbladder as the dammed-up bile stagnates. This condition requires special treatment (see Cholecystitis, next article). If you have gallstones, you are also susceptible to acute pancreatitis (see next page), because the pancreatic duct drains into the bile duct.

What should be done?

If you have a severe pain resembling biliary colic, consult your physician, who will examine you and question you as to the exact nature of the pain. If gallstones are suspected to be the cause, the doctor will probably take blood samples for analysis, and your abdomen may be X-rayed several hours after you swallow a special pill that makes the gallbladder show up well on an X-ray. This type of X-ray is called a *cholecystogram*. Sometimes either an *ultrasound scan* or a *CAT scan* can detect gallstones if they do not show up in any other tests.

What is the treatment?

Self-help: Eat sensibly. Avoid overeating and any foods that bring on pain or indigestion. If biliary colic develops, go to bed and take a painkilling drug if necessary, and do not eat but sip water occasionally. If the pain persists for more than three hours, you should call your physician.

Professional help: To relieve the colic initially, your physician may prescribe a strong painkiller. But if the tests that are done show that you have gallstones, the physician may recommend that you undergo surgery to remove the gallstones and the gallbladder (see Gallbladder removal, next page).

OPERATION: **Gallbladder removal**

Cholecystectomy

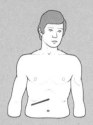

Site of incision

This operation is done when gallstones or some other gallbladder problem causes serious symptoms. It has little or no effect on the functioning of your digestive system.

During the operation Under a general anesthetic the gallbladder is cut away and removed through an incision in the upper right part of your abdomen. During the operation, which usually takes one and a half hours, the surgeon may explore the bile duct and remove any stones found there.

After the operation You will have tubes draining excess fluid from the incision site. There may also be a tube draining bile from the bile duct. This tube may stay in position for up to ten days. You will be fed *intravenously* for a few days, but then you will be able to eat and drink, and within two weeks you should be able to go home.

Convalescence The usual recovery period is two months, during which time you may gradually resume normal eating and drinking habits unless advised otherwise by your physician.

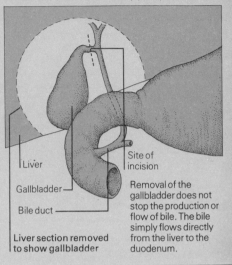

Liver

Gallbladder

Bile duct

Liver section removed to show gallbladder

Site of incision

Removal of the gallbladder does not stop the production or flow of bile. The bile simply flows directly from the liver to the duodenum.

Cholecystitis

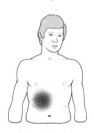

Site of the pain

In cholecystitis, the gallbladder becomes inflamed and swollen. This is usually a result of a gallstone (see previous article) that is blocking the flow of bile from the gallbladder into the intestine. Occasionally, the inflammation is caused by an infection that is spreading upward from the intestine.

The symptoms of cholecystitis itself are preceded by severe pain in the upper part of your abdomen, usually on the right-hand side. This is called biliary colic (see Gallstones, previous page). As cholecystitis develops, your temperature rises, and nausea and vomiting follow. If the condition is not treated you may develop jaundice, or yellowish skin (see p.485).

Three-quarters of the people who have this disorder have had previous gallbladder problems. If, as happens in rare cases, the gallbladder swells so much that it bursts, a particularly severe form of peritonitis (see p.470) may develop.

If you suspect cholecystitis, especially if you already have gallbladder problems, consult your physician immediately.

You may be admitted to a hospital and given an *intravenous drip* to provide you with nutrition and fluid. You may not be allowed to eat or drink for a few days. You may be given painkillers and *antibiotics* to combat any infection. Once the inflammation has subsided, tests may be done to find any gallstones that are present (see previous page). If you have had cholecystitis, you will probably be advised to have your gallbladder removed (see Box, above). In severe cases of cholecystitis, this may be done soon after you are admitted to the hospital, but some surgeons prefer that you wait until after the inflammation has subsided.

Acute pancreatitis

Why the pancreas suddenly becomes inflamed, as it does in this rare disease, is not fully understood. About half the people who develop the problem already have gallstones. Another factor that leads to the development of acute pancreatitis is excessive consumption of alcohol. Less commonly, certain drugs, a perforated ulcer (see p.468), hyperparathyroidism (see p.528) or an abdominal injury may be the cause. It can also be a complication of mumps (see p.700), but this rarely occurs.

What are the symptoms?
The main symptom is agonizing pain in the middle part of your abdomen. It often begins

12 to 24 hours after a large meal or a heavy bout of drinking. The pain bores through to the back and the chest, and over several hours it rises to a peak, accompanied by vomiting. In severe cases you become very ill and feverish, have bruise marks on your abdomen, and may even have the symptoms of shock (see p.386). If this happens, get to a hospital immediately.

What are the risks?
The main danger of acute pancreatitis is that shock, which can cause death, will develop. There is a long term risk of chronic pancreatitis (see next article). However, the majority of people who have the disease recover completely. The quicker you obtain medical help the better the outlook.

What is the treatment?
If your physician suspects acute pancreatitis, you will be admitted to a hospital immediately. The doctor's first task is to establish the diagnosis by taking *X-rays* and blood samples. Analysis of the blood samples for levels of pancreatic enzymes and other body chemicals will reveal the disease.

You will probably get painkillers and injections of drugs to reduce some of the pancreatic juices. Shock will be treated with intravenous fluids. *Antibiotics* may be necessary. As you recover, you will gradually be able to eat and drink, but you should not drink any alcohol if it caused the attack. After a few weeks tests are carried out to see if you have gallstones. If you do, arrangements may be made to remove them (see previous page).

Chronic pancreatitis

Chronic pancreatitis is a rare disease that develops over many years. It sometimes follows recurrent attacks of acute pancreatitis (see previous article), usually associated with gallstones (see p.489) or alcoholism (see p.304). In such cases, you do not recover fully between attacks. Gradually the damaged pancreas becomes less able to supply its digestive juices and hormones.

What are the symptoms?
Pain is the main symptom, although in one in ten cases there is no pain at all. It is a dull, cramping, boring pain that is aggravated by food and alcohol, and relieved by sitting up and leaning forward. As the disease progresses the attacks of pain last longer and come more frequently. Some people complain of indigestion between attacks. Additional symptoms, which do not occur in all cases, are mild jaundice (see p.485) and loss of weight. In addition, the pancreas may become unable to make the hormone insulin, so diabetes mellitus (see p.519) may develop.

If you have these symptoms, you should consult your physician. And never ignore attacks of abdominal pain (see Laparotomy and acute abdomen, p.477). If your physician

suspects a pancreatic disorder, you will undergo a number of tests to disclose the exact problem. These include blood tests, including a glucose tolerance test for diabetes (see p.519), X-rays, an *endoscopic* examination, and perhaps a *radioisotope scan* or a *CAT scan* of your pancreas.

What is the treatment?
Self-help: Once the condition is diagnosed, you should give up alcohol completely, and adhere strictly to the diet that is advised by your physician.
Professional help: Your physician may prescribe one of several painkilling drugs if your pain is particularly severe. You may also need to take tablets with each meal. These tablets contain *enzymes* that you need to digest your food but that your damaged pancreas can no longer manufacture. If you give up alcohol permanently, stick rigidly to your diet, and take the tablets of pancreatic enzymes, your chances of improvement are good.

In some cases, bouts of abdominal pain become unbearable. You may be advised to undergo surgery, during which either the damaged pancreatic tissue is removed or the nerves that carry the pain are cut.

Cancer of the pancreas

A cancerous tumor in the pancreas can cause a number of symptoms. The main ones are loss of appetite and weight, nausea, vomiting, and abdominal pain. The pain, usually in the upper abdomen, may spread to the back.

If you get the symptoms described above, consult your physician immediately. There are several possible causes, including gall-

stones (see p.489). If cancer is suspected blood tests, *X-rays*, a *barium swallow*, a *cholecystogram* and various specialized pancreas tests may be done.

If the cancer is detected in its early stages, surgical removal of the malignant tissues may cure it. Drugs and *radiation therapy* may also be used. Later, the outlook is poor.

Nutrition and metabolism

Metabolism is a general term for the chemical processes through which your body changes air, food and other materials into the substances it needs to function properly. Although in broad terms metabolism is the same for all of us, in detail it is quite individual. For example, the chemical balance in your body and the rate of your metabolism differs from those of other people. These individual differences are determined in large part by the genes you inherit.

In general, there are two types of metabolic disorders that relate to the digestive system. One type includes problems caused by poor nutrition, or eating and drinking the wrong kinds or amounts of food. This is the more common of the two types, and you can help eliminate the problems by changing your diet. The second type of metabolic disorder is genetic, that is, inherited from your parents. These disorders generally cannot be cured, but their symptoms often can be controlled by modifying your diet or environment.

There is some overlap between these two types of metabolic problems. For example, most people who are obese, or significantly overweight, can reduce their weight by eating less, though this may take discipline. Other factors such as lack of exercise, cultural patterns of eating, and psychological issues may influence your weight loss. There are a few rare individuals who actually inherit specific diseases that predispose them to becoming and then staying obese.

Other disorders of metabolism can be caused by a lack of vitamins in your diet. Vitamins play an essential role in healthy metabolism, and therefore they are a part of good nutrition. Vitamin deficiencies are also considered nutritional disorders.

This section deals first with obesity and vitamin deficiency, both of which are related to digestion and nutrition. This section also covers inherited metabolic disorders including porphyria, hyperlipoproteinemia and gout, all of which can be affected by your diet.

Obesity

Your body needs food as a source of energy, which it uses to maintain body temperature and to fuel chemical and physical functions. Food also provides raw materials for building and repairing tissues.

Food requirements vary, even among individuals of the same height, build, age and sex. The basic needs of most people are close to an average of enough food to provide about 2000 calories a day for women, and 2500 for men. However, a professional athlete or a manual laborer may need 4000 or more.

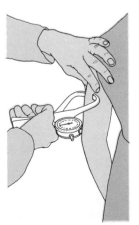

Measuring obesity
Skin callipers measure the thickness of skin, which indicates the degree of obesity.

If you eat more than you need for the energy you expend, your body stores the surplus in the form of fat. If the amount of fat becomes excessive and unsightly you may be considered obese. But obesity has not been precisely defined. Some experts feel that you are obese if you exceed the "desirable" weight (see p.28) for your height, build and age by more than 20 per cent. By this definition one in every five men and almost one in every three women in our society are obese.

What are the symptoms?
The most obvious symptom of obesity is an increase in weight. Not all people who put on weight are necessarily obese. For instance, a pregnant woman or a weight-lifter gains weight for other reasons. But an increased amount of fat in the body tissues is the commonest reason for a weight increase. Obesity is associated with a wide range of serious disorders with many other symptoms.

What are the risks?
Statistics compiled by insurance companies and health organizations indicate that obesity is associated with increases in illness and death from diabetes, stroke, coronary artery disease, and kidney and gallbladder disor-

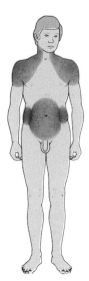

Where fat builds
up on men

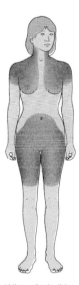

Where fat builds
up on women

ders. The more overweight you are, the stronger the association becomes. The statistics suggest that if you are more than 40 per cent overweight you are twice as likely to die from coronary artery disease as a person who is not overweight. If you are 20 to 30 per cent overweight, you may be three times more likely than a person who is not overweight to die from diabetes.

There are also some more direct drawbacks to obesity. The condition seems to contribute directly to high blood pressure (see p.382), which is, in itself, a risk factor in both heart disease and stroke. If you have high blood pressure, you may be able to reduce your blood pressure simply by doing something about losing excess weight.

Similarly, diabetes (see p.519) sometimes seems to develop as a direct consequence of obesity and to disappear when excess weight is lost. Finally, very obese persons who have surgery suffer more surgical and anesthetic complications than do their lean counterparts. Childbirth may also be more risky for both mother and child.

What should be done?

Many people can cope with this problem themselves. To lose your excess fat and keep it off, follow the self-help measures recommended below. Consult your physician if you are grossly obese and are among the minority of obese people who cannot lose weight through a balanced diet and moderate, regular exercise. If you find that you cannot control your eating at all, you may need special help, such as psychological treatment or one of several operations designed for such cases.

What is the treatment?

Self-help: If you are overweight, it is because you consume more calories than you use. This may be for any of several reasons, psychological as well as physical. Whatever the reason, it applies to you alone, so try not to make comparisons between your moderate intake of food and your slender neighbor's gluttony.

In order to lose weight, you must somehow help your own body to use up more calories than you consume. In other words, you must create an *energy deficit.* There are two ways that you can do this. First, change your diet; second, exercise more.

Any such recipe for reducing is almost too obvious to be worth repeating. There are pitfalls, however, and you must be realistic. To begin with, crash diets or a few days at a health spa seldom work if your goal is to lose weight permanently. Unfortunately, if you

lose weight that is mostly body water, the weight returns when you go back to your usual routines. Diets that are overly restrictive or strenuous exercise programs are not feasible for most people on a life-long basis.

So do not try to achieve massive weight losses in a few days. You should not try to lose more than two pounds in a week. Aim instead at a food and exercise program that gives you an energy deficit of around 500 calories a day. This will lose about $\frac{1}{2}$ kilogram (1 lb) of fatty tissue a week. This seemingly modest goal will cause you to lose about 25 kilograms (52 lb) in a year.

When you work out a diet for yourself, make sure that it is varied and balanced (see p.26), and choose foods that you like, for you want to establish eating patterns that you can maintain indefinitely. A chart that shows the calorie count of various foods is helpful in making wise selections for your diet. Such charts can be found in many readily available cook books and diet books.

Almost as important as the kind and amount of food you eat is the timing of your meals. Eat only at set intervals. This combination of carefully watching exactly what and when you eat is very useful. This is because many people are obese because they eat almost unconsciously, and hardly notice what they pop into their mouths.

Dietitians and behavioral therapists have found that such people are greatly helped by following simple rules that turn eating into a formal ritual. If you need to lose weight, it may help you to follow these rules: Never eat anything except at mealtimes; eat with a knife, fork and spoon; and never finish a mouthful of food without pausing to chew it slowly and thoroughly.

As for the second element in your weight reduction program, exercise, the rule is go slow but steady. An hour of moderate bicycle riding will burn off about 400 calories, or almost a whole day's target energy deficit.

You may have heard that exercise is self-defeating in a weight loss program, because it simply increases appetite. There is good evidence that this is untrue. In fact, some studies show that moderate exercise in previously sedentary people actually reduces appetite.

Finally, many obese people find it easier to follow a sensible diet and exercise program if they do not have to do it alone. It may help to join a weight-loss club. This can be a positive step, since it formalizes your intention to lose weight and also puts you in touch with people who share your problem.

If your reasonable efforts to lose weight do not succeed, you may be one of the few people who are constitutionally unable to lose weight on diets that normally would work for others. Some people find that their bodies adapt to a low energy intake by a significant reduction in basic energy requirement, and they fail to lose weight as expected. If this seems to be the case with you, consult your physician.

Professional help: There are antiobesity drugs, but many physicians prefer not to prescribe them because they can have major side-effects. Moreover, most such drugs are appetite suppressants, and most obese people do not suffer specifically from excess appetite. Many simply eat whether they are hungry or not. Their physicians may send them for psychological help. Newly developed drugs designed to increase the body's energy requirements are being tested, but they are still in the experimental stage.

For people who cannot lose weight in any other way and are extraordinarily obese, physicians sometimes try more drastic forms of treatment. For example, your teeth can be wired together so that you cannot open your jaws to eat. The wiring may be kept in place for several weeks, causing a dramatic loss of weight. This treatment is uncomfortable and also has some drawbacks beyond the obvious ones associated with such an experience. For example, the treatment does not produce any fundamental change in your eating habits, and your fat may return when your teeth are unwired and you begin to eat again. Also, mouth infections and dental decay can occur because your teeth cannot be properly cleaned while the wires are in place.

A more complex, and more risky, procedure that may be advised when obesity becomes life-threatening is digestive-tract surgery to by-pass part of the small intestine, or to reduce the size of the stomach by stapling. The by-pass procedure reduces the area of intestine through which food can be absorbed. It also diminishes appetite. The stomach stapling procedure limits the amount of food that you can eat at one time. These operations are done only in special medical centers, and only rarely even there because of an unacceptably high risk of death. There are also significant complications in many cases. Cosmetic surgery (see p.260), in which fat deposits are literally cut away, is another possible treatment.

About 60 per cent of obese people who are treated in one of these drastic fashions do manage to lose weight. But, apart from the greater risks, the rewards may be short lived, for a high percentage of such people eventually regain the lost weight.

Vitamin deficiency

Your body needs food for energy and for creating and repairing tissues. It also needs a variety of complex compounds that, like spark plugs in a car, provide neither fuel nor structural material but are essential for smooth running. Vitamins are such compounds. Although your body can manufacture some vitamins, notably vitamins D and K, most of these compounds are obtained in the foods you eat.

The precise function of some vitamins is not yet fully understood, but they are all known to be involved in basic metabolic activities. For example, vitamins play a role in controlling the absorption of calcium, which is needed for strong bones and for the functioning of nerves and muscles, and in regulating the supply of energy to body tissues. As a result, a lack of any one vitamin can lead to many disorders. If the vitamin deficiency is severe or prolonged, the resultant disease may be disabling or even fatal.

Vitamin deficiency is uncommon in this country, and when it occurs it is usually due to prolonged faulty eating habits, alcoholism, gastrointestinal disorders, or long-term neglect. Vitamin deficiency diseases that were once quite common here seldom occur now because many foods are fortified with vitamins, nourishing foods are available year-round, and dietary supplements are widely used. Although vitamin deficiencies serious enough to cause medical problems are uncommon, they do still occur, even in the well-fed Western world.

The accompanying table (see p.496) summarizes up-to-date facts and theories about the most important known vitamins, their sources, and their functions.

Who lacks vitamins?

In the so-called developed countries, unmistakable vitamin-deficiency diseases such as scurvy or pellagra are virtually nonexistent. These disorders can occur, however.

Vagrants often show signs of vitamin C and B-complex deficiency. Alcoholism, which sometimes goes with vagrancy, seems to exaggerate the effects of low vitamin intake. Vitamin B_6, or pyridoxine, deficiency occurs in about 20 to 30 per cent of the alcoholic population. Similarly, alcoholics commonly have deficiencies of vitamin B_1, or thiamin, and folic acid, or folacin.

Neglected, undernourished children may show the effects of vitamin C or D deficiency. Also, children who eat few fruits and vegetables may not get enough of vitamins A, C and B_2, or riboflavin. These children may not show symptoms of vitamin deficiencies because of the remainder of their diets, but they will have few reserve stores of these vitamins to help them withstand the stresses of serious illness or injury.

Moreover, some people who are neither vagrant nor deprived suffer from vitamin deficiency because of metabolic abnormalities. For instance, one form of mental retardation in infancy seems to be caused by an inability to utilize vitamin B_6. There are also occasional individuals who have anemia because their bodies cannot absorb vitamin B_{12} (see p.420). In addition, some women who use oral contraceptives may show signs of vitamin B_6 deficiency, but there is some question of whether this is a true deficiency.

You may develop a vitamin deficiency after an operation on your stomach or the bile duct of your liver. If you develop a severe intestinal disorder such as Crohn's disease (see p.473), you may become predisposed to vitamin deficiencies because your body cannot absorb needed vitamins. A crash diet may also be risky, because it may exclude an essential vitamin.

Marginal deficiency that involves relatively minor trouble, probably due to some degree of insufficiency, is more widespread than severe vitamin deficiencies. For instance, old people, who often do not eat properly, commonly have sores, and the raw, red tongue and coarse skin associated with deficiencies of the B vitamins and possibly vitamin C. Of course, there can be many other causes of such symptoms, but the condition sometimes improves when B-complex and C vitamins are added to the diet. Old people with fractured hips (a common problem of the elderly) may have a vitamin D deficiency.

Pregnant mothers and their fetuses are particularly at risk. Folic acid deficiency (see p.420) may occur during pregnancy because the woman's increased need for the vitamin is not being met adequately.

Because clear-cut cases of vitamin deficiency are now uncommon, experts tend to assume that deficiency is not a general problem. But more investigations still need to be done, and may provide more information about these disorders in the next few years.

Should you eat differently?
The chances of having a deficiency in any one vitamin depend mainly on two factors. First, how available that vitamin is in your diet, and second, how effectively your body can store it. Luckily, most vitamins are present in many foods. Vitamin A is probably less available in your diet than some of the other vitamins, since the richest sources of it are fish-liver oils. Carrots and other yellow or orange vegetables and fruits are also excellent sources of the vitamin, and fortunately, the body can store vitamin A.

If you eat the proper amounts of nourishing foods, you should be able to assure an adequate vitamin intake. The guidelines below describe food groups and the amounts you need of each group every day.

Foods can be divided into four groups on the basis of similarities in composition and nutrient content: (1) milk and its products, two or more servings per day; (2) meats, fish, poultry, dried beans and other protein-rich foods, two or more servings; (3) vegetables and fruits, four or more servings, with emphasis on good sources of vitamins C and A; (4) breads and cereals, whole grain and enriched, four or more servings. The minimum number of recommended servings will provide about 1300 calories and from 80 to 120 per cent of the nutrients needed. Active people of normal weight can, of course, have more and larger servings of these foods (plus other foods) in order to meet the need for more calories.

Vitamin C has received a great deal of attention lately, because it is important in healing wounds and enhancing iron absorption. While not all the evidence supports claims that vitamin C helps fight the common cold, there is agreement that good body concentrations of the vitamin should certainly be maintained.

Citrus fruits, including oranges, lemons, limes and grapefruit, are the main sources of vitamin C. Good quantities are present in many other foods as well; strawberries, cantaloupe, raw peppers, and even potatoes contain vitamin C. If you prefer fruit flavored drinks to fruit juices, be sure that they are fortified with the vitamin.

Vegetables also supply vitamin C, as well as other vitamins and minerals. To preserve as much of their nutrients as possible, cook them with very little water and only for a short time, or, even better, eat them raw.

Are vitamin pills effective?
Should you take vitamin pills to avoid marginal deficiency? The answer is no. Not a categorical no, perhaps, but a fairly decided no. If you eat a varied diet of fresh food and expose your skin to plenty of sunlight to

How vitamins got their names

Vitamins have been given many names and classifications as scientists have learned more and more about them. At first, they were assigned letters of the alphabet roughly according to the order in which they were discovered. As research on vitamins continued, the chemical composition of each vitamin was determined, and each one was given one or more chemical names. To add to the confusion, some vitamins that initially were considered a single substance were later discovered to include a complex, or group, of different chemicals. The vitamin B complex is the best-known, and there are several B-complex vitamins with "B" as part of their names. Even more confusing are vitamins like niacin. It is in the B-complex group, but it was discovered separately and named independently.

There is disagreement and some confusion about terminology for vitamins. The widely accepted alphabetical names commonly found on labels for special foods and vitamin pills are the ones used in this book. The chemical names for vitamins are familiar mainly to nutritionists.

increase vitamin D reserves, you will probably provide all the vitamins your body requires, as long as there are no defects in your metabolism. Vitamin pills may not harm you, but you are unlikely to need the extra-large doses of vitamins that they provide and in some cases an especially high dose can be harmful. This is particularly true of vitamins that the body can store efficiently, such as vitamins A and D. Too much vitamin A causes skin changes, hair loss, enlarged liver and various symptoms in muscles and joints. Too much vitamin D leads to excess calcium in the blood, which can cause gastrointestinal and nervous disorders. Most important, there are no known advantages to taking large amounts of these vitamins.

Mothers have been known to endanger their children's health by giving them overdoses of vitamin drops or pills. It is more sensible to rely on a good, varied diet for your child's health and to supplement the child's diet only as your physician advises.

In rare cases in which lifestyle or unalterable habits establish a diet that is clearly deficient in vitamins, vitamin pills may be necessary. To avoid an overdose, consult a physician for advice before you begin taking any vitamin pills regularly.

VITAMIN		MAJOR SOURCES
A (retinol)		Liver, fish, oils, milk, butter, egg yolks, spinach, carrots, fortified milk and margarine.
THE B COMPLEX		
B₁ (thiamine)		Pork, liver, whole grain and enriched bread and cereal, nuts, legumes, eggs, milk.
B₂ (riboflavin)		Liver, kidney, milk, cheese, eggs, legumes, breads and cereals.
Niacin		Fish, meat, poultry, whole grain and enriched breads and cereals, eggs, peanuts.
B₆ (pyridoxine)		Most foods, especially those rich in other B vitamins.
B₁₂ (cobalamine)		Animal products only, especially liver.
Folacin (Folic acid)		Liver, fresh vegetables, wheat, eggs, legumes.
C (ascorbic acid)		Fresh vegetables and fruit, especially citrus fruits.
D (calciferol)		Liver, fish oils, butter, eggs, fortified milk and margarine. (The skin also manufactures it from sunlight.)
E (tocopherol)		In most foods, especially vegetable oils; wheatgerm; dark-green, leafy vegetables; eggs; nuts.
K		Green, leafy vegetables; vegetable oils; liver.

IMPORTANCE	DEFICIENCY PROBLEMS	PEOPLE AT GREATEST RISK
Essential for good vision, particularly at night, and for growth.	Coarse, dry skin; poor night vision. (Taking excessive amounts can lead to headaches, vomiting, enlarged liver, hair loss and skin problems.)	People with cystic fibrosis (p.685) or severe liver disease (p.485).
Assists the functioning of brain, nerves and muscles.	Cardiomyopathy (p.400), numbness of hands and feet (in the severe form, called beriberi), mental confusion.	Alcoholics.
Helps break down food to provide energy.	Cracked lips, sore tongue, skin disorders, impaired vision.	Persons with other vitamin deficiencies (poor food intake).
As in B_2. Prevents pellagra.	Sore, red, cracked skin and sore mouth, general digestive upsets, diarrhea, anxiety, or even dementia. When symptoms are severe, they are called pellagra.	Alcoholics and vagrants.
As in B_2.	Irritation of the skin and dry lips, depression, nausea.	Some women taking birth control pills.
Helps produce red blood cells. Essential for healthy nerves.	B_{12} deficiency anemia (p.420).	People with Crohn's disease (p.473), strict vegetarians.
Helps produce red blood cells.	Anemia.	Pregnant women, alcoholics
Many and varied roles in growth, health of body cells and response to infection and stress.	Small hemorrhages in the skin and other tissues, stiff limbs, bleeding gums (in the severe form, called scurvy).	Elderly people on limited diets, infants fed exclusively cow's milk.
Essential for good bone structure and normal teeth. Helps in absorption of calcium and phosphorus.	In children, rickets. In adults, osteomalacia (p.543). In old people, a tendency to bone fracture.	Breast-fed infants who do not receive a supplement or exposure to sunlight. Elderly people and others who eat poorly and are confined indoors.
Probably helps to protect cells from damage and degeneration.	Deficiency is unlikely.	None.
Essential for proper clotting of blood.	Internal and external bleeding. Deficiency in pregnant women may affect the baby.	People with fat malabsorption, severe jaundice (p.485) or cirrhosis of the liver (p.487). Anyone on long-term antibiotic therapy.

Gout

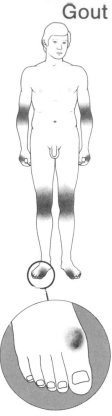

Sites of the pain

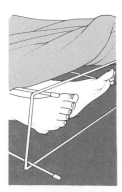

A special framework prevents sheets and blankets from pressing on a painful toe.

Uric acid, one of the body's waste products, normally passes out through the kidneys in your urine. If there is more of it than the kidneys can process, gout is a likely outcome.

In gout, uric acid accumulates and forms crystals that may lodge in areas of the body where the blood supply is too meager or sluggish to carry them away. When uric-acid crystals are caught in the spaces between one of your joints, the tissue surrounding it becomes inflamed. The inflammation irritates the nerve endings in the joint, which causes extreme pain. Sometimes the crystals also accumulate in the kidneys themselves, which may cause kidney failure.

Since all human beings produce about as much uric acid as the kidneys can handle, everyone is to some extent susceptible to gout. However, some people are more susceptible than others, for no apparent reason other than an inborn predisposition. Sometimes, however, gout develops because of an environmental factor that upsets the uric-acid balance. Such factors can include overindulgence in food or alcohol, infections, and treatment with some *antibiotics* and *diuretics*.

What are the symptoms?

The main symptom of gout is severe pain, sometimes in your elbow or knee but more often in your hand or foot, frequently at the base of your big toe. The pain usually comes without warning, though experienced sufferers may note some early twinges. Within a few hours your joint is so swollen and tender that you cannot endure even the weight of a sheet. There is often a fever of up to 101°F (about 38.5°C). The inflamed skin over the joint is likely to be red, shiny and dry.

The first attack usually involves only one joint and lasts only a few days. Sometimes there will be no more attacks, but there is usually a second, which may not occur for months or years. After the second attack, the gout occurs at shorter intervals, lasts longer, and involves more and more joints. If the disease is not treated, the inflammation of soft tissue around your joint and the irritation to the bone can lead to joint deformity. The overlying skin may degenerate, and there may be symptoms of kidney damage, such as renal colic (see Kidney stones, p.509).

Gout is a common form of joint disease. It can affect males after puberty, but women get it generally only after *menopause*, so women are less likely to be affected than men.

What are the risks?

Gout is one of the most controllable of the metabolic disorders. Left untreated, it can lead to death from kidney disease, or to high blood pressure (see p.382), a major risk factor in coronary artery disease and stroke.

What should be done?

Even though your first attack will subside on its own in a few days and there will be no immediate recurrence, consult your physician. Do not try to ease the pain with aspirin, which can slow down the excretion of uric acid. Your physician may prescribe another painkiller. Because the disease sometimes goes away permanently after a single attack, no further treatment is usually advisable at this point. But your physician will need to keep track of any subsequent attacks.

After you have had your first attack, your physician may advise you to make some changes in your eating and drinking habits. In particular, the doctor may suggest cutting down on rich foods such as red meat, sardines and anchovies. And you may need to drink less alcohol, because it, like aspirin, inhibits the excretion of uric acid. This is equally true of beer, brandy, whiskey and wine.

What is the treatment?

Self-help: To keep the weight of sheets and blankets off the painful areas, construct a protective framework (see illustration). Take no painkilling drugs other than those prescribed by your physician. Rest and abundant fluid intake can help prevent complications.
Professional help: There are three lines of treatment. The first is simply control of pain, for which your physician may prescribe an *analgesic* other than aspirin. The second treatment is control of inflammation caused by uric-acid crystals. For this your physician may prescribe an anti-inflammatory drug.

Since the symptoms may disappear after the first attack, or the disease may be dormant for months or years, your physician may not take further measures at first. If the symptoms recur, however, the disease must be attacked at its metabolic roots, and this will require the third kind of treatment. This treatment consists of taking a combination of two kinds of drugs, which you must continue to take for the rest of your life.

The first kind of drug increases the excretion of uric acid via the kidneys. Your physician may advise you to help this process by increasing your intake of non-alcoholic fluids, and perhaps by taking regular doses of sodium bicarbonate, which helps to neutralize uric acid. The second kind of drug reduces the amount of uric acid produced by your body. If you use the drugs exactly as prescribed, the disorder should not recur.

Hyperlipo-proteinemia

Hyperlipoproteinemia is the name of a wide range of disorders in which the blood contains too much fat. These maladies are sometimes called hyperlipidemia or hyperlipemia. Your body needs various kinds of lipids, or fats, as fuel, as a structural component, and, in the case of *cholesterol*, as raw material for making hormones and other vital substances. The cause of hyperlipoproteinemia is sometimes an inherited chemical defect. More often the disorder is associated with a generalized disease such as diabetes (see p.519) or hypothyroidism (see p.526) or it is simply due to an abnormal diet (or an abnormal response to a normal diet).

Research has indicated that a blood-cholesterol level of 250 milligrams (mg) per 100 milliliters (ml) poses an increased risk of coronary artery disease (see p.374). While the average level among American adults is about 200 to 230 mg per 100 ml, about 1 adult in 20 has blood-cholesterol levels above 280 mg per 100 ml.

What are the symptoms?
In most types of hyperlipoproteinemia there are no specific symptoms. In one of the hereditary types, called familial hypercholesterolemia (FH), an accumulation of lipids may form yellowish deposits beneath the skin, particularly around the elbows, in the webs of fingers, and on the Achilles tendon, above the back of the heel. FH usually affects more than one member of a family.

What are the risks?
High levels of fat in the blood are associated with developing disorders such as arteriosclerosis (see Hardening of the arteries, p.404), atherosclerosis (see p.372), heart attack (see p.379) and stroke (see p.268).

What should be done?
You are unlikely to know you are hyperlipoproteinemic unless you have a medical checkup with a blood test. If your health is good and your weight and blood pressure are normal, you probably have little reason to worry about the chemical content of your blood, unless FH runs in your family. In that case, consult your physician. Extreme forms of the disorder require medical attention.

What is the treatment?
Self-help: Your physician may suggest that you modify your diet to avoid obesity (see p.492) and to lower the concentration of fats in your blood. One of the ways to do this is to eat less saturated fat, such as that of butter, lard, most margarines and most tender meats. Use of polyunsaturated fat, which is found in the oils of sunflowers, soy beans, safflowers, and corn, seems to lower blood-fat levels. Exercise is also important in reducing blood fat levels. It appears to cause an increase in high density lipoproteins (HDL) in the blood, and these have been found to protect against coronary heart disease.
Professional help: Most often your physician will recommend a very strict diet with no fatty foods, combined with regular exercise. If the condition is secondary to another disease, it will probably respond to treatment of the underlying problem.

Porphyria

Porphyria is an inherited disease caused by an abnormality in the complex series of chemical reactions involved in your body's manufacture of the blood protein hemoglobin. As a result of this abnormality, chemicals called porphyrins accumulate in and injure the liver and digestive system, the brain and nervous system, or the skin.

What are the symptoms?
Symptoms of the disease are unlikely to appear before early adulthood. Even then they may not become apparent unless they are triggered by taking certain drugs such as barbiturates or birth control pills, drinking alcohol, becoming pregnant, or even exposing your body to sunlight. The symptoms of porphyria vary. There may be vomiting, abdominal pain, muscle cramps and weakness, psychological disorders such as manic depression (see p.298) or depression (see p.297), or skin conditions such as itching and blistering. Attacks normally subside after a few days, but some rare forms of the disease may threaten your sanity or even your life.

All forms of porphyria are notably rare. Your physician is unlikely to suspect that you have the disease unless there are known cases in your family. Chemical tests on your urine, bowel movements and blood can generally determine whether you have porphyria. Treatment is based on avoiding trigger factors and easing symptoms. The underlying metabolic abnormality cannot be corrected. You may have to avoid certain drugs, foods, or even climates. Psychiatric effects of the disorder may be minimized with tranquilizers. Women with porphyria will need advice on contraceptive methods and special care during and immediately after pregnancy.

Disorders of the urinary tract

Introduction

Your body is like a factory that contains a number of machines, all of which need energy in order to work together smoothly. The energy comes from the food you eat. The food is broken down, during digestion, into energy-containing substances that pass into your bloodstream. There, these substances circulate throughout your body and are picked up by body cells. In the cells they undergo reactions that release their energy.

As the nutrients and energy are used up, chemical waste products are produced in the cells. These wastes must be removed, because they would poison the cells if they were allowed to accumulate. The waste products are carried in your bloodstream to the two kidneys. In the kidneys they are filtered out of the blood and combined with any excess water to form urine. Thus production and excretion of urine are essential to life.

Your kidneys are situated behind your intestines and just above your waist, on either side of your spine. Each kidney contains over one million tiny filtering units called glomeruli, which remove waste material and excess water from the blood to form urine. A narrow muscular tube, the ureter, carries the slow trickle of urine from each kidney down to the bladder, a temporary storage place in the lower abdomen. From time to time the urine, expelled by the bladder, passes out of your body through another tube, the urethra. This system, from kidneys to urethra, is known as the urinary tract. It is subject to a number of disorders. Infection or inflammation of your kidneys, or even damage caused by external injury, can cause scarring of the filtering tissue. Such scarring may reduce the efficiency of the kidneys and may ultimately lead to kidney failure. Hard deposits called "stones" can form in one or in both kidneys. These stones can cause a great deal of pain as they pass down the ureters. Also, tumors can form in your urinary tract.

The structure of the urinary tract is slightly different in men and women, partly because of its close links with the reproductive system. Disorders in this section apply to both sexes. Problems specific to either men or women are covered in separate sections (see Special problems of men, p.570 and Special problems of women, p.582).

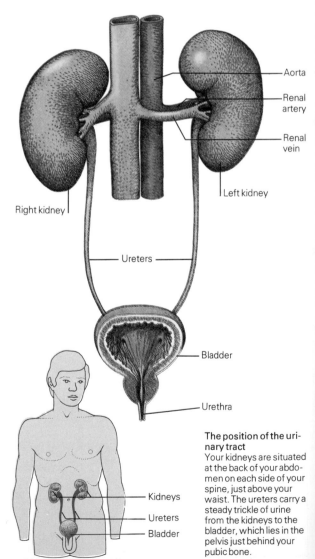

Aorta

Renal artery

Renal vein

Left kidney

Right kidney

Ureters

Bladder

Urethra

Kidneys

Ureters

Bladder

The position of the urinary tract
Your kidneys are situated at the back of your abdomen on each side of your spine, just above your waist. The ureters carry a steady trickle of urine from the kidneys to the bladder, which lies in the pelvis just behind your pubic bone.

How the kidneys function

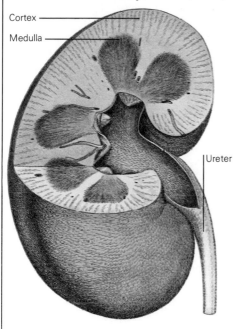

Cortex

Medulla

Ureter

Blood from the renal artery first passes through the glomeruli. These are minute, globular structures in the cortex, or outer part, of the kidney that filter a liquid containing nutrients and wastes out of the blood. The liquid then flows into the medulla, or core, of the kidney via long, thin tubes, or tubules. The tubules are surrounded by blood vessels that reabsorb the nutrients from the liquid. The blood leaves the kidneys via the renal vein and returns to general circulation. The filtered liquid, which still contains waste products from the blood, continues along the tube into the ureter and is collected in the bladder as urine.

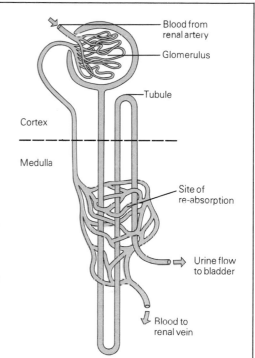

Blood from renal artery

Glomerulus

Tubule

Cortex

Medulla

Site of re-absorption

Urine flow to bladder

Blood to renal vein

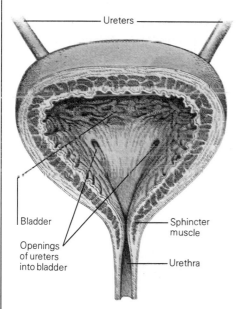

Ureters

Bladder

Openings of ureters into bladder

Sphincter muscle

Urethra

The bladder
Urine trickles down the ureters from the kidneys to the bladder. The bladder has elastic, flexible walls, which allow it to expand as it fills and then contract to expel urine when you urinate. Valves (not shown here) between the ureters and bladder prevent urine from flowing back up into the ureters.

Male and female urinary tracts
The lower part of the urinary tract is closely related to the reproductive organs, and differs in men and women. The male urethra is about 25 cm (10 in) long and provides an outlet for semen as well as urine. A woman's urethra is about 25 mm (1 in) long and lies, with the bladder, just in front of the reproductive organs. Because it is close to the anus and the entrance to the vagina, a woman's urinary tract is more susceptible to infection.

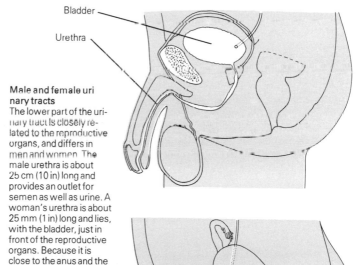

Bladder

Urethra

Ureter

Bladder

Urethra

Infections, inflammation and injury

There are no micro-organisms in a healthy urinary tract and normal urine is sterile. The urinary tract can become infected, however, and infectious agents, especially bacteria, can thrive there. These infectious agents gain access to the urinary tract from outside your body by coming up the urethra and into the bladder. They also may travel to the kidneys from another part of your body through your bloodstream. Either way, once in the urinary tract they can multiply and spread, which disrupts normal functions and causes swelling and inflammation.

Infection of the kidney itself is called pyelonephritis. This disorder can be acute, which means that it comes on quickly, or it can be chronic, in which case it recurs over many years. Infection of the bladder is called cystitis. Infection of the urethra is urethritis.

Sometimes swelling and inflammation of the kidney can occur even though there are no micro-organisms present. Glomerulonephritis, which affects the glomeruli, or minute filtering units of the kidney, is an example of this type of inflammation. Two forms of glomerulonephritis that typically affect children are described separately (see Nephrotic syndrome, p.691, and Glomerulonephritis in children, p.690).

Injury to the kidneys from a blow or wound is not common, because these organs are tucked away inside your abdomen and are protected by your rib cage. Similarly the bladder lies well protected within the pelvic, or hip, bones. So your urinary tract will probably not be damaged, except as a result of a major injury that is associated with other serious injuries and requires hospitalization.

Acute pyelonephritis

Acute pyelonephritis is the sudden development of a kidney infection. The infection and the inflammation that it causes mainly affect the tissue within which the kidney's tiny filtering units, the glomeruli, are imbedded. This occasionally occurs when infectious agents from another part of your body are carried to your kidneys in the bloodstream. In most cases, however, the infecting bacteria come from the skin around the urethral opening. Careless hygiene in this area, especially when you wipe the area after a bowel movement, can allow bacteria to enter the urethra (the tube between the bladder and the outside) and spread up through the bladder and ureter to your kidneys. This is especially likely if your normal flow of urine is partially blocked for some reason. Bacteria flourish in the resultant stagnant pool and do not wash out of the tract as easily as they do when the urine is flowing freely. Although this explains some cases of acute pyelonephritis, the disorder sometimes occurs for no apparent reason in an otherwise healthy person.

What are the symptoms?

In most cases the first symptom is sudden intense pain in your back just above your waist. Although both kidneys may be affected, the pain is usually worse on one side of your body, and it spreads around that side and down into your groin. Your temperature rises rapidly, often reaching 104°F (40°C).

This may produce chills or trembling, and may be accompanied by nausea and vomiting. You may also experience dysuria, or difficult or painful urination, and you are likely to feel that you need to urinate constantly, even when your bladder is empty. The urine itself is usually cloudy and may be light red if blood has leaked into it.

What are the risks?

Acute pyelonephritis is a common condition, particularly in women. This is because the tube through which bacteria may enter the urinary tract, the urethra, is generally shorter in women. Various conditions that reduce the flow of urine make you more susceptible. These include pregnancy (because of pressure on the ureters from the swelling uterus), kidney stones (see p.509), a tumor of the bladder (see p.508), or an enlarged prostate gland (see p.574).

With prompt treatment complications are unlikely. In an extremely young or frail person the infection may spread into the blood and lead to blood poisoning (see p.421). If you have repeated attacks of acute pyelonephritis, however, you may have a problem in your urinary tract that needs to be corrected.

What should be done?

If you have the symptoms of this disorder, consult your physician. In many cases only *antibiotics* and bed rest are needed, and the attack may subside in a day or two. After you recover, your physician may want you to have blood and urine tests, an *X-ray* of your kidneys, called an *intravenous pyelogram* (*IVP*), and *cystoscopy* for your bladder.

If you are a healthy adult, such diagnostic tests are seldom required after a single attack of acute pyelonephritis. However, for children or for persons who have had previous attacks, tests are usually advised in order to identify any underlying problems and prevent long-term damage to the kidneys (see Urinary infections in children, p.689).

What is the treatment?

The treatment for acute pyelonephritis is bed rest and a light, bland diet that includes extra fluids, particularly large quantities of water. In addition, your physician will probably prescribe *antibiotics*, which you can usually take by mouth. If you are very young or very frail, however, you may have to be hospitalized so that drugs and extra fluids can be given *intravenously*. Antibiotics generally bring the infection under control in 24 to 48 hours, although treatment may continue for 14 days, or longer in some cases.

Chronic pyelonephritis

Chronic pyelonephritis is a condition in which, over the course of many years, your kidneys become increasingly damaged by repeated, often unnoticed, infections of the urine. In most cases the condition probably starts in childhood and persists unsuspected into adulthood. Years later, symptoms of kidney trouble appear (see Urinary infections in children, p.689).

The infecting bacteria probably gain access to the urinary tract through the open end of the urethra, the tube that leads from the bladder to the outside. Usually, such invasions are confined to the lower parts of the urinary tract (see Cystitis, p.505), since the outflow of urine keeps the infection from spreading upwards. When you urinate, your bladder contracts, and squeezes urine out and down the urethra.

At the same time, the bladder muscle acts as a valve and closes off the two ureters where they enter the bladder. This prevents urine from being forced back into the kidneys. Sometimes, however, this valve-like action does not work properly, and urine flows upwards as well as downwards. This two-way flow is known as reflux. If this happens with infected urine, the infection may reach the kidneys. A combination of recurring infections and reflux is probably the cause of most chronic pyelonephritis.

Kidney stones (see p.509) may also cause the disorder. Chronic pyelonephritis may be preceded by repeated attacks of other urinary tract infections such as acute pyelonephritis or cystitis, but this is rare.

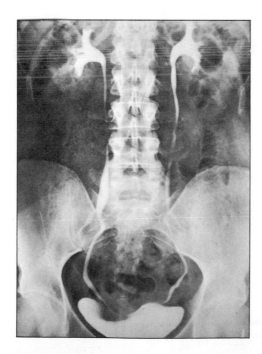

Intravenous pyelogram
An intravenous pyelogram (also known as an excretion urogram) provides a series of X-rays of the whole urinary tract. A special liquid that shows up on X-ray pictures is injected into your bloodstream. It travels around your body until it reaches the kidneys, where it becomes part of the urine. The process takes several hours and X-ray pictures are taken intermittently.

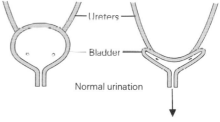

Normal urination

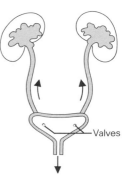

Infected urine in the kidneys
A possible cause of kidney infection is inefficiency of the valves that connect the ureters and the bladder. If these valves do not close properly when you urinate, urine may be squeezed back up the ureters. Any infection in the urine can then travel up to the kidneys.

Backflow of urine

What are the symptoms?

Chronic pyelonephritis seldom produces symptoms until the condition is well established. Eventually, though, early signs of chronic kidney failure (see p.512), also called uremic poisoning, may appear, and fatigue, nausea, or itching skin may become increasingly apparent.

In many cases the condition is discovered at a much earlier stage of its development through a blood or urine test that is given for some other reason.

What are the risks?

The main risk of chronic pyelonephritis is that the condition may develop undetected until it produces chronic kidney failure. This does not often happen today, however, since there is now more preventive treatment available for urinary infections in young children (see p.689).

What should be done?

If you have repeated mild urinary infections or any of the symptoms of chronic kidney failure, be sure to consult your physician. The diagnostic tests are generally the same as those for acute pyelonephritis. They may include blood and urine tests, an *intravenous pyelogram (IVP)*, and *cystoscopy*.

What is the treatment?

Self-help: If you discover that you have chronic pyelonephritis, but you have no symptoms, your physician may advise you to drink plenty of fluids and avoid large quantities of protein and salt. The doctor may also suggest that you have blood tests every 6 to 12 months to check on the disorder.

Professional help: Treatment depends on what stage the disease has reached when it is discovered. Although surgery to repair the faulty valve mechanism in the bladder is sometimes necessary in a child, it is not generally helpful for an adult. Any other cause of repeated infections, such as kidney stones, may respond to appropriate treatment for that condition. Otherwise, you will probably be given a prescription for an *antibiotic*. These are usually given for a short period whenever you have a urinary tract infection. Sometimes, however, the physician will prescribe a low dose of an antibiotic for six months to two years, in an attempt to keep your urine free of bacteria. Because of the sometimes slow progress of chronic pyelonephritis, some physicians will not attempt special treatment of the disorder if you are middle-aged. Instead, your physician may advise you to be alert for subsequent kidney trouble and have regular checkups.

Glomerulo-nephritis

Glomerulonephritis is the term used for several related diseases that damage the glomeruli, tiny filtering units in your kidneys. The damage is usually the result of inflammation caused by abnormal proteins that become trapped in the glomeruli.

In a healthy kidney, the blood passes through the glomeruli, and certain chemicals, not all of them waste products, are filtered out. Most of the water and certain chemicals such as glucose that are useful to the body are then returned to your bloodstream. The remaining waste materials are collected as urine and pass down the ureter to your bladder for storage until you urinate.

In glomerulonephritis, this process is adversely affected by the damaged glomeruli. Usually the most obvious disturbance is that red blood cells somehow leak through the glomeruli into your urine. Some proteins also pass from your blood into your urine. If this loss is excessive, and this occurs most often in children, it causes an illness called nephrotic syndrome (see p.691). If more and more of the glomeruli are damaged, the affected kidneys become less and less efficient as a filter and regulator of the chemical content of your blood. Waste products accumulate and cause kidney failure (see p.511).

Glomerulonephritis can occur in mild or severe forms. It may be acute, flaring up over a few days, or it may be chronic, taking months or years to develop.

What are the symptoms?

The mildest forms of chronic glomerulonephritis produce no symptoms at all. Your physician may notice the condition only when a sample of your urine is tested for some other reason. In other cases, your urine may have a smoky appearance, which is caused by the presence of small amounts of blood, or it may be bright red, which indicates larger amounts of blood.

In severe forms of acute glomerulonephritis you may feel generally unwell, with drowsiness, nausea, and vomiting. These are symptoms of impending kidney failure. You will probably produce very small amounts of urine, and fluid may accumulate in your body tissues. This is called edema; you may notice it as puffiness under your skin, particularly around your ankles. If fluid accumulates in your chest, you may become short of breath.

What are the risks?

Glomerulonephritis is not common in adults, but approximately 60 per cent of people who have end-stage kidney failure (see p.513) had chronic glomerulonephritis initially. The acute form is most common in children (see p.690).

The greatest risk of all forms of glomerulonephritis is that they may lead to chronic kidney failure. The disorder can also lead to high blood pressure (see p.382), since your kidneys play a central part in the regulation of blood pressure.

What should be done?

If you have any of the symptoms that are characteristic of glomerulonephritis, consult your physician, who will arrange for a urine test. If this suggests that you may have glomerulonephritis, you may be admitted to a hospital for a few days for further tests. These tests may include an *intravenous pyelogram* (*IVP*) and possibly a *biopsy*, in which a small piece of one of your kidneys will be removed and carefully examined.

What is the treatment?

Many forms of glomerulonephritis are so mild that they require no specific treatment. Other forms can be treated with *steroid* drugs and/or *cytotoxic* drugs.

If you have edema, *diuretics*, which increase the amount and frequency of urination, may be prescribed. If you have high blood pressure, that must also be treated, and you may need iron and vitamin tablets if you have become anemic as a result of this disorder. If glomerulonephritis leads to end-stage kidney failure, treatment is as described for that disorder (see p.513).

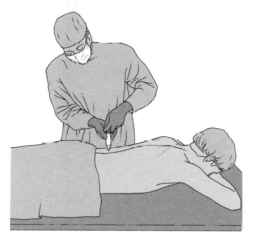

Kidney biopsy
In a kidney biopsy, a small area of skin and muscle overlying the kidney is first numbed with a local anesthetic. The doctor then passes a hollow needle through the numbed area into the kidney, and withdraws a tiny sample of kidney tissue for laboratory analysis.

Urethritis

Inflammation of the urethra, the tube that leads from the bladder to the outside, is known as urethritis. It is through this tube that urine passes to the outside. Typical symptoms of urethritis include pain in the urethral area, frequent urination and a discharge from the opening to the outside. In women, urethritis is usually the result of some bruising during sexual intercourse (see Chronic urethritis, p.601). Urethritis in males is generally caused by sexually transmitted disease (see Urethritis in men, p.578). The two most important sexually transmitted diseases that can bring on urethritis are so-called non-specific urethritis (see p.612) and gonorrhea (see p.611).

Cystitis

Cystitis is caused by a urinary infection that leads to inflammation of the bladder. The bladder is the temporary storage area for urine. The urine is released regularly from the bladder to the urethra, the tube through which the urine flows to the outside. The disorder is far more common in women than in men, because a woman's urethra is shorter, making it easier for infectious agents that enter it from the outside to reach the bladder. Cystitis rarely occurs in men unless an enlarged prostate gland or other urinary tract abnormality is present.

What are the symptoms?

The major symptom in both sexes is a frequent urge to urinate, with only a small amount of a sometimes strong-smelling, and possibly bloody, fluid emerging each time. The urine is likely to burn or sting as you pass it, and you may have a feeling of discomfort just below your navel, which is where your bladder is located. You may also have a fever.

What is the treatment?

Drinking large quantities of water will help relieve the symptoms, but you should also consult your physician, who will probably prescribe *antibiotics*. This should quickly clear up the symptoms, but you should take the medication until your physician tells you to stop. For further information, read the articles on cystitis in women (see p.600) and urinary infections in children (see p.689).

Injury to kidneys or ureters

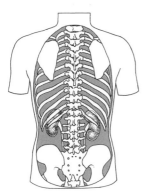

Your kidneys are well protected by your ribcage and back muscles.

The most likely cause of injury to kidneys or ureters, the tubes that carry urine from your kidneys to your bladder, is either a direct blow to the side of the body just under the ribs (from a football tackle or block, perhaps), or a crushing force (from being trapped under fallen masonry, for example). Another possible cause is penetration by a knife or bullet. In any of these cases, a kidney may be bruised or its membranous outer envelope and/or a ureter may be torn. Sometimes a large blood clot forms under the envelope and produces a lump over the kidney that can be felt through your skin. It is also possible for blood or urine to leak into your abdomen through a tear, which may cause peritonitis (see p.470).

What are the symptoms?
A mild injury to a kidney or ureter may cause pain and tenderness in the lower part of your back. You may also have a slight fever, and possibly intermittent traces of blood in your urine. You may not notice the blood until a day or two after the injury has occurred. If you have severe pain and large amounts of blood in your urine, one or both of your kidneys, and possibly the ureters, may have been seriously injured. If you have these symptoms, you should consult your physi-

cian. In particular, bloody urine is a symptom of several potentially serious conditions and should not be ignored. You will probably need to undergo an X-ray of the kidneys called an *intravenous pyelogram* (*IVP*), so your physician can assess the damage and determine whether treatment is necessary.

What is the treatment?
The ability of kidneys and ureters to heal themselves is remarkable. Even major tears and injuries seldom require treatment other than seven to ten days of rest. Unless the IVP shows that the injury is very slight, however, it is usually advisable for you to take that short rest in the hospital, where painkillers can be administered and your pulse and blood pressure can be checked frequently to see if you have serious internal bleeding. About three months after you leave the hospital, your physician will probably advise you to have another IVP to make sure there has been no permanent damage.

In the unlikely event that your kidney or ureter does not heal after a week or so of bed rest, it may be necessary to remove the kidney or repair the torn ureter surgically. Removal of a kidney is not usually a complicated operation, and you can lead a healthy, normal life with only one kidney.

Injury to bladder or urethra

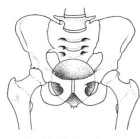

Your bladder is well protected by the circle of bones that form your pelvis.

Because the bladder, where urine is temporarily stored, lies within the abdomen, it is usually protected against injury. When damage does occur, it is generally due to a direct blow to your pelvis that fractures a pelvic bone, and causes a sharp fragment of the bone to pierce the bladder wall. Any such rupture is bound to have serious consequences because it allows urine to leak into the abdominal cavity. Rupture of the urethra, the tube that carries urine from the bladder to the outside, in men is more common but less dangerous. It can be caused by a fall or any kind of impact in the groin. Because the female urethra is very short, urethral damage is rare in women.

What are the symptoms?
If your bladder is ruptured you will have severe pain in your abdomen, and you may also show signs of shock (see p.386). A urethral injury is also extremely painful and is generally followed by an inability to urinate. Sometimes there is bloody discharge.

What are the risks?
Rupture of the bladder is dangerous because

urine leaks into the abdominal cavity and causes peritonitis (see p.470). This condition requires prompt, specialized treatment in a hospital. Damage to the urethra, on the other hand, is unlikely to lead to peritonitis. For a man, the chief risk is that the healed urethra will be scarred, causing stricture (see p.578).

If you have had an accident and you have any of the symptoms of a ruptured bladder or urethra, consult your physician immediately. A physical examination, and possibly a special X-ray of the bladder and *cystoscopy*, should allow a diagnosis.

What is the treatment?
If you injure your bladder or urethra, you will have to be hospitalized. You will probably be given *antibiotics* to prevent infection. If your bladder is ruptured, you will also need an urgent operation to repair the leak and clean out your abdominal cavity. If your urethra is damaged, you will probably have to be *catheterized*, or have a tube inserted into your bladder, for several days so that urine can drain out. Meanwhile, the urethra will usually heal of its own accord. Occasionally, however, surgery is necessary.

Cysts, tumors and stones

A growth or swelling anywhere in your body should be investigated by a physician, and the urinary tract is certainly no exception. The tract can be affected by three kinds of growths. They are cysts, tumors and stones. Cysts are usually soft, fluid-filled sacs, and tumors are more solid. Both cysts and tumors may be either *benign* (unlikely to spread) or, much less often, *malignant* (likely to spread and threaten life). Cysts and tumors are relatively uncommon in the urinary tract. The third type of growth, pebble-like kidney and bladder stones (calculi), are more commonly encountered. Although such stones may cause a lot of discomfort, they are rarely a serious threat to life.

Kidney cysts

There are two types of kidney cyst. The first is a single fluid-filled sac that develops in a kidney for no known reason. This type of cyst may slowly grow bigger over the years, but it is unlikely to cause trouble unless a cancer forms in its wall. This rarely happens. The other type of cyst is caused by an inherited disorder called polycystic disease, which is *congenital*, or present at birth. In this disorder, many cysts of varying sizes develop in both kidneys. Polycystic disease usually is not destructive and generally does not cause major problems.

What are the symptoms?
A single cyst produces no symptoms unless it becomes large enough to cause pain in the lower part of your back. In this case, you may occasionally be able to feel the soft lump in your abdomen with your fingers. Polycystic disease occasionally causes *hematuria* (blood in the urine) or repeated attacks of pyelonephritis (see p.503). Most often, though, it is symptomless unless cysts eventually replace so much normal kidney substance that you develop chronic kidney failure (see p.512). At that point, symptoms of the latter disorder will begin to appear.

The presence of kidney cysts is often discovered only when your kidneys are examined for some other reason. Many people have such cysts without knowing it. Severe polycystic disease is extremely rare, however. In the United States it causes about two per cent of all cases of chronic kidney failure.

What are the risks?
The only risk of a solitary cyst is that a malignancy may develop, and this rarely happens. Polycystic disease may lead to chronic kidney failure, but this, too, seldom occurs.

What should be done?
If you have a single kidney cyst, it will probably be discovered only when tests are done for another reason. Because of the slight possibility of cancerous cells in the cyst, your physician may want to give you further tests, such as an *ultrasound* study, or even a cyst *aspiration*, which involves piercing the cyst with a needle and withdrawing some fluid for examination. Aspiration of a kidney cyst can usually be done painlessly with a local anesthetic. If the examination of the cells in the fluid shows that they are normal, nothing further needs to be done, unless the cyst enlarges enough to cause either kidney damage or extreme discomfort.

Your physician may discover that you have polycystic disease by chance when testing you for a different disorder. But if you know the disease runs in your family, you and your family should consult a doctor about it. To prevent possible problems in the future, you should have regular checkups. Even if you feel fine when these checkups are due, be sure to go anyway, because if a cyst develops, it is best to be aware of it at an early stage.

What is the treatment?
No treatment is required for a painless, benign kidney cyst. If it becomes large enough to be painful, however, or if it is found to be malignant, surgery to remove the affected kidney will probably be necessary. Removal of one of your kidneys is usually a simple operation, and you can rest assured that you can lead a normal, healthy life with only the remaining kidney. This is true because one healthy kidney can easily take over all the work that was formerly done by two.

There is no specific treatment for polycystic disease. If cysts are discovered at an early stage, and you have regular medical checkups thereafter, your physician may be able to help you slow down the progressive damage to your kidneys in the same way as for chronic kidney failure (see p.512).

Tumors of the kidney

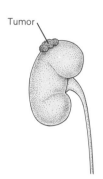

Growths on the kidney tend to be situated near the top, where they are hidden within the rib-cage. Routine examinations may not detect such a growth.

There are two major types of tumor of the kidney, both of which are *malignant* (or likely to spread and threaten life), but only one of which occurs in adults. This type, known as hypernephroma, or clear-cell carcinoma, forms on the edge of your kidney as a result of the uncontrolled multiplication of an abnormal cell. As the tumor grows, it eats into healthy kidney tissue, but because the efficiency of the kidney as a filter is affected only at a very late stage in the disease, eventual kidney failure (see p.511) is rare. The tumor more often makes itself known by causing generalized symptoms such as persistent fever, loss of appetite and weight loss. There may also be vomiting and mild abdominal pain, and your urine may be red or smoky because of bleeding from the tumor.

Hypernephromas are rare; they occur most often in men over 40, and they account for only a small percentage of all deaths from cancer. The other main type of kidney tumor, which affects only children, is called Wilm's tumor (see p.692).

What are the risks?

The main risk of a hypernephroma is that some of the tumor cells may break off into the bloodstream and spread to other parts of your body, particularly the lungs or bones.

However, hypernephromas spread less rapidly than many other types of cancerous growth, and permanent cure is usually achieved if the tumor is discovered and removed at an early stage.

What should be done?

If you have symptoms suggesting that you may have a kidney tumor, and especially if your urine looks reddish or abnormally cloudy, consult your physician, who will probably want samples of your urine for laboratory analysis. If a tumor is suspected, you will then need to undergo a series of diagnostic tests, including an *intravenous pyelogram* (*IVP*), an *ultrasound scan*, and an *angiogram* of the kidney. These tests are usually done during a short hospital stay.

What is the treatment?

If tests show the presence of a hypernephroma, the affected kidney will have to be removed surgically. However, one healthy kidney can generally compensate for the loss of the other. *Radiation therapy* and anticancer (*cytotoxic*) drugs may also be advisable to kill off any remaining cancer cells. Following this treatment, you should have regular checkups for at least five years, to make sure that cancer does not recur.

Tumors of the bladder

Tumors of the urinary bladder, like those in many other parts of your body, can be either *benign* (unlikely to spread) or *malignant* (likely to spread and threaten life). Both types originate from cells that line the bladder, and they tend to produce a growth (or, rarely, more than one) that projects inward, into the space that contains the urine. In addition, malignant tumors spread within the walls of the bladder and may, in rare cases, spread to other parts of your body. Any type of tumor near the place where the ureter, the tube that carries urine from the kidney to the bladder, enters the bladder, can block the flow of urine and cause the kidney to swell with urine. This is hydronephrosis. It damages the kidney and makes it susceptible to infection (see Acute pyelonephritis, p.502).

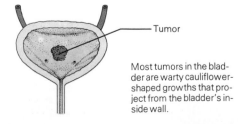

Most tumors in the bladder are warty cauliflower-shaped growths that project from the bladder's inside wall.

What are the symptoms?

The characteristic symptom of a bladder tumor is *hematuria*, or blood in the urine. The act of urinating is not usually painful, but you may have a burning feeling, and a tendency to urinate small amounts at frequent intervals. If hydronephrosis has developed, you may also have pain in the small of your back. Also, since a bladder with a tumor is especially susceptible to infection, you may have cystitis and its symptoms (see p.505).

What are the risks?

Tumors of the bladder are not common, but the disorder is most common in men over 50. A benign tumor of the bladder is easily treated. A malignant one, however, may damage a large portion of bladder tissue. If the cancerous cells spread to other parts of the body, prospects for successful treatment are not good.

What should be done?

Always consult your physician if you see blood in your urine. The doctor will take urine and blood samples for analysis, and, depending on the results, you may need to undergo other diagnostic tests. These may include *cystoscopy*, an *intravenous pyelogram* (*IVP*), or a *cystogram*. If a growth is discovered, you will probably need a *biopsy*, in which a small sample of the growth is removed and examined carefully to determine whether it is benign or malignant.

What is the treatment?

The usual treatment for all bladder tumors is to try to destroy them by burning them away with a special instrument similar to a cystoscope. This process is known as *fulguration*. The surgeon views your bladder through a system of lenses and manipulates the instru-

ment to destroy the cells. This usually clears up the problem, but you will need semiannual checkups for at least three years to make sure that the tumor does not recur.

If a tumor has affected a large area of your bladder, abdominal surgery may be necessary. In severe cases the whole bladder may have to be removed, and the ureters will then be connected to a specially made opening in the abdominal wall. Thereafter, the urine will flow into a bag (an "external bladder"), which must be emptied periodically. This is a safe and unobtrusive process. After surgery, you may need *radiation therapy* to destroy any remaining abnormal cells.

Kidney stones
(renal calculi)

The kidneys are among several organs in your body where stones are apt to form. A kidney stone normally begins as a tiny speck of solid material deposited in the middle of your kidney, where urine collects before flowing into the ureter. As more material clings to the first speck, it gradually builds into a solid object. This process can occur in one or both kidneys. Over a period of years, a stone 25 mm (1 in) or more in diameter can develop. Since most kidney stones contain calcium, it seems likely that stone formation is usually caused by an excessive amount of calcium in the urine.

Any stone with a diameter of more than about 5 mm ($\frac{1}{5}$ in) is likely to remain in your kidney, because it is too large to pass into the ureter. Such trapped stones may not be a problem if only a few are formed. Also, very

Pain from kidney stones
A kidney stone can cause severe pain (renal colic) as it travels from the kidney to the bladder. This may take several days. The location of the pain indicates the position of the stone.

— Kidney
— Ureter

— Stone traveling along ureter

— Bladder

Site of the pain

small stones seldom cause problems, since they are easily carried into the ureter and passed in the urine. A larger stone, however, may cause pain if and when it enters the ureter with urine bound for the bladder.

What are the symptoms?

If stones are too big to pass from the kidney into the ureter, you may have no symptoms or, at most, occasional mild pain as small pieces break off and are carried down the ureter. The most common symptom of troublesome kidney stones is called *colic*. This is a stabbing pain that tends to come in waves, often a few minutes apart. Colic can be caused by disorders in various parts of the body, including gallstones (see p.489) and intestinal obstruction (see p.471). Typically, it makes you "double up" with pain. Kidney pain of this type, called renal colic, can occur when a stone passes from a kidney down one of the ureters. It will subside whenever the stone stops moving or is discharged in the urine. The pain almost always occurs on one side of your body at a time, but if you have stones in both kidneys, a subsequent attack may be on the other side.

Renal colic is usually felt first in the back, just below the ribs on either side of the spinal column. Over a period of hours or days, the pain follows the course of the stone as it travels along the ureter, around to the front of the body, and down towards the groin. It may make you feel nauseous, and there may be traces of blood in your urine. After the stone reaches your bladder, it will probably pass through the remainder of the urinary tract with little or no pain (see also Bladder stones, next article).

What are the risks?

Because passage of a kidney stone often produces severe pain, the disorder is a frequent cause of hospital admissions. Fortunately, there is some evidence that the incidence of kidney stones in the Western world is declining. This may be partly because of changes in diet and lifestyle. It is known that the problem runs in families, and it is more common in hot climates. In very warm weather, people lose a great deal of body water in sweat, and they tend to produce less urine. But this urine contains a higher concentration of stone-forming calcium than it would if there was a greater volume of it.

Men seem to be more susceptible than women to the disorder, and people over 30 are more susceptible than younger people. In rare cases, children may develop a form of kidney stone that is due to a chemical abnormality in the blood.

Although most kidney stones either remain harmlessly in the kidneys or are eventually passed in the urine, an occasional stone may get stuck in a ureter and block the flow of urine on one side. Surgery is then required. Kidney stones also make you more susceptible to infections in the urine and, consequently, to attacks of acute pyelonephritis (see p.502). As a result of repeated infections, and sometimes scarring from large stones, chronic kidney failure (see p.512) may follow long-standing kidney stone disease, but this very rarely happens.

What should be done?

If you tend to suffer from kidney stones, see your physician at six-month intervals to make sure there is no permanent damage to your kidneys. If you have an attack of renal colic, your doctor will probably refer you to a hospital for blood and urine tests and an *intravenous pyelogram* (*IVP*). Such diagnostic tests will help locate stones, if there are any, and also will indicate whether further treatment is necessary.

What is the treatment?

Self-help: It is always wisest to consult your physician if you have an attack of renal colic. But you should also drink large quantities of water – at least eight to ten eight-ounce glasses a day. This should help flush any stones you may have through your urinary tract and help prevent other stones from forming. To relieve pain, you should take a mild *analgesic* such as aspirin or a stronger medication if your doctor prescribes one.

Professional help: There is no satisfactory medical treatment for kidney stones that do not pass of their own accord. However, if your body forms stones made of uric acid because you have a metabolic disorder, your physician may prescribe drugs that can prevent stones from forming in some cases. If a stone causes a blockage in the lower third of your ureter, it can sometimes be removed by manipulation during cystoscopy, using specially designed instruments. You will be anesthetized for this procedure. The physician inserts the instrument through the cystoscope, into the bladder, and up into the ureter where the stone is trapped. When the instrument is withdrawn, the stone will probably come out with it. If this procedure cannot be done, a major abdominal operation may be necessary to remove the stone.

In the unlikely event that stones have done irreparable damage to one of your kidneys, the entire kidney may have to be removed. Should this be done, your other kidney will easily take over the work of two.

In general, however, kidney stones are merely an inconvenience, though at times a very painful one.

Bladder stones
(Vesical calculi)

A kidney stone (see previous article) that has come, perhaps painfully, through the ureter (the tube that connects kidney and bladder) into your bladder will be relatively small. For this reason it can pass out of your body in the urine with comparative ease. Stones that form within the bladder itself, however, tend to be bigger than kidney stones and may remain lodged in your bladder. This may cause troublesome symptoms such as an over-frequent urge to urinate, pain when you pass urine, and blood in your urine. Often the blood seems to be "squeezed out" in the last few drops. Today, however, bladder stones are not a common problem. They are, in fact, becoming increasingly uncommon for no known reason.

If you have bladder stones that are too large to pass naturally through the urethra,

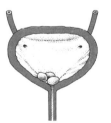

Bladder stones tend to collect at the bottom of the bladder near the urethra.

the tube that connects your bladder to the outside, they must be removed. This can sometimes be done, under a general anesthetic, by inserting a *cystoscope* up the urethra and into the bladder. The cystoscope is equipped with a device that can either draw out the stones or crush them into tiny pieces that can be washed out. In an alternative minor operation, the surgeon opens the bladder to remove the stone or stones.

Kidney failure

Kidney failure, also called renal failure, occurs in one of three forms. Acute failure is an illness in which your kidneys suddenly stop functioning, sometimes within a few days or even hours. Chronic failure could be called chronic impairment, since this condition develops over many years and may never result in actual failure. End-stage failure is the most severe kidney disorder. In this condition your kidneys function so poorly that they can no longer sustain life without the assistance of an artificial kidney machine.

Acute kidney failure

Your kidneys may suddenly stop working for any of a number of reasons. Broadly speaking, however, there are three main causes. A disease such as acute glomerulonephritis (see p.504) can abruptly damage the kidneys enough to cause their failure. A sudden drop in blood pressure, which can occur after severe bleeding or a major heart attack, can lead to an inadequate supply of blood, and thus damage the kidneys. Finally, the flow of urine may be suddenly and completely obstructed by a blockage that occurs in another part of the urinary tract (the ureters, bladder, or urethra).

As a consequence of any of these malfunctions, your kidneys cannot produce urine, and so waste products build up in your blood. Water can no longer be effectively removed from your body, and this also accumulates. Lastly, there is a dangerous imbalance of the chemicals whose concentrations are normally regulated by the kidneys.

Mild attacks of acute kidney failure are fairly common, but the more serious forms (those due to glomerulonephritis, for instance) are extremely rare.

What are the symptoms?
The most notable symptom is that you pass less urine than usual, possibly less than 0.5 liters (less than a pint) a day. Within a short time you lose your appetite, feel increasingly nauseated, and begin to vomit. If treatment is delayed, drowsiness, confusion, convulsions and coma may develop. In most cases, however, symptoms of the condition that has caused the acute kidney failure are more apparent at first than those that are due to the kidney failure itself.

What are the risks?
Much depends on the severity of the underlying problem, but acute kidney failure is a potentially dangerous condition. Even treatment with an artificial kidney machine does not always lead to recovery.

What should be done?
If you have acute kidney failure, you urgently need hospital treatment, preferably in a hospital that has a special unit to treat kidney diseases. If the cause is not obvious, you will probably have to undergo an intensive series of diagnostic tests involving blood and urine samples, an *intravenous pyelogram* (*IVP*) and possibly a *biopsy*, in which a small piece of the kidney is removed for examination.

What is the treatment?
When the cause of acute kidney failure is heavy bleeding or a heart attack, emergency treatment is usually required. The form of treatment depends on the circumstances. If the diagnostic tests show that the cause is an obstruction, you will probably need an abdominal operation to relieve the blockage. If the underlying cause is a disease of the kidneys themselves, or if, as often happens, the kidneys remain severely affected even though the basic cause of failure is successfully treated, treatment procedures vary.

An *intravenous drip* of blood or plasma, possibly with a *diuretic* drug, which increases urination, included in it, may be all that is needed to restore your kidneys to their normal function. In some instances, such as cases of acute glomerulonephritis, treatment with specific drugs may be effective. But in other cases, your physician may have to use an artificial device that performs the functions of your kidneys until they recover of their own accord. This type of treatment is called dialysis (see Artificial kidney aids, next page). Dialysis is painless, but if you have acute kidney failure you may have to stay in the hospital for several weeks before your kidneys function normally again.

While you are under treatment, you may need a special diet that is high in calories but low in protein, and may include no more than 600 ml (a pint) of fluid a day. This type of diet gives your kidneys (or the substitute machine) a minimal amount of work to do.

Chronic kidney failure

In chronic kidney failure, mild, repeated attacks of inflammation injure and scar the kidneys. This reduces their effectiveness. The inflammation may be caused by various diseases, including chronic pyelonephritis (see p.503) and glomerulonephritis (see p.504). Persistent conditions such as kidney stones (see p.509), hypertension (see High blood pressure, p.382), and an extremely rare disorder, analgesic nephropathy (see Painkillers can cause kidney failure, next page) also may cause inflammation. If you suffer from chronic kidney failure, waste products and chemicals gradually build up in your blood, your kidneys become increasingly unable to limit the amount of water in your urine, and you are likely to become hypertensive. One function of the kidneys is control of blood pressure. Hypertension can therefore be both a cause and a result of chronic kidney failure.

What are the symptoms?

Symptoms appear gradually and you may not have any for many years. Then you may notice that you are urinating more often than you used to. This is because your urine contains relatively few waste products and an abnormally large quantity of water. You may also feel progressively more tired and lethargic. If your chronic kidney failure continues to worsen, you will get the symptoms of end-stage kidney failure (see next article).

The main risk of the disorder is that the scarring in your kidneys will become progressively worse and lead to end-stage kidney failure. This happens in three out of four

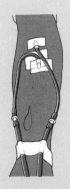

Artificial kidney aids

If your kidneys are temporarily unable to function, or if they have become badly damaged by long-standing inflammation, you will probably receive a type of treatment called *dialysis*. In dialysis the functions of the kidneys, which include removing waste products from your body and regulating the chemical and water balance, are taken over by a machine.

There are two forms of dialysis. The first, peritoneal dialysis, is carried out in the hospital. Your physician makes a small incision in your abdominal wall and threads a thin plastic tube through into the abdomen. A special fluid flows slowly through the tube and fills the peritoneal space (the space between the inner and outer layers of the sac lining the abdominal walls). Waste products seep from the abdomen into the fluid, which is then sucked out along with excess water. The process goes on continuously, sometimes for many hours.

Peritoneal dialysis is a painless procedure, though the tube may be a little uncomfortable. If you have acute kidney failure, you will gradually be weaned off the treatment as your kidneys recover. This usually takes about six weeks.

The second form of dialysis, hemodialysis, is done with what is popularly called a "kidney machine." The machine filters waste products from your blood. To do this, blood from an arm or leg artery is passed along a thin tube to the machine, through its filter, and back along another tube into an adjacent vein. A slow flow of blood trickling through the machine for six to eight hours, repeated two or three times every week, is enough to control levels of waste products and water in your body.

Everyone who begins hemodialysis treatment must first have a minor operation to enlarge a vein. Thereafter, you can insert the two needles at the start of each treatment without medical supervision. Indeed, some people have a machine at home, connect themselves up in the late evening, sleep through the night while the machine works, and disconnect themselves in the morning. This permits full daytime freedom.

It is natural to be worried at first when you realize that your life must depend on a machine. However, as most dialysis patients quickly learn how to insert the needles and run the machine, their anxiety decreases.

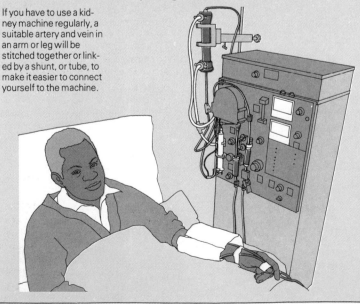

If you have to use a kidney machine regularly, a suitable artery and vein in an arm or leg will be stitched together or linked by a shunt, or tube, to make it easier to connect yourself to the machine.

Painkillers can cause kidney failure!
A word of warning: Excessive consumption of certain *analgesics*, or painkillers, can lead to a rare disease, analgesic nephropathy, which sometimes culminates in chronic kidney failure. It is not easy to develop analgesic nephropathy. You have to take nearly a dozen analgesic pills every day for several years. The preparations most likely to cause the disease are those in which several drugs are combined in a single tablet that you can buy without a prescription, such as pain-relief combinations containing a medication called phenacetin. To help avoid problems, you should discuss with your physician any use of painkilling medications, especially combination drugs.

cases. There are also the risks associated with hypertension (see p.382), and with anemia (see p.419), osteomalacia (see p.543), and hyperparathyroidism (see p.528). These last three diseases sometimes occur as a result of the ailing kidneys' inability to control the levels of blood chemicals.

What should be done?

If you find that you have to urinate with abnormal frequency and that the problem continues for more than a week without apparent cause, consult your physician, who will probably first check your blood pressure. Although most people with high blood pressure do not have a kidney problem, the combination of frequent urination and high blood pressure will suggest the possibility, especially if there is a history of kidney trouble in your family. You will then probably need to undergo blood and urine tests and another test called an *intravenous pyelogram (IVP)*.

What is the treatment?

Self-help: Be sure to follow your physician's

advice about diet. If you have kidney failure your doctor will probably advise you to eat low protein foods (see Acute kidney failure, previous article) and to drink several pints of fluid a day. Take no medicines at all without first consulting your physician about any possible danger. Also, it is important to have regular medical checkups, even if you feel well. This will allow you to become aware of and discuss any problems with your physician at an early stage, and your physician can then modify your treatment as necessary.

Professional help: No treatment can reverse the progress of chronic kidney failure, but close medical supervision can sometimes help to slow it down and counteract troublesome symptoms. Your physician may prescribe iron and vitamin pills and drugs to control your blood pressure. To prevent the development of osteomalacia, you may also need to take other supplements. With regular checkups, a carefully guided diet, and the drugs your physician prescribes for your particular problems, you should lead a comfortable life despite your kidney problem.

End-stage kidney failure

End-stage kidney failure is the most advanced form of kidney failure. It usually occurs because, despite treatment, chronic kidney failure (see previous article) progresses to the point where your kidneys can no longer sustain life. An event such as a urinary infection (see Acute pyelonephritis, p.502) often tips the balance between chronic failure and end-stage failure.

What are the symptoms?

The importance of the kidneys in maintaining health is demonstrated by the number and variety of the symptoms that occur with end-stage kidney failure. These symptoms may include lethargy, weakness, headache, a furred tongue (see p.455) and unpleasant breath, oral thrush (see p.451), nausea, vomiting, diarrhea, an accumulation of water (*edema*) in the lungs (producing shortness of breath) and just under the skin (producing generalized swelling), pain in the chest or bones, and/or intensely itchy (though rash-free) skin. In addition, a woman with end-stage kidney failure may stop having menstrual periods. This group of conditions is commonly referred to as uremic poisoning.

What is the treatment?

If you develop end-stage kidney failure, you will probably already be under treatment for chronic kidney failure. Your physician will

probably have told you to report any illness or any change in your condition.

Treatment for end-stage kidney failure is a complex team effort. The various aspects of the treatment program will be tailor-made to your individual case, and will involve physicians, nurses, health technicians, social workers and dieticians.

Many of the symptoms of end-stage kidney failure can be alleviated by drugs, but only for a short time. Because the kidney damage is irreversible, the only satisfactory form of treatment is one that will take over the kidneys' functions. This means either dialysis (see Artificial kidney aids, previous page) or an operation to transplant a healthy, donated kidney. Fortunately, one kidney can usually do the work of two. The main problems in a kidney transplant are rejection and infection (see Transplants, p.402).

Unfortunately, some patients with end-stage kidney failure are too ill for treatment by either dialysis or transplantation.

What are the long-term prospects?

End-stage kidney failure is no longer the swiftly fatal disease it once was. Well over half of those who have had it are able to live comparatively normal lives five years after the condition begins. A good proportion of transplant recipients are still well many years after receiving a new kidney.

Hormonal disorders

Introduction

Hormones are chemicals made in glands called endocrine glands. These glands are essentially hormone-producing cells clustered around blood vessels. The hormones are released directly into the bloodstream, rather than through a duct, as in certain other glands. Together with your nervous system (see p.266), your hormones coordinate and control various organs and tissues so that all parts of your body work together smoothly and efficiently.

When a hormone is released into your bloodstream it circulates to all parts of your body, but it affects only a certain part or parts of the body. Such a part is called the target organ for that hormone. Generally, the more there is of a given hormone, the more active its target organ becomes. The amount of each hormone that is released into the bloodstream depends on your body's needs. The hormone levels in your blood change in response to events such as infections, stressful situations, and changes in the chemical composition of your blood. In some cases the level of one hormone in your blood regulates the level of another. For example, several hormones produced by your pituitary gland specifically regulate the amount of other hormones released by certain other endocrine glands. Although the pituitary is just one example of such activity, it is by far the most active gland we know of in this respect. In fact, the resulting wide-ranging control of the pituitary over our hormonal system has earned for it the nickname "the master gland."

Only the more common hormonal problems are discussed in this book. This section deals with those that occur in endocrine glands found in both men and women. They include disorders of the pituitary gland, the pancreas, the adrenal glands, and the thyroid and parathyroid glands. There are several other endocrine glands that are possessed exclusively by one sex. They are the ovaries and placenta in women and the testes in men. Disorders of these glands are discussed in other sections of the book (see Special problems of men, p.570; Special problems of women, p.582; and Pregnancy and childbirth, p.616). Many hormonal disorders require the expert diagnosis and treatment of an endocrinologist, a physician who specializes in such problems.

Hormone-producing glands

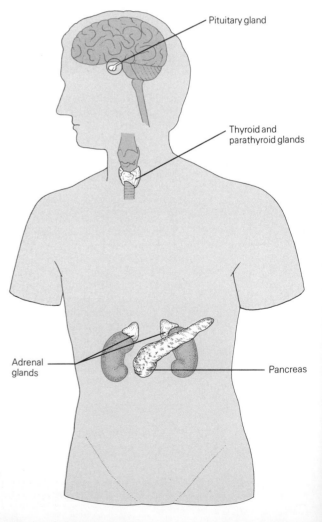

Pituitary gland

Thyroid and parathyroid glands

Adrenal glands

Pancreas

Pituitary gland

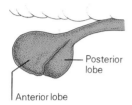

Posterior lobe

Anterior lobe

The pituitary gland has two parts, the anterior and posterior lobes

The pituitary gland, a peanut-sized organ situated just beneath the brain, is the most important of the endocrine, or hormone-producing, glands in your body. It is sometimes called the master gland, because it is like a central control switch that regulates many aspects of your body's growth, development, and everyday functioning. The gland has two distinct parts, the anterior, or front lobe and the posterior, or rear lobe.

The anterior lobe produces six hormones. Growth hormone, as its name implies, regulates the physical growth of most parts of your body. Prolactin stimulates the breasts to produce milk (see Galactorrhea, p.590). The four other hormones made by the anterior lobe stimulate four other hormone-producing glands; the thyroid and the adrenals, and the ovaries in women and testes in men. These glands, in turn, then produce hormones of their own.

The posterior lobe of the pituitary gland produces two hormones. Antidiuretic hormone acts on the kidneys and plays a large part in regulating the concentration and total quantity of your urine. The other hormone, oxytocin, stimulates contractions of the womb during childbirth and the release of milk during breast-feeding.

Disorders of the pituitary gland are rare.

Acromegaly

Typical symptoms of acromegaly include enlarged hands and head and coarser, more prominent facial features.

In this rare condition, your pituitary gland produces too much growth hormone, which causes excessive growth. However, an adult cannot grow taller, since vertical growth stops at the end of adolescence. Instead, the excess growth hormone produces acromegaly, in which your bones thicken and all other structures and organs grow larger. Overproduction of the growth hormone is usually caused by a pituitary tumor (see p.518).

What are the symptoms?
Acromegaly generally does not become apparent until middle age. Usually, the first symptom you will notice is enlargement of your hands and feet, typically revealed by the tightening of a ring on your finger, or an increase in your shoe size. After that, your head and neck grow broader, and your lower jaw, brows, nose and ears become prominent. Your skin and tongue thicken, and your features become generally coarser. Your voice may become deeper. Many people with this disorder have tingling in the hands, fatigue, increased sweating, stiffness and generalized aches. In a woman, the amount of hair on the body and limbs may increase.

In some cases of acromegaly, diabetes mellitus (see p.519) develops and causes the symptoms of this disorder. If a large pituitary tumor is present, it may cause a number of further symptoms.

What are the risks?
The longer acromegaly is left untreated, the greater the risks become. If your heart continues to enlarge, high blood pressure (see p.382), and possibly heart failure (see p.381), will develop in time. In addition, a large pituitary tumor can cause one of several problems with your eyesight.

What should be done?
If you develop the symptoms described, you should see a physician. If the doctor suspects acromegaly, you will probably be referred to a specialist for a number of tests. A blood sample will be taken to find out how much circulating growth hormone is present in your body. The usual type of *X-rays* of your skull do not show pituitary tumors. However, sometimes special tomographic X-rays, including *CAT scans*, can allow a radiologist to see the types of tumors that typically cause acromegaly.

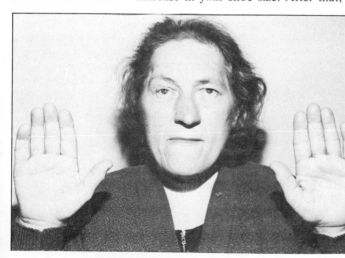

What is the treatment?

If tests show that you have a pituitary tumor, but it is no longer active and the disease has halted, then no treatment may be necessary. However, if your growth hormone level is high and cannot be reduced in a special suppression test, you should be treated as soon as possible. Your physician will probably recommend either *radiation therapy* or surgery. Drugs cannot control a pituitary tumor.

The best form of treatment depends on a number of factors, and you should be guided by your physician. You may also require treatment for other related disorders, such as diabetes mellitus, if they are present.

What are the long-term prospects?

Surgical removal of the pituitary tumor is effective in improving any problems with your eyesight. Also, tumors can now be selectively removed, leaving behind only normal pituitary tissue. You may not make a complete cosmetic recovery, however, since the changes in your bones and your appearance are largely irreversible. However, treatment will certainly halt the disease.

Gigantism

Gigantism is the same disorder as acromegaly (see previous article), except that it affects children and adolescents instead of adults. The pituitary gland overproduces growth hormone, usually because of a pituitary tumor (see p.518). This overproduction causes excessive growth of all parts of the body. The main difference between the two diseases is that acromegaly occurs when the limb bones have stopped growing, and gigantism occurs when they are still growing.

What should be done?

If a young person grows at an excessive rate, a physician should be consulted immediately. The treatment for gigantism is similar to treatment for acromegaly, and in most cases it is possible to halt the disorder.

Dwarfism

In gigantism or dwarfism the body is not only of abnormal size, but also is proportioned differently.

In rare cases, children fail to grow to normal heights because the pituitary gland does not produce enough growth hormone. More common causes of stunted growth include celiac disease (see p.684), hypothyroidism (see p.526), congenital heart disease (see p.656) and asthma (see p.355).

Deficiency of growth hormone may be present from birth or may develop at any age. Except when it is due to a pituitary tumor (see p.518), its cause is unknown. In some cases, the deficiency is accompanied by underproduction of other hormones, which leads to retarded sexual development (see Special problems of adolescents, p.706, and Hypopituitarism, next page).

What should be done?

Dwarfism in an infant is often detected at the regular checkups all babies should be given after birth. If your child seems too small for his or her age, consult the article on Growth disorders on p.687. If you think there is a problem, take your child to your family physician or pediatrician. If necessary, medical examinations and blood tests will be carried out to determine what is causing the child's slow growth. Growth hormone deficiency is extremely rare, so it is often the last cause to be considered. If it is present, it is detected by measuring the amount of growth hormone in blood samples.

No matter what causes the deficiency, the affected child will not grow normally without growth hormone replacement. Treatment consists of injections of human growth hormones until the end of adolescence. In most children, the response to this treatment is excellent and they grow normally.

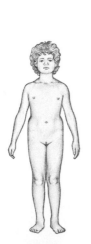

Dwarfism

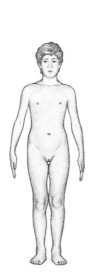

Normal

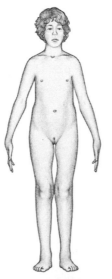

Gigantism

Diabetes insipidus

In the normal production of urine, your kidneys first filter water and other substances from your blood. The kidneys then absorb much of the water, which leaves concentrated urine ready to be passed from your body. The absorbed water is returned to the bloodstream, to maintain the correct concentrations of blood and body fluids. It is antidiuretic hormone (ADH) that stimulates the kidneys to absorb water from the urine. This substance is produced by the posterior lobe of the pituitary gland. In diabetes insipidus, there is a deficiency of ADH and your body passes large quantities of urine that contains a great deal of water.

The most common cause of the disorder is damage to the pituitary gland from a severe head injury. Other cases may be caused by an operation on the pituitary gland, or may be due to the effects of *radiation therapy* on the gland or the surrounding area. Rarely, diabetes insipidus may be caused by pressure on the gland from a pituitary tumor (see next page). More often, however, no obvious cause for the disorder can be found.

Diabetes insipidus should not be confused with diabetes mellitus, which is sometimes known as "sugar diabetes" (see p.519).

What are the symptoms?

The main symptom of this disorder is that you pass large quantities of colorless urine, as much as 20 liters (35 pts) every 24 hours. This great fluid loss results in an unquenchable thirst. You will constantly be interrupted by day and wakened at night by the need to urinate or drink. Other symptoms are dry hands and constipation.

What should be done?

As soon as symptoms appear, see your physician, who may arrange for you to have a water deprivation test. You will not be allowed to drink any fluid for 8 hours, during which time the volume of water in your urine will be measured several times. In a normal person deprived of fluid for so long, ADH would act to conserve water. If the volume of water in your urine remains high, this shows you have a deficiency of ADH. The effect of an injection of synthetic ADH on your urination can confirm an insufficient ADH level.

What is the treatment?

Self-help: Continue to drink as much water as you need.

Professional help: In some cases, when the amount of extra urination is not excessive, restriction of salt in the diet and taking certain *diuretic* tablets or other medication to help your kidneys conserve water may be all that is necessary. If the disorder is caused by a pituitary tumor, the tumor will probably have to be removed (see next page).

In other cases, the most effective treatment is with a synthetic form of ADH, given either as nose drops or by injection. How long you must take the drops or receive the injections is determined mainly by what has caused the disorder. If it was caused by a head injury, surgery, or radiation therapy, the defective gland often returns to normal within a year, which means a complete cure. If this fails to happen, you will probably have to take medication for the rest of your life. Your physician will probably want to monitor your response to the drug through regular checkups.

Hypo-pituitarism

The pituitary gland regulates body growth, general metabolism and sexual development, chiefly through the six hormones that are produced in its anterior, or front lobe (see Pituitary gland, p.515). In hypopituitarism, the anterior lobe of the gland is underactive and fails to produce adequate amounts of these six hormones. This results, ultimately, in insufficient body levels of these substances. The effects of this deficiency are wide-ranging. They include sexual underdevelopment or infertility, a prematurely aged appearance, a generalized weakness, and often general ill health.

The most common causes of hypopituitarism are serious head injury, a pituitary tumor (see next article), or the side-effects of treatment for such a tumor. Occasionally the disease develops for no known reason.

What are the symptoms?

Because the pituitary gland stimulates several other hormone-producing glands, the symptoms of hypopituitarism are a combination of the symptoms of several other disorders, each related to another affected gland. These include hypothyroidism (see p.526), adrenal underactivity (see Addison's disease, p.524), infertility (see p.607), absence of periods (see p.583) in women, and dwarfism (see previous page) in children.

What are the risks?

If hypopituitarism is not treated promptly, it can sometimes be fatal. This is mainly because when the six hormones that are provided by the pituitary gland are absent, your adrenal glands cannot respond to stress or infection (see p.523).

What should be done?

See your physician if you suspect that you have hypopituitarism. If the doctor shares your suspicion, you will probably have to have blood and urine tests. These tests, done in special laboratories to which your doctor can send some of your blood and urine, will measure the function of your anterior pituitary gland. If the tests confirm that you have hypopituitarism, you may also have further tests designed to discover whether a pituitary tumor has caused the disorder.

What is the treatment?

If you have this disorder, you will need lifelong treatment with tablets and injections that replace the hormones of the pituitary gland and the other glands that are affected. For example, injections of testosterone are given to men to make up for under-production of this hormone by the testes and thereby help to restore sex drive. Similarly, you may require substances to make up for the inactivity of your thyroid and adrenal glands, and your ovaries if you are a woman.

Pituitary tumors

Your pituitary gland is divided into two parts, the anterior, or front lobe and the posterior, or rear lobe. Pituitary-gland tumors almost always occur in the anterior lobe. Why they occur at all is unknown.

There are two types of pituitary-gland tumor. One type is an adenoma, which is *benign*, or unlikely to spread. An adenoma may cause excessive production of one of several hormones and can lead to acromegaly (see p.515), gigantism (see p.516), galactorrhea (see p.590) or Cushing's disease (see p.523). It may also enlarge and exert pressure on surrounding areas, causing other disorders, as described below.

The other type of tumor is called a craniopharyngioma. This type of tumor does not cause overproduction of any hormones, but it does progressively enlarge and can exert pressure either on the anterior lobe, which causes dwarfism (see p.516) or hypopituitarism (see previous article), or on the posterior lobe, which causes diabetes insipidus (see previous page). It can also press on the nerves to your eyes, and eventually cause headaches, double vision, and deteriorating sight (see Brain tumors, p.282).

What is the treatment?

Whenever possible, a pituitary tumor is removed or destroyed by surgery, *radiation therapy* or both.

Surgery to remove the tumor is a delicate procedure, which involves the use of extremely fine instruments. The tumor is usually reached through either a nostril or a hole made in the bridge of your nose. If the tumor is large and pressing on the nerves to the eyes, you may have to have open-brain surgery. You will probably recover quickly from the actual operation, but there is always a risk that the rest of the small, delicate pituitary gland will be damaged during the operation. If this is the case, either hypopituitarism, diabetes insipidus or both will develop as a result. However, this is usually considered an acceptable risk, because both hypopituitarism and diabetes insipidus can be treated by lifelong hormone-replacement therapy.

Instead of cutting out the tumor, the surgeon may destroy it by using extreme cold or by placing a tiny *radioactive implant* in it.

If the tumor has spread, or if it is difficult to pinpoint, radiation therapy of the whole gland may be necessary. Like surgery, radiation therapy carries the risk of some damage to the rest of the gland.

The long-term outlook depends largely on the size of the tumor, but with treatment a complete cure is possible.

Hormone-producing tumors

Normally, only the endocrine glands produce hormones. Occasionally, a tumor in an endocrine gland can produce hormones. But rarely, hormones can be manufactured by a tumor in an organ that is not normally concerned with hormone production. When this happens the excess hormone in the body causes the same symptoms as those brought on by an overactive endocrine gland. For example, a tumor of the kidney, lung, or breast can produce parathyroid hormone. This brings on the symptoms of overactive parathyroid glands (hyperparathyroidism), though the parathyroids themselves are working normally. Symptoms clear up only when the tumor is successfully treated.

Galactorrhea

Galactorrhea is production of breast milk when it is not supposed to be produced. Milk production normally occurs in a woman a few days before, and in the months following, the birth of a baby. Production at any other time in a woman, and at any time in a man, is considered galactorrhea. The problem is not a serious threat to health, though it may be irritating. However, the underlying cause of galactorrhea may be a pituitary tumor, which is more serious and may lead to other symptoms. Because the disorder most often affects women, it is dealt with under Special problems of women (see Galactorrhea, p.590).

Pancreas

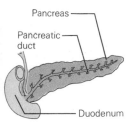

Pancreas

Pancreatic
duct

Duodenum

The pancreas is a gland about 15 cm (6 in) long. It lies close to the duodenum, and is linked to it by the pancreatic duct.

The pancreas is a long, thin gland that lies crosswise just behind your stomach. It has two major functions. The first is to produce *enzymes*, which help to digest food (see Liver, gallbladder and pancreas, p.485 for digestive disorders of the pancreas). The second major function of the pancreas is to produce the hormones insulin and glucagon. These hormones are significant in that they play a major part in regulating the glucose level in your blood.

Glucose is a form of sugar. It is found in many foods, including some that do not taste sweet. Glucose is the main source of energy for all the cells in your body. Insulin stimulates cells to absorb enough glucose from the blood for the energy they need, and stimulates the liver to absorb and store the rest. Insulin thus lowers the glucose level in your blood. Glucagon helps raise the glucose level in your body by stimulating your liver to release glucose.

Diabetes mellitus

Diabetes mellitus is a common disorder that occurs when your pancreas either totally stops producing insulin or does not produce enough of the hormone for your body's needs. This results in a low absorption of glucose, both by the cells, which need it for energy, and by the liver, which stores it. Another result is a high level of glucose in your blood.

Diabetes mellitus should not be confused with diabetes insipidus, which is a much less common disorder (see p.517). There are two main forms of diabetes mellitus. They are insulin-independent, and insulin-dependent.
Insulin-independent diabetes: In this form of diabetes mellitus, which usually affects people over 40, the insulin-producing cells in your pancreas function, but the output of insulin is inadequate for your body's needs. People who have this form of the disorder usually eat too much and are overweight (see Obesity, p.492). Their over-eating causes an excess of glucose in their blood, and the pancreas cannot produce enough insulin to cope with it. Heredity is also an important factor. In nearly a third of all cases, there is a family history of the malady. Age is also a factor, because the efficiency of your pancreas decreases with age.
Insulin-dependent diabetes: In this form of the disorder, which occurs mainly in young people, the pancreas produces very little or no insulin. The defect is caused by damage to the insulin-producing cells. Your body, unable to use glucose because of the lack of insulin, is forced to obtain energy from fat instead. This can lead to a dangerous condition called diabetic coma.

Either form of diabetes may be brought on by other diseases. Some examples of such diseases are acromegaly (see p.515), hyperthyroidism (see p.525), Cushing's syndrome (see p.523), and pancreatitis (see p.490). Such cases of diabetes are known as secondary diabetes, and in some instances the condition continues even after the main disease has been treated successfully.

What are the symptoms?
All forms of diabetes cause the same main symptoms. You urinate much more than usual, sometimes as often as every hour or so, throughout the day and night. You may notice white spots, which consist of dried splashes of glucose-filled urine, on your underwear or shoes. Micro-organisms are attracted to the sugary urine and can cause bladder infections (see p.505) and other urinary tract problems.

The excessive loss of fluid can make you perpetually thirsty, and drinking sweetened beverages increases the amount of urination and makes your thirst worse.

Your cells do not get enough glucose, so you feel extremely tired, weak, and apathetic; so much so that you may be unable to get up in the morning. Some diabetics, especially children and young adults, lose a lot of weight, since their fat and muscle are burned up to provide energy. Other symptoms that you may experience include tingling in the hands and feet, reduced resistance to infections (boils and urinary tract infections are sometimes the first signs of diabetes mellitus), blurred vision due to excess glucose in the fluid of the eye, and impotence in men (see p.614) or the absence of menstrual periods in women (see p.584).

The symptoms of insulin-dependent diabetes usually develop rapidly, within weeks or months. Those of the insulin-independent form often do not appear until many years after the actual onset of the disease. Sometimes the disorder is detected by chance at a routine medical examination, before any symptoms appear.

What are the risks?

Diabetes mellitus becomes increasingly common with age. Insulin-dependent diabetes is most common among boys and young men. The insulin-independent form occurs most often among those who are overweight, especially middle-aged and elderly women.

About one-third of insulin-independent diabetics have a relative with the disease. However, even if both of your parents are diabetic, there is only a 1 in 20 risk that you will develop the illness.

The effectiveness of modern treatment has changed this disease that once was often fatal into one from which deaths are extremely rare. However, there are still risks. Insulin-dependent diabetics risk lapsing into diabetic coma or unconciousness. This occurs when your body uses fat as a substitute for glucose to provide energy, which causes poisonous substances called ketones to form as a by-product. You may go into such a coma before your diabetes is discovered, after an infection such as influenza (see p.559), or if you neglect your treatment. You may have to be hospitalized after a diabetic coma, but you will probably recover completely.

Other complications, which can affect both types of diabetic, usually occur 15 to 20 years after the onset of the disease. Such risks include diabetic retinopathy, which is an eye disorder (see p.323), peripheral neuropathy, which is a nerve disease (see p.283), and chronic kidney failure (see p.512).

Diabetics also run a higher than average risk of developing atherosclerosis (see p.372), with its attendant risks of stroke, heart attack, and high blood pressure. The blood vessels to your legs become narrowed, which can cause cramps, cold feet, pain when you walk, and even skin ulcers or gangrene (see p.416). To avoid foot problems, you should try not to cut your nails too short, to wear shoes that fit properly, and to get treatment for such foot problems as corns or ingrown toe nails. If any cut fails to heal within ten days, you should see your physician.

What should be done?

If you suspect you have diabetes mellitus, see your physician, who will ask you to provide a urine sample to be tested for glucose and ketones. The presence of both will show that you have the disease. If only glucose is present, a blood sample will be taken to measure the amount of glucose in your bloodstream. This is done because it is possible to have some glucose in your urine without being diabetic. If there is still no clear result you will need to have a glucose tolerance test. A series of blood samples are taken before and after you swallow a glucose drink. If the level of glucose in the later samples is not normal, this shows that you are not producing enough insulin and that you have diabetes mellitus. Once the diagnosis has been established, your physician may want to give you a full physical examination before starting you on any treatment.

Your physician can give you a card to carry at all times, which gives your name and address, the fact that you are diabetic, and instructions on how to help you if you are ill. If you are so inclined, you can buy a bracelet or neck pendant that has the same information on it. Such aids are important not only to your health and safety, but also in making you feel less vulnerable and insecure.

What is the treatment?

Unfortunately, no cure has yet been found for diabetes mellitus, and you will have to have treatment for it all your life, once the disease is discovered. Since you administer most of that treatment yourself, its effectiveness will depend mainly on you.

Insulin-independent diabetes: Diet alone can control this form of the disease in many cases. The diet restricts the amount of carbohydrates you eat. If you are overweight, staying on this diet will reduce your weight significantly. The number of calories you are allowed each day will vary between 800 and 1500, depending on your weight and other factors such as height. Generally you should eat small portions of carbohydrates at regular intervals, so that there are no extreme variations in the glucose content of your blood. Do not eat sugar, candy, cake, jam, and so on. Make sure your diet contains enough fiber by eating whole grain bread and plenty of salads, fruit, and vegetables. Avoid consuming sugar-sweetened drinks and do not smoke cigarettes, because smoking can increase your risk of getting atherosclerosis.

In mild cases, merely avoiding the concentrated sugar of candy, cake, cookies, and sugar-sweetened drinks can be enough to bring your blood-glucose level down to normal. This is particularly true if you can reduce your weight and keep it within the recommended range for your height (see p.28), because then the insulin that your pancreas does produce may be enough to cope with the needs of your reduced body size.

Your progress in keeping your blood glucose down will need to be checked, and your physician will probably want to see you at regular intervals. To keep appointments to a minimum, however, you will probably be encouraged to check your own progress with a urine-testing kit. You should test your urine as often as your physician advises, and be sure to keep all your medical appointments.

Even if you keep strictly to your diet, you may find sooner or later that your tests show your condition to be getting worse. Then your physician may prescribe hypoglycemic tablets, which lower blood glucose. There are several different tablets available, and if you have unpleasant side-effects from one type, your doctor may prescribe another. In rare cases, if you take too high a dosage, hypoglycemia or low blood sugar (see next article) can result. If you have the symptoms of a

minister the injections until the child is about ten, when the child will probably be able to learn to do it independently.

You must keep rigorously to the timetable of meals and snacks advised by your physician. This keeps the supply of glucose to the blood steady, so that regular doses of insulin always act on approximately the same amount of glucose. Insulin is available in various types and strengths, and the type of insulin and the schedule that your doctor prescribes will depend on many factors, including your age and the severity of your diabetes. Always make sure that you obtain the same type and strength of insulin each time you renew your prescription.

Your physician will advise you to check on the effectiveness of your treatment by means of the same kind of urine tests that insulin-independent diabetics use. You may have to carry out the test several times each day. Today some diabetics estimate their blood glucose not by urine tests but by blood tests, which are more precise. You prick your finger to produce a drop of blood, and use a specially treated plastic strip or a small battery-operated meter to measure the level of glucose in your blood. The use of blood tests makes it possible for you to maintain a stricter control of your diabetes.

Self-discipline is essential if you are to control your diabetes successfully. You should be sure to remember to take each of the between-meal snacks prescribed by your physician. Ask your doctor if you can engage in strenuous activities such as fast-paced sports or even heavy digging in the garden, since exercise burns up glucose and may bring on hypoglycemia. Your physician may suggest that you eat extra food beforehand.

Any illness, from a cold to a heart attack, will cause stress and thus increase the amount of insulin you need. If you are unable to eat according to your usual schedule, take glucose drinks, but do *not* reduce your dose of insulin, and consult a physician as soon as you possibly can.

Diabetes can cause problems during pregnancy (see Diabetes and pregnancy, p.626) and in children. Young children may find it difficult to understand why they must stick to a diet and not have candy and soft drinks, but you must be firm in enforcing the diet. Many teenagers go through a period of rebellion, and if they are diabetics this may include a reaction against the restrictions imposed on them because of the disease.

If you are diabetic, always tell physicians or dentists before any treatment, so that they can take any necessary precautions.

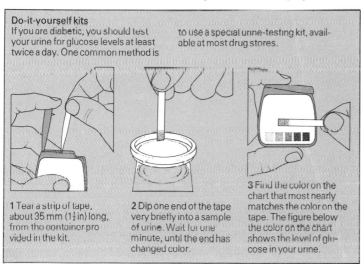

Do-it-yourself kits
If you are diabetic, you should test your urine for glucose levels at least twice a day. One common method is to use a special urine-testing kit, available at most drug stores.

1 Tear a strip of tape, about 35 mm (1½ in) long, from the container provided in the kit.

2 Dip one end of the tape very briefly into a sample of urine. Wait for one minute, until the end has changed color.

3 Find the color on the chart that most nearly matches the color on the tape. The figure below the color on the chart shows the level of glucose in your urine.

hypoglycemia attack, eat something sweet at once to avoid losing consciousness, and contact your physician about a possible adjustment of the dosage. Your doctor may recommend that you use insulin, as described below, instead of hypoglycemic tablets.

Insulin-dependent diabetes: This form of the disorder is treated with a combination of a controlled diet and daily injections of insulin extracted from beef or pig pancreas to replace the insulin that is missing.

Insulin can be taken only by injection. If you take insulin by mouth, it is destroyed by digestive juices before it can be absorbed into your bloodstream. You will be shown how to use a syringe to inject the insulin just under the skin of your thigh, arm or abdomen. Most people learn how to do this within a few days. Parents of diabetic children will need to ad-

What are the long-term prospects?
As long as you treat your diabetes sensibly, you can expect to lead a full and healthy life. You should have no problems with employment. Diabetics are found in most kinds of jobs. However, if you are taking insulin, you should avoid shift work that interferes with the regularity of your diet and injections. Also avoid heights, and do not drive buses or other public-service vehicles without the advice of your physician, because of the risk of an attack of hypoglycemia.

If you develop complications, these can be minimized by regular medical check-ups and strict control of your diabetes. Your best assurances for maximum health come from your own responsible attitudes and from following the advice of your physician.

Hypo-glycemia

Hypoglycemia is a low level of glucose in the blood. It is the opposite of diabetes mellitus (see previous article). In this disorder, the muscles and cells in your body are deprived of energy-providing glucose. The condition is almost entirely confined to people who have diabetes mellitus, especially those who are taking insulin injections or hypoglycemic tablets. Taking too much insulin, not keeping to the prescribed meal schedule, or unusually strenuous or prolonged exercise can all bring on an attack. Other causes of this disorder include stomach surgery, some types of cancer, a reaction to various drugs and foods, liver disease, pregnancy, and high fevers.

What are the symptoms?
The symptoms of hypoglycemia vary considerably from person to person, but often start with a feeling of being hot and uncomfortable, followed by profuse sweating. Other symptoms may include dizziness, weakness, trembling, unsteadiness, hunger, blurred vision, slurred speech, tingling in the lips or hands, or headache. You may become aggressive or uncooperative without knowing it, a condition that is sometimes mistaken for drunkenness. Convulsions (see p.667) may occur, particularly in children. If symptoms occur during the night, they will usually awaken you. In extreme cases you may become unconscious.

What are the risks?
Attacks of hypoglycemia are almost always treated and halted before they can become serious. The only real danger is that you might have an attack when you are swimming, operating machinery, or driving a car. If you have frequent attacks, you should not participate in these activities.

What should be done?
If you are a diabetic taking insulin, an attack of hypoglycemia may be artificially induced under medical supervision so that you can learn to recognize the form it takes in your particular case.

If you have an unexpected attack, reflect on its cause, and try to prevent another one. If you have attacks as often as once every three or four days, see your physician. The doctor may reduce your dose of insulin or hypoglycemia tablets.

What is the treatment?
Self-help: If you are prone to hypoglycemia attacks, you should always carry glucose tablets, sugar lumps, or candy. At the first sign of an attack, eat some until you feel normal again, which should be within a few minutes. Make sure your relatives and friends know about the symptoms, so that if you become disoriented or uncooperative, they can give you something sweet. Tell them that if they give you a small drink of fruit juice, or smear syrup inside your mouth, you will probably recover enough to eat properly. However, they should never try to feed you if you become totally unconscious, because this could choke you. If your hypoglycemia seems to be caused by drugs that you are taking for another disorder, discuss this with your physician, who will probably either discontinue them or suggest an alternative.

An alternative to glucose tablets that is being used more and more is an injection of glucagon, a hormone that helps raise your blood-glucose level. This is especially helpful if an attack makes you unconscious. Many people who have hypoglycemia attacks teach their relatives and friends how to inject the hormone into an arm or leg muscle.

You should instruct your friends and relatives that, if the measures described do not work, or are not available, they should summon medical assistance right away.
Professional help: The physician will give you an injection of glucose in a vein in your arm. This works so quickly that you may even regain consciousness while the injection is still in progress. You may then be admitted to a hospital for a diagnostic checkup, and the doctors will discuss with you the cause of your hypoglycemia attack and recommend ways to prevent future problems.

Adrenal glands

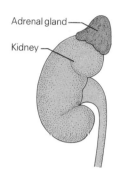

Adrenal gland

Kidney

The adrenal glands, one on top of each kidney, produce hormones that help you cope with physical and mental stress.

Your adrenal glands are about the size of grapes. You have two of them, one on top of each of your kidneys. Each one has two parts. One part is the medulla, or core, and the other is the cortex, or outer layer.

The medulla produces two hormones, epinephrine (adrenalin) and norepinephrine (noradrenalin), which play an important part in controlling your heart rate and blood pressure. Signals from your brain stimulate production of these hormones.

The adrenal cortex produces three groups of *steroid* hormones. The hormones in one group control the concentration and balance of various chemicals in your body. For example, they prevent the loss into the urine of too much sodium and water. The most important hormone in this group is aldosterone. The hormones in the second group have a number of functions. One of these is helping to convert carbohydrates, or starches, into energy-providing glycogen in your liver. Hydrocortisone is the main hormone in this group. The third group consists of male hormones called androgens and female hormones called estrogen and progesterone, which influence sexual development. Sex hormones are also produced by the testes and the ovaries. Each sex produces both male and female hormones, but androgens predominate in a man, estrogen and progesterone in a woman. Production of all steroid hormones except aldosterone is controlled by the pituitary gland (see p.515). Aldosterone production is stimulated by another hormone, renin, which is produced by the kidneys.

Cushing's syndrome

(including Cushing's disease)

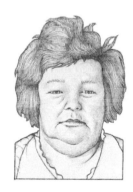

Someone with Cushing's syndrome or Cushing's disease gradually grows fatter. Also, the face can become red and moon-shaped.

In Cushing's syndrome there is an excess of *steroid* hormones in your blood. In the majority of cases it is caused by large doses of steroid drugs that are being taken for another illness, such as rheumatoid arthritis (see p.552) or asthma (see p.355). Rarely, the condition appears because the cortex, or outer layer, of one or both adrenal glands is producing excess steroid hormones. This can be caused by a tumor, either in the adrenal gland itself or elsewhere in your body, which is over-stimulating your adrenal glands. If the tumor is in your pituitary gland (see Pituitary tumors, p.518), the condition is called Cushing's disease rather than Cushing's syndrome.

What are the symptoms?

The symptoms of this disorder usually appear over several months. First, your face becomes fatter than usual, round and red. Your body also becomes fatter, and often a pad of fat develops between your shoulder blades, which makes you look round-shouldered. At the same time you lose muscle from your arms and legs. You will feel weak and tired, your skin may become spotty, and bruises sometimes appear spontaneously on your arms and legs. Your bones become thin (see Osteoporosis, p.543) and fracture easily.

Cushing's syndrome is uncommon. It affects only a very small proportion of people on long-term steroid treatment. Cushing's disease also is extremely rare. It mainly affects young to middle-aged women.

What should be done?

See your physician if you have several of the symptoms that are described above. If the doctor suspects that you have Cushing's disease you will be admitted to a hospital for tests for a pituitary tumor. On the other hand, if you are on long-term steroid treatment, your physician may be able to diagnose Cushing's syndrome right away.

What is the treatment?

If steroid drugs taken for another disorder are the cause, your physician will gradually reduce your dosage and provide other treatment. *Never* stop taking steroid drugs yourself. You could develop acute adrenal failure (see Addison's disease, next article).

When a tumor of the pituitary gland is the cause, it can be treated by either surgery or *radiation therapy* (see p.518). As an alternative, your adrenal glands may be removed. If this treatment is chosen, you will have to take medication daily for the rest of your life, to replace the missing hormones (see Addison's disease, next article). If you have a tumor on one adrenal gland, that gland will be taken out. You should, however, be able to function adequately with the remaining adrenal gland. Your physician will discuss with you the best treatment in your particular case. If the treatment is successful, you can expect to return to normal or near-normal health. However, you will probably have to take medication for the rest of your life.

Addison's disease

(including acute adrenal failure)

In Addison's disease, the production of *steroid* hormones by the cortex, or outer layer, of your adrenal glands gradually decreases over the years. The most common cause of the disease today is destruction of the cortex by the body itself. When this happens, it is probably due to an *autoimmune* problem, in which your body's immune system mistakes one of your tissues or organs for an outside invader and attacks it. Tuberculosis (see p.563) may also cause Addison's disease, but this is rare.

What are the symptoms?
The symptoms usually develop very gradually. They include loss of appetite and weight, a feeling of increasing tiredness and weakness, and anemia (see p.419). You may also have bouts of diarrhea, constipation, or mild indigestion with nausea or vomiting. In addition, your skin may become strikingly darker and stay that way.

If the disease is not treated you run the risk of acute adrenal failure. This may be triggered by the stress of even a mild infection. It causes severe vomiting and diarrhea, followed by *dehydration*, or loss of body fluids, and loss of consciousness. To prevent death, emergency hospital treatment is essential.

What should be done?
If you believe you might have the disease, be certain to consult your physician. Analysis of blood samples for low levels of steroid hormones will reveal whether you have the disorder. If Addison's disease is diagnosed, you will need to take *steroid* tablets daily for the rest of your life, to replace the hormones your adrenal glands formerly made. In some cases, injections are also necessary. The treatment will clear up your symptoms, including your darkened skin. You will be given a card that describes the treatment you need if you have acute adrenal failure. Always carry this with you. If you have any illness or infection, however minor, consult your physician, who may increase your dose of steroids to prevent acute adrenal failure. If you are having surgery, be sure the surgeon is aware that you have the disorder. As long as you take your tablets and follow the above precautions, you should be able to lead a normal, healthy life.

Pheochromo-cytoma

The hormones epinephrine (adrenalin) and norepinephrine (noradrenalin), which are produced by the medulla, or core, of each adrenal gland, work together with your nervous system (see p.266) to control your heart rate and blood pressure. Very rarely, a tumor, usually *benign* (unlikely to spread), develops in the medulla of one adrenal gland and causes it to produce excess hormones. As a result, slight exercise, exposure to cold, or a minor emotional upset will produce the racing heart, paleness, and sweating normally associated only with intense fear or overexcitement. In addition, you may feel faint and have a severe headache. During an attack your blood pressure is very high, which can lead to several problems (see p.382).

What should be done?
If you have attacks of the kind described, see your physician, who will probably arrange for you to have blood and urine tests.

If the tests show an excess of the adrenal medullary hormones, further steps, such as a *CAT scan* or an *angiogram*, may be necessary to locate the tumor. While these tests are being done, you will be given a prescription for medication that prevents further attacks.

If a tumor is discovered, it will be removed surgically, and this usually cures the disorder.

Aldo-steronism

(including Conn's syndrome)

Aldosteronism is a very rare illness in which an overproduction of the hormone aldosterone, a product of the cortex of the adrenal glands, leads to high blood pressure. Usually the condition accompanies congestive heart failure (see p.381), cirrhosis of the liver (see p.487), or one of several other long-term diseases. In rare cases it is due to a tumor, which is usually *benign* (unlikely to spread), in one adrenal gland. This form of the disorder is known as Conn's syndrome.

The main symptoms are those of high blood pressure (see p.382). Other symptoms include tingling and weakness in your limbs, muscle spasms in your hands and feet, and increased thirst coupled with excessive urination. If you have these symptoms, consult your physician, who will probably first arrange for you to have both blood and urine tests. If the results show that you have aldosteronism, you may need to have further tests to find out if a tumor is causing the disorder. If an adrenal tumor is found, it can be removed surgically, and this often cures the disorder. When the condition is caused by another disease, it is controlled by drugs.

Thyroid and parathyroid glands

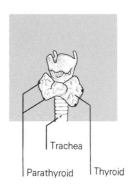

Trachea

Parathyroid Thyroid

The thyroid gland is a butterfly-shaped structure that consists of two lobes in the lower part of your neck, one on either side of the trachea, or windpipe. The lobes are joined by a thin strand of thyroid tissue. The gland makes a hormone called thyroxine or T_4, under the control of thyroid-stimulating hormone produced by the pituitary gland. Thyroxine controls the rates at which chemical reactions occur in your body. Generally, the more thyroxine that there is, the faster your body works.

Thyroxine contains the chemical iodine. Most people get sufficient iodine in their diets from fish, fish products, and drinking water. Iodine is often added to table salt and bread.

Some scientists are concerned that we may get too much iodine in our diet.

On the four corners of your thyroid gland there are four parathyroid glands, each about the size of a pearl. They produce parathyroid hormone. This hormone works with another, called calcitonin, which is made by the thyroid gland, and with vitamin D, to control the level of calcium in your blood. Your body requires calcium to develop bones and teeth. Calcium also has a role in blood clotting and the functioning of your nerves and muscles. Parathyroid hormone and vitamin D raise the calcium level both by causing your intestine to absorb more calcium from food, and by making you excrete less calcium in urine.

Hyperthyroidism

(thyrotoxicosis, toxic goiter, Graves' disease)

Hyperthyroidism is overactivity of the thyroid gland (compare Hypothyroidism, next article). Activity of the thyroid gland is normally controlled by thyroid-stimulating hormone, which is made in your pituitary gland. In hyperthyroidism, the control mechanism goes wrong. Despite normal levels of thyroid-stimulating hormone, the thyroid gland itself continuously produces large quantities of its own hormone, thyroxine. Why this happens is not well understood. Increased amounts of thyroid hormones cause a general speeding-up of all chemical reactions in your body, and this affects your mental as well as physical processes.

What are the symptoms?
There are many different symptoms typical of hyperthyroidism, but you are highly unlikely to have them all at once.

As your mental processes speed up, you become fidgety and anxious. You may be tired but unable to relax or sleep. You may feel shaky and your hands may tremble; this is especially noticeable when you are trying to write or perform other tasks that require delicate movement.

You may begin to be insensitive to cold, and to be comfortable in summer clothes even on a cold day. You may perspire most of the time and have disagreements with other people about the level of heating.

Your heartbeats may become irregular and much faster, even when you are trying to relax. This causes palpitations, or a fluttering or racing feeling in your chest. You may

become breathless after the mildest exertion. If your intestinal muscles become involved, you may have attacks of diarrhea.

Because more rapid body processes require more energy, you may eat more, yet still lose weight. Your muscles may waste away and you may become so weak that you find it difficult to walk, or lift your arms above your head. Women may have scanty or absent menstrual periods, and you may notice a swelling in your neck, due to the enlarged thyroid gland, or goiter.

The final group of symptoms concern your eyes. These symptoms are less common than the others, and they become serious in only a few cases. Your eyes may feel gritty and uncomfortable, and look wide open and protruding (see Exophthalmus, p.326). Occasionally, this can cause double or blurred vision, but more often it merely causes red and puffy eyelids.

What are the risks?
This is a fairly uncommon disorder. It can occur at any age, but it is very rare that it affects children. It is eight times more common in women than in men.

Like the symptoms, the risks of hyperthyroidism are variable. You may recover completely. However, some people have recurrent bouts of the disorder. It can be fatal if it is left untreated for many years.

If you are elderly, and already have high blood pressure (see p.382) or hardening of the arteries (see p.404), you are at the greatest risk. Additional strain on your heart and circulation can cause angina (see p.376), abnormal heart rhythms (see p.388), or heart failure (see p.381).

What should be done?

Hyperthyroidism may be confused with psychological disturbances such as anxiety states (see p.300) or depression (see p.297). If you have several of the symptoms described above, visit your physician and mention that you suspect hyperthyroidism may be responsible. After examining you, the doctor may have your blood tested for increased levels of thyroid hormone. Once the diagnosis is made, your physician may order a *thyroid scan* to see if all of your gland is affected, or only a part of it (see Thyroid nodules, next page).

What is the treatment?

Your physician will probably discuss with you the various aspects of treatment. Hyperthyroidism itself can be treated in one of three ways. Any complications that arise will also be treated.

The first possible treatment is to prescribe tablets that contain anti-thyroid drugs. In most people the disorder is brought under control in about eight weeks by this method, though you will have to continue to take the tablets for at least a year. The drugs eventually cure some people, but most of those who receive this treatment will begin to have the symptoms again, and therefore will later require some additional treatment.

The second treatment is an operation to remove either a lump in the thyroid gland, or most of the gland if it is generally overactive. Surgery cures the disorder in about 90 per cent of these cases. In a few cases, either the disease recurs or the thyroid or parathyroid may become underactive as a result of the surgery (see Hypothyroidism, next article, and Hypoparathyroidism, p.528).

The third form of treatment is the most common. It consists of taking radioactive iodine in the form of a clear, slightly salty drink. Iodine is an essential constituent of thyroid hormone, so the radioactive material ultimately becomes concentrated in the thyroid gland. There it acts on the glandular tissue to slowly control the cellular overactivity. If enough radioactivity is administered, the gland may become underactive, and you may have to take medication to compensate (see Hypothyroidism, next article).

Each of these three forms of treatment has its advantages and disadvantages, and your physician will help you determine which is most suitable for you. Despite the wide-ranging effects of hyperthyroidism, you will probably be restored to normal health.

Hypo-thyroidism

(including Hashimoto's disease)

Hypothyroidism, sometimes called myxedema, is underactivity of the thyroid gland. When it occurs, your thyroid gland produces only small amounts of thyroid hormone, and all chemical processes in your body slow down as a result.

Underactivity of the thyroid gland can be due to one of several causes, or it can occur for no apparent reason. One occasional cause is treatment for hyperthyroidism (see previous article), which carries a significant risk that the overactive thyroid gland may later become underactive. Another possible, but much rarer, cause is a lack of thyroid-stimulating hormone due to a disorder of the pituitary gland (see p.515). Hypothyroidism may also occur in the course of Hashimoto's disease, a disorder in which an inflammatory thyroid condition thought to be caused by an *autoimmune* reaction destroys your body's thyroid. In such a reaction, *antibodies*, or biochemical substances in your blood that normally protect you from infection, attack a part of your body.

Very rarely, a baby is born with a defective thyroid gland, or with no gland at all. The result is little or no thyroid hormone. If it is not detected and treated, this condition can lead to irreversible mental deficiency.

What are the symptoms?

The symptoms of hypothyroidism develop slowly, taking months or even years. Someone who has not seen you for a few months may be struck by the deterioration in your physical and mental health.

If you have hypothyroidism, your whole body slows down. You feel continually tired and worn out. You find that even simple mental tasks, such as adding up a bill, take longer. You may have general aches and pains and move more slowly than usual. Your heart may slow to 50 beats per minute or less (the normal range is usually anywhere from 60 to 100 beats per minute) and your intestinal muscles may slow down, which leads to bouts of constipation.

Because slowed-down body processes need less energy, you eat less but gain weight. You begin to feel cold more acutely, and wear far more clothing than do others. Your hair tends to become thin, dry, and lifeless. Your skin becomes dry and thickens due to a mucus-like substance that collects in it. Why this happens is not known, but it makes your face look puffy. Puffy tissue also collects on your vocal cords, which makes your voice deeper than usual and hoarse; in your ears, which causes hearing loss; and in your wrists, where it presses on the nerves going to your hands and causes numbness and tingling in them. Women may have heavy, prolonged menstrual periods, and both women and men may lose interest in sex.

In very severe cases of hypothyroidism you become very cold and drowsy, and may even tually become unconscious. This rare condition is called myxedema coma. It may be brought on by cold weather or by taking certain drugs, especially sedatives.

A baby born with hypothyroidism is lethargic and difficult to feed, has a large tongue and often also an umbilical hernia (see Hernias, p.537). Such a child often develops prolonged jaundice (see Neonatal jaundice, p.647) soon after birth.

What are the risks?
Hypothyroidism is not rare, and it can affect anyone. However, it is very rare at birth, occurring in only about 1 in 5000 births, and it is most common in middle-aged women.

A baby with hypothyroidism, left untreated, will not grow and develop properly. Instead, the child will become dwarfed and mentally retarded. In adults the disease is unlikely to be fatal unless myxedema coma develops.

What should be done?
Many people feel tired and generally "down" at some time or other. Of course, few of them have hypothyroidism. But if you notice several of the symptoms described in this article occurring together, visit your physician.

After examining you, the physician will probably take several blood samples for analysis. If they contain a low level of thyroid hormone, hypothyroidism is the diagnosis. If the samples also contain antibodies that are active against the thyroid gland, the diagnosis is Hashimoto's disease.

Hypothyroidism in infants is sometimes detected at the physical examination carried out just after birth. More often, children with congenital hypothyroidism are detected before signs and symptoms develop, through a routine screening of blood samples taken from babies in the first few days of life.

What is the treatment?
Whatever its cause, the treatment of hypothyroidism is straightforward. You will have to take tablets of artificially-made thyroid hormones every day for the rest of your life. After a few days of treatment, you feel much better, and after a few months you should have returned to normal health.

A baby with the disorder is started on the tablets as soon as possible. If treatment is started before the baby is about three months old, he or she has a very good chance of growing and developing normally. Parents must make sure that the child always takes the tablets as prescribed by the physician.

Thyroid nodules

A thyroid nodule is a distinct lump growing in an otherwise normal thyroid gland. There are four types of nodule: a soft, fluid-filled cyst; an area of bleeding called a hemorrhage; a *benign* growth (unlikely to spread) called an adenoma; and a *malignant* growth (likely to spread and threaten life) called a carcinoma. Why thyroid nodules develop, or why some people have more than one, is not known.

What are the symptoms?
Thyroid nodules usually show up as a swelling in the front part of your neck. They can be painful or big enough to make breathing or swallowing difficult, but this is rare. If you suspect you have a thyroid nodule you should consult your physician, who will probably refer you to a specialist.

What should be done?
All nodules except carcinomas are fairly common, and usually harmless. If they are small, your doctor may advise you to leave them alone. A large, unsightly cyst can be *aspirated*, or removed with a needle. If a *thyroid scan* shows that a nodule may be a carcinoma, or if it is an adenoma that is causing hyperthyroidism (see p.525), the whole gland will be removed or destroyed. After such treatment, you must take thyroxine tablets for the rest of your life. This is because with the absence of your thyroid gland your body will no longer have a natural source of this important hormone, and it must be provided artificially.

The outlook for those who get thyroid cancer is generally good. If you get it when you are young, you will probably be completely cured, either through neck surgery only or through a combination of surgery to remove the gland and subsequent series of radioactive iodine treatments.

Hyperpara-thyroidism

Hyperparathyroidism occurs when excessive amounts of parathyroid hormone are produced, in most cases because of a small growth in one of the four parathyroid glands, the glands that help control bone growth. The small growth is usually *benign*, or unlikely to spread. Occasionally the disorder occurs because of a generalized enlargement of all four glands. It is not known what causes the growth or the enlargement. The excess parathyroid hormone creates a higher than normal level of calcium in your blood, most of which is removed from your bones. In an attempt to lower the blood calcium level, your kidneys pass more calcium into your urine, but the effects of this kidney activity are limited. Over the years the calcium level gradually builds up.

What are the symptoms?

Most people do not have any symptoms unless the disorder is well advanced. However, most cases of hyperparathyroidism are detected in a routine blood calcium test, or tests for some other related disorder.

After several years, the excessive amounts of calcium that have been passing through your kidneys and into your urine can cause the formation of kidney stones (see p.509).

The excess calcium in your blood upsets your metabolism, and indigestion and/or depression may result. Loss of calcium from your bones makes them soft, generally weak, and very easy to fracture.

What should be done?

If you suspect for any reason that you have this disease, see your physician. Your doctor will arrange for you to have blood tests. If analysis of blood calcium and parathyroid hormone shows that you have the disorder, you may need to have a special *X-ray* called an *angiogram* to determine which of your glands are affected.

What is the treatment?

Surgery to remove either a growth or three out of four enlarged parathyroid glands completely cures the disorder in most cases. There is a risk that after the operation the amount of parathyroid hormone produced will not be enough to maintain a normal level of calcium in your blood (see Hypoparathyroidism, next article). Also, any kidney stones that formed before you had the operation may have to be attended to later. This will be done either with surgery or through drug treatment.

Hypopara-thyroidism

In hypoparathyroidism, your parathyroid glands, the glands that help control bone growth, do not produce enough hormones. This causes the level of calcium in your blood to fall below normal. The disorder can occur either alone or in conjunction with the failure of other endocrine gland functions (for example, those of the thyroid or adrenal glands). In either case, the cause of the defect is unknown. Hypoparathyroidism is rare, and it affects children more commonly than adults.

Hypoparathyroidism can also be caused by an operation on the thyroid gland. Such an operation is done in an attempt to control overactivity in the gland (see Hyperthyroidism, p.525). An operation on the parathyroid glands to control their overactivity (see Hyperparathyroidism, previous article), may also trigger hypoparathyroidism.

What are the symptoms?

The main symptoms are painful cramp-like spasms in your hands, feet, and throat. These spasms are known as *tetany* (not to be confused with tetanus, see p.564). Other symptoms include tingling and numbness in your face and hands, dry skin, thin hair, and often oral thrush (see p.451) or vaginal yeast infection (see p.602). If the disease is not detected in a child, he or she may have vomiting, headaches, convulsions (see p.667), and poor tooth development. The child may also become mentally retarded.

What should be done?

If you suspect that you have the disorder, see your physician, who will arrange for you to have blood tests. The results of these tests will show whether or not you have the disease.

What is the treatment?

Once the illness has been diagnosed, you will require lifelong treatment with calcium and vitamin D tablets, which will restore your blood calcium to normal levels. If you have an attack of tetany, your physician will send you to a hospital for an injection of calcium. This usually provides relief within minutes. The correct doses of vitamin D and calcium will restore you almost to normal health. However, to help check your condition and the necessary treatment, you will need to see your doctor every few months for tests on the level of calcium in your blood. To maintain maximum health, it is important that you remember to have these tests on schedule.

Disorders of the muscles, bones and joints

Introduction

Muscles, bones and joints provide your body with a supportive framework that allows flexibility of movement. All movement, including the movement of both the body itself and the organs within the body, is carried out by muscles, which can do their jobs because they are composed of tissues that can contract.

Voluntary muscles, such as those in the limbs, are under conscious control, and contract only when your brain tells them to. For example, if you want to bend your elbow, your brain instructs your biceps muscle to contract; to straighten the arm your brain signals the biceps muscle to relax and instructs the triceps muscle to contract. These brain signals are sent via your nervous system.

Involuntary muscles, such as those that are in the heart and digestive tract, normally function without conscious control or even awareness. The articles in this section deal only with voluntary muscles, mainly those of the limbs, the neck and the trunk. Disorders that affect involuntary muscles – irritable colon, for instance – are discussed in sections dealing with the organs whose movements and functions they control.

The 206 bones of your skeleton serve mainly as an important support system for the various parts of the body. In addition, some bones also encase and protect certain organs. For example, the skull protects the brain, and the rib cage and backbone shield the heart, lungs, and, to some extent, upper-abdominal organs such as the stomach, liver and kidneys.

Bones are not lifeless structures. They are composed of living cells embedded in a hard framework of minerals, mostly calcium and phosphorus. This framework acts partially as a storage and supply area for these minerals. Inside some bones is a soft core, the marrow, that manufactures blood cells (see Bone marrow, p.429, for further information).

Some bones, such as those of the skull are joined closely together by almost immovable connective fibers called *sutures.* But when most people speak of a "joint," they generally mean the special hingelike structure between certain neighboring bones that permits them to move in relation to each other.

There are several different types of joints in your body. Each of your vertebrae (backbones) can move only slightly in relation to its neighbors, but this provides enough flexibility over the whole spinal column to allow you to bend your back considerably. The knee is actually called a "hinge" joint, because it permits movement in only one direction (backwards). The shoulder is a "ball-and-socket" joint, which is more versatile. It allows the arm to bend, twist and turn, and, therefore, move in almost any direction.

Each joint is a complicated structure. It is bound together on the outside by fibrous bands called ligaments. Inside the ligaments is a fibrous joint *capsule* lined on the inside by the *synovium*, a thin membrane that continuously produces tiny amounts of fluid to lubricate the joint. Where the bone ends meet, their surfaces are covered by a smooth, flexible cartilage.

Bone tissue
Magnified bone tissue reveals many tiny cylinders. These are made of organic material impregnated with minerals, mainly calcium and phosphorus. These cylinders provide much of bone's strength.

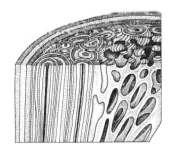

Muscle tissue
A muscle is composed of tiny filaments that move in relation to each other when stimulated by a nerve impulse. It is this movement that accounts for the contraction and relaxation through which a muscle does its work.

Relaxed

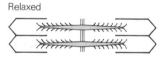

Contracted

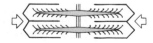

The musculoskeletal system

How the skeleton and muscles work together

Skeletal muscles are attached to two or more bones. When a muscle contracts, the bones to which it is attached move. Muscles nearly always work in coordinated groups; contraction of one muscle is accompanied by relaxation of another, while other muscles stabilize nearby joints.

Abdominal muscles

This large group of muscles assists in the regular movements made in breathing, balances the muscles of the spine during lifting movements, and keeps the intestines and other abdominal organs firmly in place.

Leg muscles

Leg muscles are among the most powerful in the body, and have strong, broad anchorage points, especially at the pelvis.

Head and neck muscles

Contraction of these muscles produces facial expressions and head movements. They are also responsible for speech and swallowing.

Arm muscles

Most of the bulk of arm muscles is at the shoulder and below the elbow. Long tendons connect the muscles in the forearm to the wrist and fingers.

Involuntary muscles

Involuntary muscles are not under conscious control. That is, they do not contract or relax in response to your decision to make a movement. Instead, they work automatically. They include muscles that propel food through the intestine and those that control sweating and blood pressure.

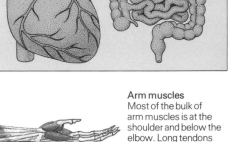

Heart   Intestine

The male and female pelvis

Most bones in the female skeleton are the same shape as the bones in the male skeleton, but usually a little smaller. One exception is the pelvis, or hip bone. A woman's pelvis is usually broader than a man's, and has a larger space in the middle. This is to accommodate the head of a baby as it passes from the uterus through the pelvis and to the outside world during childbirth.

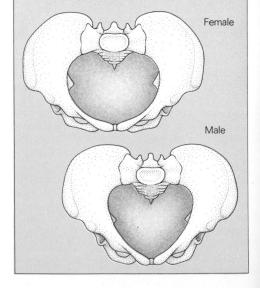

Female

Male

Protection of internal organs

Besides providing a rigid internal framework, the skeleton also provides some protection for certain vulnerable internal organs. The brain is encased in the bony box of the skull. The ribcage shields the lungs and heart, and forms a protective umbrella over upper abdominal organs such as the liver and kidneys. The bladder and (in a woman) the reproductive organs lie within a solid ring of bone, the pelvis, at the base of the abdomen.

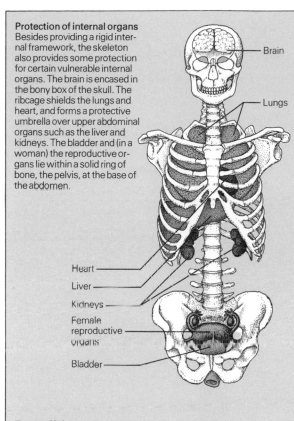

Different types of joints

Some joints, like the fibrous sutures that join the separate bones of the skull, allow little or no movement and effectively weld the bones into one rigid structure. Others permit limited movement. Each individual vertebra (backbone) can move only slightly, although this adds up to considerable flexibility over the whole vertebral column. Yet other joints – for example the shoulder joint – have a wide range of movement.

Little or no movement

Limited movement

Maximum movement

Types of joint movement

The knee joint (right) is a typical "hinge" joint. It moves on only one plane, that is, backwards and forwards. Finger and elbow joints move in the same way. A "ball-and-socket" joint such as the hip or shoulder joint (below) allows movement on two planes: backward and forward (1) and sideways (2). It also allows the limb to rotate (3). Most actions of the arm involve a combination of these movements (4). In general, hinge joints with their restricted range of movement are more stable and less easily dislocated than are ball-and-socket joints.

Plane of movement of knee joint

Planes of movement of shoulder joint

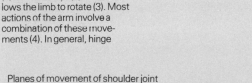

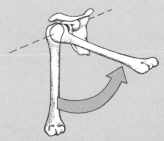

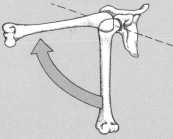

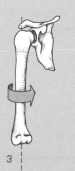

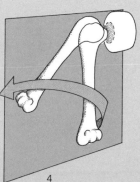

1   2   3   4

Injuries

Muscles, bones and joints are more susceptible to damage from injury than most other parts of the body. Because every muscle has a limited pulling strength, it will be torn or otherwise damaged if it is required to overcome a force too powerful for it, such as when your try to lift a weight that is too heavy for you. Similarly, bones cannot change shape in response to extreme physical pressures, so they split or snap if subjected to too much stress. Finally, each joint in the body is designed to allow a particular range of movement. If a joint is overflexed or forced to move in an unnatural direction, the ligaments or other tissues that bind neighboring bones together will be damaged.

Pulled muscle

If a muscle is over-stretched, for example by being forced to do very vigorous exercise to which you are unaccustomed, some of the fibers of which it is composed may tear. When this happens, the muscle contracts and may also become swollen because of internal bleeding. Occasionally, the muscle may be ruptured, or torn completely.

What are the symptoms?
The main symptom is pain when the injury occurs. The pulled muscle feels tender, may become swollen, and will not function efficiently until the torn fibers have healed. If the muscle is ruptured, it will not function at all. A muscle that gradually becomes stiff, painful and tender (often overnight) has probably been pulled. In addition, a few of its fibers may have been torn.

What are the risks?
Almost everybody pulls a muscle at some time. People who are active in sports are particularly susceptible. Ruptured muscles are much less common.

In most cases recovery from a pulled muscle is quick and complete, and there is no danger of permanent loss of mobility. The older you are, the greater the damage you can do and the more slowly you recover. A ruptured muscle, however, may become permanently useless unless it is successfully treated.

Thigh muscles are easily strained, especially while you are active in sports. An elastic bandage around the vulnerable area gives support.

What should be done?
If you have a pulled muscle that does not seem to be severely damaged, try the self-help measures suggested below. If you are in great pain or the affected area becomes badly swollen, consult your physician, who will probably be able to assess the extent of damage by a careful examination of the injury.

What is the treatment?
Self-help: Apply ice wrapped in a cloth or in an ice pack to the area to help prevent further swelling and to decrease the pain. Try not to use the pulled muscle for several days, or as long as the pain persists. Bandaging or strapping the affected area will give it support, but be careful not to bind it too tightly. If you do, further swelling might then interfere with blood circulation.

Professional help: Treatment depends on the severity of the injury. Your physician may prescribe a painkiller, a muscle-relaxant drug, or both. You may be advised to use crutches for a leg injury or a sling for an arm that has been hurt, or even to stay in bed for three or four days. The doctor may also recommend physical therapy. As the acute pain and swelling subside, a graduated program of exercises may be started to restore the motion and strength.

If the muscle is ruptured, the best treatment is often direct repair through surgery.

Sprain

If excessive demands are made upon a joint, the ligaments that hold the neighboring bones together and keep the joint in position may be torn. This particular type of injury is a sprain, and its severity depends on how badly the ligaments are torn. Any joint can be sprained, but the joints at the knees, the ankles and the fingers are especially susceptible to this type of injury. Many people have a tendency to call any painful injury that they get in a joint a sprain.

What are the symptoms?
The amount of pain and tenderness in the injured area varies depending on the extent of damage. A sprained joint will still function, but it will be painful to use. There may also be swelling and, later, skin discoloration. In a

sprain so severe that all supporting ligaments are torn through, the joint will be misshapen as well as swollen.

What are the risks?

There is no danger in a minor sprain. Repeated stretching and tearing of the ligaments, however, are bound to weaken any joint. This is particularly true of the ankle, which may begin to give way occasionally for no apparent reason if it is sprained often.

What should be done?

For a mild sprain try the self-help measures recommended below. If the pain is severe or persists for more than two or three days, see

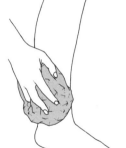

Treating a sprain
Put a cold compress or ice pack on a recent sprain to help reduce the swelling and ease the pain for the first 24 hours. Apply a firm bandage to support the joint while the ligaments heal. When a tendon is cut, the muscle to which it is attached contracts and the tendon springs away from the site of the injury. Then surgery is required to locate and join the severed ends.

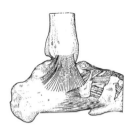

Sprained ankle
The tough, fibrous ligaments of the ankle hold the several ankle bones firmly in place. If you fall with your ankle in an abnormal position, you may put the weight of your whole body on those ligaments and stretch or tear them. This is a sprained ankle.

your physician, who will examine the joint and will probably have it *X-rayed*, since a severe sprain is often difficult to distinguish from a fracture.

What is the treatment?

Self-help: If you have a mild sprain, support the joint with an elastic bandage and rest it. An ice pack helps keep down the swelling for the first 24 hours. After a day or so, start to exercise the joint as much as possible, but without forcing it to bear weight. When you are not exercising the damaged limb, keep it in an elevated position to help drain away the fluids that cause the swelling. Soaking the sprain in warm water several times a day is also helpful.

Professional help: If you have a severe sprain, your physician may put a cast on the affected portion of the injured limb or finger. Occasionally, surgical repair of badly torn ligaments is necessary. After any such operation the limb must stay in a cast for several weeks. When the cast is removed, you will probably need to wear a supportive bandage and have physical therapy to restrengthen the joint for normal use.

Severed tendon

If you cut or injure yourself badly over your forearm, hand, calf, or foot, the cut may go partly or completely through one or more tendons. Tendons are long, fibrous cords that connect muscles and bones, such as the ones that move the fingers, thumbs and toes. The muscles that move your fingers are located in your forearms, and those that move your toes are in your calves. If you sever a tendon you will be unable to move one or more of your fingers or toes properly.

What should be done?

Get to your physician or a hospital as soon as possible if you think you have severed one or more tendons. Depending on the injury, a surgeon may attempt to sew together the two ends immediately. Tendons are under considerable tension, so when one is severed, the cut ends snap back from the cut and are difficult to retrieve. A larger cut may have to be made to find the two free ends of the tendon for repair.

Sometimes it is better to wait for the cut to heal, before the tendon is repaired. It may be necessary to use a piece of tendon from elsewhere in the body to patch the damaged one.

The results of tendon repair are usually satisfactory, though in some cases an affected digit may be stiff and less maneuverable than it was before the injury.

Locating the severed ends
When a tendon is severed, the muscle to which it is attached contracts, causing the tendon to spring away from the site of the injury. In such cases, surgery is required to locate the severed ends before they can be rejoined.

Path of tendon before cut

Cut

Cut ends of tendon

Dislocation

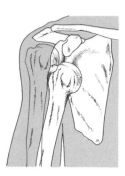

Dislocation of the shoulder
The shoulder joint is a ball-and-socket joint. The ball of the upper-arm bone fits into a cup-shaped socket in the shoulder blade. The shoulder is a very maneuverable joint, and so tends to become dislocated fairly easily.

A joint is dislocated if the bones that should be in contact are torn apart so that the joint no longer functions. The cause is usually a severe injury that exerts a force great enough to tear the joint ligaments. In addition to displaced bones, there is likely to be serious damage to the joint *capsule* (the membrane that encases the joint), and to surrounding muscles, blood vessels and nerves. Occasionally, the injury that causes the dislocation also produces a fracture (see next article) in one or both of the bones.

Dislocations that are not caused by an injury may be congenital (see p.664) or may occur as a complication of rheumatoid arthritis (see p.552). Finally, a dislocation may happen repeatedly, without apparent cause, to someone with a joint already weakened by an earlier injury. The jaw and shoulder joints are especially susceptible to this "spontaneous" type of recurring dislocation.

What are the symptoms?

A dislocated joint looks misshapen, is extremely painful, and becomes rapidly swollen, discolored and immovable. Other possible symptoms are related to and depend on the extent of damage to surrounding tissues, nerves and blood vessels.

What are the risks?

Dislocation of spinal vertebrae can damage the entire spinal cord, sometimes causing paralysis in the body below the level of the injury (see Spinal cord injury, p.278). Similarly, dislocation of a shoulder or hip can damage the main nerves to the affected arm or leg, and cause paralysis of the limb. Less dramatically, some joints that have been dislocated tend to be susceptible to osteoarthritis (see p.550) in later years.

What should be done?

Do not let anyone try to replace your dislocated joint in its normal position unless you are sure they know how. There may be a fracture or other damage that can be made worse if the problem is handled incorrectly. Simply protect the damaged area as well as you can (see within Accidents and emergencies, p.801), and get to a physician or hospital as quickly as possible. Do not eat or drink, for this is a problem if you need to have a general anesthetic to undergo *reduction* (the technical term for repositioning) of the dislocation. The physician will arrange for an *X-ray* of the joint and surrounding areas to determine the extent of the damage.

What is the treatment?

Self-help: None is feasible in most situations, but reduction without an anesthetic is possible in uncomplicated cases. To be effective, it must be done within a few minutes of dislocation, by someone who knows exactly what to do. If you have recurrent spontaneous dislocations, you may be able to learn how to reposition the joint by yourself. Even in such cases, you should see a doctor promptly to make sure the repositioning has been done properly.

Professional help: After 15 to 30 minutes a dislocated joint normally becomes so swollen and painful that repositioning may have to be done under a general anesthetic. Afterwards, if the blood vessels, nerves, and bones are in place and undamaged, the joint will probably be immobilized and splinted for two to three weeks so that other damaged tissues can heal. Follow the instructions of your physician when beginning to use the joint again. Failure to do so can result in reinjury.

Sometimes surgery is necessary to achieve satisfactory repositioning. Also, if one of your joints has become very weak because of repeated dislocation, your physician may recommend an operation to tighten the ligaments that bind the adjoining bones.

Fractures

A fractured bone is a broken bone. The break occurs as a result of the bone being stressed by physical forces greater than it can withstand. For purposes of diagnosis and treatment, different types of fractures are classified in the following ways:

A simple fracture is one in which the bone itself is broken, but the bone does not protrude through the skin. In a simple fracture, the neighboring muscles and other tissues remain largely undamaged. In a compound fracture, on the other hand, there is a considerable amount of damage that is done to surrounding soft tissues, and the bone does come through the skin.

A complete fracture is one in which the break is total and the two broken parts separate from one another. In an incomplete fracture, the break is more like a crack and does not extend all the way across the bone.

A fracture is usually caused by severe stresses on the bone from an accident or injury, but this is not always the case. Any bone weakened by old age or by a bone disease such as osteoporosis (see p.543) or bone cancer (see p.545) may break with little or no

Types of fracture

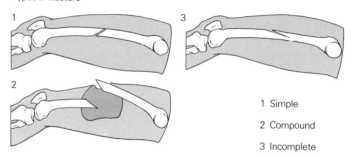

1 Simple

2 Compound

3 Incomplete

provocation. This is called a pathological fracture. Such fractures are common in the hips of elderly people, whose bones are weakened by a combination of disuse, the changes associated with aging, and sometimes disease. Another type of fracture, called a fatigue fracture, may occur in a normal, healthy bone that has been subjected to prolonged or repeated periods of excessive stress.

What are the symptoms?
A fracture makes the area around the injury look swollen, bruised, and possibly deformed. If you fracture a bone, you will probably be in severe pain, which is increased by any pressure on the area or attempt to move that part of the body. A minor fracture may cause only minor symptoms, and can be mistaken for a sprain (see p.532).

What are the risks?
Few people go through life without breaking a bone. One would have to lead a very protected life to totally avoid such injuries. The bones most likely to break are those in the wrists, hands and feet, which are often

broken during a fall. Fractures of other bones, such as the arm and leg bones and the spine and hip, are usually the result of much more powerful forces, such as those that can occur in a traffic accident.

The older you get the more likely you are to break a bone. This is because children, although they are very active and susceptible to injury, have springy, resilient bones that tend to bend rather than snap. At the other end of the scale, the bones of elderly people are fragile and brittle, and age-related problems with balance and coordination make falls more likely.

There are two main risks if you fracture a bone. The first is related to the bone itself. If a fracture is not treated, or if treatment is delayed, the broken pieces of bone may begin to rejoin out of alignment. In such cases, the bone may have to be separated and realigned surgically. In a severe compound fracture where the skin is broken, the bones may become infected. This complicates the healing process (see Osteomyelitis, p.695). And it is possible (but uncommon) for a fragment of broken bone, cut off from its blood supply, to die gradually.

The second risk that is associated with fractures is damage to neighboring tissues. Sharp bone fragments may compress or sever nearby blood vessels or nerves. Fractures of the skull or spine can damage the brain or spinal cord (see Brain injury, p.276, and Spinal cord injury, p.278). Occasionally other internal organs are damaged by a fractured bone. For example, a broken rib can puncture a lung (see Pneumothorax, p.362). Damage to soft tissues will have to be repaired surgically. Often this is done at the same time that the fracture is treated.

What should be done?
If you or someone near you suffers a possible fracture, apply first aid (see within Accidents and emergencies, p.801), and send for medical help immediately. Do not give an injured person anything to eat or drink. This may delay treatment because a general anesthetic cannot be given for several hours after a person has eaten.

Any presumed sprain that has not improved after two or three days may be a fracture. See your physician. The diagnosis of a fracture is confirmed by an *X-ray*.

What is the treatment?
The first task in the treatment of a fracture is to realign the broken pieces of bone if they are in the wrong position. The technical name for this process is *reduction*. It is often done

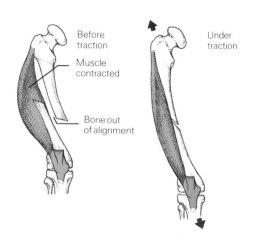

When you break your thigh bone, the strong muscles connecting it to the pelvis contract. This causes the broken ends of the bone to ride over each other, making healing difficult. Treatment stretches the muscles, thus pulling the broken bone back into the correct position. This can be done by putting the leg "in traction" in which heavy weights and pulleys provide the pulling power.

Before traction

Muscle contracted

Bone out of alignment

Under traction

Common fractures
This is a list of some of the most commonly broken bones.
1. Forearm bones (ulna and radius), broken near the wrist.
2. Bones in the hands (carpals and metacarpals) or feet (tarsals and metatarsals)
3. Ribs.
4. Fingers and thumbs (phalanges).
5. Shin bones (tibia and fibula).
6. Thigh bone (femur).
7. Skull.
8. Upper arm bone (humerus).
9. Collar bone (clavicle).
10. Backbones (spinal bones or vertebrae).

under a general anesthetic, and may involve cutting open the tissues around the fracture to reposition the bones correctly.

The second part of treatment is *immobilization*, or holding the various bone fragments together in the correct alignment while they heal. The medical term for this healing is *union*. Plaster casts or the more modern lightweight plastic or resin casts and splints are not the only ways to immobilize a fracture during the time it needs to knit together. In fact, some bones are held together naturally, and need no cast or splint. A broken rib, for example, is held by numerous chest muscles to nearby unbroken ribs. In a similar way, a fractured finger or toe can be bandaged to one next to it, to stabilize it while it heals.

The thigh bone is so buried beneath large muscles that a fracture in it cannot be held immobilized by a cast or splint. Frequently the ends of the broken bones in the thigh override each other. Such breaks are healed with the aid of *traction*. In traction, weights attached to the leg pull and hold the bones in the proper position.

In some cases, a fracture is held in position internally. An operation is performed to insert one or more metal screws, nails or plates that will hold the broken ends in place. Internal immobilization has a great advantage, because use of the injured limb can be resumed after a few days rather than in weeks or months. This is important, because it contributes to the third part of the treatment, the

rehabilitation of any joints or muscles that have not been used during the immobilization phase of treatment.

It is important that you begin to move and exercise the limb that contains the fractured bone. Particular attention is given to keeping nearby joints as active as possible. This helps to keep the immobilized area from swelling, and stimulates a good blood supply to aid healing. In addition, it keeps muscles and bones from wasting away because they are not used. But most important, it prevents the joints from becoming stiff from disuse. Discuss with your physician what exercise you should do and what limits you should observe to protect the healing bone.

The time needed for a fracture to heal depends on many factors, including which bone is fractured, and the age of the injured person. A child's broken finger may heal completely in two weeks; an adult's shin bone may take three months or longer.

Occasionally, in spite of treatment, for one reason or another, a fracture does not heal. If your physician suspects that a bone is not knitting, you may need to have additional X-rays taken of the area. Steps may have to be taken to encourage healing. The most common procedure is a bone graft, in which small pieces of bone are taken from some other site in your body (often the hip bone) and packed around the break.

If a fracture receives prompt treatment, the chances of a complete recovery are excellent.

Sports injuries

Athletes, and others who do vigorous exercise regularly run a high risk of injuring muscles, ligaments, bones or joints (see Pulled muscle, p.532, and Sprain, p.532). Such injuries are most common at the beginning of an athletic season and among people who begin to exercise after long periods of relative inactivity. If you are injured during a game, you may be eager to return to the game as quickly as possible, but treatments that allow you to do this may have long-term dangers. If the injury is a cut or bruise that does not involve serious damage to muscles or ligaments, it is reasonable for your coach or trainer to relieve pain with an ice-pack or an anesthetic spray, but if there is a possibility of muscle or ligament damage, painkillers may make it possible for you to damage the tissue further without realizing it. When the extent of your injury is uncertain, or when you become unconscious, even for only a few seconds, you should take no further part in the day's play.

Remember, professional teams often employ physicians to look after their athletes, but most people do not have such an advantage. Do not return to a game after any injury until you feel you are all right. If you are not sure, consult a physician.

Many injuries require no treatment other than rest, and possibly physical therapy to increase the circulation of blood to damaged tissues and strengthen the affected muscles. But some injuries require surgery.

If you have recurring injury, you may have to consider giving up your sport or exercise. If an injury to a ligament or bone recurs there is a strong possibility of permanent damage, and a price of not stopping the activity may be early development of osteoarthritis (see p.550) or some other joint problem. Before you reach a decision, get an accurate diagnosis of the extent of the damage. This may involve *X-rays*, *arthroscopy*, or perhaps an exploratory operation.

Hernias

A hernia is a bulge or protrusion of soft tissue that forces its way through or between muscles. Normally, body muscles are taut and firm. They press on various tissues and organs, helping to restrain them and keep them in the correct position within your body. However, for any of a number of reasons, muscles sometimes become weak or slack, because of a *strain* or a *congenital* weakness, for example. When this occurs the organs in the abdomen are able to force their way through the weak point and create a hernia.

Where do hernias occur?

Hernias can occur in many parts of the body, but they are most common in the abdominal wall. The abdominal wall is made up of flat sheets of muscle that encase the abdominal organs: the stomach, intestines, liver, kidneys

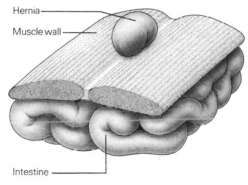

Hernia
Muscle wall
Intestine

A hernia is a bulge of soft tissue that protrudes through a weak point in a muscle wall. Injury and lack of use of the muscle are possible causes of a weak point. The hernia usually occurs due to increased pressure in soft tissue beneath the muscle wall.

and reproductive organs. Normally, these abdominal organs are held in by the firm muscles of the abdominal wall, even when the pressure inside rises, as it does when you cough, lift a heavy weight, or strain to pass urine or move your bowels. But if a weak point occurs in the wall, pressure inside the abdomen forces the muscles to part at that point. Some portion of the abdominal contents, often the intestinal tissue, is pushed through the muscles and becomes a visible bulge or sack, a hernia.

One common hernia is called a hiatus hernia. This type of hernia occurs in the sheet of muscle that is called the diaphragm, which separates the chest from the abdomen (see Heartburn and hiatus hernia, p.456). Several other hernias, all of which occur in the abdominal wall, are shown on the next two pages, along with their specific causes, symptoms and treatments.

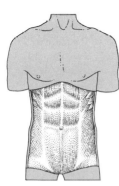

The abdominal wall is a large sheet of muscle at the front and the sides of the abdomen. It keeps the abdominal organs firmly in place.

What are the symptoms?

Usually, the only symptom of a hernia is a bulge or swelling. The bulge usually appears slowly over several weeks, but occasionally it forms suddenly, during the strain of lifting a heavy weight, for example. You may have a feeling of heaviness or slight tenderness at the site of the hernia.

Most hernias can simply be pushed back through the muscle opening into place. Such hernias are said to be *reducible*. If a hernia cannot be replaced it is called *irreducible*.

What are the risks?

If a hernia contains a length of intestine, the contents of the intestine may be prevented from moving through. This is called an *obstructed* hernia. If you have a hernia that becomes obstructed, you will have increasing abdominal pains, nausea and vomiting.

Another risk is *strangulation*, where a hernia swells and cuts off the blood supply to the loop of intestine within it. The strangulated hernia becomes enlarged, red, and very painful. An obstructed hernia or strangulated hernia needs urgent medical attention. If the condition is not treated, the result will be intestinal obstruction (see p.471), and eventually gangrene of the bowel.

What should be done?

If you suspect you have a hernia, see your physician. Any unexplained bump or swelling over a week old should be reported to your physician. A careful physical examination should confirm the diagnosis of a hernia, and your doctor will discuss with you the various methods of treatment.

In general, surgery is the best treatment for a hernia. Your physician may advise you to wear a supportive corset or truss until you have the operation, but this is usually only a temporary measure. Most hernias tend to slowly get worse, not better, and the dangers of obstruction and strangulation are present until the hernia is repaired. An obstructed or strangulated hernia is likely to require an emergency operation.

Hernias are repaired by pushing the protruding tissue back into place, and tightening or sewing together the loose muscles. You must follow your physician's advice while you are recovering from the surgery, because any sudden activity that strains your abdomen may cause the hernia to return.

Different types of hernia

These illustrations show the most common types of hernias, along with specific symptoms and treatments.

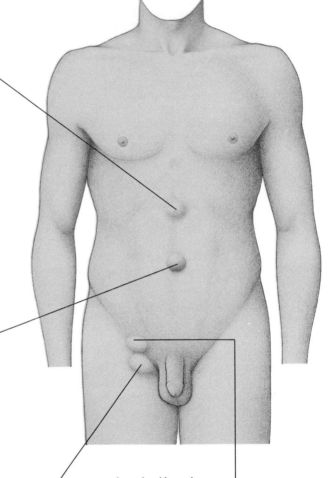

Epigastric hernia

A weak point in the fibrous tissue that joins the central abdominal muscles allows protrusion of a small piece of the fatty material that covers the intestines. It occurs somewhere on the line between the navel and the breastbone.

Symptoms: The hernia is usually small, but may be tender and cause indigestion, belching, and occasionally vomiting.

Risks: Strangulation is a possibility. It makes the lump painful, but is unlikely to be serious if the hernia contains only fat.

Treatment: If the hernia causes no problems, it may be left untreated. Otherwise surgery is usually done to repair the defect. Convalescence from surgery takes two to four weeks.

Paraumbilical hernia

A weakness develops in the abdominal wall muscles around the navel, but the soft bulge of the hernia appears to be at the navel.

Symptoms: A heavy feeling in the abdomen, sometimes accompanied by constipation and perhaps abdominal pain.

Risks: There is a risk of obstruction and/or strangulation.

Treatment: Your physician will probably recommend surgery to tighten the abdominal wall muscles, or sew them together at the site of the hernia. It usually takes four to six weeks to recover from the surgery.

Femoral hernia

This hernia occurs in a similar but slightly lower position than an inguinal hernia. It is often difficult to detect in a physical examination. The condition is most common in overweight women who have had a large number of children.

Symptoms: There are often no symptoms, and many femoral hernias go unnoticed unless they become obstructed or strangulated.

Risks: Because the hole through which a femoral hernia protrudes is small, the risks of obstruction and strangulation are high.

Treatment: The same as for inguinal hernia.

Inguinal hernia

This hernia appears as a bulge in the groin. There are two types. In a direct inguinal hernia the abdominal organs push aside weak abdominal-wall muscles that line the groin. An indirect inguinal hernia protrudes down the inguinal canal, a tube through which a testis descends from the abdomen to the scrotum, usually just before birth (see also Undescended testes, p.692).

Symptoms: None, or perhaps a heaviness in the groin.

Risks: Obstruction and strangulation are possible (but unlikely) risks.

Treatment: An operation is carried out to remove the hernia sac and shorten or sew together the weak muscles. Convalescence usually takes about four weeks, and you should avoid heavy lifting.

Umbilical hernia

This hernia appears as a soft bulge of tissue around the navel of a newborn baby. It occurs when, for some reason, the abdominal wall is not fully developed.

Symptoms: The hernia is unlikely to cause the baby any discomfort. It is most visible when the baby cries.

Risks: Because the opening is wide, there is virtually no risk of strangulation or obstruction.

Treatment: Most of these hernias heal naturally in a few years. Large hernias or persistent cases can be treated surgically. It takes the baby two to four weeks to recover from the operation.

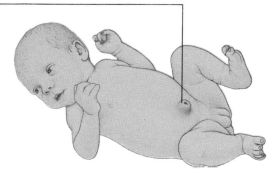

Incisional hernia

This type of hernia is an uncommon result of abdominal surgery. The cut abdominal wall muscles and fibrous layers sometimes do not heal properly, and the intestines may bulge through this weak point. If you are overweight and you remain inactive after an abdominal operation you are most likely to develop an incisional hernia. Incisional hernias also affect the elderly or very thin, weak people. Wound infections and broken stitches can also cause incisional hernias.

Symptoms: Large incisional hernias can cause constipation and sharp abdominal pains.

Risks: Strangulation and/or obstruction are unlikely.

Treatment: Sometimes a corset relieves the problem, but further surgery is usually the best solution. Because of the nature of this type of hernia, however, it sometimes recurs.

OPERATION: **Hernia repair**

(herniorrhaphy)

In a hernia repair operation, the bulge of soft tissue that has come through a weakened muscle or tissue layer is corrected surgically. This is especially important if your physician feels that the hernia may strangulate or become constricted.

During the operation Depending on the position and severity of your hernia, you will be given either a local or a general anesthetic. A small incision is made over the hernia and the bulging tissue is pushed back into place. The muscles or similar tissues are then sewn firmly together. The operation usually takes less than an hour.

After the operation You will be encouraged to get out of bed the day of, or the day after the operation. The area of the repair will be painful, so you may need to take painkillers. The length of time you need to stay in the hospital depends on the type of hernia you have.

Convalescence You should be able to return to work and continue with your normal activities within a few days, but you will probably be advised not to lift any heavy weights for up to 12 weeks.

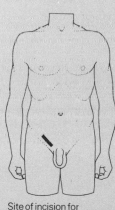

Site of incision for inguinal hernia

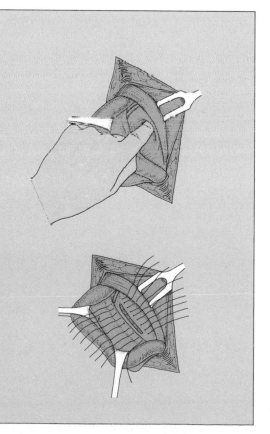

Muscle and tendon disorders

A muscle is composed of special elongated cells that contract to produce movement. At each end of most muscles there is a band of fibrous tissue that connects the muscle to a bone. In some parts of the body these bands of tissue are very short or their fibers are inextricably mixed with the muscle tissue to which they are joined. But in other areas, especially in the hands and feet, the tissue forms long, tough cords known as tendons.

Both muscles and tendons can be damaged by injury or disease. Damage from injury is discussed on p.532. The following articles deal with damage from other causes.

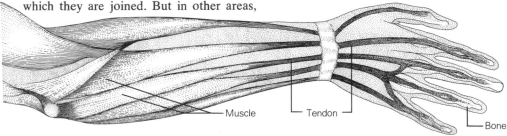

Tendons are tough, fibrous bands or cords that join some muscles to bone.

Muscle — Tendon — Bone

Cramp

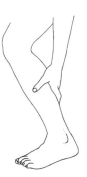

Massage the affected muscle

A cramp is a painful *spasm* in a muscle. It happens occasionally to almost everybody, and there is usually no underlying cause other than unaccustomed exercise or a prolonged period of sitting, standing, or lying in an uncomfortable position. Some people are roused from sleep quite regularly by sudden, severe cramp. In most cases there is no reason for concern. When cramps are accompanied by other symptoms, however, a more serious disorder may be causing them. If you think your cramps may be related to an underlying disease, consult the self-diagnosis chart on cramp (see p.171).

What are the symptoms?
When you try to move the cramped muscle, it contracts violently. There is usually a visible distortion of the affected area along with the sudden pain. If you feel the muscle, it seems hard and tense, and you cannot control it.

What should be done?
An ordinary cramp lasts no longer than a few minutes and will quickly clear up of its own accord. You can hasten and ease the process by massaging the muscle and gradually forcing it to function. If you are bothered by recurrent night-time cramps in your legs, try raising the foot of your bed slightly higher than it now stands. Relaxing and sipping a glass of milk just before you go to bed may also help. If you continue to have troublesome cramps, consult your physician, who may be able to discover what is causing the cramps and prescribe a helpful drug.

Tendonitis

For some reason, possibly a minor injury, a tendon, the tissue that connects muscles to bones, becomes torn and inflamed. A painful tenderness develops over the affected area, and the tendon is usually slow to heal because the muscle is constantly in use. When it does heal, the inflamed fibers may leave a painful scar in the tendon. The pain will generally disappear after a few weeks or months, but it can persist and even worsen, especially in older people. Tendonitis may occur in any place where a tendon joins muscle to bone, but it is most common at the shoulders or heels, on the outside of the elbows (where it is known as tennis elbow, though you need not play tennis to get it), or on the inside of the elbows (called golfer's elbow).

What is the treatment?
Rest the painful part for a few days, in a sling if necessary. A firm bandage and an *analgesic* such as aspirin should help relieve the pain. After a few days start to exercise the joint gradually, to prevent it from getting stiff. If the pain persists or worsens, your physician may want you to have an *X-ray* to assess the extent of the problem. The doctor may decide to inject a *steroid* drug and perhaps a local anesthetic into the affected area. This procedure may need to be repeated.

Tenosynovitis

Some tendons, particularly those that work fingers and thumbs, are sheathed in a membrane, sometimes called the synovium, that assists freedom of movement. The synovium may become inflamed and swollen, especially if you constantly use your fingers in repetitive fashion, in typing or assembly-line work, for example. In time, the synovium heals, but it may become too tight or narrow as it does so. A tight synovium restricts movement of the tendon it covers, and the result is tenosynovitis. One example of what happens is the minor disability called "trigger finger," in which a tight synovium makes it hard for you to straighten your finger once you have

Tendon — — Synovium

The synovium
The synovium membrane lines the interior of a joint. It makes and encases synovial fluid, which lubricates the joint.

bent it. The straightening mechanism is jammed for a few moments before the tendon suddenly overcomes the obstruction and the finger completes its movement with a sudden jerk. In any such case the area over the tendon will become painful and tender, and the affected finger will hurt and make a soft, crackling sound whenever you move it.

Tenosynovitis is occasionally caused not by mechanical factors but by an infection. In such cases your sore finger or thumb will become extremely painful and almost impossible to use, and you are also likely to feel generally ill.

What should be done?

If your symptoms suggest the possibility of infection, see your physician immediately. You may require treatment with *antibiotics*, and you may also need surgery to release pus produced by the invading bacteria that have caused the infection. Troublesome non-infectious tenosynovitis is sometimes cured by injections of *steroid* drugs. If the condition persists, a simple operation to slit open the constricting synovium will allow the tendon within it to move freely again.

Fibrositis
(*myofascial pain*)

Fibrositis is a term for stiffness and pain felt deep within the muscles. It may be caused by one of several factors ranging from straining a muscle or joint to emotional tension reflected in the knotting up of muscular tissues. If you have an attack of fibrositis, there is nothing basically wrong with the muscles themselves. Yet you are likely to have sharply localized pain, and you may even feel slight swellings within the affected muscles.

Fibrositis often affects the back, causing an apparent non-specific backache (see p.546). It is a common condition, especially in people past middle age, and it usually clears up within three or four days. Relaxing hot baths and *analgesics* such as aspirin should help to relieve the pain. If it persists, see your physician, who, after making sure that your symptoms are not those of a more serious disease such as rheumatoid arthritis (see p.552), may prescribe stronger painkillers or muscle-relaxant drugs.

Ganglia

Ganglia are swellings under the skin, generally in the wrist or the upper surface of the foot. A ganglion develops when a jelly-like substance accumulates in one of two places, a joint *capsule* or a tendon sheath, and causes it to balloon out. The size of ganglia varies, but they are often no bigger than peas. They may be soft to the touch or quite hard, and they are usually either painless or only somewhat bothersome.

Although ganglia are harmless, you should not ignore them. Always consult your physician about an inexplicable swelling, so that the possibility of a *malignant*, or life-threatening, growth can be excluded. Also, your physician may be able to burst the gang-

lion by pressing on it. Ganglia that are especially painful can be cut away. But since ganglia sometimes recur and frequently disappear of their own accord, such surgery is seldom recommended.

The wrist is one of the most common sites for ganglia.

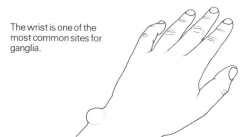

Dupuytren's contracture

In Dupuytren's contracture a layer of tough, fibrous tissue that lies under the skin on the palm of your hand thickens and shrinks. This shrinkage eventually causes your ring finger and little finger to be permanently bent at the knuckles. Although it is not painful, the condition weakens your grasp. One or both hands may be affected, and you may also have thickened skin pads over your other knuckles and on the balls of your feet. This is a common condition in men over 40 and tends to run in families. It is also found among alcoholics and in people who have epilepsy. The reason it occurs is not known, but its tendency to run in families suggests that it may be partly hereditary.

What should be done?
Because Dupuytren's contracture can make your fingers permanently useless, you should see your physician if you begin to develop it. If the condition is treated early enough, stiff fingers can be unbent by an operation that either removes or cuts through thickened tissue. With the aid of physical therapy, you can then regain the use of your hand. In some cases the condition recurs.

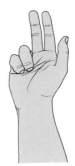

Your ring finger and your pinky bend involuntarily at the knuckles when you have Dupuytren's contracture.

Myasthenia gravis

This rare disease mainly affects women. It occurs when certain muscles become weak because of faulty transmission of nerve impulses to the muscles they control. Symptoms of muscular weakness usually appear first and most noticeably in the face. Your eyelids droop, you may see double, and you may have difficulty talking and swallowing because of an inability to control the movements of your lips and other parts of your mouth. If your arms or legs are affected, you may at times be almost unable to stand up or to carry out such simple tasks as combing your hair. The degree of weakness varies considerably from hour to hour, day to day, and even year to year. The cause of the fault in transmission of nerve impulses is complex, but it is thought to be due to an *autoimmune* problem. In such problems, your immune system, which usually protects you, turns against some of your own tissues. In about one-fifth of cases, the trouble appears to be related to the development of a growth in the thymus, a gland in your chest that plays a key role in immunity.

What should be done?
If you think you may have myasthenia gravis, consult your physician, who, after examining you, may want you to have blood tests and chest *X-rays* in order to make a diagnosis. If you have the disease, treatment with special drugs that restore transmission of nerve impulses to the affected muscles should greatly improve your condition. Surgery may be required to remove any thymus growth.

Although myasthenia gravis cannot usually be cured, treatment can minimize the symptoms of the disease so that you can lead a more normal life.

Muscle tumors

Tumors are exceedingly rare in muscles. When they do occur, they are nearly always *benign*, or unlikely to threaten life. Just why muscle tissue seems to resist serious tumors is not yet well understood. A *malignant*, or life-threatening, growth in a muscle is a rare but serious matter, since malignant muscle tumors grow and spread rapidly and are difficult to treat.

The first sign of a growth in a muscle is a detectable lump in the affected area, and usually there are no further developments. If the growth is malignant, however, it enlarges rapidly and may become painful.

What should be done?
See your physician without delay if you develop an inexplicable lump anywhere on your body. The doctor will examine you and, if the lump indicates the presence of a muscle tumor, will probably want you to have *X-rays* and a *biopsy* to make sure the growth is not malignant. In a biopsy, a sample of the growth is removed for examination. No treatment is necessary for a benign tumor. In the unlikely event of malignancy, possible treatments include injections of *cytotoxic* drugs, *radiation therapy*, and, if feasible, surgical removal of the tumor.

Bone diseases

The bones that make up your skeleton are active, living structures. They are composed of several different types of cells embedded in a hard framework primarily made of calcium and various proteins. The cells are constantly breaking down old bone and replacing it with new material, so that your skeleton is gradually but continuously renewed. If this maintenance system goes wrong, the result is one (or more) of the bone diseases included here.

Inside some bones are spaces occupied by marrow, a tissue that makes many of the blood cells found in the body. Diseases of the bone marrow therefore mostly affect the blood, and are discussed elsewhere (see Bone marrow, p.429). An injury may lead to a fractured, or broken, bone whether the bone is diseased or not (see Fractures, p.534).

Osteoporosis

Osteoporosis is the wasting, or deterioration, of bone. In healthy bone, there is a balance between the breakdown of old bone tissue and the manufacture of new, replacement material. In osteoporosis, breakdown occurs faster than replacement, and the bones become soft and weak.

Osteoporosis may occur in one or more bones after prolonged *immobilization* of part of the body, possibly because of a fracture (see p.534) or a prolapsed disc (see p.548). Some hormonal disorders (see Cushing's syndrome, p.523) may cause some osteoporosis. It may also result from a diet low in protein or calcium, which are needed to maintain healthy bones. The problem occasionally occurs in conjunction with osteomalacia (see next article). However, the most common cause is the natural process of aging. Elderly women are especially susceptible.

What are the symptoms?
Osteoporosis does not usually produce symptoms unless it occurs in the vertebrae, or backbones. If this happens you will have a backache, and you may also notice that you are becoming shorter and more round-shouldered due to the gradual compression of your weakened vertebrae. In rare cases of osteoporosis, one vertebra or a few vertebrae may collapse and you will have a sudden and extremely severe attack of back pain.

A bone weakened by osteoporosis is much more likely to fracture, or break, if you fall. The wrists and hips are the most likely to break under these conditions.

If you develop backache or a sudden, severe back pain, see your physician, because a fracture of your spine could result in paralysis. If the doctor suspects osteoporosis, you will probably need to have *X-rays* taken of your spine to confirm the diagnosis and determine the proper treatment.

What is the treatment?
Self-help: You can help to keep your bones healthy by making sure you eat a balanced diet rich in calcium. Stay active as much as possible, because exercise keeps both your bones and your muscles strong and healthy. Aspirin or another *analgesic* recommended by your physician should help relieve the pain. Take precautions to avoid falls: you should use a cane if you are unsteady on your feet; remove hazards such as loose rugs or electrical wires that may trip you; and keep your house well lit even at night (see also Special problems of the elderly, p.716).
Professional help: There is no specific treatment for osteoporosis. Your physician may prescribe calcium tablets to slow down the wasting process.

Osteomalacia

Osteomalacia is a softening and weakening of the bones because of vitamin D deficiency. If you lack vitamin D, you cannot absorb calcium and phosphorus from your food; both of these valuable dietary chemicals are required for the growth, hardening, and healthy maintenance of your bones.

A healthy person obtains vitamin D from two sources; from food, and from the natural action of sunlight on chemicals that are found naturally in the skin of all human beings. Therefore, a poor diet, lack of skin exposure to sunlight, or both can cause vitamin D deficiency. More rarely, vitamin D deficiency is caused by a specific disease such as chronic kidney failure (see p.512) or celiac disease (see p.474). Other rare causes are prolonged drug treatment for epilepsy (see p.287) and some forms of digestive-tract surgery (see also Vitamin deficiency, p.494).

What are the symptoms?
Your bones become tender and painful, causing symptoms that can be mistaken for rheumatoid arthritis (see p.552). You feel generally tired and stiff, you may have difficulty standing up, and you may have frequent muscular cramps. Depending on how severe they are, these symptoms can cause varying degrees of debilitation.

What are the risks?
Osteomalacia is common in less developed countries, but in the Western world it is a rare disease. Pregnant women are especially susceptible because of their increased need for calcium. The main risk of the disease is that weakened bones tend to break under slight stress (see Fractures, p.534).

What should be done?
A normal Western diet provides ample vitamin D, even if you are pregnant, but if you suspect you have osteomalacia, see your

physician. If you seem to have the disorder, the physician will probably question you about your diet and arrange for you to have blood and urine tests, *X-rays*, and perhaps a *biopsy*. In the biopsy, a small sample of bone is removed for examination.

What is the treatment?
Self-help: To prevent and to treat osteomalacia, make sure your diet contains plenty of vitamin D and calcium. Milk, eggs and liver are rich sources. Exposure to sunlight will also help. Avoid diets that severely restrict the types of foods you can eat, unless you first check with your physician. Be particularly wary of fad or cult diets.

Professional help: If you have osteomalacia, your physician will probably prescribe regular amounts of vitamin D and treat any underlying disease. If you are able to absorb vitamins from your digestive system you will probably receive tablets. If not, you will need vitamin D injections. Your doctor may also suggest ways in which you can improve your diet to help avoid a recurrence of the problem.

Paget's disease
(*osteo deformans*)

There is another disorder called Paget's disease that is a form of breast cancer. The disease discussed here, however, affects your bones. In this disease, the normal maintenance system that keeps your bones healthy and strong is disrupted. For no known reason, new bone is produced faster than old bone is broken down. The disease occurs in two stages. In the first, called the "vascular" stage, bone tissue is broken down but the spaces left are filled not with new, strong bone, but with blood vessels and fibrous tissue. In the second or "sclerotic" stage, the blood-filled fibrous tissue becomes hardened and bone-like, but it is weak and fragile.

Paget's disease can occur in part or all of one or many of your bones. The hip bone (pelvis) and shin bone (tibia) are the most common sites of the disorder. The thigh bone (femur), skull, spine and collar bone (clavicle) are also frequently affected.

What are the symptoms?
Paget's disease does not always produce symptoms, but when it does, bone pain is the most usual problem. The aching discomfort is virtually continuous, and is often worse at night. The affected bones become enlarged and misshapen, and they feel warm and tender. Depending on which bones are diseased, your head may enlarge, or you may appear

shorter, bent, or bow-legged, and your shoes may become too tight.

What are the risks?
Men seem to be more commonly affected than women by Paget's disease. It also has a clearly defined geographical distribution. For example, it is rare in India, Japan, Africa and South America. It is more common in Europe than in the United States. The significance of this uneven distribution is not yet understood by medical researchers.

Bones weakened by Paget's disease are more likely to break (see Fractures, p.534). Very occasionally, Paget's disease of the skull can compress the auditory nerve that carries signals from the ear to the brain, at the point where it passes through the skull. This can cause deafness. Another possible risk is heart failure (see p.381), because your heart is strained from trying to cope with the greatly increased blood flow through the diseased bones. In rare cases, a bone tumor develops (see next article).

What should be done?
If you think that you may have Paget's disease, you should consult your physician. After a physical examination, the physician will probably order *X-rays* and various blood tests to confirm the diagnosis.

What is the treatment?

There is at present no cure for the disease, but the major symptom, pain, can be relieved by an *analgesic* drug such as aspirin. If the pain is very severe your physician may advise that you have injections of a hormone that is called calcitonin. This hormone is made by your thyroid gland (see p.525), but the injections will provide you with increased quantities. Extra calcitonin seems to reduce the pain, but some people develop an allergic reaction to the injections and others feel extremely nauseated by them. In these cases, stronger painkillers are usually prescribed.

Bone tumors

Most bone tumors are secondary tumors; they develop from cancer cells that have *metastasized*, or spread, from a primary *malignant* (life-threatening) tumor somewhere else in the body. The bone tumor weakens the bone, and it breaks under the slightest strain. Once cancer has spread to bone, the outlook is poor.

Primary bone tumors, which start in the bone, are very rare. Most of them are *benign*, or unlikely to spread and threaten life, but a few are malignant. Both kinds generally appear as hard lumps on the bone. They may be painful even before the bone breaks.

What should be done?

If you develop any lump on a bone (or anywhere else on your body) you should see your physician, who will examine it and probably order *X-rays*. If the growth causing the lump is benign, nothing more needs to be done. Very rarely, however, a primary bone tumor is malignant, and amputation of the part of the body around the growth may be necessary. In addition, injections of *cytotoxic* (cancer fighting) drugs, *radiation therapy*, or both may be necessary. If the cancer is in an arm or leg and the limb is amputated, an artificial limb (see below) can be fitted.

Artificial limbs

An artificial limb is used when part or all of an arm or leg is lost. The loss may be the result of an accident, if micro surgery to repair the damaged limb was not possible. Or it may be a result of a disease such as dry gangrene (see p.415) or wet gangrene (see p.416), which may have to be treated by removing the affected limb.

After you have lost a limb, a physical therapist will teach you exercises to keep your remaining muscles strong. Then you will be given a temporary artificial limb to use for short periods until you become accustomed to it and can wear it all day. Once you are active again, an artificial limb can be designed specifically for you.

Ideally, an artificial limb should fulfill two requirements. It should provide mobility, so that you can carry on your normal life, and it should look natural, to restore your normal appearance. Unfortunately, it is difficult to meet both requirements with one artificial limb. It is important that you discuss your needs with those helping you so that the limb that is selected for you will meet as many of those needs as possible.

Once you have your new limb, your physical therapist will teach you how to use it. Many people, even those with more than one artificial limb, learn to use these devices quickly. Your age, the general state of your health, and your attitude are all factors in how quickly you can return to a normal active life. The extent of your own perseverance and enthusiasm are also particularly important.

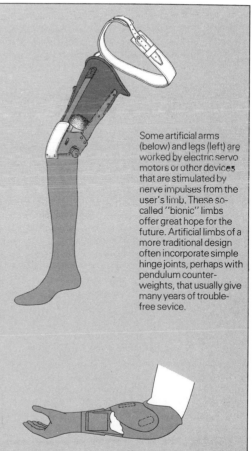

Some artificial arms (below) and legs (left) are worked by electric servo motors or other devices that are stimulated by nerve impulses from the user's limb. These so-called "bionic" limbs offer great hope for the future. Artificial limbs of a more traditional design often incorporate simple hinge joints, perhaps with pendulum counterweights, that usually give many years of trouble-free sevice.

Backaches

The spinal column, or backbone, stretches from the base of the skull to the bottom of the buttocks. It consists of more than 30 separate bones called vertebrae. The vertebrae are linked by strong ligaments, and flexible, flattened discs lie between them. Each disc is constructed of a tough, fibrous outer covering wrapped around a jelly-like inner substance, and this construction provides enough elasticity to permit some movement over the entire spinal column. It is partly the restrictions imposed by this limited flexibility that are responsible for most back troubles. If you twist the wrong way or overstrain one link of the chain, it can have a painful effect on the backbone itself, and on the muscles and ligaments that tie the vertebrae together.

Susceptibility to pain is increased by the fact that the spinal cord, which is a major part of the central nervous system, is located in a channel that runs the length of the spinal column. There are also narrow side channels through which peripheral nerves pass on their way to and from the rest of the body. Thus, any problem with a vertebra, supportive ligament, or disc may affect a far-reaching part of the nervous system. As a result, a back problem can lead to symptoms such as pain or weakness in almost any part of the body.

Non-specific backache

The vast majority of backaches are often called "non-specific" because they have no obvious cause. There are also no obvious, easy cures. Most non-specific backaches are probably due to a strained ligament or vertebral joint that causes surrounding muscles to go into painful *spasm*. In other cases, pain is due to fibrositis (see p.541) in the back muscles. In addition, some people tend to develop back pain when they are under stress, just as other people commonly develop tension headaches.

Backaches of all kinds are a major health problem. They are one of the most common causes of work days lost through illness.

Although a non-specific backache is often very painful and may make it difficult for you to continue your daily routine, there is virtually no risk of complications. Such backaches generally heal without treatment, but unfortunately they also tend to recur.

Symptoms of backache

Pain, generally along with stiffness, may de-

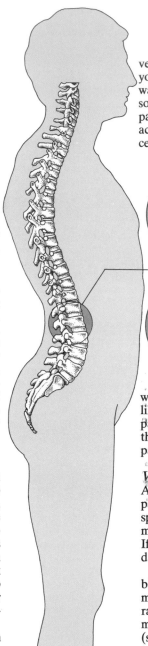

Standing correctly
To avoid back problems, try not to slouch. Stand with your head up, your shoulders straight, and your chest forward. Balance your weight evenly on both of your feet.

velop slowly or suddenly. It may begin after you lift a heavy object, fall, stay in an awkward or cramped position for some time, do some unaccustomed exercise, or for no apparent reason at all. It may be a continuous ache or it may occur only when you are in a certain position. Coughing and sneezing as

Your spinal column
Your spinal column is made up of more than 30 separate bones, vertebrae, which form a protective casing for your spinal cord.

Your spinal cord
Your spinal cord runs through a continuous canal within your vertebrae. It transmits nerve signals between your brain and your body.

well as bending and twisting the back are likely to aggravate the pain. Sometimes the pain seems to occur only in one spot. Three of the most common sites for localized back pains are shown on the next page.

What should be done?

Always protect your back (see Box, next page). If you get what seems to be a non-specific backache, first try self-help treatment (see Treatments for backache, p.548). If pain persists for more than three or four days, consult your physician.

Because of its very nature, a non-specific backache is difficult to diagnose. After examining your back, your physician may arrange for *X-rays* to be taken of your spine to make sure that you do not have spondylosis (see p.549) or a prolapsed disc (see next article). But in most cases where a physician suspects non-specific backache, you will be advised to continue with the self-help measures for a few days. The doctor may prescribe stronger painkillers or a muscle-relaxant drug, or may inject a *steroid* drug if you have a specific sensitive spot.

Massage can sometimes give beneficial results. However, an overly vigorous massage given by an inexperienced or poorly trained person may do more harm than good.

Types of back pain

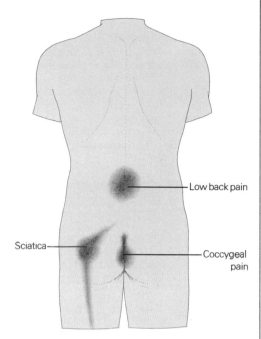

— Low back pain

Sciatica —

— Coccygeal pain

Low back pain: Low back pain is centered in the small of the back. It is often caused by unusual exertion such as moving furniture or unaccustomed heavy digging in the garden. It may develop either abruptly or overnight. Low back pain tends to be severe, and sometimes you will be completely unable to move your back. Physicians disagree about the exact cause of this problem. It is probably a mixture of pulled muscles, muscle spasm, and sprained muscles or ligaments.

Coccygeal pain: This is a term used to describe a non-specific backache (see previous page) that is located in the area of the coccyx, at the very base of the spinal column. It is a continuous ache that is worse when you are sitting down. It may be caused by a heavy fall on the buttocks or an injury from a blow. Women occasionally have pain in this area after childbirth. Some relief from the problem can be obtained by sitting on a soft cushion designed for this purpose.

Sciatica: Sciatica is a pain caused by pressure on the sciatic nerve (the biggest of all the nerves, with branches throughout the lower body and legs) as it leaves the spinal cord. The pressure is generally caused by either a prolapsed disc or spondylosis (see next two articles). You may feel a burning pain shooting into your buttocks and down along the back of your thigh. If you cough, sneeze, or try to bend your back, the pain worsens.

Whatever type of back pain you have, you should consult your physician if it persists for more than three or four days.

How to protect your back

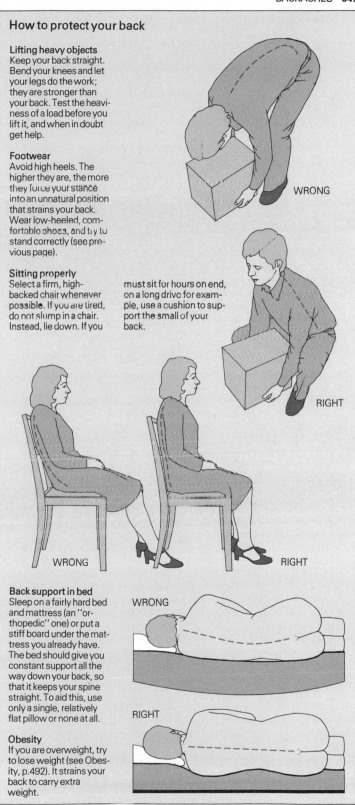

Lifting heavy objects
Keep your back straight. Bend your knees and let your legs do the work; they are stronger than your back. Test the heaviness of a load before you lift it, and when in doubt get help.

Footwear
Avoid high heels. The higher they are, the more they force your stance into an unnatural position that strains your back. Wear low-heeled, comfortable shoes, and try to stand correctly (see previous page).

Sitting properly
Select a firm, high-backed chair whenever possible. If you are tired, do not slump in a chair. Instead, lie down. If you must sit for hours on end, on a long drive for example, use a cushion to support the small of your back.

WRONG

RIGHT

WRONG

RIGHT

Back support in bed
Sleep on a fairly hard bed and mattress (an "orthopedic" one) or put a stiff board under the mattress you already have. The bed should give you constant support all the way down your back, so that it keeps your spine straight. To aid this, use only a single, relatively flat pillow or none at all.

WRONG

RIGHT

Obesity
If you are overweight, try to lose weight (see Obesity, p.492). It strains your back to carry extra weight.

Prolapsed disc
(*slipped disc*)

The term "slipped disc" is often used rather loosely. If you have a backache, you probably have a non-specific backache (see previous article), not a slipped disc. A slipped disc, more correctly called a prolapsed disc, is a specific disorder. Between each vertebra and its neighbors there is a disc made up of a fibrous outer layer surrounding a jelly-like inner substance. If a disc begins to degenerate and become less supple, because you are growing older, or because you have been overstraining your back, the disc may prolapse. In other words, the pressure squeezes some of the softer central material out through a weak point in the harder outer layer. The result is a loss of the cushioning effect of the disc, and painful pressure on a nerve at the squeezed-out portion of the disc. Any disc may prolapse, but those that are in the lower back are especially susceptible.

What are the symptoms?

If you have a prolapsed disc in the neck portion of your spinal cord, you are likely to wake up suddenly with an aching, twisted neck, which you cannot straighten out without extreme pain. You may also have numbness or tingling in an arm.

Symptoms of a prolapsed disc anywhere below the neck may start abruptly or develop gradually. On attempting to lift something, for example, you may suddenly feel intense pain in your back, often along with a searing pain down one or both legs. The sudden

Treating a backache

The exact causes of back pain are often difficult to pinpoint. Consequently, if you develop backache, it may be difficult for your physician to make an accurate diagnosis and prescribe immediate, precise treatment. Physicians know that a person with a backache will probably recover in a few days with the help of the simple self-help measures described below. But if your backache is severe, persistent, or recurrent, your physician may order *X-rays* and other diagnostic tests to discover the underlying cause of the problem. Once the cause is known, you will receive more specialized treatment for your particular type of backache.

Self-help for backache

Whatever the cause of your backache, there are measures you can take to ease pain and speed healing. Take simple painkillers such as aspirin as instructed on the package. Apply heat to the painful area to ease pain. You can use an electric heating pad or a hot water bottle wrapped in a towel. Lie flat on your back for as long as you can on a bed with a fairly hard ("orthopedic") mattress, or on an ordinary bed with a stiff board under the mattress. It may help to put a pillow under your knees. If your backache persists for more than three or four days despite these measures, consult your physician.

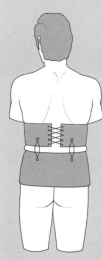

For some types of back pain, your physician may advise you to wear a special corset that supports your back. Other types of backache respond better to complete bed rest on a firm mattress that gives overall support.

Professional help for backache

Much depends on your history of back trouble and your physician's assessment of the situation. The doctor may prescribe stronger painkillers, or a muscle-relaxant drug. If you have a definable sensitive spot in the back muscles, one or more *steroid* injections may relieve it rapidly. Some physicians may recommend physical therapy, some form of *massage, traction*, a supportive belt or corset, special medications, or exercises to stretch the spine. However, the most widely used and so far most successful treatment, especially for a suspected prolapsed disc, is to lie flat on your back on a firm bed for two weeks. This may mean having meals in bed, using a bed pan, and having bed baths. If you become bored and get up, at mealtimes for example, this can ruin the treatment. It must be *complete* bed rest if it is to be effective.

Occasionally, backache is not relieved by these measures. If this happens, your doctor may refer you to an appropriate specialist for further examination and treatment. There are possible surgical procedures for back trouble, but these are usually not considered unless non-surgical treatment has failed.

As you gradually recover from your backache and cautiously resume your normal routine, the physician may advise you to do exercises to strengthen your back muscles and joints. While the problem is most likely to recur in the first few months after the first episode, you must be aware that throughout your life you will continue to be prone to backache. Therefore remember to protect your back (see previous page).

Take the proper protective measures and follow any recommended exercise routine to avoid back trouble in the future.

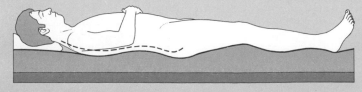

How a prolapsed disc causes pain

The flexible discs between your vertebrae act as shock absorbers to cushion the bones from each other as you move your spine. Each disc has a hard outer layer and a soft, jelly-like core. When your back is strained, pressure may push some of the soft substance through a weak point in the hard outer layer. It presses against a nerve where it leaves the spinal cord, and causes pain.

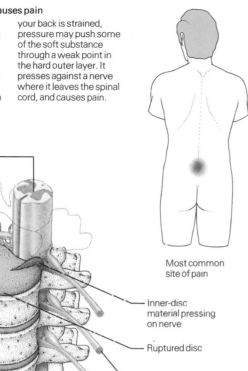

Spinal cord

Vertebra

Disc

Most common site of pain

Inner-disc material pressing on nerve

Ruptured disc

Nerves

strain has caused the prolapsed part of the disc to press on a nerve. Alternatively, you may have back and leg pains that build up over several weeks. If the prolapsed disc is in the lower part of your back, you may develop the symptoms of sciatica (see p.547).

What are the risks?

Except in the neck, attacks of pain from a prolapsed disc tend to recur, sometimes resulting in permanent backache. But the most serious risk is damage to the spinal cord, which can cause permanent paralysis of the lower parts of the body (see Spinal cord injury, p.278).

What should be done?

If you have the symptoms of a prolapsed disc, see your physician. The physician will carefully examine your back and legs, and may arrange for an *X-ray* to be taken of your spine. To locate a prolapsed or ruptured disc, the doctor may want you to undergo *myelography* or a *CAT scan*.

Treatments for a prolapsed disc vary. If the disc is in your neck, you will probably only need to wear a supportive collar for about two weeks. But much depends on your own situation and temperament, and your physician. Self-help and professional treatment procedures for back problems are summarized on the previous page.

Spondylosis

Spondylosis, sometimes called degenerative joint disease or osteoarthritis of the spine, is a hardening and stiffening of the spinal column that results in a loss of flexibility. This happens if some of the spaces between vertebrae are narrowed because the discs between the vertebrae have degenerated and lost their elasticity through age, over-use or injury. Sometimes bony outgrowths develop on the vertebrae or along the edges of degenerating discs, and these may press painfully on various nerves where they join the spinal cord. The narrowing and stiffening of intervertebral joints puts additional strain on the backbone and its supporting structures: the muscles, the ligaments, and the other discs. Every new stress then makes the back more susceptible to injury.

What are the symptoms?

Mild cases of spondylosis are usually symptomless. Thus, you may have the disease for many years, even your entire life, without knowing it. Often, however, you get intermittent pains in the part of your back that is most severely affected (see also Cervical spondylosis, p.280). Your back may become increasingly tender and difficult to bend or twist. If the lower part of your back is affected you may have the shooting pains in your buttocks and legs that are characteristic of sciatica (see p.547).

What are the risks?

If you have had frequent problems with a prolapsed disc (see previous article), you may be especially susceptible to this condition. Very rarely, a severe attack of spondylosis that occurs in the lower part of your back can adversely affect your ability to urinate, move your bowels, or walk.

What should be done?

If you think you may have spondylosis, try the recommended self-help measures (see Box, previous page). If the symptoms persist for more than three or four days, consult your physician, who, after examining you, may arrange for you to have back *X-rays* to help diagnose your problem.

Joint disorders

Because you use one or more joints every time you move, you soon notice any problems with them. It is perhaps not surprising that they sometimes go wrong; a highly maneuverable joint, such as the hip, is a complicated structure. The whole joint is bound together by fibrous bands called ligaments. Inside the ligaments is a fibrous joint *capsule* lined on the inside by the *synovium*, a thin membrane that continuously produces tiny amounts of fluid to lubricate the joint. Where the bone ends are in contact, their surfaces are covered by a smooth, firm substance that is called articular cartilage.

Most joint disorders are discussed in the following pages, but there are three main exceptions. Certain problems of the spinal column, which has a somewhat different jointed construction, are covered under backaches (see p.546). Sprains and dislo-

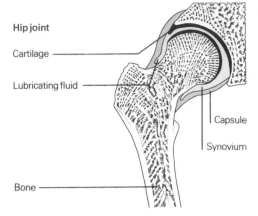

Hip joint
Cartilage
Lubricating fluid
Capsule
Synovium
Bone

cated joints are discussed under injuries (see p.532). Finally, gout, a joint disease that is affected by diet and metabolism, is discussed in the section that covers problems related to nutrition (see p.498).

Osteoarthritis

(*degenerative joint disease*)

Osteoarthritis is a condition that normally occurs as a result of wear and tear on the joints. It develops most commonly in older people, in the larger, weight-bearing joints including the hips, knees, and spine. Many physicians prefer to call the disease osteoarthrosis because the suffix "-itis" means "inflammation," and the joints of a person who has this disease are not necessarily inflamed. What happens is that the smooth lining of a joint, which is known as the articular cartilage, begins to flake and crack because of over-use, injury, or for some other reason. As the cartilage deteriorates, the underlying bone is affected, and may become thickened and distorted. Movement becomes painful and restricted, causing you to use associated muscles less often. The unused muscles may gradually waste away. This is a natural reaction of muscles that go unused anywhere in the body.

What are the symptoms?
Episodes of pain, swelling, and stiffness in the affected joint occur at intervals of months or years. Although osteoarthritis often affects several joints, it is rarely severe enough to cause symptoms in more than one or two. Pain that begins as a minor discomfort may, in a few cases, slowly become severe enough to disturb sleep and interfere with everyday life. As the joint continues to degenerate and

becomes more and more stiff and immobile, it may become less painful.

The amount of swelling in an affected joint varies. You may scarcely notice it, or the joint may become extremely knobby and enlarged. The pain itself is frequently deceptive. You may feel it directly in the area of the joint, or it may be transmitted to other parts of the body. Physicians call this not infrequent transmittal "referred pain." For example, osteoarthritis of the hip is sometimes felt most painfully in the knee.

What are the risks?
Osteoarthritis is the most common of all joint disorders, mainly because it is a natural part of the aging process. If you live long enough, you are certain to have the condition in some joints, though you may not know that you have it. *X-rays* show some degree of osteoarthritis in one or more of the joints of most people who are past the age of 40. It seldom becomes a serious problem, however, and the disease involves no life-threatening risks. Thus if you have osteoarthritis with no troublesome symptoms, there is no reason to worry about it or treat it.

Certain occupations and sports are closely associated with the eventual development of osteoarthritis. For example, many ballet dancers get it in their feet after many years of standing on their pointed toes. Football

Replacing damaged joints

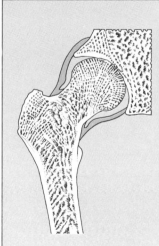

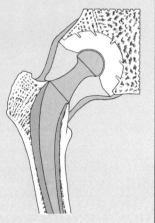

The replacement of natural joints with artificial ones made of metal or a combination of metal and plastic is a constantly developing and improving form of treatment for joints that are badly crippled by an arthritic condition. If the replacement is successful, it improves movement and relieves pain. The most common and generally satisfactory replacements are of hip joints. More than 90 per cent of these are completely successful. Other replacements are more susceptible, during or after the operation, to problems such as infection or even the working loose of the joint. But most such operations are successful.

Replacement joints are advised only for people with severe arthritis for whom the small but real risk of failure is a reasonable gamble. Other factors that have to be taken into account include age, general health, and whether or not other joints are affected.

players are also particularly susceptible to problems as a result of the repeated *trauma* and injuries that occur during games.

What should be done?

If you have occasional mild attacks of pain and stiffness in a joint, there is no cause for concern. If symptoms become troublesome, try the self-help measures recommended below. Then, if necessary, consult your physician, who will examine you and may want you to have blood tests along with X-rays of the affected joint or joints. If these tests do not indicate anything out of the ordinary, the chances are good that your problem is osteoarthritis, not a more serious disease such as rheumatoid arthritis (see next article).

What is the treatment?

Self-help: For obvious reasons the wear and tear on weight-bearing joints is greatest in people who are overweight or obese. If this applies to you, take off some of the strain by losing weight. Use a walking stick or cane, take frequent rests, and sleep on a firm bed. Keep warm, since heat generally helps to ease most kinds of joint pains.

It is important that you do not allow the muscles around your osteoarthritic joints to become weak through disuse. Regular exercise will strengthen your muscles and, in the long run, minimize your symptoms. Apart from an occasional dose of aspirin, do not use painkilling drugs other than those prescribed by your physician. Non-prescription preparations that are advertised as doing wonders for "arthritis" should be avoided unless they are specifically recommended by your physician.

Professional help: Your physician may pre-scribe a stronger painkiller than aspirin. Some *anti-inflammatory* drugs seem to ease the symptoms of osteoarthritis, though why this is so is unknown. If pain becomes severe, an injection of a *steroid* drug into the painful joint may help, but this type of treatment can do further damage to the joint cartilage if it is tried too often. The doctor may also arrange for you to have physical therapy, which usually involves exercises and heat treatments.

Surgery is sometimes both feasible and advisable. The most common operation, which is mainly recommended for people with osteoarthritis of the hip, is joint replacement (see Box above). Hip-joint replacement has proved successful in a high proportion of the cases in which the procedure has been attempted.

If you wonder whether a change in your diet might have a beneficial effect on your arthritic symptoms, the answer is simple: there is only one kind of diet that helps; a reducing diet (see p.28), since excess weight can further damage the joints and surrounding tissues. Other possible treatments, none of which can be guaranteed to help, include *acupuncture*, special kinds of warm clothing (so-called thermal wear), heat applied to the affected area, and swimming regularly in heated pools. The fact is that there are no magic cures. If you have arthritic pains caused by the natural degeneration of joints, ordinary painkillers such as aspirin should give you some relief.

Do not forget that there are many household gadgets and other aids available for those disabled by diseases such as osteoarthritis. Your physician can give you information and assistance.

Rheumatoid arthritis

Rheumatoid arthritis is a long-term disease of the joints. Its exact cause is unknown, but it is thought to be brought on by an *auto-immune* process. In this disorder the *synovium*, which is a thin membrane surrounding a joint, gradually becomes inflamed and swollen, and this leads to inflammation of other parts of the affected joint.

If the problem persists, the bones linked by the joint are slowly weakened. In severe cases bone tissue may eventually be destroyed. The joints that are usually affected are the small ones in your hands and feet, mainly the knuckles and toe joints, but rheumatoid arthritis can also occur in your wrists, knees, ankles, or neck. It occurs less often in the spine or hips, which are much more susceptible to osteoarthritis (see previous article).

In many cases the disease is not limited to the joints. It can also cause generalized inflammation in the heart muscle, the blood vessels, and in the tissues that are just beneath the skin.

What are the symptoms?

Rheumatoid arthritis may begin without obvious symptoms in the joints. Over several weeks or even months you may feel generally ill, listless, and without appetite. You are likely to lose weight and to have vague muscular pains. Only later do you develop the joint problems that are characteristic of the disease. In other cases, the joint symptoms appear suddenly, without previous symptoms of any other kind.

When the joints are affected, they become red, swollen, tender to the touch, painful to move, and stiff. The stiffness is usually most noticeable first thing in the morning. As you move about and exercise the joints, the pain and stiffness gradually become less severe.

In some people, these joint symptoms are accompanied by bursitis (see p.555). Others become anemic (see p.419). Only one or two joints may be affected, or the disease may rapidly become widespread. Some people have only one mild attack, while others have several episodes that may or may not leave them increasingly disabled. In a few cases, and it should be emphasized that these are relatively rare, continuous deterioration of joint and bone tissues produces deformities in the joints and surrounding area and makes it difficult to live an active life.

What are the risks?

Most cases of rheumatoid arthritis occur in the 40 to 60 age group, but the disease can attack people of any age. In severe cases swollen, deformed joints may collapse and become partly or completely dislocated. This can cause great discomfort and problems with walking if knee or foot joints are affected. Tendons may also become so weak that they snap, making it impossible to control certain movements.

If the neck is involved, the interlocking mechanism of the top two vertebrae may be badly weakened, and there is a risk that paralysis or death from serious damage to the spinal cord may follow.

What should be done?

If you develop the symptoms described, consult your physician, who will examine your joints, and may want you to have *X-rays* and some special blood tests. Rheumatoid arthritis can usually be identified from the results of these tests, but occasionally the only way to make a firm diagnosis is to observe the progress of the disease for several weeks or even months.

What is the treatment?

Self-help: The best thing you can do is to come to terms with what may be a permanent condition. Follow the advice of your physician, get plenty of rest, and exercise regularly and moderately. Swimming in a heated pool is good for stiff joints. A firm mattress and warm but lightweight covers help you to sleep

---

Rheumatism and arthritis

"Rheumatism" and "arthritis" are virtually interchangeable words, which are loosely used to describe disorders characterized by red, stiff, and sometimes swollen joints and muscles. Strictly speaking, however, there is no medical condition called simply "rheumatism" or simply "arthritis." The terms become medically significant only when used as part of the more definitive name of a disease – for example, rheumatic fever (see p.393) or osteoarthritis (see p.550). So, if your physician tells you that you have arthritis or rheumatism, you will be able to find out more about the condition if you ask for more details.

Many people believe that rheumatism is a milder condition than arthritis. According to this notion, rheumatism comes and goes, is often brought on by wet weather or strenuous activity, and tends to be bearable. Thus many people believe that all they need to cure their "rheumatic pains" are a hot bath and a couple of aspirins. On the other hand, arthritis is often looked upon as a more severe, perhaps crippling condition, a chronic disorder that can only be made bearable with the frequent use of painkillers and other drugs.

In fact, no such simplified distinction between rheumatic and arthritic conditions can be made. Symptoms termed rheumatic may, indeed, be milder than those normally characterized as arthritic, and although the symptoms of various arthritic disorders are occasionally severe and can become increasingly so, this rarely happens.

comfortably without putting too much pressure on your joints.

Professional help: If you have a bad attack of rheumatoid arthritis, your physician may arrange for you to be admitted to a hospital. The major element in treatment for severe cases is complete rest. You will remain in bed, probably with the affected joints encased in soft-molded splints, until the symptoms have subsided. Thereafter you may be referred to a physical therapist and/or an occupational therapist who can teach you some helpful exercises. They may also provide you with removable splints that can be strapped onto painful joints when they need rest.

Whether or not your condition is severe enough to require a stay in the hospital, your physician will also prescribe pain-relieving drugs. The basic drug is likely to be aspirin in high doses (the equivalent of 15 or 16 ordinary-sized tablets a day). But you and your physician may have to experiment for a while before finding the best possible painkiller and/or anti-inflammatory drugs for you.

This is because the many possible drugs, including aspirin, can have unpleasant side-effects, particularly on the digestive system and the urinary tract.

Occasionally, surgery may be needed to treat this disease. In the early stages of rheumatoid arthritis, a *synovectomy*, the removal of badly inflamed joint synovium, is effective if only a single joint is severely affected. In later stages it is sometimes possible to replace a severely damaged joint with an artificial one. But most physicians usually advise an operation only in severe cases where other treatment has failed.

What are the long-term prospects?
Rheumatoid arthritis is as variable in its outlook as it is in its severity. Statistics indicate that in a little less than half of all cases, the patient recovers completely after one or more episodes of painful joint inflammation. About the same number remain somewhat arthritic. Only about one in ten people who have the disease are severely disabled by it.

Infectious arthritis

True infectious arthritis is a rare disease caused by the invasion of a joint by bacteria. The bacteria may enter through a wound, spread directly from a nearby infection, or be carried to the joint through the bloodstream from a more distant infection. Once in the joint, the bacteria multiply and cause redness, pain, and swelling due to inflammation and accumulation of pus. It is unlikely that more than one joint will be affected. The infection will also cause a fever, sometimes as high as 104°F (40°C).

Many diseases, including rheumatic fever, German measles, mumps and chickenpox, can cause joints to become swollen and painful. These arthritic symptoms will clear up when the infection is over, and they are not the same as infectious arthritis.

What should be done?
If you have the symptoms of infectious arthritis, see your physician without delay. If it is not treated, the joint may become stiff and almost useless. Your physician will examine the swollen joint, and may use a needle and syringe to draw out some of the accumulated fluid. Examination of the fluid should confirm the diagnosis. If you have infectious arthritis *antibiotic* drugs in tablet form, injections directly into the joint, or both, are used to treat the problem. In addition, you may have to go to the hospital for an operation. In this operation, a surgeon opens the affected joint so that it can be drained. As the joint heals, you will be taught how to exercise it carefully but thoroughly, to prevent it from becoming permanently stiff.

Ankylosing spondylitis

Spondylitis is inflammation of the joints that link the vertebrae (backbones). In ankylosing spondylitis, the inflammation recedes but leaves behind hardened, damaged joints that effectively fuse together the separate bones of the spinal column. The cause of this debilitating disease is not known.

The first joints to be affected are the sacroiliac joints, which link the base of the spine to the pelvis, or hip bone. Bony growths fuse the normally separate bones together, and the resultant stiffness may move slowly up your

spine until it affects many, if not all, of the joints between your vertebrae.

What are the symptoms?
Ankylosing spondylitis often starts with an ache in the lower portion of the back. The ache may spread into the buttocks. The pain and stiffness are generally at their worst in the morning. You may also have stiff, painful hips and a general feeling of stiffness in your spine. Other possible symptoms are vague chest pains and, oddly, tenderness over your

heels. You will also feel generally ill, with loss of energy and weight, a poor appetite, and a slight fever. And, for reasons that are not clear, your eyes may become red and painful.

What are the risks?
This disease is much more prevalent in men than in women and occurs mainly in the 20 to 40 age group. It also seems to run in families to a limited extent.

Although the disease does not usually progress very far up the spine, it can sometimes do so, and leave you with a stiff spinal column that may cause your head to be permanently bent down onto your chest. The ribs can also become involved at the point where they join the spine, and this reduces your ability to breathe because of constriction of the lungs. Chest infection then becomes a danger. Your jaw may be stiff, which causes difficulty in eating and speaking.

What should be done?
If you have symptoms of ankylosing spondylitis, consult your physician, who will examine you with special attention to the extent of your back movements and chest expan-sion. You will probably need to have blood tests, and also X-rays of your back and pelvic area before a diagnosis can be made.

What is the treatment?
Self-help: Regular daily exercise is essential. Swimming, if possible, is especially helpful. Get in the habit of breathing deeply, sleep on a hard mattress, and do not use a pillow. Try to teach yourself to sleep on your stomach rather than on your back or side. All such measures help to keep your back muscles strong and prevent your spine from becoming permanently stiffened into a bent position.
Professional help: Your physician may refer you to a physical therapist, who will probably give you special exercises to improve your posture. The doctor may prescribe painkilling and anti-inflammatory drugs.

A very badly bent spine can be improved by osteotomy, a surgical procedure for straightening the bent, fused bones. But any such operation may damage the spinal cord and is therefore advised only in extreme cases. If your hips are badly damaged you may be advised to have the joints replaced with artificial ones (see p.551).

Bunions

A bunion is a bony protrusion from the outside edge of the joint at the base of the big toe. Bunions are usually caused by a minor foot disorder known as hallux valgus. The technical name for the big toe is "hallux," and if your big toe has grown or been forced into a position where it overlaps one or more other toes, you have hallux valgus. This tends to happen in people with an inherited weakness in toe joints. Poorly fitted shoes, especially those with very high heels and pointed toes, make it worse. One result of the deformity is that the bony base of the twisted big toe is pushed out beyond the normal outline of the foot and forms an unattractive bump known as a bunion. As this rubs on the inside of your shoes, the overlying skin toughens and thickens into a callus (see p.253).

What are the risks?
Bunions are common but not usually troublesome. Three times as many women as men have bunions, and the occurrence of the problem tends to run in families.

Sometimes the persistent pressure of a shoe on a bunion causes painful bursitis (see next article) under the pressure point. In addition, the affected joint is likely to develop osteoarthritis (see p.550) sooner than it normally would.

What should be done?
If you have a bunion that has become troublesome, consult your physician, who will examine your feet, and may treat you or refer you to an orthopedic surgeon.

What is the treatment?
Self-help: Always make sure your shoes fit comfortably and leave plenty of room for your toes. If you have developed bursitis, you can relieve pressure on the bunion and give it a chance to heal by cutting a hole in the top of an old, comfortable shoe and wearing it exclusively until the inflammation clears up.

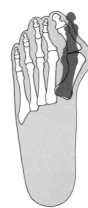

Normal position of big toe shown in brown

Professional help: If you have a severe hallux valgus, you may be advised to have an operation. Usually, after the operation you must keep the affected foot in a plaster cast for up to two months. Because of the pain and inconvenience, your physician probably will not recommend surgery unless your bunion is causing severe discomfort.

Bursitis

A bursa is a soft sac filled with a lubricating liquid that minimizes friction between body tissues that must constantly move by each other. Bursas are usually found near joints, either between the skin and underlying bones or between tendons and bones. If a bursa is irritated by pressure over it or by injury to the nearby joint, the little sac may become inflamed and fill with fluid. This is called bursitis. It is a fairly common complaint that causes pain and swelling in the area around the bursa. The condition generally known as housemaid's knee is a familiar type of bursitis that occurs around the patella, or kneecap. Other joints that are particularly susceptible to bursitis include the elbows, the heels, the base of the big toe (see Bunions, previous article), and the shoulders.

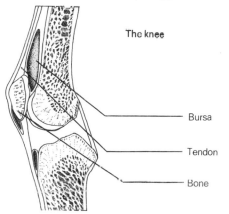

The knee

Bursa

Tendon

Bone

What should be done?

Bursitis is not a serious disorder. It usually clears up of its own accord in a week or two, especially if you are careful to keep pressure off the tender spot while it remains swollen. If bursitis persists, consult your physician, who will examine the joint to make the diagnosis. To bring down any swelling, the physician may draw off fluid with a needle and syringe, and then bandage the joint firmly. *Anti-inflammatory* drugs may be prescribed for the condition as well.

Bursitis has a tendency to recur in the same place. If it keeps coming back, it may be wise to have the affected bursa removed. This type of surgery can be done with either a local or a general anesthetic, and seldom requires more than 24 hours in the hospital. Where surgery is not feasible, as for a painful bursa lying deep in the tissues around a shoulder, the best treatment may be an injection of *steroid* medication and a local anesthetic into the most painful point.

Frozen shoulder

In a frozen shoulder, the shoulder becomes stiff and painful, making normal movement impossible. It usually starts as a slight injury or a minor problem such as tendonitis (see p.540), or bursitis (see previous article), which prevents you from using the joint. This disuse leads to more stiffness and pain, followed by more disuse, and so on. Finally you can hardly move your arm at all, and the pain is often severe enough to disturb your sleep. The pain may be localized either in the shoulder itself or (more frequently) it may spread to your upper arm, your neck, or both.

If it is not treated, the condition runs a slow course. Symptoms gradually worsen over several months. They then tend to remain the same for a few months, followed by a slow period of gradual improvement. Thereafter you usually feel no more pain, but your shoulder mobility often remains permanently impaired and may interfere with some of your activities. This is why it is important to seek professional help quickly if you think you may be developing a frozen shoulder.

What is the treatment?

A frozen shoulder should be kept in motion as much as possible. Use a painkiller such as aspirin to ease any pain. Your physician will probably prescribe antirheumatic drugs to try to decrease the inflammatory process and may also refer you to a physical therapist or an occupational therapist for treatment such as range of motion exercises. Injection of *steroid* drugs into the shoulder increases the pain temporarily, but generally proves helpful in the long run. If your problem is severe and persistent, your physician may urge you to have your shoulder manipulated as far as possible under a general anesthetic. With treatment, your chances for recovery of pain-free mobility are good.

Collagen diseases

Connective tissue is as essential part of every structure in the body. Its main component is a protein called collagen. In collagen diseases, damage to the collagen in certain areas of connective tissue causes inflammation.

Collagen diseases are regarded as *autoimmune* disorders, which means the body's natural defense mechanism, called the immune system, starts to work abnormally. In this case, it begins to attack and destroy the collagen. This damages some of the body's own connective tissue.

Scientists do not know why the immune system malfunctions in this way. Normally it attacks only things that are foreign to the body, such as bacteria and viruses. Somehow, however, the system wrongly identifies the body's own tissues as foreign in autoimmune disorders such as collagen diseases.

There are no specific cures for collagen diseases, but they can become less damaging over time and some patients show dramatic improvement. This usually takes many years. Rarely, collagen diseases are fatal.

Polyarteritis nodosa

In this disorder, the small arteries in several organs of the body become inflamed, which damages those organs.

What are the symptoms?
The heart is nearly always affected, and this causes chest pains. Many other organs can also be affected. Lung damage produces shortness of breath. Liver and intestine damage causes abdominal pain. Nerve damage causes general weakness and numbness. And kidney damage may produce blood in the urine, swelling of the face and limbs, or both. Such symptoms are generally accompanied by tiredness, aches and pains, a persistent fever, poor appetite, loss of weight, and a rapid heartbeat.

What are the risks?
Polyarteritis nodosa is extremely rare. Three times as many men as women get it. Without treatment, the disease is rapidly fatal, usually because of heart and kidney damage.

What should be done?
With treatment, some damage may be prevented. If you survive one year of the disease, you have a good chance of continuing to live for many more years.

A great number of tests are needed before a diagnosis of polyarteritis nodosa can be made. Then specific treatments, usually with drugs, are begun according to which organs have been damaged. To relieve the general symptoms, *steroids* may also be prescribed.

Systemic lupus erythematosus
(SLE)

This disease, often called SLE, inflames and damages connective tissue in any part of the body. The disease flares up periodically and varies considerably in the areas it affects and its intensity. Most commonly, SLE involves inflammation of various membranes that surround and envelop the kidneys, joints, lungs and other organs.

What are the symptoms?
In many cases the skin is affected. A rash appears on the cheeks and may spread to the entire body. Exposure to the sun aggravates the rash. Skin damage can also cause Raynaud's phenomenon (see p.412) and bald patches. In some cases the kidneys are attacked and there are symptoms of kidney failure (see p.511). Damage to joints results in stiffness and pain that are much like those of rheumatoid arthritis (see p.552). If the lungs are affected, you can become short of breath.

Apart from such variable but specific symptoms, SLE also causes more general symptoms. These include loss of appetite and weight, a slight but persistent fever, and a feeling of general ill health.

What are the risks?
SLE most often attacks women in their 30s or 40s. It is a serious disease, but most people who have it can expect at least ten years of fairly normal life.

What should be done?
If you have SLE, you will probably feel so ill that you will need to consult a physician. The disease is diagnosed from the results of blood tests. The progress of SLE can be slowed or even halted by treatments. These include various drugs – *steroids, immunosuppressives,*

and *antirheumatics* – along with physical therapy and *plasmapheresis*, a type of blood therapy. Your physician will give you regular checkups and will prescribe various drugs to combat troublesome symptoms of SLE. Al- ways inform medical workers that you have SLE before you are treated for any disorder or before you have an immunization. You should also seek prompt treatment for any infection, however minor.

Scleroderma

In scleroderma the connective tissue in and around the tiny blood vessels called capillaries becomes inflamed. As the inflammation heals, internal scarring occurs. This makes the tissue shrink and become stiff.

What are the symptoms?
The skin and the esophagus, or gullet, are almost always affected. Patches of skin become shiny and uncomfortably tight, and the esophagus stiffens.

What are the risks?
Scleroderma may also bring on kidney failure (see p.511), heart failure (see p.381), shortness of breath, and joint problems similar to those of rheumatoid arthritis (see p.552). In addition, there are usually general symptoms including a persistent slight fever, loss of appetite and weight, and feeling ill.

What should be done?
Scleroderma is a rare disease, but if you suspect you have it, see your physician. He or she will arrange for you to have blood tests and a *barium swallow X-ray*. If these tests confirm that you have the disease, many of the symptoms can be prevented with drugs. Your physician may recommend that you receive rehabilitation for this disease. Physical therapy and occupational therapy can be helpful in maintaining as independent a life as possible. The shiny appearance of the skin will probably remain, however. Unlike other collagen diseases, scleroderma does not respond to *steroid* drugs.

Polymyositis and dermato-myositis

Polymyositis is inflammation of the muscles, most commonly those of the shoulder and pelvis. The affected muscles gradually become weak. If the disease is accompanied by any skin inflammation, it is called dermatomyositis. In such cases, a rash often spreads over your face, shoulders, arms, and any bony prominences, such as the knuckles. In all cases, you feel generally sick.

Two thirds of those who get polymyositis and dermatomyositis are women. Nobody knows why the diseases occur, though they are thought to be *autoimmune* disorders. If you have the symptoms described, you should see a physician. A firm diagnosis is made based on blood tests and by *elec-tromyography*, or tests of the electrical properties of the painful muscles. A *biopsy* may also be necessary to confirm the diagnosis. In a biopsy, a small sample of tissue is removed for examination.

What is the treatment?
Treatment is aimed at minimizing the symptoms of the disease. High doses of *steroid* drugs are usually prescribed to suppress the inflammation. In some cases, *immunosuppressive* drugs are also given. A physical or occupational therapist can teach you exercises to minimize weakness and shrinkage of muscles. In many cases the disease disappears on its own after a few years.

Polymyalgia rheumatica

This rare disease causes inflammation of many of the body's muscles, particularly those of the shoulders and buttocks. The affected muscles become tender, and associated joints feel stiff, particularly in the morning. Accompanying symptoms are persistent, slight fever and a feeling of general ill health. In some cases a very similar condition, temporal arteritis (see p.414), also develops.

If you have the symptoms described, you should consult a physician, who will examine you and arrange for blood tests. The physi- cian may also order a *biopsy* of one of the temporal arteries on the side of your head, to discover if temporal arteritis is developing. In the biopsy, a small sample of tissue is removed for close examination.

If the disease is present in a mild form, ordinary painkillers and *anti-inflammatory* drugs such as aspirin are all that is needed to control the symptoms. In severe cases, *steroid* drugs are prescribed. Usually, polymyalgia rheumatica disappears of its own accord after a few years.

General infections and infestations

Introduction

The articles in this section deal with diseases caused by identifiable organisms that live in or on the human body. Infections are caused by minute organisms invisible to the naked eye that invade and multiply within the body. Bacteria, viruses, chlamydia and some fungi cause infections. In general, the body is capable of mounting an attack, through its natural defenses, against such organisms. The infections occur when this attack fails to control the organisms adequately.

The infections discussed in the following pages have generalized effects on the body. Infections that attack specific parts of the body are discussed in the relevant sections. Similarly, infections that are primarily children's diseases (mumps, chickenpox, and so on) are discussed under special problems of infants and children (see Childhood infectious diseases, p.698).

The parasites that cause infestations are larger organisms than those that cause general infections. Parasitic organisms also differ somewhat from those that cause infections in that the body generally lacks effective natural means to combat them. The problems caused by bites from some common insects are included in this section.

Many of the organisms responsible for general infections and infestations are *contagious*; that is, they spread between people in close contact.

Some diseases that could be classified as general infections are not included here because they are very rare in North America. One is leprosy, a bacterial disease that causes permanent damage to skin and nerves, but is very rarely contagious. Leprosy can be treated and eventually cured with modern medications.

Two other infections, which are extremely rare in North America, are Bornholm's disease and anthrax. Anthrax is caused by bacteria, and is sometimes fatal. Bornholm's disease is a painful viral disease that is not dangerous in an otherwise healthy person.

The two major infectious agents

Viruses, the smaller of the two major infectious agents, are of many shapes ranging from that of miniscule planetary lander space probes to tiny cut jewels. They cause their damage when they invade cells, taking over their reproductive mechanisms to make thousands of new viruses. In the process, the original cells are usually destroyed and others are invaded. Viruses cannot be controlled with antibiotics.

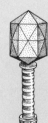
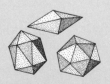

The shape of bacteria also varies. And although they are many times larger than viruses, bacteria are far smaller than the cells of your body. Bacteria live virtually everywhere, and many are harmless. The large population of bacteria in your intestines, for example, usually causes no harm. Because most bacteria can be controlled with antibiotics, many bacterial diseases are now both uncommon and easily treated.

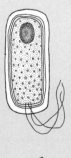

Infections

The organisms that invade your body and cause infections spread in various ways. Some are coughed or sneezed into the air. Others are transferred by direct contact. Some infect people who handle animals or animal products. If the spread of an infection can be halted, there is a chance that the disease it causes can be eradicated. This is how smallpox has been eliminated.

Once infectious agents enter your body, it takes time for them to become numerous enough to cause symptoms. This time period before symptoms appear is called the *incubation* period. The length of time this takes generally varies from a few days to several months, depending on the disease. If you get an infectious disease, and the incubation period of that disease is known, it is often possible to figure out when, where, and how you caught it.

The symptoms of an infection are caused by injury to body tissue from infectious agents, and also by the body's mechanisms for fighting infection. Your white blood cells attack invading organisms either by trying to engulf them or by producing *antibodies* to disarm or destroy them. This combat within your body causes some symptoms.

Immunization (see p.701) along with *antibiotic* and *antifungal* drugs can be used to assist your natural defenses. But antibiotics do not work against most viruses. That is why viral diseases such as influenza and infectious mononucleosis are difficult to treat.

Influenza
(flu)

Influenza, usually called flu, is caused by a virus that spreads from one person to another in the spray from coughs and sneezes. The virus enters the upper part of the respiratory tract through the nose or mouth, and it may also invade the rest of the tract, including the lungs. Symptoms appear after an *incubation* period of one or two days. The incubation period is the time between the entry of the infection into your respiratory tract and the beginning of symptoms. Influenza is usually an epidemic disease, affecting many people within a community. Usually such epidemics occur in winter or early spring.

What are the symptoms?
Among the early symptoms are chills, fever that may be as high as 104°F (about 40°C), sneezing, headache, muscular pains and a sore throat. These are usually followed by a dry, hacking cough and, often, chest pains. Later the cough produces mucus, and you get a runny nose. The fever generally lasts for two to three days, and leaves you feeling weak for another few days. If there are no complications, you should be fully recovered within one or two weeks.

What are the risks?
Epidemics of influenza occur at unpredictable intervals. Sometimes there are as many as five or six successive winters without one, but at other times there are two or three epidemics in the same community in a single year. In a severe outbreak, most people in an affected area will have at least a mild attack of the disease.

Epidemics die out when everyone who has been infected by a particular strain, or type, of flu virus becomes immune to further attack by that strain. There are several strains of influenza virus, however, and new strains are constantly developing. These new viruses are often named according to their assumed place of origin. That is why you may hear about Hong Kong flu one year and Russian flu the next. Immunity from one strain does not protect you from other flu viruses, and immunity is only temporary.

The main risk of influenza is that the infection may spread from the upper respiratory tract down to the lungs, and cause bronchitis (see p.353) or even pneumonia (see p.359). Such complications are rare, and are most likely to occur in very young children, the elderly, heavy smokers, diabetics, or people with chronic chest disorders.

What should be done?
Influenza must run its course, but you can ease the symptoms by using the self-help measures recommended below. You probably do not need to see your physician unless you are among the groups most susceptible to complications, or you seem to be the only person in your area with the illness. In an apparently isolated case of flu you may have a different disease with similar symptoms (for some examples, see Infectious mononucleosis, p.562, and Fungal diseases of the

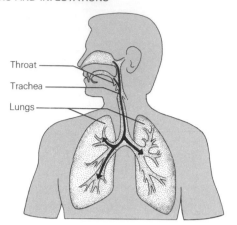

The spread of flu
The flu enters your nose or mouth, and infects the nose and throat. It then spreads down into the trachea (windpipe) and lungs. It can also spread throughout the body by entering the blood-stream.

Throat

Trachea

Lungs

lungs, next article). You may need a blood, urine, or sputum test to identify the cause of your symptoms.

What is the treatment?
Self-help: Go to bed as soon as symptoms begin, and stay there until your temperature returns to normal. Take aspirin or an aspirin substitute approved by your physician, and drink as much water or fruit juice as you comfortably can. If your fever lasts for more than three or four days or if you become short of breath while resting, call your physician. You should expect to feel weak, and possibly depressed, for about a week after your temperature drops, and you should rest as much as possible until you have recovered fully.

Professional help: There is no specific treatment for flu, since *antibiotics* are not effective against viruses. If a complication such as bacterial pneumonia develops, however, antibiotics will be prescribed, and you may have to go to the hospital.

Some physicians advise people who are most at risk from complications (those with chronic lung diseases and the elderly, for example) to have annual injections of an anti-influenza vaccine. Because of the many kinds of virus, however, it is difficult to know which vaccine to use and such inoculation cannot guarantee protection. Even against the strain for which it is effective, the vaccine protects you for only one winter or less.

Fungal diseases of the lungs

There are several diseases that are caused by different types of fungus, or mold, that primarily infect the lungs. These include blastomycosis, cryptococcosis, histoplasmosis and coccidioidomycosis. These diseases occur when you breathe in fungus spores, or seeds, that have become airborne.

The different types of fungus occur in different environments. The fungus that causes cryptococcosis is found in chicken and pigeon droppings, while the coccidioidomycosis fungus lives in semi-arid desert soil. The histoplasmosis fungus is native to the Ohio and Mississippi River valleys, and may be found between there and the east coast of the United States. It flourishes in soil enriched with bird and/or bat droppings.

Fungal diseases often clear up without treatment. However, they can spread throughout the body in the bloodstream, and cause dangerous complications.

What are the symptoms?
Most of these diseases begin like flu (see Influenza, previous article). The severity of the symptoms vary and may include fever, a cough, chest pain and muscle aches. In cryptococcosis you may have no symptoms, or you may have weight loss, night sweats and shortness of breath and the usual flu symptoms. With coccidioidomycosis some people, especially children, will also have a red, blotchy rash on their palms and soles and in the folds of the groin. Blastomycosis sometimes causes painless, warty skin ulcers on the face or arms, and can lead to prostatitis (see p.576) in men.

What are the risks?
Although most people who get one of these disorders recover in a few weeks without treatment, in some cases the disease spreads through the bloodstream to other parts of the body. People who have diabetes, chronic lung, blood, or kidney diseases, or cancer are particularly susceptible to complications. Pregnant women are especially at risk with coccidioidomycosis. The elderly and young children are also more likely to have severe symptoms and complications. Also, blastomycosis and coccidioidomycosis can lead to chronic lung disease in a few cases.

If a fungal lung disease spreads, one of the possible complications is meningitis (see p.273), an inflammation of one of the membranes that surrounds the brain. The symptoms of this serious condition include headache, confusion and lack of energy.

What should be done?
If you have flu-like symptoms that do not improve within about two weeks, see your physician, particularly if you have a chronic illness or cancer, if you are pregnant, or if you

are elderly or very young. The physician may want a sample of sputum, or phlegm, from a cough; spinal fluid; urine; or some other body fluid to test for signs of a fungal infection.

What is the treatment?
If a fungal infection is found, and if the symp-toms are severe or you are particularly susceptible to the spread of the disease, an antifungal medication will probably be prescribed. The medication may be given by *intravenous drip* if necessary. This treatment can usually be counted upon to clear up the infection within a few weeks.

Sporotrichosis

Sporotrichosis is a skin disease caused by a fungus, or mold. This fungus lives in soil and decaying vegetation, and the infectious spores are often picked up from rose thorns and splinters from rotting wood. Gardeners, farmers and children are most likely to have the disease.

The disease occurs when a contaminated thorn or sharp object punctures the skin and introduces the spores into a wound. A warty, crusting ulcer, or sore, appears within two weeks. The ulcer is painless, but it does not heal, and the infection spreads to the lymph nodes directly above it. The infected area has a large sore with a series of smaller ulcers or inflamed lymph nodes in a line above it.

If you have an infected area with this appearance, see your physician, who will probably take a sample of pus from the ulcers for laboratory tests. If sporotrichosis is diagnosed, the physician can prescribe a specific medication to heal the sore.

Staphylococcal infections

Staphylococcus aureus bacteria normally live in the nose, mouth, rectum or genital area without causing infection. When a wound or injury introduces the organism into some other part of the body, however, these bacteria can secrete substances that tunnel into tissues, destroying and dissolving matter along the way. The bacteria can produce pus-containing *abscesses* anywhere on or in the body. If you have an illness such as chronic liver or kidney disease, diabetes, or cancer, you are particularly susceptible to severe staphyloccocal infection.

Staphylococcal skin infections
Several fairly common skin infections can be caused by *Staphylococcus* bacteria. Boils (see p.251), impetigo (see p.257), cellulitis (see p.257) and paronychia (see p.264), which affects the nails, are some examples. This bacteria also causes other skin problems.
Folliculitis This staphylococcal infection is a smaller version of a boil. Small, white-headed pimples erupt around hair follicles anywhere on the body. Friction, blockage of the follicle, or injury (from shaving for example) can cause a rash-like eruption.
Staphylococcal scalded skin syndrome This infection occurs only in infants and young children. A form of the bacteria produces a substance that peels or detaches the outer layer of skin from the body. Blisters fill with fluid and dislodge the top layer of skin.
Wound complications Any skin wounds, whether they are caused by an injury or made during surgery, can be complicated by staphylococcal infections. The symptoms are the formation of pus, pain, redness and heat.

Other staphylococcal infections
Staphylococcus bacteria can infect any part of your body. In the eye, they can cause styes (see p.314), some types of conjunctivitis (see p.317) and orbital cellulitis (see p.327). In the breast they can cause a breast abscess (see p.590), which occurs frequently in nursing mothers.

Bones and joints develop staphylococcal abscesses from blood infections. As the organism circulates in the bloodstream it tends to lodge in the long bones of the arms and legs, or in the vertebrae. In the lungs, staphylococcal pneumonia can develop (see Pneumonia, p.359). This type of pneumonia may occur if the bacteria circulates in the bloodstream or if an abscess lodges on one of the valves on the right side of the heart. If *Staphylococcus* infects the inner lining of the heart, endocarditis will develop (see p.394). This disorder can cause irreversible heart damage, and may be fatal in some cases.

Staphylococcal food poisoning can occur if you eat contaminated food that contains *toxins* produced by the bacteria (see Box, p.462). *Staphylococcus* can also cause a colon infection if you take an *antibiotic* drug that kills many kinds of bacteria, including those that normally live in the digestive tract. This may upset the balance of organisms in the intestines, so that *Staphylococci* overmultiply and cause abdominal pain, a swollen abdomen and bloody diarrhea.

It is also possible to develop a kidney infection (see Pyelonephritis, p.502), or abscesses in the kidney tissue or along the outside of the kidney, if *Staphylococcus* bacteria are circulating in your bloodstream.

What is the treatment?

In mild cases of staphylococcal infection such as folliculitis or boils, cleaning the infected area with soap and eliminating the cause of the infection will often clear up the problem. If the infection persists, however, or if you have severe symptoms, you should see your physician. The physician will probably prescribe an *antibiotic* to combat the infection. In extreme cases, you may have to be hospitalized so that antibiotics can be given by *intravenous drip*. Sometimes abscesses must be surgically drained to clean out pockets of pus before the infection will heal completely.

Infectious mononucleosis
("*mono*")

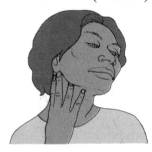

Swollen glands that can be felt in the neck are one of the most common symptoms of infectious mononucleosis.

This type of viral infection is sometimes known as "mono." It is also called "the kissing disease" because of a common belief that it is passed from one person to another through oral contact. Exactly how it does spread is not known, but it is not usually an epidemic disease such as influenza (see p.559). If you get mononucleosis, the virus may spread through your bloodstream into almost any organ in your body. The infection, therefore, can have a variety of symptoms. Some of the most common symptoms are swollen lymph glands and high fevers.

What are the symptoms?

You may think at first that you have influenza, since the early symptoms of infectious mononucleosis are similar to those of flu. These include fever, headache, sore throat, and a general feeling of illness and weakness. After a day or two you may also notice that you have painful, swollen glands in your neck, armpits, and/or groin. In addition, you may develop jaundice (see p.485) or a skin rash similar to that of German measles (see p.699). All these major symptoms usually disappear within two to three weeks, but for at least two more weeks you will probably feel weak and lack energy. You may also find that you are depressed.

What are the risks?

Infectious mononucleosis is not very common. Children and young adults are most susceptible to the disease.

Mononucleosis is not a dangerous disease, but it tends to recur, sometimes several times, during the year after you have the first attack. These succeeding attacks of the malady are usually milder than the first one, however, and once the infection has disappeared altogether, there are no after-effects. You do not gain immunity against re-infection after you have the disease.

What should be done?

If the symptoms of what you believe to be influenza persist for more than a few days, and especially if your glands are swollen, consult your physician. A blood test will probably be necessary, to determine whether you have infectious mononucleosis.

What is the treatment?

Self-help: Drink plenty of water and fruit juice, especially while you have a fever, and stay indoors. To relieve discomfort or pain, take aspirin or an aspirin substitute recommended by your physician. Rest is essential to your recovery. Do not attempt to return to your normal daily routine for at least a month after the illness begins.
Professional help: Because infectious mononucleosis is a viral disease, *antibiotics* will not be of any help. The disease, unfortunately, must simply run its course.

Shingles
(*herpes zoster*)

See p.238, **Visual aids to diagnosis, 25.**

Shingles is the result of infection by the herpes zoster virus, the same virus that causes chickenpox (see p.700). During an attack of chickenpox the virus may find its way to the root of a nerve in the brain or spinal cord. It lies dormant there, often for many years, until it is reactivated. Then the virus multiplies and produces intense, knife-like pain in the nerve where it has lodged. It also causes a rash in the form of groups of blisters to appear on the skin that lies above the nerve. It is not known what reactivates the dormant herpes zoster virus.

What are the symptoms?

Severe burning pain in the affected area often precedes the rash of blisters by several days. Almost any part of the body may be involved, but the disease is especially common on one side of the trunk, and it is most troublesome if it affects the face, especially near the eyes. Unfortunately, the pain does not stop when

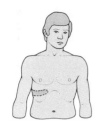

Common site of shingles

the rashes erupt. In fact, the pain often lasts for weeks after the blisters disappear. The condition is most common, and the pain is most severe, in the elderly.

Blisters caused by shingles are itchy, and they gradually become encrusted. They generally disappear after about seven days, but they leave scars like those that are caused by chickenpox (see p.700). If your facial nerve is affected by your case of shingles, you may have temporary facial paralysis. If your eyes are affected, there is a risk of damage to the cornea (see Corneal ulcers, p.316), which can be very painful.

What should be done?
If you have shingles, you can do little except apply calamine lotion to soothe the rash and take an *analgesic* such as aspirin to ease the pain. You should see your physician, however, particularly if your face is affected. The physician may prescribe a more effective analgesic. In addition, you will need professional advice on how to protect your eyes.

Tuberculosis
(TB)

Tuberculosis, often called simply TB, is a disease that develops slowly and can lead to chronic ill health and death if it is not treated. It is caused by bacteria, which are usually transmitted from one person to another through the air, but since cattle are susceptible to the disease, it can also be carried in cows' milk. The bacteria usually attack the lungs, but can also spread to other parts of the body, especially the brain, kidneys, or bones. As the bacteria multiply, they create a small area of inflammation. They may then spread to the nearest lymph nodes.

The primary, or first, phase of the infection usually lasts for several months. During this period the body's natural defenses resist the disease and most or all of the bacteria are either destroyed or walled in by a fibrous capsule that develops around the inflamed area. Before the initial attack is over, however, a few bacteria may escape into the bloodstream and be carried elsewhere in the body, where they are again walled in. In many cases the disease never develops beyond this phase. Sometimes, however, natural resistance cannot subdue the invading bacteria, and the progress of the disease is not blocked. In some cases, the disease is, at first, halted in the primary phase, but it flares up again. This can happen, often after a symptom-free period of many years, because the walling-in process does not actually kill the bacteria. They can therefore become active again if you become weak, ill, or undernourished.

The secondary phase of tuberculosis used to be called "consumption." It most commonly affects the lungs. As the number of bacteria grows, the resulting lung damage reduces your ability to breathe. Similarly, little pockets of trapped bacteria elsewhere in the body may become active again. Such secondary outbreaks of tuberculosis can usually be stopped if they are adequately treated, but they may leave disabling scar tissue wherever tissues have been damaged.

What are the symptoms?
The primary stage of tuberculosis often causes either no symptoms or a flu-like illness. You may never even discover that you have had the disease. If the infection progresses to the secondary stage, you are likely to develop a slight fever, lose weight, feel tired without obvious cause, and have various other symptoms, depending on which parts of your body are affected. Tuberculosis of the lungs, which is the most common type, causes a dry cough that eventually produces blood and pus-filled phlegm, or sputum. Sometimes shortness of breath and chest pain also develop. If any other body organ is affected, the symptoms of an infection of that organ will become apparent, but very gradually.

What are the risks?
Tuberculosis is becoming a rare disease in the United States. About 1 person in 5500 is diagnosed as having the disease in an average year. Because all cattle in the United States are routinely checked for tuberculosis, and most milk is pasteurized, milk is no longer a source of infection.

Very rarely, generally in someone whose natural resistance is abnormally low, primary tuberculosis spreads so quickly that it can be fatal unless treatment is begun early. This occurs today almost exclusively among very young or very old people. Untreated secondary tuberculosis can also be fatal, but the health of the person who has it usually deteriorates quite slowly. Even with successful treatment, infected organs may be left with severe damage.

What should be done?
You should consult your physician if you begin to lose weight, become generally ill, or develop a fever with a persistent cough. The doctor will examine you, will probably take samples of saliva for tests, and also will probably arrange for a chest X-ray.

What is the treatment?

Self-help: If you have tuberculosis, you must take the prescribed drugs regularly and eat the nourishing foods that your physician recommends. You must also be prepared to be sure you get enough rest, because rest is essential for full recovery from this disease.

Professional help: Special *antibiotics* will cure tuberculosis. Several are used together, and they must be taken continuously for several months. If an organ is infected severely it may be necessary to have the damaged part of it removed surgically. After successful treatment, you should have periodic check-ups for at least two years to make sure that the disease does not flare up again.

Tetanus
(*lockjaw*)

Tetanus is a serious and often fatal disease. It is caused by certain bacteria that live in the soil. These bacteria can invade the human body through a wound from an object that has some of them on it. The object can be anything from a nail to a thorn. A *toxin*, or poison, produced by these bacteria attacks the nerve cells in the spinal cord that control muscle activity. After an *incubation* period that may be as short as two days or as long as two weeks, your muscles become rigid and subject to extremely painful spasms.

What are the risks?

Since immunization for this disease is now routine (see p.701), tetanus is rare in this country. Only 100 or fewer cases are treated each year. Infants are immunized against the disease as a matter of course during their first year, and booster injections are normally given at ten year intervals.

In spite of *antibiotic* treatment, about 60 per cent of all tetanus cases end in death, often because of suffocation brought on by spasms of the throat and chest.

What should be done?

If anyone in your family has not been immunized against tetanus, have it done immediately. Make sure that each family member has a booster shot every ten years. It is a good idea to keep a record of dates, since some people have an unpleasant reaction to these injections if they are given too frequently. Even if you believe you are immune, always clean out small wounds with soap and water and apply an *antiseptic.* This is especially important with cuts that occur outdoors. It is also important with puncture wounds, because they are hard to clean and they also provide an environment particularly favorable to the growth of the bacteria.

If you have never had a tetanus injection and suffer an obviously dirty wound, do not delay in getting to your physician, who will probably immunize you immediately. The wound should be quickly and thoroughly cleaned to avoid any kind of infection.

If tetanus develops, hospital treatment should start immediately. It includes a course of antibiotics, along with injections of an *antitoxin.* You may be given *muscle-relaxant* drugs, and your breathing will be aided or taken over by an artificial *respirator.* The aim is to keep the body functioning for the several weeks that the disease takes to run its course.

Rabies
(*hydrophobia*)

Rabies is a viral disease of animals and humans that can be spread through a bite or scratch. If the virus reaches your central nervous system, it causes inflammation of the brain and is virtually always fatal. The earliest symptom of this dangerous disorder is a fever and a general sense of illness, as in any viral infection. After two or three days, however, you become irrational and have violent mouth and throat spasms. These spasms are made worse by the sight of water (hydrophobia means "fear of water"). Death is likely to occur within a few days.

The *incubation* period for rabies, the time it takes from infection to the appearance of symptoms, varies from ten days to eight months, but is usually one to three months. In the United States, the animals that most often carry rabies are skunk, fox, bobcat, badger, bat, coyote, dog, raccoon and cat.

What should be done?

Take no risks. If you have been bitten or scratched by an animal that may be rabid (for example, one that is acting aggressively or strangely), see a physician without delay. Any time lost may be placing you in increased danger. The animal should be captured if possible, but not destroyed. Tests can be done to determine if the animal has rabies. Meanwhile, you will probably be given a series of vaccinations to help prevent the disease from developing. You can also help prevent rabies by having your pets immunized. This will help protect both people and your pet from contracting the disease.

Chlamydial infections

Chlamydiae are a type of microscopic organism that are not bacteria, viruses or fungi. However, they are similar to bacteria in that they can be eliminated with certain *antibiotics*. Chlamydiae are responsible for several human diseases.

Trachoma Trachoma is a chlamydial infection of the conjunctiva, the moist tissue that lines the eyelids and the white portion of the eyeball. It is the major cause of blindness in North Africa and the Middle East. Trachoma does exist in North America. It is associated with poor hygiene.

Nongonococcal urethritis Chlamydiae also cause nongonococcal urethritis (NGU), a urinary-tract inflammation. Symptoms of this type of urethritis include pain on urination and a watery, mucous discharge. In men the bacteria that produce gonorrhea (see p.611) also cause a urethritis, but the chlamydial infection is milder and the discharge from the penis contains no pus.

Nongonococcal urethritis is passed on through sexual intercourse. Women may carry the organism in the cervix or vagina and develop no symptoms of the disease.

Lymphogranuloma venereum Certain strains of chlamydiae produce lymphogranuloma venereum, another disease transmitted through sexual intercourse. The organism is rare in North America, but is more common in tropical climates. Seamen, travelers, and military personnel are especially likely to get the disease.

The initial sign of infection is a painless pimple or blister that develops on the penis or the outer labia, or lips, of the vagina, 5 to 20 days after exposure. About 2 to 12 weeks later, the lymph nodes in the groin painfully enlarge, mat together, redden, and drain pus.

The infection sometimes seems to improve without treatment, but ugly *ulcers*, or sores, appear on the genitals. Later complications include scarring, which causes strictures in the urethra, vagina, or rectum. Strictures are small bridges of tissue that narrow the size of the body opening.

Psittacosis Psittacosis is a chlamydial disease that infects the lungs of people who inhale organisms from the nasal excretions, feathers and droppings of infected birds, particularly parrots and parakeets. To prevent psittacosis, the government specifies that all imported birds must be quarantined for 30 days, and all birds of the parrot family must also be treated with antibiotics.

The infection rapidly spreads from the lungs to the bloodstream. Symptoms vary from a mild flu to a severe pneumonia (see p.359) with temperatures ranging from 103° to 105°F (39.4° to 40.6°C).

What should be done?

If you have the symptoms of any of these diseases, see your physician. Chlamydial disorders are usually identified by a blood test in which the levels of certain *antibodies*, or substances that the body produces to combat infection, are measured. Once the diagnosis is made, the physician will probably prescribe an antibiotic, which clears the infection.

In cases of nongonococcal urethritis and lymphogranuloma venereum, which are transmitted sexually, all sexual partners should be treated for the disease so that the disease will not continue to be transmitted.

Rocky Mountain spotted fever

Rocky Mountain spotted fever is a disease caused by rickettsia, or microscopic organisms that are not bacteria, viruses, or fungi. Rickettsia can live inside ticks, and people are infected with them through tick bites (see p.569). However, an infected person may not notice the tick bite that caused the disease.

What are the symptoms?

About two days after the tick bite, you will have three major symptoms of the disease: severe headache; a high fever (up to 103° to 105°F or 39° to 40°C); and severe muscle aches and weakness.

Most people develop a characteristic rash. It usually begins as flat red spots or splotches on the palms of the hands and the soles of the feet, then spreads to the wrists, ankles, legs, arms and finally the trunk.

If the disease is not treated, it causes shaking chills, occasional abdominal pain, nausea, intense headache, back stiffness, mental confusion and finally unconsciousness. The later stages of the disease can damage the kidneys, liver, lungs and blood.

What are the risks?

Although ticks that harbor Rocky Mountain spotted fever rickettsia are found all over the United States, the disease today most frequently occurs in the southeast, from Maryland to Georgia. It usually appears in the spring and summer in children who are spending a lot of time outdoors.

There is a greater risk of getting the infection when a tick has remained attached to your body for several hours or if you crush the tick while removing it.

Left untreated, the infection can become severe. Seven per cent of all cases are fatal.

What should be done?

The best preventive measures are to minimize contact with ticks, avoid tick-infested areas and wear protective clothing. If you are traveling through a tick-infested area, inspect your body thoroughly several times a day and at bedtime to remove any ticks (see illustration, p.569). Consult a physician at once if, shortly after a tick bite, you develop the symptoms described.

The physician will diagnose the infection with two blood tests that measure *antibodies*. Because the second test looks for a large increase in antibodies, it is done 10 to 14 days after the illness begins. The physician must treat the infection much earlier, however, because there is a greater risk of more serious illness if treatment is delayed.

Antibiotics will usually cure Rocky Mountain spotted fever. If the disease is not treated right away, you may have to be hospitalized to be treated for the damage that may be done to your kidneys, liver, lungs and blood.

Yellow fever

This viral illness, which usually attacks the liver, is carried by mosquitoes. It usually occurs in Central and South America, and in parts of Africa. Immunization is very effective and will probably be required for anyone visiting those countries.

Attacks of yellow fever range from mild to fatal. A mild attack may have symptoms similar to those of influenza (see p.559). However, symptoms of more severe cases include nausea, vomiting, bleeding, abdominal pain and yellowing of the skin (see Jaundice, p.485). You may feel very depressed and confused, and may even go into a coma. As with many viral illnesses, there is no really effective treatment for yellow fever, but a person who has recovered from the disease is immune for life.

Smallpox

Smallpox has now been eliminated as the result of a successful worldwide vaccination campaign. Vaccination is no longer necessary and in 1980 the World Health Organization declared the disease officially extinct.

The disease was severe, highly infectious, and often fatal. People who survived it were left with varying degrees of scarring caused by the smallpox rash.

Smallpox viruses now exist only in medical laboratories, where they are controlled and maintained for research purposes.

Going abroad

If you are planning a trip out of the country, make sure you are adequately protected against any dangerous diseases that may occur in your country of destination. About six weeks before you go, find out from either your travel agent, the airline you are flying on, or the country's embassy which vaccinations are compulsory for entry into the country, and which are sensible precautions. The American Medical Association and the United States Centers for Disease Control also have booklets available. Be sure you get the latest edition, since requirements and recommendations may change. Then, at least a month before you travel, consult your physician. Discuss both mandatory and advisable immunizations, and do it in plenty of time because many vaccinations are not immediately available or must be taken in advance of your trip.

If you are going to a tropical or subtropical country ask your physician about tablets to protect you against malaria. You will probably have to take the tablets before you leave, throughout your visit, and also after you return.

Some immunizations are not totally effective. In addition, there are many other minor infections that you may catch, especially in tropical areas. While you are abroad, take some precautions. Boil water and milk unless you are certain they are safe to drink. Alternatively, there are tiny tablets that you can use to treat water and other liquids by the glassful. These are particularly useful in restaurants, when visiting people's homes, or in other situations where boiling the liquids would be inconvenient or embarrassing. Carbonated beverages such as colas from sealed cans and bottles are generally safe since the chemical composition of the liquids helps retard growth of bacteria. Avoid salads, unpeeled fruits, and reheated foods. Finally, *always* wash your hands before handling or eating any food.

Infestations

Infestations occur when parasites invade your body and live either on it (for example, lice) or in it (for example, tapeworms). Parasites that live only on the skin usually cause no symptoms other than discomfort. Some of these, ticks for example, can cause infections because they may carry disease. Those that infest the inside of the body sometimes cause vague, ill-defined symptoms that you hardly notice, so they may remain undetected. If, however, they lodge in a vital place or become extremely numerous, they can cause severe problems.

It is almost impossible to get rid of parasites without treatment. This is because the body does not normally have adequate natural defenses against them. Fortunately, most types of dangerous infestation are rare in the United States, and parasite-killing drugs are highly effective.

Malaria

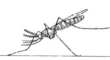

The female *Anopheles* mosquito carries the tiny organisms that cause malaria. The mosquito gets the organisms by biting a malaria sufferer, and sucking in some blood. The organisms, in the blood, multiply in the mosquito and enter the bloodstream of the next person the mosquito bites.

Malaria is caused by minute single-celled parasites called *plasmodia*, which are transferred from one person to another by the *Anopheles* mosquito. There is no other carrier of the disease, so plasmodia can only enter your bloodstream if you are bitten by an *Anopheles* mosquito that has bitten someone who has malaria. Once in your bloodstream, the plasmodia travel to the liver, where they multiply very rapidly. After several days, thousands of them flow back into your bloodstream, where they destroy red blood cells. However, many plasmodia also remain and continue to multiply in the liver cells, and some of these are released into your bloodstream at intervals. This is why a person with malaria usually has repeated attacks unless the disease is treated. Each attack signals the release of plasmodia.

A particularly dangerous type of malaria is caused by *Plasmodium falciparum*, one of the four species of plasmodia that infect humans. If you have falciparum malaria, all the organisms are released from your liver into your bloodstream at the same time. Thus there is only one bout of the disease, but that bout is extremely severe.

What are the symptoms?

Malaria causes no symptoms at first. About 8 to 30 days after the mosquito bite, depending on the type of plasmodium, a full day of headache, weariness and nausea is followed by what is called "the classical febrile paroxysm" of malaria. This lasts 12 to 24 hours. It consists of a sudden chill followed by a feverish stage with rapid breathing but no sweating, and ending with a sweating stage accompanied by a drop in temperature. Similar bouts occur whenever more plasmodia are released into your bloodstream, which generally occurs every two or three days.

If malaria is not treated, attacks can continue to occur for years, but you slowly build up a defense against the disease, and the attacks come less often. In falciparum malaria, the febrile paroxysm is likely to last for two or three days and to be exceptionally severe, but it does not recur.

Children with malaria are apt to have prolonged high fever without chills. The fever sometimes affects the brain, causing unconsciousness or convulsions (see p.667).

What are the risks?

The *Anopheles* mosquito lives in the southeastern and western United States, and is widespread in tropical and semi-tropical countries. The number of malaria cases in the United States rose sharply during the late 1960s and early 1970s due to returning Vietnam veterans and increased travel.

Since plasmodia destroy red blood cells, anemia (see p.419) may develop along with malaria. Also the damaged cells clump together in small groups, which may block blood vessels and lead to brain or kidney damage. The main risk comes from untreated falciparum malaria, which may cause massive blood-vessel blockage and possibly death.

What should be done?

If you develop symptoms of malaria, consult your physician without delay. The physician will probably arrange for you to have blood tests. Because it is not always easy to detect the presence of plasmodia, you may need to be hospitalized so that blood tests can be taken at intervals.

What is the treatment?

Self-help: To guard against the infection, if you are going to visit an area in which malaria is a problem, ask your physician to prescribe

anti-malarial drugs to protect you. You must begin to take them before you travel, and continue to take them after you return.
Professional help: Your physician will prescribe drugs to prevent malaria if you expect to be at risk. If blood tests show that you have malaria, your physician will probably pre- scribe a different drug immediately to treat the disease. New and more effective drugs to combat malaria are being developed. With proper treatment, the symptoms decrease within a few hours, but the treatment must be continued for several weeks to prevent the disease from recurring.

Tapeworm

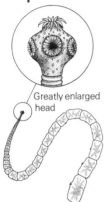

Greatly enlarged head

Tapeworms are parasites that sometimes infest pigs and cattle. They can be passed on to a human who eats infested pork or beef that has not been adequately cooked. Once in the intestines, a tapeworm can anchor itself by embedding its head end into the intestinal wall. The tapeworm then absorbs food and may grow up to 10 meters (more than 30 feet) long. Segments of the worm break off and are excreted in bowel movements. These segments look like short pieces of narrow white ribbon. If the worm remains in the intestines, it does no great harm, but it often causes mild symptoms such as slight weight loss, occasional abdominal pain, loss of appetite, and irritation around the anus.

Despite strict regulations for control of slaughter–house procedures, occasionally meat containing tapeworms gets on the market. Thorough cooking kills any worms that do exist, however.

What should be done?
If you think you may have a tapeworm, consult your physician, who will probably want to examine a specimen of your bowel movements. There are a number of drugs that kill parasitic worms, and, if necessary, your physician will prescribe one for you. The infestation will be cured when you excrete the tapeworm's head, which may take several days.

Scabies

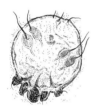

Scabies mite (greatly enlarged)

See p.248,
Visual aids to diagnosis, 67.

Scabies is caused by a mite that burrows into the skin and lays eggs from which additional mites emerge. The result is an intense but relatively harmless irritation. Scabies rarely occurs on the head or face. It most often affects the hands, wrists, armpits, buttocks, or genital area. The mites are spread through close personal contact or through contact with infested clothes or bedding, so whole families sometimes have scabies. The mites spread rapidly in overcrowded and unhygienic living conditions. They can be passed between sexual partners.

What are the symptoms?
The main symptom of scabies is itching so intense that it forces you to scratch a great deal. Continual scratching causes sores and scabs to form.

What should be done?
Although scabies occurs most commonly in unhygienic conditions, anyone can get it. If your physician diagnoses scabies, you will need to scrub all infected areas and then apply a prescribed medication to your whole body below the neck. It is important to follow the directions on the label carefully.

The mites that cause scabies do not live long if they are removed from human skin. Therefore, clothes and bedding that cannot be laundered for some reason will be free of contamination if they are left unused for at least four days.

Lice

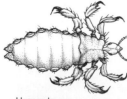

Human louse (enlarged)

Lice are tiny but visible insects that live in the hair and suck blood from the skin. Infestation is often spread among children at school. Crab lice (see p.613) live in pubic hair and are usually spread by sexual intercourse.

The eggs of lice are known as nits, and they too are visible. They look like tiny white grains clinging to the hair. The bites of lice cause itching in affected areas, and there is a slight possibility of infection. For the most part, however, these parasites simply irritate their hosts. Lice are most common among people who live in unhygienic and overcrowded conditions.

What should be done?
If you find that your child has lice, report it to the school authorities. Lice infestation is considered a public health hazard, and steps can be taken to trace them to their source and prevent them from spreading further. For treatment, whether for a child or an adult,

consult your physician, who will prescribe a special shampoo, lotion, or both. Two or three applications of the medicine are necessary to kill nits as well as lice. Hats and any other clothing where nits may be lodged should be burned.

Fleas

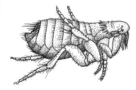

Flea
(enlarged)

See p.248,
Visual aids to diagnosis, 68.

There are many species of fleas, and each one is parasitic on a different animal. Animal fleas do not stay long on human skin. Fleas can leap great distances, and isolated flea bites on human skin can be caused by animal (usually cat or dog) fleas that have temporarily left their hosts. Flea eggs hatch in bedding about seven days after they have been laid. The fleas may then live in the bedding, and feed off their animal hosts and, occasionally, humans. Their bites cause intense irritation for up to two days. Flea infestation of humans occurs in all parts of the world, but is most common where there is close contact between people and domestic animals or where hygienic conditions are poor.

What should be done?

To avoid infestation, use anti-flea spray, powder or shampoo on your pets' skin, and spray their bedding regularly as well. If you suspect infestation in your own bedding, furniture, or carpets, you should apply a flea repellent to your skin and also spray the suspected items. In severe cases you may not be able to control the fleas, and it may be advisable to call in a professional exterminator to do the job.

Ticks

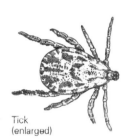

Tick
(enlarged)

Ticks are parasites that feed on blood. Tick bites are potentially dangerous because of the viruses and bacteria that ticks carry in their bodies and transmit as they feed. Infections transmitted through tick bites include Rocky Mountain spotted fever (see p.565) and encephalitis (see p.274). Some ticks also harbor a *toxin*, or poison, that paralyzes the nerves in the legs, then moves towards the trunk. The paralysis is relieved by removing the tick.

The tick embeds its head into your skin, then swells as it feeds, sometimes to several times its original size. The skin around the bite hardens into a lump surrounded by a red halo. Usually the lump subsides after the tick is removed, but it can persist.

Ticks are usually found in woods or tall grass. If you have been in the woods or fields, it is a good idea to check your body for ticks. They often lodge in your hair, around your ankles, and in the genital area, so you may have to search for them. If they are found right away, they can be removed before they become embedded in the skin.

Removal of the entire tick including the head is necessary, because any part of a tick can continue to release toxic substances, bacteria, or viruses.

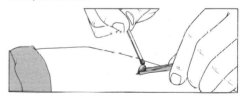

Removing an embedded tick
Place the hot end of a recently extinguished match to the tick and grab it with tweezers as it withdraws. Or use petroleum jelly, gasoline, chloroform, ether or benzene to loosen the head. If necessary, a physician can remove the head with a small incision.

Chiggers

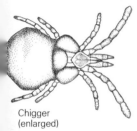

Chigger
(enlarged)

Chiggers are a type of mite, sometimes called a red bug or a harvest mite. They inhabit grasses, shrubs and vines in the southern United States and sometimes as far north as Canada. Farmers, hunters, and others who spend a lot of time outdoors are most likely to get chigger bites.

The larva, or immature mite, is only about 3 mm (about one hundredth of an inch) long. It selects a damp, moist place such as the ankles, groin, belt line, or wherever clothing is tight and attaches to a hair follicle or an area of hairless skin. The mite releases *enzymes* that dissolve the skin, then inserts a "feeding tube" to reach a supply of blood. It remains in one spot for one to four days, then drops off, engorged with blood.

The skin's response to the mite varies from an allergic skin reaction with hives (see p.255) to an itchy, red, pimple-like lump. Sometimes blisters, swelling, or large red patches develop. Usually the bites itch severely, making it almost impossible to keep from scratching. Medications for chigger bites include *antihistamines* to relieve itching, *steroid* creams to reduce irritation and allergic reaction, and *antibiotics* if a secondary infection occurs.

Special problems of men

Introduction

The male reproductive organs, which include the two testicles suspended in a sac (the scrotum) and the penis, are so closely connected with the organs of the male urinary tract that a disorder in either system often causes symptoms in the other. Each of your testicles is a gland (the testis) that produces sperm and the male sex hormone *testosterone*. A long, tightly coiled tube called the epididymis, lies behind each gland. Sperm are continually manufactured in each testis. They pass into the epididymis, where they mature over a period of two or three weeks before they are propelled into a duct called the vas deferens, which acts as a storage system.

When you have a climax, or orgasm, the sperm pass into the urethra, and are propelled or ejaculated in the seminal fluid. Your urethra, which runs from the bladder along the length of the penis, carries both seminal fluid and urine. The muscular action of urination automatically closes the passageway for seminal fluid, and vice versa.

Sperm is only a small part of the seminal fluid, which is composed mainly of secretions from a number of glands. The various secretions probably act to mobilize and nourish the sperm and provide them with additional nutrients for their journey through the male and female reproductive tracts. The largest of these glands is the prostate, which encircles the top section of the urethral channel at the point where the urethra leaves the bladder. Prostate problems, therefore, can seriously affect both the genital and urinary systems. The urethra, which is much longer in a man than it is in a woman, can become troublesome because it is surrounded in the penis by the spongy, heavily veined tissues that make erections possible. Generally speaking, however, the length of the male urethra provides an effective barrier against invasion of the reproductive and urinary tracts by infectious agents. Infections of these tracts are therefore rare in men, while they are quite common in women.

The disorders discussed in the following articles are grouped according to the part of the urinary tract or the reproductive system in which problems can occur. These are the testicles and scrotum, the prostate gland, and the bladder, urethra, penis and rectum.

The male reproductive organs

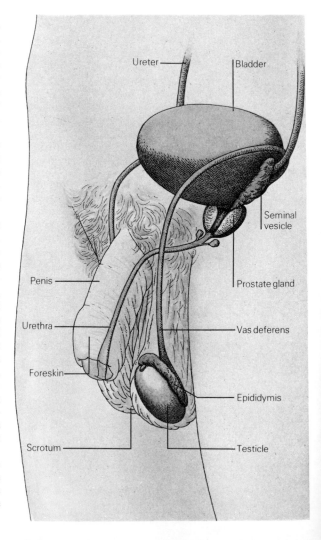

Ureter

Bladder

Seminal vesicle

Penis

Prostate gland

Urethra

Vas deferens

Foreskin

Epididymis

Scrotum

Testicle

Testicles and scrotum

The two male sex glands, the testes or testicles, develop inside the abdomen of a male fetus. Usually by the time of birth they have descended through the abdominal wall to the familiar external position, where they hang suspended in a pouch of skin called the scrotum (see also Undescended testicles, p.692). Each gland is connected to the body by a single attachment called the spermatic cord, which is composed of the vas deferens, or sperm duct, and a number of nerves and blood vessels.

The sperm that each testicle produces remain in the epididymis, a coiled tube that lies behind the testis, for about three weeks, until they mature. The fully developed sperm then pass into the vas deferens, where they are stored. If they are not eventually ejaculated, they gradually disintegrate. The following articles deal with disorders not only of the testes and scrotum but also of the closely related epididymis. The spermatic cord is not usually susceptible to disease.

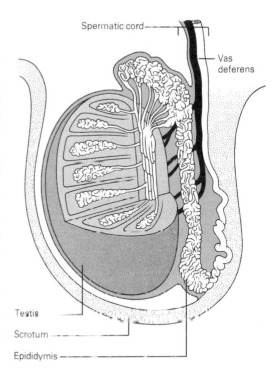

Spermatic cord

Vas deferens

Testis

Scrotum

Epididymis

Cancer of the testicle

Cancer may occur in the cells of a testicle. Unless the disease is treated in an early stage, it can spread through the lymphatic system (see p.432) to lymph nodes in the abdomen, chest and neck, and eventually to the lungs. It is not known why the disease develops. Because there is no direct lymphatic connection between the two testicles, the disease is unlikely to spread from one testicle to the other.

What are the symptoms?
The main symptom is a lump in the testicle. The lump grows slowly, and you may not be aware of it for some time since in most cases there is no associated pain. You may notice the swelling for the first time only when a minor injury to your scrotum makes you examine the area closely.

What are the risks?
Cancer of the testicle is rare. It is, however, the most common type of cancer in men between the ages of 20 and 35. Three out of every four cases occur in men under 50.

If cancer of the testicle remains undetected long enough to spread, it may reach vital points of the body, particularly the lungs. With early detection and treatment, your chances for complete recovery are excellent.

What should be done?
As a preventive measure, get into the habit of examining your testicles at least once a month. If you notice a lump, no matter how trivial it seems, consult your physician, who will probably refer you to a urologist, a physician who specializes in urinary and genital problems. The swelling may be harmless; there are often small swellings in the epididymis (see Cysts of the epididymis, p.573), and these are generally not dangerous to your health. A lump in the testis itself, however, is almost never harmless, and most such swellings should have a *biopsy* done on them. In a biopsy, a small sample of tissue is removed for examination, to determine with certainty whether cancer is present.

What is the treatment?
If you have cancer of the testicle, the only possible treatment is surgical removal of the diseased gland.

The operation usually leaves one testicle intact, so it is unlikely to have a significant effect on either potency or fertility. *Radiation therapy*, *chemotherapy*, and a procedure called a *lymphadenectomy*, in which lymph nodes are surgically removed, may be done to further treat the disease.

Torsion of the testicle

In this disorder, one testicle is twisted out of its normal position. Each testicle is enclosed in a fibrous two-layered sheath. A small amount of lubricating fluid lies between the two layers, which allows the contents to move around. These sheaths should not be confused with the scrotum, which is simply a loose pouch of skin in which the testicles hang. The sheathed testicle is attached to the spermatic cord in a way that usually prevents it from twisting out of its natural position. However, when an extreme twist, or torsion, does occur, it can cause the blood vessels that supply the testicle to become kinked. This can prevent blood flow to and from the testicle. It is quite painful, and is a medical emergency. Such torsion can happen at any time, even when you are asleep.

What are the symptoms?
The major symptom of torsion of the testicle is a sudden pain in one testicle. Your scrotum then becomes swollen, red and tender. The intensity of the pain varies from case to case, but it can be so severe that you feel nauseated and may vomit. In many cases the testicle somehow untwists by itself and if this occurs you will get immediate relief from both the pain and the swelling.

What are the risks?
Torsion of this type is uncommon. The problem occurs most often in adolescence, but it can happen at any age, even in infancy.

If the testicle does not return to normal spontaneously and you do not see a physician immediately, the sperm-producing parts of the testicle may be permanently damaged. This will significantly reduce your chances of having children, but sperm can still be produced by the other testicle.

What should be done?
Even if the problem seems to have cleared up by itself, see your physician without delay. The pain from injuries, inflammation, and even cancer of the testes sometimes can resemble torsion of the testicle, so diagnosis by a review of your medical history and gentle physical examination is especially important. If the diagnosis is torsion of the testicle, your physician may try to untwist the testicle by gentle manipulation. Even if this procedure successfully relieves the pain, however, the disorder may recur.

For this reason, surgery is necessary, and it is usually done within hours. The surgeon untwists the testicle, then stitches it into position so that the problem cannot recur.

Injury to the testicles

An injury to the testicles usually causes severe pain, but you can assume there is no serious damage if the pain subsides within an hour or so and your scrotum is not bruised or swollen. Continued pain, bruising, or swelling indicate internal injury. If you have these symptoms, go to your physician or the nearest hospital emergency room without delay. If the problem is not treated, a blood clot may damage healthy tissue. Surgery may be necessary to halt any bleeding and remove any clot.

Epididymitis

Inflammation of the epididymis is called epididymitis. It is caused by an infection that spreads from the urinary tract into the sperm duct. The first indication that you have epididymitis is often a sausage-shaped swelling that is hot, tender and very painful and is located in the back portion of one of your testicles. The swelling, which develops over the course of a few hours, is followed by a painful swelling and stiffening of the scrotum. The testicle itself may also be involved, and if so it will be sore as well.

What should be done?
If you think you have epididymitis, consult your physician without delay. Laboratory tests of your urine and secretions of your prostate may be done to identify the cause of infection. The disorder is most often caused by urinary tract infections from an infectious agent called *Chlamydia*. Treatment with an appropriate *antibiotic*, prescribed by a physician, usually cures the disorder.

It may also be necessary to treat your sexual partner, since the infection can be transmitted by sexual contact. This will help prevent continued or chronic infection in both of you. If swelling of the scrotum is especially painful, bed rest, ice packs, and elevating the area to promote drainage may be of additional help. Rarely, in particularly severe or chronic cases, surgery may be advised.

Cysts of the epididymis

Sometimes the tubes through which sperm pass from a testis to its epididymis develop *cysts*, or sacs of fluid. Although the cysts tend to increase in size because sperm accumulates in them, they are harmless. Cysts of the epididymis are quite common. Most men have at least one or two of these cysts after the age of 40. You can usually tell if any of these cysts are present because if they are, you will notice a painless swelling in the upper, rear portion of one or both of your testicles.

Rarely, these cysts can resemble tumors of the epididymis. Fortunately, however, the cysts are not life-threatening. If a physical examination, and possibly even minor surgery, do not show that you have a serious problem, you will probably require no further treatment, but you should watch carefully for enlargement. Sometimes cysts of the epididymis grow too large and cause varying degrees of discomfort. In such cases the cysts generally need to be cut away. The surgery can reduce fertility in the affected testicle, but the other one will not be damaged, so you still should be able to have children.

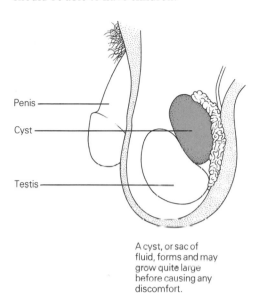

Penis ———

Cyst ———

Testis ———

A cyst, or sac of fluid, forms and may grow quite large before causing any discomfort.

Hydrocele

The normal double-layered sheath around each testicle (see Torsion of the testicle, previous page) contains just enough fluid for good lubrication. Sometimes, however, an excessive amount may be produced and a hydrocele, a soft, usually painless swelling around the testicle, forms. Hydroceles are occasionally caused by an inflammation or injury of the area, but there is usually no apparent cause. Hydroceles are harmless and quite common, especially in elderly men.

Treatment of a small hydrocele is rarely necessary. If the hydrocele becomes very large or painful, however, the fluid can be drawn off, or "tapped," with a needle. This is a simple operation that is usually done under a local anesthetic. Unfortunately, the fluid tends to re-accumulate in the same area. If you have a troublesome recurring hydrocele, your physician may advise you to have surgery to tighten or remove the fibrous sheath so that the lubricating fluid can no longer accumulate within it.

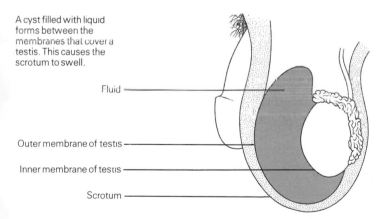

A cyst filled with liquid forms between the membranes that cover a testis. This causes the scrotum to swell.

Fluid ———

Outer membrane of testis ———

Inner membrane of testis ———

Scrotum ———

Varicocele

If the veins that drain one of your testicles become abnormally distended (see Varicose veins, p.409), you have a mild disorder called varicocele. There is usually no apparent cause for the condition, which produces a swelling around the testicle. The swelling may disappear when you lie down, but it is sometimes accompanied by an uncomfortable, dragging pain, especially in hot weather or after you have been exercising.

To relieve the discomfort, simply wear tight-fitting underwear or an athletic supporter. No other treatment is usually necessary unless the varicocele seems to be affecting your fertility. This is rare but possible. If it does occur, your physician may suggest an operation to remove the distended veins. Unfortunately, the results of this type of surgery are often not good enough to justify taking the risks that the operation presents.

Prostate gland

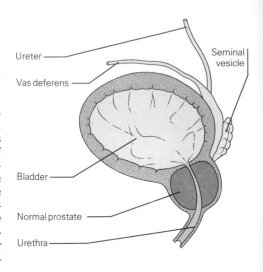

The prostate gland is not one single gland, but a cluster of small glands that surround the urethra at the point where it leaves the bladder. The glands are tubular, and have muscles that squeeze their secretions into the urethra. The exact function of the prostate gland is unclear. It is thought that the addition of prostatic secretion to the seminal fluid somehow stimulates active movement of the sperm. The main disorders that can affect the prostate are infections and growths. In elderly men, cancer of the prostate is relatively common. Because the prostate gland encircles the urethra, any kind of prostate disorder may hamper the free flow of urine, an uncomfortable and sometimes dangerous problem.

Enlarged prostate

(benign prostatic hypertrophy)

Routine tests show that nearly every man over 45 has some degree of enlargement of the prostate gland. Harmless over-growths of normal prostate tissue are a natural result of the aging process. As you grow older, small, gristly nodules gradually develop, and as they accumulate the size of the gland changes. The change may cause no problems even if the prostate becomes quite swollen. The size of a harmless enlargement matters less than the consistency of the tissue. In some men the prostate gland, which normally relaxes to permit free flow of urine from the bladder through the urethra, becomes stiff and inflexible. Even a stiffened prostate does not necessarily cause problems, however. As the gland grows more rigid, and constricts the urethra that it surrounds, the muscles of the bladder tend to compensate by becoming more powerful. This extra strength is often enough to keep the urethra open. Serious problems occur only when the bladder muscles are unable to overcome resistance caused by the rigid prostate, and the flow of urine is severely obstructed.

What are the symptoms?
Symptoms of severe prostate enlargement vary widely, but one very common symptom is a weak urinary stream. You are likely to have a frequent urge to urinate (an urge so strong that it may wake you several times a night), yet you can pass only a dribble whenever you try. You may also find that, no matter how strong the urge, it is difficult to start the sluggish stream. This may be particularly noticeable first thing in the morning.

There is almost never any pain, and there is no surface swelling or lump either, because the prostate gland is deep within the lower abdomen. Occasionally, however, there may be *hematuria*, or blood in the urine.

What are the risks?
Prostate enlargement, though it is extremely common in men over 45, rarely becomes troublesome before the age of 60. Serious urinary problems caused by this disorder affect one in ten elderly men.

The condition is not dangerous in itself, but there are three main risks. First, if your bladder is never entirely emptied, pools of stagnant urine within it can become infected (see Cystitis in men, p.577). Second, when the outflow of urine is hampered or blocked, pressure within the bladder increases and the kidneys and the ureters, the tubes that carry urine to the bladder from the kidneys, may be affected. This can lead to infection of the kidney (see Acute pyelonephritis, p.502). Finally, if severe enlargement of the prostate remains untreated, the muscles of your bladder may not be able to overcome the resistance to urine flow and may suddenly or gradually fail to function.

Sudden failure occurs when your bladder abruptly stops expelling its contents. This condition is called acute retention. It is rare, but very painful, and it requires emergency treatment. Gradual failure, which is more common, occurs when the amount of urine that cannot be expelled increases little by little. If the condition is allowed to persist, the quantity of urine left in the bladder may

An enlarged prostate can obstruct the urethra, reducing the flow of urine and causing the muscular wall of the bladder to thicken as it works harder to force urine out.

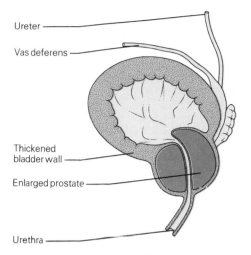

Ureter

Vas deferens

Thickened bladder wall

Enlarged prostate

Urethra

become so great that the abdomen swells as if you were pregnant. In this condition, some of the accumulated urine dribbles away whenever you cough, sneeze, or strain. The disorder seldom reaches this uncomfortable stage. If it does, and it goes untreated, it will eventually lead to either acute retention or kidney failure (see p.511).

What should be done?

If you have symptoms of an enlarged prostate, consult your physician, who will examine the gland by inserting a gloved finger into the rectum. You may be referred to a urologist, a physician who specializes in urinary and genital diseases. The urologist will observe your urinary stream, using this observation and others to determine what tests are required. You may also be given an *intravenous pyelogram (IVP)* to find out if your symptoms are due to a urinary-tract disease rather than to an enlarged prostate.

If you have the symptoms of acute retention, see your physician or go to a hospital emergency room without delay. Your bladder must be emptied with a *catheter* before treatment of the disorder can begin.

What is the treatment?

If your symptoms are mild and diagnostic tests indicate that urgent treatment is not necessary, your physician will probably take no action. In at least one in three mild cases of enlarged prostate, the symptoms clear up without treatment, so it often makes sense to wait for a while. But if the problem does not go away, if it worsens, or if tests show a serious obstruction to the outflow of urine, the tissue that is causing the enlargement of your prostate must be removed.

The operation is called a *prostatectomy*. It can be done by traditional surgery or by a method known as transurethral resection (TUR). Either method requires that you have anesthesia. To cut away the excess tissue, the surgeon makes an incision in the lower part of the abdomen. In transurethral resection no incision is made. Instead, a thin tube is passed up the penis to the prostate. In the tip of the tube is an electric cutting loop that can be guided with the help of a miniature telescope that is also in the tube to slice away the enlarged tissue. This procedure requires a hospital stay of about 10 days, as compared to about 15 days for regular surgery, and there is less post-operative pain. However, transurethral resection is not feasible in some cases.

What are the long-term prospects?

Regardless of the technique, most prostatectomies are successful. They relieve urinary difficulties, and prostate problems seldom recur. Rarely, a patient will become impotent after the operation. Others may still be able to have an erection but become sterile because their semen is expelled backwards into the bladder instead of being ejaculated. Fortunately, the age of most men who need to have this operation is such that they are not as concerned about their loss of fertility as a younger man would be. Seminal fluid in the bladder does no harm. It is simply eliminated in the urine.

Cancer of the prostate

Cancer of the prostate does not progress the same way as most cancers. Instead of spreading, this *malignant*, or life-threatening, growth tends to lie dormant, and seldom causes symptoms or health problems. In the rare cases when there are noticeable symptoms, they are indistinguishable from those of an enlarged prostate (see previous article). The fact that the growths on the gland are malignant is often discovered only during an operation for some other prostate problem.

There is a risk, however, that if the cancer is not discovered, it may *metastasize* or spread, usually to the bones. This does not happen in most cases, but when it does, the symptoms are those of cancer of the bone (see Bone tumors, p.545). It is these secondary symptoms that frequently indicate the presence of the primary prostate cancer.

What are the risks?

Cancer of the prostate is rare in the young,

but it becomes increasingly common with age. It occurs in fewer than one man in 10,000 from ages 40 to 50, but is diagnosed five times more often in men who are in their sixties. At the age of 80 virtually every male has it, although usually it is only visible when looked for with the aid of a microscope. The disorder causes the deaths of fewer than two men in 10,000. If you are over 60 when you discover you have cancer of the prostate, you will probably outlive it and die from some unrelated cause.

What should be done?

If you have the characteristic symptoms of an enlarged prostate, your physician may refer you to a urologist, a specialist in urinary and genital diseases. At first, the physician will assume that the disorder is not cancerous. If, however, a rectal examination raises a suspicion that the tissues may be malignant, you will probably be advised to have a prostate *biopsy*, in which a small sample of tissue is removed for examination. In the examination, if cancer cells are discovered, the diagnosis of cancer of the prostate can be securely made. If cancer cells are found, you may be given a *radioisotope bone scan* to find out if the cancer has spread to your bones.

What is the treatment?

Malignancy that has spread to the bones or any other part of the body will be treated in the appropriate way. In addition, any malignant tissues that remain in the prostate gland after you have had your operation for enlargement (as described on the previous page) may be treated with *radiation therapy* to try to prevent further spread of the disease. The disease may also be treated with hormone medications.

There is some disagreement among physicians about whether or not to attempt special treatment for cancer that remains confined to the prostate gland and causes no symptoms. Your urologist may advise you to do nothing except have regular checkups to make sure that the malignancy has not spread. There are two main reasons for doing nothing. First, this type of cancer seldom spreads and rarely causes serious problems. Second, alternative treatment, which is removal of the entire prostate, has unpleasant side-effects such as impotence, yet does not guarantee a cure for the basic disease. It does reduce the chances that the cancer will spread, however. Be sure to discuss with your physician the risks and benefits of both treatments before a final decision is made.

Prostatitis

Prostatitis, or inflammation of the prostate gland, is usually the result of a urinary tract infection that has spread to the prostate. As with infection and inflammation anywhere in the body, prostatitis may improve of its own accord, may fester and form pus, or may linger indefinitely and become chronic.

What are the symptoms?

An acute attack of prostatitis usually begins suddenly and can make you feel ill, with a high fever, chills, and pain in and around the base of your penis. Later, as the prostate gland becomes increasingly swollen and tender, you may find it difficult and painful to urinate, because the prostate surrounds the urethra and the swelling of the gland narrows the passageway and blocks the flow of urine. Chronic prostatitis, however, often appears slowly with some minor pain.

What are the risks?

Prostatitis is not common. Elderly men with enlarged prostates (see p.574) are most susceptible, and the disease tends to recur once you have had an initial attack.

If prostatitis is not treated, or if, as sometimes happens, treatment with drugs is unsuc-

cessful, the gland may fester, become pus-filled, burst open, and release blood and pus into the urethra. This is quite painful.

What should be done?

If you suspect you have prostatitis, consult your physician, who will probably insert a gloved finger into your rectum to feel your prostate gland and determine whether it is swollen and tender. The doctor also will probably want a sample of urine for analysis in order to identify the infectious agents that may be causing the inflammation.

What is the treatment?

If your symptoms are clearly due to a bacterial infection, your physician will probably prescribe *antibiotics.* Occasionally, however, drugs do not entirely cure prostatitis. If you do not respond to drug treatment, your physician may recommend that you try massage, soaking the area in special solutions, and avoiding spices, alcohol and sex. If pus accumulates in your prostate, your physician may recommend an operation to drain it out. Such an operation usually requires only a few days in the hospital, and usually clears up the infection completely.

Bladder, urethra, penis and rectum

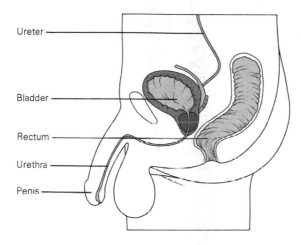

Ureter
Bladder
Rectum
Urethra
Penis

For a full discussion of the structure of the bladder and urethra and their relationships to the rest of the urinary tract, see p.500. In men, several ducts join the urethra near the point where it leaves the bladder. These ducts carry seminal fluid, or semen, to the outside during ejaculation. A group of small glands called the prostate gland (see p.574) surrounds the passageway.

In a man, most of the urethra is within the penis. The penis itself is composed mainly of spongy tissue full of tiny blood vessels. In an erect penis this spongy tissue is engorged with blood. In a relaxed penis the slightly bulbous end known as the glans is covered by a loose flap of skin, the foreskin or prepuce. In the United States, foreskins traditionally have been removed. However, this practice has recently come into question, because it may be considered unnecessary. For a discussion of the pros and cons, read "Should I have my son circumcised?" (see p.644).

The function of the rectum is described in the section of the book that deals with the digestive system (see Large intestine, p.476). The rectum is the last part of the large intestine, and it is connected to the outside of the body by the anus.

The male bladder, urethra, penis and rectum are not in themselves particularly susceptible to disease. For additional information on disorders that can affect these parts of the body but that originate elsewhere in the body, consult the sections on Disorders of the urinary tract (see p.500) and Special problems of couples (see p.606).

Cystitis in men

Cystitis, or inflammation of the bladder, is a common, often uncomfortable, but relatively harmless condition in women (see p.600). It is rare in men, but potentially more serious because it is usually caused by either an underlying urinary-tract problem such as a structural abnormality or a tumor, or by an infection that has spread from elsewhere in the urinary tract. The symptoms of cystitis include itching, burning, blood in the urine, and/or increased urination. The symptoms are probably secondary; that is, they indicate that you have some other disorder as well, so you should see your physician without delay. Although *antibiotic* drugs may cure your inflamed bladder, your physician will almost certainly want you to have tests to discover the underlying cause. Such tests will probably include *cystoscopy* and an *intravenous pyelogram (IVP)*. Once the underlying problem has been identified, further treatment will be whatever is appropriate for that disorder.

Penile warts

Warts on the penis are similar to warts elsewhere on the body (see Warts, p.252). Do not assume, however, that any wart-like growths on your penis, or just inside the urethral opening where they sometimes appear, are necessarily harmless. Rarely, but occasionally, a growth that resembles a wart may be an early symptom of either cancer of the penis (see p.579) or syphilis (see p.612). So always consult your physician if you develop what looks like a penile wart or warts. If the physi-cian confirms the diagnosis of warts and recommends or prescribes a specific type of "paint" for removing them, be sure to use exactly what the doctor suggests. Never try to treat warts on the penis with an over-the-counter preparation designed to treat warts elsewhere on the skin. Penile skin is much more sensitive than, for example, the skin on your hands or feet. It can be damaged easily by the powerful chemicals that are present in ordinary wart paint.

Like all warts, those on the penis are caused by localized areas of viral infection and are therefore to some extent *contagious*. Warts on the genital area can sometimes be transmitted to your sexual partner by intercourse. So if you have (or have had) penile warts, it is a good idea for your sexual partner to consult her physician to make sure she does not have vaginal or vulval warts (see p.603). Unless both partners are successfully treated, the virus can be passed back and forth indefinitely.

Urethritis in men

Urethritis (inflammation of the urethra) in men is usually caused by an infection transmitted through sexual intercourse with an infected partner The major symptoms are a copious, thick, yellow discharge from the tip of the penis and *dysuria*, a burning pain when you urinate. Among the many forms of male urethritis the most common are non-specific urethritis (see p.612), which is generally known as NSU, and gonorrhea (see p.611). Because these diseases can become a problem for both partners of a couple, they are discussed under Special problems of couples (see p.606).

Urethral stricture

Urethral stricture is a rare condition in which the urethra becomes scarred and narrowed as a result of the gradual shrinkage of scar tissue within its walls. The scar or scars are often caused by some sort of injury in the genital area. A common cause of urethral scar tissue used to be persistent urethritis (see previous article) due to infection, but modern treatment of diseases such as gonorrhea (see p.611) has virtually eliminated them as causes of scarring. The narrowed urethra of a man who has urethral stricture may make it increasingly difficult for him to urinate. Such problems can be painful, and can lead to urinary infections.

Scar tissue in a urethra once damaged by a disease or an accident can sometimes narrow the channel and even completely block the flow of urine.

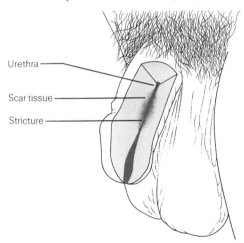

Urethra

Scar tissue

Stricture

What should be done?
If you have increasingly troublesome urethral stricture, your physician will probably refer you to a urologist, a specialist in urinary and genital diseases. The urologist may try to stretch the urethra using a long, flexible instrument called a *bougie* or *sound*. This can be inserted gently through the opening in the penis with the help of a local anesthetic. You will need a series of such treatments, which are called *dilatations*, over several weeks, and will require follow-up treatments at intervals thereafter. If this does not cure the stricture, the urologist may recommend surgery to cut the scarred tissue or to remove it and replace it with grafted tissue.

Balanitis

Balanitis is the general term for several types of inflammation of the foreskin and the underlying glans at the tip of the penis. The cause of this common problem may be infection (see Herpes genitalis, p.613), retention of a skin secretion called smegma, friction with damp garments, or irritation from chemical substances in clothing or contraceptive sheaths or creams. Diabetics are especially susceptible to the disorder because their sugary urine permits infection to flourish (see Diabetes mellitus, p.519). In some cases of balanitis the soreness and swelling that are present at the end of the penis increase because it becomes difficult to draw the foreskin back to cleanse the area.

One rare form of the disorder (called balanitis xerotica obliterans) has no known cause and does not itself cause the familiar redness and soreness of most kinds of inflammation. Instead the foreskin and/or the glans become abnormally pale and shrivelled. Although it is painless, this condition may not only make the foreskin irretractable but also may narrow the opening of the urethra, and obstruct the passage of urine.

What is the treatment?

Most kinds of balanitis will clear up if you discover the cause and remove it, and then treat the area with a soothing ointment. Your local pharmacist can recommend an appropriate one. If necessary, particularly if it is painful or difficult to draw back your foreskin, consult your physician, who may prescribe an *antibiotic* cream or tablets to relieve the inflammation. In stubborn cases the only answer may be either surgical loosening of the foreskin or circumcision, in which the foreskin is removed. If you have balanitis xerotica obliterans, you may also need a minor operation in which the surgeon widens the opening of the urethra.

Priapism

An erection that persists in the absence of sexual arousal and will not subside is known as priapism. This is a rare and painful condition. It is usually caused by a sudden, unexplained obstruction of the outflow of engorging blood from the erect penis. Occasionally, however, it may be due to disease in or injury to the nerves in the spinal cord that control erection. Whatever the cause, it is a serious matter. If the priapism lasts for three or four hours, the spongy tissues of the penis may be permanently damaged, which can make erection impossible.

What should be done?

If you have an erection that persists for no apparent reason, do not waste time trying to get it down with cold compresses or other home remedies. Call your physician or go to a hospital emergency room at once. Priapism is an emergency, and surgery to bypass the blockage, spinal anesthesia, or medications that reduce blood pressure may be used to treat it. If the condition is relieved quickly, you should eventually be able to have normal erections again and your sex life should not be adversely affected.

Cancer of the penis

This is a rare form of *malignant*, or life-threatening, growth. The cause of the disease is not known, but there is a high correlation between its development and many years of poor hygiene under the foreskin. Circumcised males are less susceptible than uncircumcised males to this problem, although if you wash your foreskin and glans regularly and thoroughly you run very little risk of developing the disease.

What are the symptoms?

The major symptom of cancer of the penis is a sore spot, an *ulcer*, or a warty lump that slowly spreads across the skin of the penis and down into deeper tissues. If it is not treated, the malignancy will *metastasize*, or spread to other parts of the body, most often via the lymphatic system (see p.432) or the bloodstream. Cancer of the penis tends to spread first to the lymph glands in the groin, and cause them to swell.

What should be done?

If you have a draining sore or any type of growth on your penis, consult your physician, who will probably want you to have a *biopsy*. In this procedure, a small sample of tissue is removed for examination. The biopsy is needed to distinguish cancer of the penis from syphilis (see p.612) and penile warts (see p.577), both of which may look similar to a cancerous growth. When cancer of the penis is discovered, surgery is usually the recommended treatment. However, *radiation therapy* is another alternative.

Hemo-spermia

"Hemospermia" means blood in the semen. The blood usually appears as pinkish, reddish, or brownish streaks in the seminal fluid. The cause of hemospermia is the rupture of a small vein or veins in the upper part of the urethra. This can happen at any time during an erection. It is quite common and usually goes unnoticed. If you or your sexual partner do notice some blood, do not be concerned. Tiny holes that occur in the veins close up within a few minutes without any special treatment. However, your semen may remain discolored for several days. There is no need to consult a physician.

If you are not sure that the blood was actually in the semen, however, and if you think it may have come from the urethra after ejaculation, you should see a physician. This is so that the possibility of bladder problems can be ruled out as a cause of the bleeding. Although hemospermia is harmless, *hematuria*, or blood in the urine, may be a symptom of serious illness (see, for example, Tumors of the bladder, p.508).

Anorectal abscesses

Abscesses, or walled off pockets of pus, can develop in the area around the anus and rectum. These infections, called anorectal abscesses, occur more frequently in men, and in persons with digestive diseases (see Irritable colon, p.478 and Crohn's disease, p.473), leukemia (see p.426) and diabetes mellitus (see p.519).

Anorectal abscesses can occur either on the edge of the anal opening, deeper in the rectum between the sphincter muscles or in the tissues even further into the rectum. The symptoms include intense rectal pain, swelling and warmth, sometimes accompanied by a fever. If the abscess is inside the rectum, it may be difficult for the physician to locate it.

What is the treatment?

If you have intense pain in the rectal area, see your physician. An anorectal abscess is treated by surgically opening the abscess and allowing the pus to drain. Abscesses near the skin's surface are easily operated on, but the deeper ones may require more exploration and probing. In such cases, a general anesthetic and hospitalization may be necessary.

Proctitis

Proctitis is an inflammation of the rectum that occurs most frequently in homosexual men. It can be caused by organisms that cause other sexually transmitted diseases (see p.611), but the symptoms are different.

If proctitis is caused by gonococcal bacteria, it produces a discharge that ranges from cloudy mucus to a pus-like material. This discharge may be accompanied by burning, itching, bleeding and painful bowel movements. Proctitis from syphilis causes a chancre, or ulcer-like open sore, either in the rectum or around the anus. The herpes virus can cause blistering ulcers inside the rectum or near the anus. Often these causes of proctitis can lead to itching and pain around the rectum and anus. Herpes can also infect the nerves that radiate from the spinal cord in the low back region and cause chronic pain in the back, thighs or buttocks; difficulty in urinating or problems with erections (see Impotence, next article). Penile warts (see p.577) can also affect the rectal area.

When proctitis is caused by these sexually transmitted diseases, it can be spread further through bodily contact. The disorder can also be extremely painful or uncomfortable. If you notice any of the symptoms described, see your physician right away. The physician may want to analyze a sample of any discharge from sores to find out what is causing the problem. If the infection is caused by bacteria, an appropriate *antibiotic* will be prescribed. Warts can be treated with a special wart paint. If the problem is a herpes infection, no proven treatment is as yet available. The infection must run its course, and it may recur in a milder form.

Impotence

Impotence is the loss of a man's ability to acquire and maintain an erection. Both psychological and physical factors can cause or contribute to this problem, and it is sometimes difficult for the physician to determine the exact nature of the cause. A man who loses sexual interest or desire will generally become impotent. Men who cannot perform sexually may still have a strong sexual drive, however, and can express great frustration about their disability.

Often temporary situations such as marital conflict, stress, fatigue or anxiety will lead to impotence. Impotence may also be a symptom of severe depression (see p.297).

When a man cannot maintain an erection for psychological reasons, he will generally continue to have erections through the night, and may have erection problems with some sexual partners but not with others. In such cases, the man would also be able to sustain an erection with masturbation.

During an erection, the penis becomes engorged with blood as blood vessels enlarge or dilate and allow an increased flow. This change is caused by nerve stimulation, and since some nerves are ultimately controlled in brain centers, a number of drugs that affect the brain can interfere with an erection. Some

---

Hygiene for men

Daily soap and water cleansing of the penile shaft and scrotum should be adequate. If you are not circumcised, be sure to cleanse the glans penis (the head of the penis) under the foreskin.

Thorough cleansing will not prevent gonorrhea (see p.611) or syphilis (see p.612), since the bacteria that produce these diseases are inside the body. However, organisms that produce minor infections such as non-specific urethritis (see p.612) and non-specific vaginitis in women may be removed by washing with soap and water.

As you wash, always look for sores, ulcers or unusual lesions that could be caused by a sexually transmitted infection.

commonly prescribed types of medication that can have this effect are those used to treat hypertension, including *diuretics*, or fluid pills. Tranquilizers and medicines used to combat depression (antidepressants) can also inhibit sexual function.

Frequently alcohol affects a man's ability to have an erection. Chronic alcoholism (see p.304) and the liver disease it often produces (see Cirrhosis of the liver, p.487) will lower the amount of testosterone circulating in the bloodstream. Testosterone, the major male sex hormone, is produced in the testes. It affects male physical characteristics such as body hair and voice, along with stimulating the sex drive and the production of sperm.

Diseased blood vessels can prevent the inflow of blood necessary to enlarge the penis. Severe arteriosclerosis (see Hardening of the arteries, p.404) in the body's lower blood vessels causes narrowing, thus restricting the inflow of blood necessary for an erection. Men who have severe, long-standing diabetes (see Diabetes mellitus, p.519) also are subject to impotence because the nerves and blood vessels may be damaged by the disease. Hypertension, or high blood pressure (see p.382), may be associated with impotence, as well as chronic illnesses such as kidney failure (see p.511).

Finally, diseases that inhibit the production or action of the male hormone testosterone can reduce sexual interest and performance. These diseases are generally unusual hormonal conditions such as tumors of the pituitary gland (see p.518) or hypothalamus, which are vital centers in the brain that regulate and produce hormones.

What should be done?

If you are consistently unable to have an erection, consult your physician. The physician will want to know whether the problem is psychological or physical. Certain clues such as erections stimulated by masturbation may suggest psychological origins. The physician will also want to know if you have a history of alcoholism or if you are taking medication for high blood pressure.

Your physician may want you to have a blood test to measure the testosterone level. If you take medications, one drug at a time may be removed from your medications list to see if the impotence improves. In this way, the physician may be able to identify a drug that is causing the problem.

Not long ago, it was thought that almost all cases of impotence had psychological causes. But recent studies have shown, through monitoring testosterone levels, that physical reasons for impotence are more common than once thought.

What is the treatment?

If psychological problems appear to be causing the impotence, and if no underlying disorder can be found, your physician may refer you (and possibly your sexual partner) to a psychiatrist, a psychologist or a sex therapist.

If a drug is found to be causing the difficulty, that drug usually can be eliminated or replaced with another.

In cases where the testosterone level is found to be low, the physician may recommend an injection to raise the level to normal. If this treatment is not successful, further testing may be necessary.

Loss of sexual desire in men

The male sex hormone testosterone stimulates the male sexual drive. If, therefore, your testosterone level is lowered, your libido, or sexual interest and capacity for arousal, is likely to diminish. The underlying cause of the drop in testosterone level may be a physical problem such as liver, kidney or pituitary disease, or it may be a side-effect of a drug you are taking. The cause also may be fatigue, stress or pain. Most often, however, the root of the problem is psychological or a combination of psychological and physical factors. Severe depression (see p.297), for example, may cause you to lose interest in sex.

A few men lose their desire for sex in general, but loss of sexual interest in a familiar partner is the most common problem. This is apt to happen when there are other problems (which may or may not be sexual) in the relationship. A disorder such as impotence (see above) or premature ejaculation (see p.614) that interferes with the enjoyment of lovemaking can cause a man to shun sex.

If self-help measures do not help you to regain sexual desire, consult your physician, who will probably examine you to look for a physical cause. If none is found, you may be referred to a sex therapist or marital counselor.

What can you do?

It may help to discuss the issue openly with your partner. This may clear up misunderstandings or uncover other problems in the relationship that may be affecting you both. If you are bored with a long-standing relationship, try mutually agreeable new ways of making love.

What treatment is available?

Treatment depends on the underlying cause, which is often difficult to determine. *Psychotherapy* can be helpful if your physician is unable to identify any physical cause. Self-help exercises, relaxation techniques, and a review of some facts about sexual arousal may also be helpful.

Special problems of women

Introduction

The problems that are dealt with in this section are mainly those that affect only women. Other sections of this book cover aspects of a woman's health that are not discussed here, such as pregnancy and childbirth, problems of adolescent girls, problems of the elderly, problems of couples (including sexually-transmitted diseases), and all the many problems that affect women in much the same way as they affect men.

The problems described in the following pages are divided into a number of categories. First, there are problems concerned with the menstrual cycle: the four-weekly cycle of egg ripening, egg release, and shedding of the lining of the uterus. The menstrual cycle is controlled by a complex system of hormones that are manufactured by and released within the body. The cycle can be disturbed if the hormonal balance is upset by any one of a number of factors, some of which are physical and others that are emotional.

Several of the other groups of articles are concerned with various structural abnormalities, infections, inflammations, and growths that can occur in female organs. These are disorders of the breast, of the ovaries, uterus and cervix, and of the vagina and vulva.

Of particular importance and interest are special boxes related to breast cancer, a major concern of women today. One box describes and illustrates the proper way to examine your own breasts for signs of cancer. As is true of any cancer, if breast cancer is detected early, the chances of controlling and even curing it are greatly improved. Self examination is one way of achieving such early detection. A second box describes mastectomy, or breast removal, an operation that is usually recommended when breast cancer strikes.

In addition, there is a group of articles that deal with problems of the bladder and urethra. They appear in this part of the book because disorders of these particular organs tend to cause different problems in women than the ones that they do in men.

If you have one of the disorders in this section, you should consult your physician. The section also contains a number of informative boxes that cover several health

The female reproductive organs

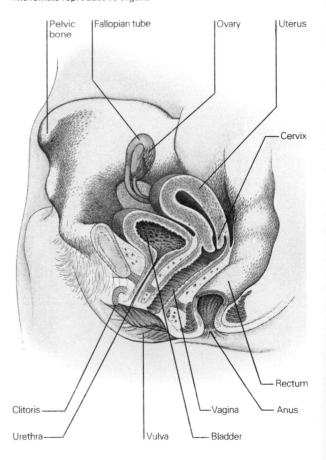

Pelvic bone | Fallopian tube | Ovary | Uterus

Cervix

Clitoris

Urethra

Vulva

Vagina

Bladder

Rectum

Anus

aspects not necessarily directly related to a specific disease. There is a box, for example, on loss of sexual desire, a problem that may have either a physical or emotional basis. Also covered in this way are menstrual care and vaginal cleansing.

Menstruation and menopause

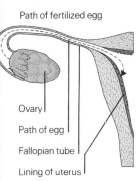

Path of fertilized egg

Ovary

Path of egg

Fallopian tube

Lining of uterus

Each month, if you are a woman in your fertile years, ovulation, or egg release, occurs. One of your two ovaries releases an ovum, or egg. The egg is a tiny single cell, barely visible to the naked eye. It travels down the fallopian tube to the uterus, or womb. This takes about five days. You can become pregnant if you have sexual intercourse within a day or two before or after the egg is released. After intercourse, sperm usually make their way up into the fallopian tubes. Sperm can live for as long as six days, so if you have sexual intercourse between five days before the release of the egg and 24 hours after, a sperm will be able to fertilize the egg.

During the few days preceding ovulation, the lining of your uterus becomes thickened and engorged with blood. This is to prepare for the possibility of fertilization. By the time a fertilized egg reaches the uterus, the lining is in a suitable condition for the egg to burrow into it and start developing into an embryo. When this happens, you are pregnant.

If the egg is not fertilized, the thickened, blood-filled lining of the uterus is not required. Both the unfertilized egg and the lining are shed about 14 days after the start of ovulation. The blood passes out of the cervix, or neck of the uterus, into the vagina, and then out of your body. This discharge, called menstruation or a menstrual period, lasts an average of five days. During the next nine days a new lining grows in the uterus, after which the process of ovulation starts again.

The entire cycle lasts an average of 28 days. But in most women the cycle fluctuates in length, sometimes by a day or two, sometimes by even longer.

Each stage in the menstrual cycle is controlled by a system of interrelated hormones and other chemicals produced in the hypothalamus, which is part of the brain, the adjacent pituitary gland, and the ovaries.

Menstrual periods usually start between the ages of 11 and 14. The first period is called menarche. Periods are irregular for the first year or two because ovulation often fails to occur regularly. Periods also become irregular, for the same reason, after the age of 45, and finally, periods cease altogether. This is known as menopause.

Problems related to the length, frequency and effect of periods are covered here.

The menstrual cycle (28 days)

Most fertile period

Egg released

Lining of uterus starts to build up

1 segment = 1 day

Menstruation

Lining of uterus shed during menstruation

Absence of periods
(amenorrhea)

The absence, temporary or permanent, of menstrual periods is known technically as amenorrhea. In some girls, periods fail to start at the normal age, which is usually between 11 and 14. This is generally known as primary amenorrhea. It is generally the result of a naturally late onset of puberty, but it can be due to some abnormality in the reproductive or hormonal system. Such abnormalities are usually not suspected except in cases where a girl has reached the age of 16 or 17 without having a period.

In a woman who has had regular periods, a delay or absence of periods is called secondary amenorrhea. It is due to a change in the balance of hormones that control the release of an egg from the ovary. One fairly obvious cause is pregnancy. The hormones may also be disrupted by emotional factors (for example, a quarrel or a new job), by a rapid weight change (see Anorexia nervosa, p.710), by illness, or by taking certain drugs. Women who have just stopped taking oral contraceptives may experience secondary amenorrhea for a few months. Less commonly, absence of periods is a result of a disorder affecting egg release (see Abnormalities of the hypothalamus, pituitary and ovaries, p.587).

Periods normally stop permanently at menopause (see p.586) or when the ovaries have been removed as treatment for some other disorder.

What are the risks?

Absence of periods is common; secondary amenorrhea occurs much more often than primary amenorrhea. Neither form presents any risk to health in itself. The only danger is that in rare cases it may indicate a more serious disorder. However, a woman with amenorrhea may not be able to have a child without special treatment.

What should be done?

If you are over 16 and have never had a period, you should consult your physician, who will examine you to make sure that you do not have an underlying disorder. In most cases there is nothing wrong and no treatment is necessary. In such an instance, you can safely wait for your periods to start natur-ally. Young women who are very thin or who are in intense athletic training programs sometimes have a delayed menarche.

If your periods have already started and become fairly regular, and a period is delayed for two weeks or more, consult your physician, who may examine you. If there is a possibility of pregnancy, your physician may recommend that you have a pregnancy test. If you are not pregnant and are otherwise well, your physician will probably advise you to wait for a few months to see if your periods will start again naturally.

If you have amenorrhea, it is important to remember that an egg may be released at any time, so if you wish to avoid getting pregnant, and you expect to have sexual intercourse, you must use some form of contraception.

If your periods have not started again within nine months, your physician may arrange for you to have various diagnostic tests to look for some underlying problem. If none is found, no treatment may be given for the absence of periods unless you wish to become pregnant. In that case, your physician may prescribe a fertility drug to restart egg release (see Infertility, p.607).

Infrequent periods
(oligomenorrhea)

Infrequent periods occur when a woman has fewer periods than the usual 11 to 13 a year. The periods are normal and are generally preceded by ovulation in the usual way, only they occur less often. Oligomenorrhea occurs most commonly in women approaching menopause (see p.586), but some women have the condition throughout adult life as a result of their particular hormone cycle (see Abnormalities of the hypothalamus, pituitary and ovaries, p.587).

Infrequent periods do not endanger your general health and do not usually require any treatment unless you wish to become pregnant. (For further information see Infertility, p.607.)

Painful periods
(dysmenorrhea)

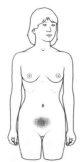

Site of the pain

Painful periods, especially menstrual cramps, are known technically as dysmenorrhea. If the pain starts within about three years of when the periods themselves start, it is known as primary dysmenorrhea. This is thought to be a result of normal hormonal changes during menstruation, and can persist throughout the child-bearing years.

If periods become painful in a woman who has been menstruating longer than three years, the condition is known as secondary dysmenorrhea. Secondary dysmenorrhea is far more likely than primary dysmenorrhea to be caused by an underlying disorder, such as endometriosis (see p.595), pelvic infection (see p.596), or fibroids (see p.593).

What are the symptoms?

Menstrual pain varies considerably. Some women have dull pain in the abdomen or back, others have severe cramping abdominal pain. Typically the pain is worse at the beginning of a period. Less commonly, there may also be nausea and vomiting.

Painful periods are very common but the majority of cases are mild and do not require medical attention. The condition itself does not endanger your general health. But it may be a symptom of a more serious underlying disorder.

What is the treatment?

Non-prescription pain-relief tablets such as aspirin may help. Your physician may recommend other medications that help control pain and reduce inflammation. Exercise also may relieve the pain. Bed rest is usually not necessary for this disorder.

Consult your physician if you develop severe menstrual pain following three or more years of relatively pain-free periods, or if the pain is worse than usual. The doctor will probably examine you to find out what is causing the dysmenorrhea, and any underlying disorder will be treated. If the pain is severe, your physician may prescribe a strong painkiller, or recommend that you start taking oral contraceptives or some other drug that will change your hormone balance in a way that will lessen your pain. Sometimes primary dysmenorrhea disappears after you have a child.

Heavy periods
(*menorrhagia*)

Unusually heavy and prolonged periods are known medically as menorrhagia. You have them if your periods last for more than seven days, if especially large clots of blood are passed, or if flooding occurs. The problem is often brought on by a spontaneous disturbance of the hormones that control the menstrual cycle. It can also be caused by fibroids (see p.593), pelvic infection (see p.596), or, rarely, endometriosis (see p.595). The presence in the uterus of an intrauterine contraceptive device (IUD) may also cause the condition.

What are the risks?
Menorrhagia is common. Some women regularly have heavy periods, and others have them only occasionally. The condition frequently occurs in young women who have not yet established regular ovulation cycles, and it is especially common in women approaching menopause.

Apart from being inconvenient, menorrhagia can be distressing. However, the condition rarely signifies a serious underlying disorder. One general risk is that if you regularly have heavy periods you may develop iron-deficiency anemia (see p.419).

What should be done?
If you have been having heavy periods for some time, consult your physician. If you have a single unusually heavy period, follow the self-help measures suggested below. If your period was late as well as heavy and there was a chance of pregnancy, you may be having an early miscarriage. In this case, see your physician immediately. The physician will question and examine you to discover the extent of the bleeding and to see if there is any abnormality of your uterus. A Pap test may be done to check for cancer, and a *biopsy* of the cervix may also be done. A blood test may be done to find out if menorrhagia has made you anemic, and to check for other blood and hormone problems that can cause the condition.

What is the treatment?
Self-help: If you have an unusually heavy period and do not believe you are pregnant, reduce your activity. If the bleeding does not lessen within 24 hours, call your physician. If your periods are always heavy, it is important to make sure your diet contains enough iron to avoid iron-deficiency anemia.

Professional help: If your uterus is normal, your physician will probably prescribe hormone tablets that contain estrogen, progesterone, or both, to reduce the bleeding. These are the same ingredients as those used in oral contraceptives. If you are already taking oral contraceptives, or if you cannot take them for some reason, your physician can prescribe another drug to reduce the bleeding. If you are using an IUD, your doctor may recommend that you change to another method of contraception. And if blood tests indicate that you are anemic, you may have to take iron tablets as well.

If this treatment does not work after a few months, your physician will probably arrange for you to have a procedure called a dilation and curettage, or D&C (see Box, p.593) to find out if an underlying disorder is causing the menorrhagia. Any such disorder will be treated accordingly. Even if nothing is found, the D&C itself sometimes clears up the problem. A D&C may also be performed if a miscarriage is suspected.

Premenstrual tension

Each month various glands in your body release hormones into the bloodstream. The two main sex hormones in women are estrogen and progesterone, both of which are made in the ovaries. They control various physical changes in your body, including the changes of the uterus during the menstrual cycle (see Menstruation and menopause, p.583), and associated physical changes such as increased breast tenderness. In addition, the monthly cycle of hormonal changes may affect your mood and produce certain mental or emotional changes. The combination of physical and emotional changes that may occur in the seven days or so before you have a period may cause the condition that is known as premenstrual tension.

What are the symptoms?
Changes of mood usually take the form of increased irritability, aggressiveness and/or depression. Physical changes may include a slight increase in weight due to fluid retention, slightly enlarged and tender breasts, bloated stomach, and lower abdominal pain. The degree of severity of these symptoms varies enormously. Usually they are either unnoticeable or moderate, and do not cause any problem. But occasionally the symptoms are so pronounced that they affect personal relationships or performance at work.

What should be done?
If you have pronounced premenstrual tension, it may help if you understand the relationship between the symptoms and the menstrual cycle. Try to avoid situations that are likely to cause stress or irritation during the days when you are affected. Reduce your salt intake to help discourage fluid retention. If the symptoms continue to be severe, consult your physician. He or she may examine you for other causes of your symptoms, and may prescribe hormone tablets to prevent ovulation for one or two cycles to relieve your symptoms. The most common hormones prescribed are estrogen and progesterone, which are the ingredients of oral contraceptives.

If your symptoms are not relieved by this treatment, your doctor may prescribe analgesics or tranquilizers to take on the days when the problem is worst. If you have severe depression, your physician may refer you to a psychologist or psychiatrist.

Menopause

Menopause is the medical term for the normal, complete ending of menstrual cycles, including both ovulation and menstrual periods. The term is often used in a broader sense to mean the months or even years before and after this natural event in a woman's life. This time is also known as the climacteric or the change of life. The last period usually occurs between the ages of 40 and 50, but can happen as late as 60. In the years leading up to menopause, your menstrual cycle is disrupted and periods may become irregular.

Menopause is a natural stage in your life. It does not signify any disease or disorder.

What are the symptoms?
About 25 per cent of women do not notice any changes at menopause, except the cessation of periods. Another 50 per cent notice slight physical and/or mental changes. The remaining 25 per cent have inconvenient or even distressing symptoms. Physical symptoms may include hot flashes, sweating, dryness of the vagina (sometimes causing soreness during sexual intercourse), palpitations, joint pains and headaches. Among the nonphysical symptoms often associated with the menopause are depression, anxiety, irritability, decreased ability to concentrate, lack of confidence and sleeping difficulties. These symptoms may last from a few weeks to more than five years.

What should be done?
If you have troublesome symptoms, bear in mind that they are not in themselves a danger to your health. Remember also that some emotional and physical problems, for example depression (see p.297) and osteoporosis (see p.543), are more common as we get older and that their symptoms may be accentuated by menopause.

It may help if you can accept unpleasant symptoms of menopause as a natural part of life and not something about which to be overly concerned. However, since diseases can occur, you should not automatically attribute all symptoms to menopause. Instead, discuss them with your physician. He or she will examine you to make sure that no other condition is causing your symptoms, and may prescribe drugs to relieve the symptoms. You should see your doctor immediately if you have any bleeding between periods, prolonged or excessive menstrual bleeding, or another period six months or more after what appeared to be the last. Any of these symptoms could indicate a *malignant*, or life-threatening, growth such as cancer of the uterus (see p.594).

What is the treatment?
Self-help: Do not add avoidable difficulties to those that may occur naturally during the years of menopause. For example, do not neglect your health or personal appearance. If you have a lot of leisure time, especially if you have children who are no longer living at home, develop new interests and friends.

If you wish to avoid pregnancy during this time, you should know that the possible period of fertility depends on your age at the time of your last period. If you are under 50, you should continue to use contraceptives for 24 months after the date of your last period. If you are over 50, you should protect yourself for 12 months after the last period.

If you are having hot flashes and sweating, remember that usually you will be the only person who is aware of them. If sweating is a nuisance at night, wear absorbent cotton night clothes. If you find that intercourse makes your vagina sore, use a lubricant such as a water soluble jelly.

Professional help: The treatment you receive will depend on a variety of factors. If you are troubled by irregular or prolonged periods, hot flashes or excessive sweating, your physician may prescribe a hormone preparation to alter your hormonal balance and reduce the symptoms. This type of treatment is often called *hormone replacement therapy.* The hormones may be a combination of estrogen and progesterone, or estrogen alone, in the form of tablets or a vaginal cream. Your physician will probably prescribe the treatment for several months, then gradually reduce the dose and eventually stop the treatment. By this time the changes in the ovaries should be complete, and symptoms should not return in severe form. If they do, you may have to take another short treatment.

There are various drugs besides hormones that act to lessen menopausal symptoms. These may be prescribed for women who are well over 50, or who have a heart or circulatory condition, or who for some other reason should not have hormone therapy. If you have mainly emotional or psychological symptoms, your doctor may prescribe tranquilizers, antidepressants or sleeping pills.

Treatment for menopausal symptoms will not usually slow down or stop the changes of menopause itself, or most other body changes associated with aging. The exception is that estrogen therapy seems to halt the progress of osteoporosis (see p.543), a bone disease. However, estrogen therapy also has a risk factor – it may increase your chances of getting cancer of the uterus (see p.594). You may wish to discuss the risks and benefits of available treatments with your physician before a treatment is selected.

Abnormalities of the hypothalamus, pituitary and ovaries

A number of problems can be caused by a disturbance of the interrelated system of sex hormones in the female body. The menstrual cycle is regulated by several hormones. Each month the hypothalamus, which is part of the brain, produces chemicals known as releasing factors. These pass into the pituitary gland and stimulate the production of pituitary hormones which in turn affect an ovary and cause ovulation, or the release of an egg. These hormones also stimulate the production of the female sex hormones estrogen and progesterone in the ovary.

This cycle can be upset by a number of factors. The hypothalamus may be disturbed by emotional factors, drug abuse, extreme weight changes (see Anorexia nervosa, p.710) or severe illness. Occasionally, it is disturbed if you stop taking oral contraceptives. Some brain disorders such as meningitis (see p.273) or a brain tumor (see p.282) can also affect the hypothalamus.

The pituitary gland is less susceptible to disturbances. Tumors of the pituitary gland (see p.518), though they are very rare, almost always cause abnormalities in sex-hormone production. Certain rare disorders of the ovary may also affect hormone production. These include some ovarian cysts (see p.592), and a very rare disorder, polycystic ovary disease. For other problems of the ovaries, see the articles beginning on p.592.

What are the symptoms?
The main symptom of an abnormality in sex-hormone production is disruption of periods (see Absence of periods, p.583). If the pituitary gland is causing the problem, there may also be other symptoms (see Pituitary gland, p.515).

In some disorders of the ovaries or adrenal glands, the production of the male sex hormone testosterone, which is produced to some extent in all women, may increase. This may cause increased hairiness (hirsutism) on the face and body, deepening of the voice and weight increase.

What should be done?
If your periods become irregular or cease altogether, consult your physician, who after examining you to see if either pregnancy or an underlying disorder is causing the problem, will probably advise you to take no further action unless you have no periods for at least six months. If your doctor suspects an underlying problem, you will probably need to have blood and urine tests to determine hormone levels in your body, and *X-rays* of your pituitary gland.

If an underlying disorder is causing your symptoms, this disorder will be treated. Otherwise, treatment is not usually given unless you indicate that you wish to become pregnant (see Infertility, p.607).

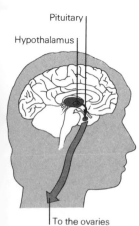

Pituitary
Hypothalamus
To the ovaries

The breast

Each of a woman's breasts consists of 15 to 20 groups of milk-producing glands embedded in fatty tissue. From each group a milk duct runs to the nipple. Around the nipple is a dark area, the areola, that contains small sebaceous, or lubricating, glands that keep the nipple supple.

During pregnancy, the release of certain hormones from the placenta and the pituitary gland causes the breasts to enlarge and, after delivery, to produce milk (see Pregnancy and childbirth, p.616). The breasts may also become a little larger, and sometimes tender, before a menstrual period.

This group of articles discusses some of the problems that can develop in the breast. Such problems may be caused by abnormal growths such as cysts or tumors. They can

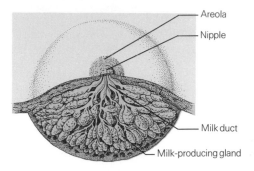

Areola
Nipple
Milk duct
Milk-producing gland

also be the result of a breast infection.

Breast cancer is the most common cancer in women. It is important that every woman examine her breasts regularly to detect any signs of possible breast cancer.

Lumps in the breast

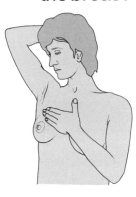

Self-examination is important because lumps in the breast usually cannot be seen and rarely cause symptoms.

Some women's breasts are irregularly shaped, uneven in texture, or have lumps in them. This is due to the make-up of the breast tissue, and is usually not a cause for concern. The appearance of a new lump is more important. There are five possible causes. The first is a *cyst*, which is a fluid-filled sac of tissue. The second is an infection; in such cases there are usually other symptoms (see Breast abscess, p.590). The third cause of a breast lump is fibro-adenosis, which is a thickening of the milk-producing glandular tissue. The fourth is a *benign* growth, which is unlikely to spread. None of these is harmful. But the fifth possibility is a *malignant* tumor, which may spread and threaten life.

Lumps in the breast may cause no discomfort at all. Sometimes a lump is slightly tender or even painful.

What should be done?
Make a regular examination of your breasts each month (see illustrations), so that you will detect a new lump early. To help you remember, decide on a specific time for the examination, such as at the end of your period, or on a specific date.

If you detect a lump that was not there before, whether it is painful or not, make an appointment to see your physician as soon as possible. Also, if you have always had a lump but it changes in some way – becomes painful, or harder, or bigger – see your physician. Your doctor will examine you and may refer

you to a specialist, probably a surgeon. The surgeon will also examine you and, depending on the results, may arrange for one or more diagnostic tests to find out the nature of the lump and to determine the cause. Tests usually include *mammography*, which is a special *X-ray* of the breast tissue, *thermography* (a heat-sensitive outline of the breast), and a *biopsy* of the lump. In a biopsy, a small piece of tissue is removed for examination.

What is the treatment?
The treatment depends on the nature of the lump. If it is a cyst, it will probably be drained through a needle into a syringe. This simple procedure may not even require a local anesthetic, and usually clears up the problem. However, you will need to have regular checkups for about two years to make sure the lump does not return.

When the cause of the lump (or lumps) is thickening of the glandular tissue in the breasts (fibro-adenosis), treatment is not essential. However, if such a lump feels tender or painful, your physician may prescribe either sex hormones or other drugs that affect your hormone balance. In addition, your physician will probably advise you to wear a brassiere that gives firm support. Certain vitamins may also be useful.

If diagnostic tests show that the lump is a tumor, you will need to go into the hospital to have it removed. The type of operation depends on the nature of the tumor. If it is

How to examine your breasts

1 Stand in front of the mirror, and look at each breast to see if there is a lump, a depression, or a difference in texture.

2 Get to know how your breasts look, and be especially alert for any changes in the nipples' appearance.

3 Raise both arms and check for any swelling or dimpling in the skin of your breasts.

4 Lie down with a pillow under your right shoulder and put your right arm behind your head.

5 With the fingers of your left hand, repeatedly press or squeeze your right breast gently and circularly from the outside to the center.

6 Squeeze your nipple to see if there is any discharge. Repeat from step 4, reversing right and left for your left breast.

benign, it is usually necessary to remove only the tumor itself. This procedure is usually done in the hospital, but may not require an overnight stay. After the operation, you will need to have regular checkups with your physician for about two years. For treatment of a malignant tumor, read the next article, which deals with breast cancer.

Breast cancer

A *malignant,* or life-threatening, tumor may develop in the breast. Why this happens is not known. At first the tumor stays in the breast. When it has grown to about 20 mm (about ¾ in) or more across, it usually sheds cancerous cells that *metastasize,* or spread, through the bloodstream and the lymphatic system to other parts of the body, where new tumors develop. In about ten per cent of cases, tumors develop in both breasts.

What are the symptoms?
A lump, which may or may not be painful, develops in the breast, most commonly in the upper, outer part. The lump is usually not readily noticeable and is most often detected in a breast self-examination. Sometimes the skin over the lump becomes dimpled or creased. There may also be a dark-colored discharge from the nipple, or the nipple may turn inwards and invert.

What are the risks?
Cancer of the breast is the most common cancer in women; about 1 woman in 15 develops the disease. It occurs most often in women in their 40s and 50s. There are several factors that contribute to the risk of developing breast cancer. It is slightly more common in women who have never breast-fed a baby, in women who have a family history of the disease, and in women who have had a late menopause (see p.586).

If it is not treated, or if it is treated too late, the disease will almost always be fatal. For this reason you should not hesitate to report any new breast lump to your physician. Breast cancer is not a common cause of breast lumps. When it does occur the outlook is good if it is diagnosed and treated early.

What should be done?
Monthly examination of the breasts will help you to detect any lump early. Read the instructions with the illustrations above to find out how to do this. If you are a woman over 50 or if several women in your family have had the disease, you should also be sure to have regular checkups with breast examinations by your physician.

Any lump that develops in the breast, even if it is painless, should be evaluated by a physician right away. If the physician confirms the presence of a lump, you will probably be referred to a surgeon, who will give you tests to determine whether the lump is due to breast cancer or one of several other disorders. *Mammography, thermography,* and/or a *biopsy* (taking a sample of the lump for examination) will probably be carried out. If these indicate that the lump is a malignant tumor, there are several methods of treatment that are available.

What is the treatment?

The most common treatment is to remove the whole breast (see Box, next page), together with the lymph glands from the armpit next to the breast. Occasionally, only part of the breast is removed. In addition to the operation, *radiation therapy* or *cytotoxic* (anticancer) drugs may be used. In some cases, radiation therapy alone can effectively eliminate the cancer. You should discuss the alternatives and the associated risks with your physician. The length of time spent in the hospital varies depending on the extent of the surgery and other treatment that is necessary.

Losing a breast is naturally distressing. However, you may be surprised to learn how many other women have had a mastectomy, since the loss can be very well concealed. A breast *prosthesis* worn in the brassiere can be matched to the other breast and is essentially undetectable. Many women who have had a mastectomy are able to adjust to it and find the problems more manageable if they undergo breast reconstruction surgery.

What are the long-term prospects?

If the tumor has been removed at an early stage, either a complete cure or many years of good health can be expected. After treatment, your physician will probably recommend annual or semi-annual checkups. If the cancer does recur, it can be held in check for many years by drugs, radiation therapy, and perhaps further surgery.

Breast abscess

An *abscess* is a pus-filled infected area of tissue. A breast abscess forms when infectious agents enter the breast tissue through the nipple and infect the milk ducts and glands. The infection usually comes from the skin surrounding the nipple, and as the infectious agents multiply they cause a red, tender, painful swelling or lump in your breast. The glands in the armpit next to the affected breast may also be tender, and you may have a fever. Breast abscesses are uncommon. In many cases the disorder occurs in women who are breast-feeding a new baby. This is because cracked nipples, a problem which may occur during the first week of breast-feeding, make it easier for infectious agents to enter the breast tissue.

What should be done?

If you are breast-feeding, you can reduce your risk of developing an abscess by keeping your nipples clean and dry between feedings, preventing irritation from clothing, and not allowing the baby to "chew" instead of suck.

Whether you are breast-feeding or not, you should see your physician if an abscess develops. The treatment is the same, whatever the cause. You will probably be given *antibiotic* tablets to fight the infection, and perhaps aspirin to reduce any pain and fever.

You will probably be advised not to continue breast-feeding from the affected breast until the infection clears up. During this time your physician may recommend that you massage the affected breast gently, to expel the milk and prevent the breast from becoming engorged.

Occasionally the antibiotic will not clear up the problem, and you will need to have the abscess drained. A small cut may be made at the edge of the areola (the brownish skin surrounding the nipple) to allow the pus to drain out. The drainage, together with antibiotics, will quickly clear up the infection, and you should have no further problems with it. No detectable scar is left by the cut.

Galactorrhea

The breasts normally produce milk only after the birth of a baby, and sometimes for a few days before the birth. If milk production occurs at any other time in a woman, or at any time in a man, it is called galactorrhea. The milk is usually produced by both breasts and is whitish or greenish in color.

Galactorrhea is very rare in women and even rarer in men. It is usually caused by excessive amounts of the female sex hormone estrogen, which can occur during pregnancy or from taking oral contraceptives. Another possible cause is excessive production of the hormone prolactin. Prolactin is made by the pituitary gland and stimulates milk production. Galactorrhea can also be caused by a disorder of the pituitary gland such as a tumor (see p.518) or by your taking certain types of tranquilizers, but may occur for no apparent reason at all. In women, galactorrhea is often coupled with an absence of periods (see p.583).

What should be done?

If you think you have galactorrhea, consult your physician. If a pituitary tumor or another underlying disorder is suspected, the physician will probably refer you to a specialist for appropriate diagnostic tests.

If tests fail to reveal any cause for the condition, you will probably not need any treatment. If the problem is caused by drugs, discontinuing the drugs will clear it up. If it is caused by a pituitary gland disorder or some other disease, your physician will probably prescribe hormone treatment to prevent milk production. The doctor will also treat the underlying problem.

Nipple problems

Most nipple problems do not affect your general health. But in rare cases, a nipple disorder may be an early sign of a serious disease. In such cases, early diagnosis means early treatment and an increased chance of a cure.

Nipple discharge

A whitish or greenish discharge is likely to be breast milk, especially if it comes from both nipples. If it occurs at any time other than just before or after the birth of a baby, it is called galactorrhea (see previous article).

Any dark-colored discharge (usually dark red or black), especially if it comes from only one breast, should be reported to your physician. Note which nipple the discharge comes from, and whether it comes from one nipple duct (the tiny holes in the tips of the nipple) or many. The coloring is probably due to blood discharge, often from a tiny benign growth called a duct papilloma. But the cause could be breast cancer (see p.589).

Your physician will examine your breasts and, if possible, analyze a sample of the discharge. You may also need other tests, including *mammography*. If a papilloma is found, it can be removed by simple surgery.

Nipple retraction

Nipple inversion, or retraction, that makes its first appearance at puberty usually affects both nipples. Such retraction is no problem to health, but it may make breast-feeding a little difficult later in life.

Recent retraction or a pulling back of the nipple or any part of the breast, especially if it affects only one breast, may be a sign of breast cancer. You should report it to your physician right away.

Cracked nipples

Mothers who are breast-feeding often find that the skin of their nipples becomes cracked and painful. See Breast problems, p.641, for how to deal with the problem.

Cysts or boils in the areola

The areola is the darker area around the nipple. It contains sebaceous glands that produce a waxy substance to lubricate the nipple. If the duct of one of these glands becomes blocked, a cyst (fluid-filled sac) forms in the duct. If the gland itself then becomes infected, a boil will result. You should consult your physician if you have such a cyst or boil. In general, treatment for a cyst or boil in the areola is the same as for a cyst or boil elsewhere (see Sebaceous cysts, p.261, and Boils and carbuncles, p.251).

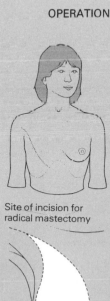

Site of incision for radical mastectomy

OPERATION: Breast removal
(mastectomy)

If a lump in the breast is found to be malignant, or life-threatening, you may be given a lumpectomy (removal of the lump only) or, if the doctor suspects that there is a danger of the cancer spreading, a mastectomy.

During the operation There are four types of mastectomy. In a radical mastectomy the surgeon removes the breast, the lymph glands from the armpit, and both pectoral, or chest, muscles. In a modified radical mastectomy, one of the pectoral muscles is left in place. In a simple mastectomy, only the breast itself is removed. In a subcutaneous mastectomy, the skin and superficial tissues are left in place, and a silicone artificial breast is inserted to replace the tissue that has been removed. You are under a general anesthetic for the entire operation, which takes between one and two hours.

After the operation You will have a drainage tube removing fluid from the site of the incision and will probably stay in the hospital for a week to ten days.

Convalescence You may be given radiation therapy or cytotoxic drugs and will have a check-up every 6 to 12 months.

Ovaries, uterus and cervix

The two ovaries and the uterus (womb) are the main female reproductive organs. Your ovaries lie one on each side of your spinal column, just above your pubic bone. They move freely within a small area. Each ovary contains thousands of eggs. During your fertile years, one egg (or sometimes more) ripens each month and is released into the fallopian tube connected to the ovary from which the egg came. As the egg travels slowly down the tube toward the uterus it can be fertilized by a sperm cell.

The uterus is a pear-shaped organ that lies at the front of your lower abdomen, behind the urinary bladder. Its walls are composed of powerful muscles, which are mainly used to push out the baby during childbirth. In the lower front end of the uterus is a narrow, thick-walled structure, the cervix, which leads into the top of the vagina.

The disorders included here are mostly structural problems and various kinds of growths or infections in the ovaries, uterus or cervix. Disorders of the menstrual cycle, which are mainly caused by hormonal disturbances, are dealt with in the articles on menstruation and menopause (see p.583).

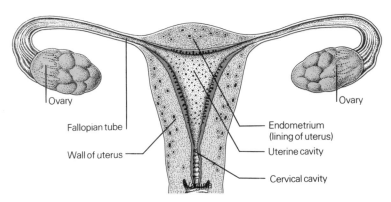

Ovary

Fallopian tube

Wall of uterus

Endometrium (lining of uterus)

Ovary

Uterine cavity

Cervical cavity

Ovarian cysts

An ovarian cyst is a sac full of fluid that forms on or near an ovary. The cyst can grow to a considerable size and in very few cases may interfere with the production of sex hormones in the ovary.

In some cases, an egg develops abnormally within the ovary and forms a small cyst. This type of cyst usually causes few if any symptoms and disappears within a month.

What are the symptoms?
Ovarian cysts often produce no symptoms, but you may notice a firm, painless swelling in the lower abdomen, or pain during sexual intercourse. A large cyst can press on the area near the bladder, causing urine retention, but this rarely occurs. When a cyst affects hormone production there may be symptoms such as irregular vaginal bleeding or an increase in body hair (see Abnormalities of the hypothalamus, pituitary and ovaries, p.587).

A cyst may become twisted. This causes severe abdominal pain, nausea and fever.

What are the risks?
Ovarian cysts are common, but seldom require any treatment. Cysts that have caused no problems are often discovered at a routine checkup. The most immediate risk is that a cyst may become badly twisted or burst, causing peritonitis (see p.470). It is also possible that, instead of being an ovarian cyst, it may be a *malignant*, or life-threatening, tumor (see next article).

What should be done?
Consult your physician if you have any of the symptoms described. If the doctor's examination reveals a mass or lump on your ovary, you may need to have additional examinations. These may include a *laparoscopy*, or a look into your abdomen through a tube.

What is the treatment?
An ovarian cyst that is not malignant can sometimes be drained through a device called a laparoscope, but the usual treatment is to remove it. Often this can be done without affecting the ovary, but occasionally the only way to ensure complete removal of the cyst is to take out the entire ovary and possibly the fallopian tube as well. Since you have two ovaries and associated fallopian tubes, you may still have children if one is removed.

If you have completed your family or are past menopause, your gynecologist may advise surgery to remove both ovaries and perhaps your uterus as well (see Box, p.594). This is because once you have had certain kinds of cysts, they are more likely to recur, and there is a slight risk that you will get cancer when they do.

Cancer of the ovary

Cancer of the ovary occurs when abnormal tissue develops, forming a *malignant*, or life-threatening, tumor. As in all cancers, there is a tendency for the disease to *metastasize*, or spread. The cause of this cancer is unknown.

What are the symptoms?

Cancer of the ovary is very difficult to detect in its early stages. This is because the ovaries are deep within the lower abdomen, so swelling often is not noticed until the disease is well advanced. At this stage there may also be lower-abdominal pain, loss of weight, and general ill-health. Sometimes the tumor produces fluid that causes the whole abdomen to swell. This condition is known as *ascites*.

What are the risks?

Cancer of the ovary is uncommon. If it is not discovered and treated promptly, it can be fatal within a few years. If the growth is discovered and removed early, there is a chance of a complete cure.

What should be done?

If you notice any of the symptoms described, see your regular physician or gynecologist right away. If the physician suspects cancer, he or she will arrange for you to go into the hospital, where a gynecologist will carry out an internal examination.

What is the treatment?

If cancer is present, an operation may be necessary to remove not only the affected ovary but also the other ovary, the fallopian tubes, the uterus, and nearby lymph glands to make sure that no cancer is left to grow and spread to other parts of your body. *Radiation therapy* or *cytotoxic* (anticancer) drugs are usually given to prevent the disease from recurring, or to slow down the progress of the disease if it has spread. Any fluid from the tumor that collects in the abdomen can be drawn off periodically with a needle and syringe. This is a swift, painless procedure known as *paracentesis*.

Fibroids

A fibroid is a *benign* tumor of the uterus. Such tumors may grow larger, but they are unlikely to spread or threaten life. The tumor develops either within the muscular wall of the uterus or attached to the uterus wall by a stalk of tissue. Some fibroids take many years to grow to the size of a pea, while others may reach the size of a grapefruit within a few years. Also, if you have one fibroid, you are likely to develop others.

Most women with fibroids have no symptoms, especially if the fibroids are small.

What are the risks?

Roughly 20 per cent of women over 30 have fibroids. They are seldom found before the age of 20, and are most common in the 35 to 45 age group. However, of the women who have fibroids, only a small proportion require medical treatment.

If your fibroids cause heavy menstrual periods, you may develop iron-deficiency anemia (see p.419) because of the extra blood lost. Occasionally, a fibroid attached to the uterus wall becomes twisted and loses its blood supply, or starts to wither away. Sudden sharp pain low in the abdomen may follow, and an emergency operation may be required to remove the fibroid. Rarely, a fibroid enlarges rapidly during pregnancy and may cause pain, a miscarriage, or obstruction during delivery.

What is the treatment?

Self-help: If your periods are heavy, you can help prevent iron-deficiency anemia by including plenty of iron in your diet. Also, the growth of fibroids is stimulated by excess estrogen, so you can help avoid problems with them by not taking extra estrogen hormones, especially after menopause.

Professional help: Small, symptomless fib-

OPERATION: D&C

(dilatation and curettage)

In this operation, the uterine lining is scraped to discover the cause of frequent or heavy periods (see Heavy periods, p.585), to terminate a pregnancy (see Unwanted pregnancy, p.625), or to treat an incomplete abortion or miscarriage.

During the operation You will probably be under general anesthetic. Your cervical opening is widened with a dilator, the lining of the uterus is scraped with a curette, and the scrapings are examined under a microscope. The operation takes between 30 minutes and an hour.

After the operation You will have bleeding from the uterus for a few days and may have some pelvic and back pain. You will probably be able to leave the hospital the same day or the next day.

Convalescence Sexual intercourse and use of tampons should be avoided for several weeks, but most normal activities can be resumed after a few days.

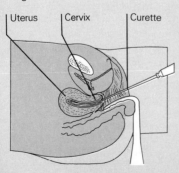

Uterus | Cervix | Curette

roids do not require treatment. You should, however, visit your physician every 6 to 12 months for an examination to see if the fibroids are growing too large. After menopause, when levels of the sex hormone estrogen usually decline, fibroids tend to get smaller or even disappear.

If your fibroids are causing problems, your physician may send you to the hospital for an examination and to undergo a procedure that is called a dilation and curettage, or D & C (see Box, previous page).

Fibroids that are causing problems are usually removed. If you do not intend to have children in the future, you may be advised to have a hysterectomy (see Box below). Otherwise, fibroids can often be surgically removed without damaging the uterus.

Cancer of the uterus

Cancer of the uterus starts in the endometrium, or lining of the uterus. After growing in the lining, the cancer invades the wall of the uterus and, if it is not treated, spreads to the fallopian tubes, ovaries and other organs. Why cancer of the uterus occurs is not known, but there are some factors that can make it more likely to occur. These risk factors include high blood pressure (see p.382), obesity (see p.492), diabetes mellitus (see p.519), and estrogen hormone medications, including some birth control pills.

What are the symptoms?
Women who are past menopause may have slight bleeding from the vagina, and women who are still menstruating may have very heavy periods, or some bleeding between periods. There may also be a discharge that ranges from a watery, pink fluid to a thick, brown, foul-smelling one. It may cause intermittent pain similar to menstrual pain.

What are the risks?
Cancer of the uterus is the second most common form of cancer of the genitals in women. (Cancer of the cervix, see p.598, is the first.) It occurs mainly between the ages of 50 and 60, and is more common in women who have not had children than in those who have.

This type of cancer grows and spreads very slowly. Therefore the risk that the tumor will be fatal is much lower than in many other cancers. If the symptoms are reported early, there is a good chance of complete cure.

What should be done?
If you have any irregular vaginal bleeding, or an abnormal discharge, it is essential that you consult your physician as soon as possible. If cancer is suspected, diagnostic tests will be done, including possibly a Pap smear (see p.599), a *biopsy* and a dilation and curettage, or a D & C (see Box, previous page) to confirm the diagnosis.

What is the treatment?
If cancer of the uterus is confirmed, the uterus is usually removed (see Box below), together with the ovaries and fallopian tubes

---

OPERATION: ## Removal of the uterus
(hysterectomy)

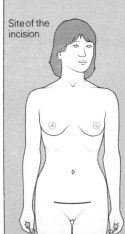

Site of the incision

The uterus, and sometimes also the ovaries and fallopian tubes, may be removed to cure several different gynecological disorders.
During the operation There are two basic methods for performing a hysterectomy. In the most commonly used method the surgeon removes the uterus through an incision in the lower abdomen. In the other method, the incision is made at the top of the vagina and the top of the vagina is stitched together after the uterus has been removed. Either operation takes between one and two hours and a general anesthetic is given.
After the operation You will probably have a drainage tube at the site of any abdominal incision, and may have some vaginal bleeding and discharge for a few days. You will be

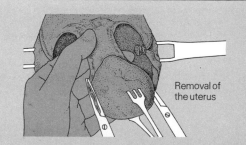

Removal of the uterus

encouraged to get out of bed and walk around a little the day after the operation and you will be able to go home after a week or two.
Convalescence Convalescence may take from two weeks up to two months, depending on your health. In a woman who has not yet reached *menopause* (see p.586), removal of the ovaries brings about an early menopause with the accompanying symptoms. Replacement hormones may be recommended.

in case the disease has spread. *Radiation therapy* and occasionally *chemotherapy*, are sometimes given instead of, or in addition to, surgery. Radiation can be given by a device called a radium implant, which is inserted in the uterus or the vagina. Another method is deep *X-ray* treatment after the operation, to halt any further growth of the tumor. If the cancer is detected at a fairly early stage, the prospects are excellent; about 80 per cent of women operated on in these circumstances are completely cured.

Tropho-blastic tumors

(including hydatidiform moles)

A trophoblastic tumor is a rare type of growth that may occur during pregnancy. It grows in the placenta, or afterbirth. If the tumor develops during early pregnancy, it prevents the fertilized egg from developing into a baby. A tumor can also grow in placental tissue left behind in the uterus after childbirth or a miscarriage. It may appear at any time up to five years after the pregnancy.

Trophoblastic tumors are either *benign* (when they are often called hydatidiform moles) or *malignant*. Both types are rare and grow quite large, so that the uterus expands as in a normal pregnancy. A physician may often suspect it is not a normal pregnancy, because the uterus expands more rapidly than a developing infant would normally grow. A benign growth remains confined to the uterus. A malignant growth, if it is not treated, rapidly invades the wall of the uterus and passes to other parts of the body through the bloodstream, thereby threatening life.

The main symptoms of a trophoblastic tumor are irregular vaginal bleeding, nausea and vomiting, and high blood pressure.

What should be done?
If you have a combination of the symptoms described, you should consult your physician without delay. An *ultrasound scan* and a urine test will probably be carried out. A trophoblastic tumor causes excessive production of the hormone HCG, which is normally made by the placenta. This hormone passes into the urine and can be easily detected (see Pregnancy testing, p.620). If a trophoblastic tumor is present, the growth is removed surgically in a way similar to a dilation and curettage, or D & C (see Box, p.593). No further treatment is necessary for a benign tumor apart from regular checkups and urine tests over the next two years to make sure it has not occurred again. Pregnancy is not advisable during this time.

If the tumor is malignant, it may be necessary to remove the uterus (see Box, previous page). Anticancer drugs will be given for several months to prevent any spread of the disease. After this treatment, regular checkups will also be necessary. The prospects for a complete cure are good.

Endo-metriosis

The tissue that lines your uterus is called the endometrium. Each month part of it grows and becomes engorged with blood, and then is shed as a menstrual period. In endometriosis, fragments of endometrium develop in other places – within the muscular wall of your uterus, in your ovaries, or (less commonly) in the fallopian tubes, the vagina, the intestine, or even in scars that have formed in the abdominal wall after surgery. Each month these fragments of endometrium bleed like the lining of the uterus. But because the fragments are embedded in tissue the blood cannot escape. Instead, blood blisters form that irritate and scar the surrounding tissue, which in turn forms a fibrous cyst, or sac, around each blister.

What are the symptoms?
In most cases endometriosis causes no symptoms, or symptoms so mild that they pass unnoticed and require no treatment. If you have symptoms, these may include abdominal and/or back pain during menstrual periods, which often becomes worse after the period is over. Sometimes periods are heavy (see Heavy periods, p.585) and sexual intercourse may be painful.

Because endometriosis is linked to menstruation, it occurs only during the fertile years. Therefore, it appears most often between the ages of 25 and 40. It occurs most frequently in women who have not had children. Endometriosis in its mild form is common. Only a few cases of the disorder are severe enough to require treatment. In very rare cases the condition causes a major problem, such as an intestinal obstruction (see p.471), which requires surgical treatment.

What should be done?
If you start to have painful periods as described, see your physician. You may need to have dilation and curettage, or D & C (see Box, p.593), and a procedure called a *laparoscopy* to confirm the diagnosis.

What is the treatment?

Your physician may prescribe the hormones that are the ingredients found in oral contraceptive pills. Taken daily for several months, these hormones reduce the blood flow in your periods. This allows your body to gradually destroy the abnormal tissues. If this is unsuccessful, large doses of the hormone progesterone may be given. They usually stop the menstrual cycle completely.

If endometriosis has affected the ovaries, the treatment will probably be similar to treatment for an ovarian cyst (see p.592). In severe cases that do not respond to treatment, you may be advised to have surgery, or, rarely, *radiation therapy*.

Pelvic infection

(*pelvic inflammatory disease, salpingitis*)

This disorder occurs when infectious agents invade the uterus and spread to the fallopian tubes, ovaries, and surrounding tissues. The infection may not have any obvious cause but it is often introduced through the vagina, during sexual intercourse. Very occasionally it occurs after an intrauterine contraceptive device (IUD) is inserted, or after a miscarriage or abortion. Pelvic infections can be acute or chronic.

What are the symptoms?

If you have an acute pelvic infection, it causes severe pain and tenderness in your lower abdomen, and probably a fever. A chronic pelvic infection causes recurrent mild pain in the lower abdomen, and sometimes backache. In both acute and chronic forms you may have pain during intercourse, your periods may be early or heavy, and you are likely to have an abnormally heavy and unpleasant-smelling vaginal discharge.

What are the risks?

Pelvic infection is not common generally, but it is most common in young, sexually active women, and least common after menopause. If the infection is neglected, an *abscess* may form in a fallopian tube or ovary, which can cause damage and scarring, and may block the fallopian tube and prevent conception. Very rarely the infection may spread quickly and cause peritonitis (see p.470) or even blood poisoning (see p.421).

What should be done?

See your physician as soon as symptoms occur, so that treatment can be started early. The physician will take a swab of material from inside your vagina. Analysis of this material helps to identify the infectious agents that are causing the condition.

What is the treatment?

An *antibiotic* is usually prescribed to clear up the infection, and *steroids* may be given to relieve the inflammation. Aspirin or possibly a stronger painkiller may be recommended or prescribed to help relieve abdominal pain. Your physician will probably recommend that you rest in bed until the symptoms have disappeared, and that you avoid sexual intercourse for three or four weeks. This treatment usually leads to a complete recovery. If there is no improvement after about five days, you may need to be admitted to a hospital for a short time, to have an internal examination under an anesthetic and perhaps a *laparoscopy* to check the diagnosis. Further treatment with another antibiotic or a combination of drugs will usually eliminate the problem. But if the examination reveals blocked fallopian tubes or an abscess, your physician may recommend surgery.

Prolapse of the uterus or vagina

Your uterus, vagina, and other lower abdominal organs are held in place by strong muscles and ligaments at the base of your abdomen. The muscles are known as the pelvic-floor muscles. Prolapse of the uterus or vagina occurs when the muscles and ligaments become extremely stretched or slackened. Slackening of the muscles may occur as a result of childbirth, and as you get older. In some cases, the muscles and ligaments no longer hold the uterus firmly in place, so it falls and causes the vagina to sag downwards. This causes the prolapse, a bulge of the front or back wall of the vagina. More rarely, the uterus may descend so far that it bulges out of the vagina, and forms a complete prolapse. The same weakness of pelvic-floor muscles can lead to stress incontinence (see p.601), or slight urine leakage.

What are the symptoms?

A lump or bulge appears in the vagina and may project outside it. This causes a feeling of heaviness and discomfort, and also backache, especially after lifting or otherwise straining your muscles. In some cases stress incontinence appears, but in others the prolapse has the opposite effect, making urination harder.

If the back wall of the vagina has descended you may find bowel movements difficult. Pushing too hard makes the problem worse by causing further prolapse.

What are the risks?
Minor degrees of prolapse are common, especially for a few months after childbirth and in later life. Prolapse can be uncomfortable and inconvenient, but there are no risks to general health unless it is allowed to worsen.

What should be done?
Exercises to tone up the pelvic muscles after childbirth may prevent prolapse. If you think you have it, consult your physician.

What is the treatment?
There is a lot you can do to make a prolapsed uterus better. Go on a diet if you are overweight. Eat plenty of high-fiber foods, so that you will be able to move your bowels without straining. You can also strengthen the muscles of your pelvic floor by doing exercises. These muscles are the ones you would use to interrupt a flow of urine in midstream. Exercise them for several minutes each day by contracting and relaxing them as though stopping and starting urination.

If there is no improvement, your physician may recommend that you have surgery to correct the prolapse or be fitted with a pessary. A pessary is a device made of rubber, plastic, or some other substance. It is inserted into the vagina to support the uterus. Tell your physician if you have any burning or itching, become constipated or fail to pass urine, or notice any vaginal bleeding.

Retroversion of the uterus
(tipped uterus)

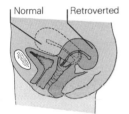

Normal   Retroverted

Normally the uterus is tilted upward and forward and lies immediately behind the bladder. In about 20 per cent of women, however, it inclines downward and backward and lies close to the anal canal. It is then said to be retroverted or tipped (see illustration). This is not a disease. In nearly all cases, the condition is completely symptomless and requires no treatment. Occasionally it causes backache, especially during menstruation.

In very rare cases, you might feel pain during sexual intercourse when your partner's penis penetrates deeply and hits tissue adjacent to an ovary. See your physician if this happens to you.

If the pain is particularly troublesome, and after ensuring that the pain is not caused by some other pelvic disease, your physician may recommend pushing the uterus temporarily into the normal position with a pessary (see previous article). If this eliminates the pain, the physician may advise an operation called a ventrosuspension, to move your uterus permanently into a new position.

Cervical erosion

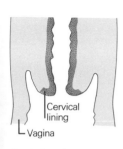

Cervical
lining

Vagina

Cervical erosion occurs when some of the cells forming the delicate lining of the inner part of the cervix, the opening between the uterus and vagina, have spread to cover the tip of the cervix at the top of the vagina.

The inner lining of your cervix is made of a delicate, mucus-secreting, red tissue called columnar epithelium. The lining normally changes at the mouth of the cervix to a stronger, pink tissue called squamous epithelium, which covers the outside of the cervix and lines the vagina. If you have cervical erosion, your uterine lining covers some of the outer part of your cervix, where it normally discharges a small amount of mucus. It is not even an actual erosion, since the area has not been made raw by friction. However, the delicate columnar lining is more susceptible to infection, and therefore pronounced cases may require treatment.

Some women are naturally susceptible to cervical erosion. In others it occurs during or after pregnancy, or while taking oral contraceptives. The extent of the condition changes with time.

What should be done?
As long as you have regular Pap smear tests (see p.599), which would detect any more serious problem, you do not need to do anything. If, however, you have a heavy vaginal discharge, or if you have bleeding after intercourse, see your physician.

After examining you to confirm the presence of cervical erosion, your physician will probably take a Pap smear to find out if you have cervical dysplasia (see next article) as well. The doctor may also take a swab of material from the upper vagina, to find out if any infection is present.

What is the treatment?
The extended uterine lining that constitutes the cervical erosion can be eliminated by *cauterization*, or destruction by heat or certain chemicals. The cauterization is painless. It is usually done in the physician's office or as an out-patient treatment in a hospital.

For about two or three weeks after the cauterization, you will have a heavy watery discharge as the tissues heal.

Cervical dysplasia

In some women who have the condition known as cervical erosion (see previous article), the delicate red skin on part of the outside of the cervix reacts to the acidic mucus produced in the vagina by changing into the thicker pink skin that lines the vagina. This change from one type of skin to another is called metaplasia. Usually it causes no problems but in some women, for no known reason, an abnormal development of cells takes place in the metaplasia area. This abnormality, which is also symptomless, is known as cervical dysplasia. Most cases do not endanger your health, but there is a risk that certain types of dysplasia may develop into cancer of the cervix (see next article) after 10 or 15 years.

What should be done?

You should have a regular Pap smear test (see next page). If the test results suggest dysplasia, you will need to have your cervix examined with a special microscope called a *colposcope*, and a *biopsy* of the cervix may also be done. In this procedure, a small piece of tissue is removed and examined. Depending on the type of dysplasia present, you may or may not need treatment.

What is the treatment?

The area of dysplasia is removed surgically (this is called a *cone biopsy*) or treated by *cauterization* or a *laser beam*. In cauterization, heat, electricity or chemicals are used to destroy the tissue treated. In laser beam treatment, the tissue is destroyed by intense, precisely focused beams of light. Both these procedures can be done during an out-patient visit to the hospital.

An anesthetic is usually given for a cone biopsy, which may involve a hospital stay, and a few days of rest at home afterwards. In very rare cases, a cone biopsy can lead to a tendency to miscarry. If you have had the treatment you should tell your physician about it if you later become pregnant. This will allow the doctor to take precautions against a miscarriage.

If you have cervical dysplasia and you have had as many children as you want, and especially if you also have heavy or painful periods, a hysterectomy (see Box, p.594) may be advised to avoid the risk of cancer.

After treatment for cervical dysplasia, you should have a Pap smear twice a year for the next two years, then once a year, so that any recurrence can be detected and treated.

Cancer of the cervix

This form of cancer most frequently develops in women who have untreated cervical dysplasia (see previous article). The cancer, if it is not treated, gradually spreads deep into the tissues of the cervix, to nearby lymph glands, and up into the uterus.

What are the symptoms?

Two main symptoms are a watery, bloody discharge, which may be heavy and foul-smelling, and bleeding from the vagina between periods, after intercourse, or after menopause. Later, there will also be a dull backache and general ill health.

What are the risks?

Cancer of the cervix, although it is one of the most common cancers in women, is an uncommon disease. It occurs mostly in women over 50. Cancer of the cervix may spread throughout the body, and eventually cause death. However, if it is detected early, it can often be completely cured.

What should be done?

See your physician regularly for a Pap smear test (see next page), to provide for early detection of cervical dysplasia. If you have any of the symptoms described, you should

see your physician. The symptoms may be caused by a relatively minor disorder, but it is unwise to take any chances. If cancer is suspected, you will probably have a Pap test and a *biopsy* of the cervix. In a biopsy, a small sample of tissue is removed for examination. If these tests show that cancer is present, a procedure called a dilation and curettage, or D & C (see p.593), will also be done to find out if the cancer has spread.

What is the treatment?

Cancer of the cervix is usually treated by removing the cervix, the rest of the uterus, the ovaries, and the fallopian tubes (see Box, p.594) and/or by *radiation therapy*. You should discuss the risks and benefits of each form of treatment with your physician before one is chosen.

What are the long-term prospects?

The chances of treatment providing a complete cure when cancer has not spread beyond the uterus are extremely good, much better than with most cancers. The treatment will probably prevent you from having children, however. Even if your reproductive organs are not removed, the radiation therapy will probably disrupt the menstrual

Pelvic examination and Pap smear test

A pelvic examination is carried out as part of a routine physical checkup, especially if you are taking oral contraceptives or if you have a gynecological problem. The examination is usually painless if you do not tense up your pelvic muscles. For the examination, you will probably lie on your back on an examining table, with your knees bent. An instrument called a speculum is inserted into your vagina to hold it open while the physician uses a light to look at the cervix and vaginal walls for any abnormalities.

A few cells are rubbed off the cervix and sent to a laboratory. There, they are examined for signs of cancer of the cervix (see previous article) or conditions that might lead to cancer. This is called a Pap smear test, or a cervical smear test. It should be done at least every three years.

After taking the cells for the Pap test, the physician removes the speculum, inserts two gloved fingers of one hand into your vagina, and carefully feels for any abnormalities of the uterus or ovaries. The physician will probably examine your rectum as well.

The results of your Pap test usually come back in a few days. They are said to be negative if the cells are normal, and positive if they are abnormal. If the results are inconclusive, the test may be repeated every three months until something definite can be determined. If the results are positive, your physician will arrange for appropriate treatment.

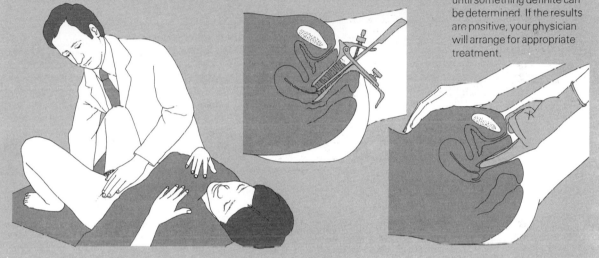

cycle. In a younger woman, the treatment may produce some symptoms of menopause.

The treatment will also cause some narrowing and shortening of the vagina, which can be corrected by regular sexual intercourse, using a lubricant jelly. For a few months after radiation therapy, there may be difficulty in retaining urine, and occasional diarrhea. After treatment, regular checkups and tests are carried out for at least five years.

Cervical polyps

A cervical polyp is a grape-like growth of the mucus-producing tissue that lines the inside of the cervix. Polyps usually occur singly, but may be multiple, and can grow up to 20 mm (almost 1 in) across. They usually produce an excessively heavy, watery, bloody discharge from the vagina, and sometimes bleeding between periods, after sexual intercourse, or after menopause (see p.586). Cervical polyps are fairly common, particularly in women who have not had children.

What should be done?

If you have the symptoms described, report them to your physician right away. Cervical polyps are harmless, but they produce symptoms similar to those that are produced by cancer of the cervix (see previous article). Do not take any unnecessary risks: Have your physician check you immediately.

Your physician will probably examine you and take a Pap smear test (see Box, above). If a polyp is present, it is removed using a quick, painless procedure. When a polyp has been causing irregular bleeding as well as a discharge, you may need to have a dilation and curettage, or D & C (see p.593). This is to ensure that some more serious disorder is not causing the bleeding.

Once the polyp is removed, it is not likely to recur and you should have no further problems with the disorder.

Bladder and urethra

The bladder is a muscular-walled bag that is located in the lower portion of the abdomen. It is in contact with the lower surface of the uterus, just above the pubic bone. Urine trickles slowly from the two kidneys down two thin tubes, called the ureters, into the bladder, where it is stored. Eventually, you eliminate the urine by squeezing it out of the bladder along a short passage, the urethra, to the outside.

Disorders of the bladder and urethra that affect both sexes are dealt with on p.500. The problems included here affect women only,

or, like cystitis, affect women and men in very different ways (see also Cystitis in men, p.577, and Urethritis in men, p.578).

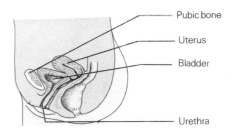

Pubic bone

Uterus

Bladder

Urethra

Cystitis in women

Cystitis is inflammation of the bladder. This is nearly always caused by bacteria that travel up the urethra and infect the bladder. There are several other urinary-tract problems that produce similar symptoms. These include chronic urethritis (see next page) and irritable bladder (see next page).

What are the symptoms?
If you have cystitis, you may feel a frequent urge to urinate, but when you try to do so only a small amount of urine comes out. This urine may have a strong smell, may have blood in it (*hematuria*), and can burn or sting as you pass it (*dysuria*). The urge to urinate is sometimes so strong that you cannot control it before you reach a bathroom. This is called urge incontinence. You may also have a fever and a dull pain in your lower abdomen.

What are the risks?
Cystitis is very common. Most women have it at some time in their lives. It is particularly common during pregnancy, especially in the first few months.

Cystitis is annoying and inconvenient, but it does not endanger your general health. Very occasionally, if it is untreated, this infection of the bladder spreads to the kidneys (see Acute pyelonephritis, p.502).

What should be done?
If you increase your intake of liquids substantially for a day, it may relieve the symptoms. See your physician if the symptoms persist or are severe. The doctor will probably give you a small container for a "clean catch-midstream" specimen of urine. You should first of all wash your vulva thoroughly with a

clean cotton ball or cloth and water. While sitting on the toilet, spread the labia (genital lips) with the fingers of one hand. Then, in the middle of urination, catch a small amount of urine in the container. The sample is sent to a laboratory for analysis to identify the agents responsible for the infection.

What is the treatment?
Self-help: Drink plenty of fluids. Try to empty your bladder completely each time you urinate, and follow the self-help measures described for chronic urethritis (see next page). Always wipe yourself from front to back after a bowel movement. Also, it is a good idea to empty your bladder immediately after you have had sexual intercourse.

Professional help: Your physician may prescribe *antibiotics* for the condition after you have provided the urine specimen. This should clear up the problem.

If you have more than two or three attacks of cystitis, your physician may refer you to a urologist, a physician who specializes in urinary-tract disorders, to see if you have any urinary-tract abnormality that is making you particularly susceptible to bladder infection. The specialist will examine you, and may ask for additional mid-stream specimens of urine. Sometimes an *intravenous pyelogram*, or *IVP*, (a special *X-ray* of the kidneys and bladder) and a visual examination of the bladder (*cystoscopy*) may also be necessary.

If these examinations and tests reveal an abnormality of the urinary tract, it will be treated. If not, the specialist may prescribe antibiotics for a month or more. This will probably solve the problem. However, cystitis often recurs.

Stress incontinence

At the base of your abdomen you have a sheet of muscles known as the pelvic-floor muscles. These muscles support the base of the bladder and close off the top of the urethra, the short channel through which you pass urine. In stress incontinence, the pelvic-floor muscles are weak. When you exert pressure on them by coughing, laughing, or lifting something, for example, you cannot help urinating a little bit. This happens only when the muscles are under stress, not when you are resting or sleeping.

What are the risks?
Some degree of stress incontinence is extremely common. The pelvic-floor muscles are weakened by childbirth, or by your being overweight. They also become gradually weaker as you grow older. Weak pelvic-floor muscles can also lead to prolapse of the uterus or vagina (see p.596).

What should be done?
If you have troublesome stress incontinence, see your physician, who will probably examine you and ask questions about the history of your condition.

You may be asked to provide a "clean catch-midstream" specimen of urine (see previous article), which will show whether a urinary-tract infection could be aggravating the condition. You may also need to have a special *X-ray* of your bladder that is called a *voiding cystogram.*

What is the treatment?
Treatment for stress incontinence usually consists mainly of exercises to strengthen your pelvic-floor muscles. If you are overweight, you will probably be advised to go on a diet (see Obesity, p.492). If these measures do not cure the condition, there are two other possible methods of treatment. You could have an operation to tighten up your pelvic-floor muscles or, alternatively, the specialist may advise you to keep a specially designed pessary, or pelvic support, in your vagina during the day.

Irritable bladder

With irritable bladder, your bladder contracts uncontrollably. You have a sudden urge to urinate, and often pass a small amount before you can reach a bathroom. You may also have to get up quickly at night to urinate. This is called urge incontinence.

Why certain people have an irritable bladder is not known, but it sometimes occurs in conjunction with stress incontinence (see previous article), prolapse of the uterus or vagina (see p.596), or, more often, an infection of the urinary tract (see p.502). It is a fairly common, inconvenient and occasionally distressing disorder, but it is not dangerous.

What should be done?
See your physician, who will examine you and arrange for you to provide a "clean catch-midstream" specimen of urine (see previous page). This will be analyzed for indications of any urinary-tract infection. The doctor may also arrange for a special *X-ray* of your bladder to be taken while you are urinating (*voiding cystogram*) and for an examination of the inside of your bladder (*cystoscopy*).

What is the treatment?
If you have an irritable bladder, your physician may advise you to try to hold back your urine for as long as possible, in order to strengthen the bladder muscles. You may also be given a drug to relax your bladder muscles or reduce the activity of the nerves that control contraction.

Chronic urethritis

This common disorder is a recurrent inflammation of the urethra, the passage through which you pass urine. It is often caused by bruising during sexual intercourse, especially if you are not relaxed. Less commonly, an infection is responsible.

What are the symptoms?
The symptoms of chronic urethritis are similar to those of cystitis (see p.505), except that they last for only one or two days. Because the symptoms of chronic urethritis and cystitis are so similar, and because the disorder is common in women who have just started having sexual intercourse, chronic urethritis is sometimes called "honeymoon cystitis."

What should be done?
Adopt the following self-help measures each time you have intercourse. Drink a glass of water before intercourse, use a water soluble lubricant, and empty your bladder completely soon afterwards. You should also see your physician so that a sample of urine can be analyzed for any infection. Any infection can usually be treated with *antibiotics*.

Vagina and vulva

The vulva is the area around the opening to the female urinary and reproductive systems. It consists of two folds of tissue (the labia) on each side of the openings from the urethra and the vagina. The clitoris and several

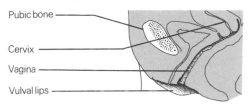

Pubic bone

Cervix

Vagina

Vulval lips

lubricating glands are also within the vulva. The vagina is the passage between the vulva and the uterus. The tissues of the vulva are similar to skin tissue, and are susceptible to skin problems such as warts or severe itching (called pruritis). The lining of the vagina and glands in the vulva produce fluid that sometimes can offer ideal conditions for infectious agents. *Benign* tumors or cysts may occur on the vulva, but they can be treated effectively with surgery. Cancer of the vulva is rare and is also treated surgically.

Vaginal yeast infection

A yeast infection occurs when the fungus *Candida albicans* grows in the vagina. Many women harbor small amounts of the fungus, but these do not cause symptoms. If vaginal conditions change and become more favorable for the fungus, it starts to grow and symptoms appear.

Normally the vagina contains harmless bacteria that produce small amounts of acid. The acid keeps the fungus under control. Anything that kills the acid-producing bacteria will allow the fungus to increase. Two things that may kill these bacteria are feminine hygiene sprays and, occasionally, *antibiotics.* Similarly, hormonal changes that occur if you are pregnant or if you take oral contraceptives can change conditions in the vagina and allow the infection to develop. Yeast infections are not dangerous.

What are the symptoms?

The main symptom of the disorder is itching and irritation of the vagina and swelling and redness of the vulva. You may notice an unusual thick, white discharge, and you may have some pain or soreness during sexual intercourse. There is a tendency to urinate more frequently than usual and the urine may sting or burn.

What should be done?

Avoid wearing nylon underpants. Unlike cotton, nylon cannot "breathe" and therefore offers a warm, moist breeding area for the infection. Do not use feminine hygiene sprays or powders, or *douche* your vagina more often than once a week.

If you develop the symptoms of a yeast infection, consult your physician, who will probably examine you and take a sample from the inside of your vagina to verify that a fungal infection is present.

What is the treatment?

The usual treatment for a yeast infection is an *antifungal* drug in the form of a vaginal suppository or cream. Using the medication for about a week usually clears up the problem. However, if you have repeated attacks, your physician may prescribe a cream for your sexual partner to apply to his penis, or tablets for you and your partner.

Trichomonal vaginitis
(Trichomonas)

Trichomonal vaginitis is infection of the vagina caused by *Trichomonas*, a tiny, one-celled organism. Symptoms of the infection are similar to those of yeast infections (see previous article), and the two infections may occur together. However, the discharge for trichomonal vaginitis is usually heavy, unpleasant-smelling and greenish-yellow in color.

Trichomonal vaginitis is common and is not thought to be dangerous, but it can be irritating and painful. And because the disease is usually transmitted through sexual intercourse, it is likely that your sexual partner also has it. The infection often does not cause symptoms in a man, but a man who has it can reinfect you.

If you have the symptoms, consult your physician, who will probably take a sample of material from the inside of your vagina for laboratory analysis. The treatment is usually a drug that your physician will prescribe in tablet form for both you and your partner.

Pruritis vulvae

Vulval itching with no identifiable disorder such as infection, allergy, or a generalized skin condition is called pruritis vulvae. It often occurs in girls before they begin to have menstrual periods, and in women after menopause (see p.586). It is thought to be related to the production of sex hormones, particularly a low level of estrogen. This is most common after menopause.

What are the symptoms?

If you have pruritis vulvae, your genital area is very sensitive, easily irritated, and intensely itchy. It may also be sore and dry, especially during intercourse. There may be a thin, white discharge.

What are the risks?

Pruritis vulvae is common, particularly in women who are over 45. There are no dangers that are directly associated with the condition, but there is a risk that white patches of abnormal skin called leukoplakia will form in the irritated area. If this happens, there is a slightly increased risk of developing cancer of the vulva (see below).

What should be done?

It is important to try not to scratch the itchy area, because scratching will only make the soreness and irritation worse. Wash with water and unscented soap once a day (no more) and apply a soothing cream recommended by your physician. Do not *douche*, or use talcum powder or feminine hygiene sprays, because they are likely to increase the irritation. A lubricant such as water soluble jelly is helpful during intercourse. Wear cotton underwear and avoid panty hose. If the condition does not improve within two weeks, see your physician.

What is the treatment?

Your doctor may prescribe a cream containing *steroids* or hormones. If there are patches of leukoplakia, you may be advised to have the patches removed to reduce the risk of cancer of the vulva.

Vulval warts

Warts are small, occasionally itchy areas of viral infection on the skin. Warts on the vulva are fairly common, and are much the same as those on other parts of the body (see Warts, p.252). Because they are believed to be caused by a mildly *contagious* virus, warts on your vulva may have spread from warts on your fingers, or perhaps from your sexual partner's warts. They spread more easily in moist and unhygienic conditions, and often appear in conjunction with a disorder that produces an increased vaginal discharge, such as a vaginal yeast infection (see previous page). Warts may also develop during pregnancy when there is a natural increase in the moistness of the vagina.

Warts neglected for many years may, in rare cases, become *malignant*, or life-threatening. If you think you have vulval warts, see your physician, who will examine you to confirm the type of warts and to see if you have any other vaginal infection. If you do, the warts may disappear when the infection is treated. A blood sample may be taken to test for syphilis (see p.612).

What is the treatment?

Your physician may treat small warts by applying a paint that kills the virus. The treatment may have to be repeated a few weeks later. If it fails, or if the warts are large or inaccessible, they can be removed in your physician's office or, possibly, in the hospital. The warts can be removed by other means such as freezing or electrical cauterization. If you got the warts from your partner, your partner must be treated as well to prevent you from becoming reinfected.

Cancer of the vulva

Cancer of the vulva starts as a small hard lump, which grows into an ulcer. The ulcer has thickened, raised edges, and may weep or bleed. It gradually enlarges and, if it is not treated, will *metastasize*, or spread. Cancer of the vulva tends to grow very slowly, and early detection and treatment usually lead to a complete cure.

What should be done?

Consult your physician if you have any lump or ulcer on your vulva. If the physician suspects cancer, you will need to have a *biopsy* of the area and possibly also a procedure called a dilation and curettage, or D&C (see Box, p.593). In a biopsy, a sample of tissue is removed for examination. The usual treatment is a vulvectomy, in which either the growth and surrounding skin are removed, or the growth, the lymph glands in the groin, and the skin between the two areas are removed. Sometimes *radiation therapy* is given as well.

Vaginal hygiene

Most physicians believe that cleansing the area around the vaginal opening (including the minor and major labia, urethra and clitoris) daily with soap and water provides the best hygiene available. Hygiene or deodorant sprays add no benefit. If you choose to use deodorant sprays anyway, follow the directions on the label. Avoid spraying them directly into the vagina, since the chemicals can irritate the vaginal lining. These sprays may also contain chemicals that irritate the labia and cause allergic skin reactions. If this occurs, you should stop using the product.

The vagina normally cleanses itself by secreting a moist discharge that flows downward, removing old cells and menstrual blood. Normal vaginal discharge is scant, clear or white and sticky, with a mild odor. It dries as a yellowish stain on underclothes. The consistency and volume may change during ovulation, or about midway between menstrual periods. Vaginal and cervical infections can produce more plentiful, creamier secretions that may be foul-smelling and cause itching.

Douching as a routine cleansing measure is no longer recommended, except as your physician prescribes it for some kinds of vaginal infections. It is not a method of birth control. Some studies have shown that regular douching may spread a vaginal infection into the uterus and fallopian tubes by forcing contaminated water upward from an infected vagina. Douching may also wash away the protective mucous plug that covers the cervix to prevent organisms from entering the uterus.

If you do douche, use gentle water pressure or hang the douche bag no more than two to three feet over your head to avoid forcing fluid into your uterus. Do not douche more than once a week, because water can irritate the vagina's membrane or lining. Some commercial douche fluids may disturb the chemical balance of your vagina. Vinegar-water douches are less likely to cause this problem. Use one or two tablespoons per quart of water.

Remember not to douche if you have a vaginal infection, because you risk spreading it into your uterus. See your physician for treatment. If you suspect a vaginal infection due to a foul-smelling or unusual discharge, do not douche for three days before your appointment. It will wash away secretions that can help diagnose the infection.

Menstrual care

Odor
To eliminate menstrual odor during your period, change pads or tampons frequently and bathe with soap and water daily. Perfumed or deodorized tampons and pads provide no additional benefit over soap and water washing, and the chemicals they contain can cause skin allergies.

Tampons vs. pads
Although almost half of American women use tampons, some misconceptions about their use still exist. For example, teenage girls and women who are virgins can use tampons comfortably and safely. However, after childbirth or surgery involving the vagina, uterus or cervix, use pads rather than tampons until healing is complete.

A disease called toxic shock syndrome has been diagnosed in some menstruating women who are using tampons. In this disorder, *Staphylococcus* bacteria from the vagina or cervix are thought to enter the uterus and then the bloodstream (see Staphylococcal infections, p.561). Tampons, particularly when they are especially absorbent and are not changed often, are thought to provide an environment in which these bacteria can multiply and produce poisons called toxins. Toxic shock syndrome is a life-threatening illness that requires hospitalization in an intensive care unit and *antibiotics*. There is a characteristic beet-red skin rash, and thin sheets of skin eventually peel from the body. The kidneys, liver, intestines, stomach, blood and skin can also be affected by the disease. If you are menstruating and using tampons, you can try to avoid the problem by changing your tampons several times a day and staying alert for flu-like symptoms that quickly worsen, especially if they are accompanied by a rash. If these symptoms appear, call your physician at once or go to the nearest emergency room.

Premenstrual syndrome and menstrual cramps
The premenstrual syndrome is a group of symptoms that occurs during the week before a woman's menstrual period. Most women are familiar with breast tenderness and fluid retention that often occurs several days before the period. However, some women have other symptoms such as headache, irritability, nervousness, fatigue, depression, crying spells and poor concentration. All of these happen without apparent reason, except that they consistently occur a few days before the menstrual period starts (see also Premenstrual tension, p.585).

The medical term for menstrual cramping is dysmenorrhea. Intrauterine contraceptive devices (IUDs) and specific disorders such as endometriosis, fibroid tumors and pelvic infections will sometimes cause a crampy, aching sensation. For more information, read the article on painful periods (see p.584).

If you have premenstrual syndrome or severe cramps, consult your physician, who can check for any underlying problem. No treatment works for everyone, but certain drugs that contain aspirin and other mild painkillers often help. Studies have shown that pills to reduce fluid accumulation are not effective during the premenstrual cycle. Some drugs are being tried experimentally but no recommendations can be made. Discuss with your physician whether one of the nonprescription medications might work for you, or if you need a prescription drug.

Loss of sexual desire in women

If you are a woman who is frustrated and unhappy with your response during sexual activity, effective treatment is available.

Many factors shape the sexual desire and response of women, including cultural conditioning and learned attitudes. Scientific investigation has begun only recently on how women's bodies (such as the blood vessels, nerves and muscles) change during sexual arousal and intercourse. A major difficulty in analyzing diminished sexual desire involves defining what is normal sexual behavior. The meaning of the term "normal" tends to fluctuate with the cultural and social climate.

Generally, only a very small number of women lose interest in the desire for sexual activity because of diseases, drugs or hormonal imbalances. This is because the diseases that alter sexual drives usually affect other body systems to such an extent that the woman is too ill to be concerned about sexual disinterest. However, depression, stress, alcohol, fatigue and some drugs can temporarily decrease sexual desire. Drugs that can have this effect include narcotics and tranquilizers. Oral contraceptives have rarely been associated with a decline in sexual desire.

Female sexual arousal

Before any woman feels sexually responsive, there are usually several conditions that must be fulfilled. Otherwise she is likely to experience a secondary loss of sexual interest. One requirement during lovemaking is that a woman must receive adequate physical stimulation to the erogenous or sensitive areas of her body, including the clitoris, if she is to respond with vaginal lubrication and finally orgasm. Lubrication is the moist, sticky substance secreted by glands that line the vagina. This substance allows the penis to glide easily in and out. An orgasm is the uncontrolled contractions of the uterus and muscles surrounding the vagina that occurs during peak sexual stimulation.

Another condition that is necessary for many women's enjoyment is a relaxed and secure environment, both physically and emotionally. Any fears of rejection, desertion or pregnancy can prevent optimal sexual pleasure.

Research has shown that the amount of time it takes to arouse a woman varies with the individual, as does the type of foreplay most women prefer. In some cases, poor communication between the sexual partners about what is pleasurable causes a loss of sexual interest. Some women find it difficult to communicate and sometimes even to identify specific prefer-

ences. This is often because they may have been culturally conditioned to be sexually passive and unassertive, allowing their partner to take responsibility for the pleasure of both of them during lovemaking.

Disorders of the female sexual response

When a woman does receive adequate sexual stimulation in a relaxed and undemanding environment and still finds herself unable to enjoy sexual activity, then there is likely to be an underlying problem. There are two general categories for these problems. One is general sexual dysfunction, which refers to women who are not aroused by erotic foreplay and subsequently do not lubricate. The other category is called orgasmic dysfunction. This refers to women who are sexually stimulated and lubricate, but do not experience an orgasm.

In both of these conditions, unconscious feelings and attitudes about sex such as shame, fear, or guilt can block all or part of the natural response to sexual stimulation. A woman may have some conflict about her sexuality of which she is unaware, or she may feel guilty about freely expressing her sexual nature. The quality of a woman's relationship with her partner also influences her ability to respond. Most women need to feel love and/or affection for their partners. Power struggles, hidden hostilities toward the partner, ambivalence, passivity, fear of losing control, fear of rejection and abandonment, a poor marital relationship, low self-esteem or psychological disturbances can inhibit a woman's sexual response.

Women with general sexual dysfunction who unconsciously block their erotic feelings and physical responses can be treated with a combination of psychotherapy (see p.299) and sex therapy. Qualified sex therapists sometimes use specially designed exercises to teach the woman how to get in touch with her body's erotic sensations. A secure and undemanding atmosphere, whether she is alone or with her partner, is important to successful treatment.

Women with orgasmic dysfunction are sexually responsive and often enjoy intercourse. However, they unconsciously overcontrol the orgasm reflex, usually because of some of the feelings discussed above. Counseling and psychotherapy often are helpful. Prescribed sexual exercises combined with psychotherapy are usually most beneficial. If you decide to seek treatment, consult your physician, who can refer you to reputable professionals with credentials and training in sex therapy.

Special problems of couples

Introduction

Problems specific to couples – that is, to sexual partners – have changed considerably in recent years. Advances in surgical methods and the discovery of new drugs have transformed the outlook for many couples who would otherwise be unable to have children, or for someone who has syphilis. But it is not only medical and surgical procedures that have changed. Attitudes have also changed, and sexual problems that would never have been considered treatable in the past can now be successfully treated, either medically or surgically.

The problems in this section of the book are divided into three groups. The first group deals with infertility and contraception. When a couple is not able to have a child, a variety of factors may be involved. Many of the causes can be treated, resulting in successful pregnancies.

If, on the other hand, you want to avoid conception, there are several reliable contraceptive techniques available, and each one has advantages and disadvantages. Some contraceptives require a prescription, while some are available over-the-counter. Be sure to discuss the possibilities and the risks and benefits associated with each one with your physician before choosing one particular method. Reliability and side-effects are two of the factors you should consider.

The second group of articles in this section is concerned with sexually transmitted diseases. The term "venereal diseases" used to be applied to such infections. The three main venereal diseases were syphilis, gonorrhea and non-specific urethritis. During recent years, however, it has been discovered that certain other disorders, among them infectious mononucleosis (see p.562) and acute hepatitis B (see p.486), can also be transmitted either by sexual intercourse itself or by other forms of intimate sexual contact. The diseases covered in this section of the book are those that are spread primarily (if not exclusively) by sexual contact.

The third group of articles deals with sexual problems. It is usually most helpful to look at these problems as difficulties for both partners to tackle. A frank exchange of views with your partner is important in these situations, and in some cases this kind of communication is all that is needed to put an end to the problem.

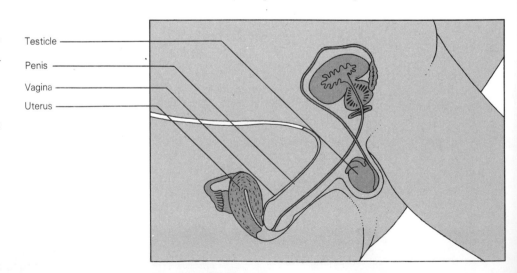

Sexual intercourse
In sexual intercourse, the man's penis, which has become erect due to sexual arousal, penetrates the woman's vagina. Sperm produced in the testicles can then be ejaculated through a series of "tubes" and out at the entrance to the uterus, an ideal location to maximize chances of fertilization.

Testicle

Penis

Vagina

Uterus

Infertility and contraception

Some couples invest a lot of energy in trying to avoid having children, while others do everything they can to try to conceive a child. Fortunately, modern medical science can be helpful in both cases. New diagnostic techniques and drugs as well as sophisticated surgical procedures are able to offer the majority of infertile couples an eventual pregnancy. Similarly, a wide variety of contraceptive techniques are also available. There is not complete freedom of choice, however. Health considerations, religious views, reliability (see Table at right) and convenience may all influence a couple's choice of a contraceptive method. Your physician may be able to help you make your decision.

Method	% chance of pregnancy
Oral contraceptives	less than 1
The IUD	2
Condom plus spermicide	3
Diaphragm plus spermicide	3
Condom alone	15
Diaphragm alone	15
Spermicide alone	25
Natural (rhythm)	25
No contraception	90

Infertility

If you plan to have a baby, make sure you know as much as possible about the best conditions for conception (for more information, see p.616).

If you have not conceived in 12 months, both partners should visit a physician. Initially the physician will try to establish whether intercourse is suitably timed to maximize your chances of conception. The doctor will also want to know if you have a psychological or sexual difficulty that could prevent conception, such as impotence.

If your problem seems to be physical, you will probably be referred to a fertility clinic for further tests. The first test is usually a microscopic examination of the male partner's semen to check the number of healthy sperm. Many factors can contribute to a low sperm count. Among them are emotional stress, overwork and fatigue, excess use of tobacco and alcohol and a raised temperature within the scrotum (sometimes caused by tight underwear). Varicocele (see p.573) is the most frequent cause of a reduced number of sperm in the semen. This problem can be corrected surgically in nearly half of the cases in which it affects fertility.

If sperm production and ejaculation are found to be normal, the next step is to make sure the female partner's reproductive system is functioning properly. A women must ovulate to become pregnant. Ovulation is the process in which an egg ripens in the ovary and migrates into a fallopian tube. This occurs about 14 days before the beginning of each menstrual period. After ovulation, the ovary produces the hormone progesterone, which alters the consistency of the mucus in the cervix and the endometrium, or lining of the uterus. For this reason, the physician may test samples of the cervical mucus and take an endometrial *biopsy* to confirm that the woman is ovulating. Also, the woman will probably be asked to keep a diary of her morning body temperatures, because temperature generally rises one or two degrees after ovulation.

If a woman does not ovulate because the pituitary gland and hypothalamus are not releasing the appropriate hormones to stimulate ovulation, a medication known as a "fertility drug" can help nudge these glands into action. Physicians prescribe these potent drugs only under specific conditions, and there are special instructions that must be followed to avoid unwanted results.

Since fertilization occurs in the fallopian tubes, they must be unobstructed for the fertilized egg to travel into the uterus and implant in the uterine wall. Previous pelvic infections can scar and block these tubes, and this can prevent pregnancy. Your physician may use a special test that is called *hysterosalpingography* to check for this problem, and tubal obstructions can sometimes be removed surgically.

Occasionally endometriosis (see p.595) or adhesions, fibrous tissue from old infections or previous surgery, may interfere with fertilization. This sometimes can be diagnosed by *laparoscopy*. The problem can usually be corrected surgically if adhesions are found.

Contraception

Oral contraceptives ("the pill")

The contraceptive pill is the most effective method of temporary birth control yet invented. Physicians know more about "the pill's" side-effects than about almost any other medication. Some of the good as well as bad side-effects of birth control pills are described here, but your physician will have the latest information about this form of birth control.

The most commonly used birth control pills are called "combined" pills because they contain both types of female hormones (estrogens and progestogens). The birth control pill works by signaling the pituitary (the "master gland" of the body) to stop causing the ovaries to release eggs.

Taking the pill Oral contraceptives are reliable as long as they are taken regularly according to the instructions on the pack. However, vomiting or diarrhea that lasts for more than 24 hours may expose you to the risk of pregnancy. At such times, continue to take the pills, but use some other method of contraception in addition until you are halfway through your next pack of pills.

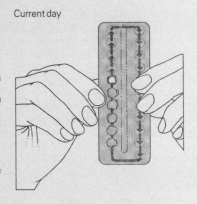

Current day

The natural female sex hormones determine the amount and time of menstrual bleeding. Because small amounts of these hormones are made by the ovaries when they are prevented from releasing an egg, most women notice changes in their menstrual cycles when they take birth control pills. One such change that almost all women notice when they take birth control pills is that their periods become shorter and lighter. In fact, a menstrual period may be so light that you may not think you have had a period at all, and you may wonder if you are pregnant. It is important to remember that, if you have been taking birth control pills regularly, pregnancy is extremely unlikely (about 1 chance in a 1,000). It is far more likely that the birth control pills have decreased menstrual bleeding so much that there is almost no blood to come out of the uterus.

A change that fewer women experience is bleeding between menstrual periods. This is called "breakthrough bleeding." This kind of bleeding usually happens only with the first few packages of pills and can be treated by taking a little extra estrogen when the bleeding occurs.

Side-effects The serious possible side-effects of taking birth control pills include heart attack (see p.379), stroke (see p.268), and thrombosis, or the formation of blood clots in veins (see Thrombophletitis, p.407). However, physicians in the United States have studied thousands of women who used birth control pills for up to ten years and have discovered that serious side-effects are very unlikely to occur in young women (under age 30). In addition, birth control pills

may be safer now than they were a few years ago, because many women are taking pills with lower doses of estrogen. However, new knowledge also shows that women 35 years or older who take oral contraceptives, especially if they smoke cigarettes, are much more likely to die of heart attacks and strokes than those who do not.

In addition to preventing unwanted pregnancy, birth control pills have other beneficial effects. A woman who takes birth control pills is much less likely to have an ectopic pregnancy (see p.629) or an ovarian cyst (see p.592) than a woman who does not, and is also less likely to have breast lumps (see p.588), anemia (see p.419), rheumatoid arthritis (see p.552) and pelvic infections (see p.596).

Women who have a history of blood clots, high blood pressure, severe diabetes or breast or uterine cancer usually should not take birth control pills.

Taking the pill Birth control pills are easy to use. Because the hormones in the pills do not last very long in the body, you must take a pill regularly at the same time every day. If a pill is missed, you should take it as soon as you notice the mistake. Most women prefer to take birth control pills before they go to bed. Your physician will probably advise you to begin taking the pills on the fifth day after your menstrual bleeding has started. Then you take a pill every day for three weeks. Some pill packages include seven inactive pills to take during the last week of the cycle. These pills may contain iron, but they do not contain hormones. These pills are a different color from the first 21 pills. When the last of the hormone-containing pills is taken, the hormone levels in your blood fall quickly, and menstrual bleeding occurs. If you miss taking a pill, the sudden withdrawal of the hormones also may cause menstrual bleeding. If you miss two or more pills from one package, you should continue to take pills from the package, but should use some other method of birth control until you begin a new package of pills.

Birth control pills should not have any effect on your ability to become pregnant after you stop taking them. There is no need to stop taking birth control pills in order to see if a "normal" period will occur. It is safer to take the pills continuously until you want to become pregnant.

The mini-pill If you cannot take the combined birth control pill, which contains estrogen and progestogen together, you may be able to take the so-called "mini-pill." This pill contains only a progestogen hormone and therefore may be safer if you have high blood pressure, diabetes, a history of blood clots, or other diseases that estrogen hormones might make worse. Because they do not contain estrogen, which helps prevent the lining of the uterus from coming off during the pill cycle, a small amount of bleeding may occur at any time. In addition, some women may go for a long time without having regular menstrual periods. The mini-pills do not always prevent the release of eggs from the ovaries, and are less effective than combined birth control pills. On average about 10 out of 100 women who use the mini-pills for a year will become pregnant.

The IUD (intrauterine device)

An IUD (intrauterine device, or coil) is a small piece of molded plastic with a string attached to it, sometimes with copper or progesten, a female hormone, added. It is inserted into the uterus through the cervix, usually during a menstrual period when the cervix is more open and the woman definitely is not pregnant. It is thought that IUDs work by causing a change in the lining of the uterus that interferes with the growth of a fertilized egg. The IUD is a very effective method of birth control (see Table, p.607).

The most common problems with wearing an IUD are increased menstrual bleeding and increased menstrual pain. Therefore, the IUD is usually not the best contraceptive method if you already have long, painful periods. Sometimes spotting occurs between periods during the first two or three months after an IUD is inserted, but this usually goes away. Menstrual bleeding usually becomes less heavy after a year or two of wearing an IUD.

The IUD must be inserted by a trained health professional using special equipment. The insertion takes only a few minutes, but it sometimes causes menstrual pain for a short time. Sometimes this pain can be relieved by giving a local anesthetic at the time of insertion. The progesten and copper-containing IUDs must be replaced every one and three years, respectively. Some physicians now believe the plain plastic IUDs should also be changed, about every five years.

Once inserted, the IUD protects you from pregnancy as long as it remains in the uterine cavity. Since any accidental expulsion of the IUD generally occurs in the first several months, for those months you or your partner should check frequently to make sure the IUD is in place. This is done by putting a finger inside your vagina and feeling for the string up against the cervix. If you can feel the string you can be confident that the IUD is in place. If you feel the hard plastic of the IUD, the device must be removed and replaced with a new one by a trained professional. If you cannot feel anything at all, the most likely explanation is that the string has slipped up inside the uterus. Then you should use a diaphragm, condom or spermicide until you are examined to make sure that the IUD is still in the uterus. After the first few months, you do not need to check the IUD as often, but you still should check it after every menstrual period.

Although cramping pain and increased menstrual bleeding are by far the most common problems with wearing an IUD, the most dangerous problems are pelvic infections (see p.596) and ectopic pregnancy (see p.629). Women who wear IUDs are more likely to have pelvic infections than women who do not. Since a very severe pelvic infection can cause sterility, your physician may recommend that you not use an IUD if you want to have children in the future. Infections are also more common in IUD users who are age 20 or younger and in women who have not had children.

Because pelvic infection and ectopic pregnancy are serious side-effects, you should see a physician if you develop pelvic pain, have an unexplained fever, have a foul-smelling vaginal discharge or believe you have become pregnant while wearing an IUD.

The condom

A condom is basically a tube-shaped piece of thin latex rubber, closed at one end, which is rolled onto the erect penis before intercourse. When you ejaculate, the sperm are trapped in the closed end of the condom. During withdrawal of the penis after intercourse, the condom should be held at the base to prevent it from slipping off and spilling the contents. For maximum reliability you should use the condom in conjunction with some form of spermicide, or spermkilling substance (see Table, p.607). Some condoms are available that are pre-lubricated with spermicide.

Condoms are easy to obtain and widely available. They come in a variety of designs, some of which may increase sexual arousal. Also, wearing a condom gives some protection against sexually transmitted diseases.

There are some drawbacks, however. Putting the condom onto the erect penis tends to interrupt love-making, and it must be done carefully to avoid accidental tearing. Also, a condom may cause reduced sensation in the penis and, therefore, reduced pleasure during intercourse.

The diaphragm and cervical cap

The diaphragm is one of the most effective "barrier" methods of contraception, in which the sperm is blocked from entering the uterus. The diaphragm is a rubber pouch stretched over a flexible wire frame. Diaphragms are usually specially fitted to each user's vaginal cavity.

Using the diaphragm correctly is very important in preventing pregnancy. It must be inserted every time before sex, but not more than six hours before. A special chemical jelly that kills sperm (see Spermicides, next page) must be put on the diaphragm every time it is inserted. A ring of jelly is put all around the edge of the diaphragm, and about ½ tsp. of jelly is placed in the center before the diaphragm is put into the vagina. Flexible spring diaphragms bend into a partial circle when they are squeezed together to be inserted in the vagina. Other diaphragms form a straight line when they are inserted. No matter what kind of diaphragm you use, you must check (or have your partner check) immediately after insertion to make sure that the rubber of the diaphragm covers the cervix and that the edge of the diaphragm is behind your pubic bone. Sometimes the diaphragm edge will rest on top of the cervix. If this happens, sperm will not be blocked from entering the uterus and pregnancy can result.

Some people use a plastic inserter to put in the diaphragm. The diaphragm is stretched along this plastic rod, which is then gently pushed into the vagina. When the rod is turned, the diaphragm is left behind. It is still important to make sure the cervix is covered by the diaphragm. Most women prefer to insert the diaphragm with their fingers, or have their partner put the diaphragm in and check its position.

After sex, the diaphragm must be left in place for at least six hours to give the chemical in the jelly a chance to kill any sperm. If you have sex again before six hours are up, put more jelly in your vagina using the plastic applicator that comes with the jelly. If more than six hours have passed,

(Continued on next page)

remove the diaphragm, wash it, put jelly on it as before and replace it in your vagina.

The diaphragm can be a good method of birth control if these directions are followed (see Table, p.607).

The cervical cap, like the diaphragm, is a barrier method of birth control. It is made of the same kind of rubber as the diaphragm, but it is much smaller because it fits tightly over the cervix (the mouth of the uterus) rather than filling the vagina. There are several types of cervical caps, but the one most commonly used attaches to the cervix by suction. The cap must be fitted carefully. Most women use the cervical cap in the same way as the diaphragm, with jelly and following the same precautions. Used in this way, the cap is about as effective as the diaphragm.

Spermicides
Spermicides are chemicals that kill sperm. They may be a cream, jelly or foam, and are inserted into the vagina shortly before intercourse. Once there, they tend to lose strength, so you should use additional spermicide for each session of intercourse. A spermicide should be used along with a condom or a diaphragm (see Table, p.607). Very rarely, a spermicide may cause an allergic reaction, with itching and redness in the genital area of either partner.

Natural, or rhythm, method
The natural, or rhythm, method of contraception is based on predicting the day in the menstrual cycle when you will ovulate, or release an egg. Intercourse for at least that day or for about a week before carries a high risk of conception. This is because sperm can live in the woman's body as long as six days after intercourse (an average of four), and an egg can be fertilized by a sperm for about the first 24 hours after ovulation. This method of birth control is the least reliable of those discussed here (see Table, p.607), because each woman's cycle may vary, so the method depends on an estimate of the time of ovulation. Also, the method's effectiveness depends on both sexual partners being willing to abstain from intercourse on the days when it is "unsafe."

To calculate your "unsafe" days each month by any of the following methods, it is necessary to keep records over several months to find out the pattern of your cycle. The unsafe days begin a week before ovulation and last for at least a day afterwards. Because cycles, sperm life-spans and egg life-spans can vary, it is best to allow a few days at each end of the time, so there would be about ten unsafe days each month for a woman whose cycle was very regular.

There are three ways to calculate the time of ovulation. Ovulation occurs in most women about 14 days before the first day of the period.

The calendar method: Keep an accurate record of the lengths of your cycles for at least 12 months. Subtract 18 from the number of days in the shortest cycle (14 from ovulation to your period, plus 4 for average sperm-life span) and 11 from the longest (14 from ovulation to your period, less 1 for egg life-span and 2 for good measure). The results are the first and last unsafe days in your cycle, counting the first day of your period as day 1.

The temperature method: In most women, body temperature rises slightly just after ovulation and does not fall again until the next period starts. To detect this temperature change, take your temperature each day as soon as you wake up, using a basal thermometer designed to show slight variations. Record it on a chart to determine your pattern of ovulation. Intercourse is safer, in terms of preventing pregnancy, if you wait at least two days after you ovulate.

The mucus inspection method: When you ovulate, the mucus in the cervix changes from thick and sparse to thin, clear and profuse. You can learn to recognize the change by examining your own mucus over several months and recording its appearance. You can use this record to determine the pattern of your cycle.

A combination of the temperature and mucus inspection methods offers greatest reliability, especially when carried out under the guidance of your physician.

Sterilization
If you are sure that, whatever the circumstances, you never want another child, sterilization offers an almost completely safe and reliable form of birth control. Most physicians recommend male rather than female sterilization to couples, because it is slightly safer and simpler.

Because sterilization is simply a sealing off of the tubes that carry sperm or eggs, it has no effect on the production of sex hormones. If you are a man, you will produce sperm-free semen. If you are a woman, you will produce eggs but these cannot reach the uterus. Menstrual periods are not affected. Sterilization does not physically affect masculinity or femininity, but for some individuals emotional problems may develop.

Male sterilization (*vasectomy*): A vasectomy is a simple operation that usually involves no hospitalization. It requires only a local anesthetic and takes only about 20 minutes. Your physician will probably ask you to wear a pair of close-fitting underpants or a jock-strap, to ease any dragging feeling you may have in your testicles, for a few days after the operation. The operation may cause some temporary bruising of the scrotum, stomach and thighs.

Some sperm may already have been stored in the testicles when the operation is done, so you will probably be advised to use some other method of contraception for the first four weeks after the operation. During that same time, you will have to bring in a specimen of semen at least twice. When two consecutive specimens have been found to be sperm-free, you are considered sterile. How soon you have sexual intercourse depends entirely on how you feel.

Female sterilization: Female sterilization can be done with either a general or a local anesthetic. The operation takes less than an hour to perform, and usually requires an overnight stay in the hospital. It can sometimes be done in a physician's office or clinic. In the most commonly performed operation, two tiny cuts that leave virtually no scars are made just below the navel. Through this a *laparoscope* is inserted, and an attachment to this instrument is used to seal off the tubes by *electrocautery*, tiny metal or plastic rings and clips, or cutting and tying off the ends of the tubes.

Sexually transmitted diseases

A sexually transmitted disease, also called a venereal disease, is an infection transferred from person to person during sexual contact. The way you are most likely to catch such a disease is by having sexual intercourse with a partner who has it. In some cases, however, other forms of sexual contact may transmit the infection. For example, gonorrhea and syphilis can be transmitted by oral or anal sex. Once the infection is established, it may spread beyond the sexual organs. Untreated syphilis, for instance, may eventually spread to the nervous system, and cause paralysis and insanity up to 20 years after the original infection was contracted.

If you suspect you have caught a sexually transmitted disease, you should consult a physician immediately. Gonorrhea and syphilis can be cured, but delaying treatment can have serious consequences. Also, you are now a potential source of infection. You should therefore abstain from sexual relationships until you are cured, and also make sure that anyone with whom you have had sexual contact seeks treatment from a physician without delay. This will help stop the chain of infection.

You can go to your own physician for treatment, or to a clinic that specializes in diagnosis and treatment of sexually transmitted diseases. In either case, your visit will be treated with the strictest confidence.

Although gonorrhea and syphilis are probably the best known sexually transmitted diseases, there are several others. These include non-specific urethritis, herpes genitalis and pubic lice, all of which are covered in this section of the book.

Gonorrhea

Gonorrhea (commonly known as "the clap") is an infectious disease caused by *Gonococcus* bacteria and transmitted through sexual contact. Most frequently, these bacteria infect the man's urethra, the tube that carries urine and semen through the penis, and the woman's cervix, the canal into the uterus.

What are the symptoms?
Men with gonorrhea commonly find it painful to urinate and have a cloudy discharge from the penis that looks like pus. Women may have a cloudy discharge from the vagina, some discomfort in the lower abdomen, or abnormal bleeding from the vagina. Sometimes a woman with the disease may also find urinating painful. Frequently, both men and women have no symptoms at all. When they do occur, symptoms will appear about two to eight days after infection.

Gonorrhea can also infect the rectum or mouth through anal or oral sexual contact. These infections often cause few symptoms. A person with rectal gonorrhea may feel rectal pain, especially during a bowel movement, or notice a cloudy discharge. With a gonorrhea throat infection, a person may have a sore throat.

What are the risks?
Untreated gonorrhea in men can spread from the urethra to the prostate gland and the epididymis, two internal structures that play roles in semen production. Often the urethra, the tube that carries urine through the penis, will become narrowed, which may make urinating difficult.

Untreated gonorrhea in a woman can infect the uterine lining or the fallopian tubes, which are portions of her reproductive system, and make her sterile or unable to bear children. The bacteria can also infect the uterus and the surrounding abdominal cavity, which causes peritonitis (see p.470).

In both men and women, untreated gonorrhea can spread through the bloodstream and infect the joints, skin, bone, tendons and other parts of the body.

What should be done?
As soon as you suspect you have gonorrhea, consult your physician or go to a clinic that specializes in treating sexually transmitted diseases. It is important not to have sexual relations until your symptoms have been diagnosed and treated. Gonorrhea usually is diagnosed by analyzing a sample of the cloudy discharge from the man's urethra or the woman's cervix.

What is the treatment?
Gonorrhea can be cured with an *antibiotic* medication. This treatment can be given as pills or by injection. Your doctor may advise you not to drink any alcohol during the course of the treatment.

Non-specific urethritis (NSU)

Non-specific urethritis (NSU), sometimes referred to as non-gonococcal urethritis, is an infection of the urethra, the tube urine goes through to pass from the bladder to outside the body. The group of organisms that cause NSU are transmitted through sexual activity, but they are less dangerous than syphilis (see next article) or gonorrhea (see previous article) since they are thought to produce no serious, long-term illnesses. The disorder is caused by a type of organism called chlamydia in about half of the cases (see Chlamydial infections, p.565).

What are the symptoms?

Many men and women who have NSU have no symptoms but pass the infection to their sexual partners. In men who have symptoms, the symptoms often resemble gonorrhea, with painful urinating and a cloudy, mucus discharge from the penis. Only an analysis of this discharge can determine which of these diseases you have.

Women with symptoms generally have symptoms resembling a urinary tract infection (see Cystitis in women, p.600), including painful, burning urination, and the need to urinate frequently without expelling much urine. A test of the urine, however, will show that no bacterial infection is present.

What should be done?

Any man who has a cloudy discharge from his penis should consult his physician or a public health clinic to find out if the problem is caused by gonorrhea. If the gonorrhea test is normal, the problem is probably NSU. Women whose urine shows no bacterial infection though they still have symptoms probably have NSU. There are few laboratory tests currently available outside of research centers to diagnose NSU.

Antibiotics, taken several times a day for about a week, usually clear up the infection. If you have NSU, you should not have sexual intercourse until you have completed the medication. This will prevent reinfection and help protect your partner from getting your infection. Your sexual partner should also go in for medical treatment.

Syphilis

Syphilis is a serious disease frequently transmitted through sexual activity. It is caused by a bacterium called *Treponema pallidum*. This organism easily penetrates the moist mucous membranes of the mouth, the vagina, and the penis's urethra, through which urine passes from the bladder to the outside.

If it is not treated, syphilis has three stages that can appear throughout a lifetime. Usually the painless skin ulcers that occur during the first and second stages are highly infectious and contaminate others through contact with the infected mucous membranes, and, rarely, through open sores. The third stage of syphilis is usually not contagious.

What are the symptoms?

The first stage Any time between one and eight weeks after infection, a small painless sore or ulcer called a chancre (pronounced "shanker") appears. Usually a chancre is red and solid and protrudes above the skin. The initial chancre usually occurs in the genital area. Chancres on the penis are usually visible, but when they occur in a woman's vagina or cervix they may not be noticed. They can occur elsewhere on the body, frequently on the mouth or rectum. The chancre heals in one to five weeks, leaving a thin scar. During this period, the syphilis-causing bacteria are circulating in the blood throughout the body.

The second stage This stage is called secondary syphilis. About six weeks after the chancre has healed, you feel generally ill, have a fever and a headache and lose your appetite. Glands in your neck, armpit and groin may swell. These symptoms are caused by the spread of the bacteria. Most people also develop a skin rash of small, red, scaling bumps that do not itch. Sometimes spots appear on the palms of the hands and the soles of the feet. Gray plaques, which are different from chancres, can occur in the mucous membranes of the mouth, vulva and penis. A rash around the rectum may also develop. All of these skin conditions are highly infectious and heal in two to six weeks.

Rarely, syphilis can also infect the liver, the eye and the meninges, or the membranes that cover the brain.

The third stage This is also called latent syphilis or late syphilis. The symptoms of the first two stages disappear for several years, and unless you have a special blood test, you have no way of knowing that you have syphilis. This final stage can last anywhere from two years to a lifetime.

During this stage, the disease flares up without warning. It can affect the brain, causing paralysis, senility or insanity, loss of equilibrium, loss of sensation in the legs and rarely, blindness. The disease can also infect the aorta (the large blood vessel that leads from the heart), weaken its walls and cause an aneurysm (see p.407). Sometimes the disease affects the normal functioning of a heart valve.

What should be done?

Anyone with a suspicious sore in the mouth or genitals should see a physician. Syphilis is highly contagious during the first and second stages, so you should notify your sexual contacts since they are likely to be infected and need treatment.

Syphilis can be diagnosed by a blood test, and is readily curable with *antibiotic* injections. If you are allergic to penicillin, which is usually used, another antibiotic can be prescribed. However, in the late stages syphilis cannot be halted once damage has been done to the blood vessels and brain.

Herpes genitalis

The herpes simplex virus can produce a painful infection of the genitals called herpes genitalis. Groups of blisters develop on one or several areas. These blisters eventually rupture and become shallow ulcers or sores. A similar virus causes cold sores in the mouth (see p.451), but herpes genitalis is transmitted through sexual activity and through contaminated hands.

What are the symptoms?

About six days after contact with an infected person, you may feel pain, tenderness, or an itchy sensation near the penis or vulva. These symptoms may be accompanied by fever, headache or a generally ill feeling.

Single and multiple blisters soon appear along a man's penis or on a woman's vulva. They sometimes also occur on the thighs or buttocks. The blisters also form in a woman's vagina or on the cervix, where they cannot be seen, so it is possible to unknowingly infect a sexual partner.

When the blisters break, they form open sores of raw exposed skin, or ulcers, which are extremely painful. The ulcers last from one to three weeks.

Since the virus may remain in the body after the blisters subside, about half of the people who get herpes genitalis will have recurrences in the following months or years. Usually they are less severe, and the problem disappears altogether with time.

What are the risks?

The major risk is infecting another person, which can only occur when you have an active infection, so avoid sexual contact until the infection clears up. The herpes virus can spread into the bloodstream and infect other organs in persons who have difficulty fighting infection, such as cancer patients and people who have kidney, lung or blood diseases.

If you are pregnant and have herpes near delivery, your physician may recommend delivery by a cesarean section (see p.640) to avoid a serious infection in your new baby.

What should be done?

Your physician can usually diagnose herpes genitalis by examining the blisters. There is no cure, but your physician can prescribe medications as well as soothing ointments to reduce the pain. Frequent warm baths may reduce the inflammation. If the sores become infected, *antibiotics* may be necessary.

Pubic lice

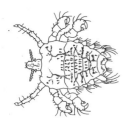

Pubic louse about 20 times life size.

Pubic lice, also known as crab lice (or "crabs"), are blood-sucking lice that usually appear only in the pubic hair and the hair around the anus. Occasionally, however, they occur on other body hair and sometimes on the eyebrows and eyelashes. The louse, which can be clearly seen if you look closely, is 1 to 2 mm across and resembles a minute, flat crab. It is slow-moving and spends most of its life clinging tightly to hair with its claw-like legs. The female's pale, white eggs, called "nits," can just barely be seen with the naked eye. They are attached so firmly to hairs that normal washing will not remove them.

Pubic lice are caught from sexual contact with someone who has them. You probably will not catch them from bedding or clothing previously in contact with an infested person.

What are the symptoms?

It may take several weeks to find out that you have pubic lice. This is how long it takes for the lice to breed and appear in noticeable numbers. Many people have no symptoms, but others have itching in the pubic region, particularly at night.

What should be done?

If you have pubic lice, go to a public health clinic or to your physician. You will be given a lotion or shampoo to kill the lice and their eggs. At the same time the physician may advise a checkup to make sure that you do not have any other sexually transmitted diseases.

Sexual problems

Sometimes a couple cannot fully enjoy sexual intercourse, or even cannot have it at all, because of physical or psychological problems. These problems are discussed separately in the following articles, but in fact many couples suffer from a combination of problems that often stem one from another. For example, premature ejaculation by a man may result in lack of orgasm for his partner, or the man's problem may cause him to become impotent. Treatment of sexually related problems is usually far more successful if it is applied to the couple rather than only one individual.

Impotence

An impotent man is one who fails to get or maintain an erection. This problem can prevent a couple from having any sexual relationship, but it can often be successfully treated. So if you are impotent, consult your physician. There are a number of courses of treatment he or she may recommend.

It was once thought that most cases of impotence had psychological causes, but more physical causes of the problem have been discovered. Among the physical factors that can cause impotence are conditions in which the level of the male sex hormone testosterone in the blood is drastically lowered. Extreme stress, fatigue, chronic illness and heavy use of alcohol can also be contributing factors in impotence.

Most men have been impotent for a day or two or longer at one or more times in their lives. The experience can be embarrassing. Worse yet, it can cause enough worry and stress about "poor sexual performance" to cause the impotence to last longer than it otherwise would. Impotence may also develop as a result of worry over other sexual problems, such as premature ejaculation (see next article).

For a detailed discussion of the causes of impotence, read the article on this topic in Special problems of men (see p.580).

Premature ejaculation

Premature ejaculation is orgasm in the man immediately after, or even before, the penis penetrates the woman's vagina in sexual intercourse. It is one of the most common sexual problems of men. Most men have probably ejaculated prematurely at least once. Some sex researchers consider it to be premature ejaculation when a man reaches orgasm before his sexual partner in more than half of his sexual experiences.

There seems to be little if any relationship between premature ejaculation and specific psychological problems. However, it is thought that some men can develop premature ejaculation through social conditioning in their early youth. For example, if a man's first sexual experiences were with prostitutes, he may have learned that it was preferable to ejaculate rapidly. Anxiety about premarital sexual activity can also lead to this problem. Also, some men develop impotence (see previous article) as a result of anxiety about premature ejaculation.

A couple in which the man has a problem with premature ejaculation should consult a physician. This type of sexual problem can lead to conflict between the partners, hostility and distrust if it is not treated. Treatment often requires the participation of both partners in order to be effective, and loving communication may be a crucial part of a successful recovery.

What is the treatment?
Although several modes of therapy are available, the "squeeze" technique is an effective method used to delay ejaculation. The woman stimulates her partner's penis until ejaculation is almost inevitable. Then she firmly squeezes the glans penis (the head of the penis) where it is joined to the shaft for about three to four seconds. The male partner should then lose his urge to ejaculate and his erection will diminish by 10 to 30 per cent. After about half a minute, the couple can resume sex play including stimulation of the penis. Should the man feel the urge to ejaculate again, the squeeze technique can be repeated. Thus this relatively simple technique allows about 15 to 20 minutes of sexual foreplay without ejaculation. The success rate for treatment of premature ejaculation is reported to be about 98 per cent by those who are experienced in treating the disorder.

Lack of orgasm

Lack of orgasm is nearly always caused by underlying psychological problems, but it may be the result of a lack of sexual interest that began with a physical problem such as damage to the nervous system by accident or disease, or a side-effect from a drug.

Lack of orgasm is rare among men. However, only about one in three women regularly reaches orgasm through intercourse alone, without additional stimulation of the clitoris. Up to ten per cent of women cannot reach orgasm, even by stimulation.

If you are dissatisfied with the frequency or ease with which you or your partner reaches orgasm, have a frank discussion about the matter. You may find that you need to change your sexual techniques. For example, it may help to spend more time stimulating each other's genitals before intercourse.

Sometimes a new position during intercourse helps. If both partners are willing, experiment with some new positions. One that some women report to be very stimulating is with the woman on top, astride her partner. In this position, the woman can control the quantity and exact location of her vaginal stimulation. Men may find the position particularly desirable when they are too tired to play a more active role.

If the problem persists, see your physician, who may refer you to a specialist clinic or a sex therapist. Drugs are seldom prescribed unless they are needed for associated problems. Sex therapy usually involves both therapy sessions and exercises devised by the therapist to be done at home.

Painful intercourse

Painful sexual intercourse, or dyspareunia, has a number of causes, and can affect both men and women. In many cases there are physical reasons that your physician can identify by asking questions and examining you.

Painful intercourse in women
There are many medical conditions that can make sexual activity painful for women. Vaginismus is one such condition. In vaginismus, natural lubrication of the vagina does not occur, and the lower vaginal muscles tighten into spasm. This prevents sexual intercourse or causes it to be painful. This condition is usually diagnosed by eliminating the other possible causes of painful intercourse. The problem occurs when a woman's natural sexual arousal is somehow inhibited for psychological reasons (see Loss of sexual desire in women, p.605).

This condition can be relieved by working with a physician or therapist trained in treating sexual disorders of women. The physician or therapist may prescribe a series of dilators or tubes of varying size. You insert the smallest one into the vagina, then the next size and so on, until you are comfortable with inserting a dilator that is the size of an erect penis. Then your partner can try inserting his penis into your vagina. This treatment may be supplemented with exercises that are designed to teach you how to contract and relax the vaginal muscles at will.

Infections or irritations of the vulva such as herpes genitalis (see p.613), cysts or boils, and rashes or allergic reactions all can also cause sexual discomfort. Vaginal infections irritate the vaginal walls and can cause painful intercourse. Sometimes episiotomy scars (see Special procedures in childbirth, p.640) also cause pain during intercourse.

Diseases that affect the uterus can cause pain when the man thrusts his penis deeply into the vagina. These include pelvic inflammatory disease (see Pelvic infections, p.596), ectopic pregnancy (see p.629), endometriosis (see p.595), and ovarian cysts (see p.592) and tumors.

Bladder disorders such as cystitis (see p.600), urethritis (see p.505) and cystocele, when the bladder loses its pelvic support and collapses into the urethral canal, all make intercourse uncomfortable. Arthritis or chronic pain in the lower back also can cause pain during intercourse. Pain from these latter two causes can sometimes be relieved to some degree by using a new position.

Painful intercourse in men
Men, too, can experience painful intercourse. The causes are usually physical. Infection or irritation of the skin of the penis, such as herpes genitalis (see p.613) or allergic rashes, can cause pain during sexual intercourse. Some spermicides that are used as contraceptives (see p.610) cause a burning sensation on the surface of some men's penises.

Infections of the prostate gland, urethra or testes can also make sexual intercourse painful. Cancer of the penis or testes, and arthritis of the lower back also make the thrusting that is done in sexual intercourse uncomfortable.

If intercourse is painful for you, consult your doctor or a urologist, a physician trained to diagnose and treat disorders of the male genitals. The physician can provide proper treatment once the cause of the painful intercourse is determined.

Pregnancy and childbirth

Introduction

If you are not yet pregnant but are planning to become pregnant, it is a good idea to read through the entire section on pregnancy and childbirth. In this way, you will understand the types of problems that can occur, and you will be prepared if anything out of the ordinary happens. Remember as you read, however, that pregnancy is a natural event, and most pregnancies and deliveries do not involve major problems.

Conception, or fertilization of one of your eggs, can occur shortly after a mature egg has been released from one of your two ovaries, approximately half-way through a menstrual cycle (for more information on ovulation see p.583). The egg travels along the fallopian tube toward the uterus. If you have sexual intercourse during this time, the millions of sperm that your partner has ejaculated travel from your vagina, through the uterus, and up to the fallopian tube. Here one sperm of many penetrates the egg-cell wall. This is called fertilization. The fertilized egg reaches the uterus, or womb, a few days later and embeds itself in the uterine lining. This happens at about the time your next period is due. By the time you are beginning to suspect that you might be pregnant, the egg has become an embryo and is already developing rapidly in your uterus.

A full-term pregnancy lasts about 38 weeks. Although conception usually occurs halfway through a woman's menstrual cycle, because the exact day the egg is fertilized is rarely known, the expected delivery date is calculated from the first day of your last period. This means that if you conceived halfway through a regular 28-day cycle you will be said to be four weeks pregnant two weeks after conception, and the entire pregnancy will be said to have lasted 40 weeks, not 38.

The articles in this section are divided into several parts. One covers general problems of pregnancy, which range from the almost universal problem of heartburn to the comparatively rare disorder of Rhesus factor blood incompatibility. Others cover disorders that tend to occur in either early, middle, or late pregnancy. The most common problems of childbirth are described, as well as the modern techniques available to assist you during pregnancy and childbirth. In the final part of the section, any problems that may affect the mother shortly after childbirth are also covered. Problems that particularly affect the newborn baby are described elsewhere, in the section called Special problems of infants and children (see p.644).

German measles and pregnancy

If you contract German measles (see p.699) during pregnancy, there is a risk that your baby will be born with a defect. The risk is highest if you have the illness in early pregnancy. When this occurs during the first four weeks of pregnancy, more than 50 per cent of babies are born with a major defect such as a congenital heart disorder (see p.656). By the 13th week, that figure has dropped to eight per cent, and the risk steadily decreases after that.

If you have already had German measles, you cannot catch it a second time. However, you should not rely on your own or a relative's memory that you have had the illness. Make absolutely sure by asking your physician to give you a blood test before you become pregnant. If the test shows you have not had the disease, your physician will immunize you against it by injecting you with a vaccine that gives you a mild form of the disorder. You should avoid conception for three months after the injection, since during that time the disease might possibly harm a developing baby.

If you do not take these precautions and you do develop German measles in early pregnancy, it may be possible to have the pregnancy terminated, and thus avoid the considerable risk of having a severely handicapped child.

The Path to Pregnancy

Egg production and ovulation

A woman has two ovaries, one on each side of the uterus, which contain many thousands of immature eggs. After puberty, a single egg normally ripens each month in one of the ovaries. The maturing egg and about 100 cells that cluster around it and nourish it together form what is called a follicle. This follicle is filled with liquid. About halfway through the menstrual cycle, the follicle bursts and the ripe egg is expelled (ovulation) and drawn into the fallopian tube nearby.

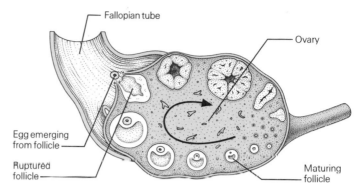

Fallopian tube

Ovary

Egg emerging from follicle

Ruptured follicle

Maturing follicle

Sperm production

Sperm are minute, tadpole-shaped cells made in the many coiled tubes, called seminiferous tubules, in the two testes. The sperm pass from the testes into the epididymis, then to the seminal vesicles where they are stored until ejaculation.

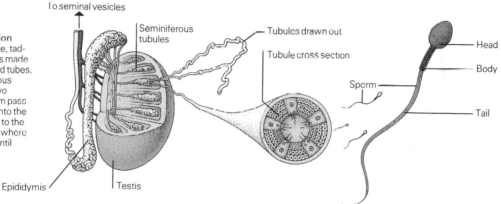

To seminal vesicles

Seminiferous tubules

Tubules drawn out

Tubule cross section

Sperm

Head

Body

Tail

Epididymis

Testis

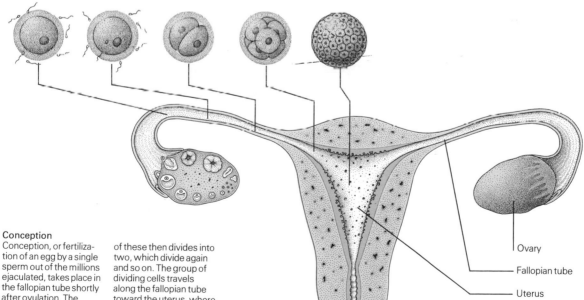

Conception

Conception, or fertilization of an egg by a single sperm out of the millions ejaculated, takes place in the fallopian tube shortly after ovulation. The sperm's nucleus joins with the egg's nucleus, combining their genetic material, and the cell divides into two cells. Each of these then divides into two, which divide again and so on. The group of dividing cells travels along the fallopian tube toward the uterus, where it embeds itself in the wall about seven days after fertilization. In a few weeks it develops into an embryo and placenta.

Ovary

Fallopian tube

Uterus

Cervix

Vagina

The growing embryo

Until about the 12th week of pregnancy, the developing baby is known as an embryo. (From 12 weeks until delivery, it is called a fetus.) The embryo develops extremely rapidly. At five weeks it is about the size of a grain of rice, but by 12 weeks it is about 6 cm (2½ in) long. At 28 days the largest, most developed organ is the heart. The limbs first develop as "buds." The nervous system, eyes and ears are all obvious by six weeks. The proportions of a developing embryo are very different from those of an adult human being. The illustrations below show the embryo (multiples of life size) at different stages of development and (in outline) at life size.

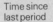
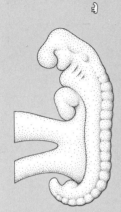
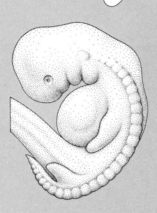
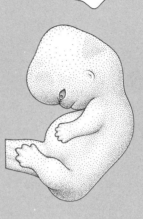
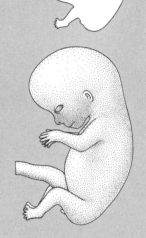

| Time since last period | 6 weeks | 7 weeks | 9 weeks | 10 weeks |

Your changing shape

During the first weeks of pregnancy, there is little obvious change in your body, although your breasts may seem a little larger and feel tender and heavy. By about the 12th week, the expanding uterus causes a bulge, and it can be felt through the abdominal wall. By the time you are 20 weeks pregnant, your abdomen may be swollen and, instead of being indented, your navel may be protruding. Toward the end of pregnancy the baby's head may move down slightly to settle in the pelvic cavity. This makes your breathing easier, but means that you may need to urinate more often than is usual, because of pressing on your bladder.

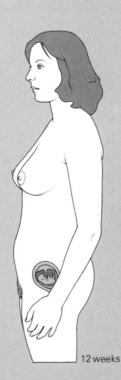
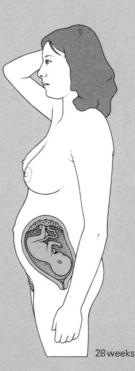
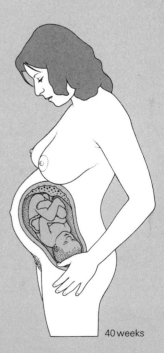

| 12 weeks | 28 weeks | 40 weeks |

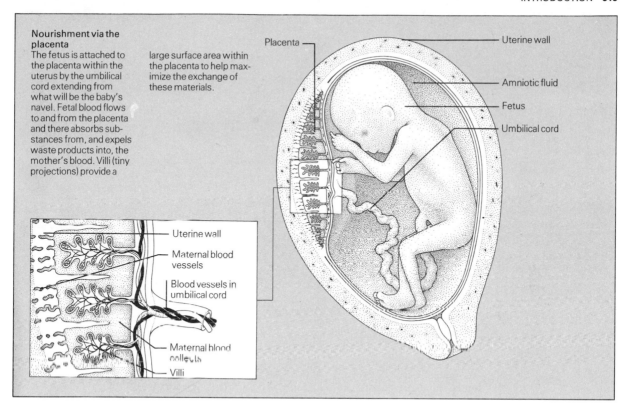

Nourishment via the placenta

The fetus is attached to the placenta within the uterus by the umbilical cord extending from what will be the baby's navel. Fetal blood flows to and from the placenta and there absorbs substances from, and expels waste products into, the mother's blood. Villi (tiny projections) provide a large surface area within the placenta to help maximize the exchange of these materials.

Placenta

Uterine wall

Amniotic fluid

Fetus

Umbilical cord

Uterine wall

Maternal blood vessels

Blood vessels in umbilical cord

Maternal blood collects

Villi

Genetic counseling

As medical understanding of inherited diseases has improved, genetic counseling services have become available from specialists in the field, often at major medical centers. The purpose of such counseling is to help couples who are concerned about the possibility of having a child with an inherited disease or defect, because of their age or family history. If you are concerned that you might have a child with an inherited disease, you should ask your physician for advice before a pregnancy begins. Your physician may refer you to a genetic counselor or to a physician who specializes in genetic diseases.

Children born with cystic fibrosis, Huntington's chorea, sickle-cell anemia, thalassemia, or certain other inherited diseases acquire them from parents who, though they are healthy, are both carriers of the disease (see Genetics, p.704). Tests are now becoming available to determine whether or not people are carriers of such diseases. If both potential parents are carriers, the risks of having children with the disease can be calculated, and you will also be told about the severity of the disease, whether treatment is available, and whether the diagnosis can be made before the baby is born. For example, if both partners are found to be carriers of thalassemia, they will be told that there is a one in

four chance that any one of their children will have the malady; that, if they decide to have a child, the mother should have tests carried out early in pregnancy because the disease is of crippling severity; and that, if the fetus is found to have thalassemia, it may be possible to have the pregnancy terminated. When parents have religious or other objections to terminating pregnancy, the tests will not be carried out, since they create a slight risk to the fetus (see Amniocentesis, p.639).

With some inherited diseases, risks are more difficult to calculate because the detection of carriers is not completely reliable, and diagnosis before birth is not possible. In these cases, the counselor will probably study the pattern of the disease over several generations before estimating the risks.

As part of the counseling, you will probably have tests to determine whether you are carriers. You will also be asked for detailed information about the health of your parents and other relatives. It will help if you have this information with you in written form when you go for counseling. In every case, the genetic counselor can only give advice: he or she cannot guarantee that a baby will be normal. The decision of whether or not to go ahead and have a child can be based on more information, but still has to be your own.

General problems of pregnancy

The problems discussed here are those that may occur at any time throughout the nine months of pregnancy. In some cases, even the diagnosis of pregnancy may not be straightforward. Many women claim that they just "know," at a very early stage, when they are pregnant. Others can only tell if they have some of the early symptoms of pregnancy. These include missing a period when you were previously regular; having a short, scanty period and tender, swollen breasts with darkened nipples; feeling nauseated; urinating more frequently; having an increased vaginal discharge; feeling tired; or suddenly losing your taste for some foods.

Diagnosis of pregnancy

If you miss two menstrual periods and your periods are usually regular, then you are almost certainly pregnant and should see your physician to confirm it. At this stage, the doctor can usually diagnose pregnancy by a pelvic examination. However, you may want to know sooner if you are pregnant, especial-ly if you have had trouble with previous pregnancies or you do not wish to have a child. In such cases, as soon as you suspect you are pregnant you should have a pregnancy test. This can be arranged through your physician, a family planning clinic, or a reputable commercial pregnancy-testing service. You can also do your own test (see Box below).

Once your pregnancy has been confirmed, and if you wish it to continue, your physician will arrange for you to have prenatal care. Appointments are usually scheduled monthly, and more frequently in the last two months before delivery. Prenatal visits should start by the 12th week of pregnancy. Your doctor may refer you to an obstetrician if he or she does not handle deliveries. Prenatal care consists of checkups and any necessary medical care before birth, and also provides you with information about labor and delivery. Many studies have shown that prenatal care helps prevent complications of pregnancy and childbirth, so keeping appointments and following your physician's advice are important.

Diet during pregnancy

When you are pregnant, what you eat also provides food for your baby, so it is more essential than usual that you eat regular, well-balanced meals. Meat, fish, cheese, beans, lentils and eggs are excellent sources of protein. Dairy products are also rich in calcium. Eggs, liver, kidneys, wholegrain or enriched bread, dried fruit and green vegetables will supply you with the iron you need to avoid anemia (see p.623). Fresh fruit and vegetables provide vitamins.

Your physician will suggest a range of weight that you should gain, usually 10 to 15 kg (about 20 to 30 lb). Either too much or too little can harm your baby.

Research indicates that alcoholic drinks can harm the fetus, and alcohol and drugs have been shown to cause many other complications and birth defects. Consult your physician before taking any medications or drugs. Smoking during pregnancy can definitely cause your baby to be underweight at birth. It also increases the risk of premature delivery. If you cannot give up smoking completely, you should at least try to cut down on the number of cigarettes you smoke.

Do-it-yourself pregnancy testing

Kits for pregnancy testing are available at many drug stores. They work by detecting the hormone HCG, which is present in the urine of pregnant women about two weeks after the first missed period. The most widely used type of kit contains a chemical solution that, mixed with a few drops of urine in the test tube provided, will almost always form a dark ring in the tube if you are pregnant. If no ring forms, you are probably not pregnant. The negative result is less reliable than the positive, especially if you are taking anti-depressant drugs, nearing menopause, or having irregular or infrequent periods.

Follow the manufacturer's instructions carefully. It is best to test urine obtained first thing in the morning, before you drink anything.

Pregnancy testing that is more reliable and not necessarily more expensive can be obtained at family planning clinics, your physician's office, or the local or county health department.

Physical activity during pregnancy

(including sex)

Exercise: You should not avoid normal physical activity while you are pregnant, unless otherwise advised by your physician. Regular exercise, especially walking or swimming, will probably help you feel well and keep you in good physical condition, although there is no evidence that it will aid the development of your baby. You should avoid strenuous sports and those that carry a danger of injury, such as horseback riding, mountain climbing, or marathon running. But as a general rule, after discussion with your physician, you can continue the forms of exercise you enjoy as long as you are careful not to overtire or overstrain yourself. It is probably also a good idea to avoid saunas, steam baths and hot tubs.

Travel: Traveling may tire you more than usual, and you should allow for this in planning any trips. Most airlines will not carry women who are in the last weeks of pregnancy, because of the risk of an unexpected delivery. If you are planning to fly, you should check with your physician and the airline before you make the reservations.

If your physician has given you any records concerning your pregnancy, you should carry these with you so that in an emergency the information will be readily available. Avoid traveling far from home if you have recently

had a threatened miscarriage (see p.628), if you are within about two weeks of the expected time of delivery, or if your pregnancy has some complication that would require special care at the time of delivery.

Work: Many women stop working at about the seventh month of pregnancy, when the increase in girth makes it difficult for them to move easily. If your physician thinks your work is too strenuous, he or she may advise you to give it up before that time. However, if you are physically well and the pregnancy has been smooth, there may be no medical reason not to continue working until much nearer the time of the birth, even up to the day of the birth. Whether you are at work or at home, be careful not to lift heavy objects. Also it is important to be sure to get plenty of rest, whether you are working or not.

Sex: If your pregnancy is normal, you can safely have sexual intercourse for the first six months. There is some evidence that intercourse during the last three months may cause early labor and delivery. Pregnancy makes some women feel increased desire for intercourse, while others may lose desire. In cases of lost interest, sexual desire almost always returns to normal after delivery.

In the last four weeks of pregnancy it is advisable either not to have intercourse or to have it while lying on your side or on top of your partner. In these positions penetration by your partner is not so deep and there is therefore less risk of precipitating premature labor. Also, you will probably find these positions more comfortable.

If you have had repeated miscarriages during the early weeks of past pregnancies, or if you have recently had a threatened early miscarriage, you should consult your physician about intercourse during your pregnancy. There is conflicting data about timing and possible ill-effects.

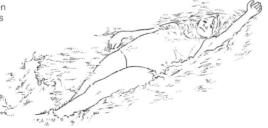

Swimming is a fine exercise for pregnant women because the water helps support the baby's weight.

Nausea and vomiting during pregnancy

(morning sickness)

Many women suffer with nausea and vomiting during pregnancy. This usually happens in the morning, often immediately after waking. The problem usually begins during the first month and continues until the 14th to 16th week. Its cause is unknown.

The vomiting is usually minor and harmless, though unpleasant. In only a small percentage of cases, it develops into severe vomiting, known as hyperemesis. This drains the body of liquids and chemicals and harms general health.

Nausea, and sometimes vomiting, occur in about half of all pregnant women in the first

three months. Almost all pregnant women have some queasiness, but very few develop hyperemesis.

What should be done?

If you have begun vomiting during your pregnancy, avoid greasy foods and do not go too long without eating. Have small frequent meals during the day instead of a few large meals. If you wake up feeling nauseated, eating some dry toast or a saltine cracker before you get up may help relieve the feeling. Do not take any drugs for your vomiting without first consulting your physician, because there is some controversy over which drugs can be harmful to the developing baby.

If your vomiting is making you miserable, see your physician. He or she will assess whether the vomiting has caused a harmful loss of body liquids and chemicals, and check on the unlikely possibility that some disorder is causing the vomiting.

Hyperemesis (severe vomiting) requires hospital treatment. Anti-vomiting drugs are given, and lost liquids and chemicals are replaced by intravenous *drip*.

Heartburn during pregnancy

Heartburn is a burning pain in the center of the chest and upper abdomen, sometimes accompanied by an unpleasant taste in the mouth or belching. Despite its name, it has nothing to do with the heart. For general information, read the article on heartburn and hiatus hernia (see p.456).

Heartburn is common during pregnancy; it affects almost half of all pregnant women. This is because during pregnancy the muscle that helps to close off the upper part of the stomach from the esophagus, or gullet, becomes lax and allows digestive juices from the stomach to re-enter the esophagus and irritate its sensitive lining. In late pregnancy the enlarging uterus (womb) presses on the stomach and aggravates the condition.

Heartburn is a harmless condition and disappears after your baby is born unless it is not related to the pregnancy.

What should be done?
You can minimize heartburn by eating small, frequent meals. This means that there is always food in your stomach to soak up much of the digestive juices. If this does not solve the problem, consult your physician, who may prescribe an antacid to take regularly, and discuss with you a diet that is nutritious but may also reduce heartburn.

Preparing for the birth

During pregnancy, the growing fetus and the hormones that nurture its growth may produce overwhelming and sometimes worrisome changes inside the body of a woman. If you are an expectant mother, it is important to learn not only about pregnancy but also about the labor and delivery of your child.

Many organizations sponsor prenatal, or before childbirth, educational classes, and your physician can recommend a suitable one. Many of these classes include teaching you techniques that use breathing patterns to help deal with uterine contractions or labor pains. To prepare for delivery, both you and your husband, or a close friend with whom you would like to share your childbirth experience (called a coach) attend several classes starting at about the seventh month of pregnancy. Most women who attend these classes have a more positive childbirth experience since they are calmer and more relaxed during delivery, and they know what to expect.

What are the options?
Trends in the care of women during labor and delivery are changing. Most women deliver their babies in hospitals, but some hospitals offer alternatives to the normal labor and delivery room. One such alternative is called a birthing center. This is a private room with windows, curtains and a large bed where a woman spends both labor and delivery. Her husband (or a friend) can share with her the time spent in labor as well as provide help and support. If any problems come up during labor, the woman can be easily moved into the labor and delivery suite, where the medical and nursing staff can manage complications more easily.

To qualify for this type of childbirth, a woman must have no medical problems that are complicating her pregnancy, and she must have adequate prenatal care. She and her husband (or friend) must also attend the prenatal classes.

Hospitals vary in their policies about caring for women and their babies. Some offer a family-centered approach in which the infant can stay in the mother's hospital room and both the father and other children in the family can visit extensively.

Some women prefer to deliver their babies at home. If any difficulty should arise that requires emergency treatment in a hospital, however, home childbirth can be a real danger. Studies are being conducted to evaluate the safety of this method in healthy, low-risk pregnant women, but results are not yet available.

If you are pregnant, many options are available to you, and you can decide how and where you want to deliver your baby. Discuss the possibilities thoroughly with your physician. In addition to where you can have your baby, you should also discuss your doctor's policy about episiotomy, pain medications during delivery, and the special circumstances that may require a cesarean section (see Special procedures in childbirth, p.640). You may also want to discuss breastfeeding (see p.641).

Anemia during pregnancy

One of the most important components of blood is hemoglobin, a protein that carries oxygen to the body's tissues. If the hemoglobin in your body falls below an adequate level, you are anemic. The most common cause of this problem is a deficiency of iron in the body (see Iron deficiency anemia, p.419). Another possible cause is an inadequate amount of folic acid (see B_{12} deficiency anemia and folic-acid deficiency, p.420).

You may not notice mild anemia, but if the condition is more pronounced, you could have any of the following symptoms: paleness, weakness, tiredness, breathlessness, fainting, and palpitations, or an abnormal awareness of your heartbeat.

Even if you have a normal amount of iron and folic acid in your diet, you may become anemic when you are expecting a baby. This is because pregnancy alters the normal processes of the digestive system. As a result the body may not absorb enough of these nutrients as they pass through the digestive system. In addition, later in pregnancy the developing baby will use more of them.

What are the risks?
Anemia in pregnancy makes you less able to cope with a sudden large loss of blood. Such blood loss can occur in a postpartum hemorrhage (see p.638). Anemia also may make you more likely to have a premature baby, and more vulnerable to infection.

What should be done?
You can help prevent anemia during pregnancy by eating foods that are especially rich in iron, such as liver, beef, wholegrain bread, eggs and dried fruits. Eat citrus fruits and fresh vegetables, because the vitamin C in them helps iron to be absorbed more efficiently. Make sure you eat plenty of green vegetables, since these are one of the best sources of folic acid

Early in your pregnancy, your physician will do a simple blood test to find out if you are anemic. Even if this shows that you are not anemic, the physician will probably prescribe iron and folic acid tablets to supplement your natural intake. If you have troublesome digestive side-effects from the tablets, tell your physician, who will probably be able to prescribe a different tablet.

If you do develop severe anemia, the treatment will be as described under iron deficiency anemia (see p.419). Other types of anemia such as sickle-cell anemia (see p.422) can cause complications during pregnancy. Discuss any family history of sickle-cell disease with your physician.

Constipation during pregnancy

Constipation is common in pregnancy, and is probably caused mainly by increased laxity of the digestive-tract muscles. In late pregnancy it is aggravated by the pressure of the enlarging uterus, or womb, on the intestines. Constipation is not a dangerous condition.

You can help to avoid constipation by eating plenty of fresh fruit and vegetables and other foods with a high fiber content (see Balanced diet, p.26), by drinking plenty of liquids, and by moving your bowels whenever you feel the need.

Do not take laxatives without consulting your physician, since some of them can irritate the intestines. If your constipation is severe, see your doctor, who will probably prescribe a medicine to soften your bowel movements.

Varicose veins during pregnancy

Many women have varicose veins (see p.409) during pregnancy. The problem is especially likely to occur in the later months. This is because when you are pregnant, your blood vessels have to accommodate an increased volume of blood in order to supply the needs of your developing baby. As the uterus enlarges, the flow of blood from the leg veins up to the pelvis slows down. This combination of factors sometimes produces pressure that causes the veins in your calves and thighs to become swollen and painful. The veins around the entrance to the vagina and rectum may also be affected, due to the same kinds of pressures.

What should be done?
Do not wear clothing that fits tightly around your waist or legs. Rest with your feet up as often as possible. If you are working and you spend a lot of time on your feet, arrange for some periodic relief from standing.

Support stockings relieve the discomfort of varicose veins considerably and can stop the veins from becoming more swollen. You can ask your physician to prescribe specially fitted stockings, or buy a serviceable substitute over the counter. Put them on first thing in the morning, *before* you get out of bed.

Varicose veins usually become considerably less swollen after you have had your baby.

Sleeping problems during pregnancy

Many women find it difficult to get to sleep or stay asleep when they are pregnant. This may be due to changes in hormone levels, the need to urinate more often, worry about the health of the baby and your ability to take care of it, and other realistic and unrealistic concerns. In later pregnancy, you may also have difficulty finding a comfortable position. Anxiety about the loss of sleep (which actually has no harmful effects) makes it even harder to fall asleep, and so a vicious cycle can develop.

What should be done?
Try the self-help measures described on p.77. It may also help if, before you go to bed, you do some relaxation exercises that you may have learned at prenatal checkups or childbirth preparation classes. If none of this works, you may have to simply accept your wakefulness. You may be able to use the time to do other things, and then try to catch up on your sleep at some other time.

If you are losing a great deal of sleep, do *not* take any drugs. Instead, consult your physician. He or she *may* prescribe a sedative, but most physicians prefer not to because of the possibility of affecting the baby. This is especially true in the first 14 weeks of pregnancy, when there is the risk that the drug could harm the baby, or close to your due date, when the drug could make the baby very sleepy after birth.

Backache during pregnancy

When you are pregnant, the ligaments and fibrous tissue that normally lock your joints firmly together become slightly more elastic. This is to allow your pelvis to expand at the moment of birth to ease delivery. However, this loosening of the joints also has an adverse effect: it makes them more susceptible to strain. This applies particularly to the joints of your spine, because during pregnancy these come under additional strain. The growth of your uterus, or womb, shifts your center of balance and your posture changes, so even standing for any length of time at all can give you what is known as non-specific backache (see p.546).

You may also get a form of backache commonly called sciatica (see Types of back pain, p.547). Some extra fluid that your body produces during pregnancy is stored inside nerve tissue, which makes the sciatic nerve become slightly swollen. The swollen tissue then presses against the bony channels of the spine. The pain of sciatica may radiate from the back and down the legs.

Many women also have abdominal pain during pregnancy, probably because of stretching of the ligaments that attach the uterus to the abdominal wall. This is called round ligament pain, and it is usually worst in the middle three months of pregnancy, when the uterus expands most rapidly.

What should be done?
You can keep the strain on your back during pregnancy to a minimum by bending your knees when you lift heavy objects and by not gaining excess weight (see Diet during pregnancy, p.620). You may learn exercises to relieve back pain in prenatal classes. For the treatment of backaches in general, see p.548.

Round ligament pain can often be relieved by lying on the aching side. Like many other problems of pregnancy, these types of pain usually disappear after your baby is born.

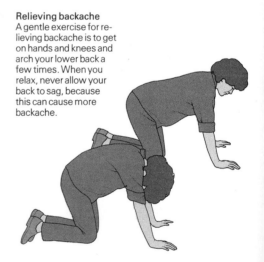

Relieving backache
A gentle exercise for relieving backache is to get on hands and knees and arch your lower back a few times. When you relax, never allow your back to sag, because this can cause more backache.

High blood pressure and pregnancy

At routine checkups in early pregnancy, some women are found to have high blood pressure (see p.382). This may have been present for some time before pregnancy, or it may be related to the pregnancy. Anxiety alone can raise blood pressure for short periods of time. If anxiety is the cause, the pressure will gradually return to normal, and stay there. It is normal for blood pressure to fall slightly during the middle weeks of pregnancy, and to rise slightly at the end. There are generally no symptoms, but extremely high blood pressure is associated with difficult childbirth and can harm the baby.

High blood pressure in late pregnancy can be a symptom of pre-eclampsia and eclampsia (see p.631). It can also lead to hemorrhage (see Antepartum hemorrhage, p.631), intrauterine death (see p.632) and intrauterine growth retardation (see p.632).

What should be done?

The earlier pre-existing high blood pressure is discovered, the greater your chances of having a safe pregnancy. That is one reason why it is important to see your physician as soon as you suspect you are pregnant. If you have high blood pressure, you should have more frequent examinations than usual. Not only will the pressure be monitored, but also blood and urine tests will be done to check on the function of your kidneys and the well-being of your baby. *Ultrasound* (see p.639) may also be used to see if your baby is developing at a normal rate.

Your physician will probably advise you to rest, and if your blood pressure is above a certain level, a drug may be prescribed to lower it. Most women with the condition can have a normal delivery, but if your blood pressure is very high, a cesarean section (see p.640) may be recommended.

Heart disorders and pregnancy

Pregnancy always involves extra work for your heart, and if your heart already has a serious underlying defect such as those caused by congenital heart disorders (see p.656) or rheumatic fever (see p.393), there is a risk of heart failure (see p.381).

What should be done?

If you know you have a heart disorder, you should consult your physician before deciding to have a baby. He or she can tell you what, if any, special risks pregnancy involves for you. If you become pregnant, you will probably be referred to a heart specialist for additional care.

Although a physician can usually tell if you have a heart disorder, sometimes such a disorder shows up for the first time under the extra demands that pregnancy makes on your body. Such disorders produce a heart murmur, which a physician can detect during a routine examination. You can have a murmur without having a disorder, however, and in fact most heart murmurs discovered in early

---

Unwanted pregnancy

The news that you are pregnant may require some serious decision-making, depending on you and your life circumstances. If you feel you cannot accept the responsibilities of motherhood and child-rearing, you have two alternatives. You can continue the pregnancy until delivery, and give the baby to an adoption agency or foster home, or you can terminate the pregnancy with an abortion.

In 1973 the United States Supreme Court ruled that an abortion could be legally obtained up to the 24th week of pregnancy, and later if the pregnancy endangered the mother's life. Up to the 12th week of pregnancy, an abortion is a private matter between a woman and her physician. After the 12th week and until the 24th week, the states have enacted different laws to govern termination of a pregnancy. There have been attempts by various groups to ban abortions in some or all cases. So far, this decision can be made by a woman and her physician.

Remember that the date of your pregnancy determines the abortion technique. This is calculated from your last menstrual period, since the exact time of conception is impossible to pinpoint.

The simplest type of abortion is called *vacuum suction*. It can be done up to the 12th week of pregnancy at a physician's office, a clinic, or in a hospital outpatient department. After dilating the cervix with slender wire-like rods, a flexible tube is inserted into the cervix from the vagina. One end of the tube is connected to a suction machine and the other end in the uterus removes the fetal tissue.

Another method for terminating a pregnancy is dilation and curettage or D & C (see Box, p.593), which may require overnight hospitalization and general anesthesia. This can be done from the 8th to the 15th week of pregnancy.

From the 16th to the 24th week, termination of a pregnancy is more complicated. Labor must be induced (see p.640) and drugs injected through the uterine wall into the amniotic fluid that surrounds the fetus. The procedure usually induces uterine contractions within 6 to 12 hours, but you must stay in the hospital for 24 hours after the abortion is completed.

pregnancy are insignificant. If, however, your physician suspects you have a heart disorder, an *electrocardiogram* (*ECG*), an *echocardiogram* and other tests may be carried out.

What is the treatment?

The main treatment is rest, so that extra strain is not placed on a heart that is already working harder than usual. You may be given *antibiotics* to take throughout your pregnancy, to prevent another attack of rheumatic fever if that is the cause of the disorder. If you develop heart failure, it will be treated as described on p.381. If you smoke, you will probably be told to make every effort to stop.

Delivery in a hospital will be necessary. When you go into labor, your physician's main goal will be to secure an easy delivery for you, one with a minimum of pushing, since this puts a strain on the heart and deprives it of oxygen. Episiotomy (see p.640), local anesthesia, and forceps (see p.640) may be used to speed delivery, decrease discomfort, and prevent tissue from tearing.

Diabetes and pregnancy

Diabetes mellitus (see p.519) can be a dangerous condition in a pregnant woman. Three to five per cent of all babies carried by women with the disorder die before or shortly after birth, despite every precaution. The risk to the mother's life during pregnancy also is higher than average. The danger to both mother and child is greater if the mother's diabetes is not carefully controlled. It is believed that the diabetes has an adverse effect on both the blood and the blood vessels of the mother, which in turn affects the baby's supply of nourishment and oxygen.

For every woman known to have diabetes before pregnancy there are several who are found to be diabetic during pregnancy.

What should be done?

If you have a family history of diabetes, if you are obese, have high blood pressure, or previously had a baby that weighed more than 4.25 kg ($9\frac{1}{2}$ lb) at birth, or if tests show that you have glucose, a form of sugar, in your urine, your physician may want you to have further tests for diabetes. You will be given a blood test, and possibly a glucose-tolerance test (see Diabetes mellitus, p.519). Glucose can be found in the urine of non-diabetic pregnant women, and in that case the tests for diabetes are a precautionary measure, and are probably no cause for concern.

What is the treatment?

If you have diabetes, you will first be given a diet to follow to control the disease. If this is not effective, you may need to take insulin (see p.520 for details). If the disease is very severe, which is rare, you may be admitted to the hospital for the last days or weeks of the pregnancy, so that the diabetes can be controlled precisely and the baby's condition can be monitored.

Rhesus (Rh) incompatibility

Rhesus (Rh) incompatibility is an incompatibility between the Rhesus blood groups of the mother and the developing baby. Blood groups are determined by the presence or absence of certain protein molecules on the surfaces of blood cells. Which and whether these proteins are present depends upon genes inherited from the parents. Rhesus incompatibility only occurs if the mother has Rh-negative blood and the baby has Rh-positive blood because it has inherited Rh-positive genes from the father. However, there is a chance that a baby may inherit Rh-negative genes from a father whose blood is Rh-positive, and have Rh-negative blood itself, in which case the problems of Rhesus incompatibility do not occur (see Genetics, p.704 and Blood groups, p.428).

When any baby is born, and also after a miscarriage (see p.628), an abortion (see previous page), or a hemorrhage (see Antepartum hemorrhage, p.631), some of the baby's blood enters the mother's circulation. An Rh-negative mother's body reacts to the baby's Rh-positive blood as foreign material, and produces *antibodies* to combat it. Because this almost always happens as a delayed reaction after the baby is born, the first baby may not be harmed. However, the mother will continue to produce these antibodies after delivery, and in any subsequent pregnancy these antibodies may pass from the mother's bloodstream into that of the developing baby and will start to destroy the baby's red blood cells, if the baby has Rh-positive blood.

What are the risks?

About 15 per cent of the white population of the United States has Rh-negative blood. The trait is less common in other races (see Table in Blood groups, p.428). Slightly over ten per cent of marriages are between an Rh-negative woman and an Rh-positive man. However, modern diagnosis and treatment have made the problems of Rhesus incompatibility rare.

Rhesus incompatibility produces no symptoms in the mother. When it occurs, the baby may develop hemolytic anemia (see p.423) and neonatal jaundice (see p.647) at birth or, in extreme cases, may be stillborn, or dead at birth. These risks increase with each Rhesus-incompatibility pregnancy.

What should be done?

At the beginning of the pregnancy you will automatically be given a blood test to determine (among other things) whether your blood is Rh-negative or Rh-positive. If your blood is Rh-negative, then the father's blood will also be tested, and if there is a chance that the baby's blood will be Rh-positive, you should have regular blood tests throughout your pregnancy.

If it is your first pregnancy, the tests are done to make sure that yours is not a rare case where antibodies develop before the baby is born. If it is a subsequent pregnancy, the tests are carried out to make absolutely sure that the treatment given after your previous pregnancies was effective. If your first pregnancy occurred before modern treatment was available, then the tests will show the concentration of antibodies in your blood. When antibodies have formed, any effect they are having on your baby can be detected in one of

two ways: by amniocentesis (see p.639), an examination of the amniotic fluid that surrounds the baby in the uterus; or by taking samples of the baby's blood.

What is the treatment?

The development of a serum for protective vaccination has almost eliminated the dangers of Rhesus incompatibility. The serum is given by injection to the mother soon after every delivery, or after a miscarriage, hemorrhage or abortion. It destroys any red blood cells from the baby that have entered the mother's circulation, before the mother's body has had time to develop antibodies. In this way, a subsequent pregnancy has the same risk as the first, but no more.

In cases where the mother does develop antibodies during a pregnancy and these are beginning to affect the baby's blood adversely, labor will be induced, or started artificially (see p.640), in the hospital if the baby is sufficiently mature. If the baby is not mature enough to be delivered, the baby may be given a blood transfusion while still in the uterus. This gives the child a chance to mature to the stage where delivery is feasible.

After delivery, such a baby will have jaundice, and if this is severe he or she may need an *exchange blood transfusion.* Since the development of specialized units in many hospitals to deal with the diverse problems of ill and premature infants, the health outlook for babies with Rhesus incompatibility has improved considerably.

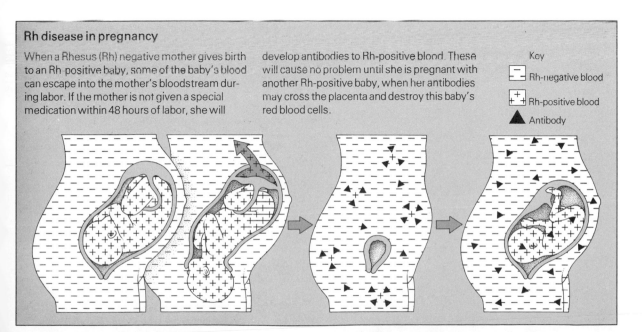

Rh disease in pregnancy

When a Rhesus (Rh) negative mother gives birth to an Rh-positive baby, some of the baby's blood can escape into the mother's bloodstream during labor. If the mother is not given a special medication within 48 hours of labor, she will develop antibodies to Rh-positive blood. These will cause no problem until she is pregnant with another Rh-positive baby, when her antibodies may cross the placenta and destroy this baby's red blood cells.

Key

Rh-negative blood

Rh-positive blood

▲ Antibody

Complications of early pregnancy

During the first three months after conception, the fetus is especially vulnerable. This time in a pregnancy is often called the first trimester. Because so much is happening to the baby during early pregnancy, any infection in the mother (see German measles and pregnancy, p.616) or unfavorable drug action can cause damage. In addition, any severe genetic defect of the fetus or disorder of the reproductive system that affects proper implantation of the fertilized egg can cause serious complications that characteristically occur in early pregnancy. One of the most common of these is miscarriage, in which the pregnancy ends spontaneously and too early. Another complication of early pregnancy is an ectopic pregnancy, in which the baby starts to develop outside the uterus.

Miscarriage

A miscarriage (known medically as a spontaneous abortion) occurs when a pregnancy ends spontaneously before the beginning of the 20th week of the pregnancy counted from the first day of the last period. After that time, the spontaneous end of a pregnancy is known as a stillbirth if the baby is born dead and a premature delivery if the baby is born alive. When a pregnancy is ended artificially, this is also known as an abortion, but the medical term is termination of pregnancy.

A miscarriage is due to the separation of the developing fetus and the placenta from the inner wall of the uterus, usually during the first 14 weeks of a pregnancy. The separation may occur because of a developmental defect in the fetus or because the placenta is not attached properly. Usually, however, the cause is not known. Miscarriages from falls or other accidents are rare, because the fetus is well protected inside the uterus.

Miscarriages can be grouped into different categories. Some women have what is called a "threatened" miscarriage in early pregnancy. There is usually a small amount of bleeding from the vagina. There is sometimes slight bleeding when the fertilized egg implants in the uterus, and this may be misinterpreted as a threatened miscarriage. About one in five women have some bleeding in the first three months, but if care is taken, the pregnancy usually proceeds normally.

An "inevitable" miscarriage occurs when the fetus has died, so nothing can be done to prevent the miscarriage.

The term "incomplete" miscarriage means that only parts of the fetus and placenta remain in the uterus.

A "missed" miscarriage means that the fetus has died in the uterus, but there are no symptoms of a miscarriage.

Any kind of miscarriage is usually followed by emotional distress.

What are the symptoms?

The first symptom you are likely to notice when a miscarriage begins is bleeding from your vagina. This can range from a few drops of blood to a heavy flow. The bleeding either starts with no warning or is preceded by a brownish discharge.

A threatened miscarriage is often painless, but an inevitable miscarriage is usually accompanied by pain in the lower abdomen or back. The pain may be either dull and constant or sharp and intermittent. At some stage during an inevitable miscarriage you may notice passing some solid material out of the vagina. Try to keep this material so that your physician can examine it.

In an incomplete miscarriage bleeding and pain may go on for several days, either constantly or intermittently. With a missed miscarriage, you may have no bleeding or pain, but the symptoms of early pregnancy will disappear. Often the only symptom is that your physician discovers that your uterus has not increased in size.

Vaginal bleeding during pregnancy

Vaginal bleeding at any time during your pregnancy can signal a serious problem, so you should notify your physician promptly. In early pregnancy about 20 per cent of women notice some vaginal bleeding (see Miscarriage, this page).

Vaginal bleeding in the final three months of pregnancy affects less than two per cent of women, but it indicates more critical problems. Contact your physician immediately if bleeding occurs late in pregnancy.

What are the risks?

Although exact figures are unknown, at least ten per cent of all pregnancies end in miscarriage, most during the first eight weeks.

Miscarriages generally do not endanger a woman's health unless the miscarriage is incomplete. If an incomplete miscarriage is not diagnosed and the uterus emptied, you will eventually become anemic and the tissue left in your uterus may become infected.

If you are pregnant and have bleeding from the vagina, with or without pain, contact your physician. If the bleeding stops or is not very heavy, the physician may simply tell you to rest at home. If the bleeding is heavy or you have severe pain, you should consult your physician immediately.

If the pregnancy seems to be continuing, even though you have had some bleeding, your doctor may arrange for you to have another pregnancy test, and perhaps an *ultrasound scan*, to confirm the pregnancy. It is best not to have sexual intercourse for a few weeks after bleeding, to give the pregnancy a chance to become more stable. Consult your physician for other precautions.

What is the treatment?

In the case of a threatened miscarriage, there is nothing that can be done medically, and you will probably be told simply to rest in bed as much as possible. At one time a drug (diethylstilbestrol or DES) was given to help prevent miscarriages. However, it is no longer used for this purpose because it was not very effective and it was linked to a number of abnormalities in babies, especially female babies.

If your miscarriage is inevitable, incomplete, or missed, you will usually have the remains of the fetus and placenta removed from your uterus by your physician, usually in the hospital but sometimes in the doctor's office or a clinic.

After a miscarriage you are likely to be depressed by your loss. However, you can safely start trying to conceive again soon afterwards. Most physicians recommend that you give your body at least six to eight weeks to return to normal. You should certainly wait until you have had at least one normal period, since then it is easier to make an accurate estimate of when the baby is due.

Ectopic pregnancy

In ectopic (or tubal) pregnancy an egg is fertilized by a sperm but develops outside the uterus, usually in one of the fallopian tubes. The placenta burrows into the surrounding tissue, which usually tears and causes internal bleeding. This tissue cannot sustain a placenta and fetus, and the pregnancy cannot continue. In this condition you will have constant, severe abdominal pain, probably followed by vaginal bleeding. You may not even suspect that you are pregnant.

About 1 in every 200 pregnancies is ectopic, and most are discovered in the first two months. You are more likely to have an ectopic pregnancy if you have had some abnormality of your fallopian tubes from birth, if the fallopian tubes were previously operated on or infected, or if you are using an intrauterine contraceptive device (see p.609).

What should be done?

If you develop abdominal pain that lasts for more than a few hours, contact your physician. Delay may cause severe internal bleeding that can lead to shock (see p.386).

Your physician will examine you carefully, since the abdominal pain of ectopic pregnancy can be similar to that of several other conditions, including miscarriage (see previous article), appendicitis, and infection of the fallopian tubes. You may be sent to a hospital. An *ultrasound scan* often allows an accurate diagnosis, but sometimes a *laparoscopy* is required.

Once an ectopic pregnancy is confirmed, any severe loss of blood is treated with a blood transfusion and an operation is performed immediately. The developing fetus, placenta and surrounding tissue are removed and the torn blood vessels are repaired.

Even if one of your fallopian tubes has been damaged by an ectopic pregnancy, it is possible to have a normal pregnancy, although the chances of conception are slightly reduced. You may also need extra checkups and tests, since ectopic pregnancies can recur.

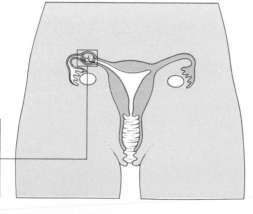

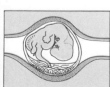

An ectopic pregnancy usually occurs in a fallopian tube when the fertilized egg does not make its way down into the uterus.

Complications of mid-pregnancy

During the middle three months of pregnancy, also called the second trimester, many women say they have never felt better. The fact that the physical changes associated with the baby's development proceed more slowly at this time may explain this feeling.

Most women start regular prenatal care by the time they are about 12 weeks pregnant. Their general health is assessed by the physician, and they are given iron and folic-acid supplements. Blood and urine are examined regularly for any signs of abnormality.

Most pregnancies continue smoothly during the middle three months. The main complications that can occur are incompetent cervix, hydramnios, intrauterine growth retardation (see p.632), urinary tract infections (see Cystitis in women, p.600), and either excessive or insufficient weight gain by the mother (see Diet during pregnancy, p.620).

Incompetent cervix

In this condition the cervix opens up during pregnancy, usually after the 14th week. The fetus and placenta escape from the uterus, which causes a miscarriage (see p.628). Weakness of the cervix may trigger this, but usually the cause is not known.

If you are known or suspected to have an incompetent cervix, a miscarriage may be prevented by an operation during early pregnancy. While you are under a general anesthetic, a piece of strong thread is sewn through the cervix and tightened to hold the cervix firm. After the operation you may be given a drug to reduce the chances that the operation will stimulate premature labor (see p.636). The thread is cut when labor starts or at about the 38th week of pregnancy if labor has not started by then.

Hydramnios

Hydramnios is a usually harmless condition that can occur in the later stages of pregnancy. It is caused by an excessive amount of amniotic fluid around the baby. In most cases, the swelling of the uterus is only slightly greater than normal, and the condition produces either no symptoms or a gradual onset of slightly more breathlessness than is usual, indigestion, and a tenseness in the abdomen. In rare cases, the swelling is pronounced, the symptoms begin suddenly and are accompanied by nausea, and there is risk of premature labor.

Hydramnios is more common than average in diabetic mothers, in women who have pre-eclampsia (see next page), and in a twin or other multiple pregnancy (see p.633).

What should be done?

For a minor case of hydramnios, your physician will probably advise you simply to rest a little more. If hydramnios comes on suddenly your doctor will probably advise you to rest completely, and may give you drugs to relax your uterus and reduce the risk of going into premature labor.

Screening for congenital defects

Women who have had children with diseases such as spina bifida (see p.654) or Down's syndrome (see p.653), or who are over 35 years old, have a greater risk of having a child with congenital, or birth, defects. They may wish to have amniocentesis (see p.639) and genetic screening to help evaluate the risks. After testing it may be possible to terminate the pregnancy if there are substantial risks.

The amniotic fluid around a fetus with a defect of the nervous system such as spina bifida usually contains a raised level of a protein called AFP (alpha fetoprotein). However, there may also be a raised level of AFP if you are carrying twins or if you are more than 18 weeks pregnant.

If tests show a raised level of AFP between the estimated 16th and 18th weeks of pregnancy, you will probably have an ultrasound scan to find out if you are carrying twins or if you are beyond the 18th week of pregnancy. If neither of these is the cause, amniocentesis can show whether your baby has a central nervous system defect.

Amniocentesis is also used to screen for Down's syndrome. The chromosomes in the sample of amniotic fluid are examined under a microscope to determine whether the baby has this disorder.

Complications of late pregnancy

Because most babies stand a better chance of survival the nearer to full term they are born, some treatment in late pregnancy is designed to prevent you from going into labor too early. This is accomplished mainly with rest and with drugs to relax the uterine muscles so that they do not begin the contractions of childbirth. However, if your physician suspects that the baby is having difficulties inside the uterus, the treatment may be designed to encourage a quick labor and birth.

It is important that you continue to keep your prenatal appointments during the last weeks of your pregnancy, so that any possible complications can be diagnosed and treated before you and your baby can be harmed.

Pre-eclampsia and eclampsia
(*toxemia of pregnancy*)

Pre-eclampsia is a disorder of late pregnancy in which the mother's blood pressure rises and there is excess fluid in the mother's body. Why this happens is not known. If, in addition, her urine contains protein, the mother is in danger of developing eclampsia, in which the blood pressure increases drastically. This condition can cause seizures, and endanger the lives of both mother and baby.

In mild pre-eclampsia you may feel perfectly well. You should therefore go to all your prenatal checkups, so that the condition can be spotted early. The symptoms of severe pre-eclampsia, which can develop during the last few weeks of pregnancy, are headaches, blurred vision, intolerance for bright light, nausea and vomiting, and salt and water retention. You may then develop eclampsia, the symptoms of which are convulsions and sometimes unconsciousness.

Pre-eclampsia seems to occur particularly in the first pregnancies of young women and in women who have high blood pressure or a family history of high blood pressure. Eclampsia is rare. Chronic high blood pressure is believed by physicians to play a role in retarded growth of babies while they are still in the uterus. This is because high blood pressure reduces the efficiency of the placenta, which provides the baby with oxygen and nutrients. In eclampsia, there is also a definite risk to the life of the mother.

What is the treatment?
Your physician may prescribe a drug to control your blood pressure. You can help lower it yourself by getting plenty of rest and by reducing your salt intake.

If you do develop the symptoms of severe pre-eclampsia or eclampsia, you should contact your physician immediately. You may be admitted to a hospital, where you will be given drugs to lower your blood pressure, remove excess fluid from your body, and prevent other complications. Delivery of the baby may be advisable, either by inducing labor (see p.640) or by cesarean section (see p.640). These procedures involve some risks, which must be weighed against the risks of eclampsia. Your physician can discuss your particular situation with you and outline the choices for treatment.

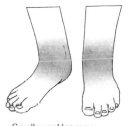

Swollen ankles may indicate pre-eclampsia.

Antepartum hemorrhage

Antepartum hemorrhage is any bleeding from the vagina after the end of the 20th week of pregnancy. Earlier bleeding is known as a threatened miscarriage (see Miscarriage, p.628).

Antepartum hemorrhage may be the result of placenta previa (see next article), a burst vaginal varicose vein, damage to the cervix, or partial or complete separation of the placenta from the wall of the uterus (accidental hemorrhage).

In most cases, mainly those that do not involve the placenta, antepartum bleeding is mild and harmless. A hemorrhage caused by placental separation can cause intrauterine growth retardation (see next page), however, and if placental bleeding is heavy it can endanger the lives of both the baby and the mother.

If you have bleeding during pregnancy, call your physician as soon as possible. You may be admitted to the hospital, and have blood tests and an *ultrasound scan*. If a considerable amount of blood has been lost, and if bleeding continues, blood will be replaced by transfusions and the baby may be delivered as soon as possible. This will be done either by induction of labor (see p.640) or cesarean section (see p.640), depending on the duration of the pregnancy.

Placenta previa

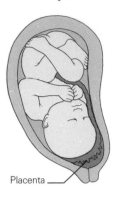

Placenta

In placenta previa, the placenta develops low in the uterus, either near, or sometimes over, the cervix. Any part of the placenta that is near the cervix is poorly supported and vulnerable to damage. The condition occurs in about 1 pregnancy in 200 that have continued past the 28th week.

In some cases, the placenta starts off low in the uterus, but as the pregnancy develops it moves up the wall of the uterus to a more normal position, and causes no problems.

What are the symptoms?

There may be no symptoms, but if the placenta becomes partly detached from the uterus, you will have sporadic, painless bleeding from the vagina, usually late in the pregnancy. If you have bleeding from the vagina during pregnancy, call your physician at once and go to bed. Do not put anything in your vagina, not even a tampon.

What is the treatment?

In the case of a slight degree of placenta previa fairly early in pregnancy, your physician may recommend that you have one or more *ultrasound scans* to determine if normal labor may eventually be possible. If placenta previa is severe, bleeding will be heavy and will require a blood transfusion, and the baby should be delivered as soon as possible. This is done by cesarean section (see p.640) to prevent further hemorrhaging of the placenta. Such bleeding can cause brain damage in the baby, or even death. It can also cause the mother to lose a dangerous amount of blood.

Premature rupture of membranes

When labor starts, the membranes that surround the baby in the uterus rupture, releasing amniotic fluid. This is called "breaking water." Occasionally the membranes rupture prematurely, before labor has begun. The main risks that are associated with premature rupture are that it may be followed by premature labor (see p.636) or allow an infection to enter your uterus.

What should be done?

If you think your membranes have ruptured prematurely, contact your physician, who will probably admit you to a hospital, where you may be given medications to prevent complications for the baby. Amniocentesis (see p.639) may also be done to find out if the baby's lungs are developed enough for the baby to survive. If your expected delivery date is in two or three weeks' time, and tests confirm that the baby is mature enough, labor may be induced (see p.640), but if the expected date is further ahead, you may be given a drug to relax the muscles of the uterus and reduce the chances of premature labor.

Sometimes a small tear in the membranes will heal naturally and allow the pregnancy to continue to a full term delivery, but the risk of infection remains, so your condition must be watched carefully.

Intrauterine death

This is the death of a baby in the uterus after the 20th week of pregnancy. In many cases this intrauterine death is caused by severe pre-eclampsia or eclampsia (see previous page), a hemorrhage (see Antepartum hemorrhage, previous page), postmaturity (see next page), or a severe abnormality of the baby. It may also be related to diabetes mellitus (see p.519) in the mother. In other cases the cause is not known.

Usually the only symptom of intrauterine death is that the mother no longer feels any movement from the baby. If the physician cannot hear any heartbeat, a fetal *electrocardiogram* (*ECG*) and other special tests are done. If these show an absence of fetal life, intrauterine death is confirmed.

If the mother does not go into labor spontaneously, labor is brought on artificially (see Induction of labor, p.640).

Except when the mother has diabetes mellitus, the outlook for any future pregnancy after an intrauterine death is usually the same as for any first pregnancy.

Intrauterine growth retardation
(retarded fetal growth)

In some pregnancies, the placenta does not supply enough nourishment to the fetus. The result is that the baby's development in the uterus is stunted. The deficiencies of the placenta in this disorder may be caused by severe pre-eclampsia or eclampsia (see previous page), high blood pressure (see p.382), hemorrhage (see Antepartum hemorrhage, previous page), placenta previa (see above), or heart disease (see Heart disorders and pregnancy, p.625) or diabetes mellitus (see p.519) in the mother.

What are the risks?

At birth, the baby will have less body fat and therefore less resistance to cold than normal, and will be susceptible to hypoglycemia (see p.522). If the baby is delivered early, he or she may have some of the complications of premature labor (see p.636), including respiratory distress syndrome (see p.647).

What should be done?

Pregnant women should keep all prenatal appointments. If you are beyond the 30th week of your pregnancy, and you think your baby is not moving as much as before, count the movements accurately. Choose two days when you are not planning to leave the house, and on each day make a note of each movement you feel between nine in the morning and five in the afternoon. Then discuss the problem with your physician. Your baby is probably perfectly well. In fact, there is a complete absence of movement in some normal pregnancies. But it is always wise to check rather than take any chances.

Your physician may recommend tests such as blood or urine tests to measure the level of your hormones, *ultrasound* (see p.639), and fetal heartbeat tests (see p.639), to check on the baby's condition.

If it is determined that fetal growth is retarded, your physician can discuss with you the best time for the baby to be delivered. If the baby is not growing well, it may actually develop better in an intensive care nursery where it won't have to depend on a placenta that may be functioning inefficiently. You may have to have the baby in a hospital that has a specialized nursery to treat such problems in newborns. Labor may have to be started artificially (see Induction of labor, p.640) or you may need to have a cesarean section (see p.640).

Postmaturity

Ideally, labor starts when your baby is fully mature and able to survive on its own. When labor does not occur until long after this stage, the baby can be harmed. This condition is known as postmaturity. An aging placenta can fail to provide a large baby with enough oxygenated blood, and this can result in brain damage or even death. The stillbirth rate in postmature babies is almost double that in babies born at the right time.

If your physician suspects postmaturity, labor will probably be started artificially (see Induction of labor, p.640). A close watch will be kept on your baby during labor, usually with special instruments, and if he or she seems to be in difficulty, delivery will be speeded up by the use of forceps (see p.640) or cesarean section (see p.640).

Twin pregnancy

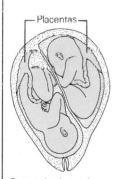

Placentas

Fraternal twins each have their own placenta.

Twins occur as the result of either the splitting of a single egg or the parallel development of two eggs. They account for 1 in 90 births in the United States. Triplets, by comparison, are very rare. They occur in about only 1 in 8000 pregnancies. Multiple births are more common among black women than white. Seven out of ten pairs of twins are binovular, which means that two eggs were fertilized by two sperms. These are "fraternal" twins. "Identical," or mono-ovular, twins develop from one egg that has split shortly after fertilization. Fraternal twins each have a placenta, but identical twins have only one between them.

The outlook for both the mother and the twins is good, particularly if the mother has adequate nutrition, rest and prenatal care. But there are risks associated with every pregnancy, and in a twin pregnancy the risks of anemia (see p.623), pre-eclampsia (see p.631), placenta previa (see previous page) and postpartum hemorrhage (see p.638) are slightly greater than in a single pregnancy. Also, about one fourth of twin pregnancies end four or more weeks early (see Premature labor, p.636).

A multiple pregnancy is usually discovered by your physician during a routine prenatal examination, and confirmed by *ultrasound* (see p.639). As with any pregnancy you should get enough rest and be sure to eat a balanced diet. To combat the risk of anemia, your physician may prescribe more than the usual number of iron and folic acid tablets.

If you have contractions in late pregnancy or have a watery discharge from your vagina, you should contact your physician. This is because you may be going into premature labor. If you are, you will be admitted to a hospital and possibly given a drug to relax the muscles of the uterus and delay delivery.

Childbirth

There are several signs that tell you when your baby will soon be born. The first sign in normal labor is contractions of the muscles of the uterus. At first these may seem like irregular bursts of indigestion-like pain or twinges of backache. As the birth approaches, however, the contractions come at more regular intervals and there is less time between each of them.

Contractions alone are not always a reliable sign that labor has started. Throughout pregnancy, the uterus has been contracting in preparation for labor, although these contractions, called Bracton Hicks contractions, are usually not noticeable until the last weeks of pregnancy. If you have contractions, but they are not accompanied by any other signs and do not increase in frequency, you are probably not in labor.

As labor starts, the mucous plug that has formed a barrier between your uterus and vagina during pregnancy will be expelled as a bloody discharge. This occurrence, which is called the "show," is no cause for concern.

Another sign of labor is the bursting of the membranes that surround the amniotic fluid in which the baby floats. When this occurs, you may have a slow trickle of fluid from your vagina or you may have a sudden gush. This is called "breaking water," and it is usually a sign that delivery is not far off.

Notify your physician when you have any of these signs of labor. You will probably be advised to go to the hospital where you have pre-registered, to be admitted. If you have planned to have your baby at home, the physician or nurse-midwife should be called to come when these signs appear.

In the hospital there is usually an admission procedure. The physician does a vaginal examination to see how far your labor has progressed and to find out the baby's position. You may also be given an enema to empty your bowels. In some hospitals, all or part of the pubic hair is shaved off as a precaution against infection.

Stages of labor

Labor usually occurs in three stages. The first stage starts with the first contractions and they help open the cervix, through which the baby leaves the uterus. With each contraction, the cervix is gradually pulled open and up, so that it becomes effaced; that is, it merges with the walls of the uterus. Then the cervix is "dilated." Full dilation is reached when the opening of the cervix with the baby's head protruding is 10 cm (about 4 in) in diameter.

The average duration of the first stage of labor is 12 hours for a first baby and 4 to 8 hours for a subsequent birth. But these are only averages. For some women who are having their first baby, the first stage can last for more than 24 hours, although every effort is made to prevent this. For some women who have already had several children it may last only a few minutes.

When the cervix is fully dilated, there is a transition period between the first and second stages of labor. In some women, labor seems to come to a temporary halt at this point. As the second stage begins, contractions become much more powerful and are usually accompanied by an urge to push the baby out and down the birth canal. As the baby moves through the birth canal, it presses on the rectum and may make you feel that you want to move your bowels.

You will be advised to push only when you are having a contraction. This is so that the two forces (your pushing and the contractions) combine to expel the baby and you can conserve energy by resting as much as possible between contractions.

The second stage of labor ends when the baby emerges completely from the birth canal. The second stage can last up to an hour for a first baby, and up to 30 minutes for a subsequent baby.

After the baby is delivered, the umbilical cord that connects the baby to the placenta while it is inside the uterus is clamped shut and then cut.

The third stage of labor is delivery of the placenta (the afterbirth). Your uterus continues to contract to expel it. During this stage there is some bleeding, and the umbilical cord moves a little further out of the vagina. To speed up this process and to try to prevent excess bleeding, the physician pulls gently on the cord while pressing on your abdomen with the other hand. The third stage of labor usually lasts about 15 minutes.

After the placenta has been delivered, you may be given a medication that will prevent excessive bleeding. Any tears or incisions that are present in the vagina are cleaned and stitched. You may be able to hold your baby while this is being done.

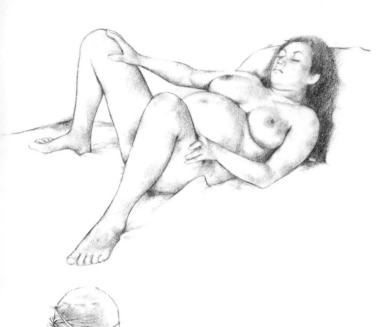

During the first stage of labor the mother has con-tractions that increase in strength and frequency.

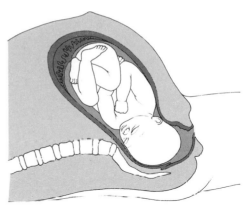

When the cervix is fully dilated, the contractions are stronger. The baby moves down the birth canal, and the head appears.

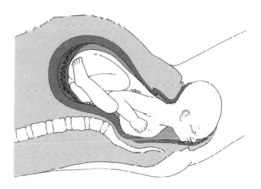

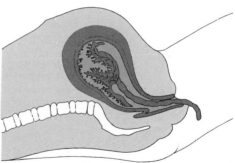

After the baby has been born, the mother's uterus continues to contract to expel the placenta, or afterbirth. This com-pletes the third and final stage of labor. While this is happening, the mother is often allowed to hold her child.

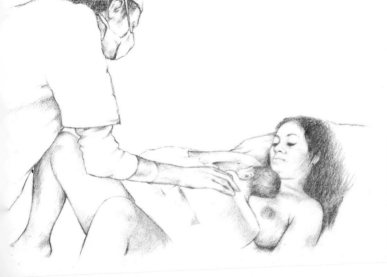

Premature labor

Labor is called premature if it occurs well before the expected date of delivery and results in the birth of a pre-term baby, which means the child has had less than 37 weeks of development in the uterus.

Severe pre-eclampsia and eclampsia (see p.631) cause about a third of all premature labors. High blood pressure during pregnancy, placenta previa (see p.632), hemorrhage (see Antepartum hemorrhage, p.631), cigarette smoking by the mother, and other causes account for some cases. About five per cent of pregnancies end in premature labor.

The earlier in a pregnancy that a baby is born, the less the baby's chances of survival. Babies who do survive are in danger of having respiratory distress syndrome (see p.647) and neonatal jaundice (see p.647). The risk of having one of these disorders is greater the more premature the birth.

What should be done?

If you think you are starting labor prematurely (see p.634) contact your physician at once. If the physician is not immediately available, arrange for immediate transportation or call an ambulance to take you to the hospital where you plan to deliver. Warn the hospital that you are coming. If the hospital is far away, call the hospital for advice. In the hospital you will be examined to see whether your labor actually has started. There are many false alarms. Amniocentesis may be done to check the baby's lung development. Medications may be given to try to increase lung maturity.

What is the treatment?

If you are in the early stages of labor, your physician may prescribe a drug to relax the muscles of the uterus and try to prevent further labor. If it is decided to let the labor proceed, you will probably have an episiotomy (see p.640) to allow a free passage for the baby's head, which is more fragile than that of a full-term baby. Forceps (see p.640) may also be used to protect the head. After birth, the baby will be placed in a special care unit. Heartbeat, respiration and temperature will be carefully monitored, and any problems treated promptly. Because of recent advances in care of premature babies, yours will have a good chance of surviving and living a normal life.

Pain relief in labor

The intensity of pain in labor varies considerably from woman to woman. It is partly governed by your expectations. If you are frightened or tense, you may feel pain more acutely. This is one reason why you, and the child's father if possible, should attend childbirth classes if they are available in your community. Some classes include breathing and relaxation exercises.

You may not need pain relief during labor, but if you do, there are various methods available. If the first stage of labor is very painful, you may be given medication to help reduce tension and pain. This is generally done only if the physician is fairly sure that delivery is not imminent. The reason is that the drug may affect the newborn baby's breathing if it is given late in labor.

Another method of relieving pain at the end of the first stage of labor and during the second stage is to have you inhale a combination of anesthetic gas and air. This provides only short-term pain relief, and is seldom used in the United States.

Vaginal pain can also be relieved by a local anesthetic injected into the tissues of the vagina. This is called pudendal block. It is often used before a delivery that will be made with the aid of forceps or before an episiotomy, in which a cut is made in the vagina to aid delivery.

Many hospitals offer a painkilling method called epidural anesthesia. This involves injecting an anesthetic into the base of your spine to numb the nerves running to the lower half of your body temporarily, so that you feel nothing. If the anesthetic is given late in the first stage of labor, its effect may still be so strong that you are unable to push the baby out, and a forceps delivery (see p.640) may be required. Another similar method called spinal anesthesia involves an injection of an anesthetic into the spinal canal.

Epidural anesthesia
The injection for epidural anesthesia is given between contractions with the mother lying on her side and curled up as much as possible to allow the anesthetist to insert the needle between the vertebrae.

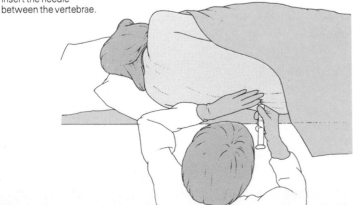

Prolonged labor

Prolonged labor is usually due to one of two things. Either the muscles of the uterus do not produce sufficiently strong or regular contractions (sometimes called "lazy" uterus), or there is an obstruction to normal delivery. Obstruction occurs in disproportion (see below), when the baby's head is too large for the bony outlet from the pelvic cavity, or malpresentation (see next article), when the baby's position makes delivery difficult.

Uterine muscles can be stimulated to contract more by *intravenous infusion* of a medication into your bloodstream (see Induction of labor, p.640). In some cases of prolonged labor, delivery will need to be by cesarean section (see p.640) or by forceps (see p.640), depending on the stage of labor and the position of the baby.

Mal-presentation

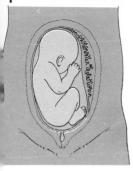

In breech presentation the baby passes into and comes down the mother's birth canal buttocks first.

The part of the baby that has settled at the outlet of the mother's pelvic cavity immediately before birth is called the presenting part. The most common presenting part is the head, with the crown settled into the cavity of the pelvis, and the face to the mother's back. This presentation positions the baby for the easiest passage through the birth canal. The baby, however, may be in one of several other positions that cause problems and are called malpresentation.

Two of the more common malpresentations are occipital posterior presentation and breech presentation. An occipital posterior presentation is head down, but with the face toward the mother's front. This puts the baby in a difficult position to travel through the birth canal, but usually the baby rotates naturally to the proper position. Delivery by forceps and rarely by cesarean section may be

necessary. Breech presentation is particularly common in premature labor (see previous page) because a baby may not assume a normal position for delivery until late in pregnancy. The baby is positioned with its buttocks down, and one or both feet may emerge first. In a buttocks-first delivery, the baby's head is more vulnerable to pressure as it passes along the birth canal, which is not sufficiently enlarged by the buttocks. Such a delivery may have to be by cesarean section or forceps.

In some cases of breech presentation, the physician can manipulate the baby into the normal presentation position during the last few weeks of pregnancy. If breech presentation persists, but there are few other problems, the physician may suggest you allow labor to start naturally, while being prepared to have a cesarean section if labor is difficult.

In occipital posterior presentation (right), the baby's chin is pushed down onto the chest, so that he or she cannot flex the neck to get around the curve of the birth canal as in the normal presentation (far right).

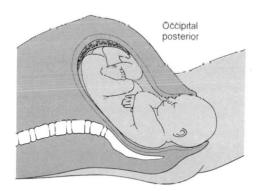

Occipital posterior

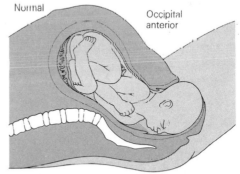

Normal

Occipital anterior

Disproportion

The term disproportion means that the mother's pelvic cavity is too narrow for the passage of her baby's head. This can happen in small-boned women and in women who are under 1.5 m (5 ft) tall. In some cases, a woman's pelvis is disproportionately small because of an injury. Disproportion may also occur if the baby's head is abnormally large, as in hydrocephalus (see p.655).

If your physician suspects disproportion, you will be given an extra internal examina-

tion late in pregnancy. If you appear to have severe disproportion, delivery by cesarean section (see p.640) may be recommended. Pelvimetry, or *X-rays* to outline the bony structure of the baby and the mother, is usually done only if labor has already begun. It is not recommended before labor since X-rays may harm the fetus. If the decision is to go ahead with a vaginal delivery, labor will be allowed to proceed, but the baby's condition will be monitored closely.

Postpartum hemorrhage

Postpartum hemorrhage is excessive loss of blood from the uterus or vagina after delivery. It often occurs when the uterine muscle does not contract firmly enough to control the bleeding produced when the placenta separates from the uterus. This problem can be caused by exhaustion of the muscles if you had a very long labor, or by previous weakening of the muscles of the uterus, which can occur when the uterus has been stretched excessively by a twin pregnancy or by a large number of pregnancies. Another possible cause is that parts of the placenta can remain inside the uterus and prevent it from tightening up sufficiently. A hemorrhage can also occur if tissues of the vagina have been torn during delivery.

Bleeding from the uterus is controlled by drugs that encourage the uterus to contract. If fragments of placenta remain in the uterus, they should be removed. If bleeding is from torn tissues of the vagina, the tear will be stitched up after the area has been numbed with a local anesthetic.

Retained placenta

Normally the placenta separates from the wall of the uterus after delivery and, with the help of the physician who presses on your abdomen and pulls gently on the umbilical cord, it is expelled. Occasionally the placenta becomes trapped in the uterus, in some cases because it has not separated completely from the uterine wall. If it has not been expelled within 30 minutes after delivery it is called a retained placenta.

If necessary, a retained placenta can be removed manually by the physician while you receive some form of anesthetic. When it has been taken out, you will be given a drug to encourage your womb to contract to prevent excessive bleeding.

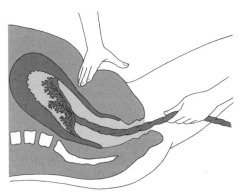

Expulsion of the placenta

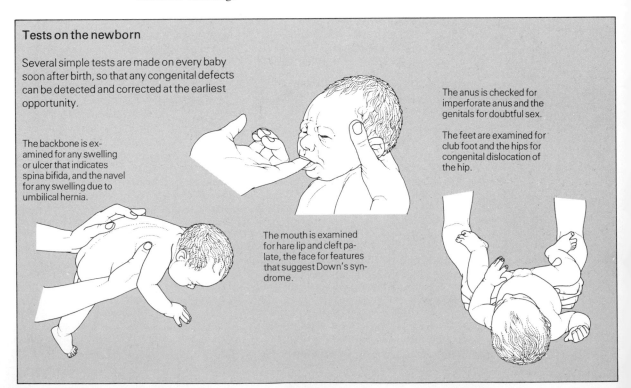

Tests on the newborn

Several simple tests are made on every baby soon after birth, so that any congenital defects can be detected and corrected at the earliest opportunity.

The backbone is examined for any swelling or ulcer that indicates spina bifida, and the navel for any swelling due to umbilical hernia.

The mouth is examined for hare lip and cleft palate, the face for features that suggest Down's syndrome.

The anus is checked for imperforate anus and the genitals for doubtful sex.

The feet are examined for club foot and the hips for congenital dislocation of the hip.

Special procedures in pregnancy

Amniocentesis

In amniocentesis the physician inserts a hollow needle through the abdomen and the uterine wall into the amniotic sac to withdraw a sample of amniotic fluid, which surrounds the baby in the uterus. Amniocentesis is done if there is a possibility that the baby has spina bifida (see p.654), Down's syndrome (see p.653), or some other serious genetic abnormality. If you have already had an abnormal child, if there is a family history of some abnormality, or if you are 35 years old or older, amniocentesis may be done between the 16th and 18th weeks of pregnancy. This procedure is also used to find out the level of maturity of the developing baby's lungs if premature labor (see p.636) is expected or if the baby will be delivered by cesarean section. Ultrasound (see below) is done first to learn the exact position of the baby and placenta, and your abdomen is numbed with a local anesthetic.

Tests of amniotic fluid can identify a great proportion of abnormal babies. The procedure involves a slight risk, so if terminating a pregnancy is not possible for any reason, you may not want to have the procedure.

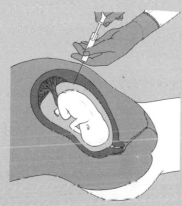

Amniocentesis, in which a sample of amniotic fluid is withdrawn from the uterus, is done if some abnormality that can be diagnosed by examination of cells shed by the baby into the fluid is suspected.

Amniocentesis coincidentally may reveal the sex of the developing child. So, if you are having amniocentesis done for some other purpose, you can ask your doctor to tell you the sex of your child in advance of his or her birth. Given this opportunity, many parents choose not to learn their unborn child's sex, feeling it somehow unnatural or less pleasurable to do so.

Ultrasound

Ultrasound is a device that transmits sound waves through body tissues, records the echoes as the sounds encounter objects within the body, and transforms the recordings into a photographic image. When used on a pregnant woman, the transmitter/recorder is moved slowly over the surface of her abdomen. The surface of the abdomen is first covered with a film of oil.

Ultrasound is a relatively new technique. As the equipment associated with it improves and those who use it learn more about how best to interpret the data it provides, ultrasound should grow in importance to medicine.

Ultrasound can already be used to measure accurately the size and shape of the fetus to help establish the stage of a pregnancy, to detect twins, to show a baby's rate of development if intrauterine growth retardation (see p.632) is suspected, to find out the position of the baby in the uterus during late pregnancy (see Malpresentation, p.637), to locate the position of the placenta if placenta previa (see p.632) is suspected, and to detect body malformations that are present in the fetus. Ultrasound is a painless procedure that does not harm either the fetus or the mother.

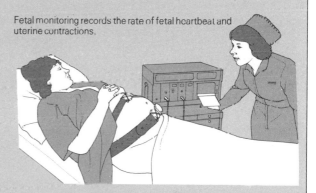

Fetal monitoring records the rate of fetal heartbeat and uterine contractions.

Fetal monitoring

This is a method used in many pregnancies to record the unborn baby's heart rate and movements and also the contractions of the uterus. These activities can be detected starting at about the 30th week of pregnancy. In the test, two flat metal recording devices linked to a monitor are strapped to the mother's abdomen. Your physician may recommend a non-stress test without drugs or a stress test in which you are given medication to start contractions. Both of these tests use fetal monitoring to predict ahead of time how the unborn baby will react to labor.

If the membranes that surround the fetus in the uterus have ruptured, an electrode may also be attached to the baby's scalp to allow more precise monitoring. Fetal monitoring is particularly helpful in cases where there are special risks for the baby. For example, monitoring may be advised if you have pre-eclampsia or eclampsia (see p.631), if *ultrasound* (see left) or other tests indicate that the pregnancy may not be normal, and also when labor is induced (see next page). Fetal monitoring is also being used more frequently when labor is expected to be normal, to detect unexpected risks to the baby that might develop. The technique gives the physician extra information about how the baby is reacting to labor. Although most pregnancies, labors and births proceed without any problems, added information should be useful in assuring a successful outcome.

Special procedures in childbirth

Induction of labor

This is deliberate initiation of labor by a physician. It is usually done when the risks of allowing the pregnancy to continue appear to outweigh the risks of induction. It is often the case in intrauterine growth retardation (see p.632) or postmaturity (see p.633). The physician first examines you internally to find out if your cervix has begun to dilate, or open. Then the doctor locates the membranes around the amniotic fluid, the liquid that surrounds the baby while it is in the uterus, and may make a small, painless cut in the membranes to drain the fluid away.

Sometimes this is enough to initiate labor. If not, a synthetic form of a hormone is slowly passed into your bloodstream by intravenous *drip*. The hormone encourages the uterus to contract as it would in natural labor. However, in about 1 in 50 inductions of labor, the uterus fails to respond to the hormone. In such cases, the baby may be delivered by cesarean section (see text, next column).

When labor is induced, the condition of the baby is watched throughout delivery by fetal monitoring (see previous page) and by frequent physical examinations. Usually labor proceeds safely to a normal delivery, but there are some slight risks involved. To avoid infection for you and your baby if labor still does not start after attempts to induce it, the baby may have to be delivered by cesarean section. There is also a chance that you will have a premature baby with the associated risks, because even the most modern methods cannot always identify the exact stage of a pregnancy.

Episiotomy

This is an incision sometimes made during labor to widen the opening of the vagina. It is often done when labor is premature, especially when a forceps delivery is necessary, because the baby's head is less than normally resistant to pressure. It may be done to avoid a tear in the vagina as the baby's head emerges from the birth canal. The cut usually is made after a local anesthetic is injected. After delivery, the cut is carefully sewn up, usually with stitches that gradually dissolve. The cut heals rapidly, although the scar may cause discomfort later, especially during intercourse.

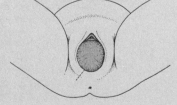

The two most common incisions (dotted lines) for an episiotomy are midline – down toward the anus – and mediolateral – to the side.

Forceps

Obstetrical forceps consist of two wide, blunt blades designed to fit around a baby's head. There are several different types, and they are used to assist delivery when, for example, your uterus is not contracting efficiently, or when the baby shows signs of asphyxia and needs oxygen as soon as possible. Forceps may be used to protect the baby's head in a breech presentation (see Malpresentation, p.637) or in premature labor (see p.636). The physician also can use them to turn the

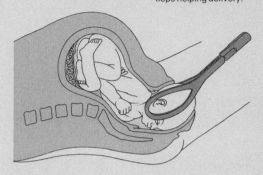

A cross-section of the birth canal, reveals forceps helping delivery.

baby's head to a more favorable position for delivery. In nearly all cases when forceps are used, you will first be given an episiotomy. The forceps are then carefully inserted into the birth canal, and the doctor pulls the baby out as gently as is possible. There are certain risks to using forceps. They range from marks on the baby's cheeks or ears that usually disappear quickly to tears or other damage to the baby or the mother.

Cesarean section

When it is impossible or unsafe for a baby to be delivered through the birth canal, a surgical incision for a cesarean section is made in the lower part of the mother's abdomen and uterus, and the baby is delivered through this instead of through the birth canal. Cesarean section is necessary if there is marked disproportion (see p.637), severe placenta previa (see p.632), unsuccessful induction of labor, signs of asphyxia in the baby, and in many cases of malpresentation (see p.637). Like any operation, this form of delivery involves some risks, so a normal vaginal birth is preferable whenever possible. Usually the mother is given a general anesthetic for the operation, but some doctors use a spinal or what is called an epidural anesthetic.

The number of cesarean sections done in the United States has been increasing in recent years. One reason for this is that women are having their first children later in life, and want to reduce the risks of late childbirth both for themselves and for their babies. Also, in general but not always, once a woman has had one baby by cesarean section, subsequent babies are delivered this way. Finally, with the new techniques of detecting potential problems of unborn babies, including fetal monitoring, more cesarean sections are being done as soon as there is evidence that the baby may be in danger.

After pregnancy and childbirth

It is easy to see pregnancy only as a preparation for childbirth and not look beyond the baby's birth. However, changes that have been taking place gradually in your body over a period of nine months are reversed after the delivery in a much shorter time. Your body is changing quite quickly while, especially if this is your first baby, you are learning how to cope with a new and demanding person. These changes can cause many women to feel depressed for the first week or two.

Before your baby was born, you probably gave some thought to whether to breast-feed or bottle-feed, and you may have received conflicting advice on the advantages and disadvantages of each. Breast-feeding has several advantages over bottle-feeding, but both arc good for the baby if done properly. Artificial milk is very similar in composition to breast milk and babies thrive on it if it is prepared in sterile containers and given in the correct quantities, but it lacks certain constituents of breast milk that are beneficial to the baby. For example, breast milk can help protect the baby against infections to which you yourself are immune. The composition of breast milk also seems to vary with the baby's needs, whereas the composition of bottled milk or formula stays constant. You can put your baby to the breast as often as he or she seems to want it, and the baby will not gain weight too quickly, but a baby may become overweight with too much bottle-feeding.

Day-to-day, there are advantages and disadvantages to each method. In most women, breast milk is always available and requires no preparation. There may be times when you need to be elsewhere at feeding time or are tired or ill. You can arrange for someone else to feed the baby either by pumping a feeding into a sterile bottle beforehand, or by substituting a bottle of formula.

Some women try breast-feeding for a few days, then give up, convinced that the baby is not getting enough nourishment. It can be difficult to develop a satisfactory routine, especially if you have never breast-fed before. A few women find that they cannot produce enough milk for their babies and have to supplement with bottle-feeding or change completely to bottle-feeding. If this happens, remember that the first few feedings will have already given your baby some immunity to infections and a good start.

About six weeks after the baby is born, you should have a postnatal checkup. Your physician examines you to make sure that your uterus and bladder are in the correct positions and that any scar tissue is healing satisfactorily. This visit also provides an opportunity to discuss any problems that you may be having in adjusting to the new baby.

Breast problems

If you are able to breast-feed your baby, it is a very good idea to do so. Breast-feeding

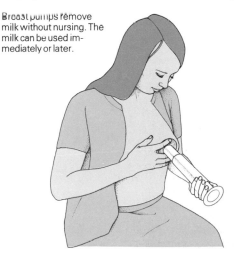

Breast pumps remove milk without nursing. The milk can be used immediately or later.

strengthens the bond between the mother and child and reduces the baby's risk of infection or salt overload. However, problems can arise to make breast-feeding difficult. Since most of these can be overcome, you should not let them deter you. Your physician will probably have advised you on care and preparation of your breasts during pregnancy. For example, an inverted nipple may have to be drawn out so that the baby can suckle from it (see Nipple problems, p.591), and you should have massaged your nipples regularly to make them supple. Even so, problems can arise during the first few weeks. They should be dealt with quickly so that breast-feeding is convenient and enjoyable.

Engorgement
In most women, the milk supply arrives quickly and forcibly a few days after delivery. The breasts become tightly swollen and sore,

and are said to be "engorged." This can also happen when you decide to stop breast-feeding and milk accumulates in the breasts. A baby cannot suckle from a swollen nipple, so some excess milk must be removed before you can breast-feed. This can be done either by hand or with a breast pump. The breasts should also be softened by bathing them in hot water. If your breasts are engorged because you have stopped breast-feeding, you should support them with a firm bra and take *analgesic* medications if necessary. After a few days the build-up of milk will prevent still more milk from being produced and your breasts will gradually become less full and less painful.

Cracked nipples

You may feel a sharp pain in your nipple when your baby is suckling, which probably means that there is a thin crack in the nipple.

This can happen if you do not dry your nipples thoroughly after each feeding. Tell your physician, who will probably recommend a soothing cream to apply to the nipple. The crack should take only a few days to heal, but in the meantime, feed the baby from the other breast.

Blocked milk duct and abscess

If you feel a small, hard lump in your breast, you may have a blocked milk duct. Try massaging the breast and bathing it in hot water. If the lump does not disappear right away, see your physician immediately. The lump may be a breast abscess (see p.590). Your physician will examine the breast and may give you *antibiotics* to treat the infection. You usually can go on feeding your baby from the affected breast. If the abscess is not caught early enough, you may have to have a minor operation to drain it.

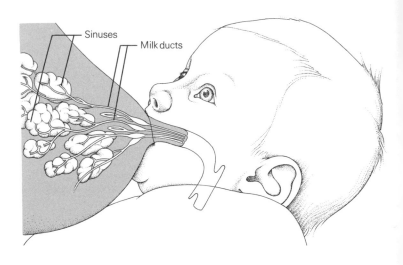

The baby's sucking stimulates milk, produced in sinuses in the breast, to flow along ducts leading to the nipple. A blocked duct may become infected, and cause an abscess.

Sinuses

Milk ducts

Puerperal fever

Puerperal fever is fever caused by an infection of the genital tract within two weeks after childbirth. Since the development of *antibiotics* and the use of *antiseptics*, puerperal fever has become extremely rare. If you have a high fever shortly after childbirth, your physician may suspect puerperal fever. If you have it, there is a slight risk that the infection can spread to the bloodstream and cause blood poisoning. It can also spread to the uterus and fallopian tubes, and cause infertility.

Samples of your blood, urine and material from your birth canal may be tested for infection. If the results show an infection, an *antibiotic* will probably be prescribed to stop the infection from spreading.

Postnatal depression

Many women feel down or miserable a few days after childbirth. This is so common that it is almost considered a normal part of pregnancy and has come to be called postnatal depression. It probably has several causes. One factor is that the sudden change in your body hormones caused by the birth can affect your mood. Also, you may have a sense of anticlimax after an event that you have looked forward to for so many months. Many new mothers are very tired, and may be a little afraid and under-confident. Postnatal depression usually goes away quite quickly with the understanding of friends and family.

It is also normal to feel mildly depressed during the first weeks of motherhood. The tiredness that is inevitable when you are looking after a new baby, the sudden change in your life style, the feeling, especially if you were working before the birth, that your horizons have shrunk, all contribute to this.

A few women do become more seriously depressed after childbirth, to the extent that they are unable to look after themselves and the baby. Such an illness (see Depression, p.297) usually starts within about a month of the baby's birth. The symptoms are tiredness, a feeling of failure and inability to cope as a mother, and quite often aggressive feelings towards the baby, possibly provoked by excessive crying (see p.651). You may lose your feelings of pride in your appearance and home. You may also withdraw from others and either lose your appetite or begin to eat compulsively.

What should be done?

It is important for a new mother to avoid becoming over-tired. Keeping your baby in the same bedroom with you is usually not recommended, because it can disturb you not only when the baby is hungry, but also when the baby moves in its sleep and makes noises while awake. You need all the sleep you can get, so you should move the baby to another room as soon as possible. This should not prevent you from hearing the baby when it is hungry. You should also arrange a shift system with your partner, so that you don't have to take care of the baby each time he or she is unsettled or distressed. Try to obtain help during the day from family or friends who are willing to do shopping for you or look after the baby while you get some rest. If you feel depressed, try to share the problems with your partner or anyone else close to you who is a good listener. Another mother with a baby can be especially understanding.

If you find that you cannot shake off your depression, and that it is coloring your whole life so that you can no longer care for yourself and your baby properly, consult your physician. He or she may prescribe an *antidepressant* drug or suggest counseling. If your depression does not respond to treatment and is very severe, the physician may suggest that you go into a hospital for treatment. If this is necessary, you and your partner should discuss who will take care of the baby and how. It is sometimes possible for you to be admitted to a hospital that has a mother and baby unit. This may be a good idea even if you feel that the baby is the cause of your illness. A separation at this stage may make it even more difficult for you to develop a close relationship with your baby.

Sex after childbirth

After a normal delivery, you should discuss with your physician when you can resume sexual intercourse. In some cases you can start intercourse a few days after the birth of a child. Most physicians prefer that you wait until the routine postnatal examination about six weeks after the birth.

Since you can become pregnant again, discuss with your physician your options if you want to avoid pregnancy. Breast-feeding and absent periods do not protect you. If you do wish to become pregnant again soon, find out from your physician the risks and benefits.

Your vagina may be extremely tender for the first ten days or so after the birth, or possibly for several weeks if you had an episiotomy (see p.640) or your vagina was torn during labor. If intercourse is painful, discontinue it for a while. See your physician again if intercourse is uncomfortable or painful after your six-week postnatal checkup. Such pain may be caused by an area of raw skin in the vagina or a stitch that has not disappeared completely. Both of these problems can be treated by your doctor.

You may find your vagina has lost some elasticity. You can tone up the muscles around your vagina that correct this by repeatedly interrupting and resuming flow in mid-stream each time you urinate.

Looking after a new baby can be extremely tiring and emotionally exhausting, and can leave you no energy for sex. Adopt the measures for avoiding over-tiredness suggested in Postnatal depression (see previous article).

Especially with a first baby, your partner may feel left out of the developing relationship between you and the child, and may need the reassurance of your continuing affection and attention. Just as he needs to realize that you are going through a difficult period of adjustment, you should make an effort to understand that he too may be feeling confused and vulnerable now that he no longer has your undivided attention. Involve him in the care of the baby and he will feel that the baby belongs to both of you. This will also give you more time to rest.

Special problems of infants and children

Introduction

Some of the problems in this section are confined to infants and children, while others can affect anybody, but require special diagnostic tests or treatment in infants or children. Also, the outlook for certain diseases is very different if they occur in the first 15 years of life rather than later in life.

The first group of articles in this section concerns special problems of newborn babies and infants up to about six months old. A newborn baby, especially if it is your first, can cause much worry. How can you tell if the child is ill? What are the signs of serious illness? Sometimes a symptom such as a skin rash, a fever, or diarrhea make it clear that the baby is unwell. At other times you will realize from changes in your baby's behavior that something is wrong, but the nature of the problem is by no means obvious. You can consult the self-diagnosis charts in Part II of this book to help you decide what to do. If your baby has a high fever, cries loudly and persistently and does not stop when picked up, or if he or she is listless or refuses to eat, call your physician. (To check your baby's development, see Milestones, next page.)

Some infants have health problems that are *congenital*, or present at birth, although they may not be discovered immediately. Such abnormalities have a variety of causes. The extent of disability from such a disorder and how the disorder is treated depends on its severity and whether or not it can be corrected.

Most of the disorders in this section are grouped according to which part or parts of the body they affect.

Nervous system and psychological disorders, as well as eye and ear problems, can have a profound effect on the child's ability to learn. Such problems interfere with either the reception or the processing of the stimuli and information that constitute the raw material used in learning.

The respiratory disorders that are included in this section are mostly common infections that account for almost half of all childhood illness. While gastroenteritis (see p.459) commonly causes digestive problems in children, the other digestive disorders included here are far less common. Like respiratory tract infections, however, they are usually easy to diagnose.

Unlike respiratory and digestive disorders, blood and urinary disorders may go undetected, because they often cause mild and varied symptoms, or no symptoms at all. Muscle, bone and joint disorders, unless they are minor, need prompt treatment.

Finally, there is a group of articles on the most common infectious diseases in children. If you think your child has one of these disorders, check the Symptom Comparison box (see p.702) or the appropriate self-diagnosis chart, and see your physician if necessary. Also, see p.698 for suggestions on how to care for a child who has one of these diseases. Nowadays, it is possible for a child to be *immunized* against most of these diseases, and you should take advantage of this protection (see Immunization schedules, p.701). An immunized child is not only safer him- or herself, but is also less likely to transmit disease and, so, safer for others to be around.

Should I have my son circumcised?

Parents often feel that their male baby needs to be circumcised to prevent disease or because they cannot pull the foreskin back over the head of the penis. If you teach your son to wash daily and keep his uncircumcised penis clean, the presence of the foreskin should not cause any risk to health. An unretractable foreskin is quite normal in a very young baby, because at birth the foreskin is still joined to the tissues of the penis, and it is only gradually that the two separate – at some time after the baby is six months old. By the time the boy is five, the foreskin should be fully retractable. It should not be forced back in order to speed up the process.

In some cases, the foreskin remains fixed, and then circumcision will be necessary. The operation is straightforward, and there are no significant risks involved. Fewer male babies are being circumcised routinely today than before. It is a matter of personal and, in some cases, religious preference.

Milestones

All children acquire mental and physical skills in much the same order. For example, a child will not stand before having learned to sit. But the rate at which these skills are acquired varies enormously, and the age given below for each milestone in a child's development is only a rough average.

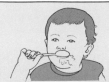

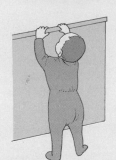

Your baby will probably be able to:

● Smile at 6 weeks

● Roll over from a sideways position on to the back at 9 or 10 weeks

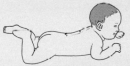

● Raise head and shoulders from a face-down position at 4 to 6 months

● Sit unsupported at 6 months

● Say simple two-syllable "words," such as "Dada" or "Mama," at 8 months

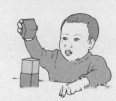

● Try to feed itself with a spoon at 8 months

● Rise to a sitting position at 9 months

● Understand simple commands at 12 months

● Stand unsupported for a second or two at 12 months

● Walk unaided at 18 months

● Make a three-brick-high tower at 18 months

● Achieve bowel control at 20 months

● Stay dry during the day at 2 years

● Talk in simple sentences at 3 years

● Stay dry through the night at 3½ years

● Get dressed and undressed (with a little help) at 4 years

● Hop, skip, and draw a figure with separate body and limbs at 5 years

For information about progress in seeing and hearing, see p.675.

Growth charts

These charts show normal heights and weights for boys (right) and girls (far right) from ages 1 to 12. Children's growth rates vary, so the charts show a normal range of height and weight for each year of growth. You can assume that your child's growth is normal if his or her height and weight fall within the shaded areas in line with his or her age.

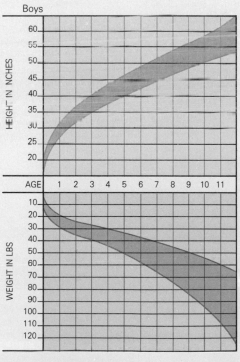

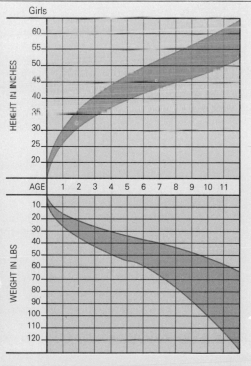

Newborn and early infants

The disorders included here most commonly affect children during the first year of life. Some, such as asphyxia and respiratory distress syndrome, occur mainly in infants who are born prematurely or who go through a difficult delivery. They are treated in the hospital. Other problems covered here, among them diaper rash and excessive crying, are extremely common and can almost always be treated at home.

Many infections that are usually not serious in adults can be much more serious in infants. Gastroenteritis, for example, usually requires special treatment. Finally, there are rare disorders such as Down's syndrome, which is caused by an abnormality in the child's chromosomes.

To see if your child is developing normally during the eventful first few years of life, see Milestones, previous page.

Asphyxia in the newborn

Some babies have asphyxia at birth – that is, they fail to breathe. The brain controls breathing, and it is failure of the baby's brain to function normally that causes the asphyxia (see Screening for congenital defects, p.630). Sometimes this is because the supply of oxygen from the mother's placenta to the baby's brain was inadequate during the stresses of labor. This may occur when the baby is undersized for the length of the pregnancy (smoking during pregnancy may cause this), or significantly overdue, or if the umbilical cord is compressed or twisted during labor.

Sometimes the brain is damaged during delivery. Also, brain function may be temporarily impaired if the mother is given a painkilling drug shortly before delivery.

What are the symptoms?
The baby fails to breathe or cry at birth. In milder cases, the baby's skin is blue and the limbs may feel quite stiff, though there may be movement in them. In very severe cases, the baby is ashen, immobile, and limp.

What are the risks?
Fewer newborn babies now need help with their breathing than before. This is because obstetric techniques have been improving steadily. However, babies born to mothers who smoked during pregnancy are more likely to be small and susceptible to asphyxia and other respiratory problems.

The risks to an affected infant are death (after about ten minutes without oxygen) and permanent brain damage (after five minutes), but these rarely occur, because obstetricians are prepared to treat an asphyxiated baby within seconds of delivery.

The risk of serious complications is higher for a home birth. This is true even when a physician is present, because, in general, only a hospital has all the equipment and personnel required to handle some emergencies.

What should be done?
In the unlikely event that you have to revive an asphyxiated newborn baby, or any baby who has stopped breathing, you should clean out any mucus from the baby's throat with your finger and then use gentle mouth-to-face resuscitation (see p.802).

What is the treatment?
Often, an obstetrician can identify a baby that is at risk for this disorder late in the pregnancy, before labor begins. Such a baby should be delivered in a hospital where full pediatric services are available. Deficiency in the oxygen supplied by the placenta is usually detected during labor, in which case the asphyxia can be prevented or minimized by an emergency delivery of the baby, perhaps by forceps or cesarean section (see p.640).

If the baby is born asphyxiated, secretions of fluid from the womb, together with mucus at the back of the baby's throat, are quickly sucked out of the baby's mouth and nose through a special tube. In mild cases of asphyxia, the baby will then gasp while inhaling oxygen, which causes the baby's brain to initiate breathing.

To treat severe cases of asphyxia, oxygen is passed into the lungs through a tube inserted into the trachea, or windpipe, and artificial respiration is initiated. The child usually begins to breathe within a few minutes. Occasionally, when the brain has been damaged during the delivery or is underdeveloped, mechanical artificial respiration may have to be continued for up to several weeks. If the baby's brain has not been deprived of oxygen for long, and action is taken immediately, asphyxia of the newborn has no after-effects.

Respiratory distress syndrome

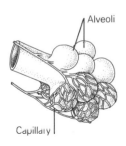

When a baby is born and takes the first breath, the alveoli (air sacs in the lungs) fill with air, and oxygen passes into the baby's bloodstream through the capillaries that surround the alveoli.

The baby in intensive care
A baby that has respiratory distress syndrome may need a mechanical ventilator to breathe properly. Neonatal intensive care units are equipped with these and other machines to treat newborn babies who have life-threatening and other extremely serious illnesses.

After a baby's first breath has expanded the lungs, the alveoli (small air sacs in the lungs) are kept open by a chemical called surfactant. This is essential, for it is at the walls of the alveoli that oxygen in breathed air enters the bloodstream and waste carbon dioxide enters the lungs to be exhaled. In other words, it is here that the major purposes of respiration are achieved.

However, in some very small, premature babies the lungs do not have enough surfactant, and the alveoli start to close up again within a few hours of birth. The baby then develops respiratory distress syndrome, which means that the child begins to have increasing difficulty in breathing.

What are the symptoms?
During the first few hours after birth, the baby's breathing becomes progressively more labored and rapid. As the baby breathes in, the chest sinks instead of expanding. On breathing out, the baby grunts.

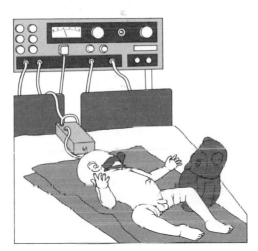

What are the risks?
The more premature a baby is, the more likely it is that respiratory distress syndrome will occur. It is very common in babies that weigh less than 1500 g (3 lb) at birth. It is also fairly common in the abnormally large babies of diabetic mothers (see Diabetes and pregnancy, p.626).

Sophisticated techniques of pediatric intensive care that have been developed in recent years have greatly improved the outlook for babies with respiratory distress syndrome, but this disorder is still a significant cause of death in premature babies.

What is the treatment?
When it is known that a birth may be premature, the adequacy of surfactant in the fetus's lungs may be determined by taking a sample of the mother's amniotic fluid (the fluid that surrounds the baby in the womb). If the surfactant is inadequate, it may be increased by giving the mother an injection of a *steroid* medication. This will not be done if the birth is imminent, because the drug takes about 24 hours to work.

A baby who has developed, or is in danger of developing, severe respiratory distress syndrome must be cared for in an *intensive care unit* specially equipped for babies. There the baby is given artificial respiration with a ventilator and the levels of oxygen, carbon dioxide, and other chemicals in the blood are carefully measured and controlled.

What are the long-term prospects?
If the baby has not suffered a serious deprivation of oxygen, the chances of normal physical and mental development are very good. In rare cases, when the baby survives a prolonged lack of oxygen, there may be permanent damage to the brain or lungs.

Neonatal jaundice

Many babies show slight jaundice, or yellowing of the skin, soon after birth. This condition usually clears up by itself within a few days. Jaundice is caused by an excess in the bloodstream of the chemical bilirubin, a normal waste product of the breakdown of red blood cells. Normally, bilirubin is removed from the bloodstream by the liver. In newborn babies, jaundice most commonly occurs when the liver is not yet functioning normally when the baby is delivered, and it, therefore, does not process bilirubin fast enough. The result is known as physiological jaundice or normal jaundice. This problem often occurs in premature babies.

In some babies, *antibodies*, which are normally protective substances, from the mother enter the baby's bloodstream and break down the baby's red blood cells. This is called hemolytic disease. The process releases an excess of bilirubin, and the baby is severely jaundiced at birth.

Another more serious type is obstructive jaundice, which is caused by the malformation or total absence of the baby's bile ducts. Bile, and with it bilirubin, cannot pass from the liver, and bilirubin builds up in the blood. Other rare causes of neonatal jaundice are neonatal hepatitis, blood disorders, and hypothyroidism (see p.526).

What are the symptoms?

In all types of jaundice, the baby's skin and the whites of the eyes turn slightly yellow. In hemolytic disease this happens within the first day after birth, in physiological jaundice after about two days, and in obstructive jaundice usually after one to two weeks. In physiological jaundice and mild hemolytic disease, the yellowness is slight and usually disappears after a few days, but in severe hemolytic disease and obstructive jaundice the discoloration grows more pronounced, and it must be treated.

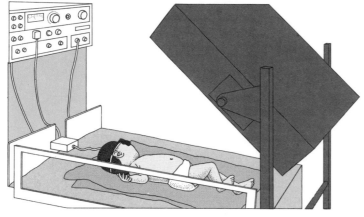

Treatment for jaundice
Rays from an ultraviolet lamp help to lower the bilirubin level in the blood. The baby's eyes will be covered to protect them from the rays.

What are the risks?

Physiological jaundice occurs in over half of all newborn babies. However, hemolytic disease is uncommon, and obstructive jaundice is extremely rare.

Jaundice carries the remote risk that a very high level of bilirubin in the blood will cause brain damage. But this almost never occurs, because once the disease has been diagnosed, the baby is treated and the level of bilirubin in the blood is checked regularly. In obstructive jaundice the blockage in the outflow from the liver will cause fatal liver damage within a few months unless it can be quickly corrected through an operation.

What is the treatment?

In most cases of physiological jaundice, no treatment is necessary. Mild cases of hemolytic disease disappear without treatment. Obstructive jaundice usually requires surgery. Otherwise, when the level of bilirubin is high, a physician may expose the baby to ultraviolet light (*phototherapy*), which helps the liver form the chemicals necessary to process bilirubin. Severe cases, especially those caused by hemolytic disease, are treated by an exchange blood transfusion, in which all the baby's blood is replaced.

Sudden infant death syndrome
(Crib death)

Sudden infant death syndrome has long been a mystery. An apparently healthy baby is laid down to sleep, and some time later dies. In nearly all cases, no explanation for the death is discovered. Research has shown that the risk of crib death is higher in the winter and may be related to immaturity of the part of the brain that controls breathing. The problem does not seem to be hereditary.

What should be done?

Losing a baby in this way can be emotionally shattering for the parents, and they generally need the comfort of relatives and friends.

Many couples find that starting another pregnancy as soon as possible helps to alleviate their grief. The reassurance of their physician that there was nothing they could have done to prevent the tragedy is extremely helpful. Psychiatric help should be sought by those who are unable to deal with their emotional problems any other way.

If an infant dies suddenly, it is essential that an autopsy be done. This may reveal the cause of the death. The information from the autopsy will be used in the research on prevention of sudden infant death syndrome, and may be used to help save future lives.

Feeding problems

Not enough mother's milk

If the baby appears to be getting an adequate amount of breast milk, but still seems to be hungry and irritable, try offering the baby a supplemental bottle of formula after the baby has nursed both breasts. If the baby takes another three or four ounces, you probably don't have enough milk and should offer a bottle. Check with your physician for further advice. He or she may be able to help if you are reluctant to stop breast-feeding.

Bottle feeding

Already prepared formula is more popular in the United States than dehydrated preparations that must be mixed with water, though both are available. Prepared formula comes in milk-based varieties and soy bean-based varieties, because some babies are allergic to cow's milk (see Lactose intolerance, p.686).

Prepare powdered and concentrated formulas exactly as specified on the container or as directed by your physician. Formula that is

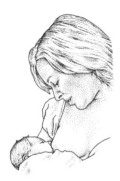

too diluted (too weak) can prevent your baby from getting enough nourishment.

Always use sterilized bottles and nipples when preparing the formula, to avoid infection (see Gastroenteritis in infants, next article). At some point in your baby's development, this precaution will probably not be necessary. Your physician can tell you when this time comes.

A baby who fusses soon after starting a bottle may be frustrated because the nipple hole is too small or clogged. If this is a problem, substitute another sterilized nipple.

Crying after and between feedings
Many babies cry for a few minutes after eating. Cuddle the baby, and if enough nourishment has been taken, the child will soon go to sleep. If the baby continues to cry, or cries a lot between feedings, it is possible that the baby has not had enough to eat. A sign of inadequate feeding is that the baby has small, firm, dark green bowel movements. Try giving the baby more. Do not worry about overfeeding. The baby knows when to stop.

Some babies cry because they are thirsty, especially in hot weather. Try giving the baby some water in a bottle.

Poor feeding
During their first few weeks, some babies start to eat actively, then drop off to sleep. When this happens, wake the baby and stimulate him or her to start eating again. The phase passes in a healthy baby, but if it continues, the baby may have an infection, and you should see your physician. Consult your physician also if your baby eats slowly for four or five days after having eaten normally.

Regurgitating after feeding
Most babies spit up a little milk, particularly when they burp. This is especially true of bottle-fed babies, because if the bottles have the wrong sized nipples the baby will swallow a lot of air. Some usually very active babies regurgitate quite a lot. This is usually nothing to worry about. Regurgitation gradually stops after solid food is introduced, when the baby is three to six months old. It usually stops completely at nine months.

Vomiting, rather than regurgitation, may be due to some disorder such as pyloric stenosis (see p.468). Check with your physician, especially if the vomit shoots some distance. This is called projectile vomiting, and it can indicate serious illness.

Gastro-enteritis in infants

When the stomach and small intestine become inflamed, a baby will have diarrhea and sometimes vomit. The disorder may be no more than a mild stomach upset, or may be a severe attack that leads to *dehydration*. Bottle-fed babies are more likely to have gastroenteritis than breast-fed babies, partly because the bottles and nipples may not be properly sterilized.

What are the symptoms?
The baby has loose, green, watery bowel movements frequently. In mild cases, the baby remains happy and eats well. In more severe attacks, the baby is miserable and irritable, eats poorly, has a slight fever, and may vomit. A baby who has as many as ten bowel movements in a day will probably become dehydrated. Signs of dehydration are a dry mouth, sunken eyes and fontanelle (the soft spot on the top of the head), lethargy, irritability, and in some cases, vomiting back all fluids. In severe dehydration, a dangerous condition, the baby's skin loses its elasticity. That is, when you pinch it between your thumb and finger, it does not immediately return to its original position. In addition, the baby refuses to eat, and may have a fever or a below-normal temperature.

Depressed fontanelle
If the soft spot on top of your baby's head seems to sink, dehydration, possibly from gastroenteritis, may have caused it. Call your physician immediately.

What are the risks?
Most cases are mild or are treated before severe dehydration can occur, and the baby suffers no ill effects. If dehydration reaches an advanced stage, it can cause brain damage or even death.

What should be done?
You can treat mild gastroenteritis yourself by adopting the self-help measures that follow in this article. But see your physician without delay if your baby has symptoms of dehydration, has three loose bowel movements in a six-hour period, and/or vomits back all feedings in a six-hour period. Once the attack is over, you should, if you are bottle-feeding your baby, make sure you are sterilizing bottles and nipples thoroughly.

What is the treatment?
Self-help: If you are bottle-feeding, cut out the baby's usual feeding for 24 hours and substitute cooled, boiled water with a level teaspoonful of sugar and half a teaspoonful of salt in each pint. On the second day, replace this liquid with the usual formula diluted to one quarter of the normal strength. Use half-strength formula on the third day, and three-quarter strength on the fourth day. During

this time, give the baby the same volume of food as usual, but feed it in small amounts every hour or so. On the fifth day, return to normal feeding.

If you are breast-feeding your baby, consult your physician for advice on how best to feed your baby when it is suffering from a mild case of gastroenteritis.

Professional help: A baby who is having a serious attack of gastroenteritis will usually have to go to a hospital. There the baby will be given special liquids to replace the lost water and vital chemicals, first intravenously and then by mouth as the baby recovers.

In most cases, the baby will return to normal and suffer no after-effects.

Diaper rash

See p.234,
Visual aids to diagnosis, 4.

Certain irritants can inflame the skin on a baby's buttocks, thighs and genitals and cause diaper rash. The irritants are chiefly chemicals in or produced by the baby's bowel movements. Most common is ammonia produced by a reaction between urine and bacteria in bowel movements. The rash this causes is called ammonia dermatitis. Another cause of diaper rash is soap or detergent left in diapers if they are not thoroughly rinsed. Most babies have diaper rash at some time, especially when they are teething. The best way to try to avoid the problem is to be sure to change diapers that are wet or soiled.

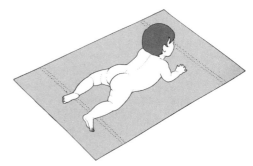

Easing diaper rash
Help to clear diaper rash by allowing your baby to spend as much time as possible with his or her buttocks exposed in a warm, dry atmosphere.

What are the symptoms?
The skin in the area covered by the diaper becomes red, spotty, sore and moist. The rash varies in severity and may smell of ammonia.

What should be done?
There are no serious risks associated with diaper rash, and it is generally a problem the parents can deal with themselves. But if the treatment described below fails to clear up the rash within a few days, see a physician.

What is the treatment?
As part of the treatment, and to ensure that the problem does not recur, sterilize and rinse cloth diapers thoroughly, and change all types promptly when they are soiled. Ordinary washing of cloth diapers is often not enough to eliminate infectious agents that originate in the baby's bowel movements, so you must sterilize the diapers. Boil them, or soak them in a solution of one of the antiseptics manufactured for the purpose. Sometimes rash is caused by fabric softeners, so these should be avoided. After washing the diapers, rinse them several times to remove all traces of soap or detergent. Using disposable diapers or a diaper service are alternative ways to make sure diapers are thoroughly cleaned and rinsed.

Babies who often get diaper rash must have their diapers changed often, especially if they have frequent bowel movements, as many babies sometimes do.

Plastic pants normally have no bearing on whether the baby gets diaper rash. If diapers are not changed often enough, however, such waterproof pants keep the rash moist, which can aggravate it.

There are several treatments for the actual rash. One is to expose the baby's buttocks to a warm, dry atmosphere. Take the baby's diaper off and lay him or her chest down, with the face turned to one side, on soft towels underlaid by a waterproof sheet. Any bowel movements or urine produced should be cleared up immediately and the rash bathed with warm water but not soap. The towels should then be changed if necessary. Afterwards, pat the affected area dry with a soft towel, and lightly sprinkle the rash with baby powder or corn starch.

You can obtain various ointments from a pharmacy to help relieve the rash. For mild rashes, use a cream that contains zinc oxide and an oil. Several rashes, particularly those aggravated by an infection, may need an antiseptic cream. Ammonia dermatitis can be relieved by using a soothing ointment that also protects against infectious agents and outside moisture. Ask your physician to recommend an appropriate preparation, and apply it liberally to all inflamed areas.

If the rash is serious or persists, see your physician, who may be able to give you more detailed practical help and a prescription ointment to speed up healing.

Seborrheic eczema

(*including cradle cap*)

See p.234,
Visual aids to diagnosis, 5.

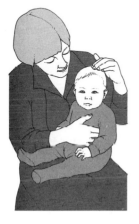

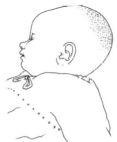

Cradle cap
The thin, dry scales of cradle cap do not bother the baby (right). They can be rubbed away gently (left) with baby oil.

This common skin disorder occurs during the first two years of life, usually during the first three to six months. The eczema occurs most commonly on the head, where it is also known as cradle cap, but it can also appear on the face, the folds of the neck, in the armpits, and in the groin.

In cradle cap, thin, dry scales appear on the scalp. Then yellow, greasy, scaly patches, which sometimes extend over the eyebrows and behind the ears, replace the initial scales. In seborrheic eczema on the face, there are small red blotches and pimples, which become redder when the baby cries, has a bath, or gets hot. Elsewhere, the eczema occurs as red, partially scaling patches.

The eczema does not bother the baby and has no effect on the baby's general health. In rare cases it becomes infected, usually because of poor hygiene. The patches become soggy, and yellowish fluid oozes out.

What is the treatment?

The disorder heals of its own accord, and there is usually no need to see a physician. Keep the affected areas clean and dry by bathing them in the normal way and drying them thoroughly. If cradle cap is unsightly, rub the scales gently with unscented baby oil. This loosens them and they can be washed away during a shampoo. Alternatively, your physician may prescribe a soothing cream. If the eczema becomes infected, your physician may prescribe an *antibiotic* cream to help clear up the infection.

For seborrheic eczema that results from diaper rash (see previous article), your physician may prescribe a mild *steroid* cream.

Be sure to consult your physician if your baby's rash and itching do not improve. Occasionally children have what appears to be an allergic reaction to various foods, clothing, infections and even vaccinations (see Infantile eczema, p.666). Together you and your physician can work to identify the irritating substance or substances and then treatment can be recommended.

Excessive crying

During the first few weeks of life the average baby sleeps a great deal but may cry loudly when fully awake. An infant who cries feebly and infrequently may be seriously ill. As the baby's awareness of his or her surroundings grows, wakeful periods without crying grow gradually longer until, at about six weeks, the baby may be awake and alert without crying for half an hour or so after some feedings. The number of quiet wakeful periods increases as the baby grows.

Babies are very different in their response and development, so there are no definite rules for how much crying is excessive. Some babies cry more than others because of differences in personality. However, some newborn babies cry for much of the time they should be sleeping, and when they are about six months old cry for much of the time they should be playing. This much crying can be termed excessive.

Much of a placid baby's contentment may come from the mother, father and whoever else is caring for the baby. In the same way, an anxious parent can transmit anxiety to the baby, who may then sleep badly and cry excessively. A vicious circle can evolve: the more the baby cries, the more anxious the parent becomes. Parents may also become angry with the baby for crying so much, which causes the baby to cry even more. Excessive crying is much more common in a first baby, because inexperienced parents may lack confidence, and communicate this to the baby. Some common explanations that are given for excessive crying are discussed below.

Colic: The word "colic" means pain. The term is often used to refer to a baby crying loudly without apparent cause. Babies with "colic" seem to be miserable and may eat poorly, act as if they have a stomach ache by drawing up their legs, and pass gas.

Infantile colic, as it is sometimes called, usually begins at two to four weeks of age. No one really knows what causes it, but the loud, continual crying of the baby can be frightening and also exhausting for the parents. In all but a few cases, colic stops by the time the baby is three to four months old.

There is no specific treatment for colic, but some babies with colic seem to do better if they sleep in a quiet room, lead a calm life, are handled very gently, and get a lot of attention from their parents. Of course, every baby, especially one with colic, should be burped thoroughly after feeding.

Teething: Babies cut their first teeth between the ages of six months and two years. Before the teeth emerge, the gums may be sore, and the baby may drool, rub the gums, and cry. Where a tooth emerges, the gum may be slightly swollen and inflamed, and the discomfort makes the baby cry. But the inflammation rapidly subsides, and even if several teeth are coming through, the baby should stop crying after a few days.

Passing urine: Sometimes a baby cries at the same time that it urinates. This leads some parents to believe that urinating is painful for the baby. In most cases, however, the crying starts a bit before the baby urinates.

In some babies who cry excessively, there is something actually wrong that needs looking after. The baby may have an infection, usually indicated by a runny nose, a cough, vomiting, diarrhea, poor eating or general *failure to thrive.* The same symptoms may also indicate a physical problem such as a hernia. Or the baby may be lonely and want comforting. This is probably the answer if the baby stops crying when you pick it up. Also, the baby may be getting unsuitable food or not enough food (see Feeding problems, p.648).

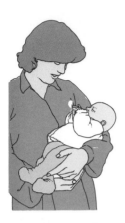

If your baby stops crying when picked up and held in your arms, the child may simply want more comfort and attention.

What should be done?

If you have made certain that your baby is not lonely, inadequately fed or uncomfortable because of a wet or dirty diaper, then you should have your physician check the child for illness. If the baby is not sick, you must realize that the baby is probably sensing and reacting to your own emotional state.

If you are tired and resentful from getting up to feed the baby at night, try to snatch a few hours of sleep during the day, while your baby sleeps. Let housework take second place to the well-being of you and your child.

Speak to other members of your family, so that they will know what is going on. Accept any offers of help, particularly from a willing spouse. If possible, treat yourself to an evening out while someone trustworthy cares for the baby. If you are breast-feeding, make sure the baby has learned to accept an occasional bottle feeding.

If you still feel under considerable strain, to the extent that you find yourself getting really angry with your baby, talk with experienced mothers or your physician at once for help in finding practical ways in which you can cope with your emotions.

Birthmarks

See p.233,
Visual aids to diagnosis, 1–3.

A birthmark is any persistent area of discolored skin that appears at birth or shortly afterwards. Discolorations that disappear a few days after birth are usually bruises brought about during labor, or forceps marks made during the delivery of the child. A birthmark may be either a concentration of tiny blood vessels in the skin called a nevus, or a discoloration on the surface of the skin called a pigmented spot.

There are three main types of nevus. A capillary nevus is a flat pink or pinkish-brown area. Most babies have many capillary nevi at birth, most of which gradually fade and disappear before the baby is 18 months old.

A strawberry nevus is a bright red, raised area up to 10 cm (4 in) across. Such birthmarks usually occur one at a time, and can occur on any part of the body. At birth a nevus is so small that it is not noticed for a few days. It grows rapidly for a few weeks, then increases in size proportionately with the baby. Occasionally, when there is fatty tissue under the nevus, the red area lies on top of a soft lump, about 1 to 2 cm ($\frac{1}{3}$ to $\frac{3}{4}$ in) above the skin. When the baby is about six months old, small, scattered white areas can be seen in the nevus. These white spots spread, gradually replacing the red tissue, and at the same time the area becomes flatter. The nevus has usu-

ally disappeared by the time the child is three, and leaves a slightly pale area of skin.

The third type of nevus is called a port wine stain, a purplish-red, often extensive and sometimes partly raised area, that generally occurs singly on the face or limbs. Generally a port wine stain persists into adult life, though it may fade slightly.

The other type of birthmark, a pigmented spot, is most commonly a flat, irregularly-shaped, coffee-colored spot. Usually there are only one or two small spots in any area, but in some cases there are many spots, large spots, or both. Pigmented spots are generally permanent. Often people consider them attractive and call them "beauty marks."

The only real problem that birthmarks may cause is disfigurement. Large, unsightly birthmarks that persist can be treated by plastic surgery or other measures when the child has reached the age of three or four (see p.260). A simple, makeshift way of dealing with a birthmark that you consider unsightly is to cover it with a special skin-colored cream that can be obtained at a pharmacy.

A large strawberry nevus occasionally bleeds, either spontaneously or if it is bumped or scratched, but pressing on the wound with a finger for several minutes usually stops the bleeding.

Down's syndrome

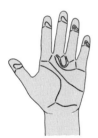

Normal hand

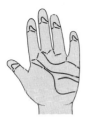

Hand of a Down's child

Before techniques for analyzing chromosomes were developed, Down's syndrome was often suspected because of distinctive crease patterns on the typically short, broad hands of an affected child.

In the normal human body all cells except egg cells and sperm cells have 46 chromosomes each (see p.704). Sometimes a child is born with 47 chromosomes in each cell. Such a child has Down's syndrome.

What are the symptoms?

Babies with Down's syndrome are recognizable at birth by their facial appearance. The eyes slope upwards at the outer corners, the face and features are small, and the tongue is large and tends to stick out. Other characteristics include a flat-backed head, sometimes a little finger curved toward the third finger, and often double-jointedness.

Children with Down's syndrome are mentally retarded (see Learning problems, p.673). But they can be happy, active participants in family life because they are responsive, loving, and even-tempered.

What are the risks?

On the average Down's syndrome affects about one or two out of every 100 babies born. But a woman is at greater than average risk of having a baby with this abnormality if she is over 35 or if she or her spouse has some rare chromosome abnormality.

When a woman of 35 or more becomes pregnant, her physician may arrange for the fetus to be tested for Down's syndrome (see Screening for congenital defects, p.630).

About a third of children with Down's syndrome also have some form of congenital heart disorder (see p.656). They also have a slightly higher than normal incidence of intestinal atresia (see p.662) and acute leukemia (see p.682). And they are particularly prone to respiratory and ear infections.

What is the treatment?

Plans for the care of a child with Down's syndrome should be discussed thoroughly with your physician at the time of birth and at frequent intervals thereafter. The best situa-

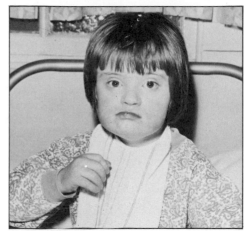

Typical facial features
Most children with Down's syndrome have upward-slanting eyes and puffy eyelids. Some- times the child's tongue protrudes slightly and the ears are abnormally shaped and set low.

tion for the child will depend on the family's emotional and financial resources. Unless parents or other family members find it a continual strain, many feel it is better to bring up a child with Down's syndrome at home rather than to send him or her to an institution. Support is often available from local social service agencies.

There are special schools or classes for children with Down's syndrome and other handicaps. These facilities are staffed by teachers trained to help such children attain their full potential.

What are the long-term prospects?

People with Down's syndrome usually can eventually be trained to do simple but useful jobs. They will always, however, need a protective environment, and they will have to be cared for either by their families or in a home for the mentally handicapped. Life expectancy is reduced if there are associated severe congenital defects.

Doubtful sex

During the first three months of pregnancy, the embryo secretes hormones (see p.514) that regulate the development of sex organs. If, for some reason, this hormone production is abnormal, then at birth the baby's sex organs will be malformed.

Minor defects in the sex organs can nearly always be corrected by surgery. But in rare cases the defect is considerably more pronounced, sometimes to such an extent that physicians are in doubt about the baby's true sex. In such cases, cells are scraped from the inside of the baby's mouth for chromosome analysis shortly after birth to find out the true sex of the child.

Once the child's sex is known for certain, plans for treatment can be made. Any necessary surgery can be carried out, usually by age two, but sometimes over a period of years, to make the appearance of the sex organs match the chromosome gender. In most cases, the surgery and any other necessary treatment assure that the child will grow up to lead a normal sex life and be able to have children.

Congenital disorders of the central nervous system

Central nervous system

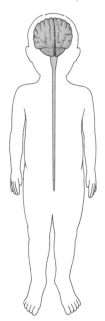

The central nervous system (described in detail on p.266) includes the brain and spinal cord. It develops in the fetus within the first two months of pregnancy, from a strip of cells running along the back of the embryo. The edges of the strip gradually curl inwards to form a tube of cells. The front part of this tube expands and forms the brain. The back part of it becomes the spinal cord. Surrounding and within the brain and spinal cord is a liquid called cerebrospinal fluid, which is produced by the brain and functions as a cushion for these delicate organs. As the bones develop, the skull and spinal column provide further protection for the brain and spinal cord.

A congenital disorder of the central nervous system is an abnormality in the brain and/or spinal cord that is present at birth. In spina bifida the spinal column and usually the spinal cord inside it are defective. In hydrocephalus, there is an excess of cerebrospinal fluid in and around the brain.

Congenital disorders of the central nervous system tend to run in families. If a couple has one affected child, or relatives who have such a child, they should discuss the risks involved in any subsequent pregnancy with a genetic counselor (see p.619).

Beginning of the spinal cord
The spinal cord begins to develop when the embryo is about 20 days old. A groove appears in the center of what will be the baby's back.

Over a few days the groove deepens and the edges curve around toward each other.

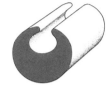

Within three days, the edges have fused and formed the tube that later develops into the spinal cord.

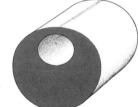

Spina bifida

In spina bifida, part of the bony spine that helps protect the spinal cord fails to develop properly. The nerves of the spinal cord in that area are exposed and unprotected and may also be defective. Usually the disorder affects the lower spine. The spinal nerves in that region control the muscles of the legs, bladder, and bowels, and a child born with the disorder will usually have some paralysis of the legs and may be unable to control the bladder and bowels. The amount of physical handicap depends on how much of a defect there is in the spine.

What are the symptoms?
The defect in the base of the spine and the consequent damage to the spinal cord varies considerably. For example, in some cases, the only visible defect may be a small dimple in the skin over the baby's spine. Other babies with spina bifida may have a large purplish-red membrane on their backs that covers a gap in the spine. In some babies the spine is also curved abnormally.

Normal spine

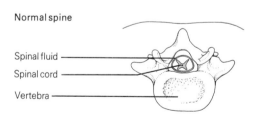

Spinal fluid
Spinal cord
Vertebra

Spina bifida

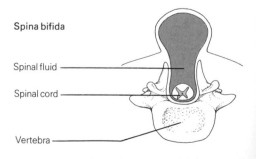

Spinal fluid
Spinal cord
Vertebra

What are the risks?

The purplish-red membrane on the baby's back is fragile, and can easily be damaged. If infection enters the cerebrospinal fluid through the damaged area, meningitis (see p.668) develops.

Infections of the bladder are common in cases of spina bifida, and these may result in kidney damage. When the baby also has hydrocephalus, which often happens, there are additional risks (see next article).

What is the treatment?

There is no cure for spina bifida. Defects in formation of the spinal cord cannot be corrected. Any paralysis will be permanent.

In many cases, an operation to repair the fragile membrane on the child's back is carried out shortly after birth. Unfortunately, little can be done to repair the defective spinal nerves.

What are the long-term prospects?

Prospects for the child with spina bifida vary considerably, according to the severity of the disorder and whether or not the child has hydrocephalus. Most children who have spina bifida will need either special braces and crutches or a wheelchair to move around. A child who has a badly deformed spine will be unable to sit up or stand, and will have to spend most of the time in a specially designed chair or bed.

From time to time, operations may be advisable to correct deformities of the legs and/or to enable a child to achieve bladder control. However, many spina bifida patients manage to achieve bladder control naturally when young.

Mentally normal children with the disorder can and should attend regular schools. This and other efforts to keep them with others will help stop them from isolating themselves.

Hydro-cephalus

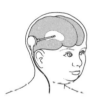

Treatment for hydrocephalus
If hydrocephalus does not clear up spontaneously, the surgeon may insert a tube, or shunt, in the child's head to drain the fluid from the brain into a vein in the neck. The tube usually remains in place for life.

The brain is bathed, inside and out, by cerebrospinal fluid. This fluid is secreted in the ventricles, or cavities, of the brain and passes into the space around the brain, where it is absorbed into a membrane that surrounds the space. If that membrane is defective in a developing fetus, or if the flow of the fluid is blocked, the fluid builds up in the cavities of the brain. The increasing pressure causes the brain to swell. To accommodate the swelling, the loosely connected bones of the skull spread apart, and the baby's head becomes larger than normal. In severe cases of hydrocephalus, also called "water on the brain," the brain is permanently damaged.

Hydrocephalus may also occur later in infancy as a result of damage to the brain from an infection or a tumor.

What are the symptoms?

Hydrocephalus may be suspected at birth if the circumference of the baby's head is significantly larger than average (35 cm or $13\frac{1}{2}$ in). If it is, the head is measured frequently for a few weeks, and if its rate of growth is excessive, X-rays and probably a CAT scan are carried out.

What are the risks?

The disorder is relatively rare and sometimes occurs in association with spina bifida (see previous article). When hydrocephalus is well advanced at birth, serious brain damage that produces extreme physical and mental underdevelopment is inevitable, and the child will probably die early from infection.

What is the treatment?

In many cases, hydrocephalus is treated surgically. The baby is given a general anesthetic and a small hole is drilled in the skull. A fine tube with a one-way valve is inserted in the hole and installed between the brain at one end and a major blood vessel leading into the heart at the other. Fluid drains from the brain into the bloodstream through this tube.

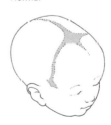
Normal

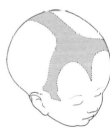
Hydrocephalic

After the operation, the size of the baby's head gradually becomes normal. During the first year the baby will need a checkup about once a month. As the child grows, the tube may become blocked, which allows pressure to build up in the brain. The child will become irritable and vomit. If this happens, see your physician immediately. The child will be hospitalized to have the blockage removed or the tube replaced.

What are the long-term prospects?

In most cases where an operation is done early, the chances of normal mental and physical development are good.

Congenital heart disorders

About 1 in every 100 babies is born with a heart abnormality of some kind. A congenital abnormality (congenital means "present at birth") may be so minor that it needs no treatment and does not affect the child's life. At the other extreme, it may be so severe that even if treatment is given immediately after birth the baby is likely to die.

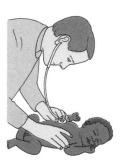

Most heart murmurs heard at birth are of no significance and do not indicate heart disease.

The development of abnormalities

The heart of a fetus starts to develop early in pregnancy and is complete by the third month. Any abnormality of development during this vital period can cause a congenital heart disorder, or possibly more than one. An abnormality may result if the mother has German measles (see p.616) or one of several other infections during early pregnancy, or if the child has defective chromosomes (see, for example, Down's syndrome, p.653). In most

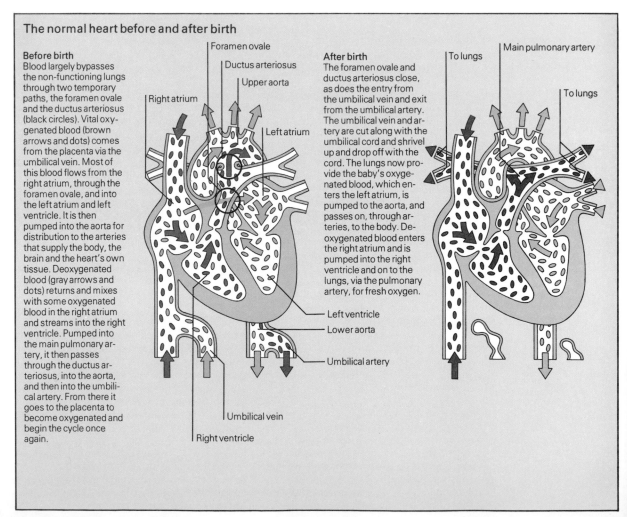

The normal heart before and after birth

Before birth
Blood largely bypasses the non-functioning lungs through two temporary paths, the foramen ovale and the ductus arteriosus (black circles). Vital oxygenated blood (brown arrows and dots) comes from the placenta via the umbilical vein. Most of this blood flows from the right atrium, through the foramen ovale, and into the left atrium and left ventricle. It is then pumped into the aorta for distribution to the arteries that supply the body, the brain and the heart's own tissue. Deoxygenated blood (gray arrows and dots) returns and mixes with some oxygenated blood in the right atrium and streams into the right ventricle. Pumped into the main pulmonary artery, it then passes through the ductus arteriosus, into the aorta, and then into the umbilical artery. From there it goes to the placenta to become oxygenated and begin the cycle once again.

After birth
The foramen ovale and ductus arteriosus close, as does the entry from the umbilical vein and exit from the umbilical artery. The umbilical vein and artery are cut along with the umbilical cord and shrivel up and drop off with the cord. The lungs now provide the baby's oxygenated blood, which enters the left atrium, is pumped to the aorta, and passes on, through arteries, to the body. Deoxygenated blood enters the right atrium and is pumped into the right ventricle and on to the lungs, via the pulmonary artery, for fresh oxygen.

Foramen ovale
Ductus arteriosus
Upper aorta
Right atrium
Left atrium
To lungs
Main pulmonary artery
To lungs
Left ventricle
Lower aorta
Umbilical artery
Umbilical vein
Right ventricle

cases, however, it is not known what causes the abnormality.

Symptoms

In many cases of congenital heart disease there are no symptoms, and the abnormality is discovered during a routine examination of the heart. In other cases, symptoms are marked. Sometimes they appear at birth, and sometimes they do not develop until childhood or much later. Symptoms are not directly related to the need for an operation; many symptomless cases require surgery to prevent trouble from occurring later in life.

A common feature of congenital heart problems is *cyanosis*, or blueness of the skin. This occurs when the abnormality has caused an excess of deoxygenated blood to circulate through the system. Mild heart failure (see p.381) in a baby may show up as difficulty in eating (because the baby must make an effort to suck and does not have enough energy to do so). This causes the baby to become underweight, and to cry less than normal. In a baby with severe heart failure, these symptoms are more pronounced. The breathing is rapid and distressed, and the baby may also have cyanosis.

Children with congenital heart disease may become breathless on exertion. Their physical development is poor, and if they have heart failure, they will be breathless even while resting, and may have cyanosis.

Heart murmurs

Diagnosis of a congenital heart disorder is most commonly made by examination with a *stethoscope.* In a perfectly healthy heart, the stethoscope picks up the sounds made when the ventricles contract and the four heart valves snap shut. Most other unexpected sounds that the heart makes are known as heart murmurs. The presence of a murmur does not necessarily mean there is an abnormality in the heart, or that the heart is seriously unhealthy. The physician can usually detect which murmurs are a sign of some abnormality and which are not. This is because each abnormality generally produces a particular type of murmur. As a result, in most cases, the doctor can tell what type of abnormality is present, before any additional testing is done.

If you have a child who has been found to have an insignificant heart murmur, you should treat that child like any other healthy child. Unless your child's physician tells you otherwise, normal activity will not do any harm at all; overprotection by the parents can be much more of a problem.

Special diagnostic tests

Once the physician has detected an abnormality, further investigations usually are carried out to find out the extent of the problem. An *X-ray* of the chest shows up certain abnormalities in the shape and size of the heart chambers. An *electrocardiogram* (*ECG*) records the electrical impulses associated with the heartbeat, and often reveals any enlargement of the chambers of the heart or abnormalities of rhythm. In addition, an *ultrasound* test is usually carried out to reveal the relative thickness of the heart chamber walls and the condition and shape of the valves. These procedures cause no discomfort, and no anesthetic is needed.

In certain cases, a test called *cardiac catheterization* is required. The baby or child is anesthetized or sedated, and a thin tube called a *catheter* is passed along a blood vessel, usually starting in a leg, until it reaches the heart. The physician watches the progress of the tube on an X-ray screen as it is manipulated through the heart and passes through any abnormal openings. The catheter also enables the physician to measure the blood pressure in each chamber of the heart, and the amount of oxygen in the blood in each chamber of the heart. Finally, an X-ray moving picture is taken while a liquid that shows up on X-rays is passed through the catheter into the heart and lungs. This procedure shows the shape and size of the chambers, valves and blood vessels.

With the information gained from these procedures, heart specialists and chest surgeons can usually diagnose the child's problem exactly and decide on and initiate an appropriate treatment.

Treatment

Most cases of congenital heart disease require an operation to correct the abnormality. Unless the disorder is so severe that it requires immediate surgery, the operation usually is delayed until early childhood, when the rate of successful correction is considerably higher than in infancy because of the greater capacity of the child's system to withstand open-heart surgery. The success rate for most heart operations on children is now high, and children who have had successful operations can, in most cases, expect to live a normal life.

When heart failure occurs in an infant, the child may need to take drugs for several years, or until surgery is possible. These drugs have two purposes: to help to strengthen the pumping action of the heart, and to reduce excess body fluid.

CONGENITAL AORTIC STENOSIS

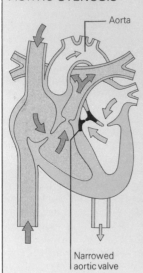

Aorta

Narrowed aortic valve

Abnormality A narrowing near the beginning of the aorta, and sometimes of the aortic valve as well, that restricts the flow of blood to the body.

Effects Usually none until later. In rare cases, the baby develops severe heart failure and *cyanosis*. The child may suffer from shortness of breath, chest pains, and blackouts. Rarely, sudden death without these symptoms can occur.

Treatment Surgery is generally performed to relieve or remove the constriction, occasionally when the child is between eight and ten, but more often when the child has grown up and is better able to withstand heart valve surgery.

CONGENITAL PULMONIC STENOSIS

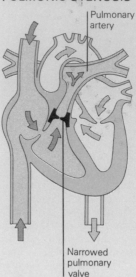

Pulmonary artery

Narrowed pulmonary valve

Abnormality A narrowing of the pulmonary valve, or, more rarely, of the upper right ventricle, that reduces the flow of blood to the lungs.

Effects Usually none. Some babies and children have shortness of breath on exertion, tire easily, and may have *cyanosis* (blueness) if the foramen ovale (see The normal heart before and after birth, p.656) is forced to reopen. In others, there may be severe heart failure.

Treatment If the stenosis is mild, no treatment is necessary. If it is moderate or severe, surgery is carried out to relieve or remove the constriction.

VENTRICULAR SEPTAL DEFECT
(*hole in the heart*)

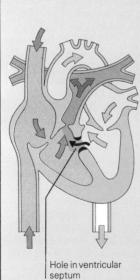

Hole in ventricular septum

Abnormality A hole in the ventricular septum, or wall, usually the upper part. Blood flows abnormally from the left ventricle into the right, sometimes in large quantities, so that excess blood passes through the lung vessels, which are served by this chamber.

Effects Most babies and children have no symptoms, but if the problem is severe, they may tire easily and have shortness of breath on exertion. Occasionally there is severe heart failure or pulmonary hypertension (high blood pressure in the lung vessels).

Treatment Usually, a small hole does not require treatment. For a larger hole, open-heart surgery is usually needed and is delayed as long as possible, often until the child is between five and ten years old. If there is an earlier danger that pulmonary hypertension may develop, a simple preliminary operation is carried out.

ATRIAL SEPTAL DEFECT

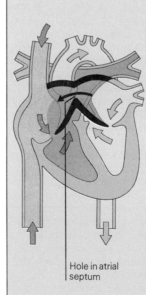

Hole in atrial septum

Abnormality A hole in the atrial septum, or wall. Blood passes from the left atrium into the right, sometimes in large amounts, so that excess blood circulates through the lungs. The hole rarely closes without treatment.

Effects Most babies and children have no symptoms, or they may tire easily and have shortness of breath on exertion. If the disorder is not detected and treated in childhood, pulmonary hypertension may develop in late adolescence or in adulthood.

Treatment Except when the hole is very small and there is, therefore, no danger that pulmonary hypertension will develop later, an operation is necessary to repair the defect. The operation is usually performed when the child is between five and ten years old.

COARCTATION OF THE AORTA

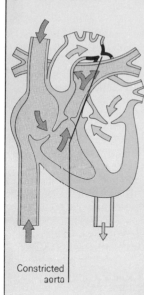

Constricted aorta

Abnormality A localized narrowing of the aorta that reduces the supply of blood to the lower part of the body.

Effects In some cases there are no symptoms. In others, symptoms such as headaches, weakness after exercise, weak or absent pulses in the groin, and sometimes coldness in the legs, appear in early childhood. These symptoms are caused by high blood pressure above the narrowed area and low blood pressure below it. In a few cases, when the aorta is extremely constricted, severe heart failure (see p.381) occurs.

Treatment Surgery is necessary in all cases, even when there are no symptoms. The constriction is removed and the two parts of the aorta are rejoined. The surgery is usually done when the child is between four and eight years old.

FALLOT'S TETRALOGY

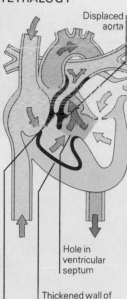

Displaced aorta

Hole in ventricular septum

Thickened wall of right ventricle

Narrowed pulmonary valve

Abnormalities Four abnormalities occur together: a hole in the upper ventricular septum, a displacement of the aorta to the right, so that blood from both ventricles enters it; pulmonary stenosis (see previous page); and a thickening of the right ventricle's wall.

Effects From birth, or shortly afterwards, *cyanosis* (blueness of the skin, particularly the lips), clubbing of the fingers and toes, and underdevelopment occur. After exercise the child is short of breath and squats to relieve discomfort.

Treatment Surgery to correct all the abnormalities usually should be carried out before the child is five.

PATENT DUCTUS ARTERIOSUS

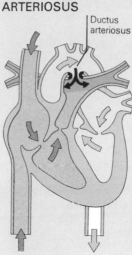

Ductus arteriosus

Abnormality The ductus arteriosus, an extra blood vessel in the heart before birth, fails to close after birth. Blood from the aorta continues to flow through it into the pulmonary artery, so that excess blood passes through the lung vessels.

Effects Usually there are no symptoms. In a few cases, the child has shortness of breath on exertion, frequent respiratory infections, and/or *cyanosis*, or blueness of the skin, particularly the lips.

Treatment In some cases, if the diagnosis is made early, the defect can be closed with a drug treatment. In most other cases, if there are no complications, a simple operation to close the duct can be carried out before the child is five years old.

TRANSPOSITION OF THE GREAT VESSELS

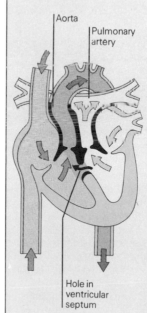

Aorta

Pulmonary artery

Hole in ventricular septum

Abnormality The aorta and pulmonary arteries are transposed, so that oxygenated blood from the lungs passes through the pulmonary artery and back to the lungs, instead of through the aorta and to the tissues. Unless there is a hole in the septum or some other passageway that allows some oxygenated blood to pass into the right side of the heart and the aorta, the baby will not survive.

Effects From birth, the child has *cyanosis*, clubbing of the fingers and toes, and underdevelopment.

Treatment In all cases an emergency procedure to create a larger hole in the septum is performed before the baby is three months old. This is done by inserting a tiny tube into the heart through a vein. In a second operation, performed before the child is five years old, the surgeon creates two artificial blood vessels which restore the circulation to normal.

Congenital disorders of the digestive system

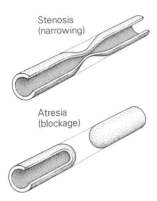

Stenosis (narrowing)

Atresia (blockage)

The digestive tract (described on p.434) is a continuous tube that digests food, absorbs nutrients from it, and eliminates what remains as waste matter. The glands connected to the tract include the salivary glands and the pancreas, which produce digestive juices, and the liver, which provides bile to aid in digestion and absorption of food (see Liver, gallbladder, and pancreas, p.485).

While it is still in the womb, the baby receives all its nutrients from the mother through the placenta and umbilical vein. It is only after birth, when the baby must start to eat, that the digestive tract is required. Any malformations of the digestive system that occurred during development, therefore, affect the baby only after birth.

The system is affected mainly by two kinds of malformation. The first is stenosis, a narrowing of a tube or duct, sometimes almost to the point of closure. The second is atresia, a gap in a tube or duct that separates it into two distinct, sealed-off sections. Why these malformations occur is not known.

Any serious abnormality in the digestive tract will affect the baby's capacity to digest and absorb food, but there are also more immediate dangers. For example, with disorders that cause vomiting there are two serious risks. One is that the baby may inhale the vomit, which can lead to choking or pneumonia, both of which can be fatal. The other is that the baby's failure to retain liquids can lead to severe *dehydration*, which can also be fatal.

The most common congenital disorders, those present at birth, of the digestive system are described in this section. They can all be treated by surgery, which has a high success rate except in the case of bile duct atresia. An infant is prepared for an operation by having the stomach washed out and by being fed with *intravenous fluid* to keep the digestive tract empty and to maintain the correct balance of water and chemicals in the body. The baby generally recovers from a successful operation within 48 hours. Usually, the baby is home within a week.

Congenital pyloric stenosis

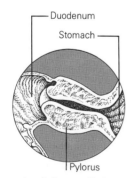

Duodenum

Stomach

Pylorus

In pyloric stenosis, the walls of the baby's pylorus are thickened, which obstructs the flow of milk from the stomach to the intestine.

The pylorus is a short muscular tube that connects the stomach to the duodenum, the first section of the small intestine. In pyloric stenosis, the muscular wall of the tube thickens, and the passageway inside narrows. As a result, little or no milk can pass from the stomach into the intestines and the baby does not get enough nourishment. The cause of this disorder is not known.

What are the symptoms?
Between two and eight weeks after birth the baby begins to vomit violently after feedings. The fierce stomach contractions made by the baby to force food through the narrowed pylorus are unsuccessful. Instead, food is forced up the esophagus, or gullet, and out of the mouth, sometimes spurting out as much as several feet away. This is called "projectile vomiting." Usually, the vomit contains a lot of milk curds and mucus and smells unpleasant. Initially the vomiting does not interfere with the baby's well-being or desire to eat. However, the baby soon begins to lose weight and becomes anxious and restless. Then, the baby eats reluctantly and becomes listless, because the constant vomiting upsets the delicate balance of body chemicals.

What are the risks?
Pyloric stenosis is more common in male than female babies and in first-born boys than in other boys. It also tends to run in families.

If the disorder is not treated, it can lead to death from starvation. In addition, there are the risks, such as *dehydration*, that are sometimes associated with vomiting.

What should be done?
If your baby is vomiting in the way described, contact your physician immediately. If pyloric stenosis is suspected, the physician will probably examine the baby and then ask you to feed the baby. During the feeding, the doctor will watch the baby's abdomen, looking for the violent contractions that are a symptom of pyloric stenosis. The contractions resemble a golf ball traveling from left to right beneath the surface of the skin. The physician will feel for the swelling of an enlarged pylorus. Several examinations, or even a *barium swallow*, may be necessary before the diagnosis can be confirmed.

You may hear the physician refer to the enlarged pylorus as a pyloric tumor. But there is no cause for alarm; the word "tumor" used in this context is unrelated to cancer.

What is the treatment?
Self-help: Until surgical treatment is obtained, feed the baby more often than usual, but reduce the volume of each feeding, so less undigested food is in the stomach.

Professional help: Relatively simple surgery is the treatment for this disorder. If the stenosis is severe, the baby will be operated on immediately. Sometimes, in mild cases, the baby is treated with drugs that are given before each feeding to relax the tightened pylorus and build up the baby's strength before the operation.

The surgeon makes a deep incision along the outside of the swollen pylorus. This immediately allows the pyloric canal to expand enough to allow food to pass through. After the operation, the amount of the baby's feedings is gradually increased until, within 48 hours, feeding becomes normal.

What is the long-term outlook?
The success rate of the operation is almost 100 per cent. The baby has no further feeding problems, and the ailment produces no after-effects either in childhood or later in life.

Esophageal atresia

In this disorder, part of the esophagus (food tube, or gullet) is missing. The top part, which leads from the mouth, is a dead-end, and there is no passageway into the baby's stomach. As a result, at birth the baby cannot swallow secretions from its mouth and nose, and instead they may enter the windpipe and partially block it.

What are the symptoms?
The blockage hinders the baby's breathing. There are continual bubbling noises in the throat, and sometimes the baby's skin turns blue from lack of oxygen. When the physician removes the secretions with a suction tube, the symptoms vanish, but they return as soon as the secretions build up again. When the baby eats it may cough, gag, or sputter. A baby with this disorder should not be given food or liquids by mouth. Special feeding techniques, which are available only in the hospital, are used to provide nourishment until the condition is treated.

What should be done?
If your child has any of these symptoms consult your physician, who may check for esophageal atresia by trying to pass a soft tube down the baby's esophagus.

What is the treatment?
Surgery is performed in one or more stages to open up and join the two separate sections of the esophagus. This procedure generally clears up the problem, and your physician will be sure to check for any other problems associated with this disorder.

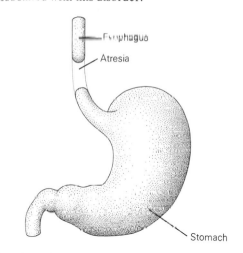

Esophagus

Atresia

Stomach

The only cure for esophageal atresia is an operation to join the separated parts.

Bile duct atresia

Bile, a liquid made in the liver, is responsible for many essential processes in the body, among them carrying a chemical compound called bilirubin from the liver into the intestine (see Neonatal jaundice, p.647). The bile travels through a series of tiny ducts in the liver and then through larger ducts outside the liver. The ducts outside the liver join to form the main bile duct that leads to the duodenum (part of the small intestine). Very rarely, a baby is born with parts of the bile ducts missing. Bile is trapped in the child's liver and escapes back into the bloodstream. This is bile duct atresia.

What are the symptoms?
There is prolonged jaundice, or yellowing of the skin, which usually starts during the second week of life. The baby may also have pale bowel movements and dark urine.

The jaundice is similar to that of neonatal hepatitis (see Neonatal jaundice, p.647), and it may be difficult to tell which of the two disorders the baby has.

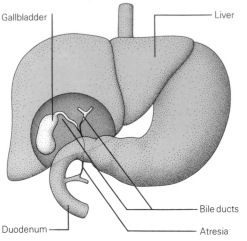

Gallbladder

Liver

Duodenum

Bile ducts

Atresia

Atresia in the bile duct below the gallbladder can be cured by joining the gallbladder to the duodenum and bypass-ing the lower part of the main bile duct. Atresia higher up the bile duct is harder to treat.

What is the treatment?

If atresia seems likely, a surgeon will carry out an operation called a laparotomy, which is performed when the baby is a few months old if possible. The inside of the baby's abdomen is examined, and if there is atresia of the ducts outside the liver, it is possible in some cases to enable bile to flow from the liver to the intestine by joining the gallbladder to the duodenum. If this procedure is not successful, cirrhosis of the liver (see p.487) will develop and cause death in early childhood.

If the bile ducts outside the liver appear normal in surgery, a small piece of liver is removed. Examination of the fragment under a microscope will show whether the baby has hepatitis (see p.687), which will eventually get better by itself in most cases, or atresia of the small bile ducts in the liver, for which there is no successful treatment. A child who is born with this type of bile duct atresia will probably succumb to cirrhosis of the liver within a year or two.

Intestinal atresia and stenosis

In the condition called intestinal atresia a baby is born with one or more parts of the small intestine missing. In intestinal stenosis part of the upper intestine is narrowed almost to the point of closure.

What are the symptoms?

A baby with either of these problems begins to vomit green within a few hours of birth. The green substance is bile, a liquid that is produced in the liver and passed into the intestine, mainly to help in digestion. The vomiting continues at intervals, and the baby's abdomen swells as gas accumulates in the intestine. Also, the child will have no bowel movements. There are two other disorders that have similar symptoms: cystic fibrosis (see p.685) and Hirschsprung's disease (see next article). Diagnosis of all these disorders may be aided by an *X-ray*.

What is the treatment?

For either of these disorders, an operation must be carried out right away. In atresia, the surgeon opens up and joins together the separate parts of the intestine. In stenosis, the surgeon widens the constricted intestine. The results of early surgery are generally excellent, and the baby usually does not have any long-term problems.

If surgery is delayed too long, the chances of its success are reduced. It is possible that the baby may even die before the operation can be performed.

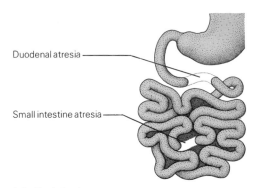

Duodenal atresia

Small intestine atresia

Intestinal atresia
When a baby is born with intestinal atresia, more than one part of the intestine may be affected, for example, the duodenum and a lower part of the small intestine.

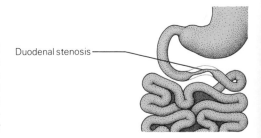

Duodenal stenosis

Intestinal stenosis
The upper intestine can be narrowed, at the duodenum for example, to such an extent that surgery to widen the intestine is needed as soon as possible.

Hirschsprung's disease

(congenital megacolon)

To produce bowel movements, the large intestine contracts and pushes its contents toward the rectum. In a few babies the lower parts of the large intestine, including the rectum, have no nerve cells to start the necessary contractions, and because they do not function normally they are narrow and rigid. This condition, which is called Hirschsprung's disease, causes severe constipation.

What are the symptoms?

Apart from noticing that the baby's bowel movements are infrequent and hard, the child's parents or physician will see that the baby's abdomen is swollen and tight. In a few cases, vomiting begins a few hours after birth (see previous article).

Diagnosis of the disease is confirmed by a *barium enema* and a *biopsy* of the rectum. In the biopsy, a small section of the rectum is removed and examined.

What is the treatment?

An operation is carried out to remove the affected part of the intestine and sew together the normal sections. The operation has a high success rate, and the long-term outlook for the child is good.

Imperforate anus

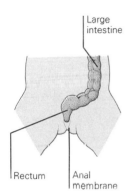

Large intestine

Rectum   Anal membrane

The anal canal is the final section of the digestive tract before the anus, the opening through which bowel movements pass to the outside. Some babies are born with the canal imperforate, or closed. Either there is a membrane stretching across the canal, or, in rare cases, the canal fails to develop and the digestive tract ends at the rectum with no connection between the rectum and the anus.

What are the symptoms?

Examination of the baby after birth will reveal the presence of the membrane across the canal. However, if the canal did not develop at all the problem is harder to detect. This condition should be suspected if, within 12 hours after birth, the baby has not, as is normal, passed a green-black substance, called meconium, which accumulates in the intestine. The diagnosis is confirmed when a finger or catheter inserted into the anus meets a blockage – the end of the rectum.

What is the treatment?

Surgery is necessary to remove the membrane or to open up the end of the rectum and join it to the anus. The operation is usually successful, and the long-term outlook is good unless the muscles of the baby's anus are weak. In such cases, the child will have either severe constipation with bowel movements of normal hardness, or poor bowel control with soft bowel movements. The child may then need an operation called a colostomy (see p.482), in which the surgeon creates a kind of artificial anus in the abdominal wall.

Dia-phragmatic hernia

The diaphragm is a large sheet of muscle that separates the chest from the abdomen and plays a major role in breathing. Some babies are born with an opening in the diaphragm, through which part of the intestine may protrude into the chest. When this happens, the child has a diaphragmatic hernia (for general information on hernias, see p.537). With this problem, the intestine can compress the lungs and make the baby breathless. This usually creates an emergency situation when the baby is delivered. The disorder is diagnosed by a chest *X-ray*.

What is the treatment?

Once X-rays have confirmed the diagnosis, surgery is performed immediately. During the operation, the chest is opened up, and the intestine is pushed into the abdomen, and the opening in the diaphragm is sewn up. The operation is usually completely successful, if it is done soon enough.

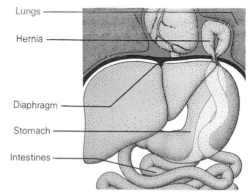

Lungs

Hernia

Diaphragm

Stomach

Intestines

Risks of diaphragmatic hernia
In congenital hernia of the diaphragm, part of the intestine protrudes through the diaphragm and presses on a lung (usually the left lung). This causes breathing difficulties. In severe cases, the baby may also turn blue. The usual treatment is an operation to reposition the intestine and repair the diaphragm.

Congenital disorders of the skeleton

The four defects included here, which are dislocation of the hip, club foot, and hare lip and cleft palate (covered together), can all be inherited but often result from an uninherited abnormality in development before birth. If the defect is slight, the baby's general health will not be affected. If it is more severe, the child will have difficulty in learning to walk or, in the case of hare lip and cleft palate, in learning to speak. Feeding problems can also result from hare lip and cleft palate. For these reasons, and because of the psychological strain on a child who must cope with such a handicap, all these disorders should be treated within the child's first few years, if possible. In the case of a dislocated hip, however, the problem may not definitely be diagnosed until later in life.

As with any deformity, special care for the child's emotional well-being may be required. If there seems to be any psychological distress, professionals who deal with such matters should be contacted. The same is true if a parent or any other family member has emotional difficulty in dealing with the child's defects. Your physician can put you in touch with the appropriate professional people to help you with such problems.

Congenital dislocation of the hip

Some babies are born with the ball-shaped head of a thigh-bone lying outside its cup-like socket in the pelvis. This is dislocation of the hip. Also, the socket is shallow and poorly formed. One or both hips may be affected. The cause of the condition is not known, but about 1 baby in 60 is born with a suspected hip dislocation. The disorder runs in families, and it occurs with much greater frequency in girls than in boys.

What are the symptoms?
When the physician manipulates the newborn baby's hip joints as a routine test, a clicking is usually heard or felt if the baby has a dislocated hip. However, clicking can also be made by movements of the ligaments, and in a few cases a congenital dislocated hip cannot be diagnosed with certainty, even after several tests.

What is the treatment?
In most cases, tests will confirm a diagnosis of dislocated hip and the physician will put splints on the baby's thighs.

The splints must usually be worn for six to nine months if they are to do their job properly. The doctor will tell you of any special care that may be required because of the temporary problems the splints may cause.

In cases when the problem is not detected until childhood, the child must have one or more operations to correct the dislocation. The patient must be hospitalized and is given a general anesthetic.

After the operation, plaster casts are put on the child's legs and must remain on them for several months. This may be a particularly trying time for the child, since the casts can be extremely restrictive and uncomfortable for a normally active youngster.

What are the long-term prospects?
If it is corrected early, the defect is often completely cured and the child is able to walk normally and suffers no adverse effects in later life. A child whose dislocation must be corrected surgically may have permanent problems in walking.

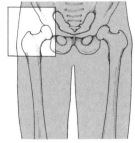

Normal hip joint
In a normal hip joint the ball at the top of the thigh bone fits neatly into the socket in the pelvis.

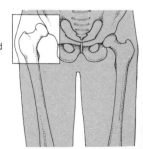

Dislocated hip joint.
In a dislocated hip joint the ball at the top of the thigh bone is not nestled into the socket.

Club foot
(talipes)

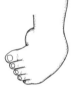

A baby with club foot is born with one or both feet bent either downwards and inwards or upwards and outwards. Many babies with normally-formed feet persistently turn them inwards, but they can be pushed back to the proper position. In club foot this is not possible. The problem sometimes runs in families.

At one time, a club foot often meant a lifelong handicap, but today nearly all cases are detected at birth and treated, and the child eventually walks normally.

What is the treatment?
If the defect is only slight, the physician will show the baby's parents how to manipulate the foot regularly each day until it settles into a normal position. In more pronounced cases, as much correction as possible is done by manipulation, then either splints or plaster casts are put on the affected foot to keep it from moving back to its former position. Periodically, the splints or casts are removed, the foot is manipulated further back toward the normal position, and new splints or casts are put on to hold it in the new position. This is repeated for a year or more, until the foot is normal.

In severe cases of club foot, the child must be hospitalized and surgery performed to correct the deformity.

Hare lip and cleft palate

A hare lip is a vertical split in the upper lip. It may be partial, or extend all the way to the base of the nose. In some children with a hare lip, the nose appears to be flattened. Sometimes there are two splits, affecting both sides of the lip. In some people with hare lips, the gap is continued down the upper jaw. This gap, called a cleft palate, runs along the midline of the palate and extends from behind the teeth to the cavity of the nose. It makes eating and swallowing difficult. In newborn infants it can be particularly troublesome, for it may make any regurgitated milk come through the nose instead of through the mouth.

Unless it is treated, a hare lip usually causes psychological distress because of its appearance. An uncorrected cleft palate later causes serious speech difficulties (see Learning problems, p.673).

These defects sometimes run in families, and may affect several children of the same parents. In most cases, the reason for the defect is unknown.

What is the treatment?
An operation to repair the abnormality is carried out when the baby is older. From birth until the time of the operation, treatment varies according to the severity of the problem. Many babies need no interim treatment, because they can eat quite well. However, some bottle-fed babies may need a larger than normal hole in the nipple, or may have to be switched to spoon feeding. The baby usually stops regurgitating milk through the nose naturally after a few weeks.

In severe cases of cleft palate, a special plate may have to be fitted on the roof of the baby's mouth before each feeding. A special brace may also be fitted on the upper gum if the gum is misaligned in the region of the mouth around the clefts.

Plastic surgery (see p.260) can be performed on a hare lip when the baby weighs about 4.5 kg (10 lb), usually at 10 to 12 weeks old. If the nose appears to be flattened, it will require additional plastic surgery later. A cleft palate can be repaired by an operation when the baby is about a year old, preferably before the child learns to speak. For each operation, the baby is hospitalized, usually for about five days, and given a general anesthetic for the surgery.

These operations usually improve the child's appearance and allow the develop-

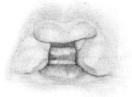

Hare lip
A hare lip can vary in severity from a small notch in the upper lip to a split extending to the nose.

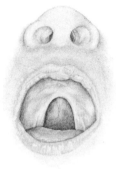

Cleft palate
A cleft palate can be an extension of a hare lip or it can occur without any corresponding damage to the lip.

ment of normal speech. If a speech defect does develop, speech therapy may be helpful. Your physician can probably help you find a good speech therapist.

Skin

Many skin problems that adults get can also affect children (see Skin, hair and nail disorders, p.250, for a general description of these problems). The two disorders discussed here occur mainly in children. Infantile eczema is an allergic reaction (see Allergies, p.705) and while it is not a serious condition, it may signal that the child will develop other allergies later in life.

Because infantile eczema results from an inborn sensitivity to certain foods or substances, it is not contagious, or catching. Ringworm, on the other hand, is a fungus infection and is extremely contagious.

Infantile eczema

See p.234, **Visual aids to diagnosis, 6.**

Infantile eczema (also called infantile atopic dermatitis) is a red, scaling, sometimes weeping, skin condition. It is a form of allergy (see p.705), and is not contagious.

What are the symptoms?
In mild cases, the skin is only slightly dry, red and scaly, and the rash only appears in small areas, particularly over the cheeks. In severe cases, the rash is more obvious and covers a greater area. In very severe cases, the rash almost covers the body.

Little red pimples appear, and as the baby scratches them, they begin to weep and join together to form large weeping areas that become encrusted.

What are the risks?
If the eczema weeps, infection may occur, particularly in the diaper area. Also, many infections that affect the skin, such as chickenpox (see p.700), can be unusually severe in children with eczema. Certain immunizations can produce widespread blistering on the skin affected by eczema, and should be postponed until treatment has reduced the rash. Certain vaccinations such as the one for smallpox should not be given to babies with infantile eczema. Consult your physician if your child is exposed to recently vaccinated persons or someone who has chickenpox or measles.

What should be done?
Mild forms of the disorder require no treatment other than applications of petroleum jelly or olive oil. For more severe cases, you should consult your physician.

What is the treatment?
Self-help: If your baby has more than a mild form of infantile eczema, try to prevent the child from becoming too hot from wearing too many clothes. Make sure that clothes in direct contact with the baby's skin are made of cotton. Do not use anything on the child's skin without first consulting your physician.
Professional help: If the baby itches badly, the physician will probably prescribe an *antihistamine*. Severe phases of the disorder are treated with *steroid* ointments or creams.

In some children infantile eczema disappears after a few months. In others, the condition comes and goes for several years. Most children outgrow the disorder by puberty.

Ringworm

See p.237, **Visual aids to diagnosis, 20 and 21.**

Ringworm is not a worm. It is a fungus called *Tinea* that infects the skin and causes scaly, round, itchy patches to develop. It usually affects the scalp, the trunk, or the feet.

When ringworm affects the scalp, bald patches develop. The skin on these patches flakes and itches. Ringworm on the trunk starts as a small, round, red patch that is scaly and itchy. The patch gradually grows bigger until it is 2 to 3 cm (about 1 in) across. As it gets bigger, the central area heals, and leaves a red ring on the skin. After a week or two, other patches may appear nearby.

Ringworm is infectious and can even be caught from a pet dog or cat with a similar condition. Generally speaking, it is not a serious condition, but it can be unsightly.

Take your child to a physician as soon as the symptoms appear. For all forms of ringworm, the doctor will usually prescribe an ointment containing a *fungicide*, to be applied at least twice daily to the affected areas. If the ringworm is on the scalp, or if the fungus is present on the trunk and is very severe, a syrup containing a strong antifungal agent may also be prescribed.

Any child with ringworm should stay away from school until the condition has been treated. You should get rid of any combs, hairbrushes or hats the child has used.

Nervous system and psychological disorders

The first three disorders discussed here are caused by an abnormality or disturbance in the nervous system (for a general description see Brain and nervous system, p.266). Three psychological disorders are also included here. They range in severity from sleeping problems, which are usually no cause for concern, to autism, which is a serious disorder and may require extensive treatment and special education.

If you are worried about your child's mental progress, consult the Milestones chart (see p.645) and read the article on learning problems (see p.673).

Convulsions in children

A convulsion is a fit, or seizure, caused by abnormal activity in nerves in the brain. Convulsions occur more often in children than in adults, because a child's developing brain is more sensitive to disturbances than the fully-grown brain of an adult.

The causes of convulsions in children vary. In most cases the cause is either unknown (idiopathic epilepsy) or related to a fever caused by a minor infection (febrile convulsion). However, convulsions may also occur in children with brain damage, cerebral palsy (see p.669), a brain tumor (see p.282), or meningitis (see next article). Alterations in body chemistry, such as those that occur when a diabetic child receives too much insulin (see Diabetes mellitus, p.519), can sometimes cause convulsions as well.

What are the symptoms?
Grand mal convulsion (also called a major seizure): This is the most common type of convulsion. The child suddenly falls to the ground unconscious, with arms and legs held stiff. After 30 seconds or so, the arms and legs, and sometimes the face, start to twitch or jerk rhythmically, often violently. The fit usually lasts for about two to three minutes, and during this time the child may urinate and, more rarely, have a bowel movement.

During the next few minutes, the child slowly regains consciousness, and is then irritable and complains of a bad headache. Soon the child falls deeply asleep, and sleeps for several hours. On waking, he or she is back to normal. Most febrile convulsions are grand mal convulsions.

One or two short-lived grand mal convulsions are extremely unlikely to be harmful, but several prolonged attacks of this kind can lead to brain damage.

Petit mal convulsion: This minor convulsion, which can occur as frequently as 20 times in one day, is often mistaken for daydreaming. The child suddenly becomes motionless, and stares ahead vacantly for a few seconds. Occasionally, he or she may totter or fall. After the convulsion the child is usually unaware of what has happened.

Nearly all children who suffer from petit mal convulsions grow out of them. A small minority do not, and will need to take drugs indefinitely to prevent the seizures or reduce the number of seizures.

Psychomotor convulsion (also called a *temporal lobe attack*): For no reason, the child suddenly starts acting violently, or laughing or crying for no reason. The convulsion, which occurs at infrequent intervals, lasts for a few minutes. Afterwards the child does not know what he or she has been doing.

Psychomotor convulsions may well continue into adult life, and if they do, drugs will be required indefinitely in order to control the seizures.

Infantile spasms: With a sudden jerk, the baby or child doubles up at the waist for only a second. This type of convulsion, which occurs several times each day, first appears at about three months old and, in a few cases, continues for several years.

What are the risks?
Convulsions tend to run in families, and are more common among mentally retarded children or children who have cerebral palsy. Convulsions are often a cause of great concern to parents, but most of them do not harm the health of the child in any way. The most serious risk is that a prolonged grand mal convulsion may result in brain damage, which will appear as mental retardation (see p.673) and/or possibly cerebral palsy (see p.669).

What should be done?
A child who has a convulsion for the first time should be seen by a physician as soon as possible. If any convulsion lasts for more than five minutes, immediate medical care is essential. If a child has a grand mal convulsion,

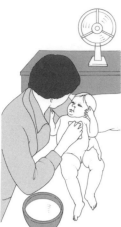

Avoiding febrile convulsions
A child who has had previous convulsions caused by a fever may have them again if he or she has another fever. Try to keep the child cool, using a sponge soaked in tepid water.

lay the child on his or her side. Do not attempt to restrain movements or to force anything between the teeth to prevent tongue biting, which is rare. For other types of convulsions, simply move aside any possibly harmful objects. Try to notice and remember the details of any convulsion to help the physician make a diagnosis later.

All first convulsions (except a first febrile convulsion, if the cause is known to be a fever) should be followed by investigative medical tests. The more severe the convulsion, the more likely it is that the child will be hospitalized for more extensive tests. These tests may include a thorough physical examination, an *electroencephalogram* (*EEG*), a skull *X-ray*, a *CAT scan*, and/or *cerebral angiography*, a specialized X-ray that shows the blood vessels in the brain.

What is the treatment?
Self-help: If your child has an infection, and has had a previous febrile convulsion, take steps to rapidly reduce the child's temperature and avoid a possible recurrence of the convulsion. Give the child a fever-reducing medication approved by your physician, and inform your physician of the fever. Take the child's temperature every two hours. If it is above 100°F (38°C), remove the child's upper clothes, sponge the face and upper body with tepid water, and set an electric fan going to keep air moving and thus aid in the evaporation of perspiration. This will cool the child's body.

Professional help: If the underlying cause of convulsions is discovered to be a brain tumor or meningitis, treatment will be for the underlying disorder. Convulsions caused by cerebral palsy or brain damage, and febrile convulsions that recur, are treated with drugs, which the child may need to take indefinitely to control the convulsions.

Depending on the frequency and type of convulsions, the physician will prescribe one or more drugs, starting with a low dose and increasing the amount until the convulsions are controlled. If side-effects occur, different combinations of drugs will be tried. Blood tests may be done to help adjust the dosage. Frequent visits to the physician will be required during this period. It is important that the child take the medications regularly as directed, and that the parents continue to work with the physician to help the child.

It is wise to inform a child's teachers about recurrent convulsions. If the child must take medication during the school day, most schools require written authorization from the child's parents to give it.

Once the frequency of convulsions has been decreased by drugs, the child should be encouraged to take part in normal activities. Supervision should be provided, but the child should not be made to feel self-conscious

In some cases, if a child under drug treatment has been completely free of convulsions for at least two years, the physician may gradually discontinue the drugs in the hope that the condition has been cured.

Meningitis in babies and children

Meningitis is a contagious infection of the three thin layers, the meninges, that cover the brain. Meningitis usually occurs alone, but occasionally it occurs as part of a general infection such as mumps (see p.700) or tuberculosis (see p.563).

It can also result from a penetrating head injury.

What are the symptoms?
The baby or child has a fever, and, if he or she is old enough to talk, will complain of a severe headache and will be miserable and irritable. The child's neck is held stiffly, or even arched backwards, and if you attempt to bend the head forward, this will be resisted. The child becomes unusually quiet and withdrawn, and turns away or tries to shield the eyes from bright lights. There may also be vomiting and/or convulsions (see previous article).

In young babies, the fontanelle (the soft spot on top of the head), instead of being slightly sunken as it normally is, may be bulging and taut.

What are the risks?
The risks for babies and young children are greater than those for older children and

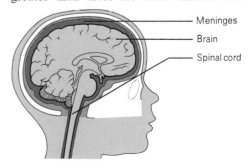

The meninges
The brain and spinal cord are covered by the meninges, which become inflamed in meningitis.

Meninges
Brain
Spinal cord

adults, because the youngster's inability to communicate may prevent the disorder from being detected early. If the infection is bacterial the meningitis may, without treatment, progress to a dangerous stage. In that case, the younger the child, the greater the chance of brain damage, which can cause mental retardation (see p.673), cerebral palsy (see next article), or even death. However, most cases of bacterial meningitis are detected early, and recovery is complete.

What should be done?

If your baby or child has the symptoms described, contact a physician without delay or take the child to a hospital emergency room. If the doctor suspects meningitis, the baby or child will probably be admitted to a hospital, where a *lumbar puncture* test may be done to confirm the diagnosis. If the infection is bacterial, *antibiotics* will probably be prescribed. If viruses are responsible, the disease will usually clear up by itself.

Cerebral palsy

Cerebral palsy is a complete or partial paralysis of the muscles (primarily those of the limbs). It is caused by a brain abnormality. The degree of the child's handicap varies. Either certain limbs are completely immobile or else the child's movements are weak and poorly controlled. Simple movements such as reaching for a cup may be jerky and only accomplished (if at all) after several attempts.

This kind of limb stiffness is called spasticity, and children with cerebral palsy are sometimes called spastics. Many of these children have some degree of mental retardation, although some others are highly intelligent. Children with this disorder may also have some degree of hearing loss, visual defects, most often crossed eyes (see p.674); and convulsions (see p.667).

For most children, the cause of cerebral palsy cannot be determined. It is definitely not inherited, and having one affected child does not increase the likelihood of having another. Cerebral palsy may result from abnormal development of the brain or from brain damage that occurred before, during, or shortly after birth. Later on, brain damage can be caused by a head injury (see p.276), meningitis (see previous article), or severe convulsions (see p.667).

What are the symptoms?

In many cases, cerebral palsy is not recognized until well into the baby's first year. Floppy muscles may be an early indication of the disorder, but many babies who have cerebral palsy do not have this symptom. The main symptom, stiffening of the limbs, does not usually occur until the baby is at least six months old. When this happens, normal muscle balance is disrupted, and the limbs settle in typical abnormal positions. For example, affected arms are usually tucked into the side, with elbows and wrists bent. Legs may be crossed like scissors, and the feet may point downward from the ankle. The baby may move very little, and what little movement there is will be clumsy. In addition, the baby may find it difficult to suck and swallow. The normal milestones in infant development (see p.645), such as walking and speech, may be delayed, sometimes considerably.

Children who walk very late or fail to walk will be unable to explore their environment and learn from their experience at a vital stage of their development. This lack of exploration is made worse if the child also has problems with hearing and/or vision.

When speech is considerably delayed, as is often the case when the child has hearing problems, it may be distorted and extremely difficult to understand. Children who have cerebral palsy and also have average or high intelligence can become extremely frustrated by being deprived of normal activity and ability to communicate, and may have emotional problems as a result.

Some children, especially those who are severely mentally retarded, may have convulsions (see p.667).

What are the risks?

Cerebral palsy is the most common crippling disorder of childhood. It is especially common in babies who are premature or under $2\frac{1}{2}$ kg ($5\frac{1}{2}$ lb) at birth.

The affected child's stiff muscles can very quickly become immobile, which further restricts the child's movements. The child may fail to walk and have to use a wheelchair.

There is a serious risk that an intelligent child will not be recognized as such, especially when movement and communication are very difficult. For this reason, it is essential that the child's mental ability and development are assessed regularly, and that vision and hearing are tested so that any problems in those particular areas can be taken into account in providing for the child's education (see Learning problems, p.673).

What should be done?

See your physician if you are concerned

Types of paralysis
Cerebral palsy may not affect the whole body. As in paralysis from any cause, if only the legs are affected, the condition is called paraplegia. If one side of the body is paralyzed, it is called hemiplegia. Paralysis of all four limbs is called quadriplegia.

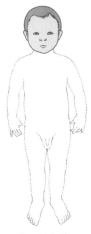

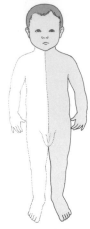
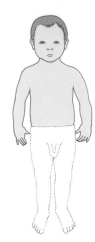

Quadriplegia   Hemiplegia   Paraplegia

about your baby's development. If you take your child for regular checkups, there is little chance that cerebral palsy will go undetected.

What is the treatment?

Abnormalities of the brain such as those that cause cerebral palsy do not get any worse, but they cannot be made any better. This certainly does not mean that nothing can be done for a child with the disorder. The aim of treatment is to determine the extent of any handicaps, whether physical, mental, visual, or auditory, and then to minimize these.

Caring for a child with cerebral palsy involves teamwork on the part of parents, physicians, physical therapists, speech therapists, teachers, and in some cases, occupational therapists.

Physical therapy is provided at special schools, clinics, and in the child's own home. Children learn how to prevent the development of fixed deformities as much as possible by relaxing stiffened muscles and finding beneficial positions for their affected limbs. With physical therapy, some children who have never been able to walk learn to do so with such aids as braces, crutches and walking frames. Speech therapy can improve not only speech but also eating abilities.

Operations done by an orthopedic surgeon can alter the fixed stiffness in some deformed limbs and make movement easier. Surgery enables some children who would otherwise be confined to a wheelchair to walk with aids. Hearing problems in many affected children can be lessened with a hearing aid. Crossed eyes can be corrected by surgery, and prescription glasses may be helpful for other visual problems. A muscle-relaxant drug is sometimes prescribed to ease limb stiffness and drugs are used to treat any convulsions.

The child with cerebral palsy should be examined regularly by a physician or other qualified health professional to assess general physical and mental progress. Sometimes a consultation with an educational psychologist or a social worker is helpful to the child's parents in determining which of the available educational arrangements would be best suited to the child.

Many children who have mild cerebral palsy have normal or near normal intelligence and can attend an ordinary school. Children who are moderately to severely handicapped by the disorder and have normal intelligence may have to attend a school for the physically handicapped, or go to special classes. A child who has sub-normal intelligence may need to attend special classes for the mentally handicapped. Different communities have different arrangements for handicapped children. The local school district can tell you what programs are offered.

Progress may be slow for a child with cerebral palsy. If you are considering unorthodox treatment for your child, be sure to discuss the matter with the professionals who have been treating him or her before making a final decision.

What are the long-term prospects?

The prospects for children with cerebral palsy depend on the degree and type of their handicap. For children able to attend an ordinary school, there should be few problems. Most of them grow up and do well. For many children who need to attend special schools or classes, there can be moderate to severe problems. However, the sophisticated devices available today to help such children communicate with others can help them interact with society.

Sleeping problems in children

Normal sleep patterns

Most babies, in the early weeks of life, wake once or twice during the night, but by the age of nine months they sleep through the night. At one year, babies will sleep an average of about 16 hours in every 24. Two to three hours of this sleep will be during the day.

By the time they have reached the toddler stage (18 months), children begin to vary enormously in the amount of sleep they need. Some toddlers will require relatively little sleep and will wake up early each morning. Leave plenty of soft toys in the child's crib overnight, to occupy the child and allow you to get your normal sleep in the early morning. Such a child is usually very active during the day, may need no day-time nap, and does not become tired until bedtime.

By the age of three, many children will have reached the same stage as the very active toddler and will have given up their daily nap. And by the age of five, nearly all children will be awake throughout the day.

Combating sleeplessness

Do not make yourself too readily available to a child during the night. Otherwise, he or she may become dependent on your attention and become sleepless if deprived of it. For example, if a baby cries after being fed at night, you should not immediately go and pick the baby up. Listen outside the door of the baby's room. In most cases, the crying will stop after a few minutes, and the baby will go back to sleep. If the crying continues, however, you should go in, because the baby may be unwell or uncomfortable.

Some children have trouble falling asleep, though they may sleep well during the night. In this case, try to make sure that the child is not disturbed by unnecessary noise such as an older brother or sister repeatedly entering the bedroom. Sometimes leaving a radio playing music softly will cover up disturbing noises. You also should not send a child to bed as punishment. If, over a period of time, the child comes to associate going to bed with punishment, he or she may fear going to bed, and, once in bed, sleep poorly.

What to do about sleeplessness

If, despite your precautions, your child finds it very difficult to get to sleep or often wakes up during the night, you may be tempted to ask your physician for a sedative for the child. (Never give a child your own sleeping medicine.) But it is unwise to treat the problem with drugs. The child may come to rely on them and acquire a habit that is hard to break. Besides, drugged sleep is not normal sleep. Most children grow out of the problem naturally within one or two months.

If, however, sleeplessness does become a persistent and unbearable problem, consult your physician, who may refer you to a child psychiatrist or psychologist.

Nightmares and sleepwalking

Nightmares usually only become a problem after the age of three. In most cases, they are caused by a disturbing incident, or a frightening story, motion picture, or television program. Occasionally, they are an indication that the child is under stress as a result of unresolved problems at home or school. They are hardly ever the result of physical illness, except a fever or occasionally an upset stomach. Some children have night terrors. They may scream, talk or babble, and appear terrified, but are difficult to wake and cannot say what has frightened them. Sleepwalking is another sign of emotional distress.

The immediate remedy for nightmares and night terrors is to comfort the child. Try to get

---

Hyperactivity

The hyperactive child is physically and mentally restless. He or she has a short attention span, is prone to temper tantrums, has apparently boundless energy and needs little sleep.

Some physicians believe that such aberrant behavior is due to "minimal brain dysfunction," which is brain damage so minimal that it cannot be detected or demonstrated by any diagnostic tests. The dysfunction is thought to be a result of birth trauma, an unspecified food allergy, or a marginal vitamin deficiency.

Treatment includes counseling with teachers, support groups and psychiatrists, and drugs.

Living with a hyperactive child often requires considerable quantities of patience and understanding. If you or anyone in the family finds this particularly difficult, it is important to realize that your feelings are normal. Air these feelings with your physician or another qualified professional familiar with the situation.

It also may be helpful to locate and speak with others who have hyperactive children in their families, since they may have already learned how to cope with behavior that troubles you.

to him or her as soon as possible, and turn the lights on to reassure the child that it was only a dream. Do not question the child about the fear on the spot, since this may only make him or her feel worse. Instead, physically comfort the child and take the child's mind off the disturbance by talking soothingly about something pleasant. A child who has a night terror will probably drift back into a peaceful sleep. Unless the terror persists, it is better not to wake the child. It is also best not to wake a sleepwalking child. Instead, guide him

or her back to bed. Once you have discovered that the child sleepwalks, fix a gate across the top of any stairs to prevent a serious fall.

If the child is old enough, it is usually a good idea to discuss nightmares or sleepwalking with the child and try to find out what the underlying problem is, so that you can deal with it. If you are unsuccessful in this and if the nightmares or sleepwalking become a serious problem, see your physician, who may arrange a consultation with a child psychiatrist or psychologist.

Autism

Autism is a child's inability from birth – or a loss of the ability within the first 30 months of life – to develop normal human relationships with anybody, even with parents. In many of its symptoms autism is similar to schizophrenia in adults (see p.295). What causes the disorder is not known.

What are the symptoms?

The symptoms of autism vary greatly, but follow a general pattern. As a baby the autistic child will have difficulty with feeding and toilet training. He or she will not give, or will cease to give, smiling recognition to the parent's face. It will become increasingly apparent that the child lives in a world of his or her own. Speech, facial expressions, or any other form of communication are absent or unintelligible. In some cases a few words are spoken, but are repeated interminably for no apparent reason. An autistic child makes no distinction among people, other living things, and inanimate objects, and treats them all in the same way. He or she cannot evaluate situations, and so reacts inappropriately to them. For example, the child may become fiercely agitated if the furniture is rearranged in the home or if he or she is taken into new but harmless surroundings, but the same child may also run across a dangerously busy road without any sign of fear.

By not communicating, the autistic child remains isolated from other family members. Such children behave unpredictably. They may be violent at one moment, and then sit completely still, in some strange position, for hours on end. Autistic children may adopt strange postures and mannerisms that can unsettle those around them. And although an autistic child may have normal intelligence he or she may give the impression of being subnormal, or in some cases deaf.

What are the risks?

Autism is far more common in boys than it is

in girls. The illness does not seem to be inherited, and there are no known predisposing factors. There is a slightly higher risk of having a second autistic child in a family that already has one.

There is always a risk that an unsupervised autistic child may be injured because of the child's inability to recognize danger.

What should be done?

If you feel that your child has always been, or has suddenly become, unreasonably withdrawn or uncommunicative, take him or her to your physician. Because a deaf child may also be unresponsive, a hearing test will probably be done. If the child's hearing is normal, and the physician suspects that the child is autistic, you and your child will probably be referred to a child psychiatrist. The psychiatrist will determine if the problem is autism.

What is the treatment?

Once autism has been diagnosed, the parents, the physician, and any specialists involved will probably meet to discuss what is best for the child. Unless the autistic child causes unbearable stress and tension in the family, you will probably be encouraged to look after the child at home. The more care, attention, and stimulation you can give the child, the more hope there is that the condition will improve. You will have support from your child psychiatrist, and any other specialists who become involved in the treatment of your child. Later the child will probably have to attend a special school for the education of autistic children.

What are the long-term prospects?

Some autistic children recover sufficiently, over several years, to grow up as relatively normal members of society and lead productive lives. Unfortunately, most do not, and when they grow older, they usually need to be cared for in special institutions.

Learning problems

Every normal parent wants his or her child to live as happily and harmoniously as possible. To do this, the child must learn early in life not only what is taught in school but also what goes on in the environment in which he or she is growing up. Such learning actually begins at birth, but it may be only later, when a child fails to perform measurable tasks as well as friends or siblings do, that parents are alerted to possible learning problems.

If your child is having trouble learning to speak, read or write relative to other children of the same age, it may be that he or she is slow to develop these skills, and will eventually catch up. It is possible that the situation is more serious. Besides slow development, there are three major causes of learning problems.

Mental retardation

The first possible cause is that the child's intelligence, defined as the ability to understand and benefit from experience, is below normal. Many such children can be educated in regular schools. Children who are severely mentally retarded may have to be educated in special classes or even in special schools.

If a series of tests and assessments indicate that your child is mentally retarded, a team of professionals from your local school district will discuss with you what programs are available in your community, and which of them would be most beneficial for your child. The school staff and your physician may be able to provide you with support and assistance in coping with a retarded child, or they may refer you to another professional or agency for specific problems. Today most parents are advised to steer a middle course between over protecting the child at home and putting him or her in an institution.

Speech and hearing problems

The second major cause of learning problems is difficulty in speaking and hearing. In order to learn to speak, a child must be able to hear other people speaking. The child must be exposed to a variety of words and word combinations in the speech of those nearby. In time, the child comes to associate a particular sound with a particular person, or an object such as a favorite toy or a household pet. Finally, the child must be able to convert an idea into the organized sounds we call speech. This is accomplished by stimulating the various parts of the mouth and pharynx to produce the desired sound. If any part of this process does not work, the child will have trouble learning to speak.

Most speech problems are related to hearing problems. If your child is slow to develop speech (see Milestones, p.645), or if you are worried about your child's hearing (see Can my baby see and hear properly? p.675), consult your physician. Once any hearing problem is corrected, you will probably be referred to a speech therapist. Regular therapy sessions, sometimes daily, enable many children to catch up with their friends or classmates and then progress normally. Become familiar with your child's problem, whatever it is, and find out what you can do to help.

Visual and reading problems

Visual and reading problems are the third major cause of learning problems. A young child learns most about the world by looking at it. But in order to do this, the child must first be able to see clearly. Most visual problems in children are due to crossed eyes (see next page), cataracts (see p.319) or nearsightedness (see p.310), all of which can be improved or corrected, or to some degree of blindness. If you are concerned that your baby's vision is not normal, consult your physician as soon as possible. Vision tests can be done at a very early age.

As with learning to speak, your child must be supplied with sufficient stimulation to be able to use his or her eyes to learn about the world. You can help by talking about pictures in illustrated books, magazines or newspapers, and by encouraging your child to explore the world visually by describing what you see when you are doing things together.

Finally, your child must be able to understand what he or she sees. Reading problems are often problems of understanding what is read; that is, of translating visual images into ideas. While such problems exist before a child learns to read, they are often identified at school by the child's teacher. In some cases a child's reading problem may be caused by severe nearsightedness, which hampers reading even from a book on the desk top. In a very few cases, reading difficulties can lead to a diagnosis of mental retardation. But for a child with a true reading disorder, learning to read is difficult and slow. One such disorder is dyslexia, in which the child sees words and letters reversed. Reversing letters such as "b" and "d" occurs as a part of normal development. A diagnosis of dyslexia is made only when this pattern persists. Most reading problems require specific treatments. Discuss your child's reading difficulties with the specialist or teacher, and find out how you can best help your child to overcome them.

Eyes and ears

A child learns about the world largely by watching, listening and touching. Even a minor problem with either the eyes or ears, if it is not treated, may interfere with the child's development (see Learning problems, previous page). Therefore it is vital to check the development of your baby's vision and hearing. Be certain to take your baby to a physician or clinic for routine eye and ear tests during the first year. You can check that your baby is progressing normally by doing some simple tests (see Can my baby see and hear properly?, next page).

If your child has crossed eyes, itching eyes, or a discharge from or crusting around the ear, or seems inattentive, take him or her to your physician. Many childhood eye and ear problems, particularly crossed eyes or ear infections, can be cured completely with early diagnosis and treatment.

Crossed eyes

Crossed eyes are rarely obvious in a newborn baby. They usually become more apparent as the baby learns to use the eyes.

In someone who is cross-eyed, the two eyes do not look in the same direction. One eye focuses on what the person wants to observe, and the other eye looks elsewhere (usually

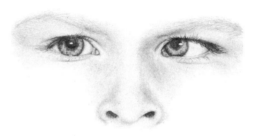

inward, but occasionally outward or even upward). This happens because the muscles in the eyes are not properly aligned. The condition is fairly common.

Crossed eyes usually appear first in infancy or early childhood, when eyesight is in the process of developing. It occurs because the muscles that control the movement of the eyes are unbalanced and misaligned. Usually only one eye is affected. The problem may be constant or it may come and go. Most children with crossed eyes do not see double, because their brains ignore what is seen by the errant eye. This eye will become amblyopic, or "lazy." That is, because it is not being used, the eye will become weak, and as it does so, it will discern less and less detail.

What should be done?
If a baby under three months old has eyes that become crossed every now and then, there is no need to see a physician. The baby is simply still learning to use his or her eyes. In cases of occasional crossed eyes past this age, and in all cases of constant crossed eyes, you should take the baby or child to your doctor for an examination. The child may not have an actual problem. Many young children have a fold of skin over the inner corner of each eye that covers the colored part and often gives the illusion of crossed eyes.

If the physician suspects true crossed eyes, then you and your baby will be referred to an ophthalmologist, who will carry out tests to discover the cause (if any) and advise you on an appropriate treatment.

What is the treatment?
If one eye is lazy, then a patch is placed over the good eye for at least several hours each day, which forces the child to use the lazy eye. This treatment is usually effective only before the age of seven or so. After this, the problem of habitually avoiding use of the lazy eye becomes ingrained and the condition is very difficult to cure. Eyeglasses may also be prescribed if the child is near- or far-sighted. In most children, the combination of a patch and glasses completely clears up the problem within a few years.

If a child has severely crossed eyes, surgery may be carried out, both to help the child use the lazy eye and to improve the child's appearance. In the operation the surgeon shortens the muscles that move the eyeball. Usually the child only has to stay in the hospital for a few days. Whatever the treatment, it may be accompanied by special eye exercises, to build up the eye muscles. The child learns the exercises under the supervision of an ophthalmologist.

What are the long-term prospects?
The prospect of cure is very good if treatment is carried out before the age of seven. After this age, remedying the problem is still possible, but there is an increased risk that the affected eye will become completely blind.

Medical myth

A child with crossed eyes soon grows out of it.

Wrong. You should not expect persistently crossed eyes to disappear naturally. It is never too early to show possible crossed eyes to your physician. The sooner treatment is started, the better the prospects of a total cure.

Chronic middle ear infection

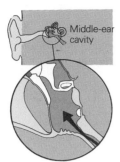

Path of infection
along eustachian tube

Some children have repeated infections of the middle ear (see p.332), which usually occur because an infection of the nose and throat such as a cold passes along the eustachian, or auditory, tube from the back of the nose to the middle ear cavity. Attacks are more frequent in children than they are in adults, because a child's eustachian tubes are relatively short, and this makes it easy for infectious agents to cross them and reach the middle ear. A sticky fluid produced by the infection may gradually collect in the middle ear. The fluid cannot drain away along the eustachian tube because this passage has become swollen and blocked.

What are the symptoms?

The main symptom of chronic middle ear infection is hearing loss in the affected ear. This is rarely total. In most cases sounds can be heard, but they are muffled or faint. The hearing loss occurs because the sticky fluid prevents the eardrum and middle-ear bones from vibrating freely. The child may also have a sensation of fullness in the head.

If your child seems unusually inattentive or is having trouble at school, it could be because of partial hearing loss from a chronic middle ear infection.

What are the risks?

If the condition is not detected and treated after several months, there is a danger that the bones of the middle ear may become cemented together. Since these bones and their movement are crucial in carrying sound to the inner ear, such a development can cause a person to suffer permanent hearing loss in the affected ear.

If the child is at a stage when speech is developing, the hearing problem may slow down this development and, later, affect performance at school (see Learning problems, Speech and hearing problems, p.673).

What should be done?

If you even suspect hearing loss after any ear infection, see your physician, who will examine the affected ear with an *otoscope*. This instrument is used to measure the fluid level behind the eardrum.

What is the treatment?

In mild cases, when there is not much fluid present in the ear and hearing loss is minimal, the physician will probably prescribe a decongestant, an *antihistamine*, or both. These drugs reduce the swelling of the eustachian tube, which allows the pent-up fluid to trickle down the tube and into the nose and throat, from which it can be eliminated.

In more severe cases, the child must have the fluid removed. This is usually done in the hospital. A general anesthetic may be given, and then either a very fine needle is passed through the eardrum and the fluid is sucked out with a syringe, or a small cut is made in the eardrum (myringotomy). Usually, tiny plastic tubes are inserted into the hole in the eardrum to allow air to enter and dry out the middle ear. They are generally left in place for several months, after which they drop out or are removed, and the hole in the eardrum heals naturally.

If the adenoids (see p.677) are acting as a breeding site for repeated infections, or are blocking the entrance to the eustachian tube, they may have to be removed.

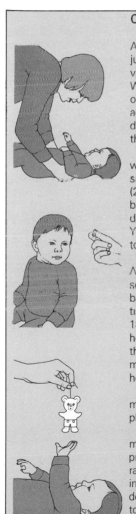

Can my baby see and hear properly?

All babies should receive a general examination just after birth, so that any apparent defects of vision and hearing can be detected immediately. When the baby is between four and six weeks old, the vision and hearing should be tested again. To check your baby's progress yourself during the first few months, try the simple tests that are outlined below.

All babies are near-sighted during the first few weeks of life. At four to six weeks, your baby will smile if you bring your face to within about 50 cm (20 in) of the baby's face. You can test your baby's vision progress at three months old by dangling a familiar toy about 20 cm (8 in) away. Your baby should follow the movement of the toy with his or her eyes.

Your newborn baby is also sensitive to sound. A loud noise will startle a baby, and the sound of somebody talking will be soothing. When your baby is three months old, crinkle up a piece of tissue paper out of sight, 30 to 45 cm (about 12 to 18 in) from the baby's head. A baby with normal hearing will react to the sound by blinking, or by throwing out the arms as if startled. By four months old, your baby should turn his or her head to look for the source of a sound.

If your baby seems to be developing slowly, mention this at the next routine visit to your physician.

Although it is true that many parents worry so much about their children that they imagine problems, it is better to check out any doubts rather than take a chance of neglecting an important problem. It will be difficult for you to detect any partial handicap yourself, so be sure to keep all regularly scheduled appointments with your doctor or health department.

Respiratory system

The most common cause of respiratory system disorder in children is infection. Because a child's respiratory tract is shorter than an adult's, infectious agents can pass more easily from one part of the system to another. This is why recurrent coughs and colds in babies and children often lead to infections elsewhere in the respiratory tract. (For a discussion of the respiratory system in general, see p.340.)

Before the widespread use of antibiotics, many respiratory infections that are now considered minor, such as tonsillitis, often led to very serious complications. Today even pneumonia, which at one time was often fatal for children, may be treated at home.

The major risk of respiratory infections is that your child will have difficulty in breathing (see Croup and stridor, p.678). If your child is short of breath and starts to turn blue about the lips (*cyanosis*), get to a hospital emergency room immediately (see also within Accidents and emergencies, p.801).

Tonsillitis in children

The two tonsils, at the back of the throat, are very small at birth. They enlarge gradually, and reach maximum size at age six or seven. Thereafter they usually shrink, but they do not disappear as the adenoids do (see next article). The tonsils are relatively large by the time a child reaches early school age and the respiratory tract begins to be attacked by a variety of infectious agents. The tonsils then serve to keep infections away from the lower respiratory tract.

Tonsillitis is an acute viral or bacterial infection of the tonsils that sometimes causes them to become abnormally large as well as inflamed. The disorder occurs both in school-age children, and in adolescents and adults (see p.351). It can occur either alone or as part of a upper respiratory infection that is much more widespread.

What are the symptoms?
The illness starts suddenly with a sore throat and difficulty in swallowing. Within a few hours the child becomes feverish and may seem quite ill. The painful irritation in the throat makes some children vomit and/or cough. In a very few cases, the child has a febrile convulsion (see p.667). Young children with tonsillitis often complain of stomach pain. Glands on either side of the neck often swell, especially at the angle of the jaw, and feel tender. They can be felt as small, knob-like lumps. Sometimes these swellings persist for several weeks after the main symptoms have subsided.

What are the risks?
Virtually every child has one or more attacks of tonsillitis, which is very infectious and is usually associated with infections of the adenoids (see next article). Those who get frequent attacks usually begin to get fewer after the age of seven as resistance develops to the infectious agents that cause the disorder. Tonsillitis is not dangerous today. Before antibiotics were discovered, it could readily lead to rheumatic fever (see p.693) or glomerulonephritis (see p.690).

What should be done?
Use a flashlight to look in your child's mouth. You can hold the tongue down with a spoon handle. You will see the bumpy tonsils on each side of the throat. If there are white spots on the tonsils, or if the tonsils are swollen over the opening of the throat, call your physician. If the tonsils are just red, try the self-help measures recommended below. If fever and reluctance to eat because of pain last for more than 24 hours, consult your physician, who will examine the child's tonsils and determine what treatment is needed.

What is the treatment?
Self-help: The child should be kept indoors, but not necessarily in bed, in a warm – not overheated – room. Symptoms can usually be relieved with medications recommended by your physician and plenty to drink. The fluids should be sipped regularly. Older children should be given at least a pint a day of extra liquids. Do not force the child to eat or drink. There is no harm in cold desserts such as ice cream to cool the throat. A cooling fan, or frequent sponging of the face with tepid water, helps to reduce the child's temperature. In most cases, children with tonsillitis respond quickly to this treatment.
Professional help: The physician will probably prescribe a ten-day supply of an *antibiotic*, and the symptoms of tonsillitis will usually clear up in a few days. Even if the child seems

Medical myth

Surgical removal of tonsils is a safe, minor operation, which would benefit most children.

Wrong. Like any operation, a tonsillectomy involves risk. Although the risk is small, it increases with age. Except in severe cases of recurrent tonsillitis, or if swollen tonsils interfere with swallowing or breathing, the operation is usually not necessary.

OPERATION: **Tonsils removal**
Tonsillectomy

The tonsils are removed in cases where recurrent attacks of tonsillitis are interfering with general health or education. The operation is usually done when the child is six or seven. It becomes more difficult as the patient gets older.
During the operation After a general anesthetic is administered, the child's mouth is held open and the tongue is pulled forward to reveal the tonsils. The tonsils are cut away, and the cut area is left to heal naturally.
After the operation There may be some bleeding of the cut areas, but this is not usually serious. The child should be out of the hospital within a few days, and back to normal within two weeks. Plenty of ice cream serves to both soothe the sore throat and cheer up the child.

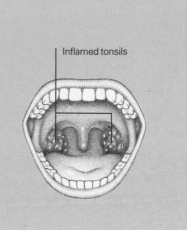

Inflamed tonsils

to be completely well, however, be sure to use the entire prescription according to your doctor's instructions.

If tonsillitis attacks are so severe and frequent that they affect the child's general health or interfere with schooling, hearing, or breathing, surgical removal of the tonsils (tonsillectomy) may be advised (see above). However, most physicians recommend that this be done only as a last resort.

The child often is given a general anesthetic for the operation and is hospitalized. There is little risk in the operation, and it can clear up the problem permanently.

Adenoids

Adenoids, which are swellings at the back of the nose, above the tonsils, are found almost exclusively in preadolescent children. They assist the body's defenses against respiratory-tract infections and are only troublesome if they grow too large. Normally, they begin to enlarge at about the age of three, probably to give extra protection to the lungs and chest when the child is particularly susceptible to infection. At about five years old, the adenoids begin to shrink, and they disappear at puberty. In a few cases, however, they grow instead, and eventually obstruct the airway from the nose to the throat, the opening of the eustachian tubes from the middle ear to the nose, or both. If either or both obstructions develop, problems usually occur.

What are the symptoms?
If the airway from the nose is blocked, the child breathes mainly through the mouth, snores, and may speak with a nasal twang. The flow of secretions at the back of the nose is obstructed, and the adenoids become infected. Infected secretions drip from the child's nose during the day. At night, or whenever the child lies down, these secre-

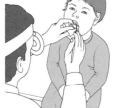

A physician looks for enlarged adenoids. The procedure is not painful, but some children find it very uncomfortable.

tions drip back down into the throat, causing an irritating cough. If the infection is not cleared up, it may spread to the middle ear.

What are the risks?
There are no serious risks if infection is kept under control. If infections are neglected and followed by chronic ear infections (see p.675), some hearing loss may result.

What is the treatment?
If your child repeatedly has a blocked nose, earaches, or an irritating cough at night, consult your physician, who will probably want to examine the adenoids. This is done by reflecting a light onto them from a mirror held at the back of the throat.

Infections caused by abnormally enlarged adenoids are treated with *antibiotics* when it is necessary. Surgical removal of the adenoids (adenoidectomy) is not required often, because the adenoids shrink of their own accord as the child reaches puberty. However, when repeated earaches interfere with a child's education or persist despite antibiotic treatment, adenoidectomy may be advised. The operation is not complicated, and involves little risk.

Croup and stridor

Croup is a problem associated with a condition called stridor. Stridor is a shrill wheezing or grunting noise that a child makes who is breathing through a narrowed larynx or trachea. The narrowing is usually due to swelling caused by a respiratory infection, often a cold (see Recurrent colds in children, p.680).

What are the symptoms?

In addition to the characteristic sound of stridor, a child with croup will have other symptoms of the associated respiratory infection, especially a harsh, barking cough, and hoarseness. Older children may complain of discomfort around the larynx or somewhere in the front of the chest.

Usually attacks of croup occur at night. The child awakes and breathes with a sudden loud crowing noise, which becomes louder when he or she inhales. The child is likely to be alarmed and bewildered. In most cases, the attack subsides in a few hours. A child who suddenly develops stridor, possibly with a fit of coughing, and does not have a respiratory infection, may have inhaled a foreign object (see box).

What should be done?

If your child has difficulty in breathing and turns bluish, especially around the lips, get the child to a hospital immediately.

What is the treatment?

Self-help: During an attack of croup, be calm and reassure the child, who may be frightened. Panic, whether your own or the child's, will only make the situation worse. Your physician may encourage you to use a steam kettle, a vaporizer, or steam from a hot shower to help relieve the congestion. Always be sure to be careful when you are using steaming-hot water.

Professional help: If the child has an underlying respiratory infection that may be caused by bacteria, *antibiotics* may be prescribed.

A child who is having difficulty in breathing may need to be admitted to a hospital. *X-rays* may be taken of the larynx to determine the amount of obstruction.

The child is usually given antibiotics and oxygen, and put in a room with a humid atmosphere. If the air passage is seriously obstructed, it will be necessary either to pass a tube through the mouth into the throat or, in the most severe cases, to make an incision in the throat and insert a tube to enable the child to breathe. The tube is usually removed within 24 hours. Rarely, breathing has to be maintained artificially with a mechanical respirator. Most children admitted to a hospital for this treatment recover completely within a few days.

Inhaled foreign object

If a child inhales a foreign object such as a bead or a peanut, it can block the air passage. If your child has sudden difficulty in breathing and/or turns bluish about the lips (*cyanosis*), get the child to a hospital emergency room immediately (see also within Accidents and emergencies, p.801).

If an inhaled foreign object causes only a partial blockage, the child will develop sudden stridor (see above) and possibly a cough. In this case, see your physician, who will arrange for *bronchoscopy* to look for the inhaled object and, if possible, remove it.

Occasionally an inhaled foreign object passes further down into the lungs, and causes a small area of inflammation and infection (see Pneumonia in children, next page). The object must be removed with a bronchoscope, and *antibiotics* may be given to treat or prevent infection.

Bronchiolitis

A large part of the lungs consists of millions of tiny tubes called bronchioles, which convey air between the larger airways, the bronchi, and the tiny air sacs called alveoli. In bronchiolitis, the lining of the bronchioles is infected, usually by a virus that first causes a cold and then spreads. The infected lining swells, and almost completely blocks the passage of air into and out of the alveoli.

What are the symptoms?

The baby has a cold and cough that suddenly becomes worse after a day or two. The baby then starts to breathe quickly and with difficulty. In some cases, the baby's chest fails to expand when breath is drawn in. The baby goes limp, is unable to eat, and may even turn blue from lack of oxygen.

Bronchiolitis is not a common disorder, and practically all cases are quickly diagnosed and promptly treated. In rare cases, heart failure (see p.381) and/or pneumonia (see next article) can result.

What should be done?

If your baby shows any of the symptoms described, consult your physician immediately. You should be especially watchful if your baby has a cold that suddenly gets worse after two to three days and if the baby's breathing becomes quickened and labored.

What is the treatment?

Getting to a hospital is vital. If *cyanosis*, or blueness of the skin, has developed, the baby will be put into a humid oxygen tent im-

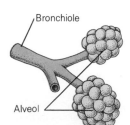

Bronchiole

Alveol

mediately. In most cases, the baby is fed with liquids passed through a tube that leads into the stomach via the nose. In severe cases, the liquids are given by *intravenous drip. Antibiotics* are often prescribed to prevent secondary bacterial infection.

In very severe cases, the baby's breathing may have to be maintained artificially with the aid of a mechanical respirator. With prompt treatment, most previously healthy babies recover completely from bronchiolitis in two to three days.

Pneumonia in children

Pneumonia (see also p.359) is an inflammation of the lungs, usually caused by an infection. This is most commonly a viral infection that has started in the upper respiratory tract. It produces patchy inflammation, sometimes called bronchopneumonia, usually in the lower parts of both lungs.

Bronchopneumonia can also develop as a complication of measles (see p.699), whooping cough (see p.701), and chickenpox (see p.700) and is common in children with cystic fibrosis (see p.685).

Some older children get what is sometimes called lobar pneumonia, which is an infection of one or more lobes, or sections, of the lung, usually by the *Pneumococcus* bacterium. Pneumonia can also be caused by an inhaled foreign object (see previous page).

What are the symptoms?
A child who contracts bronchopneumonia starts by having a cold for two or three days. The child's temperature then rises to about 101°F (38.5°C) and he or she develops a dry cough, starts breathing more rapidly than normal, and, in some cases, may wheeze. In very serious cases the child may develop *cyanosis*, or blueness of the skin. Cyanosis typically may be seen around the lips.

The onset of lobar pneumonia is quite different. There is no cold. The child becomes ill suddenly, and his or her temperature rises quickly to about 104°F (40°C). Breathing is rapid, and the child has a dry cough. Occa-

sionally, pleurisy (see p.361) develops, and causes pain in the chest.

What are the risks?
Bronchopneumonia is much more common than lobar pneumonia, but is still uncommon. It develops in only a small percentage of upper respiratory tract infections.

The high temperature that is a symptom of pneumonia can cause a febrile convulsion (see Convulsions in children, p.667), but this is unlikely. On rare occasions, the inflamed areas of the lungs are replaced by fibrous scar tissue, and this may lead to bronchiectasis (see p.363) if it occurs extensively. Fatal pneumonia in children is very rare.

What should be done?
If your child develops a temperature and starts breathing with difficulty, call your physician. This is a matter of urgency if the child is less than six months old.

Most cases of pneumonia in children can be treated at home. Hospitalization is only necessary in very severe cases.

What is the treatment?
Self-help: If it is decided that the child can be treated at home, there are several things you can do to relieve the symptoms and hasten recovery. The child's high temperature can be lowered by giving a fever reducing drug recommended by your physician, removing the child's pajamas, and sponging the body with tepid water. Give plenty of liquids; for older children, at least a pint more than usual each day. And have the child rest quietly as much as possible.

Professional help: It is mainly the child's own resistance to the infection that brings about a recovery. *Antibiotics* act only against bacteria and have no effect on viruses, which cause bronchopneumonia. Antibiotics are prescribed for lobar pneumonia, and when there is some doubt about whether a virus or bacterium is responsible for the infection. Antibiotics are usually given by mouth, unless the infection is very severe.

An otherwise healthy child will nearly always recover completely from pneumonia, usually after about a week.

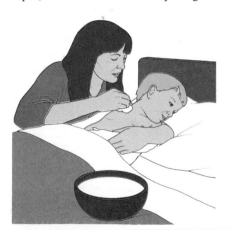

Lowering a fever
To drive a feverish child's temperature down, sponge the body with tepid water. A high temperature can lead to convulsions.

Recurrent colds in children

It is quite common for a young child to have a number of coughs and colds, especially in winter, and it is not something you need to worry about. Most children keep catching colds during the first few years of school, because at school the child is exposed to all kinds of new viruses. Gradually, however, the child acquires increasing immunity to them.

A child's cold is often accompanied by a cough, chiefly because, instead of blowing mucus into a handkerchief, the child tends to sniff it down into the throat. The mucus irritates the throat, so in an attempt to get rid of it the child coughs. Abdominal pain is also common in a child with a cold.

When to consult your physician

In rare cases, recurrent coughs and colds are a symptom of a serious underlying disorder. If that is the case, the child will appear generally unwell most of the time, even without having a cold. If this is the case with your child, you should take him or her to your physician.

In some children, cold symptoms are caused by an allergy rather than a cold. If your child sneezes and has a runny nose and watering eyes during the warm months, he or she probably has hay fever, an allergy to tree or other plant pollen. If the symptoms occur throughout the year, the child may be allergic to dust. Allergies may start when the child is a toddler (see Allergic rhinitis,

p.344). If your child has such summer "colds" or cold-like symptoms all year long, consult your physician.

If a recurrent cough is not accompanied by a cold, or if it is accompanied by wheezing, it may indicate asthma (see p.355), or in rare cases cystic fibrosis (see p.685), and you should consult your physician.

If a baby with a cold cries continually, refuses to eat, is restless and has a hot skin, develops an earache or pain in the face or forehead, runs a high fever (above 102°F or 39°C), or is persistently hoarse and has a dry painful cough, consult your doctor.

What you can do

In some cases, a child with recurrent colds will cough a lot at night. This may be because the child's room is too cold and the air is irritating the throat, or because it is too warm and the air is making the throat dry. Adjusting the temperature or humidity may solve the problem.

Babies with colds sometimes have trouble eating. This is no cause for concern if the problem lasts no more than a day or two. You can help by keeping the baby's nose clear of obstructing mucus by using a small bulb syringe available in many drugstores.

Try to give an older child a drink before bed, to help clear the back of the nasal passage. Your physician may suggest a mild cough syrup.

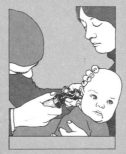

Respiratory infections often travel along the eustachian tube, and cause middle ear infections. Ear infections should be treated promptly, because they can lead to persistent ear trouble.

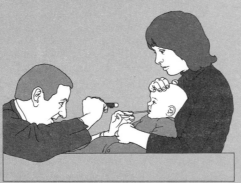

The doctor's examination Your physician will examine the child's throat to see if the tonsils or adenoids are inflamed. Although neither tonsillitis nor enlarged adenoids are usually dangerous, they can lead to breathing difficulties. If your child has been wheezing or grunting, the doctor may suspect stridor and want to see how far the inflammation has spread before making a diagnosis.

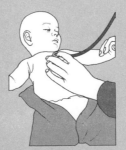

A chest examination is made to see if your baby's cold is developing into a serious disorder such as bronchopneumonia or bronchiolitis.

Blood disorders

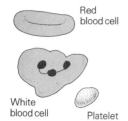

Red blood cell

White blood cell

Platelet

The blood disorders discussed here vary greatly in their effects on a child. These disorders, because their symptoms are varied and usually mild, may go undetected. For a child with iron deficiency anemia or allergic purpura, a delayed diagnosis is not likely to have any permanent ill effects, and the disorder is treated in the usual way. But a child who has leukemia, a cancer that affects white blood cells, has the best chances of recovery if the disease is discovered early. Recent progress in the treatment of leukemia has improved the prospects for children with the disease. Even so, leukemia requires intensive treatment, often in a hospital. This serious disease may put a great strain on both the affected child and his or her family (see Cancer in children, p.695).

Allergic purpura

(anaphylactoid purpura)

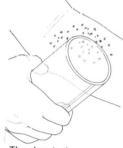

The glass test
Purpura can be diagnosed by pressing a glass against the rash. A rash that remains visible under pressure is probably caused by purpura.

In allergic purpura, a rash appears just beneath the surface of the skin. This is thought to be due to an abnormal reaction between *antibodies*, or biochemical molecules that normally protect against infection, and blood vessels. The vessels become inflamed or burst, which produces the rash. In some cases, it is thought that the antibodies are produced to combat an infection caused by *Streptococcus* bacteria. They can also be produced in reaction to a food, a drug, or possibly a virus. The disorder most commonly affects children.

What are the symptoms?
Usually the child will have a sore throat two weeks before the onset of the rash. The rash, which causes no discomfort, consists of purplish-red, irregularly shaped spots that vary in size and appear on the ankles, shins, buttocks and elbows. When the spots appear, some children feel generally unwell and have a slight fever. The rash tends to come and go.

Some children may also have swollen joints, and/or a stomach ache that is often severe and persistent. Occasionally, an affected child may have bloody bowel movements, which indicates bleeding in the bowel, or bloody urine, which signifies kidney damage (see Glomerulonephritis, p.690).

The disorder is very rare. It is more common in boys than in girls.

The main risk faced by a child with this disorder is permanent kidney damage. Two other, extremely rare, dangers are intussusception (see p.683), and massive bleeding in the bowel and other internal organs.

What should be done?
If your child has any of the symptoms described, consult your physician. Treatment will not be required in most cases, because the disorder will clear up spontaneously after a month or two. In some children, however, the problem recurs for up to two years before it finally disappears.

Iron deficiency anemia in children

Anemia is an insufficiency of hemoglobin, a protein in the blood that carries oxygen to the tissues of the body. Iron deficiency anemia (see p.419) is the most common type of anemia in children. The most likely cause of this disorder is inadequate iron in the diet. In most babies, it does not matter that the milk or formula that they are fed contains little iron, because they can draw on stores of iron built up before birth. Premature babies, however, may have low stores and may therefore have iron deficiency anemia. Other susceptible children are babies who are weaned onto a solid diet deficient in iron, and older children who do not eat enough iron-rich foods. Unfortunately, the disorder may diminish appetite, making the problem worse.

Less common causes of iron deficiency anemia in children are failure to absorb iron in the diet, as in celiac disease (see p.684), and insidious internal bleeding, such as the bleeding caused by hookworm.

What are the symptoms?
Mild anemia may produce no obvious symptoms. Signs of more pronounced anemia (of any type) include several or all of the following: paleness, especially in the hands and on the lining of the lower eyelids; tiredness; weakness; and, less commonly, fainting; breathlessness; and palpitations. These symptoms, when present, are all especially apparent on exertion. Other possible symptoms are inactivity and loss of appetite.

What should be done?

If your child is less active than playmates, and breathlessness follows minimal activity, see your physician. Do *not* treat anemia yourself with iron pills or tonics.

The physician will probably take blood samples for analysis. Further tests may then be required.

What is the treatment?

If, as is most common, the diagnosis is iron deficiency anemia caused by lack of iron in the diet, the doctor will probably prescribe iron for three months or longer, usually in liquid form. The doctor will also make recommendations about diet. Any underlying disorder will also be treated.

Leukemia in children

Leukemia is a cancer that affects white blood cells, which protect the body against infection. Acute lymphocytic leukemia is the type that appears most often in children. (For a full definition of leukemia and a description of the disease in adults, see p.426).

Acute lymphocytic leukemia affects the lymphocytes, white blood cells that are produced in the lymph glands (see p.432). The cancerous cells overflow from the lymph glands and circulate in the bloodstream. They can affect any or all of various parts of the body, including the liver, the spleen, bone marrow, and the surface of the brain and spinal cord. In the bone marrow, the leukemic cells seriously interfere with the marrow's production of red blood cells, platelets, and a type of white blood cells known as neutrophils.

What are the symptoms?

The main symptoms of acute lymphocytic leukemia are anemia, marked by progressive paleness, tiredness, and general illness; thrombocytopenic purpura (see Thrombocytopenia, p.425), characterized by a purplish-red rash; pains in the limbs; severe headaches; swollen glands in the neck behind the angle of the jaw; an enlarged spleen, which the physician will be able to feel in the upper left portion of the abdomen; susceptibility to infections, especially pneumonia (see p.679); and the development of sores and ulcers in the mouth and throat.

What are the risks?

Any form of leukemia in children is uncommon. Most of those affected are under ten years old, but some teenagers also get the disease. Because of recent advances in treatment, children with leukemia have a better outlook than ever before. But the treatment itself involves a risk that the child may contract a serious infection, in particular, blood poisoning (see p.421), which may be fatal.

What should be done?

If you are worried that your child might have leukemia, take him or her to a physician, who will examine the child and take a blood sample for analysis, and probably be able to relieve your worry on the spot. If the possibility of leukemia cannot be ruled out immediately, the doctor will arrange for further tests that may include a bone marrow *biopsy*. In a biopsy, a small amount of bone marrow is removed and examined through a microscope. The results of these tests will show whether or not the disease is present.

What is the treatment?

Treatment is carried out in a hospital. The basic treatment is *cytotoxic*, or anticancer, drugs and *steroid* drugs. Some are given as tablets, others by *intravenous drip*.

In many cases, *radiation therapy* is also used on the head, and an anticancer drug is injected through the lower spine into the fluid that surrounds the brain and spinal cord. Any infection that develops is treated with large doses of *antibiotics*.

To protect your child against the risk of serious infection, he or she may be isolated from other patients, and when you visit, you may have to wear a mask and a gown to avoid the spread of any germs that you might bring into your child's room. A young child may be bewildered and upset, and you must try to overcome your own distress so you can offer as much reassurance as possible. An older child will probably realize the seriousness of the illness (see Cancer in children, p.695).

In nearly all cases, treatment causes the symptoms to diminish after several weeks. Then the child is allowed to go home. Over the next year or so, the child is given frequent regular checkups and doses of drugs to ensure, with your essential help, that he or she leads as normal a life as possible. If symptoms recur or worsen, your child may need to be re-admitted to the hospital.

What are the long-term prospects?

A cure for the disease now seems possible. About half of the children who have received treatment for acute lymphocytic leukemia have survived for at least five years and some for a much longer time.

Digestive system and nutrition

Several of the disorders described here occur because the digestive system is unable to handle certain foods (see p.434 for a full description of the digestive system).

Most of these disorders are usually tested for and detected soon after birth, to prevent the child from ever eating the foods that can be harmful. If your child has such a disorder, your physician will prescribe a strict diet and suggest any specially-prepared foods.

A healthy digestive system and a balanced diet are essential for a growing child. If you are concerned about your child's growth, see Growth disorders (p.687).

Intussusception

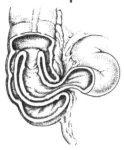

In intussusception, two parts of the baby's intestine telescope together.

In this rare disorder a part of the baby's intestines, usually the small intestine, telescopes into another part of the intestine. What causes the telescoping is not known. It happens most often in babies four to six months old, and for some unknown reason is more common in boys.

What are the symptoms?

A previously healthy baby suddenly screams violently as a wave of muscular contraction passes along the telescoped intestine. The screaming may continue for several minutes. The baby then becomes pale and limp. Vomiting may occur, and a bowel movement of bloody mucus, like red jelly, may be passed. The screaming recurs every few minutes.

What should be done?

Call your physician as soon as these symptoms occur. By feeling the child's abdomen, the physician may be able to make a tentative diagnosis of intussusception.

The baby will be admitted to a hospital for a *barium enema* examination. This will confirm the tentative diagnosis of intussusception, and may also, as the barium is forced along the intestine, push the telescoped intestine back into place. If the barium does not do this, the baby will probably have to undergo an operation in which the abdomen is opened and the intestine is pushed back into its normal position. The results of the operation are usually excellent. After the operation, the baby should have no further problems.

Encopresis

In encopresis, children who are old enough to be toilet-trained still regularly soil their underclothes, even though they have no underlying disease. In most cases, this occurs because large amounts of hard bowel movements accumulate in the rectum and lower bowel (where you can sometimes feel them as a lump in the abdomen), and a liquid material that may contain mucus trickles past the blockage. Because the material that comes out of the child is liquid, parents often think that the child has diarrhea and do not realize that the problem is actually constipation (see Constipation in children, p.688). They also often do not understand that the child cannot control the passing of this liquid.

In a few cases, another type of encopresis develops in which the child soils his or her underclothes with solid bowel movements. This is nearly always due to an emotional disturbance, either within the family or at school. Parents who mistakenly think that the child is purposely soiling clothing in this way and react with anger, may make the problem considerably worse.

What is the treatment?

A child with encopresis should be taken to a physician to make sure the problem is not caused by an underlying disorder, and to obtain appropriate treatment. One treatment is *enemas or suppositories* given to clear the rectum and lower bowel. Your physician may be able to do this in the office or clinic, but usually it is done in the hospital.

Once home, the child must be encouraged to move his or her bowels at least once a day, at a regular time. In some cases, the doctor may prescribe daily laxatives, sometimes over a long period. It is important to understand that the problem is probably far more distressing to the child than it is to you. For this reason, you should try to continually show the child that you understand the problem and are anxious to help in whatever ways you can.

You may be able to cure a child who cannot control bowel movements by instituting the toilet routine described above. If the problem persists, see your physician who may refer you to a child psychiatrist.

Celiac disease

(gluten enteropathy, non-tropical sprue)

Celiac disease is an allergy that affects the small intestine. In this disorder, when the small intestine comes in contact with gluten, a protein present in most grains, the membrane that lines the intestine loses its fluffy texture and becomes smooth. As a result, the intestine is usually less able to absorb nutrients (see Malabsorption, p.475). The disease is nearly always discovered and diagnosed in infancy or early childhood.

What are the symptoms?

Symptoms usually start within a few weeks after cereals are introduced into the baby's diet at two months old or later. The baby gains weight more slowly or may even lose weight. To increase the problem, he or she may have a poor appetite. The baby will have loose, pale, bulky, very offensive-smelling bowel movements, together with a lot of gas, several times a day. The gas is produced in such abundance that it may make the baby's abdomen swell, and this will contrast with his or her undernourished appearance. In some cases, ulcers develop in the baby's mouth. Anemia and vitamin deficiencies may also occur as a result of celiac disease.

What are the risks?

Celiac disease is rare. A child with a relative who has the disorder is at slightly more than average risk of being born with it. In the very rare cases when a mild form of the illness is not detected in infancy, the child's growth may be permanently stunted.

What should be done?

If your child has the symptoms described, see your physician. If the doctor suspects celiac disease, the child will probably have tests on the blood and bowel movements. If these tests show evidence of the disease, a *biopsy* of the lining of the small intestine is carried out. In a biopsy, a small amount of tissue is removed and examined. This test will confirm whether the child has celiac disease or not.

What is the treatment?

Wheat, rye, and other grain that contains gluten must be excluded from the baby's diet. Your physician may arrange for you to discuss this with a dietician. Rice and corn are safe for the child to eat, but he or she will need special bread and crackers, and you will have to make cakes or pastry with a special gluten-free flour. Within a few weeks of starting the diet, the child's symptoms usually clear up and the child begins to thrive again. To maintain good health, it is essential that the child continues with the diet. The child may also need iron or vitamin supplements.

The child should be included in discussions of the treatment, so that he or she will know the importance of avoiding certain foods, especially at school or friends' homes.

What is the long-term outlook?

A person with celiac disease can look forward to a normal life, apart from the diet. The diet is restrictive, but many interesting and flavorful foods can be prepared within its limits.

Recurrent stomach aches and headaches

Some children who are otherwise well have sudden stomach aches or headaches every few days, weeks, or months. They may look pale and often want to lie down. Generally the pain lasts a few hours, but it can last all day. When asked to locate the stomach pain, children usually point to the navel. Sometimes stomach aches are accompanied by vomiting, diarrhea, a slight fever, or all three.

Many children stop having these problems by puberty. Others continue to have them in adult life.

Only a small proportion of children who have recurrent stomach aches have an underlying physical problem. This can be kidney trouble, or, more rarely, a peptic ulcer, which is almost entirely confined to boys. Food allergies such as lactose intolerance (see p.686) may cause the pains in some children. But in the great majority of cases, the cause is unknown, but may be psychological.

Headaches, too, are seldom a symptom of a serious underlying disorder. Most recurrent headaches in children are the result of emotional stress at home or in school. Stress can be caused by events such as the birth of a new baby and the subsequent shift in the parents' attention, or the approach of important exams.

In some cases, one or both parents may have frequent headaches or migraines, and may have had the same sort of stomach aches as children. It is not known whether the tendency is inherited or whether it is simply the result of parental influence.

What should you do?

If your child has recurrent stomach aches, recurrent headaches or a headache that lasts for more than one day take him or her to a physician, to make sure that there is no physical cause for the pain. If there is no physical cause, the doctor may suggest that you note whether the pains occur consistently after the child has eaten a particular food. For a severe headache, give the child a pain-reducing medication approved by your physician.

If the problem persists, it is likely to be psychological or emotional. Discuss the matter again with your physician who may refer you to a child psychiatrist.

Cystic fibrosis

In this uncommon hereditary disease, the pancreas, a gland below the stomach, fails to produce any *enzymes*, or digestive juices that are necessary to break down food. The result is that the child's food is only minimally broken down, by a small number of enzymes that are produced by the intestinal wall and the salivary glands. As a result of this, the food retains its fats and most of its nutrients as it passes through the body (see Malabsorption, p.475).

In cystic fibrosis, the glands in the lining of the bronchial tubes in the lungs also malfunction. Instead of producing the normal thin mucus that traps germs and is then coughed up, they produce a thick, sticky mucus that tends to stagnate in the tubes. Germs multiply in this mucus, and cause respiratory infections, including pneumonia (see p.679).

What are the symptoms?

Symptoms sometimes occur immediately after birth. Mucus secretions in the baby's intestines make the baby's first bowel movement after birth too thick and sticky for the baby to pass, which can cause intestinal obstruction (see p.471).

In all cases, the child gains little weight right from birth, because failure of the pancreas to produce its enzymes means that

Teething problems

A baby's first teeth, the incisors, or front teeth, usually appear during the first year and seldom cause problems. The gum may be a little inflamed, there may be more drooling than usual, and the baby will probably chew a lot on the fingers or a teething ring. There may be a change in the baby's feeding, sleeping and bowel habits, but the baby probably will have very little discomfort.

The first and second molars, which are usually cut between the ages of one and three, are much more likely to cause problems. The gum may be tender and make eating painful. The cheek on the affected side of the mouth may be hot and flushed, and the child will probably be miserable for a few days. Unfortunately, there is little that can be done. Rubbing the gum gently, and giving the child a cool drink from a cup, may ease the pain a little, but teething is generally a stage that the child just has to live through.

It is possible to overlook real illness in a child by attributing all symptoms to teething. If a child of teething age shows signs of distress, you should see your physician. Clutching one side of the face, for example, may be a sign not of teething but of an ear infection (see p.675).

Average ages for teeth to appear

Age	Baby teeth
6 months	First incisors
7 months	Second incisors
12 months	First molars
18 months	Canines
2–3 years	Second molars
	Full set: 20 teeth

Age	Permanent teeth
6–8 years	First incisors
6–7 years	First molars
7–9 years	Second incisors
9–12 years	Canines
10–12 years	First and second premolars
11–13 years	Second molars
17–20 years (or never)	Third molars (wisdom teeth)
	Full set: 32 teeth

Baby teeth

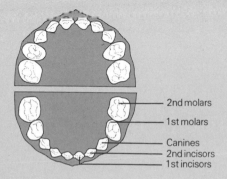

- 2nd molars
- 1st molars
- Canines
- 2nd incisors
- 1st incisors

Permanent teeth

- 1st and 2nd premolars
- 1st molars
- 2nd molars
- 3rd molars (wisdom teeth)
- 1st incisors
- 2nd incisors
- Canines

FULL SET: 32 TEETH

There are considerable variations in the ages at which teeth appear, and the ages given should be considered only as averages. Some children have one tooth or more at birth. Others have none at a year. Early or late teething has no effect on the child's general health and development.

hardly any nutrients are absorbed. The food the child eats passes out of the body as large, pale, greasy-looking bowel movements that float in water and have a foul smell.

A child with cystic fibrosis may have recurrent respiratory infections, accompanied by a cough and fever, that are more severe and persistent than is normal. This is the result of the thick, sticky mucus that is typical of the disease and tends to trap and hold germs in the bronchial tubes.

Children with cystic fibrosis often have large appetites and eat a great deal. In spite of their malnutrition, they are not in pain and do not generally feel ill.

What are the risks?

Repeated bouts of pneumonia are common in children with the disease, and usually lead to bronchiectasis (see p.363), which in turn makes the lungs even more susceptible to pneumonia. Eventually, this may prove fatal. However, modern treatment with *antibiotics* is enabling more and more children who have the disease to survive into early adulthood. Because cystic fibrosis is a hereditary disorder it may affect several children in the same family (see Genetics, p.704).

What should be done?

If cystic fibrosis is known to run in the family, the baby's bowel movements will probably be tested at birth to check for the disease. If the disorder is diagnosed this early, immediate treatment can lessen respiratory infections and lung damage, and will also lengthen the child's life expectancy.

In other cases, when abnormal bowel movements and failure to put on weight are obvious soon after birth, the physician will be aware of a possible problem and check for the disease. But in some cases respiratory infections are the predominant symptom of the disease and these may not develop until some weeks after birth. Then the parents may be the first to discover that something is wrong. If this occurs, you should consult your physician as soon as possible. Diagnostic tests will then be carried out on the child. These will indicate the presence of cystic fibrosis.

Although the child will grow up underdeveloped and tend to miss school frequently, you should not over-protect the child and should encourage him or her to be as active and live as normal a life as possible.

If cystic fibrosis runs in your family and you are considering having a child, or if you want another child after having had one who has the disease, you should consult a genetic counselor (see p.619). The counselor can tell you what the risks are of your having another child with the disease. Your doctor will be able to tell you how to contact a genetic counselor.

What is the treatment?

Extracts of animal pancreas, in powder or granule form, are prescribed to replace the missing enzymes from the pancreas, and the amount of fat in the child's diet is reduced. With this treatment, the child begins to put on weight and the bowel movements become much more normal.

To keep the lungs as free of mucus as possible, the child may need to have daily respiratory physical therapy, which includes postural drainage (see Bronchiectasis, p.363). This program can be carried out at home. The physical therapist will show you and your child what to do. Any respiratory infections that arise are treated with large doses of *antibiotics.*

Lactose intolerance

Enzymes are substances important to the body's chemical reactions. One enzyme, lactase, which is produced in the lining of the small intestine, breaks down lactose, the sugar in cow's milk. Most blacks, Orientals, and American Indians, and some whites, have little or no lactase, and have difficulty digesting cow's milk. This disorder is called lactose intolerance.

A severe attack of gastroenteritis (see p.649) in any baby can sometimes temporarily damage the intestinal lining, which then produces little or no lactase. The result of this is a temporary form of lactose intolerance. The baby may have no symptoms at first, because until the diarrhea and vomiting caused by the gastroenteritis stop, the baby is often taken off milk and given water instead. It is only when cow's milk is reintroduced that a reaction occurs and diarrhea reappears. The diarrhea is often frothy, and may cause diaper rash (see p.650) and be accompanied by vomiting.

If lactose intolerance is present at birth, it causes persistent diarrhea immediately, and the affected baby does not gain weight.

What is the treatment?

If a physician who is treating a baby for recurrent diarrhea suspects temporary lactose intolerance, the doctor will probably put the baby on a formula that contains little or no lactose. Soy bean-based formulas are commonly used because they supply needed protein without lactose. If the new food improves the condition, the baby continues with this formula. The small intestine will eventually return to normal and usually cow's milk can be introduced again later.

If the condition is present at birth, or if there is a history of lactose intolerance in your family, discuss alternative formulas with your physician. Anyone who has lactose intolerance from birth should realize the condition is probably permanent, and should continue to avoid drinking cow's milk.

Hepatitis in children

Hepatitis is inflammation of the liver. In children it is usually caused by a virus that enters through the mouth and is carried to the liver in the bloodstream. Of the various forms of hepatitis, the one that is most likely to affect children is acute hepatitis A (see p.486). The disease, which develops between two and six weeks after the initial infection, is milder in children than in adults. It frequently occurs in crowded living situations.

What should be done?
A child who develops the symptoms of hepatitis (see p.486) should see a physician, who will usually advise bed rest as the only treatment necessary. One symptom of the disease is severe loss of appetite. To make sure the child has some nourishment, give him or her frequent small feedings of whatever the child will take. Encourage him or her to drink fluids that are high in calories, such as milk shakes. After about two weeks in bed, the child usually feels well enough to get up, and after two more weeks he or she can return to school.

Hepatitis is an infectious disease, so the child who has hepatitis, together with the other members of the family, should avoid contact with other children. The family should be more careful than usual about washing hands after using the toilet and before meals. And the toilet bowl, the bathroom sink and any potties should be cleaned several times a day with an antiseptic.

What are the long-term prospects?
The outlook after recovery from the disease is excellent. In children there are usually no after-effects of the disease except the beneficial one of immunity from further attacks.

Growth disorders

Published figures for the average height and weight of children of any given age worry some parents whose child's size differs from the average. They think there may be something wrong with the child. However, this is unlikely. If you look at the charts provided here (see p.645), you will see that there is a wide range of height and weight in normal, healthy children. The differences are due mainly to hereditary factors. Usually, it is only if your child's size falls outside the total normal range for his or her age that one of these growth disorders may be responsible.

Nutritional disorders
The most common nutritional problem among children in the Western world is being overweight, or obesity (see p.492). Obesity should be treated not because it is immediately harmful to the child's health, but because it often persists into adult life. In adults, obesity increases the risks that accompany many diseases. Malnutrition is the opposite extreme. It may be due to social factors or illness. Among the disorders that can limit growth are celiac disease (see p.684) and cystic fibrosis (see p.685).

Delayed puberty
Puberty normally starts in girls at about 11½ and in boys a year or two later. Delay in its onset is often hereditary. If you are concerned about delayed onset of puberty in your child, consult your physician.

Hormonal disorders
These illnesses are usually caused by inadequate or excessive hormone production by the pituitary gland (see p.515) or the thyroid gland (see p.525). They are the least common of the growth disorders. They include gigantism (see p.516), dwarfism (see p.516), and hypothyroidism (see p.526).

Other causes of growth problems
Permanent impairment of growth may also occur as a side-effect of certain severe chronic diseases. Some examples are congenital heart disorders (see p.656), sickle-cell anemia (see p.422), thalassemia (see p.422), chronic kidney failure (see p.512), and rheumatoid arthritis (see p.552).

What should be done?
If you have consulted the charts (see p.645),

and you are still concerned about your child's size, or if there has been a change in the pattern of the child's growth, take him or her to your physician. After an examination, your doctor will either be able to reassure you that there is nothing wrong, prescribe treatment for an obvious problem such as obesity, or arrange for diagnostic tests.

Phenyl-ketonuria

To develop and function, the body needs protein, which is made up of chemicals called amino acids. Normally, excess amounts of any amino acid taken into the body are broken down or excreted, but in phenylketonuria (PKU), the body, through an inherited defect, lacks the means to break down one of these amino acids, phenylalanine.

If excess phenylalanine accumulates in the spinal fluid and blood, it damages the nervous system. This happens in rare cases when a baby with PKU develops in the womb of a mother who herself has the disorder. The baby is born with a small, deformed brain, and, in some cases, also a deformed heart. If, as is usually the case, the mother is only a "carrier" of the disorder, the baby with PKU is normal at birth.

How genetic defects such as the one that causes PKU are inherited is described elsewhere (see Genetics, p.704).

The disorder is extremely rare, but it is becoming slightly more common as more people who have the disorder reach adulthood and have children.

What should be done?
A test for PKU should be given to all babies shortly after birth. This is usually done as a matter of course. If the test shows that the baby has PKU, a special diet will be prescribed immediately so that the baby's brain will not be damaged.

What is the treatment?
The baby is immediately put on a special formula that is low in phenylalanine. (Some must be included because a certain amount of the amino acid is essential to the body.) Breast-feeding is not possible. When the baby begins to eat specially selected solids, the special formula is retained as the child's protein source. The child with PKU must stay on a vegetable and salad diet that, to provide the necessary protein, vitamins and minerals, includes a number of special foods that are available commercially. The diet is expensive and requires imagination and careful preparation so that the child will not find it monotonous. For this reason, physicians are anxious to establish whether at a certain age the nervous system is sufficiently well-developed to resist damage caused by high levels of phenylalanine, so that the child can safely change to a normal diet.

Trials indicate that this may occur when the child is between 10 and 12 years old. A woman with treated phenylketonuria who has returned to a regular diet should revert to the special low-phenylalanine diet before becoming pregnant to try to protect the health of the unborn child.

Constipation in children

A child should be regarded as constipated only if he or she persistently does not have a bowel movement for four days or more and if the bowel movements are hard when they do occur.

A diet deficient in fiber is responsible for many cases of constipation. Be sure that your child has enough fiber by including fruit, vegetables, and whole grains in the diet (see Balanced diet, p.26). Babies six months old or older can be given fiber in the form of whole wheat cereals.

Another common cause of constipation is an anal fissure (see p.484), a small tear in the anus that makes bowel movements so painful that the child avoids having them.

A child may also become constipated during an acute infection, through drinking far less than usual or through losing liquid by sweating more than usual. To prevent this, encourage the child to drink as much as possible.

Severe constipation that lasts for two weeks or more may be a symptom of Hirschsprung's disease (see p.663) or of hypothyroidism (see p.526).

If your child is severely constipated, consult your physician. Do not try to cure the condition yourself by giving the child laxatives.

Urinary tract and sex organs

The urinary tract consists of the two kidneys, the two tubes called ureters that lead from the kidneys to the bladder, the bladder itself, and the tube that leads from the bladder to the outside, which is called the urethra (see p.500 for a detailed description of the urinary tract). Closely linked to the tract are the sex organs (see Special problems of men, p.570, and Special problems of women, p.582).

Urinary problems in children should always receive medical attention. Abnormal-looking urine, especially, should be reported to your physician to avoid kidney failure (see p.511) later in life.

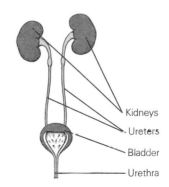

Kidneys
Ureters
Bladder
Urethra

Bed-wetting
(*enuresis*)

Medical myths

1. Children who wet the bed sleep more deeply, and generally pass more urine, than other children.

Wrong. Children who wet the bed sleep as deeply and pass as much urine as other children.

2. Cutting down on drinks before bedtime helps prevent bed-wetting.

Wrong. The amount of liquid the child drinks has no effect on the problem.

By the age of three and a half, about three-quarters of all children stay dry at night. The other quarter continue to wet the bed, and in a few cases also wet themselves during the day. The medical term for this problem is enuresis, and it is sometimes called incontinence. If the child becomes enuretic after a long period of dryness following successful toilet training, it is called secondary enuresis.

The cause of enuresis, especially secondary enuresis, can be psychological. It may be caused by stress from, for example, the arrival of a new baby, or separation from the mother. In a small minority of cases, there is an underlying illness, such as spina bifida (see p.654), or unrecognized or untreated diabetes (see p.519), which is usually marked by constant thirst. But in most cases, the cause of bedwetting is unknown.

The problem can continue for several years. It is slightly more common in boys than in girls, and it often runs in families.

What should be done?
At some time after the child goes to sleep, wake the child and have him or her urinate. If the child is of school age, he or she may be able to deal with the problem by setting an alarm clock to go off in the middle of the night. Also, try to make clean pajamas and bed linens available so the child does not have to wake you for assistance. If, after a few weeks, this fails to have any effect on the problem, consult your physician to make sure there is nothing physically wrong with the child. The doctor will probably take a sample of urine for analysis, and, in rare cases, the child may need to have further tests.

The same principles that apply to toilet training should also be used to deal with bed-wetting. Praise the child for any dry nights and encourage him or her to keep a record of them, but never scold or punish the child for wet nights, or make a record of them. This can deeply hurt the child, who, after all, has no control over the problem, and it may also make the bed-wetting worse.

If the child is seven or over, your physician may suggest the use of an alarm that rings loudly as soon as the first drop of urine touches the bed. This has the eventual effect on many children of making them wake up whenever they feel the need to urinate, before they have passed any urine. Whatever measures are used, the problem will nearly always clear up before adolescence.

Urinary infections in children

In a urinary tract infection, infectious agents, usually bacteria, gain access to and multiply in the urinary tract. The process of infection and the symptoms produced are much the same in children as in adults (see Acute pyelonephritis, p.502). Young girls are especially prone to infections because their urethra, which is the tube leading from the bladder to the outside, is relatively short. This makes it easier for germs from the outside to make their way to the bladder.

What are the risks?
Infections of the urinary tract are quite com-

mon during childhood. But, there are few risks from one or two bouts with such infections. However, if the problem recurs, it may be a sign that the child has some underlying abnormality of the urinary tract (see Chronic pyelonephritis, p.503). It is essential that any such abnormality be detected and corrected as soon as possible in order to prevent the development of chronic pyelonephritis and, eventually, chronic kidney failure (see p.512). Take your child to your physician if you suspect a urinary infection. Abnormal-looking urine, especially, should always be reported as soon as possible.

What should be done?

The physician will probably have a sample of the child's urine tested. The next step, if the infection recurs, will probably be to arrange for two special *X-rays*: an *intravenous pyelogram* (*IVP*) and a *voiding cystogram*. For these, a special dye is injected into a vein in the child's arm. The dye shows up on the X-ray, and outlines any abnormalities in the structure of the urinary tract or in the flow of the urine through it.

Remember that even a young child can be very sensitive about the parts of the body involved in urinary infections. If the child is embarrassed, indicate that you understand the embarrassment and sympathize. Since the child's feelings are normal, it is wise to tell him or her that nearly everyone feels as he or she does and must overcome it.

What is the treatment?

Self-help: Be sure that the child carries out the doctor's instructions about drinking extra liquids. Encourage the child to empty his or her bladder completely when going to the toilet. Going again a few minutes later will help this. And although symptoms subside a few days after starting to take the prescribed drugs, the treatment must be completed.

Professional help: The infection itself is treated with *antibiotics* in tablet or, for younger children, in liquid form.

If X-rays have revealed any underlying abnormality of the urinary tract, then corrective surgery may be necessary. The outlook is better for children whose urinary tract problems are diagnosed and treated early.

Glomerulo-nephritis in children

There are several forms of the disease called glomerulonephritis (see p.504 for a general description, and also Nephrotic syndrome, next article). One acute form develops in a child who has had a streptococcal (bacterial) infection, usually a sore throat, two to three weeks earlier. It is called post-streptococcal glomerulonephritis, or sometimes simply "nephritis." The body produces substances called *antibodies* to fight the invading bacteria, but through some fault in the body's immune system the antibodies persist after the bacteria have been destroyed, and they begin to harm the kidneys. The kidneys become inflamed, reduce urine production, and allow blood to leak into the urine.

What are the symptoms?

The symptoms appear over a few days. One main symptom is a reduced amount of urine. The urine that is produced looks smoky or reddish-brown because it is bloody. The main symptom is accumulation of fluid throughout the body because of the reduced urine output. The excess fluid (*edema*) appears as swellings around the eyes and face, or even over the whole body. In addition, some children suffer from a headache and fever.

What are the risks?

This type of glomerulonephritis is rare; it complicates only a small fraction of streptococcal infections. Most children recover completely from acute glomerulonephritis. During the illness, the build-up of fluid in the body may cause heart failure (see p.381). Also, the child's blood pressure may rise dramatically, and this produces a severe headache, vomiting, and perhaps convulsions (see p.667). Consult your physician without delay if this happens.

In a few children, abnormalities of the kidney persist. The result after many years could be chronic kidney failure (see p.512).

What should be done?

Acute glomerulonephritis is a problem that requires medical attention. Abnormal-looking urine or abnormal amounts of urine, in particular, should always be reported to your physician. If after a physical examination the doctor suspects acute glomerulonephritis, blood and urine samples will be collected. Laboratory analysis of these will indicate whether the diagnosis is correct.

What is the treatment?

The physician will usually advise that the child rest quietly, in bed if he or she is very ill. In addition, the child will be put on a diet that restricts the intake of salt, liquids, and, sometimes, protein (meat, fish, eggs). The diet is designed to ease strain on the kidneys and to counteract accumulation of fluid in the body.

Antibiotics in tablet or liquid form may be prescribed to eradicate any remaining infection. A *diuretic* drug may be given to increase the volume of urine thereby eliminating excess fluids from the body.

Children with any problems that increase the risks associated with the disease will be admitted to the hospital. There, with a staff of physicians, support personnel and modern equipment, any complications can be treated immediately. The child's blood pressure is checked regularly. If it rises to a dangerously high level, drugs may be prescribed to control it (see High blood pressure, p.382). Even with complications, the prospects for a full recovery within several weeks are excellent.

Nephrotic syndrome

Nephrotic syndrome is a disorder of the kidney that affects children. The tiny filtering units of the kidneys, the glomeruli, are damaged. When this happens, one result is that proteins leak out of the blood into the urine. A second result is that the volume of urine is much reduced, so fluid that should be passed out of the body accumulates in the tissues just under the skin. It is this fluid that produces the symptoms of the disorder.

What are the symptoms?

There are two main symptoms of nephrotic syndrome. The first is the gradual appearance, over several weeks, of generalized swelling throughout the child's body. This is due to accumulation of fluid (*edema*). The swelling is especially noticeable around the eyes and face.

Edema in children
A child with a kidney disorder may develop edema, a condition characterized by a puffy face and swollen abdomen and ankles.

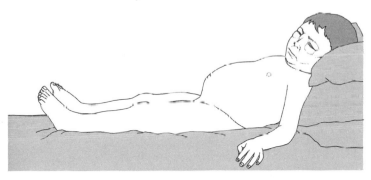

The second main symptom is a much reduced amount of urine, perhaps as little as one fifth the normal amount. The urine usually looks normal.

What are the risks?

Nephrotic syndrome is uncommon. About 80 per cent of the cases occur in children who are between the ages of one and six. Of these cases, most occur in children between two and three. Boys are more likely than girls to get nephrotic syndrome.

A child with the syndrome is vulnerable to a variety of infections, including peritonitis (see p.470). But the main risk is that in a few cases the condition persists, despite intensive treatment. As these children grow up, most of them also develop chronic glomerulonephritis (see p.504), which can lead to kidney failure (see p.511).

What should be done?

Consult your physician if your child appears to be developing edema. The doctor will carefully examine the child and have samples of urine and blood sent for laboratory analysis. If results of the analysis suggest nephrotic syndrome, further tests on samples of blood and urine, and possibly a *biopsy* of the kidney, will be needed to confirm the diagnosis. In a biopsy, a small amount of tissue is removed and examined.

What is the treatment?

Self-help: Although the condition often requires hospital treatment, you can help your child by ensuring that he or she keeps to the prescribed special diet and takes any drugs exactly as advised by the physician. Food should be cooked and served without salt, and the food itself should contain plenty of protein – fish, meat, eggs and low-salt cheese. The doctor may also instruct you to restrict the child's liquid intake.

Professional help: Usually the child is sent to the hospital, where treatment by diet and drugs can be more easily supervised. The drugs often used are *diuretics* and *steroids*. The steroids are given in high doses at first but the amount is gradually reduced to none after about six to eight weeks. The symptoms usually clear up by the end of the second week, and the child is allowed to go home to recuperate further.

In some cases there is complete recovery with no after-effects. In others, the child will have another attack of the condition after several weeks or months. Treatment as described will again relieve the symptoms. In a small proportion of cases, attacks continue to recur, and a prolonged course of steroid drugs or other drugs may eventually eliminate the condition.

692 SPECIAL PROBLEMS OF INFANTS AND CHILDREN

Wilm's tumor

In this disorder, which almost exclusively affects children who are under five years old, a *malignant*, or life-threatening, tumor forms in one of the kidneys.

What are the symptoms?
The main symptom of the tumor is a hard lump in the abdomen. There may also be blood in the urine and/or abdominal pain.

What are the risks?
The disorder is very rare. However, for those children who get Wilm's tumor, the risks are those of all cancers. The malignant cells may spread to other parts of the body and initiate secondary tumors that are also life-threatening. Fortunately, despite this, recent advances in treatment have greatly improved the outlook for children with this disease.

What should be done?
If you notice the symptoms described, consult your physician. If the doctor suspects a tumor, the child probably will be given special *X-ray* tests; an *intravenous pyelogram* (*IVP*) and a *CAT scan*. If Wilm's tumor is diagnosed, the affected kidney will have to be removed surgically to control the spread of the cancer. The remaining kidney will be able to take over the work of the missing one. The child will also be given *cytotoxic*, or anti-cancer, drugs to destroy any remaining cancer cells. *Radiation therapy* may also be used for this purpose.

Undescended testes
(*cryptorchidism*)

In boys, the testes, the male sex glands, develop inside the abdomen from the same embryonic tissue that becomes the ovaries in girls. Normally, by a month before birth, both testes have descended through the abdominal wall into the sac called the scrotum.

In a very small proportion of boys, one testis or both testes fail to descend by birth, for reasons that are not known. The condition does not cause any pain or problems with urinating, but there may be an associated inguinal hernia (see p.538).

What are the risks?
Usually, the testis or testes descend during the boy's first few years, and regular medical checkups reveal when this has happened. Undescended testes after this age may eventually cause the boy to become infertile if the problem is not corrected.

What is the treatment?
If either or both testes have not descended by the time the boy is five years old, an operation known as an orchidopexy is carried out to lower the testis or testes into the correct position, within the scrotum. Any hernia that is present is repaired at the same time.

Once the testes are descended, there should be no further problems. However, in some instances it is discovered later that the boy grew up to have decreased fertility.

Vulvovaginitis

Vulvovaginitis is redness, itching, and soreness of the vulva, the moist, normally pink fold that surrounds the opening to the vagina. It affects only a small proportion of girls, usually those who have a particularly sensitive vulva. In many cases, no cause can be found for the condition. In other cases it is caused by infectious agents in bowel movements, or by a skin allergy to wool, nylon, fabric softeners or detergents. Bed-wetting (see p.689) or pinworms (see p.703) are also possible causes. Very rarely, the discomfort is caused by the child inserting a foreign object into her vagina. In such cases, there is usually a foul-smelling discharge. The disorder may occur at any age.

The soreness can produce a frequent desire to urinate, and this urination is sometimes quite painful. This symptom may lead to the mistaken conclusion that the child has a bladder disorder.

What should be done?
In all cases, a physician should be consulted. If the doctor suspects that an object in the vagina is causing the problem, the vagina will be examined and any object removed.

In most cases, careful hygiene solves the problem. After a bowel movement, girls should wipe the anus in a backward direction only. This assures that the soiled toilet paper will not touch the vaginal area. A girl with this disorder should have a bath every day, and the vulva should also be washed after each bowel movement. After all bathing, the area should be dried thoroughly but gently, dusted carefully with medicated powder and covered with a protective ointment, also called a "barrier cream."

The child's underwear should be changed daily. The underwear should be made of cotton or, at least, have a cotton insert or panel, and be loose-fitting.

Muscles, bones and joints

The most common cause of the muscle, bone and joint problems that occur in children is injury (see p.532). Fortunately, most childhood injuries heal quickly and completely. However, in addition to injuries, there are a few disorders that are especially troublesome in children. Rheumatic fever is very rare now, but severe or recurrent bouts can lead to valvular heart disease (see p.392). It does not cause permanent joint problems, however.

An infection of the bone, osteomyelitis, can also have serious complications, but is usually treated successfully. Juvenile rheumatoid arthritis, a rare *autoimmune* disorder, will usually have run its course by the time the child reaches puberty. Muscular dystrophy is an inherited disease that causes progressive wasting of the muscles. Intensive research is being carried out to find a cure for this disease.

Rheumatic fever in children

Rheumatic fever is a disease that most commonly attacks children of school age, particularly those six to eight years old. It is usually, but not always, characterized by a painful swelling of certain joints. The disease originates, one to six weeks before its characteristic symptoms begin, in a throat infection caused by a particular strain of *Streptococcus* bacterium. The body produces specific *antibodies* to destroy the bacteria, but in some children these antibodies also attack the tissues of the joints. Less commonly, they attack the tissues of the heart, or the tissues of both heart and joints. Inflammation of the joints has no long-lasting effect, but inflammation of the heart occasionally causes permanent damage to the heart valves.

Few children infected by the *Streptococcus* bacterium develop rheumatic fever. Their susceptibility is at least partly hereditary, and is intensified if their living conditions and medical care are not adequate.

What are the symptoms?

If the joints have been affected, one or more become red, swollen, hot and painful to move. The child also has a fever, loses appetite, feels generally unwell, and may be pale and sweaty. The inflammation of the joints usually disappears after about 24 hours, but if by this stage the disease has not been treated, other joints may in turn become temporarily inflamed. The wrists, elbows, knees and ankles are the joints most commonly affected. The hips, shoulders, fingers and toes are also occasionally involved, but rarely without other joint involvement.

If the heart alone has been affected and the disorder is mild there are often no obvious symptoms, only vague ones such as tiredness, paleness and general illness. This is why in many cases a physician is not consulted and the condition remains undiagnosed. But in severe cases there are definite symptoms. The chief one is breathlessness, especially during exertion or when the child is lying flat. Also, fluid accumulates under the skin of the legs and back, often causing swelling.

In some cases of rheumatic fever a rash appears, usually on the chest, back and abdomen. The rash consists of reddish circles with pale centers. They are a few centimeters (1 to 2 in) across and keep changing in shape. The rash does not itch.

Nodules, or little swellings, sometimes appear, particularly when the heart is affected, just below the skin, over bony prominences such as the elbows, knees and knuckles, and the back of the head. They are round, about 5 to 10 mm ($\frac{1}{4}$ to $\frac{1}{2}$ in) across, firm and painless.

What are the risks?

The disease is no longer as widespread and serious a problem as it used to be. Within the last 20 years the number of cases has decreased substantially. This change has occurred partly because of *antibiotic* treatment of infections and partly because of a general improvement in living conditions, diet and hygiene. These factors have made the bacterium responsible for the disease less common and increased children's resistance to it.

Unless it is severe, a single attack of rheumatic fever is unlikely to lead to valvular heart disease (see Mitral stenosis, p.395, and Aortic incompetence, p.399). The risk of heart disease increases with one or more additional attacks. At one time, a child who had rheumatic fever once was more likely than other children to have an attack in the future, but today the life-long prescription of antibiotics for a child who has had an attack should protect against further streptococcal throat infections. The child who still runs a risk of developing heart disease is the one whose attack of rheumatic fever has not been diagnosed and treated.

In very severe cases of rheumatic fever that affect the heart, there is a slight risk of heart failure (see p.381).

What should be done?

If your child has any of the symptoms described, put him or her to bed and consult your physician. If the physician suspects rheumatic fever, a *throat culture* and a sample of the child's blood may be taken for laboratory analysis. The physician will also examine the child carefully to discover whether the heart has been affected.

What is the treatment?

If the attack of rheumatic fever is mild, the child can rest in bed at home until tests show that the attack is over.

In more severe cases, the child is admitted to the hospital. There the pain and swelling of inflamed joints may be quickly eased with fairly high doses of aspirin. When the heart is also affected, the drug may be continued in smaller doses even after the joint inflammation has disappeared.

In particularly severe cases, especially when the heart is seriously affected, more powerful anti-inflammatory drugs such as *steroids* may be prescribed.

In the rare event of actual heart failure, drugs that strengthen the heart's pumping action may be given. A *diuretic* may also be prescribed in such cases. This type of drug stimulates urination, eliminating some of the excess liquid that typically accumulates in the body in cases of heart failure. Whenever the heart is affected, the child will be more comfortable propped up in bed with pillows. This eases any breathlessness that might occur. In all cases of rheumatic fever, an *antibiotic* is prescribed to fight any bacteria that remain from the original throat infection and to prevent further attacks.

What are the long-term prospects?

Today the long-term prospects are good. After any attack of rheumatic fever, mild or severe, physicians now prescribe a low dose of an antibiotic to be taken daily to prevent another attack. Even when valvular heart disease does develop, whether it is because of undiagnosed attacks of rheumatic fever, or a repeated attack because of a failure to take the prescribed medication regularly, with available modern treatment most people who have had rheumatic fever can lead a normal or near-normal life.

Muscular dystrophy

Muscular dystrophy is a progressive wasting and weakening of the muscles. There are several forms of the disease, but all of them are very rare. The most common and well known type, which this article discusses, is Duchenne muscular dystrophy. This disease starts during early childhood, usually before the child reaches the age of five, and initially affects the muscles of the shoulders, hips, thighs and calves. In time, it spreads to all muscles and causes progressive crippling and immobility. Then the child becomes susceptible to serious chest infections.

Like hemophilia and color blindness, the disorder affects only boys and is generally inherited through female carriers of the disease. Although it is inherited, in 30 to 50 per cent of cases the disease occurs in a family that has no history of muscular dystrophy.

What are the symptoms?

The boy toddler develops a waddling gait, with his feet wide apart. He has trouble climbing stairs, falls easily, and finds it difficult to get up. Also, he can scarcely raise his arms above his head. The affected muscles sometimes look larger than normal. This is because fat replaces wasted muscle. In most cases, the limbs and spine become deformed, so that by the time he reaches adolescence the boy is confined to a wheelchair.

If your son shows any of the signs of muscular dystrophy, see your physician immediately. Special tests, perhaps including a muscle *biopsy*, will show whether the boy has the disease or not. In the biopsy, a small amount of muscle tissue is removed for examination under a microscope.

Any woman from a family with a history of the disease should consult a physician or a genetic counselor before deciding to have a child. If a carrier gives birth to a boy, there is a 50 per cent chance that the child will have muscular dystrophy. If the woman decides to go ahead and have a child, its sex can be tested during early pregnancy (see Screening for congenital defects, p.630). If you may be a

A distinctive sign of muscular dystrophy is that the child has difficulty getting into an upright position.

carrier, and the test indicates that you are going to have a boy, you may wish to consider terminating the pregnancy. Your physician will no doubt be able to tell you how to contact a genetic counsellor if you feel you need a thorough explanation of the genetic aspects of the disease and want help in determining what course of action might be best for you to follow.

What is the treatment?

No cure has yet been found for muscular dystrophy, and the physical therapy given is aimed at minimizing deformities. These deformities will always be pronounced, and the boy may need to attend a school for the physically handicapped. Eventually, by about age 20, the boy will get a chest infection such as pneumonia, which will prove fatal.

Osteomyelitis in children

Osteomyelitis is an infection of bone and bone marrow. Despite its apparent inertness, bone is an active, living tissue and is honeycombed with blood vessels that deliver the oxygen and nutrients that the bone needs if it is to survive.

Bacteria from, for example, a contaminated skin wound, can get into the blood and start an infection in the bone. The area becomes inflamed and pus forms just as in a skin infection such as a boil (see p.251). Why the bone infection develops is unknown. Usually only a single area in one of the limb bones near a joint is affected, but rarely, and especially in children, more than one bone becomes infected.

What are the symptoms?

Symptoms usually develop over two or three days. The main one is pain and excruciating tenderness in the affected area, particularly when the joint near it is flexed. An infant or young child will be reluctant to move an arm or a leg, and will probably scream with pain if the limb is touched or moved in any way. If a leg bone is infected, then the child is extremely reluctant to walk and, if forced to do so, has a pronounced limp.

A generally ill appearance and a high fever accompany the pain of osteomyelitis, and if the condition is not treated within another day or two the skin over the infection becomes red, swollen and tender.

Cancer in children

If your child has symptoms that cause you to suspect cancer, see your physician, who will probably be able to assure you that cancer is not present and put your mind at ease.

If your child is one of the few who does have a malignant disease, your physician will probably discuss with you the nature of the disease, the course of treatment, and the outlook for your child. You should know from the outset that cancer is not *contagious* (catching), and it is almost never hereditary. Nobody knows exactly what causes it, but it has nothing to do with the way you have raised the child.

Most children with malignant diseases are treated in a hospital that has access to the latest advances in treatment. If your child has to remain in the hospital for some time, he or she will demand much of your time, care and love. Being in a hospital will probably frighten the child. To make a strange place seem more familiar, bring the child a favorite toy or picture. After some time, your child may be allowed to go home, and probably return to school. Try to maintain as normal a home life as possible, and, within reason, do not lower your expectations of the child, either at school or at home.

Because you know your child best, you are probably the best judge of how much to tell him or her about the illness. If you are not sure how to explain the illness, discuss the problem with the physicians or nurses. Your doctor may agree to help you tell your child what is necessary, if you feel it would make things easier. Once you feel ready to approach your child, do not delay in doing so. It is clearly better for the child to learn about the illness from you and the doctor than to be told by someone who is less concerned for him or her, or to imagine something worse than the truth.

In most cases, the chances are greater than 50 per cent that your child will recover. But whatever the outlook, the months ahead will probably be difficult ones for your whole family. Do not keep your worries bottled up inside. Feel free to discuss your feelings with the team of professionals who are treating your child. Talking things over with friends and relatives may also help. Ask your physician to put you in touch with self-help groups of parents whose children have had cancer. Learning how other parents have coped may help you and your child to come to terms with the illness.

What are the risks?

Osteomyelitis is a rare condition in the Western world. In children it seems to occur most frequently between the ages of 5 and 14, and more often in boys than in girls.

In the extremely unlikely event that the condition is completely neglected, the bacteria can spread and multiply in the blood, and cause blood poisoning (see p.421). A more likely, though still rare, risk is that the infection will eat away a considerable area of bone and may even spread into the neighboring joint. If this happens, the result is likely to be permanent stiffness or deformity of the infected joint.

Another risk is that the infection will spread upwards and break through to the skin surface. This appears as an *abscess*, which discharges pus and will not heal until the underlying bone infection is treated.

What should be done?

If your infant or child has symptoms of osteomyelitis, consult your physician without delay. If the doctor's examination confirms that the child has the disease, the child will probably be hospitalized right away. To confirm the diagnosis, blood tests and *X-rays* of the infected area will be carried out.

Although osteomyelitis is rare, it is a good idea to guard against it. Cleanse all wounds thoroughly, and protect them with a clean dressing until they are completely healed.

What is the treatment?

The main treatment is a course of *antibiotic* drugs, given in tablet or liquid form (or perhaps at first in an *intravenous drip*) for about six weeks.

If necessary, a minor operation is carried out to drain and clean out the abscess. In some cases, the physician may decide to immobilize the affected limb in splints or a plaster cast. Once the infection is healing, the child will be allowed to go home, but your physician's instructions regarding antibiotics and exercise must be followed until the condition is cured.

Juvenile rheumatoid arthritis

(Still's disease)

Juvenile rheumatoid arthritis is believed to be an *autoimmune* disorder, or an intermittent malfunctioning of the body's defense mechanism. *Antibodies*, which are produced to combat invading infectious agents, attack the body's own tissues. These antibodies cause inflammation of organs, joints and other parts of the body. The disease starts most commonly between the ages of two and five and comes and goes over a number of years, usually disappearing by puberty. The attacks each last for an average of a few weeks, and tend to lessen in severity.

What are the symptoms?

The child usually has a fluctuating temperature, which often swings from normal in the morning to about 103°F (39.4°C) in the evening. Appetite is poor, causing weight loss. A blotchy, red rash may break out over the trunk and limbs. Anemia often develops.

Sites of inflammation vary considerably from case to case. The front of one or both eyes may become red and painful, the lymph glands in the neck and armpits may swell, or the outer membrane of the heart may be inflamed, and cause chest pain (see Acute pericarditis, p.401). The joints, most commonly the knees, ankles and elbows, and the joints of the neck, may become swollen, stiff, and painful, usually gradually, but sometimes abruptly. In a few cases, the joints become deformed over the years.

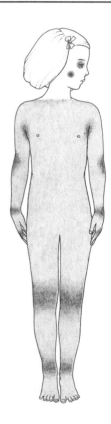

Sites of rash (gray) and other possible visible symptoms (dark gray)

What are the risks?

Juvenile rheumatoid arthritis is uncommon, and girls are affected about four times as often as boys. In a small proportion of cases, inflammation of the joints leads to partial or crippling deformity, and inflammation of the eyes to partial or complete blindness.

What should be done?

If your child has any of the symptoms described, see your physician. A physical examination and blood tests are usually sufficient to make a firm diagnosis. If only the joints are swollen and there are doubts about the cause, a *biopsy* of the membrane that encloses one of the joints may be carried out. In a biopsy, a small amount of tissue is removed for examination.

What is the treatment?

Self-help: The child should have plenty of rest but should be allowed to get up when he or she feels like it. Encourage the child to eat, and provide a nutritious, balanced diet (see p.26) that contains plenty of protein. For children who have inflammation of the hand joints, special cutlery may help. If your child cannot get to school, contact your local school district for help.

Professional help: This is the same as for adult rheumatoid arthritis (see p.552). Aspirin and anti-inflammatory drugs will probably be prescribed.

In addition, physical therapy exercises are prescribed when the joints are affected. These are exercises both for the parents to perform on the joints and for the child to do alone. It is important that you make sure the child does the exercises. This is because they are crucial to minimizing the pain and the crippling effects of rheumatoid arthritis.

What are the long-term prospects?

With treatment, most children and young adults who have the disease will recover and function normally. However, in a few cases the child is severely disabled by the disease, and a very few die from it.

Flat feet, bow legs, and knock knees

From the time most children begin to learn to walk, until the onset of puberty, their legs and feet gradually change shape. Flat feet, bow legs and knock knees are stages through which almost all children pass to some degree, and they are usually no cause for concern.

Normal feet

Flat feet

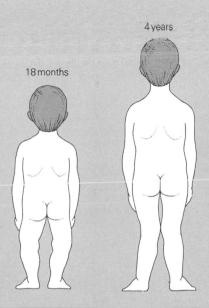

18 months

4 years

A child with flat feet has no arches and therefore makes a different footprint from a child whose arches have developed.

At birth, a normal baby has flat feet. Arches develop slowly over the first six years. Until the age of two, the child tends to have bow legs. That is, when the ankles touch each other, the knees do not. As the child learns to walk, this tendency is increasingly reversed until, at the age of three or four, he or she tends to be knock-kneed. When the child stands with the knees together, the ankles do not meet. Over the next few years, the knees and ankles become more aligned, until by the teens the legs and feet appear normal.

In the vast majority of children with flat feet, bow legs or knock knees, no treatment is necessary. Be sure that your child's shoes fit well, and that there is plenty of opportunity for the child to exercise his or her growing feet and legs. In some children one or more of these variations in posture may persist into adolescence and adulthood. Usually they are inherited, and only rarely are they caused by a disease. If your child's feet and/or legs seem to be developing abnormally, or your child's progress in learning to walk seems slow (see Milestones, p.645), consult your physician.

Childhood infectious diseases

An infectious disease is a disease caused by infectious agents that enter the body and multiply within it. Certain infectious diseases are usually caught during childhood and, once you recover, you are very unlikely to catch the same disease again. Measles, German measles, chickenpox, mumps, whooping cough, scarlet fever and diphtheria are described in the following articles. All of these except chickenpox and scarlet fever can be prevented by immunization.

The childhood infectious diseases described here are *contagious*; that is, they spread from one person to another. The causative agents can live outside the body for only a few hours, and are usually spread in tiny droplets coughed or sneezed into the air and by direct contact. Such diseases often spread through a school as a minor epidemic.

Infectious agents enter the body through the thin lining of the respiratory or digestive tract. Once inside, there is an "incubation period" during which they are not sufficiently numerous to cause symptoms, and the child cannot usually infect others.

As the infectious agents increase in numbers and spread through the bloodstream and the lymphatic system (see p.432), symptoms begin to appear and the disease is contagious.

Meanwhile, the body is fighting the infection in various ways. One way is to manufacture *antibodies*, special substances that disarm or destroy the invaders. Each disease initiates the manufacture of a particular kind of antibody. Gradually the body's immune system overcomes the invaders.

Once you have had a particular infectious disease, your body can recognize any reinfection immediately, and antibodies destroy the infectious agents before they can cause symptoms. So once you have had the disease, you become immune. That is, you cannot have measles, German measles, mumps, or chickenpox more than once. This is called natural immunity. Sometimes a child's body is able to destroy infectious agents even before they cause symptoms. Such children are immune afterwards, although they apparently have not had the disease. Also, the body can be stimulated to produce antibodies against a certain disease by injecting a specially-prepared, harmless version of the infectious agent concerned. This process is called immunization (see p.701).

Caring for a child with an infectious disease

There are aspects of health care that apply to all the childhood infectious diseases. This information is summarized here.

General risks of childhood infectious diseases
One rare, though possible, result of an infectious disease is encephalitis, or inflammation of the brain (see p.274). Its symptoms are drowsiness or sleepiness so pronounced that it is difficult to wake the child fully; headache; sensitivity to bright lights; and, perhaps, unconsciousness. Encephalitis is serious. It usually comes on a week or so after the original disease has cleared up.

Other risks include febrile convulsions (see p.667), ear infections such as acute infections of the middle ear (see p.333) and respiratory tract infections such as pneumonia (see p.679). Become familiar with the symptoms of these complications, and if they occur, consult your physician without delay.

Children at special risk
Any child who develops an infectious disease risks having complications, but certain children are at special risk. They include infants under one year old, children who are taking *steroid* drugs, and children who already have a long-term disease, such as diabetes mellitus, asthma, or cystic fibrosis.

If you feel your child is at risk, inform your physician as soon as symptoms of an infectious disease appear, or if you know that such a child has been exposed to an infectious disease. For some diseases, such as measles and chickenpox, the physician may give the child an injection of *antibodies* called *gamma globulin*. This may either prevent the symptoms from developing or make them much less severe.

How to look after the child
There are ways that you can ease the symptoms of an infectious disease and make your child more comfortable. Here is a list of them (see also Caring for the sick at home, p.754):

To avoid spreading the infection and to help your child rest and recuperate, keep your child at home until your physician recommends that the child return to school.

If your child has a fever, contact your physician for a recommended anti-fever drug. Since some research links aspirin to Reyes' syndrome (a type of encephalitis) under certain conditions, the doctor may recommend an aspirin substitute.

Do not force your child to eat or stay in bed. Encourage rest, but light activities such as reading, coloring, or watching television can be helpful both to you and your child.

Do provide plenty of liquids to drink.

Measles

Measles is a highly *contagious* disease caused by a virus that spreads throughout the body but affects chiefly the skin and respiratory tract. The incubation period (see the introduction to this section, previous page) is 7 to 14 days.

Measles is much less common than it once was, due to an immunization program introduced in the late 1960's. The Public Health Service is attempting to eradicate measles completely in the United States, because it is the most serious of the preventable childhood infectious diseases. Measles has a high rate of complications, including pneumonia (see p.679) and encephalitis (see p.274).

What are the symptoms?
The following are typical measles symptoms.

On days one and two the child becomes miserable with a fever, runny nose, red watering eyes, dry cough and perhaps diarrhea. By day three the temperature falls and tiny white spots, like grains of salt, appear on the lining of the mouth. On days four to five, the temperature rises again and a characteristic skin rash appears. It starts on the forehead and behind the ears as small (2 to 3 mm, or about $\frac{1}{16}$ in) dull red, slightly raised spots. The spots gradually spread to the rest of the head and body. As they spread, the spots get bigger and join together. By day six the rash begins to fade quite quickly and usually by day seven all symptoms have gone.

Some children with measles complain that light hurts their eyes. Usually this is no cause for concern, but mention it to your physician. Rarely, it can indicate meningitis (see p.668).

See p.239,
Visual aids to diagnosis, 26.

What should be done?
Prevention is most important. Have your physician or the public health department in your area immunize your child against measles at the proper age (see Immunization, p.701). Notify your physician if you suspect your child has measles. If there is a local epidemic, your physician will know of it, and a telephone description of the symptoms may be enough for a diagnosis. Otherwise, the physician may want to see the child. At the first sign of any complications, consult your doctor without delay.

What is the treatment?
Self-help: There are several ways to make your child more comfortable and guard against possible risks (see Caring for a child with an infectious disease, previous page). Because measles is so contagious, it is not practicable to try to prevent other members of the family who are not immune from developing it.

Professional help: Prevention by immunization is important. However, if you or members of your family have not had the disease or been immunized, and have been exposed to measles, in some cases your physician may try to prevent or modify the disease. This is done by giving you an injection of *antibodies* called *gamma globulin.* Your physician is unlikely to prescribe *antibiotic* drugs, because they do not work against viruses. They may be prescribed, however, if bacteria-caused complications develop.

In most children, measles disappears within seven to ten days.

German measles
(rubella)

German measles is a *contagious* disease that is caused by a virus. It is a very mild infectious disease. In the majority of children who catch it, German measles causes no more inconvenience than a common cold (see p.342). Once inside the body, the virus has an incubation period (see the introduction to this section, previous page) of 14 to 21 days.

What are the symptoms?
For the first two days the child has a slight fever, and perhaps swollen glands behind the ears, down the side of the neck and on the nape of the neck. A rash appears on the second or third day. It consists of flat, reddish-pink spots about 2 to 3 mm ($\frac{1}{16}$ in) across, on the head and/or body. The rash does not itch, and lasts for only a day or two. By the fourth or fifth day all of the symptoms have faded away.

See p.239,
Visual aids to diagnosis, 27.

What are the risks?
German measles is slightly less common than measles (see previous article), and it is not as highly contagious and so does not spread through a school in quite the same way.

Because German measles is such a mild disease, little specific treatment is required (see Caring for a child with an infectious disease, previous page). But although the patient is at very little risk, the disease is known to cause damage to a baby developing in the uterus. It is therefore essential to contact any pregnant woman who has been exposed to German measles, either during the disease itself, or up to one week before the rash appears. There is an immunization available (see Immunization, p.701).

In general, all children should be immunized. Women of childbearing age who have not previously been vaccinated for German measles, and who either are not pregnant or will avoid pregnancy for at least three months, should be immunized as well to help prevent birth defects. If you think you have had German measles in the past, your physician can have you take a blood test to confirm your immunity (see also German measles and pregnancy, p.616).

Chickenpox
(varicella)

This mild infectious disease is caused by the herpes zoster virus, sometimes called varicella zoster. This is the same virus that, after years of dormancy, may cause shingles in adults (see p.562). The virus chiefly affects the skin and the lining of the mouth and throat. After it gets into the body, there is an incubation period (see the introduction to this section, p.698) of 7 to 21 days.

What are the symptoms?

See p.239,
**Visual aids to
diagnosis, 28.**

The main, and often the first, symptom of chickenpox is a skin rash. Groups of small, red, fluid-filled spots appear on many parts of the body. After a few days the spots burst or dry out, and then crust over. They are very itchy, and it is difficult to resist scratching them. Spots in the mouth, around the eyes, or in the vagina, may be quite painful.

In addition to the rash, a child may also have a slight fever, but in general does not appear ill. However, adults who catch the disease often have flu-like symptoms (see Influenza, p.559) for two or three days before the rash appears. Children recover very quickly, within seven to ten days, but adults are more likely to develop complications, and take longer to recover.

What are the risks?

Because there is no general vaccine for it, chickenpox is a fairly common and very contagious childhood disease. It is rare in adults.

If the spots are scratched excessively they may become infected and produce yellow pus. Your physician may prescribe antibiotic ointment or tablets if this happens.

What is the treatment?

A soothing cream or lotion applied to the spots will help relieve itching. If spots in the mouth or around the eyes are painful, your physician will prescribe appropriate treatment to relieve the pain. An *antihistamine* may be prescribed in severe cases. Read Caring for a child with an infectious disease (p.698) for general treatment.

Chickenpox is a mild, though irritating, disease. You can expect a complete recovery and consequent life-long immunity.

Mumps

Mumps is a common infectious disease that is caused by a virus. After an incubation period (see the introduction to this section, p.698) of 14 to 28 days, the salivary glands (see p.453) begin to swell. The parotid gland, which is located in the angle of the jaw, is particularly affected.

What are the symptoms?

The parotid gland on one side of the face under the ear begins to swell. After another day, the parotid gland on the other side may also swell. The swellings are usually accompanied by a fever, diarrhea, and a general feeling of being ill. Occasionally, the salivary glands under the jaw also swell, and it may be painful to open the mouth or to swallow.

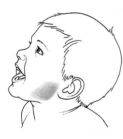

A child developing mumps will probably feel generally ill, then develop a tender swelling between the ear and the angle of the jaw.

What are the risks?

Mumps is a common childhood infectious disease. It is not very *contagious*, so it is uncommon for more than one member of a family to develop the disease at any one time. It is less common than it used to be, because a vaccine is now in widespread use.

A fairly common risk of mumps is swelling and inflammation of the testes in a boy or of the ovaries in a girl, which occurs three to four days after the neck glands swell. This is even more common when the disease occurs in adults. A boy will notice the swelling and it can be very painful for a day or two, but a girl may just have discomfort in her lower abdomen. The swelling goes down after a few days, and usually leaves no after-effects. In rare cases the swelling causes sterility.

In some cases, mumps is complicated by meningitis (see p.668). Another risk is acute pancreatitis (see p.490), which is felt as a stomach ache that usually passes within two to three days. Other risks of mumps, and general treatment for the disease, are described in Caring for a child with an infectious disease (see p.698). Mumps is generally a mild disease. Contact your physician if the salivary glands (or the testes) are very painful. You can help to ease the pain by applying warmth to the swollen area with a hot water bottle wrapped in a thick towel. Complete recovery within about ten days is usual.

Immunization

Immunization is the process by which people are made immune, or resistant, to specific disease-causing organisms, commonly known as "germs." There are two ways to become immune to disease. If you catch an infectious disease such as measles, your body produces *antibodies* that attack and destroy the measles-causing organisms. Your symptoms disappear, and you recover from the disease. If you are exposed to measles-causing organisms again, the antibodies you have already produced will destroy them before they can cause any symptoms. Therefore, you will not have measles a second time. This is called natural immunity.

You can also be made artificially immune to a disease without ever having it. Artificial immunity can be temporary or permanent. If you need temporary immunity, for example if *steroid* treatment makes you more prone to infection, your physician may inject you with antibodies. This passive, or temporary, immunity can last up to several months. To ensure active, or permanent, immunity, the physician will give you a *vaccine*, which is made with dead or harmless versions of the particular infectious agent, by injection or by mouth. Your body will produce antibodies to fend off these agents, and while you do not suffer the symptoms of the disease (except, in some cases, a slight fever), you become immune to it. This is called *vaccination* or immunization.

Today, largely because of advances in immunization, many childhood infectious diseases that used to cause serious illness and often death are now extremely rare. One

Age	Routine vaccine	Method
2 months	DTP* Poliomyelitis	Injection By mouth
4 months	DTP Poliomyelitis	Injection By mouth
6 months	DTP	Injection
15 months	Measles Mumps German measles (rubella)	Injection
1½ years	DTP Poliomyelitis	Injection By mouth
4 6 years	DTP Poliomyelitis	Injection By mouth
14–16 years	DT**	Injection

*DTP=Diphtheria, tetanus, and pertussis (whooping cough) vaccine
**DT=Diphtheria and tetanus vaccine

disease, smallpox (see p.566), has been completely wiped out. The chart above shows how a child's immunizations are usually scheduled, to offer maximum protection against serious infectious disease. These recommendations may change as new vaccines are developed and other discoveries are made, so consult your physician for the most current schedule. Vaccines are also available for influenza, pneumonia, typhoid fever, and other diseases, but these are given only in special circumstances.

If your child has ever had convulsions (see p.667), be sure to tell your physician before the child's immunizations begin. You should also tell the doctor if your child is ill at the time scheduled for an immunization. If the illness is simply a cold, the physician will probably proceed with the immunization or simply delay it a short time.

Whooping cough
(pertussis)

Whooping cough is a contagious disease that chiefly affects the respiratory system. Bacteria called *Bordetella pertussis* infect the lungs, and cause the air passages to become clogged with thick mucus. The extremely severe bouts of coughing characteristic of the disease are the body's attempts to clear the lungs of mucus. Symptoms develop after an incubation period of 7 to 14 days.

What are the symptoms?
The early symptoms are like those of an ordinary cold (see p.342): runny nose, dry cough and slight fever. But unlike an ordinary cold the symptoms do not improve after a few days. Instead, they worsen. The nasal discharge thickens, and the coughing becomes more severe until it occurs continuously in bouts up to a minute long. Because the child cannot breathe in during a bout of coughing,

his or her face turns deep red, or even blue (*cyanosis*), from lack of oxygen. At the end of each bout, as the child gasps for breath, he or she makes a "whooping" noise that gives the disease its name. Babies tend to whoop less loudly than older children.

Quite often vomiting occurs after a bout of coughing. The severe coughing phase of the disease can last from two to ten weeks. Gradually the coughing and vomiting become less severe and less frequent, though the cough may persist in a more ordinary form for several months.

What are the risks?
There is an effective immunization available for whooping cough, so the disease is uncommon. But if the number of children protected against whooping cough should fall, the disease will become more common.

Symptom comparison of infectious diseases

	Incubation period (days)	Fever	Skin rash	Swollen glands	Cough
Measles	7–14	Day 1 to 5	Day 4, dull red blotches	Slight	Day 1
German measles	14–21	Day 1 and 2, slight	Day 2 or 3 flat, light red spots	Day 1, neck and back of the head	None
Chickenpox	7–21	Slight	Day 1, groups of itchy, red spots that become blisters	None	None
Mumps	14–28	Day 1	None	One or both sides of the face	None
Whooping cough	7–14	Week 1	None	None	Week 1, becoming worse; week 2 severe bouts and characteristic whoop

There are several dangerous risks associated with whooping cough. Bursting of blood vessels in the brain during a bout of coughing, or asphyxia (lack of oxygen) can cause death. Although these are rarely lethal, they can also produce permanent brain damage. Another risk, pneumonia (see p.679), can produce permanent lung damage (see Bronchiectasis, p.363).

What should be done?
A child who has been immunized against whooping cough (see Immunization, previous page) may get a mild case at some time, but is unlikely to be seriously ill with the disease. Immunization should be carried out on young children because any risks associated with it are minimal compared with the risks of the disease itself.

If your child is not protected by immunization, and he or she develops a cough that does not clear up within a few days and seems to get worse, consult your physician.

What is the treatment?
Self-help: Most children can be cared for at home with a physician's supervision (see Caring for a child with an infectious disease, p.698). Get medical help without delay, however, if you notice that the child turns blue during a bout of coughing.

Do not give the child cough-suppressant medicines, because the cough, though distressing, does prevent mucus from clogging the lungs. You can counteract the tendency to vomit after coughing by feeding the child smaller, more frequent meals, and not giving any food just after a bout of coughing.

During a bout of coughing a baby is best lying face down with the foot of the crib raised. Children usually prefer to sit up and lean forward. There is little else you can do except comfort and reassure the child.

Professional help: *Antibiotics* may sometimes reduce the severity of the coughing phase. If the cough is very severe, babies especially are admitted to the hospital, where oxygen can be given with a face mask or a *ventilator.* Children who tend to panic during coughing bouts should be seen by a physician.

Scarlet fever

In this infection, certain *Streptococcus* bacteria enter the body through the pharynx, or throat, and cause an attack of tonsillitis (see p.676). Without *antibiotic* treatment, the bacteria multiply and produce a *toxin,* or poison, that circulates in the blood. After an incubation period of one to seven days, the amounts of toxin are sufficient to cause the symptoms of scarlet fever.

What are the symptoms?
The following is a description of a typical case of scarlet fever. The symptoms do vary slightly from person to person.

On day one the child develops a high fever (as high as 104°F, or 40°C), a red, sore throat and tonsils, and a furred tongue (see p.455). Sometimes a whitish coating covers the tonsils and the child may vomit.

On day two a bright red (scarlet) rash appears on the child's face, except for just around the mouth. By day three this rash, which may itch, has spread to cover the rest of the body and the arms and legs. Meanwhile the child's temperature starts to fall and the tongue becomes bright, strawberry-red.

By day six the rash has faded. Both skin and tongue may begin to peel, leaving a red, raw surface underneath. Peeling can last another 10 to 14 days.

Scarlet fever now has become rare. The two main risks, both very rare and occurring about two to three weeks after the rash, are rheumatic fever (see p.693) and a form of glomerulonephritis (see p.690).

Contact your physician if you suspect your child has scarlet fever. Follow the advice in Caring for a child with an infectious disease (see p.698). Also, your physician may prescribe an *antibiotic.* Make sure that the child takes the entire prescription, and you can expect a full recovery with no after-effects.

Diphtheria

Diphtheria is a dangerous disease that still occurs in less developed parts of the world. But thanks to an extensive immunization program the disease occurs very rarely. To insure the program's continuing success, it is essential that your infant receive the appropriate series of injections for life-long protection (see Immunization, p.701).

The symptoms of diphtheria include fever, rapid pulse, enlarged neck glands and, occasionally, a thick, yellow discharge from the nose. But the characteristic symptom is a greyish membrane on the throat and tonsils. This membrane can be very dangerous. It may become large enough to cause croup (see p.678) or even prevent breathing.

Inform your physician at once if these symptoms appear in a member of your family. If diphtheria is diagnosed, all personal contacts will be traced and tested for immunity to the disease. Treatment requires a hospital stay of three months or more. It involves injections of powerful *antibiotics* and *antitoxins*, and, if breathing is blocked, a temporary tracheotomy may be necessary to prevent suffocation. Damage to the heart, kidneys and nervous system, which can be caused by a toxin that is released from the bacteria causes death or permanent disability, even in treated cases.

Tuberculosis in children

Tuberculosis (TB) is an infectious disease caused by the tubercle bacteria. It occurs in two stages. At one time, the first stage mainly affected children, but today it is much rarer, and develops chiefly in young adults. The second stage occurs in adults. Because the two stages are interlinked, they are described in full in one article (see p.563).

While tuberculosis is less common today than it once was, it is still very much present in North America. Should your child develop a cough, fever, fatigue, poor appetite and weight loss, or any lumps or swellings that do not clear up, consult your physician.

Also, if your child has come into contact with someone who has active tuberculosis, take the child to your physician, who will check to see whether or not the child is infected. If the skin test is positive, chest *X-rays* may be needed, and antituberculosis drugs may be prescribed for a prolonged period to prevent the disease from progressing.

Pinworms

Pinworms are tiny white worms, about 1 cm (less than $\frac{1}{2}$ in) long, that are much more common in children, especially school-age children, than they are in adults. The worms' eggs can enter the body when swallowed by the child in food, or from clothing, toys, or even a sandbox contaminated by an infected child. The eggs hatch in the intestine, and young worms quickly begin to grow into adults. About two weeks later, a now-mature female worm lays eggs around the child's anus during the night. This may cause irritation, and if the child scratches the anus, he or she picks up some eggs on the fingers. Sucking the fingers or eating without washing them thoroughly will then cause reinfection. By contaminating food, drinking glasses, sheets and towels, the child may pass pinworms on to other family members.

Scratching the anus may make it more inflamed. The small, white, threadlike worms can sometimes be seen in bowel movements or around the child's anus at night. In some cases, the child has no symptoms.

If you see pinworms, or the child's anus constantly itches, the entire family should visit a physician. You can confirm the presence of pinworms by placing a strip of easily removable sticky tape across the child's anus in the early morning, preferably just before a bowel movement. Eggs in the area should stick to the tape, and you should give the tape to the doctor to confirm the diagnosis.

What is the treatment?
Self-help: The whole family should exercise scrupulous hygiene. Hands should be washed after going to the toilet, after handling a pet, which may also be infected, and before touching any food. Fingernails should be clipped short to lessen the chance of eggs being trapped under them. Sheets, pillowcases, nightwear, and underwear should be changed frequently, washed in very hot water or boiled, and ironed to kill worms or eggs. If you have a pet, consult a veterinarian about ridding the animal of the worms.
Professional help: The entire family will be treated, even those who have no symptoms. They may take one of several possible medications for a short time. The treatment is often repeated after two weeks. Anal inflammation may be relieved by cream or ointment, which may also contain a substance that kills the eggs. These measures should clear up the problem.

Genetics

Genetics is the scientific study of the process of biological inheritance. Its findings explain how and why certain traits such as hair color or blood types run in families.

Every baby develops from a single cell, the fertilized egg, which contains the information necessary for the development of inborn mental and physical characteristics. This information is carried in 23 pairs of rod-shaped *chromosomes*. Every pair of chromosomes includes one contributed by the mother and one by the father, and each chromosome contains thousands of genes. The genes are the factors that determine specific physical features of the child such as blood type and the color of eyes and hair. What those features will be depends on how the chromosomes from each parent were shuffled as the sperm and egg matured, and how the genes in one chromosome of a pair link up with their opposites in the other chromosome. To understand how certain disorders are caused by genetic transmission rather than by outside agents such as bacteria, it is essential to first understand the distinction between two types of genes: *dominant* and *recessive* genes.

To say that a gene is dominant means that the feature it determines will appear in the next generation regardless of the character of the corresponding gene in the other chromosome of the pair. Features determined by recessive genes will not show up in a child unless both parents contribute chromosomes that contain a recessive gene for that feature. For example, blue eyes are recessive and brown eyes are dominant, so a child will inherit blue eyes only if both parents contribute a gene for blue. If one parent contributes blue and the other brown, the child will have brown eyes. If both you and your spouse have blue eyes there are *no* genes for brown in either of you, since a gene for brown, because it is dominant, would have given you brown eyes. Therefore, your children *must* have blue eyes. On the other hand, even if both of you are brown-eyed, there may be genes for blue eyes in the chromosomes of each of you, so you could have blue-eyed children.

Single-gene disease

Most serious genetic disorders are caused by a single defective gene, which is usually recessive. In other words, the condition will not occur in a child unless both parents contribute the disease-determining gene to the fertilized egg. An example of this kind of disorder is cystic fibrosis (see p.685). About 1 in every 20 persons carries a gene for cystic fibrosis, usually without being aware of it. Only if two carriers have a child (a chance of 1 in 400) can the disease occur in the next generation, but the next generation *can* include carriers of the disease (see the accompanying diagrams for more details).

The pattern is complicated when, as in hemophilia (see p.424), the defective gene is carried in one of the chromosomes that determine the sex of the child. Females have two identical sex chromosomes (known as X chromosomes). Males have one X chromosome and one that is differently structured (known as a Y chromosome). If the sperm that fertilizes an egg carries an X chromosome, the

Cystic fibrosis is known to be caused by an inherited genetic abnormality involving a single defective gene. The defective gene is recessive, which means that only someone who inherits it from both parents will have cystic fibrosis. Most people have two normal genes (NN), one on each of the chromosomes, but a person with cystic fibrosis always has two cystic fibrosis genes (CC). In people with one C gene and one N gene, the N dominates the recessive C. But such people, though they are free of the disease themselves, are "carriers." That is, they can transmit the disease to future generations.

If two carriers have a child, it may not have the disease or be a carrier.

However, the baby may inherit genes for the disease from both parents (CC), in which case the child will have cystic fibrosis. The diagram at right shows the possibilities.

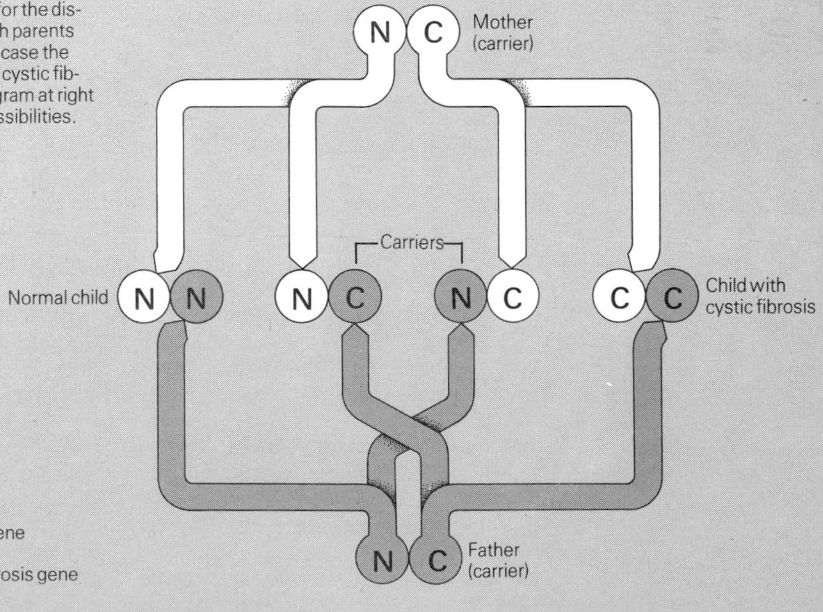

N = Normal gene

C = Cystic fibrosis gene

Mother (carrier)

Normal child

Carriers

Child with cystic fibrosis

Father (carrier)

baby will be a girl. If the sperm carries a Y chromosome, the baby will be a boy. Hemophilia is a sex-linked disease because the gene that governs the clotting ability of blood is carried in the X chromosome. Until very recently, few boys who had hemophilia survived to become fathers, so it was almost unknown for both parents to contribute a defective X gene to the fertilized egg. More usually, the mother (the carrier) contributed an X chromosome that contained the defective gene, and the father contributed a Y chromosome. There are some inevitable results of this gene combination.

1. The offspring will be a boy, because there is one X and one Y chromosome.

2. Although the abnormal gene is recessive, it cannot be overcome by a dominant gene since there is no gene for blood clotting on the differently-structured Y chromosome. Therefore, the boy child will have hemophilia. It also follows that:

1. All daughters of a man who has hemophilia will be carriers of the disease.

2. Only *some* of the daughters of a carrier may be carriers, since they can inherit the normal X chromosome rather than the one with the defective gene.

3. A man with hemophilia cannot pass the defective gene on to his sons because they will inherit his Y chromosome, on which there is no gene for blood clotting.

In a few single-gene diseases the defective gene is not recessive but dominant. This means that anybody who inherits that gene from either parent is bound to have the condition. For an example read the article on Huntington's chorea (see p.293), which is particularly tragic in that symptoms usually do not appear until middle age. For this reason, many people who have the disease do not know they have it until after they have had children and possibly passed the abnormal gene to them. Alternatively, knowing that Huntington's chorea runs in one branch of their family, they may decide not to have children and then discover, too late, that they themselves have not inherited the disease and would not have passed it on.

Multiple-gene disorders

Single-gene diseases are a relatively simple example of how inheritance works. Many disorders, however, are inherited not through a single gene but through more than one, and here the picture becomes much more complex. It can be said of many disorders that they "tend to run in families" (see, for instance, Coronary artery disease, p.374 and Asthma, p.355). What that vague phrase means is that there is probably a genetic element present in susceptibility to the disorder, but that it is difficult to isolate and define. Furthermore, the interaction between genes may be influenced, or their effects modified, by environmental factors such as upbringing and diet.

If you suspect or know that you and/or your sexual partner might pass an inherited disease along to your children, consult a genetic counselor (see p.619).

Allergies

An allergy is a physical disorder caused by hypersensitivity to substances that are eaten, inhaled, or brought into contact with the skin. This hypersensitivity results from a misdirected response by the body's natural immune system. Your immune system is designed to protect you from infection by invading organisms such as bacteria or viruses (see General infections, p.558). It does this by making *antibodies* that kill or neutralize the invaders. In people with allergies, the antibodies apparently attack normally harmless substances, which are called *allergens*.

The form that an allergy takes depends on both the type of antibody and the part of the body in which the battle between antibody and allergen takes place. In food allergies, for example, the allergen may cause symptoms that affect the intestines (as in celiac disease), or it may be absorbed into the bloodstream and come into conflict with antibodies in the blood vessels, which may cause a headache, or in the skin, which may cause a rash. In the type of allergic rhinitis known as hay fever, airborne pollens cause the reaction in the nose. In asthma, inhaled dust or pollen causes a reaction in the lungs.

In an allergic reaction, the cells of the immune system release irritant chemicals that cause the various symptoms characteristic of allergy attacks, including headaches, excessive production of mucus, and skin conditions such as redness, swelling and itching.

Who is susceptible?

Some people develop one or more allergies in infancy and have them all their lives. Others "outgrow" their allergies, while still others develop them later in life. Susceptibility seems to run in families (see Genetics, previous article), but there is no way to predict whether a particular member of a family will have allergies.

What is the treatment?

Theoretically the best "treatment" is total avoidance of exposure to the allergen. This is feasible only in certain cases, such as when you know you are allergic to a particular food or drug. More often the allergen is difficult either to identify or to avoid. Pollen and animal dander are examples of this type of allergen. When an allergen has been identified, it is sometimes possible to "desensitize" you with a series of injections that acclimatize the body to increasing doses of the substance. Desensitization is a less popular treatment than it used to be, however, because it occasionally causes dangerous reactions. Also, the end result is often disappointing.

The mainstays of modern treatment for allergies are drugs such as *antihistamines* that reduce or counteract allergic reactions. For further details consult the articles dealing with allergy-based disorders, which include asthma (see p.355), allergic rhinitis (see p.344), eczema and dermatitis (see p.253), farmer's lung (see p.365), hives (see p.255), celiac disease (see p.684) and some forms of conjunctivitis (see p.317).

Special problems of adolescents

Introduction

Adolescence, the period of transition from childhood to adulthood, is generally considered to last roughly from *puberty* to age 18 or 20. Puberty is the period of life when a person first becomes able to reproduce sexually. Though individual variations in when adolescence begins and ends are great, it makes practical sense to use the words "adolescent" and "teenager" interchangeably.

Many of the characteristic problems of adolescence stem from changes in the type and pattern of hormones present in the body (see Hormonal disorders, p.514, for more detailed information about hormones). These changes normally begin to occur soon after the age of 10 or 11 in girls, and soon after the age of 12 or 13 in boys. Growth toward physical maturity tends to reach a plateau soon after the age of 17 or 18 in both sexes. In the

intervening years there are physical, mental and emotional pressures that can make adolescence a particularly difficult time.

Some of the problems discussed here are primarily physical, and others are primarily psychological, but it is difficult to make sharp distinctions between the two. For example, an adolescent who has acne, a nearly universal physical problem, may react in a highly emotional way.

It is frequently hard to say whether the teenagers themselves or their parents are most affected by concerns such as the temptations of sexual experimentation, drugs and alcohol. Therefore, these articles are sometimes addressed to adolescents and sometimes to their parents. The key to a healthy passage towards adulthood is very often a good relationship between the generations.

Early or late development

Although the hormonal changes that indicate the onset of puberty usually begin at about the age of 10 or 11 in girls and about 12 or 13 in boys, there are wide variations in adolescent growth patterns, and most of these can be considered normal.

An adolescent's development is affected by a number of factors. One important factor is heredity. For example, a girl whose mother started her periods comparatively late is likely to begin menstruation late herself. Similarly, a boy's development is likely to follow the same pattern as his father's development.

Whether an adolescent develops early or late is also affected by his or her general health. Undernourishment or illness during childhood may delay the onset of puberty. In addition, a child who is smaller or thinner than average is likely to develop relatively late.

Very early or late developers may be made uncomfortable by their peers. This is often unavoidable, but parents can ease the pain by being understanding and reassuring. Such children should be reminded that their "differences" are only temporary.

Reaching physical maturity
Many girls reach sexual maturity by the time they are 16. Their breasts have developed and the pelvis has broadened, underarm and pubic hair has grown, and fatty deposits have been laid down to create a typically female shape.

Most boys are sexually mature by the age of 17 or 18. Their genitals have grown, facial and body hair have appeared, the voice has deepened, and there have been important changes in the bones and muscles.

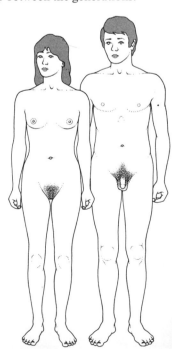

Normal adolescent development

Physical development in adolescent girls

	Average age when change begins	Average age when noticeable change usually stops	Remarks
Increase in rate of growth	10 to 11	15 to 16	If conspicuous growth fails to begin by 15, you should consult your physician.
Breast development	10 to 11	13 to 14	Noticeable development of breasts (one of which may begin to "bud" before the other) is usually the first sign of puberty. If change does not occur by 16, there may be cause for concern.
Emergence of body hair	Pubic hair: 10 to 11 Underarm hair: 12 to 13.	Pubic hair: 13 to 14 Underarm hair: 15 to 16	Age at first appearance of body hair is extremely variable. Pubic hair usually darkens and thickens as puberty progresses.
Development of apocrine sweat glands	12 to 13	15 to 16	The apocrine sweat glands are responsible for increased underarm sweating, which causes a type of body odor not present in children.
Menstruation	11 to 14	15 to 17	Menstruation often begins with extremely irregular periods, but by 17 a regular cycle (3 to 7 days every 28 days) usually becomes evident. If menstruation begins before 10 or has not begun by 17, consult your physician (see also Absence of periods, p.583).

Physical development in adolescent boys

	Average age when change begins	Average age when noticeable change usually stops	Remarks
Increase in rate of growth	12 to 13	17 to 18	If conspicuous growth fails to begin by 15, you should consult your physician.
Enlargement of genitals	Testicles and scrotum: 11 to 12 Penis: 12 to 13	16 to 17 15 to 16	As testicles grow, the skin of the scrotum darkens. The penis usually lengthens before it broadens. Ability to ejaculate seminal fluid usually begins about a year after the penis starts to lengthen.
Emergence of body hair	Pubic hair: 11 to 12 Underarm hair: 13 to 15	15 to 16 Underarm hair: 16 to 18	Development of hair is extremely variable and largely dependent on genetic inheritance. The spread of hair up the abdomen and onto the chest usually continues into adulthood.
Development of apocrine sweat glands	13 to 15	17 to 18	See remarks in the accompanying table for girls.
Voice change	Enlargement of the larynx, or voice-box, begins at 13 to 14, and the voice deepens at 14 to 15	16 to 17	Growth of the larynx may make the Adam's apple more prominent. The voice may change rapidly or gradually. If childhood voice persists after 16, consult your physician.

Medical disorders

Adolescent boys and girls are susceptible to almost any of the general illnesses in this book. The four disorders discussed here, however, are almost exclusively adolescent. Disorders that anyone can get but which seem to be more common in teenagers or young adults are discussed in the sections that deal generally with those problems. Some examples are infectious mononucleosis (see p.562), Hodgkin's disease (see p.433), and leukemia (see p.426 and p.682).

Teenagers and/or parents who are worried about whether or not physical development is proceeding normally should study the tables on the previous page. Note the broad range of ages within which changes such as the growth of body hair, the beginning of menstruation, or *menarche*, and maturation of bodily structures occur. Many boys and girls begin to develop the characteristic signs of adolescence somewhat earlier or later than the average ages that are indicated in the tables. Unusually early development toward physical maturity is not a cause for concern. In cases of unusually late development, however, it is generally wise to see a physician.

Acne

(acne vulgaris, common acne)

See p.240, **Visual aids to diagnosis, 30**.

Almost every part of your body is covered with hairs, most of them virtually invisible. Each hair grows from a follicle, or tiny pit in the skin, and within each follicle is a sebaceous gland that produces an oily substance to keep the skin lubricated. If there is an overproduction of oil and some of it becomes trapped in a follicle, bacteria can multiply in the blocked pit and cause it to become inflamed. The result is a pimple, which may be just a red lump or may become a pus-filled whitehead. Most people occasionally get a blemish or pimple somewhere on the body. You may be said to have acne, however, only if you have a number of such spots, and they come and go over a period of months or years. In some adults this condition is thought to be caused by prolonged exposure of the skin to grease, which can occur in some restaurant jobs. It can also be caused by taking certain drugs such as *steriods* or anti-epilepsy medications. Usually, however, acne is a problem of adolescence. It begins at *puberty* (when sexual reproduction becomes possible) and usually clears up in the late teens or early twenties.

The reason why so many adolescents have acne is that the level of male hormones in the body rises when a boy or girl reaches puberty, and this stimulates the sebaceous glands to increase their production of an oily substance called sebum. For more about male hormones, which are present in small amounts in females as well as males, read relevant articles in Special problems of men, p.570.

What are the symptoms?
Pimples are usually concentrated on the face, but there are often additional eruptions on the nape of the neck, the back, the chest, the buttocks, and in some cases the upper arms and thighs. If a pimple becomes more infected, it develops into a tender red lump with a white, pus-filled center. This tends to occur if you squeeze or pick at the eruptions, which is, unfortunately, a common reaction to unsightly and raw areas of skin. As individual acne pimples heal, others appear. Each healed pimple leaves behind a purplish mark, which usually fades away. Severely infected pimples may take many weeks to clear up and may leave noticeable scars.

One symptom of adolescent acne that frequently persists for years is not physical but psychological. Many young people feel resentful and are embarrassed by this unattractive disorder that seems to be inflicted upon them without cause. As a result, they may over-react emotionally to comments (however sympathetic) made by parents or other people, and this often increases the existing tension both within the individual and within his or her family.

What are the risks?
Almost all male adolescents aged 14 to 18 have some acne. It is slightly less common in adolescent girls, many of whom tend to develop pimples mainly around the time of their periods. Severe acne that leads to permanent scars is rare.

Acne does not endanger your general health, but pimples may cause extreme psychological distress to yourself and your family. It may help you if you realize that adolescent acne is really neither a disorder nor shameful. It is a normal accompaniment to the development of sexual maturity.

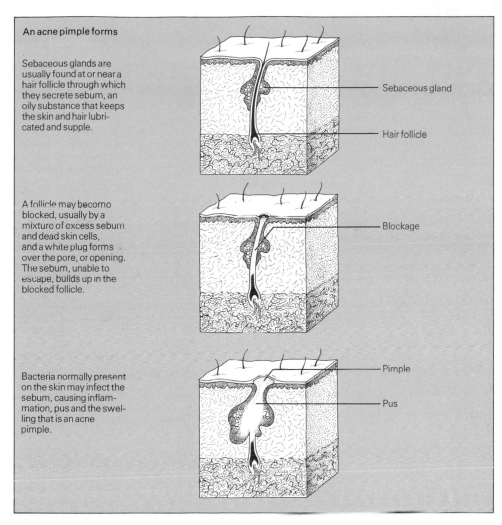

An acne pimple forms

Sebaceous glands are usually found at or near a hair follicle through which they secrete sebum, an oily substance that keeps the skin and hair lubricated and supple.

A follicle may become blocked, usually by a mixture of excess sebum and dead skin cells, and a white plug forms over the pore, or opening. The sebum, unable to escape, builds up in the blocked follicle.

Bacteria normally present on the skin may infect the sebum, causing inflammation, pus and the swelling that is an acne pimple.

Sebaceous gland

Hair follicle

Blockage

Pimple

Pus

What should be done?

If you have mild acne, the self-help measures suggested below should keep it under control. If it becomes severe, with a great many festering pimples on large areas of your body, consult your physician. Remember that your pimples will often seem uglier to you than they do to other people. Try hard not to pick at your face. Over-vigorous treatment of any kind is likely to do more damage to your skin than just leaving it alone.

What is the treatment?

Self-help: Above all, keep your skin clean. Wash it with an unscented soap twice a day, but not more often unless it becomes abnormally dirty or oily. Do not use creams or lotions unless they are prescribed or recommended by your physician. Most such preparations are ineffective, and some may irritate sensitive skin. Instead, because sunshine helps in many cases of acne, spend as much time in the open air as possible. Girls should avoid foundation make-up. If you feel you must wear it, use a non-greasy type, and clean your face thoroughly afterwards. Finally, remember that squeezing and picking at pimples is more likely to increase your problem than to relieve it.

Professional help: If your acne is severe enough to warrant professional help, your physician will probably prescribe a special ointment that makes the skin peel and may also prevent new pimples from forming. If this treatment does not work, the doctor may prescribe small, regular doses of *antibiotics* for up to six months. This usually produces a gradual improvement. While no treatment can promise a complete cure for adolescent acne, you should follow your physician's instructions exactly. This can improve the condition considerably.

Anorexia nervosa

Anorexia nervosa is a refusal to eat that can lead to extreme loss of weight, hormonal disturbances, and even death. It is primarily an illness of adolescent girls. Though it is generally treated as a disease in itself, anorexia nervosa is often a symptom of a psychological problem closely associated with family background. Anorexic girls tend to come from families that frequently think and talk about the "right" amounts or kinds of things to eat, and these girls may use their refusal to eat as a tool for manipulating their parents, whose increasing concern gradually turns each mealtime into a battle.

In other cases the illness arises from a subconscious desire to retreat from sexual maturity. The adolescent girl diets in an attempt to make her body retain its preadolescent shape. This rejection of the normal sexuality that is developing may be triggered by an early sexual experience that has led to feelings of guilt. Sometimes an emotionally insecure girl will overhear a casual comment that she is too fat, and decide she must lose weight to gain friends. Even if she becomes skeletally thin, she still sees herself as overweight and will not eat sensibly.

What are the symptoms?
The illness usually starts with normal dieting to lose weight, but the girl eats less and less every day. She gives false reasons for doing so, insisting, for example, that her legs or arms are still too fat. The less she eats, the less she wants. Sometimes, however, she may go on binges, in which she gobbles up quantities of a particular food and then vomits. To counter family pressure, she may take food and throw it away, claiming she has eaten it. When her weight drops to about 12 kg (about 26 lb) below normal, she may stop having periods (see Absence of periods, p.583) and her body may become more hairy.

A girl who has anorexia nervosa is often abnormally energetic. She may cook large meals for others while starving herself, and she will insist that she feels fine. But her skin may begin to look sallow and thin and she eventually will become very obviously ill. Whether or not she is constipated, she may take large doses of a laxative in the belief that by hurrying food through her system she will keep from growing fat. In later stages of the illness she may lapse into severe depressive illness (see Depression, p.297).

What are the risks?
Anorexia nervosa fortunately is a rare disease. It appears almost exclusively in adolescent girls. Many teenagers go through a temporary phase of excessive dieting, but only a minority develop anorexia nervosa. Of those who do, up to 15 per cent die of starvation or from secondary infections caused by undernourishment, *dehydration* caused by excessive use of laxatives, or suicide because of depression.

What should be done?
If your adolescent daughter has an unrealistic image of herself as being too fat and seems to be dieting excessively, see your physician without delay. Treatment of anorexia nervosa becomes increasingly difficult as the condition progresses. After examining the girl, the physician may decide that she is not actually ill, and may simply give you and her some advice on how to avoid problems with excessive weight loss. If her condition is diagnosed as anorexia nervosa, the doctor will probably arrange for immediate hospitalization.

What is the treatment?
Even in the early stages, anorexia nervosa is best treated in a hospital. Your physician can discuss the illness with you and your daughter and help her to decide on a suitable weight. They will then agree on the type of diet she should have in order to gain weight at a healthy rate. It is usually wise for a girl to have her own room where she can be closely supervised, and she will probably need regular doses of an appetite-stimulating drug. While in the hospital she will also be given *psychotherapy*, and it often helps if the psychotherapist tries to get to the root of the problem in the presence of the girl's parents. The more that personal and family problems

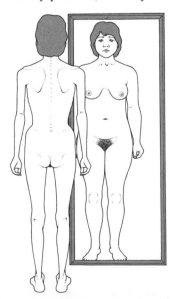

Advanced anorexia nervosa
Even after dieting to the point where she is extremely thin, a girl with anorexia nervosa still sees herself as overweight.

come out into the open, the better the chance of solving them.

When the patient has made suitable progress in treatment and no longer seems reluctant to accept physical and emotional maturity, she is permitted to go home. Before she leaves the hospital, the hospital staff usually advises the girl's family on how to treat her and how to recognize another attack of the disorder if one should occur.

What are the long-term prospects?
For a year or two after an apparent cure, a girl who has had anorexia nervosa should visit her physician periodically. This is because many girls who seem to have recovered from anorexia nervosa have further problems with the condition. Although many parents assume that this disorder is a phase of adolescence, there is often an underlying psychological problem that must be resolved.

Abnormal curvature of the spine
(Scoliosis)

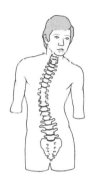

Sideways curvature of the spine that causes the rib cage to lose its symmetry is called scoliosis. The distortion may be due to a congenital abnormality of the spinal column, to paralysis or weakness of the spinal muscles, or to abnormal growth of the spine associated with a disorder such as dwarfism (see p.516). But in most cases the cause of the curvature is not known. Scoliosis becomes a noticeable problem mainly in the adolescent years and is much more common in girls than it is in boys.

What should be done?
A minor degree of sideways spinal curvature in your daughter or son may not be serious, and you may not even notice it. But if you do notice a possible problem, you should consult your physician, since the curve is often much greater than it appears to be, and early treatment can be important to the ultimate out

come. The problem may get worse and, as a consequence, the lungs may be affected to the point where the adolescent has recurrent chest infections and shortness of breath. Once scoliosis has become noticeable, the physician will probably want to examine the spine periodically in order to monitor the progress of the curvature.

What is the treatment?
If scoliosis is caused by spinal abnormality, the underlying problem must be diagnosed and treated. Sometimes, all that is needed is physical therapy, which will concentrate on improving posture and toning up spinal muscles. If this fails to correct the curvature, you may have to wear a spinal brace. Such braces are fitted by an orthopedic surgeon, are kept in place for at least a year, and help straighten the curvature. Surgery may be necessary for treatment as well.

Phimosis
(tight foreskin)

"Phimosis" is the technical term for a tightness of the foreskin that prevents it from being comfortably drawn back over the glans at the tip of the penis. The difficulty cannot generally be detected before an uncircumcised boy reaches the age of about five, because the foreskin is normally small and tight in the very young. Most commonly, phimosis is discovered in adolescence, when it may

become extremely painful or make it impossible for the boy to have an erection.

What should be done?
Never use force to pull back a tight foreskin. Force can damage the tissues. Consult your physician, who will probably recommend that the boy have a circumcision. This is a relatively minor operation.

Circumcision
Most boy babies are circumcised shortly after birth in the United States. Among those who are not, a tight foreskin is normal until about three or four years of age. Circumcision is usually recommended if it is a problem later. A general anesthetic is usually given and the foreskin is cut away from around the glans.

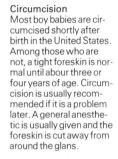

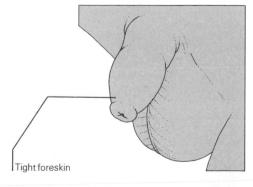

Tight foreskin

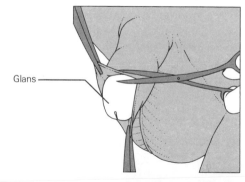

Glans

Psychological and behavioral problems

Significant changes in body chemistry inevitably affect your mental outlook. In adolescence the emotional ferment that accompanies drastic physical changes is increased by the conflicting pressures that come from other teenagers, the family and society in general. There are many books available about the psychological and behavioral problems of teenagers. The brief articles in this section can only summarize the most common problems and suggest a few ways of trying to cope with them.

Unfortunately, this is one of the most controversial areas in medicine. Whether you are a teenager or a teenager's parent or guardian, do not expect to find easy answers either here or in your physician's office. The following articles are designed only to give you some basic facts about problems that are complex and extremely difficult to solve.

Rebelliousness

The hallmarks of adolescence are self-consciousness, self-awareness and self-centeredness. Coupled with these is an inner conflict that seems to be a prerequisite of growing up. A stubborn determination to assert independence conflicts with a continuing need to rely on adult support in both emotional and financial aspects of life. The typical adolescent demands the right to question and criticize parental behavior and standards, and resents parental efforts to shape and control his or her own behavior.

Adolescent children are unlikely to reject their parents' values completely, but they will not completely accept them either. Quiet, cooperative teenagers often have as much inner conflict as their outwardly rebellious brothers or sisters, and they may have underlying disorders or developmental problems. Some clashes between parents and normal teenage children are inevitable. This problem usually becomes especially troublesome in the turbulent middle years of adolescence, between 13 and 16.

What are the symptoms?
Teenagers are often moody and sullen. They tend to act as if they know everything, to reject advice from their elders, and to see situations from only their own viewpoint. Yet, and this is one reason for the sullenness, they are inwardly much less confident than they seem. For instance, they tend to attach extreme importance to outward appearance. Their adoption of outrageous fashions or "in" hair styles may seem to their elders to be an unpleasant flouting of convention. In fact, however, it is more likely to be an acceptance of the conventions of their peers. Lacking the self-confidence to be themselves, most teenagers need the security of dressing and behaving like the rest of their group.

The same self-consciousness may also make them acutely aware of any of their physical defects, which they may magnify out of all proportion to reality. Parents whose teenagers are convinced that life is in ruins because of acne or curly hair may find it almost impossible to persuade their children that straight hair or clear skin is not necessary for happiness. At this age apparent physical imperfections can sometimes lead to serious disorders such as anorexia nervosa (see p.710), anxiety (see p.300), or intense depression (see p.297).

Since they have a continuing need for adult support, some adolescents form close relationships with adults who do not belong to the school and family circle. The adult may be a respectable neighbor or youth leader, or may be someone of whom the parents would disapprove if they knew of the relationship. This yearning to confide in someone who is unlike the parents rarely leads to harmful results. It generally lasts for only a short time.

Toward the end of adolescence, between the ages of 16 and 18, rebelliousness usually fades. The teenager will still be critical, but criticism gradually becomes more constructive and is aimed at matters other than those of direct personal concern. A degree of intolerance of older people's ways may continue, but the unpredictable turbulence and moodiness of mid-adolescence almost always is replaced by a more mature willingness to compromise and accept differences as the adolescent approaches 20.

What should parents do?
Successful relationships between parents and adolescents depend on communication, and this is not always easy. Adolescents cannot be expected to be patient and tolerant and to treat their parents like equals. It is the parents

who must bear these burdens, so the following paragraphs are directed to older people. If you are an adolescent, however, do not skip what follows. You can help your parents through these difficult years just by knowing that they want to help, not hinder, you as you try to become mature and independent.

The basic question for many parents is this: should you continue to enforce your old standards, with disciplinary measures to back them up if necessary, or should you relax the rules, after discussing them reasonably with your adolescent son or daughter? Too much parental concern is an irritant, but too little may be interpreted by the teenager as a lack of interest. You must base your decisions on standards for behavior and discipline in your particular family situation, but there is one rule for parents that should not be broken: mothers and fathers should present a united front to their teenage children. Begin by agreeing on the issues in two areas. First, decide what you both consider vital for the teenager's health and safety, which may include wanting to know where adolescents are at a given time, or insisting that they do not drive a car after drinking alcohol. Second, agree on other limits that you both feel strongly about, such as the level of rudeness you are prepared to tolerate. Then, once you have agreed on the ground rules, try to be flexible in other areas such as dress or speech habits, which, although they may irritate you, do not matter in quite the same way.

Teenagers' anxieties about appearance tend to focus mostly on hair, skin, or weight. Provide any practical help that you can. If your daughter is really overweight, for example, help her to modify her diet. Whatever the problem and however trivial it may seem, do not laugh it off. It is only in very late adolescence that the confidence comes to accept oneself as one really is, and to believe that others can do the same.

What is abnormal behavior?

Adolescent rebelliousness very seldom reaches a point so critical that professional help should be sought. But there are some situations in which such help becomes essential. Refusal to go to school, which can come from unreasonably high parental expectations, is one example. Once a pattern of truancy is established, it can be virtually impossible to reverse, so you should consult a teacher at the school, and preferably a guidance counselor also, if the problem arises in your family. Similarly, if your child rejects your guidance so completely that his or her behavior seems to be approaching the limits of the law, quickly contact a counselor, a social worker, or your family physician.

Occasionally, the stresses of adolescence may precipitate mental illness. Short periods of depression are common, but if a teenager's mood remains somber for more than a few days, and if symptoms of depressive illness such as insomnia, loss of appetite, and/or withdrawal from both friends and family begin to appear, you should consult your physician without delay. Occasionally, the swings of mood that are a common feature of adolescence may become so extreme that medical help should be sought (see Manic depression, p.298). Finally, a very few adolescents are unable to cope with what they see as a disastrous situation, often the break-up of a love relationship, and may take drastic action to escape harsh reality. Adolescents tend to resort to alcohol, physical violence including suicide, and drug abuse and overdose. Medical help is essential for any teenager who threatens or resorts to such drastic and destructive measures.

Addictions in adolescents

Anyone who drinks, smokes, or takes drugs may become dangerously addicted (see Alcoholism, p.304; Drug addiction, p.305; and the section on cigarette smoking in Part I of this book). The danger is most acute among teenagers, who tend to be attracted to assertive, "sophisticated" gestures, and who tend to think that they will live forever. Fortunately, fewer adolescents are likely to experiment with "hard" drugs such as heroin, if only because they are more difficult to get. The use of "soft" drugs, however, is quite common. In many circles marijuana or hashish (cannabis) are easily obtained and casually used. Cigarettes and alcohol are also available at many teenage gatherings. Parents therefore, do have some cause for worry.

Adolescence is characterized by a desire to experiment, a sense of almost limitless powers and possibilities, and a need to test oneself to the utmost. Adolescents, too, are particularly susceptible to pressures from their peers. They need to feel part of a group. If the group pattern involves the use of drugs, alcohol and/or cigarettes, it is often difficult for a teenage boy or girl to resist the temptation to conform. And as one experiment frequently leads to a second, experimentation can easily become habitual use, if not addiction. Most smokers, for example, began to smoke in adolescence. Statistics suggest that young people who do not smoke before the age of 20 are unlikely to start, but many of those who do smoke while still teenagers become thoroughly "hooked."

What should parents do?

Where drugs are concerned, the best thing you can do is to make sure that the adolescent knows the risks he or she is running. The fact that hard drug addiction can present more immediate danger of dying than smoking or drinking may make your appeal to your child seem convincing. Assume that all adolescents are exposed to temptation at one time or another, and discuss with them the best way to refuse any offer of drugs, including alcohol. Your advice will carry most weight if it is supported with facts. To make clear the hazards of taking hard drugs, recommend a careful reading of the article on addiction (see p.305), with special attention to the facts on the accompanying chart. Recent studies have associated the habitual use of cannabis with brain, heart and lung damage. Although marijuana use may not be as risky as the use of some hard drugs, it also can lead to a lack of motivation. It impairs judgement and is especially dangerous while driving a car. There is also a real danger of becoming psychologically dependent on smoking cannabis, and any such dependence is bound to be harmful. Finally, use of marijuana is illegal in most states.

Efforts to discourage young people from smoking cigarettes have not been very successful. It is hard to combat the constant exposure to advertising, which portrays smokers as successful, suave, and in happy control of their lives. Whether or not adolescents start to smoke depends largely on their social surroundings and on the availability of cigarettes. Friends who smoke are the main influence, but family environment is also important to the adolescent's decision about whether to smoke or not. Teenagers are quick to resent double standards. You are in a poor position to point out the evils of tobacco with a cigarette in your hand. The best way to encourage your children not to smoke is not to smoke yourself.

Some non-smoking parents refuse to permit their children to smoke at home even though they realize that parental control stops at the front door. If teenagers agree to such an arrangement, and surprisingly enough, many do, it has the advantage that it cuts down their consumption of cigarettes. If they do not acquiesce, there is sometimes a danger that adolescents may feel driven out of their own homes by the ban.

If you think your child may be drinking, the article on alcoholism (see p.304) may provide him or her with some thought-provoking reading. But most people, and especially adolescents, need to learn most things for themselves by experience. Most teenagers sooner or later discover how alcohol affects them. It is important for parents to emphasize that drinking does not make someone grown up. In fact, quite often the reverse of this is true. A warm, supportive family relationship and moderate, restrained parental drinking will almost always lead to intelligent restraint in the drinking habits of the maturing, but still younger, generation.

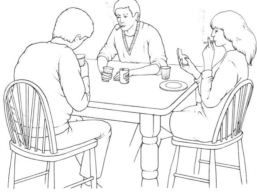

Smoking
Many teenagers begin to smoke to appear more adult, cover up a feeling of social inadequacy, or just to conform. Whatever the reason, the smoking often soon becomes an addiction.

Initial sexuality

In the early years of adolescence (ages about 12 to 15) the closest friendships are often made with people of the same sex. However, the teenager usually becomes increasingly aware of himself or herself as either male or female and begins to seek relationships with people of the opposite sex. An increasing number of teenagers in the United States have sexual intercourse at least once. Some studies put the figures as high as 7 out of 10 girls and 8 out of 10 boys by the age of 19. About ten per cent of those who have had intercourse have had it often, and with more than one partner.

Parents and children tend to have unrealistic views of each other's sexuality. Adolescents may find it difficult to believe that their parents are still interested (or indeed were ever interested) in sex. Parents often feel strongly that, even though their teenage children may be able and eager to have sexual relationships, they are not emotionally ready

Interest in and attraction to the opposite sex is a normal part of adolescence.

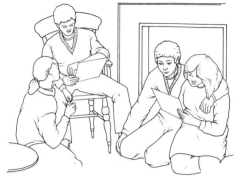

for sex. Adolescence is a time for experimenting, however, and most adolescents are going to experiment to some extent in this area as in any other. If your children seem sensible and responsible in other ways, they will probably be responsible sexually as well, but it is increasingly likely that they will have some type of sexual experience by the time they finish high school.

What should parents do?

The period of sexual transition is easier for everyone involved if you can come to terms with your children's sexuality, show that you trust them, and be prepared to give them any help or advice they may need. To begin with, do not worry about masturbation. It does not involve any risk to health, and you should not do or say anything to cause guilt feelings

about it. Masturbation is probably a universal practice and a harmless one. On the other hand, do not hesitate to speak out about the real risks of irresponsible sexual intercourse, including unwanted pregnancy and venereal disease (see Sexually transmitted diseases, p.611).

You have a responsibility to make sure that your adolescent children know the facts of life, including those that you find difficult to discuss. If you find it impossible to talk to them yourselves, check to make sure they have received adequate information about sex at school, ask your physician to talk with them, or give them a book on the subject. They should know about all available contraceptive techniques and about how to get contraceptive advice, and they should know that condoms not only guard against conception but also protect against sexually transmitted diseases. Another protection against the spread of venereal disease is to make sure that teenagers know where they can be treated for it. They should also know the importance of reporting cases to their physician so that the source can be located and treated as well. It may be helpful to stress that such reports are kept strictly confidential.

At best, your own attitudes should encourage confidence in your teenage boys and girls. Confidence, along with an understanding of the complexities of sexual relationships, almost always leads to a sense of responsibility.

Adolescent pregnancy

Details about various methods of contraception appear elsewhere in this book (see Infertility and contraception, p.607). If you intend to start a sexual relationship, however, it is important to get some direct personal advice. Do not hesitate to consult your family physician, who will not tell your parents about the consultation without your permission. If you prefer to talk about contraception with someone other than your own doctor, you can try a family planning clinic.

If you are a girl, remember that pregnancy is a possibility even if your periods have not yet started. The first egg is released before the first period. The timing of your menstrual cycle may not be the same each month, and sperm can remain alive for up to seven days after intercourse, so it is not wise to rely on "rhythm," or timing intercourse with your cycle, to avoid getting pregnant. Remember, too, that the consequences of a pregnancy may be unpleasant not only for you but also for your baby. Unplanned birth to an unmarried teenage girl is a poor start

in life. Moreover, there are higher risks, both for mother and baby, attached to having a baby when you are a teenager. So if you have intercourse, always use a contraceptive. Any contraceptive is better than none.

If you are a boy, you are just as responsible for the child as your partner is. You have an obligation to participate in planning related to the pregnancy, and support of the child after it is born.

If you become pregnant, or if you are responsible for a pregnancy, it is important to tell your parents at once. The girl should see her family physician without delay. The earlier help is sought, the more options are open to you. Continuing the pregnancy and either raising the child or arranging for adoption are possible choices. If you decide to terminate the pregnancy, it is safer and easier to do so earlier in pregnancy. There may be legal restrictions, however, especially if the girl is under 18. Also, an abortion should only be done by a licensed physician in a reputable clinic or hospital.

Special problems of the elderly

Introduction

Like all aging machines, a human body that has been functioning for a number of years tends to work less efficiently than it did when it was "new." This does not mean that illness is an inevitable part of old age. Certainly your lungs, kidneys, heart and other organs will be less efficient at 60 that they were at 20, but aging should not be equated with unavoidable breakdown of body systems. You should neither expect nor accept illness as a necessary part of growing old.

The problems that are discussed in this section are those that affect only the elderly, or affect the elderly primarily. If you have symptoms, check the self-diagnosis charts that start on p.68. Two of the charts deal specifically with problems of the elderly (see Chart 98, Incontinence in the elderly, and Chart 99, Confusion in the elderly). To acquaint yourself with other disorders that often occur in older people but are not covered in this section, read the articles or groups of articles recommended in the box, Problems more common in the elderly, p.726.

How old is an "old" person? There is some truth in the saying that "you're as old as you feel." Many people of 75 or 80 years and beyond are as alert and active as they were at 60, but some 60-year-olds appear to have already reached senility. Yet all of us can benefit from the advances being made in medicine and health care. There is movement toward positive solutions for some problems of aging, and more attention is being given to providing social support for the increasingly elderly population. Hopefully these efforts will provide the elderly, not only with better prospects for a healthier and longer life, but also with the promise of a more interesting and happier one.

The physical and mental disorders that mainly affect old people sometimes pose as great a problem for their families as they do for the elderly. For this reason, most of the following articles include suggestions for concerned relatives intermingled with direct information for older people. Also, if you have family members who are over 65, you should find out about organizations in your community that specialize in providing assistance and advice for old people.

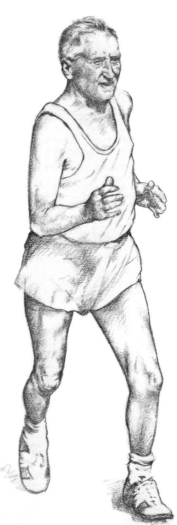

Aging and the body

The effect of age on different tissues and organs varies, but all become more susceptible to fatigue and disease.

Over the years, a gradual loss of elastic tissues causes skin to wrinkle and sag.

Between the ages of 30 and 75, the heart's efficiency decreases by about 30 per cent and the lungs' by about 40 per cent.

The liver's efficiency decreases by 10 per cent, the kidneys' by about 40 per cent.

Bones become lighter, and more brittle. They break more easily.

Planning for retirement

Now that many people retire earlier and live longer, it seems likely that the majority of the population will spend much of their adult life in retirement while remaining physically and mentally active for a good deal of this time. Yet some people approach this major period of their lives with no idea of how they are going to manage financially or with what activities they will fill their new free time.

Financial planning for your retirement is essential. If possible, work out at least five years in advance how much you will have to live on. If this amount seems less than or only just adequate, seek professional advice, perhaps from your lawyer, accountant, or banker, about how best to manage any investments as well as your social security and other retirement income.

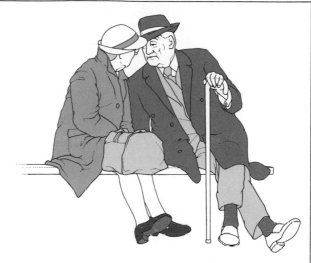

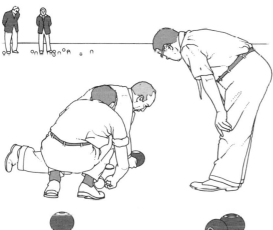

Activities

Retirement will give you the opportunity to devote more time to interests such as hobbies. It will also allow you to pursue new interests. Explore your local library, watch your newspapers and contact any nearby schools that give adult education classes if you need to search out new interests. Some communities offer senior citizen programs that may interest you. You may wish to do some limited work that will earn some extra money. Speak to a tax accountant about how this will affect any pension or retirement income. You may want to do volunteer work, for which there is no payment.

Relationships

Friends, relatives and neighbors are one of the best insurance policies for a happy old age. Think of this before moving to another area when you retire, it you might find it difficult to make new friends and fit into a new community as you become less active.

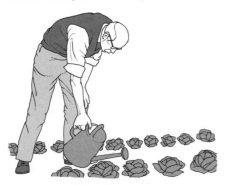

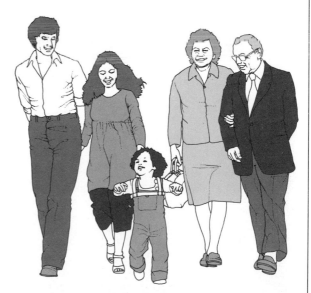

Incontinence

Incontinence is the uncontrollable, involuntary discharge of urine, bowel movements, or both. Incontinence in the elderly, like incontinence in the young, is usually caused by some underlying condition, such as a urinary-tract disorder or a problem with the nerves that control the bladder or bowels. Incontinence is not an unavoidable part of growing old, and should not be accepted as such. It is, however, much more common in the elderly than in the young. This is because the efficiency of muscular *sphincters* and the tone of ligaments connected with the urinary and digestive tracts diminish with age.

In general, incontinence will disappear if the underlying condition is treated successfully. For example, a urinary tract infection (see Infections, inflammation and injury, p.502) or problems with the prostate gland (see p.574) may cause urinary incontinence. Similarly, certain gastrointestinal diseases or too little *fiber* in the diet are often responsible for loss of bowel control. In such cases, treatment of the causative condition should cure the incontinence.

A few people who are incontinent have a more severe disorder such as stroke (see p.268), spinal-cord injury (see p.278), or senile dementia (see p.724). In at least some of these cases the disorder causing the incontinence may not respond to treatment. The accompanying incontinence will then be dealt with as a problem in itself.

The great majority of those elderly people who are incontinent have urinary incontinence only. Some can no longer go several hours without urinating. If their bladders are full they may dribble urine when they cough or sneeze. This is called stress incontinence. Others may have an uncontrollably powerful urge to urinate even though there may be hardly any urine to pass. This problem is called urge incontinence.

Only a few people have bowel incontinence. This problem can be a sign of depression. One specific type of bowel incontinence that tends to occur mainly in the elderly is caused by a bowel or *fecal impaction*, or the accumulation of a hard mass of waste matter somewhere in the bowel. The partial blockage upsets the mechanism by which bowel movements are regularly expelled, but it is not complete enough to prevent the more liquid portion of bowel contents from seeping past and leaking out. If the blockage becomes big enough it can press on the bladder and cause urinary incontinence as well.

What should be done?

Regardless of your age, you should consult your physician if you cannot control your bladder or bowels. Depending on the circumstances, your physician may want you to have specific diagnostic tests to find out whether the incontinence is due to an underlying condition such as urinary infection. If it is, and the condition is reversible, you will be treated for it. If, however, the cause turns out to be irreversible, much can still be done to reduce the unpleasant effects of incontinence.

What is the treatment?

Self-help: You may be able to re-establish some control over your bladder and bowels by going to the bathroom at frequent, regular intervals. Make sure your living and sleeping quarters are close to a bathroom, and keep a bedpan or commode within reach of your bed. Make sure your garments are easy to remove. All bathroom facilities should be made as easy as possible to use. Hand-rails alongside the toilet may help.

If you are becoming somewhat forgetful, you can use memory aids or even an alarm clock to remind you to follow a routine of regular visits to the bathroom. For urinary incontinence, drink sparingly at bedtime. For bowel incontinence, eat plenty of high-fiber foods and remember that uncontrollable bowels tend to produce bowel movements about an hour after every meal.

Professional help: Your physician may be able to prescribe a drug that stabilizes activity of the bladder so that urination times are fewer and further apart. Unfortunately, effective bowel-stabilizing drugs have not yet been developed, but taking laxatives or other medications for a specified period of time may improve the incontinence temporarily. If you have a bowel or *fecal impaction* or long-term constipation, consult your physician.

There are a number of body-worn incontinence aids. Your physician or the nurse in your physician's office can tell you about them and may be able to help you get any that will help you.

A typical example is specially designed underwear that soaks urine up into a porous outer layer and neutralizes the odor, leaving the inner layer (next to the skin) relatively dry. Another aid, which is designed specifically for men, is a condom catheter, which is worn over the penis and is connected by a tube to a bag that can be emptied at intervals. In some difficult cases of urinary incontinence a treatment called indwelling catheterization is used. In this procedure, a plastic tube is inserted into the bladder and drains urine into a bag. The bag can be emptied and cleaned periodically.

Accidental falls

Everyone has an occasional fall, but falls among adults are common and especially serious in people over 65. Many such older people neglect the precautions listed in How to guard against falls (see next page) and live in a home full of potential booby traps including slippery floors and stairs. Some elderly people have poor vision and poor general health, and some slowing of the reflexes is inevitable with age. Unfortunately, your bones also become more brittle as you age. In addition, you become increasingly susceptible to disorders such as Parkinson's disease (see p.291) and various circulatory disorders (see Circulation, p.403) and arthritic conditions (see Bone diseases, p.543 and Joint disorders, p.550) that may affect your ability to retain your balance. Finally, the drugs prescribed to control these disorders sometimes cause dizziness as a side-effect.

What are the risks?

Falls are by far the most common type of accident in those over 65. This is because of the factors described above. Deaths from falls, or from complications directly related to falls, account for more than half of all accidental deaths of old people. In a typical orthopedic, or muscle and bone disorder ward of a hospital, about half the patients are likely to be elderly women with broken bones. The corresponding proportion of elderly men is lower, probably because women's bones tend to become more brittle than men's and because there are more elderly women than there are elderly men.

Many falls, even of people over 65, cause nothing worse than a bruise. However, fragile skin and small blood vessels make bruising more serious and extensive in the elderly after even a minor fall. There is always a risk, moreover, of falling against or on something that is itself dangerous. Half of all deaths from burns in this country, for instance, occur among the aged, who tend to have accidents such as stumbling into heating appliances or grabbing for support at the handles of pots of boiling liquid. And if you hit your head on the floor or pavement, what is an apparently gentle blow may cause dangerous delayed bleeding within the skull (see Subdural hemorrhage and hematoma, p.272).

One common result of an old person's fall is a fractured bone or bones, and those most frequently broken are much the same as the ones listed for the general population (see Fractures, p.534). But among these frequently broken bones are some that are especially likely to break in the elderly. For example, so-called broken hips, which are in fact thigh bones (femurs) that are broken near the top, are particularly common in the elderly. The chances of a hip fracture resulting from a fall apparently increase significantly after the age of 50.

Apart from the injuries of the fall itself, there may be several indirect consequences of an accidental fall. If, as sometimes happens, a solitary victim lies immobilized and undiscovered for hours or days, the result may be hypothermia (see p.723), pneumonia (see p.359), psychological problems, or even death. Moreover, if broken bones necessitate hospitalization, the resultant possible long period of enforced immobility may further weaken aging bones and muscles, and other vital organs as well. And some old people who have had serious falls become permanently frightened and lose confidence in their ability to get around. They become less and less active, and therefore less and less confident. This vicious circle can lead prematurely to becoming bedridden or, at least, home bound.

What should be done?

Guard against falls by following the recommendations in the accompanying box (see next page). If you live alone, work out some way of alerting others quickly in case you have an accident. Some elderly people always carry a noise-making device such as a whistle. Some have understandings with neighbors based on certain regular habits, such as a daily hour for raising a blind or taking a stroll. The neighbor can check for a possible accident whenever the habitual act is omitted. A word of warning, however: be careful not to develop a routine or set of signals that can be useful to housebreakers. It is also wise to have a regular schedule of telephone calls or visits to and from friends and relatives, who will know enough to be alerted if the schedule is disrupted without any prior warning.

Remember that even a few days in bed may cause weakness and stiffness of your muscles and joints, and make your balance less steady. So stay as active as you can. If you begin to feel that you are less steady on your feet than you ought to be, consult your physician. Since there are several possible causes of unsteadiness, the physician may order a series of tests, including blood tests and X-rays, to determine whether your problem is caused by a treatable underlying disorder. Always see your doctor, too, if you have had a bad fall, even though there seem to be no ill-effects. It pays to be cautious.

If you are present when someone falls, or if you find someone who is apparently im-

How to guard against falls

Because anyone can have a bad fall, the following suggestions are worth considering regardless of your age. Except for toddlers, the people most susceptible to falls are the elderly. If you are over 65 or if you are in any way responsible for the well-being of an elderly person, try to follow as many of these recommendations as are applicable in your situation.

1. If you need glasses, wear them, but never walk around with glasses on that are meant only for reading. Take them off before moving around.

2. If you are even slightly unsteady on your feet, use a walking stick or cane. Do not hesitate to use a walker or support frame outdoors as well as in the house if you feel safer with one or your physician recommends one.

3. Wear well-fitted shoes with low heels or slippers with non-slip soles. Avoid long shoelaces, which can easily come undone and trip you.

4. Make sure carpets and other floor coverings are secured around the edges, and tack down worn spots. Never use loose mats and rugs on shiny, polished floors.

5. See to it that potentially hazardous spots such as stairs are brightly lit. White paint on either side of a flight of stairs can help.

6. A strong banister running along all indoor and outdoor steps is essential. Be sure to install one wherever such a support is not already in place.

7. Have a bedside lamp or low-wattage night light in your bedroom so that you never have to grope around in the dark when getting out of bed at night.

8. Fit secure handrails in convenient places near the bath-tub and toilet, and use non-slip mats both inside and alongside every bath or shower.

9. Do everything possible to minimize clutter in rooms frequented by the elderly. Children's toys, especially those on wheels, are particularly hazardous.

10. Do not permit wires from electrical appliances to run loosely along the floor. Wherever possible, wires should be secured to walls or moldings.

11. Store frequently used clothes and other items in places where you can reach them without standing on a stool or chair. If you must climb up to get something, use a stable stepladder or sturdy chair. Better still, get someone to do the reaching for you.

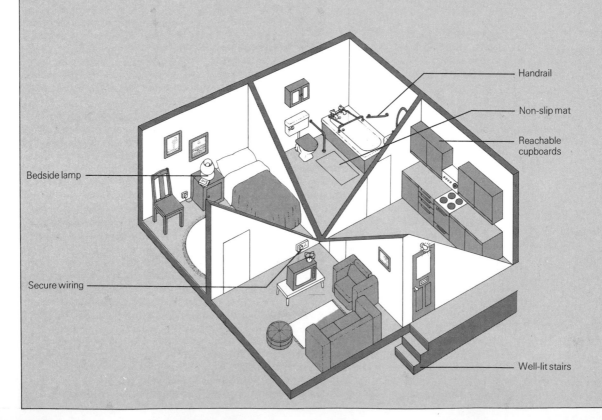

Handrail

Non-slip mat

Reachable cupboards

Bedside lamp

Secure wiring

Well-lit stairs

mobilized by a fall, carry out appropriate first-aid measures (see within Accidents and emergencies, p.801). An elderly person who is in pain should be seen by a physician without any undue delay. If you find anyone unconscious, you should summon medical help at once. If a doctor or someone else who is trained in first aid is not available, get someone to call for an ambulance. Someone should stay with the unconscious person until medical help arrives.

What is the treatment?

Self-help: The pain and discomfort of a fall, even if no bones have been broken, may be considerable. (If there is any doubt about broken bones, get confirmation from a physician.) It is important to relieve the pain as quickly as possible so that the person can keep moving. Bed may seem to be the most comfortable place, but it is too easy for someone who is already stiff and sore after a fall to become bedbound and immobile. Painkilling medications may be needed. Cold compresses for the first 24 hours, and warm compresses thereafter, reduce the pain and swelling of bruises. Application of heat from a hot water bottle or electric heating pad can relieve muscle stiffness. See also within Accidents and emergencies, p.801.

For treatment of fractures see p.534. Elderly people who have been treated in the hospital for broken bones (or any disabling disorder) should inquire about visiting nurse services and housekeeping help for a recovery period after their release.

Aging and the senses

The senses, most notably sight and hearing, are likely to deteriorate with age. Often, however, declining sensitivity turns out to be at least partly caused by factors other than aging. Such cases can be treated. Even when the problem cannot be reversed, modern technical aids can significantly improve your ability to see and hear, so consult your physician about how you can take advantage of them.

The eyes

By age 50 most people have come to rely on glasses to read, walk, or drive. Most people over 65 have presbyopia (see p.311), in which the lens of the eye focuses less easily on nearby objects. There is no cure for such changes, but you should visit an ophthalmologist regularly (see Box, p.312) for a checkup. A new pair of glasses may help you or, even more important, an examination may reveal an underlying, treatable disorder such as a cataract

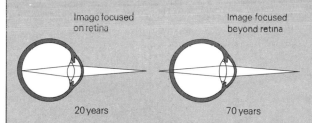

Image focused on retina	Image focused beyond retina
20 years	70 years

(see p.319) or glaucoma (see p.320). If you are diabetic, you should be especially aware of any changes in your vision (see Diabetic retinopathy, p.323).

The ears

Many people have trouble hearing, but have not sought medical help. This is unfortunate because increasing hearing loss may be due to an easily treated underlying cause such as an accumulation of wax in the ear. Wax accumu-

lates faster as you get older (see Wax blockage, p.330), so ask your physician about the possibility of flushing out your ears whenever you notice that your hearing seems to be impaired. Another possible cause of hearing loss that can be treated is otosclerosis (see p.332).

There is no magic cure for the gradual impairment of hearing due to natural deterioration of the hearing mechanisms in the ear. Do not hesitate, however, to ask your physician to prescribe a hearing aid, and persevere in its use until you have learned how to make the most of it. Do not buy a hearing aid without first consulting your physician, since there are untrained and unscrupulous sales people who will sell you a hearing aid that will not help your particular problem. For information on types of hearing aids, read the box on page 335.

Other senses

Among other senses that often become less sharp as you grow old are taste, smell and balance. Do not worry if food tastes and smells less appetizing than it used to. Just continue to eat a sensible and varied diet. Balance is a more serious matter, since unsteadiness can lead to accidental falls (see previous article).

There is one other kind of sense perception, sensitivity to changes in temperature, that can be life-threatening if it deteriorates. The skin of healthy young adults can detect a temperature drop of only 1°F (about $\frac{1}{2}$°C) in the surrounding air. In old age this sensitivity can diminish, and you may fail to notice a drop of up to 9°F (about 5°C). That is one reason why elderly people tend to be susceptible to hypothermia (see p.723). If you cannot afford to heat your home adequately, your physician may be able to refer you to a social service agency for assistance.

Altered sensitivity to temperature can also be caused by disorders of the thyroid gland (see Thyroid and parathyroid glands, p.525), so if you are warm when others are cold, or cold when they are warm, consult your physician.

Skin problems of the elderly

(including senile purpura)

One reason why aging skin becomes increasingly thinner, more wrinkled, and less flexible is that there is a gradual change in the nature of the fibrous and elastic elements that keep your skin supple and smooth. This and other physical changes are irreversible, and as the aging process continues, the skin may also become more susceptible to some skin disorders (see Skin, hair and nail disorders, p.250). In addition, many blotches and oddly pigmented patches tend to appear in old age. Often called age spots, they may come and go and usually are not a cause for concern.

Senile Purpura

Reddish-brown or purplish areas, sometimes as large as 5 cm (about 2 in) across, may appear anywhere on the body. They are usually most noticeable on the legs, the forearms, or the back of the hands. These markings are caused by bleeding under the skin. Blood seeps slowly from tiny vessels that have become damaged by loss of elasticity in the skin. Although the blood is gradually reabsorbed, the underlying defect is irreversible, and so the spots are likely to recur.

Most such spots are harmless, but you should see a physician about any unexplained spot because there is a possibility of skin cancer. For more information, read the articles on basal cell carcinoma (see p.258), malignant melanoma (see p.259) and squamous cell carcinoma (see p.259). Most skin cancer can be cured if it is treated early.

Itching

Another irritating by-product of old age may be the development of extremely dry, itchy skin. If you are bothered by constant itching, see your physician, who will examine you for a possible underlying condition such as jaundice (see p.485). If there is no cause other than age, the doctor may recommend an ointment or lotion to relieve the itching.

Trigeminal neuralgia

(tic douleureux)

This kind of neuralgia ("neuralgia" means pain from a damaged nerve) almost never affects anyone under 50 except in cases of multiple sclerosis (see p.292), and is more common among people over 70. The trigeminal nerve is a major nerve in the face. If it is damaged the result is severe pain, which is usually felt on only one side of the face. It is not known what causes the nerve damage or why the condition occurs almost exclusively in older people. Although it is not a life-threatening disorder, trigeminal neuralgia can be very distressing and disabling.

What are the symptoms?

The pain of trigeminal neuralgia shoots through one side of the face along the length of the nerve. It may last for a few seconds or as long as a minute or more, and while it lasts it can be excruciating. It may be triggered just by touching a sensitive place somewhere on the face or even by sitting in a draft. Sometimes attacks occur for no apparent reason every few minutes during several days or weeks. They may then fade, but stabbing pains usually return at decreasing intervals, and attacks may eventually become almost continuous. In some cases occasional muscular spasms accompany the pain and cause a facial tic, or twitching.

What should be done?

If you have what seems to be trigeminal neuralgia, consult your physician, who may carefully examine your sinuses and ears and may also suggest that you see your dentist before making a firm diagnosis. This is because infections of the sinuses, ears, or teeth often cause facial pain that is very similar to neuralgia. If you have trigeminal neuralgia, your physician may prescribe a drug that can help prevent attacks. It must be taken exactly as prescribed. If drugs are not effective, your physician may recommend an operation to destroy the trigeminal nerve either by cutting through it or by injecting alcohol around it. But because destruction of the nerve leaves part of the face permanently numb, surgery is not usually advised except in cases of extreme, persistent pain.

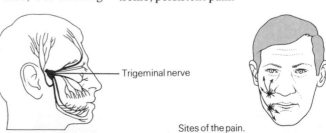

The trigeminal nerve supplies sensation to the face, teeth, mouth and nasal cavity and triggers the muscles that move the jaw.

Trigeminal nerve

Sites of the pain.

Hypothermia

In hypothermia, body temperature falls more than 4°F (about 2°C) below the healthy norm of 98.6°F (37°C). Death is a real possibility if hypothermia persists for more than a few hours, and anyone whose body temperature drops below 90°F (about 32°C) has anywhere from a 17 per cent to 33 per cent chance of dying. Anyone can become hypothermic and freeze to death if exposed to extreme cold for some time without adequate protection. So hypothermia is a risk for anyone who lives in a cold climate or spends a lot of time outdoors in winter weather.

The elderly are susceptible to hypothermia in less extreme temperatures, however. There are two main reasons for this. First, the aging body becomes progressively less able to maintain an even temperature when subjected to external cold. Second, the body mechanism that normally detects a drop in its own temperature gradually loses its sensitivity as you age. As a result, some old people do not realize that they are dangerously cold in frosty air (see Aging and the senses, p.721) and may even die without warning.

If you are over the age of 60, it is a good idea to purchase a thermometer that reads body temperatures *below* as well as above normal (98.6°F or 37°C). Take your temperature occasionally, especially during cold weather. If you have poor eyesight and cannot read the thermometer, have a friend or relative read it for you. Some people always have a temperature below 98.6°F (37°C), and this is "normal" for them. However, if your temperature suddenly or gradually falls in cold weather, consult your physician.

What are the symptoms?

If you find an old person sitting listlessly in a cold room or outdoors in cold weather, you should suspect hypothermia even if he or she is covered by several blankets or layers of clothing. Early symptoms of hypothermia are likely to include drowsiness, mental confusion and pallor. Loss of consciousness follows. The hypothermic individual's hands and feet may feel cold to the touch, but a much more telling indication of hypothermia is a cold abdomen.

The best way to determine whether someone's body temperature is dangerously low is to use a thermometer.

What should be done?

To begin with, take preventive measures if you have elderly relatives or neighbors. Visit them as often as you can in cold weather, and do everything possible to ensure that they have plenty of warm clothes and blankets, that they eat well, and that their living quarters are kept at a temperature at which they are comfortable.

Make certain, too, that they are taking advantage of any available government services or benefits, such as fuel-bill subsidies, that they may require. Consult a physician for help in preventing and treating hypothermia. In addition, there are many organizations such as local aging councils, visiting nurse associations, some hospitals, and community food programs (sometimes called "meals on wheels") that are prepared to assist the elderly in a variety of ways.

If you find an old person in what appears to be an early stage of hypothermia, take him or her to the nearest hospital or physician, or call for medical help. If the person is unconscious, the unconsciousness may be due to some other condition such as a stroke or heart attack, and emergency treatment is necessary in any case. While waiting for professional help to arrive, do what you can to warm the cold person slowly. Additional coverings and a warm, non-alcoholic drink may help if the person is still conscious. Be gentle, calm and understanding. Do not pile very heavy coverings on the person, and do not try to force them to eat or drink. Do not rub their hands or feet roughly in an attempt to restore warmth. Also, contrary to some popular "wisdom," alcohol is one of the worst things to take on a cold day. It both reduces and wastes vital body heat.

The key to treatment of hypothermia is gentle, gradual re-warming of the chilled body, and this is what is done by the physician. The treatment *must* be gradual because too rapid application of heat can cause sudden enlargement of blood vessels at the surface of the body. If this happens, a rush of blood into the swollen vessels may rob vital inner organs of the blood they need in order to continue to function.

Preventing hypothermia
Elderly people may become dangerously cold without realizing it, so they should be encouraged to keep their living quarters warm. Financial help may be available if heating bills are too high.

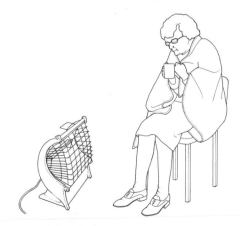

Senile dementia

Dementia is a disorder in which a formerly normal mind ceases to function normally and a person becomes forgetful, confused, and out of touch with the real world. The condition is very rare among people who are under 65, but senile dementia, or dementia that affects the elderly, is common. Deterioration of the mind is sometimes due mainly to the progressive wasting of irreplaceable brain cells and sometimes to gradual narrowing and hardening of the arteries that carry blood to the brain (see Hardening of the arteries p.404). The blood supplies the brain cells with the oxygen and nutrients they require to remain healthy and function normally. Without it, the cells malfunction or die.

Senile dementia is by definition progressive and incapacitating. Do not assume, however, that signs of confusion or impaired intellectual capacity in someone over 65 are always due to senile dementia. There may be an underlying, and treatable, cause. It has been estimated that 10 to 20 per cent of people over 65 who have an intellectual impairment have reversible conditions. For example, chest infections (see Lungs and chest, p.353) or urinary-tract infections (see p.502), stroke (see p.268), heart attack (see p.379), depression (see p.297) and hypothermia (see previous article) can result in mental confusion, and so can a low blood-sugar level (see Hypoglycemia, p.522) or the use of certain types of medications. Symptoms that resemble senile dementia are sometimes caused by long-term abuse of alcohol or drugs or by vitamin deficiency (see p.494), hypothyroidism (see p.526), syphilis (see p.612), or brain disorders such as tumors (see p.282) or subdural hemorrhage and hematoma (see p.272). Very often many of these symptoms will lessen when any such condition is properly treated.

The following paragraphs deal with senile dementia, in which the symptoms begin slowly and increase gradually. It has no known cause, though the damage to brain cells is apparent in many autopsies. Many elderly people in an early stage of the condition realize that they are beginning to lose their mental abilities, but they can do little to stop its progress. This article is therefore directed to close relatives and friends rather than to those who have the condition.

What are the symptoms?
The first symptom of senile dementia is a gradual loss of memory, particularly of recent events. You may notice that the elderly person cannot remember what has happened a few hours (or even moments) earlier, al-

though he or she can recall what happened many years ago. As weeks and months pass, powers of reasoning and understanding dwindle, and there also may be a loss of interest in all familiar pursuits, even in such simple activities as watching television or seeking news of relatives and friends. Eventually there may be a complete disintegration of the personality.

Senile dementia often culminates in emotional and physical instability. Some people tend to swing between moods of apathetic withdrawal and over-active aggressiveness. They may behave in uninhibited and anti-social ways. Table manners may deteriorate, personal cleanliness is sometimes neglected, and usual politeness abandoned. Some people may even become violent if impulsive behavior is frustrated. A few old people lose their sexual inhibitions, too, and this can lead to embarrassing physical approaches to young persons of either sex. Any or all such symptoms lead slowly but progressively towards the general decay of a person's intellect and emotion.

What are the risks?
The older the age group that a person falls into, the greater is his or her likelihood of getting senile dementia. About ten per cent of the over-65 population has some intellectual impairment, and it is estimated that there are about 650,000 people in the United States who have senile dementia. In the general population, about one family in every ten includes at least one elderly member who has this condition.

There are risks whenever mentally impaired people live alone, especially after they have progressed beyond an early stage of senility. Because of forgetfulness and a decreased ability to concentrate, there is a danger of fires, falls and other accidents. Combined with possible physical disabilities such as impaired hearing or vision, mental confusion makes it difficult for some elderly people to take medicines as prescribed, to cross streets safely, or even to use the bathroom. Without some supervision a senile person may eat poorly and neglect personal hygiene. It also can be distressing if, as often happens, the person becomes incontinent (see p.718).

If a relative of yours who is in the early stages of senile dementia insists on traveling around alone, you can help minimize the danger involved. Be sure that he or she always carries some identification such as a bracelet inscribed with his or her name and address or, at the very least, a piece of paper

Drugs and the elderly

Even the minor disorders of old age often need treatment, at least in part, with tablets, pills, or liquid medicines. As a result, you could be taking several different drugs at one time, probably in different forms and on different schedules. It is very easy to become confused about which medicines to take at which intervals, or to forget whether the correct dose of a given drug is one, two, or three pills. Research studies have shown that about four in every ten people who are under a physician's care do not take their medicines as prescribed. This is a remarkable figure when you consider the total number of people that are involved and the potential danger of skipping or taking too much of some drugs.

The following list of DOs and DON'Ts should help you to avoid making serious mistakes. The list has been compiled primarily for the use of people who are over 65, but it contains good advice for anyone who uses drugs for medical reasons. If you use medicines regularly, keep this list easily available and review it every now and then.

Do

Use memory aids to help you remember dose times. For example, a once-a-day drug might always be taken at bedtime, and a three-times-a-day drug after each meal. Write down a checklist of all the drugs you are taking, and update the list whenever there are changes. It will also help if you prepare your list in the form of a calendar so that you can mark off each dose of each drug as you take it. Another aid is to use an egg carton and put each required dose of medication in a separate section.

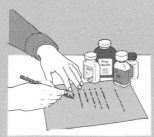

Ask your physician to give you a drug in the easiest possible form to take. For instance, if you find it difficult to pour a liquid medicine into a measuring spoon without spilling some, it may be possible to get the same drug in tablet form. Sometimes, however, this is not possible, because different forms of drugs are absorbed differently into your body.

Make sure that all containers are clearly labeled with their contents and when they should be taken. If you have trouble reading a label, ask to have it rewritten in larger, clearer characters. Also, you can request an easy-to-open container if child-proof containers are difficult for you.

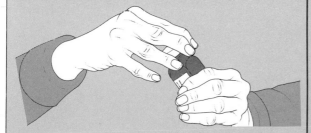

Be sure to inform every physician who treats you about *all* the drugs you are taking. Show them your checklist if you can, or bring in the containers for the drugs you are taking. This will help prevent double treatment or dangerous interactions of drugs.

Don't

Don't be a drug hoarder, or permit unused pills to accumulate in your medicine cabinet. Keep drugs that you are currently using, and those you use occasionally such as antihistamines or aspirin, and discard partially used supplies of all others.

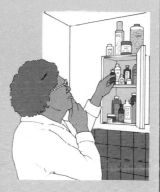

Don't start taking a drug again after a long interval without consulting your physician. Your present symptoms may be due to an entirely different disorder from the one for which last year's drug was prescribed. Moreover, some drug that you may now be taking could interact dangerously with the old one. Also, many drugs have a limited "shelf life," after which they become less effective or even harmful.

Don't keep containers of pills on your bedside table unless it is absolutely necessary. There is too much risk of taking either the wrong medicine or an overdose of the right one when you are sleepy. This can happen especially if, instead of switching on the light, you trust to your sense of touch.

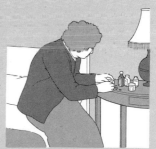

Don't leave similar-looking drug containers grouped together. To avoid confusion, ask your pharmacist to change the packaging of a drug if necessary. You yourself should not transfer the contents of one container to another without making absolutely sure that the new container is correctly and clearly labeled.

or card with your own address and telephone number on it.

What should be done?

If you suspect that an elderly relative or close friend is getting senile dementia, you should gently persuade (or take) him or her to see a physician. After taking a personal history, making a physical examination, and testing memory and reasoning power, the physician will probably look for symptoms of an underlying disease, such as the pallor of Vitamin B_{12} deficiency, that might be causing mental deterioration. Further laboratory tests and *X-rays* will also be necessary.

All cases of senile dementia should be investigated, since some can be cured and some can be helped to some extent. Unfortunately, some cases do not respond to treatment.

Some practical help can be given to both the person with senile dementia and those who care for him or her. In the early stages of impairment, when many old people are still able to live alone, their friends and relatives can help by organizing memory aids such as lists and routines, and by making sure that adequate food and warmth are provided. Activity, discussion of current events, and involvement with friends and family should be encouraged. Assistance from a visiting nurse, visits from church or synagogue volunteers, and regular help from services such as so-called "meals on wheels" and home health agencies, can help many people to maintain some degree of independence and to remain comfortably and safely in their homes.

If you feel responsible for the well-being of a relative with senile dementia, you should take as much advantage of community services as you can. In many places, for instance, there are day-care centers where old people are looked after for several hours and provided with lunch and some kind of occupational and activity therapy. Your physician may also be able to arrange for an elderly person to be admitted to a hospital or nursing home for brief periods so that you can have an occasional holiday. Rehabilitation hospitals also may be helpful in upgrading an elderly person's physical and mental abilities. The physician can advise you how to cope with such specific problems as incontinence.

Eventually, however, your elderly relative may require the skilled and constant care that is available only in high-quality nursing homes. If the doctor strongly recommends this form of care, you may be doing the patient the best possible service by accepting the recommendation.

Problems more common in the elderly

Problems that are more common in, but not exclusive, or even nearly exclusive, to the elderly are covered in various other parts of this book. They include Vascular disorders of the brain, p.268; Structural disorders of the brain, p.276; Depression, p.297; Lung and chest disorders, p.353; Major disorders of the heart, p.372; Circulation disorders, p.403; Leukemia, p.426; Hormonal disorders, p.514; Disorders of the muscles, bones and joints, p.529; Special problems of men, p.570; and Special problems of women, p.582. The Visual aids to diagnosis section, which begins on p.233, should also be helpful.

Special care for the elderly

The combined effects of disease and increasing age can be an inability to cope, either mentally or physically, with everyday tasks. Many old people are fiercely independent and may try to hide any disability because they are afraid of being put into a nursing home. However, only about five per cent of old people are in residential care – either state-run or private. The other 95 per cent are either largely independent, dependent on friends or relatives, or being supported in some way by community services.

Many old people prefer an arrangement where they are cared for by relatives who live with or near them. However, this can be a tremendous burden on the families involved. The family physician may be able to make arrangements for day care or short-term holiday care. The elderly person goes to a special center or residential home for a week every few months, or for one or two days every week.

Full-time residential care, run either privately or by a government agency, is usually recommended only for old people for whom the alternatives are impractical. Many old people adapt well to institutional life after an initial upheaval, but in some cases it has been found that loss of independence leads to loss of initiative, intellect and personality. Sheltered homes that are now being provided in some communities may be the answer for the many old people who need a certain amount of daily care but want to retain a measure of independence.

The decision to send a relative away from home for care is very difficult for some people to make. It is best to discuss such a decision with your physician and all family members. Then, if you must send the person for care, you can be more secure that the move is best for everybody concerned, including the person being moved.

Part IV

Caring for the sick

The American health care system

Introduction

Few people are aware of just what elements make up the American health care system, the extent of it, how best to make use of it, and many other particulars related to it. In the United States, about seven million people work in the system. Approximately one-half million of them are physicians.

The amount of money involved is enormous. More than two hundred billion dollars a year, or over nine per cent of the gross national product, is spent on health care in the United States.

Could any single area be worth so much expenditure of human energy and money? Opinions might vary, but there is no denying several pertinent facts. Today more Americans are healthier and are living longer than ever before. Life expectancy at birth is continuing to rise. Death rates from heart disease, cancer and stroke are decreasing, and so is the infant mortality rate. How much of this improvement is due to modern medical care and how much is due to other factors, such as changes in diet and exercise, is a matter of debate, but few disagree that major improvements have been made in recent decades in the general health of Americans.

Modern technical training

At the heart of the health care system is the physician. Each physician participates in long and difficult training, which never really ends. In addition to attending college, the aspiring physician must go to medical school for three or four years. The medical degree (M.D.) is awarded on graduation from medical school, but residency training, which is preparation for entry into a specialty area of medicine, may require from three to nine additional years.

To practice medicine legally, a physician must pass standardized examinations. Successful completion of these examinations allows the physician to become licensed by the state in which he or she wishes to practice. But even after a doctor is licensed, his or her study and training goes on, for continuing education is part of the physician's professional obligation.

Most physicians are associated with hospitals, and hospitals also have a mechanism for reviewing physicians' competence. The hospital's credentials committee reviews the training and fitness to practice of everyone on the medical staff. Similar requirements and reviews exist for the hospitals themselves and also for nurses, physical therapists, social workers, physician's assistants, and the more than 200 other types of health workers. All of these health workers have had special training ranging in length from several weeks or months to up to six years.

Ethics and Compassion

Fine technical training can produce a technically competent physician, but that is not enough. From the beginning of a physician's professional education, ethical behavior and compassion for those who require medical care are emphasized. Dealing with death and disability on a daily basis can sometimes lead to stress and distance. Still, a fair, friendly and sympathetic approach to people in addition to the highest possible technical competence is every physician's goal.

Using the health care system

With all the well-trained people and with thousands of health care facilities in the United States, it is important to learn how best to make use of them. How do you choose a physician, or, for that matter, drop one? What are the differences in different kinds of practices? What special services are available to those who are sick at home? What health programs specifically can benefit you? How do you pay medical bills? What are nursing homes like and how does one differ from another? What happens during an operation? What are your rights and obligations as a hospital patient? What is "alternative medicine"?

This section contains answers to these questions and many more that you might ask. Reading it will help you maximize the benefits that the fine health care system of this country has to offer. It will also benefit the system itself. This is because an informed person who enters the system as a patient, or as a concerned friend or relative of a patient, will know what to expect and how to achieve what is required more efficiently and perhaps also at a lower financial cost.

Physicians' ethics

Because physicians are responsible for the very lives of their patients, it is no surprise that they are expected to live up to ethical principles as high or higher than those of any other profession. By living up to these principles, a physician can set an example for those in other health-related professions. As a patient, you have the right to expect the highest ethical behavior from a physician (see Choosing a physician and Evaluating your physician, p. 735). An example of what is expected of a physician in this respect is contained in the following Principles of Medical Ethics of the American Medical Association:

"Preamble:

The medical profession has long subscribed to a body of ethical statements developed primarily for the benefit of the patient. As a member of this profession, a physician must recognize responsibility not only to patients, but also to society, to other health professionals, and to self. The following Principles adopted by the American Medical Association are not laws, but standards of conduct which define the essentials of honorable behavior for the physician.

1. A physician shall be dedicated to providing competent medical service with compassion and respect for human dignity.

2. A physician shall deal honestly with patients and colleagues, and strive to expose those physicians deficient in character or competence, or who engage in fraud or deception.

3. A physician shall respect the law and also recognize a responsibility to seek changes in those requirements which are contrary to the best interest of the patient.

4. A physician shall respect the rights of patients, of colleagues, and of other health professionals, and shall safeguard patient confidences within the constraints of the law.

5. A physician shall continue to study, apply and advance scientific knowledge, make relevant information available to patients, colleagues, and the public, obtain consultation, and use the talents of other health professionals when indicated.

6. A physician shall, in the provision of appropriate patient care, except in emergencies, be free to choose whom to serve, with whom to associate, and the environment in which to provide medical services.

7. A physician shall recognize a responsibility to participate in activities contributing to an improved community."

Philosophies of medicine

Medicine as we know it in this and other Western nations is based on the theory that identifiable physical factors are responsible for disease, and that drugs or other specific treatments can help provide a cure. This "mechanistic" view differs from the "vitalist" view of health and disease, in which spirits or gods are the cause of illness, and magic or faith is the only important force for cure.

The discovery of bacteria and viruses, and their association with diseases in the nineteenth century played a crucial role in bringing people in industrialized nations to believe that these organisms and other physical forces cause disease. Some people in non-industrialized nations in Asia, Africa and South America still view illness as related to their religious and cultural beliefs.

Although at one time Westerners tended to think of our view of medicine as clearly superior, this is no longer true. Currently, physicians in Western cultures are expressing an interest in many aspects of Eastern philosophies of health and illness.

Orthodox medical practice in the Western world is also called "allopathic" medicine, which prescribes treatment to counteract the symptoms of a disease. A primary treatment is with the use of drugs.

The success of "modern medicine" with its powerful drugs, advanced surgery, new vaccines and public health measures (clean water and sewage management, for example) was, and remains, remarkable. It has made inroads against infectious diseases that once caused an incredible amount of death and human misery. Smallpox, yellow fever, typhoid fever and a host of other infections came totally or largely under control. And all this strengthened our belief in traditional Western medical ideas.

Soon, however, we discovered that non-infectious diseases such as cancer, heart and blood vessel disorders, congenital problems, and environmentally triggered diseases were quickly replacing infectious diseases as a major source of human suffering.

These non-infectious diseases do not respond to "standard treatment." This tends to lead our thinking toward the vitalist view of health and illness. "What are we doing to deserve this?" is a question that the Ancients asked themselves. Modern science is looking at this question again, this time in terms of the limitations of the human body rather than the anger of the gods. As everyone agrees, we still have a good deal to learn about both health and illness.

Medical specialties

Most people have, at one time or another, been seen and treated by a physician "specialist." Yet only a very few people are aware of the number and nature of special fields of study within medicine that exist. A sampling of both specialties and subspecialities appears below. A complete list is not possible in the limited space that is available.

Adolescent medicine is concerned with adolescent patients, who are sometimes considered too old for pediatric care (see Pediatrics) and too young for "adult" medicine.

Allergy involves the treatment of persons who have allergies or "reactions" to irritating agents, called *allergens*.

Anesthesiology is concerned with anesthesia, or the loss of sensation, and use of anesthetics, or agents that cause such a loss.

Cardiovascular diseases is the specialty concerned with the heart and circulation and related diseases.

Cardiovascular surgery is a surgical subspecialty that involves operating on the heart and related blood vessels.

Clinical pharmacology deals with the action of drugs in the treatment of disease.

Colon and rectal surgery is a surgical subspecialty that concentrates on surgical treatment of the lower intestinal tract.

Dermatology is concerned with the diagnosis and treatment of skin disorders.

Emergency medicine requires special training in handling emergency situations such as heart attacks and accidents.

Endocrinology is the specialty that deals with the organs and tissues that produce hormones, and the treatment of hormonal disorders and diseases.

Family medicine/general practice is a medical specialty in which the physician cares for the medical problems of all the members of a family, so it is not necessary to have a different specialist for each problem, or for each family member by age-level or sex. Physicians who practice in this specialty are called family physicians. They see themselves also as advocates for good patient care in a complex health care system.

Gastroenterology deals with the esophagus, stomach and intestines.

General surgery is a surgical subspecialty for treatment of a wide variety of problems including those in the abdomen, the hormone system, the breast and the circulation.

Geriatrics is the branch of medicine concerned with disorders of the elderly.

Gynecology deals with disorders and diseases of the female genital and reproductive system. A gynecologist may also be an obstetrician. See Obstetrics.

Hematology deals with disorders of the blood.

Immunology is concerned with the body's ability to handle infectious or irritating substances that threaten it with disease, and with how the body's "immune" systems work.

Infectious diseases deals with diseases that are caused by viruses, bacteria and other organisms, and are *contagious*.

Internal medicine is concerned with the medical (rather than surgical or obstetrical) diagnosis and treatment of diseases of adults. Physicians in the specialty are called internists. There are several subspecialties within internal medicine in which the physician has particular training in diagnosis and treatment of a particular organ, system or type of disease.

Neonatal-perinatal medicine involves the study, support and treatment of newborn and prematurely born babies and their mothers.

Nephrology is the specialty concerned with diagnosis and treatment of kidney disorders.

Neurology deals with the nervous system, its disorders, and their diagnosis and treatment.

Neurosurgery is a surgical subspecialty concerned with the brain and nervous system.

Nuclear medicine is a specialty field in which radioactive substances are used for the diagnosis and treatment of disease.

Obstetrics is concerned with pregnancy, labor, delivery and care of the mother and child immediately after delivery.

Oncology involves the diagnosis and treatment of *malignant*, or life-threatening, tumors.

Ophthalmology involves diagnosis and treatment of eye and vision disorders and diseases by a variety of techniques including surgery.

Orthopedics is a surgically-oriented branch of medicine that is concerned with the bones and associated structures.

Osteopathy is an approach to medical practice based in part on the theory that the normal human body is capable of making its own remedies if its physical and physiological integrity is intact. Thus, the focus of osteopathic treatment is to restore that integrity by manipulation, surgery or medication.

Otolaryngology deals with disorders of the ear, nose and upper respiratory tract. It includes head and neck surgery.

Pathology is the branch of medicine concerned with the laboratory study and diagnosis

(*Continued on next page*)

of disease, including its causes, development and consequences.

Pediatrics is concerned with the care and development of children, the maintenance of their health, and the treatment of childhood diseases. It includes several subspecialties such as pediatric nephrology (kidney diseases in children), pediatric hematology-oncology (blood diseases and cancer in children), and several others.

Physical medicine and rehabilitation is concerned with the diagnosis and treatment of disorders and disabilities of the neuromuscular system. A physician in this specialty is called a physiatrist. He or she uses the physical elements such as heat, cold, water, electricity and exercise to help restore physical function and independence.

Plastic surgery is a surgical subspecialty concerned with correction of the loss or deformity of tissues, including skin.

Preventive medicine is the branch of medicine concerned with preventing disease and disability. Analysis of present health services and planning for future medical needs are part of preventive medicine, as are occupational medicine and public health.

Proctology is concerned with the diagnosis and treatment of diseases of the anus and rectum.

Psychiatry involves the diagnosis and treatment of mental and emotional disorders.

Pulmonary diseases is the branch of medicine concerned with diseases and disorders of the lungs.

Radiology is the specialty in which X-rays are used for the diagnosis and treatment of disease. There are several subspecialties within this branch of medicine, including diagnostic radiology and therapeutic radiology.

Rheumatology is concerned with joint and tissue diseases, including arthritis.

Surgery is the branch of medicine that involves the treatment of disease, injury or deformity by means of surgical operations. It includes several subspecialties, some of which appear in this list.

Thoracic surgery is a surgical subspecialty concerned with the treatment of the chest, including the lungs.

Urological surgery is a surgical subspecialty concerned with treatment of the female urinary tract and the male urinary and genital tracts.

The health care team

This is a partial list of health professionals who work with physicians to provide medical care. They are sometimes called allied health workers.

Emergency medical technicians (EMTs) provide immediate care to critically ill or injured patients in emergency situations.

Health services administrators manage nonmedical aspects of health care delivery in hospitals and other health care facilities.

Home health aides provide nursing and other household services for patients who are homebound or disabled.

Licensed practical nurses (LPNs) are trained and licensed to provide basic care for patients. They are supervised by physicians and RNs.

Medical records personnel analyze patient records and keep them complete, up-to-date, accurate and accessible only to those authorized to use them.

Medical technologists perform laboratory tests to diagnose medical disorders and to help identify their causes and extent.

Nurse-midwives are nurses who have special training in prenatal and postnatal care, labor and delivery.

Nurse practitioners or nurse clinicians are RNs who have been specially trained to provide health services such as preventive care, monitoring of chronic conditions, physical examinations and health counseling, under the supervision of a physician.

Nurse's aides and orderlies assist nurses in hospitals, nursing homes and clinics.

Nutritionists apply knowledge of proper diet to maintain health and also to treat certain diseases. This group includes dieticians and food researchers.

Occupational therapists help disabled patients adapt their daily activities and job skills to their particular problems. This may include helping a patient relearn ordinary activities such as dressing or cooking, and also helping to modify the environment so that tasks can be done more easily.

Orthotists and prosthetists make and fit braces and artificial limbs to replace limbs damaged or lost due to disease or injury.

Pharmacists are trained and licensed to make
(Continued on next page)

up and dispense drugs as directed by a physician's prescription.

Physical therapists provide services designed to help prevent loss of function and restore or develop physical strength and mobility in patients already physically disabled. PT uses exercise, heat, cold, water and electricity to relieve pain and restore function.

Physician assistants (PAs) work under a physician's supervision to do tasks such as performing physical examinations, prescribing certain drugs and providing counseling and education.

Psychologists are trained in human behavior, and provide testing and counseling services related to mental and emotional health.

Recreational therapists provide programs for patients to enhance physical and emotional well-being through art, music, dance and other artistic and recreational activities.

Registered nurses (RNs) are registered and licensed by a state to care for the sick and also to promote health. RNs supervise hospital care, give drugs and treatments as prescribed by physicians, monitor patient progress, and provide health education. RNs work in hospitals, nursing homes, physicians' offices, clinics, people's homes and schools.

Respiratory therapists treat respiratory problems under a physician's direction.

Social workers are trained to help bring about change in individuals and society. A medical social worker helps patients to handle social problems such as finances, housing and family problems that occur as a result of illness.

Speech pathologists diagnose and treat disorders of speech and communication.

Vocational rehabilitation counselors work with disabled patients to help them return to (or begin) satisfying jobs.

Alternative medicine

In recent years, the growth of "alternative medicine," or those treatments generally not considered to be "orthodox," has accelerated. Such treatments appeal to many people, particularly some who are deeply dissatisfied with modern medicine, its cost and its emphasis on the scientific rather than the spiritual approach to treatment.

The following are a few examples of alternative medicine that are available in the United States today. They are by no means the only ones, but they are among the best known. The list and descriptions are intended purely as a source of information, not as an endorsement.

Wholistic health care

This approach to health care, also called holistic health care, is a philosophy of medical care that attempts to focus on the entire, or whole, person. This is not really radical, since health workers traditionally have a person's total welfare as a top priority. Also, physicians and all other trained health professionals are fully aware that physical conditions do not exist in total isolation from a person's mental, emotional and spiritual states. However, the tendency toward medical specialization also has increased as the amount of medical knowledge has expanded. It is not surprising, therefore, that there is renewed emphasis on the "whole patient" and not just the tumor, the heart or the damaged nerve that is being treated. Wholistic health care is an attempt to combine scientific treatment of medical problems with treatment of psychological and spiritual problems.

Herbalism

In herbalism, plants are used in treatment, including prevention (rosemary as an insect repellant), cures (garlic as a germ killer) and relief of pain and discomfort (aloe vera for arthritis pain).

Centuries ago, herbs were the only available medications for many poorly understood diseases. Today, however, the modern pharmacy stocks many examples of purified herbs in the form of pills, pastes or liquids as well as medications synthesized to treat specific diseases. In herbalism, the number of plants that are used medically is diverse and further complicated by the differing effects of barks, leaves, stalks, roots, flowers and seeds.

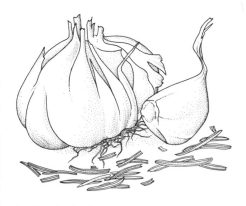

Traditional herbs of herbalism include garlic as a germ killer and rosemary as an insect repellant.

Chiropractic

Chiropractic does not use drugs or surgery, nor is it intended to treat diseases as such. Instead, it attempts to maintain the structural and functional integrity of the nervous system. According to the theory of chiropractic, this is accomplished by massage, spinal manipulation and adjustment of joints and soft tissues.

Acupuncture

Chinese medicine considers a cycle of energy called "chi" (pronounced "chee") to be essential to health. This cycle of energy is thought to flow through the human body in meridians, or channels, each day.

Acupuncturists deal with 12 to 14 of these meridians and some 500 to 1000 points along them. After a diagnosis of an imbalance of the energy flow, an acupuncturist may use the insertion of thin needles (acupuncture), the heating of points with burning mugwort (moxibustion) or finger point pressure (Shiatsu or acupressure) to treat a patient, most often for pain. Theoretically, this treatment works by adjusting the energy flow along the meridians.

Naturopathy

Naturopathy is a therapeutic system that was introduced in the United States in the 1890s. This system attempts to use natural forces to maintain health and treat disease. Such remedies include sun bathing, diet regimens, steam bathing, exercise, manipulations and a number of others. High vegetable consumption is encouraged in naturopathy as is abstinence from salt and stimulants.

Spiritual healing

The term spiritual healing refers to the restoration of physical, mental, emotional or spiritual health by prayer and other religious practices. Through the ages, most of the recognized religions have practiced some forms of spiritual healing.

Some other semi-spiritual groups that do healing border on the magical or occult. Be very cautious if a healer asks you to suspend your own religious values or relinquish large amounts of money or property to participate in a form of therapy.

Homeopathy

Homeopathy is a form of medical practice in which the practitioner administers remedies that cause reactions in a person that are similar to symptoms of illness. The philosophy is in marked contrast to conventional modern medical practice, which makes use of medica-tions to counteract the symptoms of disease. An example of homeopathy is treating diarrhea by giving the patient a very small dose of a laxative.

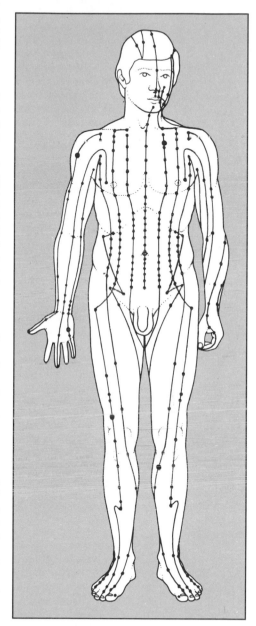

Meridian lines are dotted with the points at which acupuncturists insert needles to influence the flow of energy to various body areas.

There are 14 main lines covering the body, each representing an internal organ. If the organ is diseased according to acupuncturists, its particular energy flow will be disturbed, and the needles can correct the flow.

Needles inserted in the proper points can also sometimes dull pain as does an anesthetic.

Broad types of health care

There are many ways to categorize the various types of health care. One approach is to look at the ultimate goal. This creates four categories: preventive, curative, rehabilitative and palliative.

Preventive medicine refers to health practices and medical care that prevent disease, disability and suffering. Public health measures that insure clean water, adequate sewage disposal and sanitary food handling are a part of preventive medicine.

Immunizations are a more recognized part of preventive medicine as are periodic checkups, screening for important and treatable illness, and early treatment of serious illnesses such as cancer. Stopping smoking and using seat belts are just a few examples of preventive medicine that everyone can and should practice.

Curative medicine is a term for medical care that leads to a cure. A complete recovery is the goal of most health care in America today, and billions of dollars are invested in research as well as the diagnosis and treatment of diseases.

Rehabilitative medicine is directed at those who are disabled by disease or injury. Its goal is to restore the person physically and mentally to as full a life as possible. Many factors influence the choice of treatment.

A variation of this approach for a person who has been ill or disabled from birth is called habilitative medicine. Again the goal is the optimum physical, intellectual and emotional development of the individual.

Palliative medicine or palliation, is used when neither a cure nor a return to full function is possible. It includes measures that seek to keep a patient comfortable. One important time for palliation is in the treatment of painful, terminal or end-stage disease. Pain-killing drugs, radiation therapy and supportive nursing care are some common examples of palliative medicine.

Levels of health care

Modern medicine is organized into a complex system with different levels of care. The levels most commonly referred to are primary, secondary and tertiary care.

Primary care is care given to maintain and monitor normal health. Minor health problems are diagnosed and treated at this level, which is sometimes called "first-contact" care. Examples of this level of care include regular checkups for babies, immunizations, prenatal care in a normal pregnancy, treatment of minor injuries, diagnosis and treatment of minor disorders such as sore throat, as well as the monitoring and treatment of chronic conditions such as high blood pressure and diabetes.

At one time, nearly all physicians dealt with such problems, and most of these physicians were GPs, or general practitioners. A GP usually had one year of formal training beyond medical school. In recent years new specialties that are called family medicine or family practice and general internal medicine have developed. A medical student who wants to be a family practitioner or a general internist must complete all the training that is required to become a physician, enters a three-year residency program and then takes a qualifying test.

Part of the job of a primary care physician is to make sure that his or her patients get the appropriate care from the right specialists if a referral to another level of care is necessary. Your primary care physician can act as your advocate and adviser.

Secondary care usually involves a specialist who is an expert in one particular group of diseases, group of organs or body system. For example, a specialist may deal exclusively with the treatment of allergies. Family practitioners would refer patients whose allergies are extensive or do not respond to the usual medication to such a specialist. Dermatologists, who specialize in skin problems, and ophthalmologists, who are experts in treating diseases of the eye, are also considered secondary level practitioners. Many people go to such physicians without being referred by another physician.

Tertiary care is care that is highly specialized and oriented toward unusual and complex problems. It usually requires sophisticated equipment, even more years of training for the physician, and hospitalization of the patient. Tertiary care physicians include such subspecialists as pediatric psychiatrists and neonatologists (physicians trained to deal with diseases of newborn babies). Tests such as *CAT scans* and *cardiac catheterization* are considered tertiary care, and often can only be done in certain hospitals that have the necessary equipment and staff.

These levels of care sometimes overlap. A physician who usually does primary care may be trained to do a particular procedure that is considered a secondary level procedure, while a physician who is trained in a surgical subspecialty that is usually considered tertiary care may sometimes also provide primary care if necessary.

Choosing and using physicians

Everyone wants his or her physician to be well trained and competent. Compassion and high ethical standards (see Physicians' ethics, p.729) are also universally sought. These are the basics of good health care. But there are characteristics beyond these obvious ones that you should consider in choosing or evaluating a physician. One goal might be to obtain the best possible care with a physician you respect, trust and like as a person. Once you find such a doctor, you will probably have little desire to change and will find yourself seeing other physicians only on your own doctor's recommendation, if you need specialized care (see Levels of health care, previous page) or a second opinion.

Choosing a physician

In choosing a doctor you should examine your own preferences and know what you want in a physician. For example, would you prefer a physician who is older than you are, or one who is close to your own age? Do you want a physician who is the same sex as you are? Do you prefer a person who appears warm and personally concerned about you, or would you be willing to do without warmth if you are impressed by a physician's technical knowledge? In general, both patient and physician are happiest and the care is most successful when both participants feel good about and comfortable with each other.

Unfortunately, a comfortable relationship does not necessarily assure high quality care.

The quality of care is difficult to measure, but there are certain factors that you can look for in attempting to do so.

Local and state medical societies may provide the names of any physicians who are taking new patients in or near your area. In addition, many hospitals are offering physician referral services to those who inquire.

Other indications of the high quality of a physician are an excellent reputation among other physicians or health workers, an association with a hospital with a good reputation, recommendations from friends, an association with teaching or university programs, and advanced residency training and specialty board certification.

Evaluating your physician

Once you have chosen a physician, or if you already have one, how can you assess the quality of the care you are receiving? Modern medicine is far too complex, and so is the human body, to base such an assessment only on results and outcomes. Some conditions are more difficult to diagnose and to cure than are others, and of course some diseases cannot be cured. What follows are four areas that you can use as rough indicators of your physician's performance and your satisfaction with the care you are receiving.

First, you can look at how well the physician's practice is organized. This is important because a well-organized practice allows for effective follow-up, accurate record-keeping, a minimum of waiting time before appointments, and adequate time for the physician to spend with you and other patients. It is also important that the physician has set up an effective system for after-hours and weekend care in emergencies, and that the practice allows for taking care of patients who do not have appointments if there is an urgent need. This should be arranged with a minimum of disruption of the schedule for those who do have appointments.

Second, think about how the physician treats you personally. Do you feel that the doctor spends enough time with you to assess a problem? Are physical examinations done carefully, and with adequate respect for your modesty? Does the doctor explain both what is wrong with you and what the treatment is in such a way that you can understand it? If you do not understand, do you feel that you can ask questions? Does the doctor give you a chance to explain your symptoms in your own words, before asking a lot of questions? Does he or she explain the reasons for any diagnostic tests that are ordered? Do you find out what you can expect from treatment, and do you feel free to call to ask about drug side-effects, changes in your condition, or questions that you thought of after you left the office? Do you feel that the physician is really listening to everything that you have to say when he or she is with you?

A third area that you can evaluate is the physician's willingness to consult with other physicians if your problem is outside his or her area of expertise, or if it appears to be especially complex. The physician should explain to you why the consultation is needed, and should provide adequate information for the other doctor to evaluate your situation. Your physician should also make an effort to send you to the most appropriate specialist available, and should be concerned to learn what that other physician found.

If your physician is concerned, he or she can also be an advocate for you or a coordinator of care if you have complex problems that require the attention of several different medical specialists.

Finally, a good physician should be willing to discuss with you any questions you have about your treatment, especially in cases where a disease has been under treatment for a long time and no apparent progress is being made. The doctor should also discuss alternative treatments with you when there are choices, and be able to tell you the relative advantages and disadvantages of each, so that you can make intelligent, informed choices.

In turn you must accept your fair share of responsibility for your health. Your doctor is your partner in the effort to maintain health, but you will have to pay for your physician's advice and follow it to get the best results.

Second opinions and changing physicians

If you have chosen a physician on the basis of your general preferences and evaluated his or her qualifications to your satisfaction, give the relationship a chance. If you have one unsatisfactory appointment, it may have been just a bad day for one or both of you. But if there is still not good communication about your problem or problems after several attempts and your condition is not improving, it may be in your best interest to either seek the opinion of another physician or change physicians. Although this is a wise and rational decision, many people are reluctant to make it. A common reason is fear that the physician's feelings or pride may be hurt. This should not be a consideration, however, for two reasons. First, most physicians understand and accept such developments fully. Second, your first concern must be with your health and the best way to protect and maintain it.

In general, it is better if your regular physician knows about any outside consultation with another doctor so that the second physician can get a copy of your medical records and the results of any tests that have already been performed. This can save you much time and money. Do not fear that the first physician will talk the second into believing his or her diagnosis or even personal opinions about you if you feel the first physician is wrong about either of these things. Doctors are trained to look at such matters independently and reach their own conclusions.

There is a caution against changing physicians under certain circumstances. For example, if your health problem is very unusual or quite rare and you are receiving care from a specialist, there may not be any other physicians available who are capable of treating your problem better. Switching doctors in this situation could end up being unwise, for you risk a loss of both specialized expertise and continuity of care.

If you are unhappy with the care you are receiving, discuss this with your physician. If you cannot work out any problems you may be having, both you and your physician will probably welcome and benefit from a change. (See Choosing a physician, previous page.)

Second opinions on surgery

Since most operations are not emergencies, you will usually have ample time to get a second opinion if you or your physician feel one is warranted. Getting second opinions for a relatively trivial problem can be both costly and confusing. The help of a good family physician in arranging your referral to a surgeon may be your best and easiest route to good surgical care. But even in cases of simple surgery for a small problem, you may not be happy without a second opinion. In such a case, get one for your peace of mind.

Your need for a second opinion on surgery is greatest when the problem you have can be treated without an operation, is particularly complex or rare, or is especially dangerous. In addition to providing information about whether the surgery is necessary, a second surgical opinion in these situations provides an opportunity for you to get the names of and ask about several surgeons. Then, if there is agreement that the surgery is necessary, you can decide which surgeon you prefer.

When choosing a surgeon, consider which one has more experience in performing the particular operation. Also be sure that the surgeon will do the operation in a hospital where such operations are done frequently.

Medical care at home

When you feel sick, what is more comforting than crawling into your own bed to recover? Indeed, home was the place that most health care was given until the last few decades, when hospital care became the norm. Currently, health professionals and planners are looking to medical care at home as one possible answer to the question of how to keep people out of hospitals and nursing homes, where expensive, around-the-clock, professional care is provided.

It seems reasonable to expect that medical care delivered in the home will be emphasized and encouraged in the coming years. For example, rather than going to the hospital for several days for relatively minor surgery such as hernia repair or the stripping of varicose veins, you may be sent home on the same day or the next day after surgery. This saves hospital costs, but it also means that more home nursing skills will be needed. Although this may sound difficult, many families have been and are dealing successfully with illness and disability in their own homes (see Caring for the sick at home, p.754). Guidance and support are available from health professionals including your physician and through community agencies that help serve the needs of the patient at home. However, more of these kinds of service are needed.

Your ability to provide the best possible care for a sick person at home depends on several factors. A few of the most important ones include efforts to draw together the advice of all the health professionals involved, to divide care duties and to determine what outside services are available, useful and affordable.

Team care

In the hospital, a team of health professionals may meet with the patient and family members to discuss plans for meeting the patient's medical needs. This meeting, often called a "family conference," may be impossible for a family to assemble at home. But patient and family can weigh, coordinate and use the suggestions, recommendations and evaluations of all health workers to help make important decisions, such as whether an operation should be performed.

For the everyday care of the patient at home, a team other than the health professionals is required. This other team is made up of those who live where the patient will be, usually his or her family. Members of this team must divide and share the added work that is involved when a sick person is cared for at home. If each person does his or her share, no one person will be burdened excessively, and all can feel the satisfaction of helping a loved one at a time of need.

The home team
The care of an ill person at home can be shared by all family members.

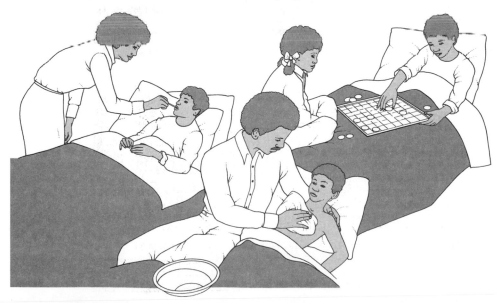

Home services

The following are services to help provide the sick and the disabled with excellent medical care at home:

Home health services are medical services that are provided in a patient's home under a physician's direction. The visiting nurse association or the county or city health department, for example, may provide a variety of types of physician-directed care. These might include home visits by nurses to give injections, change bandages, monitor symptoms, give medications and teach family members to give such care to the patient.

In many areas, one or more home health agencies may provide physical therapy, occupational therapy, speech therapy, general health assessment, social work services, counseling and nutrition programs. If an agency has home health aides or homemakers on staff, a patient can receive help with personal and household tasks. A modest fee schedule for these services may be established. Many of these fees may be paid by Medicare, Medicaid or others (see Paying for medical care, p.752), so often you can get some of these important services even if you are someone who cannot afford to pay for them with your own money.

Friends and relatives can be of great assistance to a family that is caring for someone at home. When they ask what they can do to help, take a minute to think of what needs to be done this week and next (errands, phone calls, letters, meals and home management) and then offer a couple of suggestions from which they can choose. Do not feel you are imposing on them. They are probably very concerned and anxious to help.

Organizations to which you belong, such as a church or a social group, may ask to help in some way. Accept the offers, because such relationships can be important to the patient and to you in the future.

Physicians and other health workers, especially social workers, are familiar with public and private agencies that can provide specialized services the patient may need. A social worker will often spend time with both the patient and the family while the patient is still in the hospital, to gather information and make suggestions about how anticipated problems might be solved. In addition, the social worker can help you identify and contact the agencies that provide the specific services you need.

Drug stores and medical supply houses stock sick room equipment and supplies. Try to rent, rather than buy, the items you need. This may be particularly economical if there is only a temporary need for expensive de-

vices. Renting is also useful so a patient can try out several types of a device that may later be purchased. Often businesses renting and selling such equipment and supplies will deliver, a welcomed service when shopping hours and abilities are few.

Hospice is the name of programs that are specially designed for the terminally ill and emphasize relief of pain and the security of a caring environment. The goal is to have the dying patient's time spent with family, friends and his or her interests.

Adult day care programs may provide either supervised medical and rehabilitative service or recreational and social activities. These programs are primarily for the elderly who need extra help during the day in order to remain at home instead of living in a nursing home. Adult day care may be available for just one day a week, or for as many as five days, depending on the program. Your physician should be able to tell you how to apply for this service.

Day hospital care is similar to the medical type of adult day care. Programs are located in a hospital. This care may be available to adults of all ages as well as to the elderly.

Door-to-door transportation for the elderly and disabled at minimal cost is available in some cities and can be very useful. Ask the visiting nurse or your physician if such a program exists in your area.

Chore services are available in a few states. This program provides trained people to do difficult home chores for the handicapped or the elderly. Occasionally churches or church-related groups have such services available on a limited basis.

Local voluntary health organizations such as the American Cancer Society and the Easter Seal Society may be able to lend specialized equipment and provide you with information. These organizations often have programs that benefit the ill or disabled.

Vocational rehabilitation programs provide guidance, training and job placement assistance with the goal of enabling a person to obtain or maintain employment. There are eligibility requirements for these programs, which may be supported in part by community, state and federal funds.

Recorded information is available by telephone through some hospitals and medical societies that subscribe to libraries of recorded medical information. You can dial a message from the hospital or from your home on a variety of topics such as how to deal with a urinary catheter, the tube through which an ill person's urine is sometimes drained, or how to care for a person with diabetes.

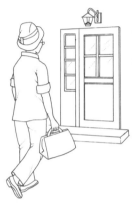

Visiting nurse

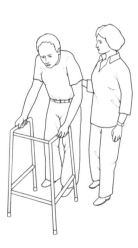

Physical therapist

Office and clinic care

People in the United States average almost five visits to a physician per year. Much of this care is provided in what is known as "ambulatory care settings." The term ambulatory care means walk-in care that does not involve one or more nights spent in a hospital or other health care facility. Examples include the care that is given in a physician's office, in the outpatient department of a hospital including an emergency room, or in a free clinic, a health center or an agency that is not physically attached to a hospital. It also includes all the many home care services (see previous page). While there are many different types of ambulatory care and new ones are always developing, the following material will focus only on the more common forms of walk-in medical care.

Office-based practice

There are three major ways physicians organize their office-based practices. They are solo practices, partnerships and group practices.

Solo practices: As the name implies, a solo practice is one in which the physician works alone. He or she usually owns the office equipment, and hires staff such as an office nurse, a billing clerk and/or a receptionist. A solo physician will sometimes share some of the expenses with other physicians in what is called an association. Such an arrangement does not necessarily involve any other obligations between the physicians. Some physicians work this way because they find it simpler to work alone, and others because there are no other physicians in the community. Solo practice is becoming less popular with physicians, partly because it requires taking on a great deal of extra responsibility for patients, such as being expected to be available 24 hours a day, 365 days per year.

Partnerships: A partnership involves a specific type of legal agreement between two or more physicians to share income, office space and equipment. In some partnerships, one or two physicians own the practice and hire others who are paid a salary initially and may eventually become full partners.

Some of the advantages of a partnership over solo practice include that the physicians can help each other with after-hours care, consult each other with difficult cases, and otherwise share some of the responsibility of care where appropriate. It is also sometimes more economical to share staff and various other office expenses.

Medical care at work

Until quite recently, most companies limited their health care responsibilities for employees to providing health insurance programs and reviewing job safety. Workers seemed satisfied with this, for labor contracts emphasized medical care insurance packages. Recently, however, the costs of medical care have risen to the point that efforts have begun to bring routine health care services and health maintenance activities closer to the job. Some employers, for example, have added health and exercise facilities (gymnasiums or swimming pools) to the work place, while others provide a medical clinic.

The health care professional who is particularly concerned with health in the workplace is the preventive medicine specialist. He or she may also be trained in occupational medicine. Occupational medicine involves expertise in a variety of areas including the safety of the workplace.

The science of studying disease in groups or populations is called epidemiology. Epidemiology in the workplace is becoming more important today since businesses can save money as well as increase their productivity if workers stay healthy. Today, health care on the job is expanding to include some specific health promotion programs. Programs to combat alcoholism are one example. Alcoholism in the workplace can affect anyone. It also has implications for job safety and productivity. Alcoholism is a serious disability and anyone who suffers from it deserves support and treatment. Other programs being tried by some companies include incentives for workers to stop smoking. Many programs are extremely worthwhile for both the employees and the companies who have started them. For example, heavy smokers as a group miss more days at work than do nonsmokers. Successfully combatting smoking means fewer workdays lost.

Group practices: A group practice is a voluntary association of three or more physicians in medical practice who use common facilities and share income and expenses in an agreed upon manner. Such a practice often has many of the same advantages as does a partnership. A group practice is often based on a less formal and more flexible agreement than a partnership. Groups that are made up of physicians who are all in the same medical specialty are called single specialty groups, and groups that include physicians that are in a variety of medical specialities are called multi-specialty groups.

Health maintenance organizations (HMO) and independent practice associations (IPA) are group practices that are organized to provide complete care for patients on a prepaid basis. Each patient (or his or her employer) pays a set amount each month, and the group provides, at no extra charge or sometimes a nominal charge, care for any illness or accident and preventive care such as checkups. Hospitalization and referral for services that the group cannot supply directly are also covered by the monthly fee. The services that are covered by a particular prepaid plan vary, depending on the contract with patients.

Hospital clinics

Some physicians have practices that are located in hospitals. They see patients either in the outpatient departments, in clinics, or in the emergency room. In large cities, hospital outpatient clinics have been a major source of medical care for the poor. However, in communities where there is a medical college, university teaching hospitals may serve all income groups in their clinics. Depending on the hospital, the patient may receive care from residents who are supervised by more senior specialists, or may see the specialists themselves. Contrary to some popular opinion, the care received in a hospital clinic, particularly in a fine hospital, can be of the highest quality.

Ambulatory surgery centers

These centers are sometimes called "surgicenters." They may be either independent facilities or part of a hospital. They are equipped for doing surgical procedures that do not require overnight hospitalization. Surgicenters provide facilities where minor surgical procedures can be done efficiently and at a reduced cost. A surgicenter does not require the same sophisticated and costly equipment that is necessary in an operating room where all kinds of complex surgical procedures can be done. It also does not need to have as many beds, staff and services. If you need surgery, you can ask your physician if having it done at an ambulatory surgical center is possible.

Mental health and counseling

Mental health and counseling services may be located in hospitals, clinics, offices, schools and small independent practice units. There are a variety of health workers in this field, including psychiatrists (physicians), as well as clinical psychologists and social workers. Some mental health practices are specialized. For example, a psychiatrist may limit his or her practice to psychoanalysis while another may emphasize marriage counseling.

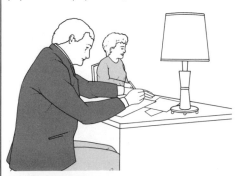

Psychiatric care

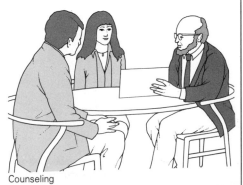

Counseling

Community, or public, health

Community health, sometimes referred to as public health, includes a variety of services provided by county health departments, city health departments or other publicly supported agencies.

Preventive medicine, which is important for maintaining a high level of health, requires effort that is well beyond the capacity of any single health worker. Thus, this area of medicine is often considered to be a part of community health. In most states health departments are organized to serve a city, town, county, or region.

The organization and function of state health agencies varies, but state health departments usually have been responsible for coordinating current public health activities and for planning for the future. Local and county health departments often are organized to deliver more direct services. These may include school health, health screening, immunization programs, rodent and insect control, nutrition programs, maternal and child health and similar programs.

School health

In many communities, nurses and other health professionals are assigned to the schools and work with students, parents, community physicians and school staff. A variety of services may be provided by such a person, including consultation with administrators, teachers and parents in matters of physical and emotional health; home visitation to assist parents in planning follow-up medical treatment for their children; educational support for teachers, students and parents in health-related subjects; screening programs for dental, vision and hearing problems; and checking immunization records. A school nurse may also plan and/or participate in health conferences and classes.

Health screening

In health screening large numbers of people are tested for disease, so that early treatment can be given to prevent the disease from worsening or spreading. Local health departments can usually provide information on voluntary health screening agencies in the community, and may also offer such services. Screening may include testing for infectious diseases, or chronic ailments such as high blood pressure, diabetes and foot troubles. Such programs may also help with such matters as diet or medication problems.

For children, there are programs available for the early screening, diagnosis and treatment of many diseases. These screening programs include a health history, vision and hearing tests, a dental examination, immunizations and a blood test for anemia.

Neighborhood and primary health care centers

These programs were first developed in the late 1960s with federal funding and, in some cases, with funds that were obtained from private foundations. They were set up to provide ambulatory, or out-of-hospital, care in areas of the United States where there were not enough physicians and other medical services to adequately provide for the population. These are called "underserved areas" and are generally found in the poor areas of cities and in rural areas, where physicians are not likely to settle and open new practices. The centers are often staffed by physicians and nurses from the National Health Service Corps, a branch of the Public Health Service that recruits medical personnel to work in underserved areas.

Some of the centers are set up in order to serve the poor, and the services that are provided are paid for in part by Medicare and Medicaid. Other such centers are intended to serve the entire community in areas where only a few or no other medical services are available to the residents.

Another program that has sometimes been combined with these health care centers is the Migrant Health Program. It was established specifically to serve migrant farm workers and their families.

The range of services that are provided by these centers depends on the funds available, the number and type of expertise of the staff of the center, and what other services are present in the community.

Maternal and child care

Maternal and child care programs are available in many neighborhoods and communities. These federally funded programs are aimed at upgrading maternal and child health by providing food of specific nutritional value. The program serves pregnant women, new mothers, infants, and children up to the age of five whose weight is low for their age or who are anemic or near-anemic (see Anemia, p.419, and Anemia during pregnancy, p.623). You must be below a certain income level to qualify for this care.

In many communities, you can request a home visit from the health department for help in determining your and your family's health needs. Instruction and guidance may be given in prenatal care, infant care, nutrition, family planning and others.

Disease prevention and control

Immunization clinics are available in many communities. The immunizations available are those to protect children against diphtheria, tetanus, whooping cough, polio, measles, German measles (rubella) and mumps (see Immunization, p.701).

Community tuberculosis control activities are also frequently available (see Tuberculosis, p.563). Some departments of health have a chronic disease program to screen people for tuberculosis. Sexually transmitted, or venereal, disease control and quarantines may also be administered by the local health department (see Sexually transmitted diseases, p.611).

Communicable diseases that pose problems for the population at large are called "reportable diseases," because health workers are supposed to report cases to the local health department.

Mental health

Community health programs include services for both the mentally ill and the mentally handicapped. State-administered institutions and community-based day programs are included in these activities.

Community mental health programs are designed to prevent, detect and treat mental illness. Services of local mental health departments include diagnosis and referral to treatment programs.

Staff members for these programs may be either part-time or full-time psychiatrists, psychologists, social workers, community health nurses, pharmacists, and other mental health personnel. These trained mental health workers may provide services that include consultation for detention centers and departments of social service, educational support for civic and fraternal groups and schools, alcoholic and drug addict rehabilitation programs, and emergency care for the mentally ill.

Local services for the mentally handicapped usually are administered by voluntary associations and boards of education. State hospitals for the mentally handicapped emphasize training and education.

The term developmental disability is currently used to describe the problems of persons whose mental and/or physical development has been impaired. State institutions for the severely developmentally disabled provide a wide range of services.

Churches and voluntary organizations have a tradition of building and administering institutions for the severely mentally or physically handicapped. Although the quality of care given is usually good, these institutions are too few in number to meet the entire need for such residential or institutional care.

Other services

There are several other services that may be provided by a local or county health department or by other local government and private agencies. One such service is protecting the population from health problems that are caused by deterioration of the environment. This responsibility includes dealing with the hazards of tainted water, sewage, garbage, rodents or insects. To do this requires regular testing for pure air and water; a program for inspecting hotels, restaurants, swimming pools, recreation facilities and food stores; and careful monitoring of radiation levels. Some local health departments have laboratory services for performing some or all of the tests that are related to disease control and the quality of the environment.

In some communities, the health department conducts dental surveys in the schools, distributes fluoride tablets where they are needed to help protect children's teeth, and may provide a dental clinic. Finally, some have programs for nursing services and home health services.

The hospital

Recently we have seen a major shift of emphasis away from hospital care and toward care in the physician's office and at home. Two reasons stand out among the many that help explain this change. One reason is the effectiveness of modern drugs and other treatments. The other reason is that some kinds of health care can be provided more cheaply out of the hospital. Nevertheless, sooner or later most of us must go to a hospital, and it remains an important part of the medical care system. Therefore, it is important to learn about different types of hospitals and the services offered within them.

Few people are aware of what mechanisms exist to assure quality care in a hospital or what a patient's rights are in a hospital. And what about the patient's obligations as a hospital patient?

A frequent reason for entering a hospital or outcome of hospital examinations and tests is the need for surgery. Many people have never had an operation or even seen the inside of a typical operating room. They and many who have had one or more operations know little or nothing of what specialists will be present and working during the operation and what each one's particular job is. And what of all the machines and other equipment? Will they be used? How many of them? What do they do? Most people also are not well-informed about intensive care in the hospital, yet each year, millions of people require such care. And then there is the frightening possibility that you might die in the hospital. What happens then?

These are some of the areas covered and questions answered in the articles that follow.

Defining a hospital

Most hospitals, whether large or small, public or private, for profit or not-for-profit, can provide, at a minimum, basic services for patients who need many different types of medical and surgical diagnosis and treatment. To fit the definition of a hospital, an institution generally has the following:
- Patient beds for at least overnight stays.
- Operating rooms, X-ray and clinical laboratory services.
- A board or other governing body that is legally responsible for the institution, plus a professional medical staff.
- An administrator who operates the hospital following the policies set by the governing body.
- Supervision of medical care for each patient by a physician on the medical staff.
- Nursing services that are supervised by registered nurses.
- A pharmacy, supervised by a registered pharmacist, which provides drugs for treatment.
- A food service that is equipped to provide adequate nutrition for patients and that also can prepare special diets as needed for treatment
- Complete medical records for all patients.

Types of hospital

Hospitals can be characterized on the basis of ownership, type of services provided, length of hospital stay, type of health care providers (for example, medical doctors or osteopaths) and as teaching or non-teaching hospitals. However, the variety within these types is so great that any classification system has exceptions. The two most important groups by size and volume of care provided are the voluntary, short-stay, general community hospitals and nonfederal, long-term hospitals.

In terms of their ownership, there are government-owned hospitals and privately-owned nongovernment hospitals. Government hospitals include federal short-term, or short-stay, hospitals and state and local (county or municipal) short-term hospitals. Short-term state hospitals are typically run by state medical schools as teaching hospitals.

There are also six major types of community or voluntary short-stay hospitals. These include religious, community, cooperative, proprietary, osteopathic and organizational.

Religious hospitals may be owned and/or run by a religious group or they may be sponsored or supported by a religious faith.

Most voluntary hospitals today are so-called community hospitals. These hospitals are independent, nonprofit associations of citizens who form a corporation that includes a board of directors or trustees that is responsible for the hospital's actions.

Cooperative hospitals are those owned by the users and/or potential users of those hospitals. The hospitals of large health maintenance organizations (see Office-based practice, p.739) are examples of cooperatively-owned hospitals.

Proprietary hospitals are operated for profit by an individual or by a corporation. The number of such hospitals is rapidly growing, although these hospitals now account for only 15 per cent of all community hospitals. In the past, most were owned by a physician or a group of physicians. Today several investor-owned corporations are running existing hospital chains, as well as building new hospitals and nursing homes.

Osteopathic hospitals are those in which osteopathic physicians work together. They can be either nonprofit community hospitals or proprietary hospitals.

Organizational hospitals include those run by companies or certain other groups. Railroads, large companies and labor unions still run a few hospitals. Fraternal societies such as the Shriners (The Ancient Arabic Order of Nobles of the Mystic Shrine of North America) own and operate a number of hospitals for crippled children.

Emergency care

Although not every hospital has an emergency room, those that do provide a great deal of a community's emergency care. They also sometimes give routine medical treatment. Generally care received in emergency rooms is substantially more expensive than care received in a clinic or a physician's office. In addition, emergency room treatment usually does not provide for continuity of care by a single physician, and the most seriously ill or injured patients must be taken care of first, no matter when they arrived. For these reasons it is best to go to an emergency room only for truly urgent problems.

Recently, specialized centers for emergency care have been developed in some hospitals, particularly in large cities. Such centers include those that deal with burns, accidents, heart attacks and so forth. These centers are staffed with specialists in the particular problem treated and have sophisticated, specialized and expensive equipment.

Quality of health care

The modern hospital is subject to continuous reviews to help maintain the quality of care that it provides. The hospital regulations that are designed to assure quality care are complex. They involve ongoing internal mechanisms as well as external reviews. Some reviews are required by government regulations, and some are voluntary.

The major voluntary mechanism for reviewing a hospital and its performance is the accreditation process of the Joint Commission on Accreditation of Hospitals. Hospitals are accredited, or approved, by the Commission for no more than three years at a time. Unaccredited hospitals may receive accreditation whenever they meet the standards of the Commission. Accredited hospitals usually post the certificate of accreditation in a prominent location where anyone who is interested can see it.

All hospitals have a set of medical staff by-laws. These rules and regulations are developed by the medical staff, to assure the high quality of their work. In addition, a credentials committee reviews all physicians on the medical staff on a regular basis.

Hospital review mechanisms also include committees that regularly examine the appropriateness of hospitalization of patients, written reports on surgical specimens, patient complaints, the quality of medical records, frequency and control of infections, and the use of drugs. These committees meet regularly to discuss their findings and make recommendations. Minutes of all of these meetings are kept on file.

Services and departments

In addition to the medical staff, a typical, large, community, general hospital provides many other services that serve the patients either directly or indirectly. Some of the major ones are described below.

Nursing services: The nursing department usually has the single largest staff of a hospital. This is because nurses are needed for three shifts, around-the-clock and seven days a week. Nurses are assigned to specific stations, often on hospital wards (separate floors or sections of floors) or on specialized units such as surgical, cardiac care, and intensive care units. Nurses are responsible for the constant, day-to-day care of hospitalized patients. They supervise nurse's aides, give drugs and other treatments as prescribed by physicians, monitor the progress of patients, and provide information to patients about their conditions and treatments. The nursing staff also assists with surgical procedures that are performed in the operating rooms or ambulatory surgical units.

Clinical support services: Providing medical treatment and care requires support services from other departments of the hospital. Patients are often totally unaware that such services exist. These services are often called ancillary services. They include radiology (*X-ray* department), anesthesiology, and the clinical pathology laboratories where tests are done on blood and tissue. Clinical support services also include laboratory tests on bacteria and urine and other body liquids. The staff of the anatomical pathology laboratory examines tissue specimens, performs autopsies and maintains the morgue.

Other clinical support services include physical therapy, occupational therapy, respiratory therapy, dietetics, pharmacy, blood bank, *electroencephalography* (*EEG*), *electrocardiography* (*ECG*), renal *dialysis*, audiology, social services, the library and providing for patients' religious needs. Larger hospitals have even more clinical service sections to evaluate less common problems that are referred to specialists who are on the staff.

Administrative and nonclinical support services: These areas of hospital management are the responsibility of the hospital administrator and his or her staff. These services include admissions, food service for patients and staff, a business office, hospital volunteers (auxiliaries), public relations, central supply, medical records, housekeeping, maintenance, purchasing and stores, a messenger and transport service, laundry and linen, and a telephone switchboard.

Patient's rights

Patients who receive hospital care have a number of freedoms they can exercise. They have the right to refuse or withdraw from care. They must give their consent to treatment, and have a right to have any risks and alternatives explained clearly.

Although a patient's medical record is a legal document and not his or her property, the patient has a right to review it. Before you review your own medical record, however, you should consider whether you are physically and psychologically prepared to deal with whatever information you find.

Assuring confidentiality of medical information is extremely important, and a variety of mechanisms exists to assure that no one has access to an individual's medical record except as necessary to serve the interests of the patient or to improve medical care.

Patients may, and indeed should, bring problems relating to their care to the attention of their physicians and other hospital staff. Most hospitals have a mechanism for registering and reviewing the complaints and concerns of patients. Quality review committees in hospitals (see Quality of health care, previous page), for example, are interested in the complaints of patients.

Patient's bill of rights
The American Hospital Association issued a bill of rights for patients in 1973. Essentially, its main points are:
1. The patient has the right to considerate and respectful care.
2. The patient has the right to obtain from his physician complete current information concerning his diagnosis, treatment and prognosis in terms the patient can reasonably be expected to understand.
3. The patient has the right to receive from his physician information necessary to give informed consent prior to the start of any procedure and/or treatment.
4. The patient has the right to refuse treatment to the extent permitted by law, and to be informed of the medical consequences of his action.
5. The patient has the right to every consideration of his privacy concerning his own medical care program.
6. The patient has the right to expect that all communications and records pertaining to his care should be treated as confidential.
7. The patient has the right to expect that within its capacity a hospital must make responsible response to the request of a patient for services.
8. The patient has the right to obtain information as to any relationship of his hospital to other health care and educational institutions insofar as his care is concerned.
9. The patient has the right to be advised if the hospital proposes to engage in or perform human experimentation affecting his care or treatment.
10. The patient has the right to expect reasonable continuity of care.
11. The patient has the right to examine and receive an explanation of his bill regardless of source of payment.
12. The patient has the right to know what hospital rules and regulations apply to his conduct as a patient.

Having an operation

Before any operation you will have to sign a consent form. If there is anything you do not understand in the form, ask your physician about it before you sign.

On the morning of the operation you will not have anything to eat or drink. The reason for this is that if your stomach is not empty, the anesthetic may cause you to vomit while you are unconscious, and this could be dangerous. Any necessary shaving, to remove hair from the area to be operated on, may be done at this time or earlier. You are then dressed in a clean gown to minimize the risk of infection. An hour or so before the operation is scheduled, you are given an injection that makes you sleepy. The anesthetic is given in the operating room.

Except when blood vessels are being stitched, internal and membranous areas that have been cut or injured will be closed with dissolving stitches. Small skin incisions will usually be closed with nylon thread or clips, and larger incisions may be held together by large supporting stitches.

After any surgery, the patient goes immediately to a recovery room for about half an hour to two hours, to be watched quite closely until the staff permit a transfer to the patient's regular hospital room. If the patient is very ill or the surgery extensive, he or she may be sent to an intensive-care unit (see next page).

After some types of surgery, particularly abdominal surgery, you may have to be fed or given fluids through an intravenous drip, or a tube inserted into a vein, for a day or two. Other tubes (drainage tubes) may also be used to drain off fluids and pus.

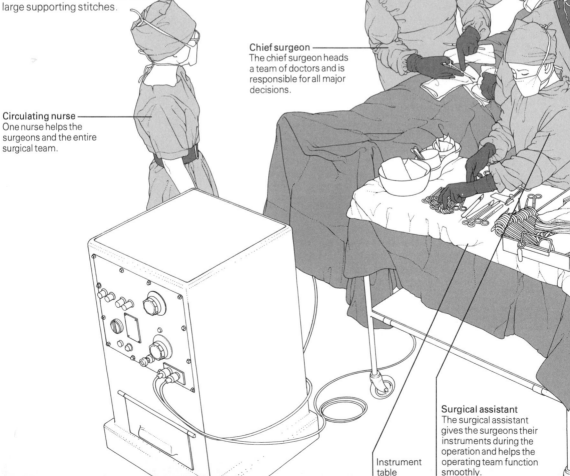

Anesthesiologist
The anesthesiologist administers anesthetics and is an expert in treatment of surgical shock, maintenance of life support and relief of the pain that follows the operation.

Surgical resident
The surgical resident obtains experience in the operating room and gets further training in surgical techniques.

Chief surgeon
The chief surgeon heads a team of doctors and is responsible for all major decisions.

Circulating nurse
One nurse helps the surgeons and the entire surgical team.

Surgical assistant
The surgical assistant gives the surgeons their instruments during the operation and helps the operating team function smoothly.

Instrument table

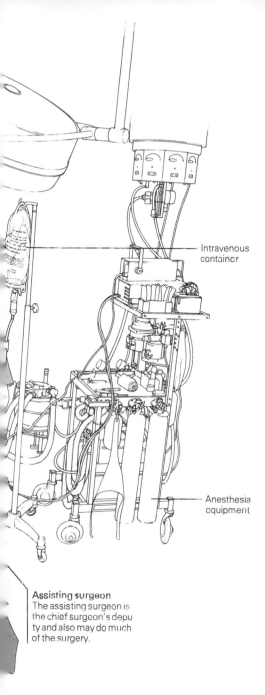

Intravenous container

Anesthesia equipment

Assisting surgeon
The assisting surgeon is the chief surgeon's deputy and also may do much of the surgery.

Intensive care

After some major operations and during some serious illnesses, the patient may need breathing aid from an artificial ventilator or may have to breathe with the help of extra oxygen. Continuous electronic monitoring of blood pressure, heart rate and other vital body functions may also be required. The equipment necessary to provide intensive care after an operation is usually concentrated in a unit where the patients are cared for by specialist medical and nursing staffs. Most patients remain in this intensive-care unit, under constant supervision, for only a few days. They are then transferred to a less intensive hospital unit to continue their recovery.

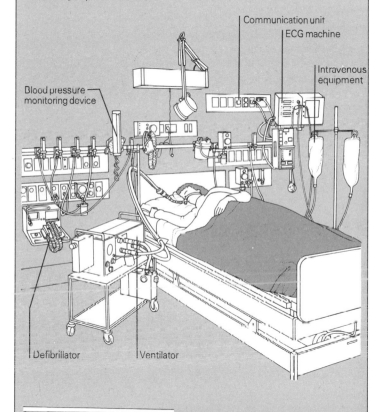

Communication unit
ECG machine
Intravenous equipment
Blood pressure monitoring device
Defibrillator
Ventilator

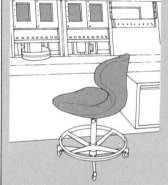

Central control station
An intensive-care unit often has a central console, which allows a single member of the nursing staff to keep a check on all the patients in the unit. The recordings made of each patient's vital functions are shown on the console, and the instruments are fitted with automatic alarms that indicate any emergency.

The patient's role

Your role in your hospital care is a most important one. If you understand the goals of your health care team and how you can help, it can make a surprising difference in how long your recovery will take. There may be complex technical factors involved in your treatment, so take notes when necessary as you speak with members of your health care team, and write down any questions you may have. It is one of the obligations of the professionals on the hospital staff to answer these questions to the best of their ability.

Try to stay in the hospital no longer than is medically needed. Where possible, consider outpatient care (care out of the hospital) if your physician tells you your medical problem would allow it safely. The rising cost of medical care is partly due to inefficient use of hospital services, so don't be surprised if you are encouraged to use outpatient care or be discharged as early as possible.

If you notice ways in which your care could be improved, pass the word along. If you have been pleased, the hospital staff would like to know that as well. A number of hospital routines may seem strange and sometimes inappropriate. Usually there is a good reason behind the practice or policy, but it is also possible that some things should be changed.

Hospitals exist to serve the larger community. Good communications about the quality of a hospital's services can help everyone. This includes exercising your right to complain (see Patient's rights, p.745). Complaints, of course, are always most welcome when made calmly and rationally.

In order to function well, hospitals need well-trained people to work with them. Well-trained people start out as students who need to develop their skills. Your willingness to allow students to witness your care and assist where they can is vital to maintaining excellence in medicine. So, if students seem to be prying or awkward, remember that they are still learning, and that you are performing a very valuable public service when you permit them to participate. Moreover, their interest may help insure high quality care.

If you die

Because hospitals serve many patients who are very seriously, even terminally, ill there are people who die in the hospital. If you know that you might die in the hospital, as frightening and unpleasant as that realization may be, there are certain special things that might concern you. For example, you should consider donating organs and tissues should you die. Eye transplants involve removing the cornea, the covering over the eye, and transplanting it onto someone else's eye to restore their vision. This operation must be performed soon after the donor's death if the transplantation is to be effective.

Another commonly transplanted organ is the kidney. Kidney transplantation, when successful, allows a person with kidney failure to live without frequent special treatments. For kidneys to be suitable for transplantation, they must still be able to function normally, so they must be "alive." In most cases, the kidney donor is a person who has irreversible, untreatable brain injury. The kidneys are removed if the donor has previously agreed or after permission is given by the immediate family. This is done before life-support measures, such as heart-lung machines, are withdrawn from the donor. Donation of kidneys in this manner has allowed many people to remain alive.

You may wish to think about your feelings on these matters and share them with your family. More and more human tissues such as bone, pancreas and skin are being used in this way. If you have already thought about donations of this type and have decided that you want to make such donations, you can make arrangements for it now (see Medical use of the body, p.773).

Whole body donations and permission for *post mortem* examinations or autopsies are also needed by medical schools and others (see Autopsies, p.773). Cadavers, or bodies used to educate physicians and other health professionals about anatomy, are important for medical education. For more information about donating your body for this purpose, write to the department of anatomy or the dean's office of any medical or osteopathic school. Generally, bodies used for this purpose are cremated, or burned to ashes at high temperatures, after they are dissected.

Granting permission for a *post mortem* examination, or autopsy, can be a difficult decision for many people. In the past, autopsies were performed more commonly than they are today because it was often more difficult to determine the cause of death. Today autopsies are still important, since they provide unique material for the study of the disease or disorder that caused the death. Such study may yield new information or teach a lesson that may be of help to the family and medical science. The examination is performed by pathologists who are experts in the changes tissues undergo as a result of disease.

Nursing homes

Families are still the major caretakers of older, dependent or disabled persons in the United States. However, the number of people over 65 in nursing homes is rising, because the population in that age group is increasing. Although many people now live longer, healthier lives, this longevity has increased the need for services of nursing homes and long-term care facilities.

A "long-term care facility" is a building or group of buildings that is staffed by trained workers and suitable for people who need medical care for a longer period of time than is usually possible in a general hospital. Thus, a nursing home is only one type of long-term care facility. Long-term care (LTC) is also given in tuberculosis hospitals, chronic disease hospitals, mental retardation hospitals, rehabilitation hospitals and psychiatric hospitals. Nursing homes accommodate patients with serious illnesses and disorders that are *congenital*, or present at birth, and also patients who have been severely injured in accidents or who have chronic disabling diseases. Nursing homes, however, are primarily populated by the elderly.

Circumstances may allow an elderly or disabled person to live at home. However, if continuous nursing care of a demanding nature is required, and in-home services are scarce, many families find that a nursing home is needed.

Choosing a nursing home, like choosing any new place to live, is an important decision. It is difficult to make the decision quickly, but disabling illness can occur suddenly. The person who will be moving to the nursing

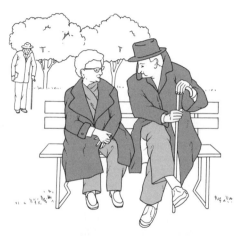

home should be consulted about his or her wishes, and in a medical crisis he or she may not be able to make preferences known. So it may be wise to look into possible nursing homes before anything happens to force a quick decision.

Nursing home accommodations are in short supply in some areas, and the patient may have to go on a waiting list. The cost of the nursing home is also important, and early exploration allows a greater chance of finding one within your family budget.

Family decision-making is very important and requires time. It may not be possible to find a facility that meets all the needs of the patient and the family, but knowing the needs and wishes of all family members involved will go a long way toward making a decision.

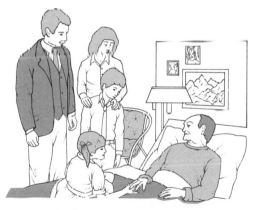

Moving into a nursing home may occur from the person's home, another family member's home, from a hospital or from another long-term care facility. If the patient requires nursing home care after hospitalization, the medical care team will assist in the planning. The hospital social worker is familiar with area nursing homes and can suggest alternatives and place the patient on waiting lists if necessary.

Often elderly people dread moving into a nursing home. They may feel they are going "to wait to die." And they may fear not only abandonment by family and friends, but also having to adapt to a totally new environment and new people. Everyone should do what they can to reassure such a person. Many elderly and disabled people adjust extremely well to nursing homes and find a new freedom and enthusiasm for life in an environment designed for persons like themselves.

Types of nursing homes

There are many types of nursing homes, and health professionals tend to use initials to refer to them. It may help you to choose an appropriate home if you are familiar with the types and terminology.

A residential care facility (RCF) provides meals and sheltered living (little or no housekeeping responsibilities for the resident) and some medical monitoring (keeping track of symptoms and signs of illness). This type of facility is appropriate for someone who must or wants to give up major household chores, but does not need continuous medical attention. Some RCF's have exercise, social and recreational programs.

An intermediate care facility (ICF) provides room and board and regular nursing care (not around-the-clock) for patients who cannot manage independent living. Physical, social and recreational activities may be provided and some have rehabilitation programs. The cost of care in an ICF may be covered by some government programs.

A skilled nursing facility (SNF) provides physician coverage and 24-hour nursing care by registered nurses, licensed practical nurses and nurse's aides. An SNF is the right place for someone who requires intensive nursing care and rehabilitation services such as occupational therapy, physical therapy and social work services. SNF's may be paid for by both Medicare and Medicaid programs, but there are eligibility conditions that may change from time to time. Up-to-date information can be obtained from your nearest Social Security office.

Determining the quality of care

Quality of care is, of course, of utmost importance in choosing a nursing home. There is no substitute for "shopping around," just as you would when considering a move to a new area. Talking to nursing-home residents and their families and to health workers who have had experience with a long-term care center, reading written material such as brochures, speaking with administrators and visiting the facilities are often necessary to make a decision. Discussing what is learned with other family members and the patient is also important. What is a priority for the patient may not be for the family. For example, orderliness can be interpreted as positive (clean and safe) or negative (over-efficient and impersonal).

Official certification of a nursing home as a skilled nursing facility or an intermediate care facility is important and signifies that the home has met state standards for that type of facility. Although certification is not in itself a guarantee of high quality care, lack of certification is a signal that the facility could have serious problems.

Other considerations

Does the person entering the home consider the range of services, outside of the basics, to be important? If so, ask about activities and recreation programs, volunteer programs, and the availability of medical equipment such as walkers and wheelchairs. Does the home offer rehabilitation programs such as physical therapy, occupational therapy, speech therapy and social work services?

Physical appearance affects the patient, the nursing-home personnel and the family. Picture yourself visiting. Are there places to visit in private or take a walk? Can you share a meal with the resident or participate in any of the home's group activities?

Affordability is another important part of the decision. You must know the exact costs involved in long-term care. Usually there is a basic cost for room and board per month, with additional charges for special medical care including medications. Ask how often the basic charge has been raised in the past few years. A home that raises prices frequently may soon be out of financial reach. There may be public funds available in some cases, such as when care has used up a person's financial assets. Start working early with the nursing home administrator or social worker to learn when a patient may need financial support in order to pay the cost of the care that is provided.

Will special medical equipment and a rehabilitation program be available?

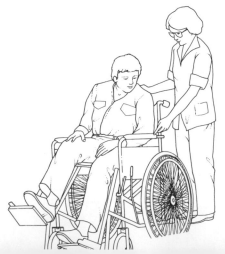

Medical care organizations

Medical care organizations usually are not, interestingly enough, organizations that deliver medical care. Some do deliver such care, however. The National Institutes of Health (NIH) in Bethesda, Maryland is one example of such an organization. At this huge center for health records, any citizen of the United States can get medical care free if his or her problem is being studied there.

Medical care organizations can be classified into three categories. These categories are federal, professional and voluntary.

Federal organizations

There are two types of federal medical organizations. One type is administrative, and is not directly involved in delivering health care. Some of these organizations administer funds that are appropriated by the government to pay for services delivered to qualified persons by nongovernment organizations such as hospitals. The two major government programs of this type are Medicare and Medicaid (see Medical insurance, p.752). Programs of this type have had a profound impact on providing medical care to the poor and elderly. They also have serious problems, since their costs are enormous.

Other non-delivery health organizations in the federal government include the Food and Drug Administration, the Centers for Disease Control and the Center for Health Statistics. There are also many others in areas of health education, research, agriculture, labor, environment, child care, vocational rehabilitation, health services regulation and health care planning.

The second type of federal medical organization does actually deliver medical services. One of these organizations is the United States Public Health Service. Other federal medical organizations that deliver medical services are the National Institutes of Health and the Veterans Administration.

Professional organizations

There are hundreds of professional medical organizations. They range widely in size, function and requirements for membership. Some of the largest include the American Medical Association, the American Public Health Association, and medical specialty organizations such as the American College of Surgeons. Most of these organizations have two roles, to provide professional and continuing education for their members and to represent them to the public and sometimes to legislative bodies.

In addition to holding national and regional meetings, many of the larger organizations publish scientific journals. This helps their members keep up with current developments in health-related research in their areas of expertise and interest.

Voluntary organizations

Voluntary health organizations are usually formed by citizens who have an interest in a specific disease or disorder. Such associations bring the energy and interest of the general public to the ongoing needs of patients with serious and/or chronic diseases. Physicians and other health workers often join these organizations as well. Voluntary health organizations exist to assist those with many diseases and conditions, including alcoholism, bleeding disorders, blindness, cancer, arthritis, autism, diabetes, kidney disease, developmental disabilities (*congenital* disorders or diseases that hinder development), mental and emotional illness, muscular dystrophy, over- or under-eating, occupational diseases, cystic fibrosis, facial deformities, hearing and speech disorders, hereditary diseases, Parkinson's disease, spinal cord injuries and other diseases and injuries that cause paralysis, epilepsy, respiratory diseases, cerebral palsy, mental retardation and multiple sclerosis.

These associations are usually, but not always, nation-wide, state-wide or regional, with local chapters in cities and large towns. The activities of these groups include services such as providing public information, working toward related legislation, providing information for patients and families, providing research funds, and supporting programs that supplement care already available.

Paying for medical care

There are several ways that medical care is commonly paid for. Because modern medical care, like almost everything today, is expensive and becoming more so, it is important to understand as much as possible about methods of paying medical bills. Most of the existing methods were created to help individuals meet their medical needs without personal financial crisis.

In the coming years, it appears that both government and private insurers, the two major sources of health care payments, will be attempting to reduce health care costs. It is possible that the pressures this produces may also reduce the range of services and benefits. Unfortunately, a reduction in the quality of care could be a result. One of the challenges facing American medicine is how to maintain and improve the health care system while spending less, despite inflation. This will be a difficult task since elderly and aged people tend to need more medical care and this population is expanding. Because of these developments, each individual person may have fewer choices for care and will almost certainly pay for more services out of his or her own pocket.

The terms that are used in association with many of the methods of paying for medical care today are as difficult as many medical terms for a layperson to understand. Since there is no avoiding this technical jargon when discussing various methods of payment and types of insurance, the terms are used in the following pages in ways that should make their meanings clear.

Individual payment

A traditional and time honored way of paying for medical care is out-of-pocket. If you have no health insurance or if your insurance policy does not pay for the service given (a more likely possibility since most people in the United States have some health insurance), you must pay out of your own income or "pocket." Many people still pay for visits to their family doctor in this way. Today, however, the cost of hospital care has risen to the point where other methods may be available to make sure that health care can be paid for, especially in the event of disabling accidents and illnesses.

Medical insurance

With medical or health insurance, either you, your employer, or both pay a set monthly premium. If you need medical care, the insurance company pays the allowable cost of the services delivered to you out of its total resources. If you do not need care, the premium that is paid for you becomes part of the company's total resources. While the specifics may differ, most insurance plans are based on this approach.

Benefits and costs
Services covered by a health insurance policy are said to be "in the benefits package." A health insurance policy that has all treatments for all diseases in the benefits package will be much more expensive than a policy that has fewer treatments or diseases covered in its package. People generally like to have a wide range of benefits or services, just in case they need them. This tends to drive up total medical costs and increase the amount of services rendered. This is partly because people with insurance coverage tend to demand more services more often, since they do not have to pay for them directly.

Coinsurance
Many health economists and government experts are convinced that the demand for medical services would be reduced if individual patients had to pay some of their hospital charges and physician's or medical clinic's fees out-of-pocket, even if their insurance then paid the remainder of the bill.

Payment of part of a fee by a patient and part by insurance is a form of coinsurance. Many people prefer to have "first-dollar coverage." That is, they would rather have an insurance company pay the whole bill from the first dollar, without having to pay either a deductible amount or part of the fee. To contain medical costs, however, it is likely that coinsurance will be encouraged in the future. This could produce problems if people respond by neglecting medical problems that require attention. There is little evidence, however, that reasonable coinsurance would cause this response, and there is evidence that it may provide incentives to reduce unnecessary use of health care services.

Breadth of coverage

If a health insurance plan covers nearly all services and diseases it is said to have a comprehensive benefit package. If the plan only pays for certain diseases such as cancer, it is disease specific and, therefore, less expensive. One problem that remains for the health insurance industry and for some unfortunate people and their families is a catastrophic, or major, medical problem that may generate medical bills of several thousands of dollars. Most health insurance policies, even comprehensive policies, do not offer unlimited coverage. Rather there are ceilings, or upper limits, to what they will pay.

A catastrophic, or "major medical," health insurance policy is one that picks up costs that exceed the ceiling of most policies. If you are concerned about overwhelming medical expenses, investing in such a policy, sometimes called major medical coverage, is a good idea and relatively inexpensive. This is because the chances of having a catastrophic medical problem are small, so the insurance company seldom has to make a payment on a major medical policy. Having such a policy can lead to peace of mind, however.

Experience-rated and community-rated policies

The difference between these two is important for those who are primarily interested in getting as much insurance coverage as possible for their money. If you are young and healthy, and if you increase your chances of maintaining good health, by using seat belts and not smoking for example, you are not likely to need as much health care as some other people. A group insurance policy that offers coverage to such low-risk individuals is called an experience-rated policy. The cost of such a policy is based on the experience of similar groups – that is, on how much health care they have actually used in the past. Since the risks of the younger, healthier group are lower than those of the general public, premium costs can be lower. A community-rated policy, on the other hand, covers expenses for anyone living in the community, regardless of their health.

Prepaid care

In a prepaid health care plan, you pay a clinic or health care group regularly, with the understanding that if you become ill they will provide the required care themselves. For more information about these plans, read the group practice section of the article on Office-based practice (see p.740).

Medicare and Medicaid

With the exception of earlier government reimbursement policies for crippled children (known as Title V), the government first got into health insurance in a major way in 1965 with the passage of the Social Security Amendments. Title XVIII, Health Insurance for the Aged, is commonly known as Medicare. It was amended in 1972 to include benefits for chronic kidney disease.

Part A of Medicare pays for hospital charges and Part B pays for professional services and supplies thought necessary by your physician. This system is financed by taxes on the earnings of employees, employers and people who are self-employed.

Medicaid is another major program in government health care financing. Medicaid, or Title XIX, consists of grants to states for medical assistance to the disabled and needy. States participate in this program to a differing extent, so specific information about what benefits are included in your state must be obtained from state agencies.

Medicare, Medicaid and other government health programs pay for almost half of the total costs of the American health care system. These programs have greatly reduced the unmet need for medical care services in the United States. However, the range of benefits varies greatly, depending on the state and on the type of coverage an individual has. For further information, contact your local Social Security office.

Private insurance

More than half of the health insurance in the United States is provided by private (nongovernmental) companies. The major insurer is Blue Cross-Blue Shield. Blue Cross covers hospital expenses while Blue Shield covers physicians' bills.

The premium that you and/or your employer will pay for Blue Cross insurance depends on what Blue Cross Plan covers the area where you live and work. Plan rates are determined by a number of factors, including data gathered by Blue Cross each quarter on how many health care services are used by members of the plan, and how much those services cost in that city or region. Blue Shield rates are determined in a similar fashion. Each plan has its own benefit package, so be sure to find out what is covered in your plan.

Many other private insurance companies also offer health insurance.

Caring for the sick at home

Introduction

Today, it is recognized that the sick and injured should be cared for, whenever possible, in their own homes. Besides keeping costs down, this keeps hospital beds and services more available to those who must have them. In addition, home care can be more reassuring and pleasant for the patient. Therefore, it often can be more conducive to a speedy recovery. At some time or another, almost every family will need to provide home nursing care for a family member for some reason.

You may have to take care of a person who is severely disabled and bedridden. Such a patient may need full-time care and attention. More often the problem will be simpler and more temporary, like the expected bouts of "flu" and childhood infectious diseases.

You should not feel intimidated at the prospect of having to take on the role of a home nurse, even if you have had no previous experience. Home nursing calls for a mixture of common sense and a caring approach that virtually anyone, whether a man or a woman, is able to provide. Difficult nursing procedures and sophisticated equipment are rarely necessary in home nursing. The basic nursing skills such as taking a temperature, making a bed, preventing bedsores, and knowing the best way to move an immobile patient are all procedures that are easily learned. Usually these skills are all that is needed. Many such routine nursing procedures are described and illustrated in this section. Do not underestimate the effect they will have on your patient.

Your principal goal is to keep the patient comfortable and clean. When horizons are limited to bed and bedroom, small problems tend to be magnified. However ill the patient feels, he or she can be made to feel better on fresh, cool, unwrinkled sheets. If you are caring for someone who is likely to be bed-bound for some time, one or two pairs of no-iron (but *not* nylon) sheets will make your task of laundering bed-linen much easier. Special diets are seldom necessary. The physician will tell you if there are any particular foods the patient should have or avoid.

If you are caring for a sick member of your family, do not try to do everything. If more complex care is needed than you are able to give, the doctor can often arrange for professional assistance through a visiting nurse association or a home health agency. These organizations can provide someone to carry out special procedures such as injections or changing dressings, or simply give you guidance and teach you procedures you can do yourself.

Long-term sickness or disability can be a great strain on the whole family, particularly on the person who has to do most of the nursing care. But it is important that the nurse's responsibility does not become overwhelming. An exhausted helper is unlikely to be an efficient one, so the whole burden of care should not fall on one person. Every member of the family can bring and return things, help with bed-making, and provide company to the sick person. Outside agencies, too, should be called upon if their help is needed. Consult your physician for helpful services (see also Home services, p.738) including home health, for example, and meals on wheels. Financial assistance may also be available for those who are nursing the sick or disabled. Equipment can often be rented or borrowed. Commodes, bedpans, urinals, and other nursing aids, for example, may be rented from medical supply companies.

Children and the elderly pose special nursing problems, the former because they make by far the most demanding patients, both emotionally and physically; the latter because of the special risks attached to enforced physical inactivity in the elderly. Information given in this section and elsewhere in the book may help you to deal with the difficulties involved in caring for both the young and the old (see also Special problems of infants and children, p.644, and Special problems of the elderly, p.716).

Convalescence can be an even more difficult time than illness for both patient and nurse. The better the patient feels, the more irritable and impatient for recovery he or she is likely to become. On occasion, however, the reverse may be true. A patient who has been well taken care of may be reluctant to abandon the "security" of his or her ailment. So it is vital that you try to encourage your patient to do whatever he or she can manage throughout the illness. This will make it easier for the patient to recover former independence and self-sufficiency as health returns to normal.

Home health care in general

The following pages include many practical hints on how to care for a sick person at home. Give some thought to the day's routine, and the arrangement of furniture and items of equipment, so that problems are minimized for both you and your patient. The physician or a visiting nurse can provide you with much additional help and guidance.

Planning the sick-room

If you are nursing someone who is likely to be ill for some time, plan the sick-room carefully. In a two-story house, it may be better for the sick-room to be a living room on the first floor rather than an upstairs bedroom, so that the sick person will not feel isolated, and you will not have to make as many trips up and down the stairs.

Your main goal in arranging the room should be to make things comfortable for the sick person and convenient for yourself. A single bed is easier to make. If possible, the bed should be accessible on both sides. This will make it easier for the patient to move or be moved, and for those who are giving the care to reach the patient. If you can, place the bed so that the sick person can see out of the window. The coming and going of people and birds and other small animals provide welcome distraction and a feeling of being connected with the outside world. Have a bedside table to hold medicines, water, tissues, a bell (so that you can be summoned if you are needed), and other items. If the sick person is allowed out of bed but cannot easily get to a bathroom, a commode chair (a chair with a chamber-pot in it) is essential. You can rent or buy them from medical supply stores. Also, local community health agencies or volunteer organizations may have such equipment available to loan to those in need.

As long as there is reasonable air circulation in the sick-room, a sick person does not "need" fresh air, but he or she may feel more fresh and comfortable if a window is left slightly open. This is a matter of individual preference. Whether the room is ventilated or not, it should be kept free from drafts and comfortable for the patient, who may be dressed only in pajamas.

Giving medicines

It is essential for medicines to be taken exactly as prescribed by the physician. This includes both the number and timing of doses per day and the total length of time that the doctor directs. You should not stop giving a sick person medicine just because he or she appears to be getting better, since this may encourage a relapse.

For example, if a medicine is prescribed four times a day, ask the doctor if all the doses can be given during waking hours or if the patient should be awakened to take it. Measure the dose of a liquid medicine, using a special spoon if it is provided, to ensure accuracy. When you pour the medicine, hold the bottle with the label upward so that any overflow does not make it illegible. If a sick person finds it difficult to swallow tablets or capsules that have been prescribed, a glass of water or a small dish of applesauce or ice cream usually helps.

Drugs can have predictable side-effects, and the physician will probably warn you about them. But very occasionally, a sick person has an unexpected allergic response to a drug. Penicillin and related *antibiotics* are among the most common drugs to cause an allergic reaction, and the most usual reactions are a rash, hives (see p.255), itching, or wheezing. If, after taking a medicine, a sick person develops symptoms that seem to be unrelated to his or her illness, call the physician to find out if you should withhold the drug (see also Drugs and the elderly, p.725).

Taking a temperature

Normal body temperature is about 98.6°F (37°C), but it may vary by about 1 to 2° (0.5 to 1°C) during the day. It is usually at its lowest in the early hours of the morning. A rise in temperature (a fever) is not in itself dangerous unless it exceeds 106°F (41.1°C), and the body's own temperature-control system will usually prevent it from reaching this level. A rise in temperature is usually caused by an infection. Often while the temperature is rising the sick person feels cold and shivery.

You can take a person's temperature with a thermometer orally (in the mouth), under the arm, or in the rectum. Rectal thermometers have a short, stubby bulb at the end, and oral thermometers (also used under the arm) have a long, narrow bulb.

The thermometer: A sickroom thermometer is a small glass tube that has a mercury-filled bulb at one end and is marked with a temperature scale. Normal body temperature is marked with an arrow. As the mercury is heated in the sick person's mouth, armpit, or rectum, it expands and rises up the tube to a point on the scale that indicates the body temperature. A small kink in the tube prevents the mercury from sinking back into the bulb when the thermometer is removed from the mouth or armpit. Before you buy a thermometer, examine it carefully to be sure that the mercury column and the markings on the scale are easy to see.

°FAHRENHEIT

°FAHRENHEIT	°CELSIUS (CENTIGRADE)
109	43
108	42
107	
106	41
105	
104	40
103	
102	39
101	
100	38
99	
98	37
97	36
96	
95	35

Temperature conversion scale

A thermometer in the mouth gives the most accurate reading of body temperature. But it may be easier to take the temperature of a young child by putting the thermometer in the armpit. In this case, add about 1°F (0.5°C) to the reading you get, to determine what temperature you would have gotten with an oral thermometer.

Another method is to use a special rectal thermometer. Insert the bulb end of the thermometer just a short way into the child's rectum while gently holding the child down, if necessary, with your forearm. A rectal temperature reading will be about 1°F (0.5°C) higher than an oral reading.

Never leave a young child alone with a glass thermometer, since both the glass and the mercury can be harmful if the thermometer is broken.

In addition to glass thermometers, there are also electronic thermometers and temperature strip thermometers. These are used most often in institutions. They have disposable elements that increase costs, and their reliability and accuracy have been questioned. In general, it is best to have a glass thermometer and know how to use it.

Whether you use a glass thermometer or a strip, do not take a temperature immediately after the sick person has had a bath, a meal, a hot drink, or a cigarette, since you may then get a false reading.

If a sick person has a fever, do not try to "sweat it out" by keeping the room too warm or by putting extra blankets on the bed. This may make the person's temperature rise even further. Instead, to help bring the temperature down, give the person aspirin or an aspirin substitute recommended by the physician. While the person's temperature is falling, he or she may sweat a lot. To replace the

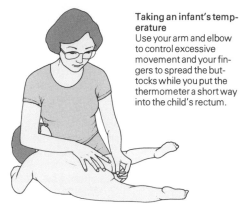

Taking an infant's temperature
Use your arm and elbow to control excessive movement and your fingers to spread the buttocks while you put the thermometer a short way into the child's rectum.

body fluids and salt lost in this way, you should give the person plenty of water, soup, fruit drinks and gelatins.

Bed-making
Sheets for the sick person's bed should be of cotton, which will absorb sweat, not of nylon. No-iron sheets can save much work.

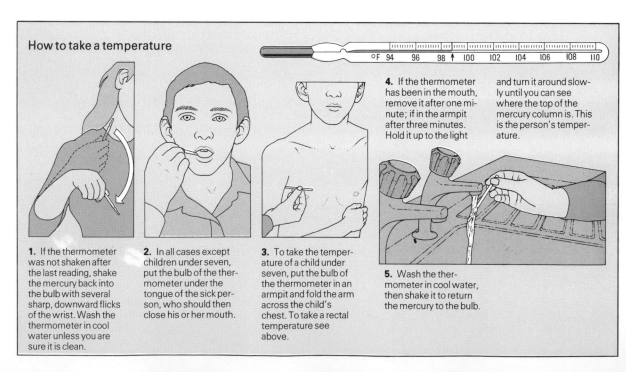

How to take a temperature

°F 94 96 98 ↑ 100 102 104 106 108 110

1. If the thermometer was not shaken after the last reading, shake the mercury back into the bulb with several sharp, downward flicks of the wrist. Wash the thermometer in cool water unless you are sure it is clean.

2. In all cases except children under seven, put the bulb of the thermometer under the tongue of the sick person, who should then close his or her mouth.

3. To take the temperature of a child under seven, put the bulb of the thermometer in an armpit and fold the arm across the child's chest. To take a rectal temperature see above.

4. If the thermometer has been in the mouth, remove it after one minute; if in the armpit after three minutes. Hold it up to the light and turn it around slowly until you can see where the top of the mercury column is. This is the person's temperature.

5. Wash the thermometer in cool water, then shake it to return the mercury to the bulb.

A bed-bound person needs his or her bed made twice a day (morning and evening) and tidied in between. Change the sheets every four to five days, and more often if the sheets become soiled, if the person is sweating a lot, or if you want to give him or her a small but appreciated treat. Always draw the bottom sheet tightly over the bed so that there are no wrinkles, and tuck it in well. Arrange the pillows so that they support the shoulders as well as the head. The most comfortable arrangement for someone who is forced to lie on his or her back is two pillows placed at an angle to each other with a third lying across them. If the sick person prefers only one pillow, pull it well down so that the neck and shoulders as well as the head are supported and kept comfortable.

Once the sick person can sit up he or she will need either a back rest (which can be

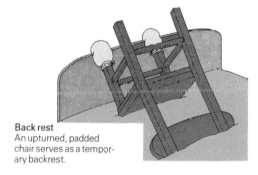

Back rest
An upturned, padded chair serves as a temporary backrest.

improvised from an upturned kitchen chair) or at least extra support with more pillows. Also provide something to brace the feet against to prevent the person from sliding down toward the foot of the bed.

If the sick person cannot get out of bed at all, you can still change the bottom sheet. First, turn the person to face away from you and roll one half of the old sheet lengthwise up against his or her back. Then roll one half of the clean sheet lengthwise and put it on the

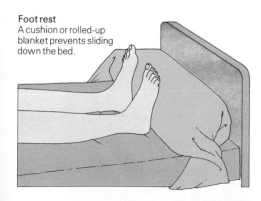

Foot rest
A cushion or rolled-up blanket prevents sliding down the bed.

Changing the sheets

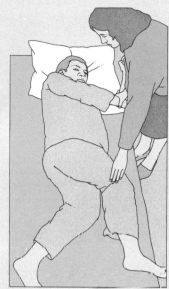

1. If the sick person cannot get out of bed at all, there is still an easy way of changing the bottom sheet. First, turn the person on one side.

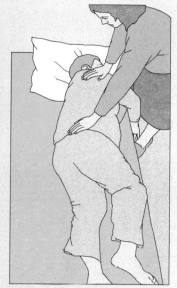

2. Move the person to the edge of the bed, making sure that he or she is lying in a stable position.

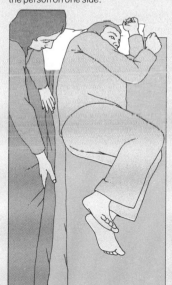

3. Roll one half of the old sheet lengthwise up against the person, then roll one half of the clean sheet lengthwise and put it on the bed with the rolled up half in the center of the bed.

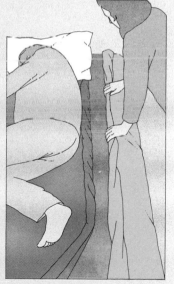

4. Roll the person on to this clean half, and take off the old sheet. Finally, unroll the rest of the clean sheet, stretch it tight, and tuck it in.

Drawsheets

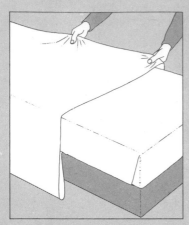 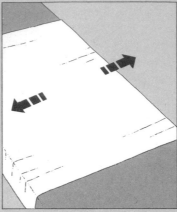

A drawsheet is an ordinary sheet folded and positioned so that it can provide the sick person with a clean, unwrinkled sheet to lie on without your having to remake the bed. Fold the sheet in half lengthwise and put it over the bed crosswise, so that it extends from the sick person's head to his or her knees, and overlaps the bed more on one side than the other. Tuck one end in, pull the sheet tight, and tuck in the other end. When you want to provide a clean area beneath the patient, untuck both ends of the sheet, pull it into a fresh position, and tuck in both ends tightly again. For the comfort of the patient, make sure the drawsheet is kept very taut.

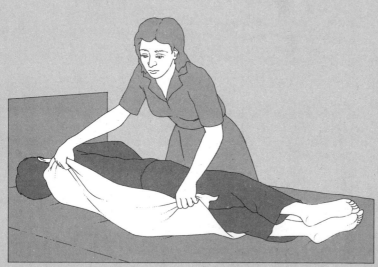

A drawsheet can also be used as an aid to moving an immobile or very weak person. If you want to move the person sideways, first untuck the end of the drawsheet opposite to the side of the bed to which you want the person to move. Then cross to that side of the bed, lean across the bed, and hold onto the free far end of the drawsheet. Use that end to roll the person toward you.

To move the person up the bed, you need another person's help. Both ends of the drawsheet are untucked, each of you holds one end, and the person is lifted on the drawsheet to the desired position.

Hospital corners

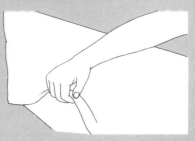

1. Hospital ("mitered") corners make a neat and comfortable finish to the sickroom bed. Place the bottom sheet in position and tuck in at the ends. With one hand, lift the side of the sheet about 40 cm (16 in) from the head of the bed.

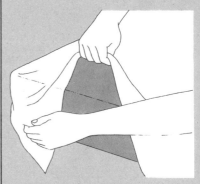

2. Tuck the flap of sheet that hangs between the side of the bed and your hand under the mattress with your other hand. Then let the side of the sheet fall to form a fold at the side of the bed.

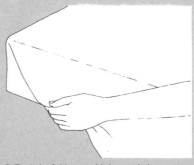

3. Tuck the fold smoothly beneath the mattress. Repeat on the other side of the head of the bed, then repeat for the top sheet and blankets. Finally, repeat with the two corners at the foot of the bed, lifting and tucking sheets and blankets together.

bed with the rolled half in the center. Roll the person onto the clean half, and take off the old sheet. Finally, unroll the rest of the clean sheet, stretch it tight, and tuck it in on both sides to complete the job.

Giving food, drink and special diets

Remember that meals may be the highlights of a monotonous day for a bed-bound person, so make them as tempting and attractive as you can. Bear in mind, too, that unless the physician advises a particular kind of diet, you can safely give the sick person a normal, balanced diet along with many "treats." Remember, however, that many snack foods such as potato chips and peanuts are high in sodium, so check to be sure the patient is not on a low-salt (low-sodium) diet before giving these foods. Small helpings of simple food will probably be all that the patient wants until his or her appetite returns to normal. Give the patient plenty of liquids.

If the physician has ordered a special diet, and if you will have to provide it for quite a long time, you may want to get a special cook book on the subject. The physician may recommend a good one, or may refer you to a nurse or dietician who is knowledgeable about that particular type of diet.

Low-salt diet: The physician may recommend a low-salt diet for someone who has heart disease (see p.372), liver disease (see Liver, gallbladder and pancreas, p.485), kidney disease (see Disorders of the urinary tract, p.500), or high blood pressure (see p.382). In North America almost everyone routinely eats much more salt than the body requires. This usually can be reduced substantially simply by adding no extra salt at the table, and cut even further if no salt is added to food during cooking. Another possible source of extra salt in the diet is a water softener on the cold water line. This can be eliminated if necessary, or other water can be used for cooking and drinking.

If the doctor considers it necessary to restrict the salt intake even further, he or she will advise you on how to provide food that does not contain salt. For example, cured or tenderized meat or smoked fish, cheese, canned food other than fruit, food made with bicarbonate of soda or baking powder, and most butter and margarine contain salt. The flavor that a salt-free diet lacks can be provided by using a salt substitute. Also, after several weeks on a low-salt diet, many people find they do not miss the salt. If the sick person has kidney disease, check with the doctor to see if you should choose a salt substitute that is also free of potassium, which is unsuitable in some cases of kidney disease.

Low-protein diets: A low-protein diet may be recommended for some kidney disorders. Such a diet will involve reducing the intake of meat, fish, eggs, dairy products and other protein-rich foods. Because protein provides a part of the body's energy needs, extra sugar or glucose is needed to make up for this loss.

Feeding a sick person: A sick person who is elderly or very ill may need to be spoon-fed. If so, feed the person with well-cut, minced, or pureed foods, since these are the easiest both to give and to swallow. Make sure the person is in a comfortable position before you start, and tuck a napkin under his or her chin. Taste the food yourself to be sure it is at a comfortable temperature. Spoon-feeding often takes a long time, and you may find that the food stays hot longer if you use a special child's dish with a hollow base that you fill with hot water, or a similar type that is warmed electrically. When giving fluids, provide an angled straw (available from drugstores) rather than trying to use a cup. The straw allows more control over intake, which is especially important if the person is lying flat on his or her back.

Someone who is seriously ill may be able to take only liquid foods. To contain enough nutrition, a liquid diet should include milk, eggs, sugar, and fruit juices or fruit purees.

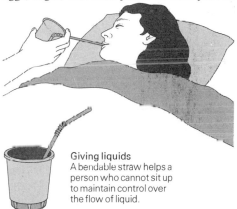

Giving liquids
A bendable straw helps a person who cannot sit up to maintain control over the flow of liquid.

There are special foods and other feeding techniques that may be helpful for extremely impaired patients. The physician can suggest some alternatives if you are having problems with feeding. Check with the doctor also if the patient seems to be losing any weight.

If a stroke has paralyzed one side of a person's body, food may tend to collect in the paralyzed cheek. If the person cannot remove the food with a finger, wipe it away with a cotton-tipped swab while holding the cheek gently away from the teeth.

Giving a bedpan

A toilet or commode chair (a chair that incorporates a chamber-pot in its seat) is the most comfortable and the easiest way for sick people to move their bowels and urinate. But if a person is too ill or disabled to get out of bed, a bedpan, and for a man, a bed urinal, will have to be used. Most people who are not used to a bedpan find it inhibiting, especially if someone else is present, so make sure the person has complete privacy, and give him or her enough time to let bowels and bladder relax. Keeping the sick person's sensitivity in mind on this matter is part of good care. Such thoughtfulness often can contribute to a more rapid recovery.

Before you give a bedpan, warm it in hot water, dry it well, and sprinkle the rim with talcum powder to make it easier for the pan to be slipped under the buttocks. If the person cannot lift himself or herself up in the bed, let the person use the pan lying down. Lift the person's hips while you maneuver the pan beneath the buttocks, with the open end toward the feet. The easiest way to give a bedpan to a totally helpless person is to turn the person on his or her side, put the pan against the buttocks, press the pan down into the bed as much as possible, and roll the person back on top of it. When the pan has been used, hold it firmly and roll the person off, away from you.

After use, bedpans and urinals should be washed thoroughly in a disinfectant diluted with water. Always put them back in the same place so that they can be found in a hurry. A urinal should be left within easy reach of the bed so that the sick person has no need to call or ring for it. Keep it in a plastic bowl or bucket to lessen the possibility of spills, especially at night.

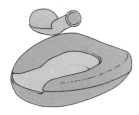

Bedpan and urinal
These items are essential for anyone who is likely to be in bed for some time. You may be able to rent them from a medical supply company.

Giving a bedpan
One person lifts the patient's buttocks while the other places the pan in position.

Preventing bedsores

Anyone who is confined to bed for a long time is liable to develop bedsores, especially if movement is restricted or if sensation is impaired. The sores occur on those parts of the body that bear the weight of the body or rub constantly against the bedclothes. The most common sites are the elbows, knees, shoulder blades, spine and buttocks.

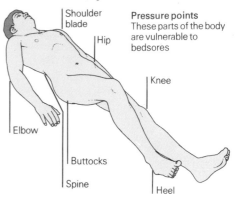

Shoulder blade · Hip · Knee · Elbow · Buttocks · Spine · Heel

Pressure points
These parts of the body are vulnerable to bedsores

A bedsore begins as a patch of tender, reddened, inflamed skin. Later, it can become purple. Then it breaks down and an ulcer or sore develops. If any skin redness or inflammation occurs, consult the physician right away. The ulcers generally take a long time to heal and are quite uncomfortable and harmful to the patient's health.

Bedsores can be prevented. Someone confined to bed can still get a kind of exercise unless he or she is paralyzed or otherwise immobile. Every hour or so, a period of wriggling the toes, rotating the ankles, flexing the arms and legs, tightening and relaxing muscles, and stretching the whole body will both stimulate circulation and prevent joint *contracture*, or stiffening. If the sick person cannot move or is very weak, gently bend and straighten the joints manually at least once a day. Also, change his or her position as often as you can – at least every two to three hours, but more often if possible – so that the pressure of the body on any particular area is relieved. This is most easily done, especially if the sick person is a great deal heavier than you, by using a drawsheet (see p.758) or by rolling the person from side to side. Otherwise, lift the person into a new position (enlisting someone else's help if necessary). Dragging the person may damage the skin and increase the chances of bedsores.

Use a bed- or foot-cradle (frames that raise the covers) to keep the weight of the bedclothes off the sick person's legs and feet. You should be able to borrow or rent one. If not, you can improvise by using a stool or a wooden box with two opposite sides cut out. If the person is lying permanently on his or her side, support the upper-arms and thighs with soft pillows to keep the elbows and knees apart, and put a pillow between the ankles to keep them from rubbing against each other. The person will still have to be turned frequently to prevent bedsores.

Relieving pressure
Use plenty of soft pillows or cushions to relieve pressure that leads to bedsores.

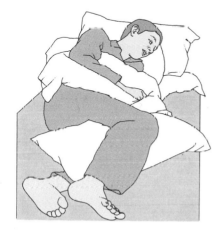

Make sure that the sheets are always clean, dry, crumb-free, and pulled as tight as possible to prevent wrinkling. If the sick person is likely to be bed-ridden for a long time, you may want to get a fluffy sheepskin (preferably a synthetic, washable one) for the person to lie on, to help cushion the whole body. Sheepskin bootees can be bought also, to protect the heels and ankles.

Also, wash the sick person frequently and keep the skin on places that are vulnerable to bedsores particularly clean and dry. If you notice any reddening, keep pressure off that area and let the physician know that a bedsore is beginning to form.

In addition to adequate turning, movement, exercise and cleanliness, a balanced diet helps to prevent bedsores.

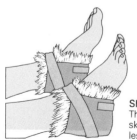

Sheepskin bootees
These help to protect the skin of the heels and ankles from bedsores.

Moving an immobile patient

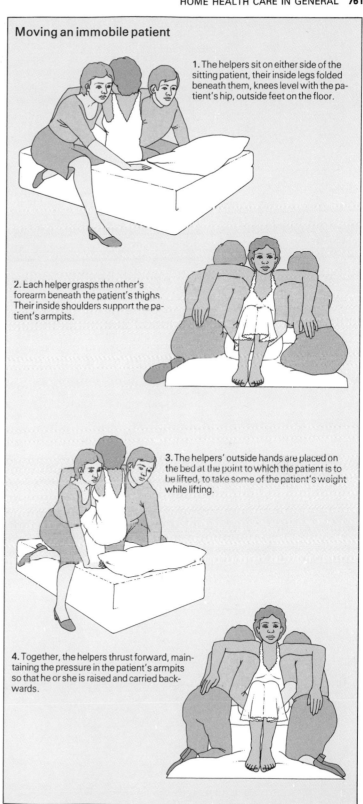

1. The helpers sit on either side of the sitting patient, their inside legs folded beneath them, knees level with the patient's hip, outside feet on the floor.

2. Each helper grasps the other's forearm beneath the patient's thighs. Their inside shoulders support the patient's armpits.

3. The helpers' outside hands are placed on the bed at the point to which the patient is to be lifted, to take some of the patient's weight while lifting.

4. Together, the helpers thrust forward, maintaining the pressure in the patient's armpits so that he or she is raised and carried backwards.

Dealing with vomiting

Most people prefer to be left alone while they are vomiting, but others find it comforting to have their forehead supported by someone's hand. If a sick person has asked for your presence in this way, offer him or her some water afterwards to rinse out the mouth and sponge the face.

After a vomiting attack, do not give the person solid food for several hours, but do give water or fruit drinks to replace body fluids. If the person is vomiting repeatedly, call the physician for any additional treatment. The doctor will probably advise you to give soup, tea, fruit drinks or gelatins if the sick person can tolerate them. Let the sick person's own inclinations about food guide you as his or her appetite returns, but make sure the person gets plenty of liquids, and also that he or she is urinating periodically.

Coping with incontinence

Some loss of bladder control is common in elderly people or in those who are paralyzed below the waist. For a full description of the problem and how to cope with it, see Incontinence in the elderly, p.718.

Relieving congestion

While a stuffy nose can be relieved by giving an inhalant, overuse of these medications can actually lead to more nasal congestion, and also to other problems. Consult your physician if an inhalant seems to be making the problem worse. The physician may recommend that you use the more traditional method of steam inhalation. Pour boiling water into a bowl or pot. Sit the sick person at a table if possible. If he or she cannot get up, put the container of hot water into a flat-bottomed dishpan to catch the boiling water if it should spill out. Drape a towel over the sick person's head and the container of water.

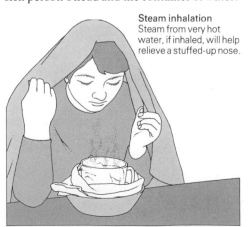

Steam inhalation
Steam from very hot water, if inhaled, will help relieve a stuffed-up nose.

The inhalation should last for ten minutes.

Another way to relieve congestion is with a hot or cool vaporizer.

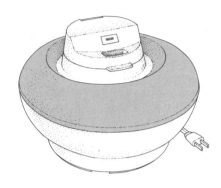

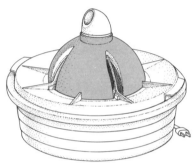

Using humidity
Vaporizers help clear congestion by humidifying the whole room.
One type (top) works by heating water to create steam.

Another (above) sprays tiny droplets of water into the air without heating the water.

Keeping a sick person clean

A sick person should be encouraged to keep clean. The face and hands should be washed and the teeth brushed twice a day, and the body should be washed once a day. This is not only a matter of hygiene. Feeling clean and fresh boosts the patient's morale and may play a part in hastening recovery. Even bed-bound people, unless they are extremely ill, can usually manage to keep themselves clean. Before giving a bed-bound person a basin of water and toiletries, place a large towel beneath the person to protect the bed. If the person is going to have a sponge bath, make sure the room is warm, and provide a second large towel to be draped over the parts of the body that are not being washed, so that the person does not become chilled.

Washing hair

Having clean hair will also boost a sick person's morale. If the person cannot get up, it is possible to give him or her a shampoo in bed.

The techniques for washing short hair and long hair differ. If the person has short hair, first protect the bottom sheet with a plastic cover overlaid by a towel. Move the person down the bed, raise his or her shoulders on a pillow, and place a bowl beneath the head. To wet the hair before shampooing and to rinse it, pour jugs of water over it. Long hair is easier to wash if the person rests his or her head on the edge of the bed so that the hair hangs over a bowl on the floor. Place one end of a large tray under the person's head and the other end in the bowl. Wet and rinse the hair as for short hair. The water will run down the tray into the bowl.

After washing the person's hair, dry it thoroughly with a warm towel and finish with an electric hair dryer.

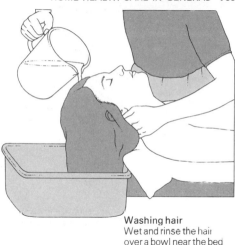

Washing hair
Wet and rinse the hair over a bowl near the bed

Giving a bath in bed

If the sick person is unable to give himself or herself a bath, you can give one. Be sure that the room is warm before you remove the person's pajamas. Cover his or her body with a large towel and place another one beneath the body to protect the bedclothes. If the person is immobile or heavy, you can get the second towel into position in the same way that you can a clean bottom sheet (see p.757).

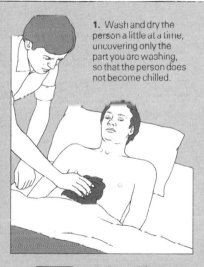

1. Wash and dry the person a little at a time, uncovering only the part you are washing, so that the person does not become chilled.

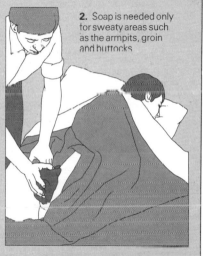

2. Soap is needed only for sweaty areas such as the armpits, groin and buttocks

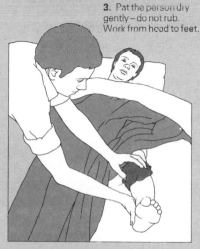

3. Pat the person dry gently – do not rub. Work from head to feet.

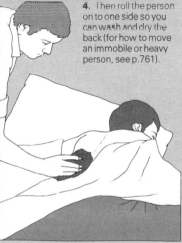

4. Then roll the person on to one side so you can wash and dry the back (for how to move an immobile or heavy person, see p.761).

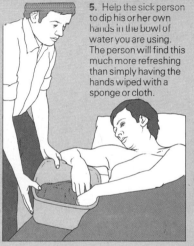

5. Help the sick person to dip his or her own hands in the bowl of water you are using. The person will find this much more refreshing than simply having the hands wiped with a sponge or cloth.

Caring for sick children

In general, children do not become as severely ill as adults and older people, but when they are sick they take up far more time than virtually any other kind of patient. You should be prepared for this or you may find yourself resenting the time and effort involved in caring even for your own child. The sick child needs at least one "nurse," preferably one of his or her parents, on hand almost constantly in order to raise morale and promote a speedy recovery. For specific information on the various childhood illnesses, read the section entitled Special problems of infants and children (see p.644).

Should you keep the sick child in bed?
Unless the physician has told you the child needs to stay in bed, you can let the child decide whether he or she feels well enough to be up and around.

The child who is not very ill but is not yet well enough to be permanently up will make the most demands on your time and company. In these circumstances, it may be helpful to make up a bed on the first floor (in a multi-story house) or in a living room, so that you do not have to keep climbing the stairs and so that the child has your household activities as a distraction. You also may want to put a television set near the child's bed. But keep track of what the child is watching if you object to certain types of programs, such as those that include a great deal of violence.

Giving medicines
It is important that a sick child takes all the medicine prescribed by the physician. Because small children often cannot swallow pills easily, their medicines are usually prescribed in liquid form. Be sure to measure out the exact dose as prescribed. It can be difficult to get a child to take an unpleasant-tasting medicine. It may help if you sit the child on your knee, give him or her a pleasant drink to hold, ready to be swallowed after the medicine. Also, because most taste buds lie at the front of the tongue, tip the medicine into the child's mouth as far back as you can. Show by your manner that you assume the child will take the medicine. If the child senses that you expect trouble, he or she will probably provide it. Sometimes "bribery" helps, in the form of a favorite treat put beside you and promised as soon as the child actually has taken the medicine.

If the child refuses to take the medicine, try mixing it with a spoonful of something he or she likes, such as jam, ice cream, or even chocolate frosting. If you still have no success, ask the physician if the medicine can be given in tablet or capsule form. A child of three or older may be able to swallow a tablet or capsule whole with the aid of a drink. If the child cannot do this, you may be able to get him or her to take a tablet by crushing it (this cannot be done with a capsule) and sandwiching it between layers of jam, chocolate frosting, or whatever else the child likes, in a spoon. With luck, the spoonful will slip down and the child will not even taste the medicine. One trick that often works in this situation is to follow the first helping of the treat immediately with a second helping. Eagerness for the second helping often causes the child to "bolt" down the first before tasting the medicine in it.

Dealing with a fever
A fever is not dangerous and only very rarely has any harmful effects. In a few susceptible children, however, a high temperature may cause febrile convulsions (see p.667).

Unless a child's temperature is higher than 102°F (38.9°C), all you need to do is make sure that the child drinks plenty of liquids and keep him or her lightly clothed or covered. Forget what you may have heard about "sweating a fever out" by covering the patient with lots of heavy blankets.

Above 102°F, you can, if the child seems miserable or uncomfortable, give him or her a child's aspirin or an aspirin substitute as recommended by your physician. When it is time for a subsequent dose, first take the child's temperature again. If it has started to fall, do not give the medicine. If the child is asleep, do not wake him or her up; the sleep will do as much good as the medication.

If the child's temperature continues to rise in spite of the medication, and reaches 104°F (40.0°C) or higher, call the physician and in the meantime relieve the discomfort of the fever by fanning the child or by sponging his or her face, neck, arms and legs with warm water and leaving them to dry naturally. The evaporation of the water cools the skin.

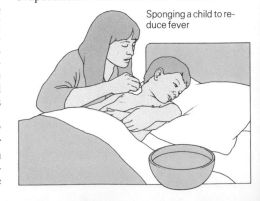
Sponging a child to reduce fever

If your child has had a febrile convulsion in the past, make sure the physician knows about this. In such cases, the doctor will probably recommend that you try to lower the child's temperature at an early stage by giving medications at the first sign of a fever and sponging the child as soon as he or she feels at all hot.

Feeding the sick child

Unless the physician has recommended a special diet, let the child eat what he or she feels like, within reason, rather than give what you think is suitable. Provide smaller helpings than usual, and do not worry if the child does not eat much. In cases of fever, vomiting, or diarrhea, it is important that the child is given plenty to drink. Again, let the child choose. If he or she wants carbonated beverages or sugary drinks, this is not too important. The amount of liquid is what matters, not the content.

Dealing with vomiting

Children vomit much more easily than most adults do. Often they will vomit without warning, at the beginning of an illness. A vomiting child will need your comforting and help. Support the child's head with one hand pressed against the forehead and, with the other hand, hold a bowl in which to catch the vomit. If the child can hold the bowl, put the other hand firmly on his or her stomach to support it. Afterwards, give the child a glass of water to rinse out the mouth and a bowl to spit in, and then wash the child's face.

Keeping the sick child occupied

Sick adults usually like to be left alone, but sick children, unless they are very ill, usually want company or entertainment. The younger the child, the greater will be the demands on your time, because the child will be more dependent on you for amusement.

Generally, a sick child will not feel like concentrating on one thing for very long, and will not want to do anything intellectually demanding. He or she will probably want to play with familiar toys and games rather than learn something new. Children tend to regress a little when they are ill and may prefer toys and activities meant for a slightly younger age-group. A child who is confined to bed will need a flat surface such as a bed-table or a large tray for toys and games, and to serve as a drawing board.

The following suggested activities for a sick child are absorbing, undemanding, and suitable for doing while the child is in or out of bed.

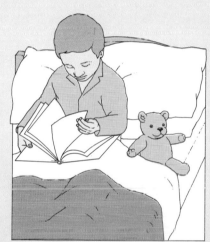

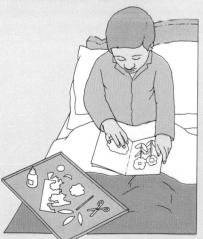

1. Sticking pictures in a scrapbook. Instead of buying a scrapbook, you may be able to make one yourself from rolls of old wallpaper or large sheets of heavy paper. Give the child the book, a stack of old magazines, round-ended scissors, and a stick of solid glue.

2. Making felt pictures. Glue a piece of felt onto a sheet of stiff cardboard. Using differently colored pieces of felt, cut out the shapes of figures, animals, houses, trees and other objects, or draw the outlines on the pieces of felt for the child to cut out. The felt cut-outs stick naturally to the felt base, and the child can arrange them to create various pictures.

3. Cardboard modeling. Provide old cardboard cartons, tubes, and other containers, a pair of round-ended scissors, and a stick of solid glue, so the child can make models of animals, vehicles or buildings.

4. Dough modeling. Mix equal parts of flour and salt with enough water, and food coloring if you like, to make a stiff dough. Give the child a rolling pin and pastry cutters and, if he or she is in bed, cover it with a plastic tablecloth.

Caring for old people

The increasing likelihood of illness in old age means that elderly people tend to spend more and more time at home, perhaps in bed. Many families with aging relatives can obtain practical advice and assistance from local community health agencies. Consult your physician for helpful health services that may be available in your community (see also Home services, p.738). For details on some of the specific illnesses that affect old people, see Special problems of the elderly, p.716.

Food
The appetite of an old person who is sick will probably be small. It is therefore important that the food that is served is nutritious. Each day give at least one meal that includes high-protein foods such as meat, cheese, fish or eggs, about half a pint of milk, and some high-fiber foods such as fruit, vegetables, or bran cereal. Unless there is a medical reason not to, encourage the person to drink plenty of liquids to avoid *dehydration*, in which body tissues become dangerously dry.

Coping with mental confusion
Many old people remain mentally alert and independent to the end of their lives. Some, however, become both mentally and physically feeble (see Senile dementia, p.724). If you are looking after a sick person who is confused or disoriented, make the fullest possible use of visiting nurse and home health services. It may be possible for you to use meals on wheels and a laundry service, and to get help once or twice a week to help you give the sick person a bath and injections. If the person you are caring for is incontinent, you may also need assistance in maintaining a bowel and bladder program.

Caring for the convalescent

After a long illness, it takes a certain amount of time for a person to recover and to get back to former routines and activities. This transitional time, when the patient is neither ill nor fully recovered, is called convalescence. During this period all strenuous activities, including physical and mental activities, and sports and leisure pastimes as well as work, must be resumed gradually. This slow but steady return to everyday life is essential if there is to be a good recovery.

General care
People who are convalescing from an illness often become bored and frustrated by their enforced inactivity, especially if they were very active before their illness. Radio, television, newspapers, books, puzzles and the company of other people will help to occupy such a person's mind and lessen the frustration. If the person's work can be done at home, it may be helpful for him or her to ease back into this activity.

However, there is another side to this. The convalescent may feel that he or she is more fully recovered than is actually the case, and may consequently tackle too much too soon. This may overtax his or her strength. The person may become depressed by an unaccustomed loss of concentration, and have a setback in convalescence. It is important to try to prevent this. Ask the physician what the convalescent can reasonably do, and if the person shows signs of going beyond this limit, gently but firmly persuade him or her to stop. The doctor will also tell you if the convalescent needs a special diet and, if necessary, can also organize professional help for you in caring for the person.

The dangers of inactivity in the old
It may be possible for an elderly person convalescing from an illness to become unnecessarily bed-bound. With such inactivity comes a rapid physical deterioration. Unused muscles become weak and flabby, joints stiffen, and constipation, bedsores, and weak bladder and bowel control may develop. The bed-bound patient is also more prone to *thrombosis* or *embolism* and more likely to have severe respiratory infections such as pneumonia (see p.359). Mental confusion also seems to occur more easily in the bed-bound. You should therefore encourage the convalescent to get up and about as soon as possible and to stay active, within the limits recommended by the physician.

Getting out of bed
Anyone who has been ill and bed-bound for some time will feel weak and probably dizzy when getting out of bed for the first time. Persuade the person to first sit on the edge of the bed for a few minutes before attempting to stand. Put a chair covered with a blanket beside the bed. When the person feels steady, stand in front of him or her so that the person can use your body as a support while standing up, and provide extra support by holding the person under the armpits. Then help to lower the person onto the chair and wrap the blanket around him or her if necessary. Once the convalescent feels stronger, a few steps can be tried, using your arm as a support.

Physical therapy

Someone who has been weakened or temporarily disabled by illness or injury may need physical therapy, sometimes called PT, during convalescence, to enable him or her to regain muscle strength or flexibility of the limbs. Physical therapy usually includes exercises and massage, and sometimes heat or electrical treatment. It is usually arranged through your physician and given in a hospital, a nursing home or a medical clinic. In some cases, a physical therapist can visit a home-bound patient for treatment once a week. Some private and public health insurance programs will pay for home physical therapy if it is ordered by a physician and if the goal of the treatment is to increase the patient's ability to function independently.

Active exercises are those that the sick person can carry out under the therapist's direction. Passive exercises are those given if the person cannot move his or her own limbs. The therapist will manipulate them instead, to prevent joint and muscle stiffness. If you are caring for someone in this condition, ask the physical therapist to show you how to give these passive exercises.

Other professional services

Anyone who has had a long illness or a lengthy stay in a hospital may be helped at home by occupational therapy to recover lost skills and to adjust to living in the outside world again. The physician can arrange for this service. An occupational therapist can help make the patient more independent by showing him or her how to use mechanical aids to perform a great many activities of daily living such as bathing and dressing. If the person is in a wheelchair and the home needs to be modified to accommodate it, the therapist can also give advice on how to do this; for example, by widening doors and converting stairways to ramps.

A social worker can be helpful in exploring possible sources of financial aid for equipment and home modifications for a homebound or disabled person. A speech therapist can help a person who has had a stroke or another type of brain injury relearn how to speak or communicate in other ways. The physician can arrange for these allied health professionals to work with you, to help you to restore the patient to as much independence as is possible.

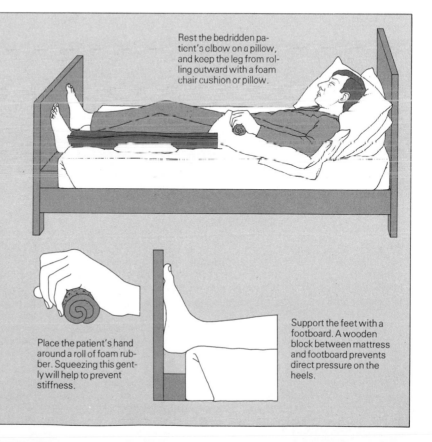

Preventing limbs from stiffening

A period of bedrest is often necessary after a major illness or operation. Although sick people tend to prefer to stay in a position they find comfortable, they should be encouraged to move around in bed as much as possible, to prevent the joint stiffness and loss of muscle tone that may follow prolonged inactivity. You can help to prevent joint stiffness, first of all by carefully placing and supporting the patient's limbs in the most comfortable, natural and strain-free positions and resting them on pillows, cushions, or foam-rubber rolls. Encourage the patient to exercise each joint through its whole range of motion several times each day. If he or she is immobile, you can help the patient do this. Gently bend and straighten each elbow and wrist, and the fingers and thumb of each hand. Raise each leg in turn, bending and straightening the knee and ankle.

Rest the bedridden patient's elbow on a pillow, and keep the leg from rolling outward with a foam chair cushion or pillow.

Place the patient's hand around a roll of foam rubber. Squeezing this gently will help to prevent stiffness.

Support the feet with a footboard. A wooden block between mattress and footboard prevents direct pressure on the heels.

Dying and death

Introduction

Most of us hope for a long life and a quick death, but only a minority of the population has this wish fulfilled. Most people die gradually over a period of weeks or months. Even though a slow death may seem like a burden to both the dying person and those around him or her, it often allows everyone concerned time to come to terms with death and prepare for it.

Those close to a dying person have to bear the emotional, and perhaps physical, strain of looking after the dying person, and, eventually, the complex practical procedures that are necessary after death. The articles that follow deal with these matters, and also give some information about helping the bereaved, including those who have to cope with the death of a child.

Death rates in the United States

The following statistics show the hard and impersonal facts about death that we often do not want to consider. The numbers serve as a reminder that it is possible to die at any age from a variety of causes. These figures show how many people died out of every 100,000 men and women in the United States in a recent year. One table gives the death rate by sex and age, the other by sex and the ten most common causes of death. Both tables are based on figures from the United States Census Bureau.

Major causes of death in the United States

Cause of death	Male deaths (per 100,000 population)	Female deaths (per 100,000 population)
Heart diseases	377	290
Cancer	200	159
Stroke and related disorders	74	94
Accidents	68	28
Pneumonia and influenza	26	21
Diabetes mellitus	13	17
Cirrhosis of the liver	19	10
Hardening of the arteries	11	15
Suicide	20	7
Diseases of early infancy	13	9

Death rates by age

Age in years	Male deaths (per 100,000 in age group)	Female deaths (per 100,000 in age group)
Under 1	1,659	1,304
1–4	77	61
5–9	41	27
10–14	44	26
15–19	146	56
20–24	202	65
25–29	194	71
30–34	193	90
35–39	260	135
40–44	393	221
45–49	626	346
50–54	999	529
55–59	1,524	785
60–64	2,431	1,217
65–69	3,474	1,691
70–74	5,230	2,767
75–79	8,153	4,740
80–84	11,364	7,394
85 and over	17,299	13,542

Terminal illness

Most people who are terminally ill prefer to know the truth about their condition, and physicians feel it is their duty to tell the patient if he or she wants to know. Sometimes the family finds it hard to accept this open approach because of their own psychological responses to death and dying. However, many dying people know, or strongly suspect, that they have a fatal disease.

When and what to tell the dying person

Let a person with a terminal illness decide the timing and extent of any discussion of death. If the patient does ask questions about the possibility of dying, this indicates that he or she has been thinking about the subject and has, to some extent, already come to terms with it. If no questions are asked, knowledge should not be forced upon the dying patient. This does not mean, however, that you should hold out any false hopes of recovery. Someone who is misled in this way will be unable to understand why he or she is growing weaker instead of stronger, may lose confidence in the medical treatment and may miss the chance to put his or her affairs in order. Worst of all, if the patient suspects the truth, he or she will be denied the opportunity to discuss fears and seek reassurance. Bear in mind that uncertainty may be even more difficult to deal with than an unpleasant truth.

A dying person will usually make it clear how much he or she wants to be told. Someone who is terminally ill usually seeks some reassurance, however, and you can give a comforting answer that is not dishonest.

One common question physicians are asked is how much time the dying patient has left to live. Usually only a very approximate answer is possible, such as "anything from a couple of weeks to several months." A more precise answer than this often is impossible for the doctor to give.

A person who is terminally ill may find it easier to talk about his or her death with someone who is not a relative, such as a member of the medical staff. This usually does not indicate any lack of affection or trust. It may be because of a desire to spare the other person pain. The closer the relationship, the more each partner may want to protect the other, and the more difficult it may be to talk freely together. For the terminally ill patient, this may cause difficulties. Members of the hospital staff are often too busy to spend much comforting time with the dying person, and they may find it difficult to talk about dying anyway, since they see their primary role as being curative. Some hospitals have tried to help deal with this problem

by having professional staff members trained to work with terminally ill patients and their families. Another approach is to have pastoral counseling programs both in the hospital and outside, and to encourage frequent visits from the clergy.

A terminally ill patient may find that the family physician is the best person to help with this problem. A doctor who knows something about the whole family can sometimes help the person and his or her relatives to break down any barrier that the prospect of death may have erected between them.

Care at home or in the hospital

It is rarely true that nothing more can be done for a dying person. When curative treatment is no longer appropriate, the dying person still needs relief from troublesome symptoms and pain, along with understanding and comfort. Sometimes this kind of care is best provided in the dying person's own home rather than in a hospital. At home, the person can remain more independent, feel more like an individual, still take a limited part in family life, and avoid some feelings of isolation. The general hospital is much more geared to curing the acutely ill patient than to caring for the dying one. If a choice is offered between home, nursing home and hospital care, home care may be the best choice. It is not usually physically demanding, pain relief seldom has to be given by injection, and many cases of terminal illness do not require difficult nursing care. Even if they do, such care will usually be needed only for a few weeks.

If you do plan to look after a terminally ill relative at home, regular visits from the family physician will be essential, together with support from family and friends. Visiting nurse services will also be helpful if they are available. Many hospitals have a home-care service to support any family that wants to care for a dying relative at home.

Hospices

These are small units (often associated with a general hospital) that have been set up especially to care for the dying and to help their families. These facilities are becoming increasingly widespread.

In a hospice a dying person usually is not troubled with hospital routines such as temperature-taking and pulse-taking. The efforts of the staff are concentrated on relieving pain and any other problems, along with comforting both the person and his or her family. One might think that to see others dying around them would be depressing for terminally ill people, but most are reassured rather than distressed because the deaths occur peacefully.

Physical pain

Pain is often the most feared problem of terminal illness. Continuous, long-term pain will usually wear a sick person down, permeate his or her whole being, and will sometimes block thoughts of anything else.

But such suffering, even in some of the most painful forms of cancer, now seldom occurs. *Analgesics*, or painkilling drugs, can be given before the pain builds up to a level where the sick person needs to ask for the medication. When analgesics are given in this way, the dose can usually be kept low, so that the person remains not only virtually pain-free but also alert.

In the terminally ill, severe pain is usually controlled by an opium-like drug. The risk of addiction to the drug is more than outweighed by the relief that the drug provides.

Emotional pain

A terminally ill person may have to face emotional pain at the thought of dying, as well as physical pain. Anger is a common reaction to the prospect of death; so is depression. Some people may have feelings of guilt or dissatisfaction when they look back on their lives and achievements. But in the end, given loving support from those around them, nearly all terminally ill people come to terms with the prospect of death, in their own way and their own time.

Often dying people resent their growing helplessness and fear a loss of dignity. For this reason, someone who is dying should be given the opportunity to manage his or her own affairs for as long as possible and should be encouraged to do as much as possible for himself or herself. The terminally ill person should be consulted on family matters, and should help the family to plan for their future.

Many dying people fear that the moment of death will be unpleasant and violent, and many are afraid of being left to die alone. This fear may make them seem overdemanding sometimes to those who are caring for them, but try to be understanding and reassuring. You can dispel the first of these fears quite honestly, by telling the person that in nearly all cases the person feels an overwhelming drowsiness just before the end, lapses into unconsciousness, and dies in his or her sleep.

The approach of death

Toward the very end, the dying person may become restless, or his or her breathing may become labored, partly because of a constant trickle of saliva into the windpipe that cannot be coughed up, partly because the lungs may become waterlogged as the heart fails. If you are at home with the patient and these symptoms occur, call the physician, who can give medications to help make the patient more comfortable. If the patient is still alert, you can make breathing easier either by propping him or her up in a sitting position with pillows, or by laying the patient on his or her side, with the top arm and leg drawn out a little for support and a single pillow beneath the patient's head.

You should assume that right until the end the dying person can hear what you say. You may feel helpless in the presence of a person near to death, but it is the very fact of your presence that is so important. Often nothing more is necessary than to hold the person's hand, so that he or she does not feel alone.

Death

Death essentially occurs when both heartbeat and breathing have stopped. It usually is easy for a physician to determine that this has happened, if the patient is not on a *ventilator*, or a life-support system. In such cases, the doctor carries out a specific series of tests to determine if the brain is dead or if the patient is simply unconscious. If the brain is dead, physical death is established and life support is discontinued.

Delaying death

In order that their lives can be prolonged, people who have certain serious diseases such as cancer may need to undergo treatment that is unpleasant and uncomfortable. However, as the periods of relative health between such treatments become shorter and shorter, the treatments may just prolong the process of dying. At this stage, usually by agreement between the patient, the family and the physicians involved, the treatments may be stopped and only painkillers and any other comfort-inducing drugs may be given. In this way, a suffering person may be allowed to die more peacefully.

Unconscious people who are able to maintain their own breathing and heartbeat but for whom there is no prospect of regaining consciousness are fed by medical staff to keep them alive. But with the informed consent of the family or a legal representative, the medical staff may be asked not to give life-saving measures. In these circumstances it may be best to withhold only "heroic efforts" and refrain from interfering with the natural process of death.

Criteria of death

As described above, death occurs when both breathing and heartbeat have stopped. In the case of serious injury, from a traffic accident, for example, when life-support equipment is not immediately available, it may be possible to maintain breathing and heartbeat for a short time with emergency first-aid procedures (see Absence of breathing, p.802). Eventually, however, if the heart and lungs do not begin to function on their own, first-aid measures will not be effective.

In a modern hospital, sophisticated equipment is available to maintain breathing and heartbeat functions and therefore, apparently, life itself. But breathing and heartbeat may cease when the equipment is disconnected. If they do, this shows that the brain stem, which connects the brain and the spinal cord, is damaged. The brain stem controls breathing and, to some extent, heartbeat. If it is substantially damaged, it will not recover and death is inevitable. An *electroencephalogram* (*EEG*) of brain activity may not necessarily help establish death, either. The EEG mainly measures brain waves in the cerebral hemispheres, the parts of the brain that deal with "higher" activities such as speech and memory (see Disorders of the brain and nervous system, p.266). For this reason, the test is not considered to be a reliable indicator of whether the brain stem itself is still active. Under such circumstances "death" is determined by a series of tests carried out by physicians to confirm that brain death actually has occurred.

The practicalities of death

When someone dies, there are several legal formalities to be dealt with before the funeral can be held. They include obtaining a medical certificate of the cause of death (the death certificate), registering the death, and engaging an undertaker to organize any funeral and burial arrangements. There will be other formalities if the death has to be reported to the medical examiner or coroner, if the body is to be cremated rather than buried, or if the body is to be donated for medical research or to have organs removed for transplant.

In this article it is assumed throughout that you are either the next of kin of the dead person or his or her executor – that is, someone appointed by the dead person to carry out the person's will.

The death certificate

Only a licensed physician can certify that someone is dead and state the cause of death. So the first thing to do if someone dies at home is to call the family physician or the police. In most cases the physician will have been looking after the person during his or her last illness and will usually have no difficulty in identifying the cause of death. If the doctor has seen the person within an amount of time specified by state law he or she is not legally obligated to examine the body before filling in the medical certificate of cause of death. However, in practice, most family physicians do visit and see the body before making out the certificate. If the doctor has not seen the person within the time specified, the case may have to be referred to the coroner or medical examiner. Also, the physician must see the body if it is to be cremated, so if a cremation is planned, tell the physician. You should also tell the physician if the dead person had asked that his or her body be used for medical research or organ donations, or if you wish this (see Medical use of the body, p.773).

If the person has died in the hospital, one of the physicians who has looked after the person will fill in the death certificate. A member of the hospital staff will tell the relatives of the death and arrange for them to claim the dead person's possessions. If a person has died in an accident and been brought to a hospital, the police will ask the relatives to identify the body. If the dead person has donated certain organs to be used as transplants, or if you wish to donate them, the organs can usually be removed for transplantation only when the person dies in a hospital, since removal should be carried out promptly after death. If organs are to be donated, you should tell the hospital physician if he or she has not already asked if they can be given.

Once the physician has filled in the death certificate, it usually will be picked up by the undertaker, who will file it with the appropriate authorities.

Referral to the medical examiner or coroner

Depending on the state and/or county, one of two offices are authorized to investigate deaths, the medical examiner or the coroner. A coroner may be appointed or elected. A medical examiner usually holds office as part of the civil service structure.

Mention of the coroner or medical examiner usually worries people because of the implication that foul play is suspected. In fact, most of the circumstances in which the coroner must be informed of a death are quite innocent. In most states, a death is reported to the coroner or medical examiner by a physician or the police if no physician attended the person during his or her final illness. Other circumstances in which such a report is required vary from state to state. The physician, a lawyer or the police department will be able to tell you if such a report is necessary. In general, investigation is required when the cause of death is not known, or when a death is known or suspected to be caused by violence.

The medical examiner or coroner may require that a *post mortem* examination or a medicolegal autopsy be carried out on the body to establish the exact cause of death (see Autopsies, next article). If the results of the *post mortem* are satisfactory, a certificate of death is issued.

Inquests
If the *post mortem* does not reveal the cause of death, and in cases when the death was violent, unnatural or due to an accident, there may be an inquest, or public court hearing. Procedures for inquests and investigations of deaths vary depending on state and local laws. If there is a public hearing, some people may be ordered to attend as witnesses. Anyone with an interest in the death can attend, and may be represented by an attorney if he or she wishes. This is probably a good idea if compensation claims are being considered. Sometimes a jury is also convened.

Once a verdict has been given and the inquest is over, the medical examiner or coroner issues a certificate of death. An order allowing burial or cremation may be given. This usually occurs as soon as the body has been identified. If the investigation is going to take a long time, the inquest may be formally opened, and then adjourned. Once the inquest has been opened, you may be able to get a letter confirming the fact of death, which will serve in place of the death certificate as proof of death for social security and insurance claims.

Acting as an executor
If the dead person has left a will, the person appointed as executor, often a spouse or other close relative, has the duty of arranging the funeral. If there is no will, the duty of being an executor usually falls on one of the dead person's close relatives anyway.

To deal with the dead person's financial and other affairs, the executor must apply to the local probate court for a grant of probate or letters of administration. Procedures depend on state law and on the size of the estate.

Any instructions left by the dead person that he or she should be cremated or not cremated are not necessarily legally binding on the next of kin, but should be observed if at all possible.

The funeral
It is sensible to contact an undertaker or funeral director soon after the physician has signed a death certificate. Even though you may not feel like it, it is wise to obtain quotations for the fee from more than one undertaker. It is also a good idea to have someone who was not as personally involved with the dead person as you are, such as a member of the clergy, a lawyer or a close friend, accompany you to the undertaker to help you decide on the arrangements. Such a person may be able to help you to objectively make arrangements that are appropriate for your financial resources.

Most funeral establishments offer funerals ranging from simple to elaborate. Often there is a flat fee that includes the coffin, preparation of the body for burial, and routine procedures such as filing the death certificate and putting appropriate notices in the newspapers. Be sure to find out what is included in the price, what costs extra, and what other arrangements and details you must take care of yourself. You will have to make decisions about the type of coffin, the type and location of the burial service and who is to conduct it, whether the body is to be embalmed, whether or not you want to have an open casket and viewing of the body, and whether the body is to be buried or cremated.

It is possible to make arrangements for your own funeral before your death. There are consumer organizations called "memorial societies" that can help you make such plans. These usually non-profit organizations are not affiliated with any particular funeral home, but they can provide information about funeral homes that will allow payment in advance for a funeral, and those that will provide the simplest of funerals if that is what you want. This can save money in some cases, and can spare your relatives from having to make these arrangements after your death.

A funeral is usually held two to four days after death. Many funeral ceremonies are performed either at a church or at a funeral home and have two parts, the religious ceremony and the committal ceremony at the graveside. Those who want a non-religious ceremony can arrange for it with the undertaker. Another possibility is to have a memorial service. The difference is that the body is not present at a memorial service. This may change the emphasis of the ceremony so that the focus is on the person's life rather than on death. It also means that the ceremony can be held at any time and in a variety of places.

Burial and cremation

If the body is to be buried, you will need to find out whether the dead person has bought a cemetery plot or if there is a family plot. If he or she has not made arrangements for a grave site, you will have to pay for a plot.

If a body is to be cremated instead of buried, additional formalities are involved. This more complex procedure is to prevent destruction of the body before the possibility of a crime has been discounted. The funeral director will explain what forms you need to fill out and where to obtain them. After the cremation, you can either collect the ashes to keep, bury or scatter yourself, or you can ask the crematorium to dispose of them for you.

Paying for the funeral

The funeral expenses are the first claim on the dead person's estate. However, the person responsible for the funeral will not be able to obtain the money from the estate until he or she has obtained a grant of probate or letters of administration from the local probate court. Procedures vary depending on state law. Some people have life insurance policies that are intended to cover funeral expenses. Also, some trade unions, credit unions and fraternal organizations have death benefits that can be used to help pay for a funeral. Be sure to find out if any such benefits are available, and how to apply for them. If the dead person was eligible for social security benefits, he or she may also be eligible for a death benefit from that source.

In some states, local government is required to arrange a funeral if no one else will do it. A hospital, too, may arrange the funeral of anyone who dies in the hospital and whose relatives cannot be traced or cannot afford to pay for the funeral.

Medical use of the body

If a person has (either in writing or verbally before two witnesses) forbidden that his or her body be used for medical research or that the organs be removed for transplantation, those instructions must be followed when the person dies. However, under the Uniform Anatomical Gift Act, it is possible to leave instructions for your body, organs or both to be donated after your death. One way to leave these instructions is to complete a Uniform Donor Card, which you can carry with you so that your wishes are known in the event of an accidental death. The card should be signed by two witnesses in the spaces provided. It will be considered a legal document in most states. These cards are available from the American Medical Association and several other sources.

In some states, however, a surviving spouse or next of kin can refuse to allow your instructions to be carried out. If you have not left instructions either way, your relatives are allowed to donate the body or organs for medical use, provided no close relative forbids it (see also Autopsies, next article). If the death has been reported to the medical examiner or the coroner, permission is needed before the body or organs can be donated.

If a dead person's body is to be donated for research, you should telephone the appropriate local organization or medical school as soon as death has occurred.

Autopsies

An autopsy is a detailed examination of a body after death. It is also called a *post mortem* examination. There are two different kinds of autopsies. One is ordered by the legal authorities. This kind is called a "medicolegal autopsy." The purpose of such an autopsy is to establish the cause of death and to gather information about the death to be used as evidence in any legal proceedings that may follow. This is done to be sure that crimes that involve deaths are detected, and that, if a crime has been committed, the appropriate persons are prosecuted. It may also be done to investigate possible industrial hazards or contagious diseases that may endanger the public health, or to establish the cause of death for insurance purposes.

The second type of autopsy is done for medical or educational reasons, usually in the hospital where the person died, and may be requested by the attending physician or the family. Such an autopsy cannot be done unless the family gives their permission. Procedures for giving such permission vary from state to state. The general purposes of this type of autopsy are to increase medical knowledge and to provide the family with a more exact cause of death.

Both types of autopsy are usually done before the body is embalmed, and afterwards the body is given directly to the funeral director hired by the family, so that the funeral can be held as soon as possible.

Medicolegal autopsies

When the coroner, the medical examiner or a judge orders an autopsy, the family has no choice but to agree. If there is any question about the order, consult an attorney.

Such an autopsy can range from a minute examination of the appearance of the body and the situation in which it was found, to a study of the entire body and all its parts, including the structure of the individual cells. The thoroughness of the autopsy depends on what is being investigated. A pathologist, or a physician who does autopsies and studies of tissues and organs, must make extremely careful records of everything that is done, in case the information is needed as evidence for legal proceedings.

Medical and educational autopsies

Until about the 13th century, very few autopsies were done for any reason. However, in the 13th and 14th centuries scientists began to perform autopsies to learn about the structure and functions of the human body. Much of the basic medical knowledge we have today was discovered and confirmed through autopsies. Since that time, more and more medical students have learned about human anatomy by dissecting an actual human body.

New discoveries are still being made from autopsies (see Box, right). In diseases such as cancer and heart disease, an autopsy study of diseased organs or systems provides information that can be used to help improve treatment of the disease, and also to expand medical knowledge about it.

Autopsies are also done sometimes as a check on the accuracy of diagnosis and the appropriateness of treatment. If a patient dies unexpectedly or if the symptoms are puzzling, the physician concerned with the case may want an autopsy to find out exactly what happened. The family may want to know as well. In some cases, the family may want information about possible inherited diseases (see Genetics, p.704), and this kind of information can sometimes be obtained from an autopsy.

If you are asked to permit an autopsy on a relative who has died, there are several things to remember. First, you can order a limited autopsy; that is, you can specify what parts of the body can be investigated. The pathologist is legally obligated to follow the family's instructions. Second, an autopsy need not show on the body, because in most cases the marks will be covered by clothing. Third, autopsies are done with respect for the body and in a carefully regulated and confidential setting. Finally, much can be learned from an autopsy, both for the benefit of medical science and in many cases for the benefit of the family.

Disorders discovered by autopsies

Listed below are a few of the diseases and disorders that have been discovered in recent years as a result of autopsy studies.

Collagen diseases	Hyperparathyroidism
Radiation injury	Viral hepatitis
Effects of potassium	Industrial hazards
deficiency on kidneys	Effects of toxic
and heart	chemicals

Bereavement

Immediately after the death of someone close to them, many people simply feel numb and empty. For a while they behave almost as if nothing has happened, until they are eventually stricken with intense grief. During this period immediately after a loss, delusions of seeing the dead person are common, and quite normal. There is also a tendency to forget that the person is dead and act as though he or she were still alive. Idealization of the dead person and feelings of guilt for not doing more for the person when he or she was alive are also common. Guilt feelings (and intense grief) are much more common in cases when the person died unexpectedly than after a death that occurred after a long illness, when the bereaved person was able to both provide care and anticipate the loss.

If someone close to you dies, try to acknowledge the loss rather than attempting to shut it out of your consciousness. Although it is painful, talking about the dead person to relatives and friends and sorting out the person's possessions will help you to come to terms with the loss.

The intensity of grief usually starts to wane after about six weeks, and is sometimes replaced by a more general state of depression and apathy. Grief is usually minimal by six months, although it will probably recur occasionally in the years that follow. By the end of a year, most bereaved people have recovered from their loss and have started building a new life for themselves.

Occasionally, however, grief is so prolonged or intense that it cannot be relieved without help from a medical professional such as a psychiatrist. Bereaved people most likely to need such help are those whose personalities make them particularly prone to grief, those whose relationship with the dead person has left them with strong feelings of guilt or anger, and those who tend to be socially isolated.

In recovering from the death of someone close to you, it often is important to interest yourself in new activities that will not remind you of the person who has died, and to meet some new people. Give yourself time to accept the fact of your loss, allow your feelings of grief to come out, and then begin to rebuild a life that allows you to forget the loss at least some of the time. If you need help, do not be afraid to ask for it.

Helping the bereaved

A bereaved person will need practical help at first to continue a normal day-to-day existence, and, perhaps, to make any necessary decisions. Apart from that, it may seem to you that there is little real comfort you can offer, but this is not so. In allowing the person to talk to you about his or her loss, you encourage an outlet for the expression of grief that can only be beneficial.

You should take any threat of suicide seriously. Call a physician, a hospital emergency room, or a suicide "hot line" (if there is one in your community) to get immediate professional advice and assistance.

Do not give your help only over the first few difficult days and then withdraw it. The bereaved person will need support throughout the lonely months that follow. The first anniversary of a death, or the first holiday spent alone, can be a particularly miserable time, and a visit or an offer of hospitality from you may be needed and welcome.

Children and death

Until about the age of three, children have no concept of death at all. By age nine, most children are able to understand that death is really the end of life and is inevitable.

The bereaved child

Children should be allowed to grieve in their own way and not made to conform to adult ideas. Young children often appear to recover from a bereavement quite quickly, especially if they can attach themselves to a substitute for the dead person.

Adults should not try to suppress their own grief in front of a child, since a child can often sense feelings that are unexpressed, and such suppression can make him or her feel excluded. Give the child every opportunity to ask questions about the death. Some children feel that the death may be their fault in some way, and they may need to be reassured that this is not the case.

Even if a child shows minimal signs of grief after the death of a close relative, it is best to try to avoid any other major changes in the child's life for about six months, if that is possible. Stability and a feeling of security are important to a bereaved child.

The dying child

A child may be able to face the prospect of his or her own death better than the parents can. More than death, the child may fear painful treatment, and, if admission to the hospital is necessary, separation from his or her parents. It will usually help a child to come to terms with death if he or she is told about the nature of the disease and if death is not treated as a forbidden subject. The most important thing that the parents can give the child is security, physically by their presence and mentally by their candor and openness.

It is important that a fatally ill child leads as normal a life as possible for as long as possible. Avoid treating him or her in any special way that will make the child feel different from his or her friends. School work, seeing friends, and normal family activities and discipline should be continued for the child for as long as possible.

If it can be done, it is much more comforting for a terminally ill child to be looked after at home rather than in a hospital. However, it is necessary that parents who take on home care have a telephone and a family physician who can be called on in any circumstances and will arrange hospital admission if the parents can no longer cope, or if the child needs more sophisticated medical care.

The death of a child

The death of a child can easily cause more grief than the death of an adult, for added to the normal sorrow of loss is misery and perhaps even rage that a life has been cut off that had scarcely begun. Sudden death is often even more difficult to bear than death that comes at the end of a long illness. For that reason, parents should enquire about the likely outcome at the beginning of a serious illness, because if the disease is potentially fatal they will have time to try to adjust to the possibility of their child's death.

Drug index

The purpose of this drug index is to provide some basic information about specific drugs and classes of drugs that your physician may prescribe or that you may purchase without a prescription. Because new drugs constantly are being discovered, and due to the large number of drugs available, this index cannot cover them all. An attempt has been made to include the most commonly dispensed drugs, including their generic and trade names, known to the American Medical Association Division of Drugs. Inclusion in this list should not be considered an endorsement for any drug, and there are many drugs on the market that are not included due to lack of space.

If you have questions about any medications you are taking you should consult your physician. Prescription drugs should not be taken without a physician's advice. Except for minor symptoms such as occasional cough or headache, it is usually best to let your physician prescribe all the medicines you need.

There are three types of entry in the alphabetical index:
1 **General categories**, listed according to function – for instance, ANTIBIOTICS or ANTIANXIETY DRUGS.

These entries describe the major groups of drugs, giving their uses, some possible side effects, and information on how the drugs are to be taken (as tablets, liquids, etc.). Other significant facts about the general category (such as the advisability of avoiding alcohol during treatment) are also included.

2 **Generic names** of specific drugs – for instance, diazepam.

The generic-name entry relates the drug to its general category and may also give details of its specific effects; whether, for instance, a particular drug has an unusual side-effect.

3 **Trade names** – for instance, Valium (a trade name for diazepam).

Entries for trade names are simply identified according to their basic chemical ingredient(s), which are given in parentheses, and the general category to which they belong. The initial letter of a trade name is capitalized so that you will know it is not a generic name.

Drugs that can be bought without a prescription are marked with an asterisk (*).

A

acetaminophen* A non-narcotic ANALGESIC and ANTIPYRETIC that can be taken in tablet or liquid form, and is less likely than aspirin to cause stomach irritation. Higher-than-normal doses can damage the liver irreversibly. Anyone who has a liver or kidney disorder should not take this drug without consulting a physician.

acetazolamide A CARBONIC ANHYDRASE INHIBITOR. Possible side-effects (in addition to those common to the group): loss of appetite, depression.

acetohexamide A HYPO-GLYCEMIC.

acetylsalicylic acid Another name for aspirin, a non-narcotic ANALGESIC. See aspirin.

Achromycin (tetracycline hydrochloride) An ANTIBIOTIC.

Actidil* (triprolidine hydrochloride) An ANTIHISTAMINE.

Actifed (triprolidine hydrochloride and pseudoephedrine hydrochloride) A DECONGESTANT.

actinomycin D A CYTOTOXIC used as an ANTINEOPLASTIC, given only by injection.

Adriamycin (doxorubicin) A CYTOTOXIC.

Adroyd (oxymetholone) An

anabolic steroid. See SEX HORMONES (MALE).

Afrin* (oxymetazoline) A DECONGESTANT.

agar gel A bulk LAXATIVE.

Agoral, plain* A liquid mixture of mineral oil and agar gel. A LAXATIVE.

Agoral with phenolphthalein* A liquid mixture containing phenolphthalein (a stimulant LAXATIVE) and mineral oil (a bowel movement softener).

albuterol A BRONCHODILATOR.

Aldactazide (spironolactone and hydrochlorothiazide) A DIURETIC and ANTIHYPERTENSIVE.

Aldactone (spironolactone) A DIURETIC.

Aldomet (methyldopa) An ANTIHYPERTENSIVE.

Aldoril (hydrochlorothiazide and methyldopa) An ANTIHYPERTENSIVE.

Alkeran (melphalan) A CYTOTOXIC.

allopurinol A drug taken in tablet form to treat gout. Possible side-effects: rashes, fever, nausea, diarrhea, abdominal pain, drowsiness. Patients are usually advised to drink at least 2 liters (4 pts) of liquids a day while under treatment with allopurinol.

Alu-Cap* (aluminum hydroxide) An ANTACID.

Aludrox* (aluminum hydroxide) An ANTACID.

aluminum hydroxide* An ANTACID. Common side-effect: constipation.

aluminum phosphate* An ANTACID.

Alupent (metaproterenol sulfate) A BRONCHODILATOR.

amantadine A drug used mainly to treat Parkinson's disease. It also is used as an ANTIVIRAL to treat shingles and prevent influenza. Possible side-effects: nervousness, insomnia, dizziness, swollen ankles.

amcinonide A CORTICOSTEROID.

aminophylline A BRONCHODILATOR. Possible side-effects (in addition to those common to the group): nausea, insomnia, increased urination, increased heart rate.

amitriptyline hydrochloride A tricyclic ANTIDEPRESSANT, also used for treatment of enuresis.

amobarbital A barbiturate, used as a SLEEPING DRUG.

amoxapine An ANTIDEPRESSANT.

amoxicillin A broad-spectrum ANTIBIOTIC.

Amoxil (amoxicillin) An ANTIBIOTIC.

Amphogel* (aluminum hydroxide) An ANTACID.

amphotericin B An ANTIFUNGAL. Possible side-effects: headache, loss of appetite, fever, physical weakness, diarrhea.

ampicillin A broad-spectrum ANTIBIOTIC.

Amytal (amobarbital) A SLEEPING DRUG.

ANALGESICS Drugs that relieve pain. There are two main types: non-narcotic analgesics for mild pain, and narcotic analgesics (based on opium) for severe pain. Most non-narcotic analgesics contain aspirin (or aspirin-like substances) or acetaminophen, and are also ANTIPYRETICS. Some are ANTI-INFLAMMATORIES as well. Many trade-name products are a combination of non-narcotic analgesics, sometimes with codeine, a weak narcotic analgesic. Although these are more costly, they are rarely more effective than single-ingredient preparations. For further information and possible side-effects, see entries on specific drugs. Narcotic analgesics may be taken as tablets or by injection. Possible side-effects: nausea, constipation, dizziness, inability to urinate. All narcotic analgesics cause gradual development of some degree of tolerance and are habit-forming. The risk of becoming addicted to weaker narcotics such as codeine is much lower than it is with powerful morphine derivatives. Narcotic analgesics are not prescribed for anyone who is taking monoamine oxidase inhibitors (a type of ANTIDEPRESSANT) or who has low blood pressure, asthma, liver damage, or head injury.

Ancef (cefazolin sodium) An ANTIBIOTIC.

Antabuse (disulfiram) A drug used to treat alcoholism.

ANTACIDS Drugs that relieve indigestion and heartburn by neutralizing the effects of stomach acid. Antacids are taken in tablet or liquid form, or as a powder mixed with water. Liquid preparations or powders are most effective. Possible side-effects: constipation (from aluminum compounds), diarrhea (from magnesium compounds). In preparations made by combining different antacids, the side-effects may neutralize each other. Antacids may be combined with an ANTISPASMODIC to treat peptic ulcers. Anyone who has damaged or inefficient kidneys should not take preparations that contain magnesium or sodium bicarbonate. Antacids are taken between meals, and because they interfere with absorption of many drugs, they should not be taken with other medicines.

Anaprox (naproxen sodium) An ANALGESIC ANTI-INFLAMMATORY.

naproxene

✓ **ANTIANXIETY DRUGS** Drugs (sometimes called anxiolytics, sedatives or minor tranquilizers) that suppress anxiety and relax muscles. Some are also used as SLEEPING DRUGS or for relief of premenstrual tension. Possible side-effects: drowsiness, dizziness, confusion, unsteadiness (especially in the elderly). Because they can become habit-forming and users develop tolerance, antianxiety drugs are usually prescribed for periods of no more than four months of continuous use. To avoid withdrawal symptoms, usage should be halted gradually, not stopped abruptly. Effects last for several hours, and driving or working with potentially dangerous machinery is not recommended during that time. The effects of alcohol may be dangerously increased by the drugs.

ANTIARRHYTHMICS Drugs used to control irregularities of heartbeat. The oldest antiarrhythmics are digitalis and quinidine, both of which are plant extracts. More recently introduced antiarrhythmics include BETA-BLOCKERS, such as propranolol.

ANTIBACTERIALS Drugs used to treat infections. See ANTIBIOTICS.

ANTIBIOTICS Drugs made from naturally occurring and synthetic

substances that combat bacterial infection. Some antibiotics are effective only against limited types of bacteria. Others, known as broad-spectrum antibiotics, are effective against a wide range of bacteria. Possible side-effects: nausea, vomiting, diarrhea, and, especially from the use of broad-spectrum antibiotics, secondary infections such as yeast infections that are due to an upset in the balance of natural bacteria within the body. Allergic reactions, particularly to penicillin and its many derivatives, may occur. Among them are rashes, fever, painful joints, body swelling, wheezing, and some blood disorders. Individuals who discover they are allergic to a particular antibiotic should ask the physician for a change of treatment. Once treatment begins, the prescribed course should be completed even if the infection seems to have been cured. Failure to take the entire prescription may allow relapse of the infection and may increase the chances of bacterial resistance to further treatment with the drug.

ANTICANCER DRUGS See CYTOTOXICS.

ANTICOAGULANTS AND THROMBOLYTICS Anticoagulants prevent blood from clotting. Possible side-effects: bleeding from nose or gums, bruising, smoky or pink urine, bleeding into the intestinal tract. Because anticoagulants interact adversely with many other drugs, including aspirin, users should carry a warning card and take other medicine only under a physician's direction. Thrombolytics help dissolve and disperse blood clots and may be prescribed for patients with recent arterial or venous thrombosis.

ANTICONVULSANTS Drugs that prevent epileptic seizures. In certain types of epilepsy, once the patient has remained free of seizures for two or three years, the dose may be gradually reduced, and in some cases may eventually be stopped altogether. However, in many types of epilepsy, medication must be continued for life. Possible side-effects: drowsiness, rashes, dizziness, headache, nausea. Abrupt withdrawal can precipitate a convulsion. Drinking alcohol, taking ANTIHISTAMINES, or operating potentially dangerous machinery are not recommended while taking anticonvulsants.

ANTIDEPRESSANTS There are two main groups of mood-lifting antidepressants: tricyclics and monoamine oxidase inhibitors (MAOIs). Beneficial effects may take three to four weeks to de-

velop, so patients may need encouragement from relatives and friends to continue the treatment. Possible side-effects of tricyclics: drowsiness, dry mouth, blurred vision, constipation, difficulty in urinating, faintness on standing, sweating, trembling, rashes, palpitations. Possible side-effects of MAOIs: dizziness, faintness on standing, headache, trembling, constipation, dry mouth, blurred vision, difficulty in urinating, rashes. The MAOIs interact adversely with other drugs and several foods and are usually prescribed only if depression fails to respond to tricyclics. Individuals taking MAOIs are advised to carry a warning card. Drinking alcohol, driving or using complex machinery are not recommended after taking any antidepressant.

ANTIDIARRHEALS Drugs used for the relief of diarrhea. Two main types of antidiarrheal preparations are simple absorbent substances (for instance, kaolin, chalk or charcoal mixtures) and drugs that slow down the contractions of the bowel muscle so that the contents are propelled more slowly. Antidiarrheals are available in tablet and liquid form. Because treatment of diarrhea can lead to constipation, using antidiarrheals for prolonged periods is not recommended.

Reglan

✓ **ANTIEMETICS** Drugs used to treat nausea and vomiting. Certain ANTIHISTAMINES and ANTISPASMODICS are also commonly used as antiemetics for prevention of motion sickness. Vomiting caused by underlying disease, radiation sickness, bacterial toxins, cytotoxic agents, or surgical procedures are most often treated with antipsychotic drugs that have antiemetic properties. Antiemetics are usually taken as tablets, but may be taken in liquid or suppository form or given by injection. For possible side-effects see ANTIHISTAMINES, ANTISPASMODICS, and ANTIPSYCHOTICS. Driving, using potentially dangerous machinery, or drinking alcohol are not recommended after taking an antiemetic. Antiemetics are not recommended in cases where the cause of vomiting is not known, and should not be taken by pregnant women without a physician's advice.

ANTIFUNGALS Drugs used to treat fungal infections, the most common of which affect the hair, skin, nails or mucous membranes. Antifungals may be taken in tablet form or applied locally as creams, ointments or suppositories. Internal fungal infections are treated by

antifungal drugs given by injection. For possible side-effects, see entries for specific drugs.

ANTIHISTAMINES Drugs used primarily to counteract the effects of histamine, one of the chemicals involved in allergic reactions. They are used with variable success to treat hay fever. Many antihistamines are also beneficial for relief of stuffy or runny nose, nausea and vertigo (dizziness). They are therefore common ingredients of COLD REMEDIES and are used to prevent motion sickness. Possible side-effects: drowsiness, blurred vision, dry mouth. Driving, operating potentially dangerous machinery, or drinking alcohol are not recommended after taking an antihistamine.

ANTIHYPERTENSIVES Drugs that lower blood pressure. The two groups that are most commonly used are BETA-BLOCKERS and DIURETICS, but other categories also are prescribed and these agents are referred to in this index simply as antihypertensives. Antihypertensives are usually taken as tablets, but may be given by injection for rapid effect. For possible side-effects see entries for specific drugs.

ANTI-INFLAMMATORIES Drugs used to reduce inflammation – the redness, heat, swelling and increased blood flow found in infections and in many chronic noninfective diseases such as rheumatoid arthritis and gout. Three main types of drugs are used as anti-inflammatories: ANALGESICS such as aspirin, CORTICOSTEROIDS and nonsteroidal anti-inflammatory drugs such as indomethacin. The analgesics that are especially effective for treating rheumatic conditions also reduce the fever and inflammation of the joints, and may help correct some of the blood abnormalities found in those disorders. Nonsteroidal drugs similar to indomethacin have little effect on pains such as those from a toothache or a bruise, but are very effective in relieving the inflammation, and therefore the pain, of diseases such as gout. CORTICOSTEROIDS may be applied locally as cream or eye drops for inflammation of the skin or eyes, but they are not generally prescribed for rheumatic conditions unless such disorders have failed to respond to treatment with nonsteroidal drugs.

ANTINEOPLASTICS Drugs used to treat cancer. See CYTOTOXICS

ANTIPSYCHOTICS Drugs used to treat symptoms of severe psychiatric disorders. These drugs are sometimes called major tranquilizers. Some antipsychotics also may be useful in treating migraine headaches. They may be taken in tablet, liquid or suppository form, or given by injection. Possible side-effects: faintness on standing, dry mouth, constipation, abnormal face and body movements.

ANTIPYRETICS Drugs that reduce fever. Those most commonly used are aspirin and acetaminophen, which are both also ANALGESICS. This double action makes them particularly effective for relieving the symptoms of illness such as the flu.

ANTIRHEUMATICS See ANTI-INFLAMMATORIES and ANALGESICS.

ANTISPASMODICS Drugs for reducing spasm of the bowel to relieve the pain of conditions such as irritable colon or diverticular disease. Some antispasmodics are used, in combination with ANTACIDS, to treat peptic ulcers. A few are also used as ANTIEMETICS. Antispasmodics may be taken in tablet or liquid form or by injection. Possible side-effects: dry mouth, palpitations, difficulty in urinating, constipation, blurred vision.

Antivert (meclizine hydrochloride) An ANTIEMETIC. Also used to treat vertigo (dizziness).

ANTIVIRALS Drugs used to treat viral infections or to provide temporary protection against infections such as influenza. Few viral disorders respond to drugs, and those that do respond, such as cold sores and shingles, will do so only if treatment is started early. For further information, see entries for specific drugs.

Anturane (sulfinpyrazone) A drug used to prevent gout.

Anusol* A cream or suppository used to treat hemorrhoids or anal itching.

APERIENTS See LAXATIVES.

Apresoline (hydralazine hydrochloride) An ANTIHYPERTENSIVE.

Aristocort (triamcinolone) A CORTICOSTEROID.

A.S.A. Enseals* (aspirin) An ANALGESIC. A form of aspirin that has been coated for intestinal release.

ascorbic acid (vitamin C) Used to treat vitamin deficiency (scurvy). See VITAMINS.

Ascriptin* (a combination of aluminum and magnesium hydroxides and aspirin). An ANALGESIC.

Asendin (amoxapine) An ANTIDEPRESSANT.

aspirin* A non-narcotic ANALGESIC, also used as an ANTIPYRETIC or ANTI-INFLAMMATORY drug. Aspirin is an effective treatment for headache and muscle and joint pains. Although usually taken as tablets, it is less likely to irritate the stomach in soluble form. Buffered aspirin and tablets with a special protective coating that is not broken down until the tablet reaches the intestine, may also reduce stomach irritation. Possible side-effect: stomach pain. High or prolonged doses may cause hearing loss, noises in the ear, nausea or headache. Aspirin is available in reduced strength tablets for children, but is not recommended for infants under one year. Aspirin is not recommended for anyone who has abdominal pain, nausea, vomiting, a peptic ulcer or a bleeding disorder. Anyone who is being treated with ANTICOAGULANTS AND THROMBOLYTICS should not take aspirin.

Atarax (hydroxyzine hydrochloride) An ANTIANXIETY DRUG.

Ativan (lorazepam) An ANTIANXIETY DRUG.

Atromid-S (clofibrate) A drug used to reduce the blood-cholesterol level.

atropine sulfate An ANTI-SPASMODIC. Not recommended for anyone who has glaucoma, or anyone with a tendency to urinary retention, such as men with prostate disorders.

Aventyl (nortriptyline) An ANTIDEPRESSANT.

azathloprine A CYTOTOXIC used primarily as an IMMUNOSUPPRESSIVE. Possible side-effects (in addition to those common to the group): rashes, wasting of muscles.

Azene (clorazepate monopotassium) An ANTIANXIETY DRUG, also used as a SLEEPING DRUG.

B

bacampicillin hydrochloride A broad-spectrum ANTIBIOTIC.

bacitracin An ANTIBIOTIC used in preparations applied to the skin and other surface areas.

Bactrim (sulfamethoxazole and trimethoprim) An ANTIBIOTIC.

BARBITURATES See SLEEPING DRUGS.

belladonna An ANTISPASMODIC that contains atropine.

Benadryl* (diphenhydramine hydrochloride) An ANTIHISTAMINE.

bendroflumethiazide A DIURETIC.

Benemid (probenecid) A drug used to prevent gout.

Bentyl (dicyclomine hydrochloride) An ANTISPASMODIC.

benztropine mesylate A drug used to treat Parkinson's disease. Given by injection. Possible side-effects: dry mouth, visual difficulties, rapid heartbeat, constipation, urine retention in the bladder.

BETA-BLOCKERS Beta-adrenergic blocking agents, or beta-blockers for short, reduce the oxygen needs of the heart by reducing heartbeat rate. They are used as ANTIHYPERTENSIVES and ANTIARRHYTHMICS, to treat angina due to exertion, and to ease symptoms such as palpitations and tremors in patients who are troubled with anxiety states. They are used occasionally for migraine headaches. Beta-blockers may be taken as tablets or given by injection. Possible side-effects: nausea, insomnia, physical weariness, diarrhea. Overdose can cause dizziness and fainting spells. Discontinuation of treatment with these drugs should be gradual, not abrupt. Beta-blockers are not prescribed for people who suffer either with asthma or heart failure.

Betadine (povidone-iodine) A skin antiseptic.

betamethasone A CORTICOSTEROID.

bethanechol chloride A drug used to treat urinary retention disorders. Possible side-effects: abdominal cramps, nausea, increased salivation, sweating. The drug should not be taken by people with asthma.

bisacodyl* A stimulant LAXATIVE. Possible side-effect: abdominal cramps.

Bicillin (penicillin G benzathine) An ANTIBIOTIC.

Bicillin C-R (penicillin G benzathine and penicillin G procaine) An ANTIBIOTIC.

bismuth subgallate* An ANTIDIARRHEAL. Also used topically to treat skin conditions.

bisomycin sulfate A CYTOTOXIC, given only by injection.

bran* A bulk LAXATIVE, made of fibrous wheat and taken as tablets.

Brethine (terbutaline sulfate) A BRONCHODILATOR.

Brevicone A combination of a progestin and an estrogen used as an oral contraceptive. See SEX HORMONES (FEMALE).

Bricanyl (terbutaline sulfate) A BRONCHODILATOR.

bromocriptine A drug used to treat Parkinson's disease, also used to suppress milk production and to treat some hormonal disorders. It is generally taken in tablet form. Possible side-effects: nausea, constipation, headache, drowsiness, confusion, dry mouth, leg cramps, hallucinations.

brompheniramine maleate An ANTIHISTAMINE.

BRONCHODILATORS Drugs that open up the bronchial tubes within the lungs when the tubes have become narrowed by muscle spasm. Bronchodilators ease breathing in diseases such as asthma. They are most often taken as aerosol sprays, but they are also available in tablet, liquid or suppository form. In emergencies such as severe asthma attacks, they may be given by injection. Effects usually last for three to five hours. Possible side-effects: rapid heartbeat, palpitations, tremor, headache, dizziness. Because of the possible effects of bronchodilator drugs on the heart, prescribed doses should never be exceeded. When asthma does not respond to the prescribed doses of these drugs, emergency medical treatment is needed.

Bronkosol (isoetharine hydrochloride) A BRONCHODILATOR.

busulfan A CYTOTOXIC used as an ANTINEOPLASTIC. Possible side-effect (in addition to those common to the group): skin pigmentation.

butabarbital A BARBITURATE used as a SLEEPING DRUG and to treat anxiety.

Butazolidin (phenylbutazone) An ANTI-INFLAMMATORY.

Butazolidin alka (phenylbutazone, aluminum hydroxide and magnesium trisilicate) An ANTI-INFLAMMATORY.

Butazone (phenylbutazone) An ANTI-INFLAMMATORY.

C

Cafergot (ergotamine and caffeine) A preparation used to treat migraine headaches. Possible side-effects: nausea, vomiting, tingling sensations or cold in the fingers or toes, chest pain. All side-effects should be reported to the physician.

caffeine A mild stimulant used as part of an ANALGESIC mixture.

calamine* A soothing skin preparation in cream or liquid form used mainly to treat sunburn and mild rashes or sores caused by insect stings, poison ivy, etc.

Cantil (mepenzolate bromide) An ANTISPASMODIC.

caramiphen edisylate A cough medicine. See COUGH SUPPRESSANTS.

carbamazepine An ANTICONVULSANT, also used for relief of trigeminal neuralgia. Possible side-effects (in addition to those common to the group): dry mouth, double vision, drowsiness, dizziness.

carbidopa A drug used to treat Parkinson's disease.

CARBONIC ANHYDRASE INHIBITORS Drugs used to decrease pressure within the eye in the treatment of glaucoma. Possible side-effects: loss of appetite, weight loss, nausea, vomiting, diarrhea, weakness, depression, dizziness.

cascara* A stimulant LAXATIVE. Possible side-effects: abdominal cramps, red-tinged urine. It should not be taken by nursing mothers.

Catapres (clonidine hydrochloride) An ANTIHYPERTENSIVE.

CCNU (lomustine) A CYTOTOXIC.

Ceclor (cefaclor) An ANTIBIOTIC.

Cedilanid-D (deslanoside) A drug used to treat heart disease, including heart failure and arrhythmias.

CeeNU (lomustine) A CYTOTOXIC.

cefaclor A broad-spectrum ANTIBIOTIC.

cefamandole nafate A broad-spectrum ANTIBIOTIC.

cefazolin sodium A broad-spectrum ANTIBIOTIC.

cefotaxime sodium A broad-spectrum ANTIBIOTIC.

Celestone (betamethasone) A CORTICOSTEROID.

Cellothyl* (methylcellulose) A bulk LAXATIVE.

cephalexin A broad-spectrum ANTIBIOTIC.

cephalothin A broad-spectrum ANTIBIOTIC.

cephradine A broad-spectrum ANTIBIOTIC.

Cerubidine (daunorubicin hydrochloride) A CYTOTOXIC used as an ANTINEOPLASTIC.

chloral hydrate The oldest synthetic SLEEPING DRUG. Possible side-effects: rashes, stomach irritation, bad breath. The drug should be taken well-diluted.

chlorambucil A CYTOTOXIC used as an ANTINEOPLASTIC.

chloramphenicol An ANTIBIOTIC used as an ointment or in drops for ear and eye infections. Also used orally or by injection for certain extremely serious, possibly life-threatening infections.

chlordiazepoxide An ANTI-ANXIETY DRUG.

Chloromycetin (chloramphenicol) An ANTIBIOTIC.

chlorothiazide A DIURETIC.

chlorotrianisene An estrogenic SEX HORMONE (FEMALE) most commonly prescribed for men as an ANTINEOPLASTIC.

chlorpheniramine maleate An ANTIHISTAMINE.

chlorpromazine hydrochloride An ANTIPSYCHOTIC, also used as an ANTIEMETIC. Possible side-effects (in addition to those common to the group): muscular stiffness, constipation, difficulty in urinating, faintness on standing, menstrual disturbances, rashes.

chlorpropamide A HYPOGLYCEMIC.

chlorthalidone A DIURETIC.

Chlor-Trimeton* (chlorpheniramine maleate) An ANTIHISTAMINE.

chlorzoxazone A MUSCLE RELAXANT.

Choledyl (oxtriphylline) A BRONCHODILATOR.

cimetidine A drug used to treat peptic ulcers. Possible side-effects: diarrhea, dizziness, rashes.

cisplatin A CYTOTOXIC used as an ANTINEOPLASTIC. Possible side-effects (in addition to those

common to the group): hearing loss that may progress to deafness, kidney damage.

Claforan (cefotaxime sodium) A broad-spectrum ANTIBIOTIC.

Cleocin (clindamycin) An ANTIBIOTIC.

clidinium bromide An ANTISPASMODIC.

clindamycin An ANTIBIOTIC. Patients are usually advised to discontinue use of clindamycin if severe diarrhea occurs.

Clinoril (sulindac) A nonsteroidal ANTI-INFLAMMATORY.

clofibrate A drug used to reduce blood-cholesterol level, usually taken in tablet form. Possible side-effects: nausea, diarrhea, aching muscles. Clofibrate is not generally prescribed for people with liver or kidney disease.

Clomid (clomiphene) A drug used to treat infertility in women.

clomiphene A drug taken in tablet form to treat infertility in women. Possible side-effects: hot flashes, abdominal discomfort, blurred vision, nausea, vomiting, depression, insomnia, breast tenderness, weight gain.

clomipramine hydrochloride A tricyclic ANTIDEPRESSANT.

clonazepam An ANTICONVULSANT. Possible side-effects (in addition to those common to the group): muscular weakness, clumsiness, mood changes.

clonidine hydrochloride An ANTIHYPERTENSIVE, also used for prevention of migraine attacks. Possible side-effects: dry mouth, drowsiness, depression, swollen ankles. Abrupt withdrawal should be avoided.

Clonopin (clonazepam) An ANTICONVULSANT.

clorazepate dipotassium or chlorazepate monopotassium An ANTI-ANXIETY DRUG, also used as a SLEEPING DRUG.

clotrimazole An ANTIFUNGAL. Possible side effect: local irritation.

cloxacillin An ANTIBIOTIC.

codeine phosphate A mild narcotic ANALGESIC also used as a COUGH SUPPRESSANT and ANTIDIARRHEAL. Taking codeine phosphate shortly before, during or after drinking alcohol is not recommended. The drug also is not recommended for infants under one

year. Possible side-effects: nausea, dizziness, drowsiness, constipation.

Cogentin (benztropine mesylate) A drug used to treat Parkinson's disease.

COLD REMEDIES Although there is no drug that can cure a cold, the aches, pains and fever that accompany a cold can be relieved by aspirin or acetaminophen, taken with plenty of liquid. Cold remedies are often available in fizzy or fruit-flavored preparations. Many preparations also contain ANTIHISTAMINES and DECONGESTANTS, for dealing with nasal symptoms. However, taken by mouth, these drugs are unlikely to be effective unless swallowed in doses high enough to produce side-effects that outweigh the benefits. Possible side-effects: drowsiness, giddiness, headache, nausea, vomiting, sweating, thirst, palpitations, difficulty in urinating, weakness, trembling, anxiety, insomnia. Cold remedies should be avoided by people who have angina, high blood pressure, diabetes or thyroid disorders, and by anyone who is taking monoamine oxidase inhibitors, a type of ANTIDEPRESSANT. Driving or using potentially dangerous machinery are not recommended after taking a remedy that contains an ANTIHISTAMINE.

Cologel* (methylcellulose) A bulk LAXATIVE.

Combid (isopropamide iodide and prochlorperazine maleate) An ANTISPASMODIC, also used as an ANTIEMETIC.

Compazine (prochlorperazine) An ANTIPSYCHOTIC.

conjugated estrogens A combination of estrogens used to treat menopausal or postmenopausal women. See SEX HORMONES (FEMALE).

Corgard (nadolol) An ANTIHYPERTENSIVE, also used to treat angina attacks.

CORTICOSTEROIDS These hormonal preparations are used primarily as ANTI-INFLAMMATORIES in arthritis or asthma or as IMMUNOSUPPRESSIVES, but they are also useful for treating malignancies or compensating for a deficiency of natural hormones in disorders such as Addison's disease. They are effective for many types of dermatitis, when applied to the skin. Corticosteroids may be taken as tablets, applied locally as cream or eyedrops, or given by injection. Possible side-effects of overuse: swollen ankles, raised blood pressure; fat deposits on face, shoulders and abdomen; hairiness; flushing; acne; disturbance of menstrual patterns; muscle weakness; mood changes; peptic ulcers; cataracts. Corticosteroid tablets also reduce the body's resistance to infection, and they may suppress growth in children. Given as eyedrops, they may cause glaucoma; as creams, they may cause rashes, acne and other skin problems. In all forms, these drugs should be used sparingly and for limited periods only. Discontinuation of treatment should be gradual, not abrupt. People who are taking corticosteroid tablets are advised to carry a warning card, and anyone who has been under corticosteroid tablet treatment within the past two years should inform any new physician, nurse or dentist.

Cortisporin Otic (hydrocortisone, neomycin sulfate and polymyxin B) An ANTI-INFLAMMATORY and ANTIBIOTIC.

Cosmegen (dactinomycin) A CYTOTOXIC.

COUGH SUPPRESSANTS Simple cough medicines, which contain substances such as honey, glycerine or menthol, soothe throat irritation but do not actually suppress coughing. They are most soothing when taken as lozenges and dissolved in the mouth. As liquids they are probably swallowed too quickly to be effective. A few drugs, notably dextromethorphan and codeine, are actually cough suppressants; that is, they can help to control a dry, unproductive (nothing coughed up) cough. For possible side-effects, see entries for specific drugs.

Coumadin (warfarin) An ANTICOAGULANT.

cromolyn sodium A drug used to prevent attacks of asthma. Taken by inhaling a powder. Possible side-effects: throat irritation and cough, chest tightness, breathlessness.

Crystodigin (digitoxin) A drug used to treat heart disease including heart failure and arrhythmias.

cyclacillin A broad-spectrum ANTIBIOTIC.

Cyclapen (cyclacillin) A broad-spectrum ANTIBIOTIC.

cyclizine* An ANTIHISTAMINE primarily used for relief of nausea and vertigo (dizziness).

cyclobenzaprine A drug used to relieve muscle spasms. Possible side-effects: drowsiness, dry mouth, dizziness.

Cyclocort (amcinonide) A CORTICOSTEROID.

cyclophosphamide A CYTOTOXIC used as an ANTINEOPLASTIC and IMMUNOSUPPRESSIVE.

cyproheptadine hydrochloride An ANTIHISTAMINE used to treat allergic disorders.

cytarabine A CYTOTOXIC used as an ANTINEOPLASTIC, given only by injection.

Cytosar U (cytarabine) A CYTOTOXIC.

Cytoxan (cyclophosphamide) A CYTOTOXIC.

CYTOTOXICS Drugs that kill or damage cells. Cytotoxics are used as ANTINEOPLASTICS (drugs used to treat cancer) and also as IMMUNOSUPPRESSIVES. They are taken as tablets or given by injection, and several cytotoxics with different types of action may be used in combination. Possible side-effects: nausea, vomiting, loss of hair. Because cytotoxic drug action can affect healthy as well as cancerous cells, these medications may also have more dangerous side-effects. For example, they can damage bone marrow and affect the production of blood cells, causing anemia, increased susceptibility to infection, and hemorrhage. Therefore, frequent blood counts are recommended for anyone who is having such treatment.

D

Dactil (piperidolate hydrochloride) An ANTISPASMODIC.

dactinomycin A CYTOTOXIC used as an ANTINEOPLASTIC, given only by injection.

Dalmane (flurazepam hydrochloride) A SLEEPING DRUG.

danthron* A stimulant LAXATIVE. Possible side-effects: abdominal cramps, red-tinged urine, diarrhea in infants if taken by nursing mothers.

Daranide (dichlorphenamide) A CARBONIC ANHYDRASE INHIBITOR.

Daraprim (pyrimethamine) A drug used to prevent malaria.

Darvocet N (propoxyphene napsylate and acetaminophen) An ANALGESIC.

Darvon Compound (propoxyphene hydrochloride, aspirin, phenacetin and caffeine) An ANALGESIC.

Datril 500* (acetaminophen) An ANALGESIC and ANTIPYRETIC, in tablet form.

daunorubicin hydrochloride A CYTOTOXIC used as an ANTINEOPLASTIC, given by injection.

DDAVP (desmopressin) A HORMONE used to treat diabetes insipidus.

Decadron (dexamethasone) A CORTICOSTEROID.

Deca-Durabolin (nandrolone decanoate) An anabolic steroid. See SEX HORMONES (MALE).

Declomycin (demeclocycline) An ANTIBIOTIC.

DECONGESTANTS Drugs that reduce swelling of the mucous membranes that line the nose by constricting blood vessels, thus relieving nasal stuffiness. Decongestants are best taken as a nasal spray or drops. Overuse can lead to increased stuffiness. They can also be taken by mouth as one ingredient of COLD REMEDIES, but they are less effective in this form. Large doses taken by mouth may adversely affect heart rate.

DEHYDRATING AGENTS See DIURETICS.

Delatestryl (testosterone enanthate) An androgen. See SEX HORMONES (MALE).

Delta-Cortef (prednisolone) A CORTICOSTEROID.

demeclocycline A broad-spectrum ANTIBIOTIC. See tetracycline; this preparation is similar.

Demerol (meperidine hydrochloride) An ANALGESIC.

Demulen A combination of progestin and estrogen used as an oral contraceptive. See SEX HORMONES (FEMALE).

Depakene (valproic acid) An ANTICONVULSANT.

Depomedrol (methylprednisolone) A CORTICOSTEROID.

desipramine hydrochloride A tricyclic ANTIDEPRESSANT.

deslanoside A digoxin-like drug used to treat heart disease including heart failure and arrhythmias. It is given only by injection. See digoxin for side-effects.

desmopressin A HORMONE, given either as nasal drops or by injection, used to treat diabetes insipidus.

Dexadrine (dextroamphetamine sulfate) A stimulant drug.

dexamethasone A CORTICOSTEROID.

dexbrompaeniramine maleate An ANTIHISTAMINE. Most probable side-effect: drowsiness.

dextroamphetamine sulfate. A stimulant drug with limited medical usage in treating obesity (overweight), hyperkinetic states (a nervous disorder characterized by agitation and non-purposeful physical activity) and narcolepsy (an uncontrollable desire to sleep). The drug is addictive.

dextromethorphan hydrobromide* A cough medicine. Possible side-effect: constipation. See COUGH SUPPRESSANTS.

Diabinese (chlorpropamide) A HYPOGLYCEMIC.

Diamox (acetazolamide) A CARBONIC ANHYDRASE INHIBITOR.

Dianabol (methandrostenolone) An anabolic steroid. See SEX HORMONES (MALE).

diazepam An ANTIANXIETY DRUG, also used as a SLEEPING DRUG.

diazoxide An ANTIHYPERTENSIVE, given only by injection.

dichlorphenamide A CARBONIC ANHYDRASE INHIBITOR used to treat glaucoma. Possible side-effects: loss of appetite, depression.

dicyclomine hydrochloride An ANTISPASMODIC, often used to treat infantile colic. Not recommended for anyone with glaucoma or anyone who has a tendency to urinary retention, such as men with prostate disorders.

digitoxin A digoxin-like drug used to treat heart disease such as heart failure and arrhythmias. See digoxin for side-effects.

digoxin A plant-derived drug that increases the force of contraction of the heartbeat and may be used to treat heart failure. It is also called an ANTIARRHYTHMIC. Possible side-effects: nausea, palpitations, confusion.

Dilantin (phenytoin) An ANTICONVULSANT and ANTIARRHYTHMIC.

dimenhydrinate* An ANTIHISTAMINE primarily used for relief of nausea and vertigo (dizziness).

Dimetapp (brompheniramine maleate, phenylephrine hydrochloride and phenylpropanolamine hydrochloride) A DECONGESTANT.

diphenhydramine hydrochloride An ANTIHISTAMINE.

diphenoxylate hydrochloride An ANTIDIARRHEAL.

dipivefrin hydrochloride A drug used to treat glaucoma.

dipyridamole A VASODILATOR used to treat angina.

disopyramide phosphate An ANTIARRHYTHMIC. Possible side-effects: markedly dry mouth, blurred vision, urinary retention and associated discomfort.

disulfiram A drug taken in tablet form to treat alcoholism. If taken before, during or after drinking alcohol, disulfiram may cause throbbing headache, palpitations, nausea, vomiting and even severe shock. It is these uncomfortable and even dangerous reactions that are relied upon to keep the patient from drinking.

DIURETICS Drugs that increase the quantity of urine produced by the kidneys and passed out of the body, thus ridding the body of excess fluid. Diuretics reduce waterlogging of the tissues caused by fluid retention in disorders of the heart, kidneys and liver. They are useful in treating mild cases of high blood pressure. They are usually taken as tablets. Possible side-effects: rashes, dizziness, weakness, numbness, tingling in the hands and feet.

Diuril (chlorothiazide) A DIURETIC.

Docusate* A bowel movement-softening LAXATIVE.

Dolophine (methadone hydrochloride) An ANALGESIC.

Donnatal (hyoscyamine sulfate, hyoscyamine hydrobromide, atropine sulfate and phenobarbital) An ANTISPASMODIC.

Dopar (levodopa) A drug used to treat Parkinson's disease.

Doxan* A combination of danthron (a stimulant LAXATIVE) and docusate sodium (a bowel movement softener).

doxepin hydrochloride A tricyclic

ANTIDEPRESSANT.

doxorubicin A CYTOTOXIC used as an ANTINEOPLASTIC, given only by injection.

doxycycline A broad-spectrum ANTIBIOTIC. See tetracycline; this preparation is similar.

Dramamine* (dimenhydrinate) An ANTIHISTAMINE and ANTIEMETIC.

Drixoral (dexbrompheniramine maleate and pseudoephedrine sulfate) A DECONGESTANT.

Dulcolax* (bisacodyl) A stimulant LAXATIVE.

Durabolin (nandrolone phenpropionate) An anabolic steroid. See SEX HORMONES (MALE).

Duration* (oxymetazoline) A DECONGESTANT.

Durel-Cort (hydrocortisone) A CORTICOSTEROID.

Dyazide (triamterene and hydrochlorothiazide) A DIURETIC and ANTIHYPERTENSIVE.

Dymelor (acetohexamide) A HYPOGLYCEMIC.

E

Edecrin (ethacrynic acid) A DIURETIC.

E.E.S. (erythromycin) An ANTIBIOTIC.

Efudex (fluorouracil) A CYTOTOXIC.

Elavil (amitriptyline hydrochloride) An ANTIDEPRESSANT.

Eldodram* (dimenhydrinate) An ANTIHISTAMINE.

Empirin with codeine (aspirin and codeine phosphate) An ANALGESIC.

E-Mycin (erythromycin) An ANTIBIOTIC.

Enduron (methylclothiazide) A DIURETIC.

Enovid A combination of progestin and estrogen used as an oral contraceptive. See SEX HORMONES (FEMALE).

ephedrine hydrochloride A BRONCHODILATOR and DECONGESTANT.

epinephrine or epinephrine bitartrate A BRONCHODILATOR and DECONGESTANT.

Equanil (meprobamate) An ANTI-

ANXIETY DRUG.

ergotamine or ergotamine tartrate A drug used to treat migraine headache. Possible side-effects: nausea, vomiting, diarrhea, numbness in the hands and feet, disturbances of heart rhythm. All side-effects should be reported to the physician.

Erythrocin (erythromycin) An ANTIBIOTIC.

erythromycin An ANTIBIOTIC.

Esidrix (hydrochlorothiazide) A DIURETIC.

Estinyl (ethinyl estradiol) An estrogen. See SEX HORMONES (FEMALE).

estradiol An estrogen. See SEX HORMONES (FEMALE).

estriol An estrogen. See SEX HORMONES (FEMALE).

ESTROGENS See SEX HORMONES (FEMALE).

estrone piperazine sulfate An estrogen. See SEX HORMONES (FEMALE).

ethacrynic acid A DIURETIC.

ethinyl estradiol An estrogen. See SEX HORMONES (FEMALE).

ethleterone A progestogen. See SEX HORMONES (FEMALE).

ethosuximide An ANTICONVULSANT used primarily to treat petit mal epilepsy. Possible side-effects (in addition to those common to the group): clumsiness, mood changes.

ethylestrenol An anabolic steroid. See SEX HORMONES (MALE).

EXPECTORANT A drug that stimulates the flow of saliva and promotes coughing to eliminate phlegm from the respiratory tract.

F

fenoprofen An aspirin-like ANALGESIC, ANTIPYRETIC and ANTI-INFLAMMATORY used mainly to treat rheumatic disorders. For further information see aspirin.

ferrous sulfate An iron supplement used to treat certain types of anemia and to maintain iron supply.

Fiorinal (butalbital, caffeine, aspirin and phenacetin) An ANALGESIC and SLEEPING DRUG.

Flagyl (metronidazole) A drug used to treat infections.

Flexeril (cyclobenzaprine) A drug

used to relieve muscle spasms.

fluorouracil A CYTOTOXIC used as an ANTINEOPLASTIC.

fluphenazine decanoate An ANTIPSYCHOTIC, given by injection to treat schizophrenia.

fluphenazine hydrochloride An ANTIPSYCHOTIC.

flurazepam hydrochloride An ANTIANXIETY DRUG, used primarily as a SLEEPING DRUG.

FUNGICIDES See ANTIFUNGALS.

Fungizone (amphotericin B) An ANTIFUNGAL.

Furadantin (nitrofurantoin) An ANTIBIOTIC.

Furan (nitrofurantoin) An ANTIBIOTIC.

furosemide A DIURETIC.

Fybranta* (bran) A bulk LAXATIVE.

G

Gantrisin (sulfisoxazole) An ANTIBACTERIAL drug used primarily to treat kidney infections.

Garamycin (gentamicin sulfate) An ANTIBIOTIC.

gentamicin sulfate A broad-spectrum ANTIBIOTIC (one that is effective against a broad range of infectious agents), usually given by injection or used topically as an ointment. Possible side-effects: hearing loss, kidney damage.

globin zinc insulin injection An intermediate-acting insulin preparation.

glyceryl guaiacolate* An EXPECTORANT. See also COLD REMEDIES.

Glysennid* (senna) A stimulant LAXATIVE.

gramicidin An ANTIBIOTIC used in preparations applied to the skin and other surface areas.

Grifulvin (griseofulvin) An ANTIFUNGAL.

griseofulvin An ANTIFUNGAL. Possible side-effects: headache, nausea, rashes, sensitivity to light.

guaiacosulfonate potassium An EXPECTORANT.

guaifenesin* An EXPECTORANT. See also COLD REMEDIES.

guanethidine sulfate An ANTI-

HYPERTENSIVE. Possible side-effects: faintness, swollen ankles, diarrhea and, in men, failure to ejaculate.

Gynergen (ergotamine tartrate) A drug used to treat migraine headache.

H

Haldol (haloperidol) An ANTIPSYCHOTIC.

haloperidol An ANTIPSYCHOTIC.

heparin An ANTICOAGULANT, given only by injection.

HORMONES Chemicals produced naturally by the endocrine glands (thyroid, adrenal, ovary, testis, pancreas, parathyroid). In some disorders, for example, diabetes mellitus, in which too little of a particular hormone is produced, synthetic equivalents or natural hormone extracts are prescribed to restore the deficiency. Such treatment is known as hormone replacement therapy. For other uses of hormones, in particular the CORTICOSTEROIDS and SEX HORMONES, and for side-effects, see appropriate entries in this index.

Hormonin A combination of estriol, estron, and estradiol, all estrogen compounds. See SEX HORMONES (FEMALE).

hydralazine hydrochloride An ANTIHYPERTENSIVE. Possible side-effects: palpitations, swollen ankles, faintness, headache, nausea, vomiting.

Hydrea (hydroxyurea) A CYTOTOXIC.

hydrochlorothiazide A DIURETIC.

hydrocortisone A CORTICOSTEROID.

Hydrocortone (hydrocortisone) A CORTICOSTEROID.

Hydrodiuril (hydrochlorothiazide) A DIURETIC.

hydroxyurea A CYTOTOXIC used as an ANTINEOPLASTIC.

hydroxyzine hydrochloride An ANTIHISTAMINE used as an ANTIANXIETY DRUG and ANTIEMETIC.

hydroyzine pamoate An ANTIHISTAMINE used as an ANTIANXIETY DRUG and ANTIEMETIC.

Hygroton (chlorthalidone) A DIURETIC.

hyoscine hydrobromide (scopolamine hydrobromide) An ANTISPASMODIC, also used as an ANTIEMETIC. Not recommended for people with glaucoma or a tendency to retain urine, such as men with prostate disorders.

hyoscyamine sulfate or hyoscyamine hydrobromide An ANTISPASMODIC.

HYPNOTICS See SLEEPING DRUGS.

HYPOGLYCEMICS (ORAL) Drugs that lower the level of glucose in the blood. Oral hypoglycemic drugs are used in diabetes mellitus if it cannot be controlled by diet alone, but does not require treatment with injections of insulin. Possible side-effects: loss of appetite, nausea, indigestion, numbness or tingling in the skin, fever, rashes, jaundice. If the glucose level falls too low, weakness, giddiness, pallor, sweating, increased saliva flow, palpitations, irritability and trembling may result. If such symptoms occur several hours after eating, this indicates that the dose is too high, and the symptoms should be reported to the physician.

I

ibuprofen A non-steroidal ANTIINFLAMMATORY. Also has ANALGESIC and ANTIPYRETIC actions.

idoxuridine An ANTIVIRAL for herpes infections, usually taken as an ointment or eye drops.

Ilosone (erythromycin estolate) An ANTIBIOTIC.

Ilotycin (erythromycin) An ANTIBIOTIC.

imipramine hydrochloride A tricyclic ANTIDEPRESSANT, also used to treat enuresis.

IMMUNOSUPPRESSIVES Drugs that prevent or reduce the body's normal reaction to invasion by disease or by foreign tissues. Immunosuppressives are used to treat autoimmune diseases (in which the body's defenses work abnormally, and attack its own tissues) and to help prevent rejection of organ transplants. Most drugs used in this way are CYTOTOXICS or CORTICOSTEROIDS.

Imodium (loperamide hydrochloride) An ANTIDIARRHEAL.

Imuran (azathioprine) A CYTOTOXIC.

Inderal (propranolol hydrochloride) A BETA-BLOCKER.

Indocin (indomethacin) An ANTIINFLAMMATORY.

indomethacin An ANTIINFLAMMATORY, taken in tablet, liquid or suppository form. Possible side-effects: headache, dizziness, loss of appetite, nausea, indigestion, diarrhea.

Insulin A HORMONE, produced by the pancreas, that controls both the breakdown and storage of sugar in the body and thereby regulates the production of energy. As a drug, insulin is used to treat most young diabetics, and some older diabetics whose illness cannot be controlled by diet or by oral HYPOGLYCEMICS. Most insulin preparations are extracted from pork or beef pancreases. Single component insulins are obtained from a single animal source and are valuable if an allergy develops to one species (usually beef insulin). Many specially purified insulins are also available and these are less likely to cause an allergic reaction. If allergy is a severe problem, a "human" insulin may be given, which is synthesized by microorganisms or by chemical modification of a single component insulin. Insulin is always given by injection, as it is destroyed by the digestive juices. Some preparations act rapidly but have only a short duration, others begin to act more slowly and last longer. The type given depends on an individual's needs, and often a mixture is necessary. Initial treatment may be given in a hospital so that the correct dosage can be established. Possible side-effects: hypoglycemia (which may occur if too high a dose is given, or if the person misses a meal, eats too few carbohydrates, or exercises more than usual), with weakness, giddiness, pallor, sweating, increased saliva flow, irritability, trembling, confusion and coma. Allergic reactions: rashes, itching, swelling of the face and throat, local irritation or lumpiness of the skin at the site of the injection.

insulin injection A short-acting insulin preparation.

Intal (cromolyn sodium) A drug used to prevent attacks of asthma.

ipecac fluidextract* An emetic (produces vomiting).

ismelin (guanethidine sulfate) An ANTIHYPERTENSIVE.

isocaboxazid A monoamine oxidase inhibitor ANTIDEPRESSANT.

isoetharine hydrochloride A BRONCHODILATOR.

isoniazid An antituberculosis drug.

isophane insulin suspension An intermediate-acting insulin preparation.

isopropamide iodide An ANTISPASMODIC.

Isoptin (verapamil) An ANTIARRHYTHMIC.

Isordil (isosorbide dinitrate) A VASODILATOR.

isosorbide dinitrate A VASODILATOR.

isosuprine hydrochloride A VASODILATOR.

K

Kabikinase (streptokinase) A THROMBOLYTIC. See ANTICOAGULANTS AND THROMBOLYTICS.

Kaodene (codeine phosphate and kaolin) An ANTIDIARRHEAL.

kaolin* An ANTIDIARRHEAL.

Kaopectate* (kaolin) An ANTIDIARRHEAL.

karaya gum* A bulk LAXATIVE.

Keflex (cephalexin) An ANTIBIOTIC.

Keflin (cephalotin) An ANTIBIOTIC.

Kefzol (cefazolin sodium) A CORTICOSTEROID.

Kenacort (triaminolone) A CORTICOSTEROID.

Kenalog (triamcinolone acetonide) A CORTICOSTEROID.

ketoconazole An ANTIFUNGAL.

L

Lanoxin (digoxin) A drug used to treat heart disease including heart failure and arrhythmias.

Larodopa (levodopa) A drug used to treat Parkinson's disease.

Larotid (amoxicillin trihydrate) An ANTIBIOTIC.

Lasix (furosemide) A DIURETIC.

LAXATIVES Drugs that increase the frequency and ease of bowel movements, either by stimulating the bowel wall (stimulant laxative), by increasing the bulk of bowel contents (bulk laxative), or by lubricating them (stool-softeners, or bowel movement-softeners). Laxatives may be taken by mouth or directly into the lower bowel as suppositories or enemas. Bulk laxatives must be taken with plenty of water. If laxatives are taken regularly, the bowels may ultimately become unable to work properly without them.

lente insulin An intermediate-acting insulin.

levodopa A drug usually taken in tablet form to treat Parkinson's disease. Possible side-effects: loss of appetite; nausea; vomiting; dizziness; faintness on standing; palpitations; involuntary tongue, jaw or neck movements; abdominal pain; difficulty in urinating; mental disturbances; insomnia. Levodopa is not generally prescribed for anyone who has acute glaucoma.

levothyroxine A HORMONE taken in tablet form to treat hypothyroidism. Possible side-effects: angina, palpitations, muscle cramps, headache, restlessness, excitability, flushing, sweating, diarrhea, weight loss.

Leukeran (chlorambucil) A CYTOTOXIC.

Librax (chlordiazepoxide hydrochloride and clindinium bromide) A drug used in conjunction with ANTACIDS in ulcer therapy. Possible side-effects: dry mouth, constipation, drowsiness.

Librium (chlordiazepoxide) An ANTIANXIETY DRUG.

lomustine A CYTOTOXIC used as an ANTINEOPLASTIC.

Limbritrol (chlordiazepoxide) An ANTIANXIETY DRUG.

Lincocin (lincomycin hydrochloride) An ANTIBIOTIC.

lithium carbonate A drug used to help prevent the disorders associated with manic-depressive states.

Lomotil (diphenoxylate hydrochloride with atropine) An ANTIDIARRHEAL.

loperamide hydrochloride An ANTIDIARRHEAL.

Lopressor (metaprolol tartrate) a BETA-BLOCKER.

lorazepam An ANTIANXIETY DRUG.

Lotrimin (clotrimazole) An ANTIFUNGAL.

Ludiomil (maprotiline hydrochloride) An ANTIDEPRESSANT.

Luminal (phenobarbital) An ANTICONVULSANT.

M

Maalox* (magnesium and aluminum hydroxides) An ANTACID.

Macrodantin (nitrofurantoin) An ANTIBIOTIC.

magnesium carbonate* An ANTACID. Possible side-effect: diarrhea.

magnesium hydroxide* An ANTACID.

magnesium trisilicate* An ANTACID. Possible side-effect: diarrhea.

magnesium sulfate* A fast-acting bulk LAXATIVE. Tablets act within two hours if they are taken with plenty of water and on an empty stomach.

Mandol (cefamandole nafate) An ANTIBIOTIC.

Maltsupex* (methylcellulose) A bulk LAXATIVE.

maprotiline An ANTIDEPRESSANT.

Marezine* (cyclizine) An ANTIHISTAMINE used as an ANTIEMETIC.

Marplan (isocarboxazid) An ANTIDEPRESSANT.

Matulane (procarbazine hydrochloride) A CYTOTOXIC.

Maxibolin (ethylestrenol) An anabolic steroid. See SEX HORMONES (MALE).

Maxitrol (dexamethasone, neomycin and polymyxin B sulfate) An ointment or liquid used to treat inflammation of the eye.

Meclan A drug used to treat acne.

meclizine hydrochloride* An ANTIHISTAMINE used to treat motion sickness.

meclocycline sulfosalicylate A drug used to treat acne.

meclofenamate sodium An ANTIRHEUMATIC.

Meclomen (meclofenamate sodium) An ANTIRHEUMATIC.

mechloretamine hydrochloride A CYTOTOXIC used as an ANTINEOPLASTIC. Given only by injection.

Medihaler-Epi (epinephrine bitartrate) A BRONCHODILATOR.

Medrol (methylprednisolone) A CORTICOSTEROID.

medroxyprogesterone acetate A progestin. See SEX HORMONES (FEMALE).

Mellaril (thioridazine hydrochloride) An ANTIPSYCHOTIC.

melphalan A CYTOTOXIC used as an ANTINEOPLASTIC.

mepenzolate bromide An ANTISPASMODIC.

meperidine hydrochloride An ANALGESIC.

meprobamate An ANTIANXIETY DRUG, also used as a SLEEPING DRUG.

Metamucil* (psyllium hydrophilic colloid) A bulk LAXATIVE.

metaproterenol sulfate A BRONCHODILATOR.

methacycline hydrochloride A broad-spectrum ANTIBIOTIC. See tetracycline; this preparation is similar.

methadone hydrochloride A powerful narcotic ANALGESIC, also used in the withdrawal detoxification of morphine and heroin addicts.

methandrostenolone An anabolic steroid. See SEX HORMONES (MALE).

methicillin sodium An ANTIBIOTIC, given only by injection.

methocarbamol A MUSCLE RELAXANT. Possible side-effects: dizziness, allergic reaction, nausea. This drug should not be taken by pregnant women.

methotrexate A CYTOTOXIC used as an ANTINEOPLASTIC and for the systematic relief of severe psoriasis.

methyclothiazide A DIURETIC and ANTIHYPERTENSIVE.

methylcellulose* A bulk LAXATIVE.

methyldopa An ANTIHYPERTENSIVE. Possible side-effects: dry mouth, drowsiness, depression, diarrhea, swollen ankles.

methylprednisolone A CORTICOSTEROID.

methyltestosterone An androgen. See SEX HORMONES (MALE).

metoclopramide An ANTISPASMODIC, also used as an ANTIEMETIC. Possible side-effects (in addition to those common to the group): drowsiness, constipation, tremor.

metolazone A DIURETIC and ANTIHYPERTENSIVE.

metoprolol tartrate A BETA-BLOCKER.

metronidazole A drug used mainly to treat nonbacterial infections such as trichomonas and amebic dysentery, but used also for certain bacterial infections. Possible side-effects: nausea, indigestion, diarrhea, unpleasant taste in the mouth.

Micatin (miconazole) An ANTIFUNGAL.

miconazole An ANTIFUNGAL. Possible side-effects: itching, rashes.

Micronor A progestin-only oral contraceptive. See SEX HORMONES (FEMALE).

Migral (ergotamine tartrate, cyclizine hydrochloride and caffeine) A preparation used to treat migraine headache.

Miltown (meprobamate) An ANTIANXIETY DRUG.

mineral oil* A bowel movement-softening LAXATIVE. Prolonged use is not recommended. Possible side-effect: seepage, which may cause anal irritation.

Minipress (prazosin hydrochloride) An ANTIHYPERTENSIVE.

Minocin (minocycline) An ANTIBIOTIC.

minocycline A broad-spectrum ANTIBIOTIC (one that is effective against a broad range of infectious agents). See tetracycline; this preparation is similar. Minocycline can be taken only in tablet form. Possible side-effect (in addition to those common in the group): vertigo (dizziness).

MINOR TRANQUILIZERS See ANTIANXIETY DRUGS.

Monistat (miconazole) An ANTIFUNGAL.

Monoamine oxidase inhibitors See ANTIDEPRESSANTS.

morphine A powerful narcotic ANALGESIC.

Motrin (ibuprofen) A nonsteroidal ANTI-INFLAMMATORY.

Movicol* (karaya gum) A bulk LAXATIVE.

Multi-Vites* A multivitamin preparation.

MUSCLE RELAXANTS Drugs that relieve muscle spasm in disorders such as backache. ANTI-ANXIETY DRUGS, which also have a muscle-relaxant action, are used most commonly. This term is applied also to drugs such as curare that are used only during surgery.

Mycifradin (neomycin sulfate) An ANTIBIOTIC.

Mycolog (triamcinolone acetonide, neomycin, gramicidin and nystatin) An ANTIBIOTIC and ANTIFUNGAL, used to treat skin infections.

Mycostatin (nysyatin) An ANTIFUNGAL.

Mylanta* (magnesium and aluminum hydroxides and simethicone) An ANTACID.

Myleran (busulfan) A CYTOTOXIC.

N

nadolol An ANTIHYPERTENSIVE and VASODILATOR used to treat angina.

Naldecon (phenylephrine hydrochloride, phenylpropanolamine hydrochloride, phenyltoloxamine citrate and chlorpheniramine) A DECONGESTANT.

Nalfon (fenoprofen calcium) An ANALGESIC, ANTIPYRETIC and ANTI-INFLAMMATORY.

nalidixic acid An ANTIBIOTIC used primarily to treat urinary-tract infections. Possible side-effects (in addition to those common in the group): joint and muscle pains, visual disturbances. Sunbathing is not recommended during treatment.

nandrolone An anabolic steroid. See SEX HORMONES (MALE).

Naprosyn (naproxen) A non-steroidal ANTI-INFLAMMATORY.

naproxen An aspirin-like ANALGESIC and ANTI-INFLAMMATORY used to treat rheumatic disorders. For further information see aspirin.

Nardil (phenelzine sulfate) An ANTIDEPRESSANT.

Naturetin (bendroflumethiazide) A DIURETIC.

Navane (thiothixene) An ANTI-PSYCHOTIC.

Negram (nalidixic acid) An ANTIBIOTIC.

Nembutal (pentobarbital sodium) A SLEEPING DRUG.

neomycin sulfate An ANTIBIO-

TIC, usually used as an ointment or in drops for infections of the skin, ears and eyes. Possible side-effects (in addition to those common to the group): loss of balance, hearing loss, kidney damage.

Neosporin ointment (polymyxin B sulfate, bactracin and neomycin sulfate) An ANTIBIOTIC.

Neosporin Ophthalmic Solution, Sterile (polymyxin B sulfate, neomycin sulfate and gramicidin) An ANTIBIOTIC for the eye.

neostigmine A drug used to treat myasthenia gravis. Possible side-effects: abdominal cramps, nausea, increased salivation, sweating.

Nilstat (nystatin) An ANTIFUNGAL.

Nitro-Bid (nitroglycerin) A VASODILATOR used to treat angina.

nitrofurantoin An ANTIBACTERIAL used primarily to treat urinary-tract infections.

nitroglycerin A VASODILATOR.

Nitroglyn (nitroglycerin) A VASODILATOR.

Nitrostat (nitroglycerin) A VASODILATOR.

Nizoral (ketoconazole) An ANTIFUNGAL.

Noctec (chloral hydrate) A SLEEPING DRUG.

Nolvadax (tamoxifen citrate) A CYTOTOXIC.

norethindrone A progestin. See SEX HORMONES (FEMALE).

Norgesic Forte (orphenadrine citrate, aspirin, phenacetin and caffeine) An ANALGESIC.

Norinyl A combination of progestin and estrogen used as an oral contraceptive. This mixture also is used to treat menstrual disorders. See SEX HORMONES (FEMALE).

Norlestrin A combination of progestin and estrogen used as an oral contraceptive. This mixture also is used to treat menstrual disorders. See SEX HORMONES (FEMALE).

Norlutin (norethindrone) A progestin. See SEX HORMONES (FEMALE).

Norpace (disopyramide phosphate) An ANTIARRHYTHMIC.

Nor-Q.D. A progestin-only oral contraceptive. See SEX HORMONES (FEMALE).

nortriptyline A tricyclic ANTIDEPRESSANT.

NPH Iletin (isophane insulin suspension) An intermediate-acting insulin preparation, given by injection.

Nydrazid (isoniazid) An ANTIBIOTIC.

nystatin An ANTIFUNGAL used primarily to treat yeast infections. Possible side-effects if taken as tablets: nausea, diarrhea.

O

Ogen (piperazine estrone sulfate) An estrogen. See SEX HORMONES (FEMALE).

Oncovin (vincristine sulfate) A CYTOTOXIC.

opium alkaloids, concentrated A powerful narcotic ANALGESIC.

ORAL CONTRACEPTIVES See SEX HORMONES (FEMALE).

Oratrol (dichlorphenamide) A CARBONIC ANHYDRASE INHIBITOR.

Orinase (tolbutamide) A HYPO-GLYCEMIC.

Ornade (chlorpheniramine maleate, isopropamide iodide and phenylpropanolamine) A DECONGESTANT.

orphenadrine citrate An ANTIHISTAMINE and MUSCLE RELAXANT.

Ortho Novum A combination of progestin and estrogen used as an oral contraceptive. See SEX HORMONES (FEMALE).

Otrivin Hydrochloride* (xylometazoline hydrochloride) A DECONGESTANT.

Ovcon A combination of progestin and estrogen used as an oral contraceptive. See SEX HORMONES (FEMALE).

Ovral A combination of progestin and an estrogen used as an oral contraceptive. See SEX HORMONES (FEMALE).

Ovrette A progestin-only oral contraceptive. See SEX HORMONES (FEMALE).

Ovulen A combination of progestin and estrogen used as an oral contraceptive. See SEX HORMONES (FEMALE).

oxamniquine A drug used to treat schistosomiasis, a parasitic blood infection.

oxazepam An ANTIANXIETY DRUG.

oxtriphylline A BRONCHODILATOR.

oxycodone A powerful narcotic ANALGESIC.

oxycodone hydrochloride or oxycodone terephthalate A powerful narcotic ANALGESIC.

oxymetazoline* A DECONGESTANT.

oxymetholone An anabolic steroid. See SEX HORMONES (MALE).

oxytetracycline A broad-spectrum ANTIBIOTIC. See tetracycline; this preparation is similar.

P

PAIN KILLERS See ANALGESICS.

Panmycin (tetracycline) An ANTIBIOTIC.

Pantopon (opium alkaloids, concentrated) An ANALGESIC.

Parafon Forte (chlorzoxazone and acetaminophen) An ANALGESIC.

Parlodel (bromocriptine) A drug used to treat Parkinson's disease and hormonal disorders, and to suppress milk production.

Parnate (tranylcypromine sulfate) An ANTIDEPRESSANT.

Penbritin (ampicillin) An ANTIBIOTIC.

penicillin G or penicillin G benzathine An ANTIBIOTIC.

penicillin G procaine An ANTIBIOTIC that is given only by injection.

penicillin V or penicillin V potassium An ANTIBIOTIC.

pentaerythritol tetranitrate A VASODILATOR, used to treat angina.

pentazocine A mild narcotic ANALGESIC. Possible side effects: visual hallucinations, nausea, vomiting, dizziness. Injection of this drug may cause tissue damage.

pentobarbital or pentobarbital sodium A barbiturate SLEEPING DRUG.

Pentritol (pentaerythritol tetranitrate) A VASODILATOR.

Pen-Vee K (penicillin V potassium) An ANTIBIOTIC.

Percocet-5 (oxycodone hydrochloride and acetaminophen) An ANALGESIC.

Percodan (oxycodone hydrochloride, oxycodone terephthalate, aspirin, phenacetin and caffeine) An ANALGESIC.

Perdiem* (psyllium and senna) A stimulant LAXATIVE.

Periactin (cyproheptadine hydrochloride) An ANTIHISTAMINE.

Peritrate (pentaerythritol tetranitrate) A VASODILATOR used to treat angina.

Permitil (fluphenazine hydrochloride) An ANTIPSYCHOTIC.

perphenazine An ANTIDEPRESSANT and ANTIEMETIC.

Persantine (dipyridamole) A coronary dilator that is used to treat angina.

Pertofrane (desipramine hydrochloride) An ANTIDEPRESSANT.

Petrogalar with phenolphthalein* (phenolphthalein and liquid mineral oil) A combination of a stimulant LAXATIVE and a stool-softener, or bowel movement-softener.

phenacetin An ANALGESIC and ANTIPYRETIC.

Phenaphen with codeine (acetaminophen and codeine) An ANALGESIC.

phenelzine sulfate A monoamine oxidase inhibitor ANTIDEPRESSANT.

Phenergan (promethazine hydrochloride) An ANTIHISTAMINE.

Phenergan Expectorant (promethazine hydrochloride, potassium guaiacolsulfonate, ipecac fluid extract, citric acid and sodium citrate) An ANTIHISTAMINE and EXPECTORANT mixture used to treat an unproductive cough; that is, a cough in which no phlegm (mucus) is coughed up.

Phenergan Expectorant with codeine (promethazine hydrochloride and codeine) An ANTIHISTAMINE with a COUGH SUPPRESSANT. See also COLD REMEDIES.

Phenergan VC Expectorant with codeine (promethazine hydrochloride, phenylephrine hydrochloride, ipecac extract, potassium guaiacolsulfonate, citric acid, sodium citrate and codeine) A DECONGESTANT and COUGH SUPPRESSANT. See also COLD REMEDIES.

phenobarbital An ANTICONVULSANT. Possible side-effects (in addition to those common to the group): drowsiness, restlessness, confusion (particularly in the elderly).

phenolphthalein* A stimulant LAXATIVE. The effects of the drug may continue for several days. Possible side-effects: abdominal cramps, red-tinged urine, rashes.

phenylbutazone A non-steroidal ANTI-INFLAMMATORY, taken as tablets or suppositories, used especially to treat gout and ankylosing spondylitis. Possible side-effects: nausea, indigestion, ulceration, and bleeding from mouth and digestive tract, swollen ankles, insomnia, dizziness. This drug is prescribed by physicians only in limited quantities and only for short periods of time.

phenylephrine hydrochloride A DECONGESTANT, also used to dilate the pupil of the eye.

phenylpropanolamine hydrochloride A DECONGESTANT.

phenyltoloxamine An ANTIHISTAMINE.

phenytoin An ANTICONVULSANT, also used as an ANTIARRHYTHMIC. Must be taken only in controlled doses. Possible side-effects: acne, excessive hairiness, gum growth. Signs of overdosage, which should be reported to the physician: drowsiness, weight loss, blurred vision, eye movement, unsteadiness.

Phosphaljel* (aluminum phosphate) An ANTACID.

THE PILL Oral contraceptives. See SEX HORMONES (FEMALE).

pilocarpine Eye drops to relieve glaucoma.

piperazine* A drug used to treat pinworms and roundworms that is available in liquid or tablet form. Possible side-effects: nausea, diarrhea, itching.

piperidolate hydrochloride An ANTISPASMODIC.

Platinol (cisplatin) A CYTOTOXIC.

polymyxin B or polymyxin B sulfate An ANTIBIOTIC.

povidone iodine A skin antiseptic.

prazocin hydrochloride An ANTIHYPERTENSIVE. Possible side-effects: faintness, drowsiness, physical weakness. Abrupt withdrawal should be avoided.

prednisolone A CORTICOSTEROID.

prednisone A CORTICOSTEROID.

Premarin (conjugated estrogens) A combination of estrogens, which are female sex hormones, used to treat menopausal or post-menopausal women. See SEX HORMONES (FEMALE).

Pro-Banthine (propantheline bromide) An ANTIHISTAMINE.

probenecid A drug taken in tablet form to prevent gout. Possible side-effects: nausea, frequent need to urinate, headache, flushed skin, dizziness, rashes. Persons taking this medication should drink extra liquids.

procainamide hydrochloride An ANTIARRHYTHMIC. Possible side-effects: nausea, diarrhea, rashes, fever.

procarbazine hydrochloride A CYTOTOXIC used as an ANTINEOPLASTIC. Drinking alcohol while under treatment with procarbazine is not recommended.

prochlorperazine A weak ANTIPSYCHOTIC that is used primarily as an ANTIEMETIC.

Progelan (progesterone) A progestin. See SEX HORMONES (FEMALE).

progesterone A progestin. See SEX HORMONES (FEMALE).

Prolixin (fluphenazine hydrochloride) An ANTIPSYCHOTIC and ANTIEMETIC.

Proloprim (trimethoprim) An ANTIBIOTIC.

promazine An ANTIPSYCHOTIC.

promazine hydrochloride An ANTIEMETIC.

promethazine hydrochloride* An ANTIHISTAMINE used as a mild sedative and to treat allergic disorders, nausea and vertigo (dizziness).

Pronestyl (procainamide hydrochloride) An ANTIARRHYTHMIC.

propantheline bromide An ANTISPASMODIC.

Propine ophthalmic (dipivefrin hydrochloride) A drug used to treat glaucoma.

propoxyphene napsylate or propoxyphene hydro-

chloride An ANALGESIC.

propranolol hydrochloride A BETA-BLOCKER.

Prostigmin (neostigmine) A drug used to treat myasthenia gravis.

Protamine, Zinc and Iletin (protamine zinc insulin suspension) A long-acting insulin preparation.

protamine zinc insulin suspension A long-acting insulin preparation.

Provera (medroxyprogesterone acetate) A progestin. See SEX HORMONES (FEMALE).

pseudoephedrine hydrochloride A BRONCHODILATOR and nasal DECONGESTANT.

PURGATIVES See LAXATIVES.

puromycin hydrochloride An ANTIBIOTIC.

pyrazinamide An ANTIBIOTIC used primarily to treat tuberculosis. Possible side-effects (in addition to those common to the group): fever, loss of appetite, jaundice.

pyrilamine maleate* An ANTIHISTAMINE.

pyrimethamine A drug used to prevent malaria. It is available in tablet form, and should be taken weekly, starting a week before entering a malaria zone and continuing for four to six weeks after leaving the area. Possible side-effect: rashes.

Q

Quibron (theophylline and guaifenesin) A BRONCHODILATOR.

quinidine An ANTIARRHYTHMIC.

R

Reglan (metoclopramide) An ANTISPASMODIC, also used as an ANTIEMETIC.

Regular Iletin (insulin injection) A short-acting insulin preparation.

reserpine An ANTIPSYCHOTIC.

Retin A (tretinoin) A drug used on the skin to treat acne.

Rifadin (rifampin) An ANTIBIOTIC.

Rifamate (rifampin and isonizid) An ANTIBIOTIC.

rifampin An ANTIBIOTIC primarily used to treat tuberculosis. Possible side-effects (in addition to those common to the group): loss of appetite, jaundice, orange-red urine, reduced effectiveness of oral contraceptives.

Rimactane (rifampin) An ANTIBIOTIC.

Robaxin (methocarbamol) A MUSCLE RELAXANT.

Robitussin* (guaifenesin) An EXPECTORANT. See also COLD REMEDIES.

Romilar CF* (dextromethorphan hydrobromide) A COUGH SUPPRESSANT.

Rondomycin (methacycline hydrochloride) An ANTIBIOTIC.

S

scopolamine hydrobromide (See hyoscine hydrobromide.)

secobarbital A SLEEPING DRUG.

SEDATIVES See ANTIANXIETY DRUGS.

senna* A stimulant LAXATIVE. Possible side-effects: abdominal cramps, red-tinged urine.

Senokot* (senna) A stimulant LAXATIVE.

Septra (sulfamethoxazole and trimethoprim) An ANTIBIOTIC.

Ser-Ap-Es (reserpine, hydralazine and hydrochlorothiazide) An ANTIHYPERTENSIVE.

Serax (oxazepam) An ANTIANXIETY DRUG.

SEX HORMONES (FEMALE)
There are two groups of these hormones (estrogens and progestins), which are responsible for development of female secondary sexual characteristics. Small quantities are also produced in males. As drugs, female sex hormones are used to treat menstrual and menopausal disorders and are also used as oral contraceptives. Estrogens may be used to treat cancer of the breast or prostate, progestins to treat endometriosis. Sex hormones may be taken as tablets, given by injections, or implanted in muscle tissue. Possible side-effects: nausea, weight gain, headache, depression, breast enlargement and tenderness, rashes and skin pigmentation, changes in sexual drive, and abnormal blood clotting, which can cause heart attack, stroke or venous thrombosis. Estrogens are usually not prescribed for anyone who has circulatory or liver disorders, and estrogen treatment must be

carefully controlled for people who have had jaundice, diabetes, epilepsy, or heart or kidney disease. The risk of clotting disorders and strokes is greater in patients who smoke, and also increases with age. Progestin treatment is usually not prescribed for people with liver disorders and must be carefully controlled for anyone who has asthma, epilepsy, or heart or kidney disease.

SEX HORMONES (MALE)
Androgenic hormones, of which the most powerful is testosterone, are responsible for development of male secondary sexual characteristics. Small quantities are also produced in females. As drugs, male sex hormones are given to compensate for hormonal deficiency in hypopituitarism or disorders of the testes. They may be used to treat breast cancer in women, but either synthetic derivatives called anabolic steroids, which have less marked side-effects, or specific anti-estrogens are often preferred. Anabolic steroids also have a "body building" effect that has led to their (usually nonsanctioned) use in competitive sports, for both men and women. Male sex hormones (androgens) and anabolic steroids can be taken as tablets, given by injection, or implanted in muscle tissue. Possible side-effects: edema, weight gain, weakness, loss of appetite, drowsiness, nausea. High doses in women may cause cessation of menstruation, enlargement of the clitoris, deepening of the voice, shrinking of the breasts, hairiness, or male-pattern baldness. These hormones are usually not prescribed for people with kidney or liver problems and must be carefully controlled for anyone who has epilepsy or migraine headaches.

simethicone A drug used to combat gas in the stomach and small intestine.

Sinemet (levodopa and carbidopa) A drug used to treat Parkinson's disease.

Sinequan (doxepin hydrochloride) An ANTIDEPRESSANT.

SLEEPING DRUGS The two main groups of drugs that are used to induce sleep are ANTIANXIETY DRUGS and barbiturates. All such drugs have a sedative effect in low doses and are effective sleeping medications in higher doses. ANTIANXIETY DRUGS are used more widely than barbiturates because they are safer, the side-effects are less marked, and there is less risk of eventual physical dependence. Possible side-effects of

all types: "hangover," dizziness, dry mouth, and (especially in the elderly) clumsiness and confusion. Sleeping drugs are habit-forming, should be taken for short periods only, and should be discontinued gradually. Broken, restless sleep and vivid dreams may follow withdrawal and may persist for weeks. Driving, operating potentially dangerous machinery, and drinking alcohol are not recommended until the effects of a sleeping drug have completely worn off.

Slo-phyllin (theophylline) A BRONCHODILATOR.

Slow-K (potassium chloride) May be prescribed to compensate for excess potassium loss during diuretic therapy.

Sparine (promazine hydrochloride) An ANTIEMETIC.

sodium bicarbonate* An ANTACID. Preparations that contain sodium bicarbonate are not recommended for prolonged use for anyone on a salt-restricted diet or with severely decreased kidney function. Possible side-effect: belching.

somatropin A HORMONE given only by injection to treat undersized children.

Somophyllin (aminophylline) A BRONCHODILATOR.

Sorbitrate (isosorbide dinitrate) A VASODILATOR used to treat angina.

Spectrobid A broad-spectrum ANTIBIOTIC.

spironolactone A DIURETIC.

Stelazine (trifluoperazine hydrochloride) An ANTIPSYCHOTIC and ANTIEMETIC.

stanozolol An anabolic steroid. See SEX HORMONES (MALE).

STEROIDS See CORTICOSTEROIDS.

Streptase (streptokinase) A THROMBOLYTIC drug. See ANTICOAGULANTS AND THROMBOLYTICS.

streptokinase A THROMBOLYTIC drug, given only by injection. Possible side-effects: rashes, hemorrhage, fever, allergic reactions. See ANTICOAGULANTS AND THROMBOLYTICS.

streptomycin An ANTIBIOTIC given only by injection. Possible side-effects (in addition to those common to the group): disturbance of hearing, loss of balance, kidney damage.

Sudafed* (pseudoephedrine hydrochloride) A BRONCHODILATOR and DECONGESTANT.

sulfadiazine An antibacterial sulfonamide that is given only by injection.

sulfamethizole An antibacterial sulfonamide used primarily to treat urinary-tract infections.

sulfamethoxazole and trimethoprim An ANTIBIOTIC.

sulfinpyrazone A drug, taken in tablet form, used to prevent gout. Possible side-effects: nausea, abdominal pain. This drug should be taken with an increased amount of liquids.

sulfisoxazole An ANTIBIOTIC.

sulindac An ANTIRHEUMATIC used to treat gout.

Sumycin (tetracycline) An ANTIBIOTIC.

Surmontil (trimipramine maleate) An ANTIDEPRESSANT.

Symmetrel (amantadine) A drug used to treat Parkinson's disease and as an ANTIVIRAL.

Synthroid (levothyroxine sodium) A HORMONE, used to treat hypothyroidism.

T

Tace (chlorotrianisene) An estrogen. See SEX HORMONES (FEMALE).

Tagamet (cimetidine) A drug used to help heal peptic ulcers.

Talwin (pentazocine) An ANALGESIC.

tamoxifen citrate A CYTOTOXIC used as an ANTINEOPLASTIC.

Tegopen (cloxacillin) An ANTIBIOTIC.

Tegretol (carbamazepine) An ANTICONVULSANT.

terbutaline sulfate A BRONCHODILATOR.

Terramycin (oxytetracycline) An ANTIBIOTIC.

testosterone An androgen. See SEX HORMONES (MALE).

tetracycline A broad-spectrum ANTIBIOTIC (one that is effective against a broad range of infectious agents). Must be taken between meals, and not with milk, antacids, or iron preparations. Because it may cause staining of developing teeth, tetracycline should not be taken by pregnant women or children under eight years of age.

Tetracyn (tetracycline) An ANTIBIOTIC.

Tetramine (oxytetracycline) An ANTIBIOTIC.

Theo-Dur (theophylline) A BRONCHODILATOR. See also aminophylline.

Theolair (theophylline) A BRONCHODILATOR.

theophylline A BRONCHODILATOR.

thiroidazine hydrochloride An ANTIPSYCHOTIC.

Thiosulfil (sulfamethizole) An ANTIBIOTIC.

thiothixene An ANTIPSYCHOTIC.

Thorazine (chlorpromazine hydrochloride) An ANTIPSYCHOTIC, also used as an ANTIEMETIC.

THROMBOLYTICS See ANTICOAGULANTS AND THROMBOLYTICS.

thyroid A natural product prepared from the thyroid gland and used to treat hypothyroidism. Taken in tablet form. Possible side-effects: angina, palpitations, muscle cramps, headache, restlessness, excitability, flushing, sweating, diarrhea, weight loss. (See levothyroxine.)

Tigan (trimethobenzamide) An ANTIEMETIC.

timolol maleate A BETA-BLOCKER.

Timoptic (timolol maleate) A drug used on the eye to treat glaucoma.

tobramycin An ANTIBIOTIC.

Tofranil (imipramine hydrochloride) An ANTIDEPRESSANT.

tolazamide A HYPOGLYCEMIC.

tolbutamide A HYPOGLYCEMIC.

Tolectin (tolmetin sodium) An ANTI-INFLAMMATORY.

Tolinase (tolazamide) A HYPOGLYCEMIC.

tolmetin sodium An ANTI-INFLAMMATORY.

Trancopal (chormezanone) An ANTIANXIETY DRUG.

TRANQUILIZER This is a term commonly used to describe any drug that has a calming or sedative effect. However, the drugs that are sometimes called minor tranquilizers should be called ANTIANXIETY DRUGS, and the drugs that are sometimes called major tranquilizers should be called ANTIPSYCHOTICS.

Tranxene (clorazepate dipotassium) An ANTIANXIETY DRUG.

tranycypromine sulfate A monoamine oxidase inhibitor ANTIDEPRESSANT.

tretinoin A drug used on the skin for acne.

triamcinolone or triamcinolone acetonide A STEROID.

triamterene A DIURETIC that must not be taken with potassium supplements.

Triavil (perphenazine and amitriptyline hydrochloride) An ANTIDEPRESSANT.

trifluoperazine hydrochloride An ANTIPSYCHOTIC, also used as an ANTIEMETIC.

Trilafon (perphenazine) An ANTIPSYCHOTIC and ANTIEMETIC.

trimethobenzamide hydrochloride An ANTIEMETIC.

trimethoprim An ANTIBIOTIC used primarily to treat urinary-tract infections.

trimiperamine or trimiperamine maleate An ANTIDEPRESSANT.

Trimpex (trimethoprim) An ANTIBIOTIC.

triprolidine hydrochloride* An ANTIHISTAMINE.

Tuinal (amobarbital with secobarbital) A SLEEPING DRUG.

Tuss ornade (caramiphen edisylate, chlorpheniramine maleate, phenylpropanolamine hydrochloride and isopropamide iodide) A DECONGESTANT cough syrup. See also COLD REMEDIES.

Tylenol* (acetaminophen) An ANALGESIC and ANTIPYRETIC, in tablet or liquid form.

Tylenol with codeine (acetaminophen and codeine phosphate) An ANALGESIC.

U

Urecholine (bethanechol chloride) A drug used to treat urinary retention disorders.

V

Valisone (betamethasone valerate) A CORTICOSTEROID.

Valium (diazepam) An ANTIANXIETY DRUG.

valproic acid An ANTICONVULSANT. Possible side-effect (in addition to those common to the group): temporary loss of hair.

Vanceril (beclomethasone dipropionate) A CORTICOSTEROID used to treat asthma, given by inhalation.

Vancocin (vancomycin) An ANTIBIOTIC.

vancomycin An ANTIBIOTIC. Possible side-effects (in addition to those common to the group): chills, fever, rashes, ringing in the ears.

Vansil (oxamniquine) A drug used to treat schistosomiasis, a parasitic blood infection.

Vasodilan (isoxsuprine hydrochloride) A VASODILATOR.

VASODILATORS Drugs that dilate blood vessels. These medications are used to prevent and treat angina, but they are also useful for treating heart failure and certain circulatory disorders. Vasodilators are taken as tablets, often dissolved beneath the tongue for rapid action. Possible side-effects: headache, palpitations, faintness, nausea, vomiting, diarrhea, nasal stuffiness.

V-Cillin-K (penicillin V potassium) An ANTIBIOTIC.

Velocef (cephradine) An ANTIBIOTIC.

Ventolin (albuterol) A BRONCHODILATOR.

verapamil hydrochloride An ANTIARRHYTHMIC. Possible side-effects: nausea, faintness.

Vibramycin (doxycycline) An ANTIBIOTIC.

Vi-Daylin A multi-vitamin preparation.

vincristine sulfate A CYTOTOXIC used as an ANTINEOPLASTIC, given only by injection. Possible side-effects (in addition to those common to the group): odd skin sensations, muscle weakness, constipation, abdominal pain.

Vistaril (hydroxyzine pamoate) An ANTIANXIETY DRUG.

Vitacee* (ascorbic acid) Vitamin C. See VITAMINS.

VITAMINS Chemicals essential for good health. Some vitamins are not manufactured by the body, but adequate quantities are present in a normal diet. People whose diet is inadequate or who have digestive-tract or liver disorders may need to take supplementary vitamins. These are generally available without a prescription, in either tablet or liquid form.

vitamin B$_{12}$ A drug used to treat pernicious anemia.

Viterre E* (vitamin E) See VITAMINS.

W

warfarin An ANTICOAGULANT, taken in tablet form.

Winstrol (stanozolol) A SEX HORMONE (MALE).

X

X-Prep* (senna) A stimulant LAXATIVE.

xylometazoline hydrochloride* A DECONGESTANT.

Z

Zarontin (ethosiximide) An ANTICONVULSANT.

Zaroxolyn (metolazone) A DIURETIC and ANTIHYPERTENSIVE.

Zomax (zomepirac sodium) An ANALGESIC.

zomepirac sodium An ANALGESIC.

Zyloprim (allopurinol) A drug used to prevent gout.

Glossary

A

Abscess A collection of pus, caused by a local infection, that builds up under pressure and may eventually burst.

Accommodation Adjustment of the eye to see objects at various distances. Contraction of muscles in the eye adjusts the lens to bring close objects into focus. Relaxation of the muscles adjusts the eye to see objects that are at a distance.

Acuity A term that means sharpness or clearness of vision.

Acupuncture A system of treatment in which needles are inserted into the skin and either left or manipulated for several minutes. The treatment is used most widely in China. Acupuncturists are not usually medical doctors, but there is evidence that acupuncture is an effective form of treatment for a number of disorders, particularly for painful conditions such as sciatica.

Adhesion Fibrous scars that form when tissues heal and cause adjacent organs to stick to each other. Adhesions in the abdomen may be painful when pulled or stretched, because fibrous tissue is not elastic.

Allergen A substance, such as food, animal fur, pollen grains or dust, that is normally harmless but causes an allergic reaction in susceptible individuals.

Amnesia Partial or complete loss of memory.

Analgesic A pain-killing drug. For further information see Drug index.

Angiogram See Angiography.

Angiography A technique for examining the interior of blood vessels by injecting a solution visible on X-rays into them, usually through a catheter, or tube. The passage of the solution can be followed on a television screen at the same time a recording is made on film of the progression of pictures. This record is called an angiogram.

Anopheles A type of mosquito found in tropical parts of the world. It can transmit malaria, an infectious disease that destroys the red blood cells.

Anoxia Lack of oxygen. Anoxic tissues cannot function properly. If they are completely deprived of oxygen for more than a few minutes, tissues will die. See also Cyanosis.

Antibiotic A drug, usually derived from living organisms, that combats bacterial infection. For further information see Drug index.

Antibodies Complex substances formed to neutralize or destroy foreign substances or organisms (antigens) in the blood. Each individual type of antibody recognizes only the substance or organism that provokes its formation. Antibody activity normally fights infection, but can be damaging in allergies and a group of maladies that are called autoimmune diseases.

Anticoagulant A drug that prevents the formation of blood clots. For further information see Drug index.

Anticonvulsant A drug used to prevent or relieve seizures. For further information see Drug index.

Antidepressant A mood-lifting drug. For further information see Drug index.

Antiemetic A drug that prevents or alleviates nausea or vomiting. For further information see Drug index.

Antifungal A drug that combats fungal infections such as thrush. For further information see Drug index.

Antigen Any substance, for example, a poison produced by an infectious agent, that can be detected by the body's immune system. Detection of an antigen usually stimulates production of antibodies to combat it.

Antihistamine A drug to counteract some types of allergy. For further information see Drug index.

Anti-inflammatory A drug for reducing the redness, heat and swelling that occur in infections and in other disorders such as rheumatoid arthritis and gout. For further information see Drug index.

Antirheumatics Another term for anti-inflammatory drugs. For further information see Drug index.

Antiseptic Any substance for killing infectious agents that is too powerful to be swallowed or injected into the body.

Antiserum Serum rich in antibodies, obtained from animal blood or human blood. It is used to combat specific types of infection providing a temporary supply of antibodies.

Antispasmodic A drug that relieves spasm. For further information see Drug index.

Antithrombotic A drug that prevents the formation of blood clots. For further information see Anticoagulants in the Drug index.

Antitoxin A substance that neutralizes the effects of a toxin, or poison.

Apicectomy A dental procedure used to treat chronic tooth abscesses. Under anesthetic an incision is made in the gum below the infected tooth, the infected root tip is cut away, and the remaining root of the tooth is filled.

Appendectomy Surgical removal of the appendix, a small organ located where the large and small intestines join. If the appendix becomes inflamed, it may rupture, spread pus through the abdomen, and cause peritonitis.

Arrhythmias Variations in the regular rhythm of the heartbeat. Arryhthmias may cause serious conditions such as shock and congestive heart failure, or

even death. They may be treated with drugs or electrical current. A pacemaker may be implanted to correct the problem.

Arteriogram See Arteriography.

Arteriography Angiography of an artery (see Angiography in this glossary). The resultant pictures are known as arteriograms.

Arthroscopy Examination of the interior of a joint with an instrument that illuminates the area.

Ascites An abnormal collection of fluid within the abdominal cavity due to disease of the heart, liver or kidney.

Aspiration A procedure in which fluid is sucked from a body cavity using an instrument such as a syringe. The cavity may be a natural one (the abdominal cavity, for example) or one made by a disease (a kidney cyst, for example).

Ataxia Lack of coordination in body movements due to some form of nerve or brain damage.

Atheroma Fatty tissue that develops in an arterial wall and forms a patch that narrows the artery.

Autoimmune A term used to describe a condition in which the body manufactures antibodies against its own tissues, and damages itself. Such a defect in the immune system produces symptoms of autoimmune disease (see, for instance, Rheumatoid arthritis).

B

Barium enema An enema containing the metallic chemical barium, which shows up on X-ray pictures. A series of pictures taken while the enema is retained in the bowel reveals the lining of the colon and rectum. The procedure takes about an hour.

Barium meal or swallow A palatable liquid containing the metallic chemical barium, which is visible on X-rays. The

liquid is drunk and its progress down the digestive tract is recorded on a series of X-ray pictures. The procedure is used to detect diseases of the digestive tract. A barium swallow shows the esophagus, while a barium meal shows the upper digestive tract.

Benign A term used to describe an abnormal growth that will neither spread to surrounding tissues nor recur after removal. Compare Malignant.

Beta-blocker A drug that slows heart activity and thus lowers blood pressure. For further information see Drug index.

Biofeedback A method of training individuals to control an involuntary body function such as blood pressure or temperature by means of a sight or sound signal on a recording instrument wired to the person. When alerted by the signal to a change in pressure or body temperature, the person makes an effort to somehow produce more of the change. A further signal informs him or her when the desired effect has been produced. Patients who train in biofeedback often carry the learned abilities into daily life.

Biopsy A small piece of tissue removed from anywhere in the body for microscopic analysis. Biopsies are usually done in order to determine whether an abnormal growth is malignant or benign.

Blood tests Analyses of blood samples obtained by puncturing an ear or finger or by putting a needle into a vein. A blood sample can be tested for red and white blood cell counts, syphilis or other infections and hemoglobin concentrations. The sedimentation rate can be checked to see if the small arteries are inflamed. Also levels of cholesterol sugar and triglycerides (fat-like substances) can be determined. The process of clotting can also be tested.

Bolus The technical name for a ball of chewed food as it passes from the mouth through the gastrointestinal tract.

Bordetella pertussis A tiny organism that produces a poison and causes whooping cough. Vaccination and antibiotics are effective against the disease.

Botulism A rare type of food poisoning caused by a bacterium usually found in improperly canned or preserved foods. Early symptoms – vomiting, abdominal pains, double vision – begin hours after eating the contaminated substance. Severe breathing difficulties may develop later and risk of death is high.

Bougie A tube or rod-like instrument made of a flexible or rigid material. Bougies are useful for either exploring body passages or dilating narrow passageways (as, for instance, in esophageal stricture).

Bronchodilator A diagnostic procedure in which a flexible endoscope with a lighting system (a bronchoscope) is passed down the throat to examine the air passages (bronchi) of the lungs. Modern bronchoscopes are thin and flexible, and the procedure usually causes little discomfort.

C

Calculus A hard white, cream, or brown deposit that forms on tooth surfaces. Calculus is composed of dental plaque that has become hardened by deposits of calcium compounds, probably from the saliva.

Candida A group of yeast-like fungi that may produce infection in the mouth, intestines, vagina, skin, or (rarely) the entire body.

Candida albicans A yeast-like fungus that causes an infection called oral thrush. It also infects the vagina (vaginal yeast infection) or the intestinal tract.

Capsule 1. An oval or cylindrical pill containing a liquid, granular, or powdered drug within a soluble plastic-like coating. **2.** The tough fibrous tissue that encloses an organ or surrounds a joint.

Carcinogen Any substance that can cause cancer.

Carcinoma A malignant growth composed of abnormally multiplying surface tissues such as those of the skin, linings of internal organs (the bladder or intestines, for instance), or linings of glands (the breast or prostate, for instance). Carcinomas, the most common type of cancer, can often be treated successfully if discovered early.

Cardiac catheterization A diagnostic procedure in which a catheter, or tube, is passed along a blood vessel into the heart in order to investigate the heart at work. The procedure is done using a local anesthetic where the catheter is inserted. It is usually virtually painless.

Caries Tooth decay or "cavities." Bacteria act on food trapped between the teeth and produce acid. This progressively attacks the enamel, dentin and pulp of the tooth, and can eventually destroy it.

Carotid arteriograms X-ray pictures of the blood vessels of the brain, used as a diagnostic aid in stroke. An opaque dye is injected into the carotid artery in the neck. The dye moves through the artery and a rapid series of X-rays shows how the blood is moving through the brain.

CAT scan An abbreviation for computerized axial tomography, a painless diagnostic procedure in which hundreds of X-ray pictures are taken as a camera revolves around the area being examined. The pictures are fed into a computer, which integrates them to reveal extremely detailed views of structures within the body.

Catheter A flexible tube used to withdraw liquid (or air) from or to squirt fluid into a part of the body such as the bladder or a blood vessel.

Cauterization The destruction of tissue by burning it away with a caustic chemical, a red-hot instrument, or electricity. Cauterization is most often used to remove growths on the skin or mucous membrane such as warts.

Cerebral angiography Angiography of blood vessels that supply the brain. The resultant pictures (cerebral angiograms) can indicate the presence of disorders such as tumors and aneurysms.

Chemosurgery Removal by chemical means of diseased or unwanted tissue.

Chemotherapy The treatment or control of cancer by the use of medications including drugs that kill cells (cytotoxic drugs). These drugs are either injected into the bloodstream or they are taken by mouth.

Chlamydia A type of microorganism that causes a wide variety of diseases in man and animals, including psittacosis, trachoma and conjunctivitis.

Cholesterol A steroid-like chemical present in some foods, notably animal fats, eggs and dairy products. An overhigh level of cholesterol in the blood is associated with atherosclerosis, and excess cholesterol in the bile may cause gallstones. However, some amount of cholesterol in the body is necessary for healthy functioning.

Chromosomes The thread-like structures in a living cell that contain the cell's genetic information. Each chromosome is composed of thousands of genes, and all cells in complex organisms, except reproductive cells, contain paired sets of chromosomes (one from each parent). Chromosomes in reproductive cells are not paired.

Clubbing A condition in which fingertips become thickened and nails unnaturally curved. Clubbing itself is harmless and needs no treatment, but it is a common symptom of disorders such as bronchiectasis and congenital heart disease.

Colic Abdominal pain that comes in waves separated by relatively pain-free intervals. The precise site of pain depends upon the cause. Biliary colic, for example, affects the upper right area of the abdomen, near the gallbladder while the colic of gastroenteritis generally spreads out broadly and encompasses the whole abdomen.

Colonoscopy Examination of the colon by means of a fiberoptic endoscope. A long flexible tube on the instrument transmits light (and therefore images). This allows the physician to make a direct visual examination of the colon to diagnose disorders.

Colposcope A special microscope with a lens that can be inserted in the vagina to examine the interior. Colposcopy is useful for detecting cervical conditions.

Cone biopsy A surgical procedure in which a cone-shaped portion of the cervix is removed for laboratory examination.

Cones Nerve endings in the retina that detect color and are responsible for vision in normal light and fine details. See also Rods.

Congenital A term used for a disease or condition that is present at birth.

Congestive A term applied to heart failure when both left and right sides of the heart are affected.

Contagious A term applied to diseases that can spread from person to person, usually by personal contact rather than indirectly.

Contracture An abnormal shortening of a muscle, a tendon or scar tissue, which produces deformity or distortion. Joint contracture often affects the hips, knees and shoulders of elderly people, because of lack of use of the joint.

Coronary arteriography Angiography of the heart muscle done during cardiac catheterization. The resultant pictures, called coronary arteriograms, can show the location of patches of atheroma, blockage due to thrombosis, and other problems in the arteries of the heart.

Cryosurgery The use of extreme cold to destroy tissues. Cryosurgery is used to freeze away excessive or abnormal tissue not necessarily due to a growth. It is an effective treatment in some cases of hemorrhoids, cervical erosion, and certain kinds of brain disorders.

Curettage A procedure involving the removal of a thin layer of skin or internal lining (e.g. from the uterus). The purpose of curettage is either to remove abnormal tissue or to obtain a sample of tissue for microscopic analysis.

Cyanosis Blueness of skin caused by a lack of oxygen in the blood. This condition can be caused by respiratory or heart problems, and is often a sign of serious illness.

Cyclothymic An inborn tendency to experience repeated swings of mood from elation to depression not directly related to external events. People with cyclothymic temperaments are not necessarily mentally ill.

Cystogram See Cystography.

Cystography A diagnostic procedure in which an X-ray (cystogram) of the bladder is obtained by injecting a solution visible on X-rays into the bladder.

Cystoscope A type of endoscope (a tube equipped with a light and viewing lenses) designed to be used in examining the bladder.

Cystoscopy Endoscopy of the bladder using a cystoscope (see above) passed through the urethra. Cystoscopy is usually done under a general anesthetic and requires an overnight stay in the hospital.

Cytotoxic A drug that destroys cells, which is used to treat cancer. For further information see Drug index.

D

Dehydration A physical condition caused by the loss of an excessive amount of water from the body, often due to severe vomiting or diarrhea. Easily recognized signs of dehydration are sunken eyes, wrinkled skin, dry mouth and in babies a sunken fontanelle (area at the top of the head).

Delirium tremens A group of symptoms that may occur if an alcoholic abstains from drinking for a day or so (or even, in rare cases, without abstention). Symptoms range in severity from shaking limbs to hallucinations, often of insects crawling over the person's body.

Dialysis A technique for artificial removal of waste products from the body by clearing either the blood (hemodialysis) or the digestive tract (peritoneal dialysis). Dialysis is a way to compensate for the inadequate functioning of diseased kidneys. All artificial kidney machines use some form of dialysis.

Diastolic The lower reading obtained when blood pressure is measured. Diastolic refers to diastole, the part of the heart's cycle when the ventricles are relaxing and refilling with blood. Compare Systolic.

Diathermy The use of high-frequency electric current to heat body tissues. Current passed through a small electrode can burn away the tissues it touches and may be used as a form of bloodless surgery. Applied over a large area, diathermy relieves pain.

Dilation or dilatation The widening of a passageway or body opening either intentionally, as with a bougie or drug (see Bougie in this glossary), or by involuntary relaxation of constricting walls or encircling tissue.

Diuretic Any substance that increases urine production, thus reducing fluid content of the body. See also Drug index.

Dominant A term used in genetics to describe a gene that will always determine an inherited trait when it is paired with a recessive gene.

Douche A stream of fluid or gas projected onto part of the body or into a cavity in order to cleanse or provide superficial treatment.

Drip The common name for an intravenous infusion. A liquid substance is introduced into the body by letting it drip down into a vein from an elevated sterile container, through a tube inserted into a vein. The rate of flow is measured by counting the rate at which the liquid drips through a transparent chamber.

Dyspepsia A more technical name for indigestion, which is a group of symptoms that may include nausea, heartburn, upper abdominal pain, gas, belching, or a feeling of extreme fullness after a meal.

Dysuria Painful or difficult urination.

E

Echocardiogram See Echocardiography.

Echocardiography The use of ultrasound waves to examine the structure of the heart. The waves are directed at the heart through the chest, with findings recorded graphically on an echocardiogram.

Echogram See Echography.

Echography A diagnostic procedure that utilizes ultrasound waves to detect possible abnormalities in the chest area. The ultrasound pattern can help identify types of tumors for example, whether it is a fluid-filled cyst or a solid tumor. The recording is called an echogram.

Edema The swelling of body tissue due to excess water content. The swollen tissue may "pit," or remain indented, when you press it with your finger.

Effusion A collection of fluid in space between neighboring body tissues that

are normally in contact, for instance, between the lung and pleura or where bones meet within a joint.

Electrocardiogram (ECG) See Electrocardiography.

Electrocardiography A painless procedure for making a graphic recording (electrocardiogram, abbreviated ECG) of the electrical impulses that pass through the heart to initiate and control its activity. Electrocardiography is done by placing metal plates called electrodes on body surfaces. These plates are attached to a recording device, and they pick up the electrical impulses of the heart. Small changes occur as the heart beats, and the normal form of these is altered by heart disease.

Electrocochleography A diagnostic test in which a probe is inserted into the cochlea in the inner ear to measure and record electrical activity. Certain kinds of distortions may indicate the presence of disease.

Electroencephalogram (EEG) See Electroencephalography.

Electroencephalography A painless procedure for recording electrical impulses of the brain. A variety of patterns normally produced by nerve cells are altered in recognizable ways by abnormal conditions such as epilepsy. Electroencephalography is done by placing metal plates called electrodes on the head. The electrodes are attached to a recording device that reproduces the activity graphically. The recording is called an electroencephalogram (EEG).

Electromyography A diagnostic procedure in which metal probes are attached to or inserted into the skin in order to detect the electrical activity of contracting muscles. Such activity is altered in recognizable ways by diseases that affect either muscles or nerves that supply the muscles.

Electroshock therapy (EST) A treatment for depression in which an electric current is passed through the brain

while the patient is under a general anesthetic. Drowsiness and some loss of recent memories are possible side-effects of the treatment.

Electroversion A procedure for restoring normal, efficient rhythm to a heart with an irregular beat by passing an electric current through it. Defibrillation is one form of electroversion.

Embolectomy Emergency surgery to remove an embolus that has caused an embolism, or blockage, in a blood vessel. A successful embolectomy restores the flow of blood to deprived tissues.

Embolism The sudden blockage of a blood vessel caused by an embolus.

Embolus A blood clot or other material such as a fragment of fat or a piece of tumor tissue that is carried along in the bloodstream. Compare Thrombus.

Endodontics The branch of dentistry that is concerned with the causes, prevention, diagnosis, and treatment of diseases and injuries that affect the teeth.

Endoscope An instrument that enables a physician to look into a body cavity, photograph the interior, and (if desirable) take a sample of tissue or remove a small growth. The basic instrument is a tube equipped with a lighting and lens system. A claw-like attachment can be passed through the tube for cutting. Endoscopes designed for use in certain parts of the body have special names such as cystoscope or bronchoscope.

Endoscopy Any procedure involving the use of an endoscope. As most generally used, however, the term refers to examination of the esophagus, stomach or duodenum. Special names are usually given to endoscopic procedures involving other parts of the body.

Enema A liquid drained into the rectum through a tube or syringe and held for a set time before release by defecation or by being drained away. Enemas are used either for treatment (as in relief of constipation) or for diagnostic purposes (as in a barium enema).

Energy deficit In weight reduction, using up more calories than a person consumes. Such a condition is achieved by eating less, exercising more, or both and results in lost weight.

Enzymes Substances in the body necessary for accomplishing chemical changes such as burning up sugar to produce energy or breaking down food within the intestinal tract. Many of the enzymes in the body are found in digestive juices.

Estrogen One of the main sex hormones responsible for female sexual characteristics. In women, estrogen is produced in the ovaries. In men, small amounts of this hormone are produced in the testes. For further information see Sex hormones (female) in Drug index.

Exchange blood transfusion Repetitive withdrawal of small amounts of blood and addition of donated blood, until most of the blood in the patient's body has been replaced.

F

Failure to thrive An infant's lack of normal growth and development, due to some physical problem or simply its need for more comfort and attention.

Fecal impaction Hard masses of bowel movements that block the passage of waste out of the body.

Fiber 1. Any body tissue composed mainly of threadlike structures – for example, nerve fibers, muscle fibers, connective tissue. **2.** The indigestible components (mostly cellulose) of plant cell walls. Eating fibrous fruit and vegetables may relieve constipation, and may also reduce the risk of cancer of the colon. Dietary fiber is also known as roughage.

Fibrin An insoluble protein formed in blood as it clots. Fibrin is the substance that unites blood cells to close any damage to blood vessel walls.

Fluorescein angiography A procedure for the study of disorders of the eye. A fluorescent dye is rapidly injected into an arm vein. As the dye reaches the blood vessels in the retina, a series of X-ray pictures reveals the passage of the dye through the retinal arteries, veins and capillaries.

Fulguration The use of high-frequency electric current (diathermy) to burn away abnormal tissues such as protruding cancerous growths on the bladder lining or within the rectum.

Fungicide A drug used to treat fungal infections. See Antifungals in Drug index.

G

Gamma globulin A type of blood protein that includes antibodies. Gamma globulins can be extracted from donated blood and used to prevent or treat infections such as hepatitis.

Gastrectomy The surgical removal of all or part of the stomach.

Gingivectomy A dental procedure that involves removal of diseased areas of the gums. The resultant wound may be covered with a protective dressing, which is left in place for several days while it heals.

H

Hematoma A swelling that contains blood, usually clotted, in an organ, space or tissue. A hematoma is caused by a break in the wall of a blood vessel.

Hematuria The medical term for blood in the urine.

Hemorrhage A medical term for bleeding, which may be either internal

(within a body cavity) or external (from the skin or an opening).

Herpes simplex A virus that causes cold sores around the lips and mouth, and painful blisters on the genitals, and in the pubic area, thighs and buttocks.

Herpes zoster A painful, viral disease of the nerves commonly known as shingles.

Histamine A chemical that is released into the body when an allergic reaction occurs, and causes various symptoms. One common symptom is dilation and leakage of small blood vessels, as a result of which the surrounding tissues become swollen and ooze fluid. Another common symptom is itching.

Hormone replacement therapy The giving of hormones, in drug form, to replace those that are no longer made naturally. Hormone replacements may be given either by injection or in tablet form, and must be taken regularly, often for life. The most familiar example of hormone replacement therapy is the treatment of diabetes with insulin.

Hyperbaric A term used to describe a pressure greater than normal atmospheric pressure.

Hysterosalpingography A process in which an X-ray picture is taken of the uterus and fallopian tubes after injecting an opaque liquid.

I

Immobilization Fixing fractured bones or damaged joints in correct position and holding them in place so that they will heal properly. The procedure usually involves the use of splints, casts and/or slings, but it sometimes requires an operation in which fractures are repaired with metal splints fixed directly to bones. See also Traction.

Immunized Made immune or resistant to a disease through the body's natural mechanism for recognizing and destroying foreign material or infectious agents. The mechanism can develop naturally, as a result of your getting the disease, or artificially, through innoculation with small doses of the infectious agent.

Immunosuppressive A drug that hampers the body's mechanisms for immunity. This is particularly useful in the treatment of autoimmune diseases in which the immune system mistakenly attacks the body's own tissue, and after organ transplants. For further information see Drug index.

Incubation period The time lag between the moment of infection and the appearance of symptoms. During this period infectious agents are multiplying but are insufficient in number to cause symptoms or infect other people. Incubation periods range from a few days (for example, in influenza) to months (for example, in certain types of hepatitis).

Intensive care unit (ICU) A section in most hospitals in which intense surgical and medical care can be given to patients with heart disease, accident victims, premature babies, burn victims, patients who are recovering from major surgery, and others who are seriously ill. ICUs are commonly equipped with monitoring devices, respirators, defibrillators and other lifesaving equipment.

Intravenous drip See Drip

Intravenous fluid Such essentials as water, salt, sugar, protein, minerals, and vitamins, which are given a patient intravenously, in liquid form often following surgery.

Intravenous infusion Another name for intravenous drip.

Intravenous pyelography (IVP) A diagnostic procedure involving the injection into a vein of a solution visible on X-rays. This test is used to examine the urinary system. The result is a series of pictures known as pyelograms. An IVP takes 1–2 hours and is painless, but

patients often feel faint for a few minutes after the injection.

Involuntary A term applied generally to any physical activity not subject to conscious control. In particular, muscles not consciously controlled, such as those that propel food through the digestive tract, are known as involuntary muscles.

Irreducible A term applied to a hernia, fractured bone, or dislocated joint that cannot be treated by reduction (see Reduction in this glossary).

Isotope scan Also called a radio-isotope scan, this diagnostic procedure is used to help detect a variety of disorders including tumors and strokes. A radioactive material is injected into a vein and as it passes through the blood vessels of any body organ, a "scanner" is used to detect the pattern of radioactivity. It is this pattern through which a diagnosis can be made.

K

Keratin A horny, or hard substance present in skin, hair, nails and teeth.

L

Laparoscopy Examination of the inside of the abdomen by means of a laparoscope (an endoscope) inserted through a small slit made near the navel. Laparoscopy is done under general anesthetic, and usually involves an overnight stay in the hospital.

Laser beam An intensified, controlled beam of light powerful enough to cut, destroy, or fuse body tissues. Laser beams can be precisely focused for use in delicate operations such as eye surgery.

Lobectomy Surgical removal of a lobe, or section of an organ such as the thyroid, liver, brain or lung.

Lumbar puncture A procedure for in-

vestigating or treating diseases of the nervous system by inserting a needle between the vertebrae at the base of the spine to tap cerebrospinal fluid and occasionally inject drugs. Lumbar puncture is done under local anesthetic and takes about 20 minutes.

Lymphadenectomy Surgical removal of a lymph node.

Lymphangiogram An X-ray test to examine lymph nodes, particularly in the pelvis and the abdomen, to look for cancer. A liquid that will show up on an X-ray is injected into each foot and moves through the lymphatic system to the site to be examined.

M

Malignant A term applied to a cancerous growth to indicate that it is likely to penetrate the tissues in which it originated to spread further (metastasize), and eventually cause death. Because of their pervasive qualities, malignant growths sometimes recur after apparent removal, and complete eradication may be impossible. Compare Benign.

Mammography A procedure for detecting breast cancer by means of X-rays. The rays are directed through the breast onto an external surface that is sensitive to the changes in their strength as they pass through the breast tissue. The photographic results are known as mammograms. Mammography takes only about half an hour and can be done without hospitalization.

Massage Stroking, rubbing, and/or kneading the body in order to relax muscles. Massage sometimes relieves backaches, headaches, and the pain of injuries caused or worsened by muscle tension.

Menarche The first menstrual period.

Meninges The membranes that cover the brain and spinal cord. When they are inflamed (meningitis), stiff neck, persistent headache, vomiting, and fever result.

Menopause Technically, the end of the final menstrual period. As commonly used, the word denotes the time of life around the age of 50 when menopause occurs. The technical term for what is popularly called "change of life" is "climacteric."

Metastasis A term usually applied either to a malignant growth that develops in one part of the body as a result of the spread of abnormal cells from another part, or to the process by which such a transfer occurs. Cancer that has spread from one tissue to another is said to have metastasized.

Metastasize See Metastasis.

Muscle relaxant A drug that relaxes tense muscles or muscles in spasm. Many antianxiety drugs have this facility. For further information see Antianxiety drugs in Drug index.

Mycoplasma An organism that causes a respiratory disorder known as mycoplasma pneumonia, or atypical pneumonia. Mycoplasmal organisms are resistant to penicillin but can be treated with other antibiotics.

Myelogram See Myelography.

Myelography A diagnostic procedure for X-raying the fluid-filled space around the spinal cord in order to detect disorders such as prolapsed discs or growths on the cord. The basic method involves a lumbar puncture and injection into the space of a solution visible on X-rays, after which the patient is tilted in various ways so that the movement of the solution can be recorded on a series of pictures known as myelograms. Myelography is done under sedation, takes about an hour, and may be uncomfortable.

Myringotomy A surgical procedure in which a small cut is made in the eardrum to release fluid trapped in the middle ear.

N

Nasogastric A term applied to a thin, flexible tube that can be passed through a nostril into the stomach via the throat. Nasogastric tubes are used either for passing nourishment into the digestive tract or for draining away digestive juices. This may be helpful when intestines are not working properly, for example, when you are recovering from an abdominal operation.

Neurotic A person who is predisposed to over-reactions to mental and emotional stresses, but is unlikely to lose contact with reality.

O

Obstructed A term meaning blocked. It usually refers to a passageway from one part of the body to another. A common example is blockage of part of the intestine because of a hernia. Another example is obstructed labor, in which the fetus cannot pass out of the uterus because it is too large for the mother's birth canal.

Occlusion A term that dentists apply to a patient's "bite," or the way in which upper and lower teeth come together as the mouth closes.

Omentum A membranous flap formed from the lining of the abdominal cavity that hangs down from the stomach and covers the front of the intestines.

Ophthalmoscope An instrument that includes a source of light used to view the tissues of the interior of the eye.

Ophthalmoscopy Examination of the interior of the eye with an ophthalmoscope.

Orifice The entrance or outlet of any body cavity; an opening.

Osteoma A benign growth of hard, bony tissue, which needs treatment only if it causes problems, for example, by obstructing the passageway between the external ear and the ear-

drum. Troublesome osteomas are removed surgically.

Osteotomy A surgical procedure involving the cutting and repositioning of bones in order to treat diseased or deformed joints or the bones themselves.

Otoscope An instrument used to look at internal parts of the ear from the outer ear canal through the slightly transparent ear drum.

P

Paracentesis A diagnostic or therapeutic procedure for draining fluid from part of the body (especially the abdomen). Paracentesis involves puncturing the affected area and may in some cases require a local anesthetic, but the procedure is usually painless.

Paranoid Suffering from a mental illness characterized by extreme oversensitivity and a deluded sense of being constantly persecuted.

Patch test A test done to identify substances that cause allergic reactions in an individual. Small amounts of substances that may cause a reaction (redness and swelling) are applied to your skin to determine whether or not you are allergic to them.

Peak-flow meter An instrument used to determine lung efficiency by measuring how swiftly a person can expel air from the lungs. Peak-flow meters are useful for diagnosing respiratory-tract diseases or for assessing recovery rate during treatment of lung disorders.

Percuss To administer short, sharp taps on the body with the fingers. The technique is used to map out the area of an organ and detect possible changes in the consistency of its tissues.

Perforation A hole formed in the wall of an organ or passageway such as the digestive tract that occurs as a result of erosion caused by a condition such as duodenal ulcer or appendicitis.

Pericardectomy Surgical removal of the pericardium (the membranous bag around the heart). The incision is made between the ribs. Loss of the pericardium does not impair functioning of the heart.

Peristalsis The rhythmic, wave-like contraction of digestive-tract muscles that propels food along the tract. Peristaltic action occurs from the moment of swallowing to the expulsion of waste matter from the rectum.

Pertussis The technical term for whooping cough.

Photophobia The sensation that light is painful to the eyes. Photophobia is a significant symptom of certain nervous system diseases such as meningitis.

Phototherapy The treatment of disease by exposure to ultra violet rays for set periods of time over several days or more. Severe jaundice in the newborn and psoriasis in adults are sometimes treated by phototherapy.

Piles A common name for hemorrhoids.

Placenta The plate-shaped organ that nourishes a baby while it is in the womb, and that also produces hormones responsible for many of the changes in the mother's body during pregnancy. When the baby is born, the placenta is expelled. An expelled placenta is commonly known as the afterbirth.

Plaque (arterial) A patch of atheroma, or fatty tissue, on the inside lining of an artery.

Plaque (dental) Coating on the teeth made up of mucus, food particles and bacteria. Plaque builds up rapidly without regular, effective brushing, and leads to tooth and gum diseases.

Plasmapheresis A procedure in which blood is removed from a vein and spun in a centrifuge to separate plasma from blood cells. The cells, along with re-placement plasma, are then re-injected into the patient's vein. Plasmapheresis takes about two hours and, apart from the discomfort of insertion of needles into veins, is virtually painless.

Plasmodia Parasites that enter the red blood cells as a result of a bite from an infected mosquito, and cause malaria.

Plasmodium falciparum A particular type of plasmodia that cause especially serious cases of malaria in man (see Plasmodia in this glossary).

Pneumococcus A bacterium that causes one type of acute pneumonia, a serious respiratory disease.

Pneumonectomy The surgical removal of an entire lung or of one or more lobes of a lung.

Polyp An outgrowth of tissue from the skin or a mucous membrane that appears as a short stalk with a knob on the end. Polyps are often caused by inflammation and are rarely malignant (see Malignant in this glossary).

Polyunsaturated A chemical term for fats that are thought to be least likely to encourage the production of arterial plaque when eaten in quantity. See Plaque (arterial) in this glossary. Polyunsaturated fats tend to be more liquid than saturated fats and are found mainly in vegetable oils such as sunflower oil and corn oil, and in margarines that contain these oils.

Post mortem Examination of a dead body in order to discover and document the cause of death. Also known as an autopsy.

Proctoscopy Endoscopy of the anus and rectum by means of a proctoscope, which is a short, stumpy form of endoscope (see Endoscope in this glossary). The procedure is done without anesthetic. It is uncomfortable, but usually not painful.

Prolapse Partial or full slipping of a body organ or structure (the uterus, or a disc, for example) from its normal position. Prolapse is usually due to the weakening of surrounding supportive tissues.

Prophylactic A substance or procedure that helps to prevent disease – for example, an antimalarial drug or an immunization.

Prostatectomy Surgical removal of the prostate gland.

Prosthesis An artificial appliance used to replace lost natural structures. Common prostheses are dental bridges and plates, artificial arms, legs or breasts, and glass eyes.

Psychosis A general term for any major mental disorder of organic and/or emotional origin (such as paranoia) characterized by derangement of the personality and loss of contact with reality.

Psychotherapy Any form of nonsurgical treatment for mental disorders except drug treatment.

Psychotic Incapable of reasonable behavior in certain, or sometimes in all, situations. Unlike neurotic people, psychotics actually lose contact with reality when they are mentally ill.

Puberty The age when children begin to develop adult sexual characteristics, capabilities and feelings. Puberty usually occurs somewhere between the ages of 10 and 14.

Puncture wound A deep hole or other perforation in the flesh made by a pointed instrument or object, such as a nail or an ice pick.

R

Radiation therapy Treatment of disease by either radioactivity or X-rays. Radiotherapy (another term for the same procedure) is mainly used to destroy malignant or cancerous growths and prevent their spread.

Radioactive fibrinogen A radioactive chemical that is incorporated into blood clots so that a clot forming in the body – for example, a deep-vein thrombosis – can be detected on a scan.

Radioactive implant A pellet of radioactive material such as radium that is inserted into a cancerous tumor as a treatment. The pellet, usually implanted under general anesthetic, is left in place for several days and then removed.

Radioisotope scan A diagnostic procedure that uses a radioactive isotope, or form of a chemical element, to view a body organ and examine some aspect of its structure or function. The isotope, when introduced into natural body substances, can be detected and followed with specialized equipment. Findings of radioisotope scans are recorded either in individual photographs or on a screen.

Recessive A term used in genetics to describe genes that usually cause the presence of a characteristic or trait in a child only if they are contributed by both parents. See also Dominant.

Reducible A term applied to a hernia, fractured bone, or dislocated joint that can be successfully treated by reduction (see Reduction in this glossary).

Reduction A medical term for 1. the manipulation into correct position of a dislocated joint or fractured bone, 2. the pushing of a hernia back into its proper place.

Refraction The process by which light and images entering the eye are bent (refracted) by the cornea and the lens to bring the image into sharp focus on the retina.

Rehabilitation 1. Restoration of movement and strength to a limb in which a bone or joint has been immobilized after an injury. Such procedures are generally carried out by physical therapists. 2. Preparation of a patient recovering from an accident or serious illness for a return to domestic and working life. This type of treatment is largely carried out by occupational therapists and vocational rehabilitation counselors.

Respirator A machine, sometimes called a ventilator, that regularly pumps air in and out of the lungs to compensate for the loss of natural breathing.

Respiratory failure Failure of the lungs, which may be either acute or chronic. In either case insufficient oxygen is extracted from the air for the body's needs.

Rods Nerve endings in the retina that serve for night vision, recognition of general shapes, and movements seen from the "corner of the eye." See also Cones.

Root canal The narrow passageway beneath the pulp chamber of a tooth through which the root of the tooth extends into the gums.

S

Salmonella A type of bacteria that causes food poisoning, gastrointestinal inflammation, or disease of the genital tract.

Sarcoma A malignant tumor composed of diseased connective tissue. Sarcomas originate in bones, cartilage, or fibrous or muscular tissues. All types are rare and tend to be difficult to treat.

Saturated A term applied to fats that are thought to encourage production of arterial plaque when eaten in quantity. See Plaque (arterial) in this glossary. Among saturated fats are animal fats, dairy products, and such vegetable oils as coconut and palm oils, which are often used in margarines. Compare Polyunsaturated.

Sclerosant An irritant substance, such as phenol, sometimes used to treat hemorrhoids and similar conditions. Sclerosants heal by causing the formation of thick scar tissue.

Sensory A term applied to nerves or body organs that relay information about the senses to the brain. The areas of the brain that receive this information are known as sensory centers, and provide you with knowledge of your environment.

Shigella bacillus An acid-producing type of bacteria that causes acute inflammation of the intestines.

Sialogram See Sialography.

Sialography A diagnostic procedure for examining the ducts in a salivary gland. A solution that is visible on X-rays is injected into the gland, and pictures (sialograms) are taken while the solution is in place. The procedure takes about 30 minutes and is usually painless.

Sigmoidoscopy Inspection of a segment of the colon through an instrument called a sigmoidoscope, which is a type of endoscope (see Endoscope in this glossary).

Sound An instrument like a flexible rod or tube that can be introduced into a cavity to detect a foreign body or blockage or to widen the passage.

Spasm An uncontrollable contraction of one or more muscles.

Sphincter A ring of muscle that narrows or closes off a passageway by contracting. Examples of sphincters are those at the anus and at the opening from the bladder to the urethra.

Splenectomy Surgical removal of the spleen. The incision is made in the upper part of the abdomen. Emergency splenectomy becomes necessary if the spleen is accidentally ruptured. Planned splenectomies are usually done as partial treatment for a disease of the blood. The spleen is not essential for life.

Stapedectomy A surgical procedure for restoring hearing by removing a diseased stirrup bone (stapes) from the middle ear and replacing it with an artificially made substitute. The operation is performed under general anesthetic.

Staphylococci See Staphylococcus.

Staphylococcus A group of bacteria that can cause serious infections in various parts of the body, including the heart, bones, bowel and blood. Symptoms include boils, carbuncles, cramping pain, nausea and diarrhea.

Staphylococcus aureus The most virulent variety of staphylococcus and a frequent cause of boils, sties, abscesses, bone marrow infection and sometimes pneumonia.

Status asthmaticus Asthmatic shock, or a sudden, intense and continuous aggravation of a state of asthma, marked by shortness of breath to the point of exhaustion and collapse. This condition does not respond to the usual treatments for asthma.

Steroid A group of chemicals, many of which are normally found in the body. Most steroids are hormones and greatly affect body processes such as the overcoming of inflammation from whatever cause. Steroids given as drugs decrease inflammation and inhibit immune reactions.

Stethoscope An instrument for monitoring the activity of various organs, especially the lungs and heart. Internal sounds are picked up by the bell-shaped end, which rests on the body surface while the physician listens through the ear-pieces for unusual or abnormal sounds that may indicate disease.

Strain To exercise to an extreme or harmful degree, for example, overstretching or overexerting a particular muscle or group of muscles.

Strangulation 1. Prevention of respiration by compression of the throat. 2. Prevention of circulation by compression of blood vessels. This type of strangulation occurs if, for example, a swollen hernia blocks the flow of blood through the muscular gap through which the hernia protrudes. Such hernias are called strangulated hernias.

Streptococcus A group of bacteria responsible for diseases such as bacterial pneumonia, scarlet fever and rheumatic fever. They also cause "strept" throat, a severe sore throat that is relatively common in children and is sometimes found in adults as well.

Suppository A soluble medicated tablet that can be inserted into the rectum or vagina to act directly on the surrounding area or to be absorbed in much the same way as a swallowed drug.

Suture 1. Thread for sewing up wounds or surgical incisions. Stitches fashioned from the thread are also called sutures. The stitching process is known as suturing. 2. The interlocking joints that unite the bones of the skull, holding them firmly in place.

Sympathectomy An operation to inactivate some portion of the sympathetic nervous system (the part of the nervous system that, among other functions, controls the diameter of blood vessels). The nerves are cut or injected with a chemical, causing dilation of the affected blood vessels. An increase in the blood supply to a given part of the body follows.

Synovectomy Surgical removal of a diseased synovium (see Synovium in this glossary). Synovectomy relieves pain but is not practical if several joints or tendons are affected. The operation is done under general anesthetic. The type of operation and length of hospital stay depend on the site of the affected synovium.

Synovium A membrane that lines the tough layers surrounding a joint or tendon. Synovial membranes normally produce small amounts of fluid to lubricate, and probably nourish, adjoining surfaces.

Systolic The higher of the two readings obtained when blood pressure is measured. Systolic refers to systole, the period when the ventricles of the heart contract, and blood is pumped into the arteries. Compare Diastolic.

T

Temporal lobe attack A medical term for a type of convulsion in which a person becomes unreasonably angry, laughs for no apparent reason, or otherwise acts strangely. The person usually is not aware of these inappropriate actions. Such an attack is also called a psychomotor convulsion.

Testosterone A male sex hormone. For further information see Sex hormones (male) in Drug index.

Tetany Muscle twitchings and cramps caused by a lack of calcium in the blood. Tetany is especially apt to affect the hands, feet, and/or throat muscles. It should not be confused with tetanus, a disease that causes similar symptoms for different reasons.

Thermography A diagnostic procedure for detecting certain conditions, such as varicose veins and breast tumors, by focusing a heat-sensitive camera on overlying surfaces of the body. The camera records small variations in temperature on photographs (thermograms). Slight alterations in normal temperature patterns indicate the possible existence of various underlying problems.

Thorascope An endoscope that is used for examining the cavity that holds the lungs (see Endoscope in this glossary). The instrument is inserted into the cavity through a space between the ribs.

Throat culture The laboratory examination of a sample of mucus from the throat to detect the possible presence of infectious agents. The sample, or specimen, is used to start a colony (or culture) of the infectious organism in an artificial medium under controlled conditions.

Thrombi See Thrombus.

Thrombolytic A drug that acts to dissolve blood clots. For further information see Anticoagulants and thrombolytics in Drug index.

Thrombosis Formation of a blood clot (thrombus) on the lining of a blood vessel or the heart. A thrombus that breaks away and is carried along in the bloodstream is one type of embolus (see Embolus in this glossary).

Thrombus A blood clot that forms within the heart or a blood vessel and remains attached to its point of origin.

Thyroid scan See Radioisotope scan.

Tonsillectomy Surgical removal of the tonsils.

Toxic Poisonous.

Toxin A poisonous substance produced by bacteria, other infectious agents, and some plants and animals.

Traction A treatment for broken legs, broken vertebrae, prolapsed discs, and other bone disorders, in which damaged parts that have become compressed together are pulled apart and held in the correct position until they heal. Compare Immobilization.

Trauma Any wound or injury, whether physical or mental.

Tremor An involuntary trembling or quivering, most often in the outstretched hands. Tremors may be caused by a disturbance in the brain, diseases such as Parkinson's or multiple sclerosis, the effects of alcohol or other drugs on the nervous system, or emotional disorders.

Trichomonas A type of parasite that causes infections in the urinary or genital tracts.

U

Ulcer An open sore on any external or internal surface of the body. The tissues of an ulcerous area rot away, and pus is likely to ooze from the sore.

Ulceration The formation or development of an ulcer.

Ultrasound High-frequency sound waves, which are absorbed and reflected to different degrees by various body tissues. Ultrasound is useful for both diagnostic and treatment procedures. The reflections may be recorded pictorially to reveal the interior of such organs as the heart (see Echocardiography). Also, high-powered doses of ultrasound can be used to destroy abnormalities such as bladder stones.

Ultrasound scan See Ultrasound.

Union The process of healing, or growing together, of the parts of a broken bone.

Upper gastrointestinal (GI) series
Diagnostic tests during which the patient swallows a special drink (barium sulfate) that shows up on X-rays. Progress of the barium can be followed with a fluoroscope and X-ray pictures can be taken, revealing structures and possible abnormalities of the esophagus, stomach, and duodenum. For a lower GI series, a barium enema is used.

V

Vaccine A solution containing a killed or altered strain of a disease-producing organism. Vaccines, usually given by injection, create resistance to the diseases they cause. Administration of a vaccine is called vaccination.

Valvotomy Surgery to separate the flaps of a heart valve when they have become fused together by rheumatic heart disease. The operation is done through an incision made either along the center of the breastbone or alongside a rib.

Varicella A virus that can infect humans, most commonly causing chickenpox and thought to be involved with shingles (see Herpes zoster).

Vasoconstrictor Any substance, whether a drug or a chemical naturally produced by the body, that causes blood vessels to narrow. For further information see Decongestants in Drug index.

Vasodilator Any substance, whether a drug or a chemical produced by the body, that causes blood vessels to widen. For further information see Drug index.

Venography A technique for viewing the interior of a vein by injecting a solution visible on X-rays. Passage of the solution through the vein is recorded on a series of pictures (venograms). Venography is used to detect conditions such as deep-vein thrombosis.

Ventilator See Respirator.

Voiding cystography A diagnostic procedure for examining the bladder during urination. In the test, X-rays are taken of the bladder using specially sensitized film. The result is called a voiding cystogram.

Voluntary A term applied generally to any physical activity subject to conscious control. In particular, muscles such as those that move the arms and legs are known as voluntary muscles.

X

X-rays Rays with a short wavelength that enables them to pass through body tissues. An X-ray photograph resembles a negative of an ordinary photograph, with dense tissues such as bones showing up as white shapes. X-rays with very short wavelengths, which can penetrate tissues deeply enough to destroy them, are used in radiation therapy.

Accidents and emergencies

First aid

The goals of first aid are: to help the injured or sick person recover, or at least prevent the injury or illness from worsening; to provide reassurance; to organize help; and to make the person as comfortable as possible.

For many minor injuries, first aid may be all that is needed. More serious injuries may require professional medical attention and further treatment. Sometimes first aid is needed to deal with life-threatening injuries that may even involve resuscitating someone whose breathing has stopped. Correct and rapid assessment of what should be done is therefore crucial, and this assessment often requires using common sense. There is little point, for instance, in diving in to save a person who may be drowning in deep water unless you yourself can swim. It is equally important to know what must be done first, so a priority checklist is provided below.

The more knowledge you have immediately at hand, the more useful you can be in an emergency. The following pages will supply you with valuable information, but they cannot substitute for the practical experience you can gain if you attend classes in first aid. Also this book does not include instruction in cardiopulmonary resuscitation (CPR). This technique should not be attempted except by a trained person.

FIRST-AID INDEX

Priority checklist for life-threatening emergencies

If you have to deal with an emergency on your own, follow these steps *before* arranging for professional help. If possible send someone for help while you give the treatment.

1. Check breathing. If victim is choking (see p.803), clear airway. If breathing has stopped (see p.802) carry out resuscitation.

2. If breathing is still absent, check heartbeat. If heart has stopped (see p.804), do cardiopulmonary resuscitation (CPR) if you have been trained to do it.

3. Attempt to control any severe bleeding (see p.806).

4. If the victim is unconscious but breathing, place in recovery position (see p.805).

5. Deal with any severe burns (see p.808) or fractures (see p.810).

6. Guard against shock (see p.807).

Absence of breathing

If someone's breathing has stopped, artificial respiration is needed as soon as possible. A delay in breathing for over six minutes can cause death.

When someone has stopped breathing there is no rise-and-fall movement of the chest or abdomen, the face becomes a bluish-gray color, and you can feel no exhaled breath. As soon as you realize that someone is not breathing, start artificial respiration. Do not waste time going for help or loosening clothing around the neck (unless strangulation is obviously the cause). Continue to give artificial respiration about 14 to 16 times per minute until normal breathing resumes.

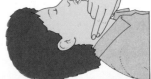
GET MEDICAL HELP NOW!

How to resuscitate babies and children

The method of resuscitating a baby or small child is the same as the method of resuscitating an adult, except that you will probably find it easier to seal your mouth over both the mouth and nose of the child. Do not tip the child's head back very far, because a child's neck and airway are more fragile than an adult's. Blow gentle breaths of air into the lungs, one breath every two to three seconds (20 to 30 breaths per minute). Stop each breath when the child's chest starts to rise.

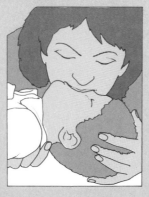

Mouth-to-nose resuscitation

A facial injury may prevent you from breathing easily into the victim's mouth. In such cases, follow steps 1 and 2 at right, then take a deep breath and seal your mouth around the victim's nose. Close the mouth by lifting the victim's chin. Blow strongly into the nose. Remove your mouth and hold the victim's mouth open with your hand, so that air can escape. Repeat as for mouth-to-mouth resuscitation, every five seconds.

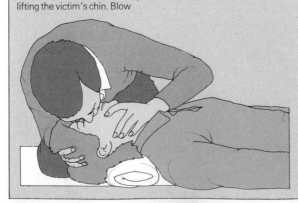

Mouth-to-mouth resuscitation

The simplest and most effective method of artificial respiration is to exhale your breath into the victim's lungs. Mouth-to-mouth resuscitation can safely be given to someone whose breathing, while regular, is very weak, shallow or labored. Time your exhalations with the victim's inhalations.

1 If possible send someone to call for medical help, but you should start first aid immediately. Lay victim on his or her back on a firm, rigid surface. Quickly clear the mouth and airway of foreign material.

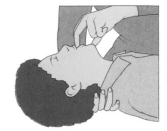

2 Tilt the victim's head backward by placing one hand beneath the head and lifting upward. Place the heel of the other hand on the victim's forehead and press downwards as the chin is elevated.

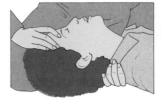

3 With the hand on the victim's forehead, pinch victim's nostrils using your thumb and index finger. Take a deep breath. Place your mouth tightly over the victim's mouth and give four quick breaths. Then give about 12 breaths per minute (one breath every five seconds). Each breath should cause the victim's chest to rise.

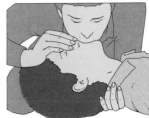

4 Stop blowing when the victim's chest is expanded. Remove your mouth and turn your head towards the victim's chest so that your ear is over the victim's mouth. Listen for air leaving his or her lungs and watch the chest fall. Repeat breathing procedure.

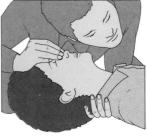

5 Check wrist or neck artery for a pulse. If no pulse is present, begin cardiac compressions *if* you are trained in cardiopulmonary resuscitation (CPR). This *must* be done in conjunction with artificial respiration. Continue until medical help arrives or victim begins breathing on his or her own.

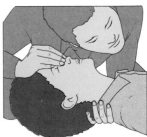

Choking

Obstruction of the airway by a piece of food or any object is an emergency. If the airway is only partly blocked, a choking person will probably inhale enough air to be able to cough effectively, and as long as the person is coughing and has good color (not bluish) you should not offer help. However, if someone is coughing only weakly and is having difficulty breathing, first aid is needed. A person whose airway is totally blocked will be unable either to speak, cough or breathe. He or she may look bluish or clutch at the throat and after a minute or so will become unconscious. If the upper airway is blocked, sweeping a finger deep inside the mouth and dislodging a piece of food may be enough to clear the obstruction. Be careful not to force a blocking particle deeper.

Note: Any choking person who has been revived as the result of an abdominal thrust (see step 2 below) should see a physician. Very occasionally the abdominal thrust can damage internal organs, but you should not be unwilling to use the thrust because of this.

GET MEDICAL HELP NOW!

1 Get behind the victim and slightly to one side. Lean the person forward and support the chest with one hand. With heel of your other hand, give four hard thumps between the shoulder blades. The victim can be standing or sitting.

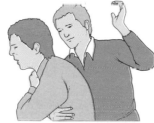

2 If this is not enough, hold the victim up in a standing position from behind, with one fist against the victim's waist area, keeping the thumb inside. Hold your other hand over the fist and quickly thrust hard, in and up, above the belt line.

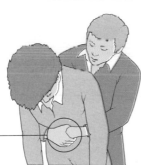

3 This abdominal thrust should dislodge the obstruction. If it does not, repeat three times. Then, if the obstruction is still there and the victim has lost consciousness, roll him or her toward you and repeat four back blows. If the obstruction is dislodged give mouth-to-mouth resuscitation (see previous page).

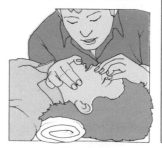

Drowning

In almost all cases of drowning, speed in starting artificial respiration is essential. *Do not* waste time either getting help or trying to clear the victim's lungs of water. You may need to blow quite hard, but the air you breathe into the victim's lungs will pass through any water in them.

If you are alone and the victim is in shallow water, start resuscitation (see previous page) on the spot. If helpers are available start resuscitation while they carry the person out of the water and make him or her comfortable. Do not stop respirations even while moving the victim.

GET MEDICAL HELP NOW!

1 Start mouth-to-mouth resuscitation (see previous page). Do not stop until the victim breathes regularly again or medical help arrives.

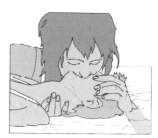

2 Once the victim is breathing naturally, place in the recovery position (see p.805), and keep warm

How to revive a choking baby or child

Sit down and lay the choking child face downward across your knee. Give several thumps with the heel of your hand between the child's shoulder blades, more gently than you would on an adult. A baby can be held face down, supported by one hand under the chest, while being thumped with the other hand. A small child can also be held upside down by the ankles.

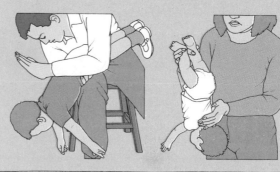

Heart attack

A heart attack is a life-threatening emergency. It occurs when there is not enough blood and oxygen reaching a portion of the heart due to a narrowing or obstruction of the coronary arteries that supply the heart muscle. If this lack of blood and oxygen is prolonged, a part of the heart muscle will die (see also p.379).

The symptoms of heart attack may include some or all of the following: pain in the central chest that is severe, crushing (not sharp), constant and lasts for several minutes; chest pain that moves through the chest to either arm, shoulder, neck, jaw, mid-back or pit of the stomach; heavy sweating; nausea and vomiting; extreme weakness; anxiety and fear; pale or bluish-gray skin, and blue fingernails; and/or shortness of breath (mild to severe). The pain of a heart attack may be mistaken for indigestion. If you are in doubt, treat it as a heart attack to be safe. Follow the first aid directions given below, and get medical help at once.

Treatment of a heart attack is different depending on whether the person is conscious or unconscious.

GET MEDICAL HELP NOW!

Unconscious victim who is not breathing

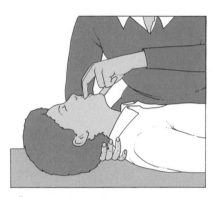

1 If possible, send someone to call for medical help, but you should start first aid immediately. Lay victim on his or her back on a firm, rigid surface. Quickly clear the mouth and airway of foreign material.

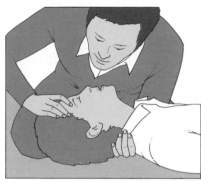

2 Tilt the victim's head backward by placing one hand beneath the head and lifting upward. Place the heel of the other hand on the victim's forehead and press downward as the chin is elevated.

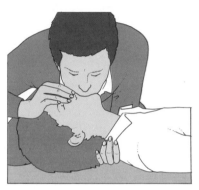

3 With the hand on the victim's forehead, pinch victim's nostrils using your thumb and index finger. Take a deep breath. Place your mouth tightly over the victim's mouth and give four quick breaths. Then give about 12 breaths per minute (one breath every five seconds) until you see the victim's chest rise.

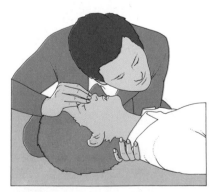

4 Stop blowing when the victim's chest is expanded. Remove your mouth and turn your head towards the victim's chest so that your ear is over the victim's mouth. Listen for air leaving his or her lungs and watch the chest fall. Repeat the breathing procedure.

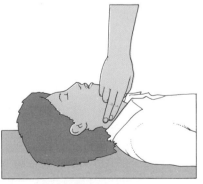

5 Check wrist or neck artery for pulse. If no pulse is present, begin cardiac compressions *if* you are trained in cardiopulmonary resuscitation (CPR). Artificial breathing *must* be continued during CPR. Continue until medical help arrives or victim begins breathing on his or her own.

Conscious victim

1 Gently place victim in a comfortable position, either sitting up or partially sitting. Lying down makes breathing more difficult.

2 Loosen tight clothing, particularly around the neck, and keep the victim warm with a blanket or coat.

3 Calm and reassure the victim, but do not give anything to eat or drink.

4 Call an ambulance or paramedics and inform them of possible heart attack and need for oxygen, or go to nearest hospital emergency room.

5 Follow these steps also if an unconscious victim regains consciousness and resumes breathing. The same basic instructions apply if you have a heart attack when you are alone.

Unconsciousness

Unconsciousness refers not only to a coma, but also to a state where the patient is drowsy, confused and unable to respond to your presence. It may result from brain damage (head injury or stroke), loss of blood, lack of oxygen in the blood (drowning), or chemical changes in the blood.

Note: If you suspect a possible spinal injury, do not move the victim into the recovery position (right) *unless* he or she is vomiting. Then move him or her without flexing the spine. Turn the head and body simultaneously but keep them in exactly the same relationship to each other.

GET MEDICAL HELP NOW!

How to treat unconsciousness

When consciousness is lost, the body's normal reflexes disappear and the muscles may lose their tone and become floppy. The main danger is obstruction of the airway, either because the lower jaw and tongue have flopped limply backwards, blocking the airway, or because the person can no longer cough to clear vomit or other matter from the back of the throat. Even after treating an unconscious person, never leave him or her unattended. A person who goes into a coma may stop breathing and the heart may stop as a result.

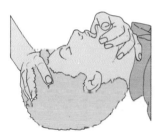

1 Bend the victim's head well back. If the person is not breathing, start artificial respiration (see previous page).

2 If breathing sounds noisy or gurgling, sweep a finger around deep inside the victim's mouth. Remove any loose or false teeth.

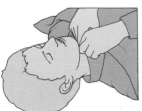

3 Loosen any tight clothing around the person's neck and chest once normal breathing is established.

4 Place the victim in the recovery position (right), if possible on a blanket to minimize heat loss. Cover with a coat or blanket and stay close.

The recovery position

Note: *Do not* use the recovery position if you suspect a spinal injury.
When you have done everything you can to alleviate the victim's condition (see priority checklist, p.801), place the person in the recovery position while waiting for help to arrive.

In the recovery position, the head hangs forward so that the person can breathe freely and liquids can drain easily from the mouth. The bent limbs support the body in a stable and comfortable position, with the victim's body weight evenly distributed.

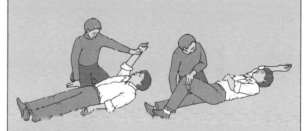

1 Kneeling at the victim's side, straighten the arm and hand nearest to you and place it behind the head.

2 Cross the far arm over the chest, and the far leg over the near one at the knee.

3 Grasping clothing at the hip, pull the victim gently over toward you with one hand, rotating the head with the body and protecting the face with the other hand.

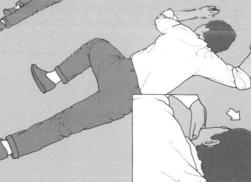

4 Draw up the upper arm and thigh until each one forms a right angle with the body, bent at the elbow and knee.

5 Tilt the head well back so that the chin juts forward, but is lower than the body. Keep the person warm, and stay close.

Severe bleeding and wounds

GET MEDICAL HELP NOW!

Blood can be lost very rapidly from a severed or torn artery. Severe blood loss can lead to shock and unconsciousness, and if the bleeding is not stopped may be fatal. If an adult loses more than 1½ pints of blood or a child loses as little as half a pint, blood loss is considered severe.

The natural response of a damaged blood vessel is to contract, thereby reducing loss of blood. This combines with formation of a blood clot to seal the wound (see Bleeding and bruising, p.424). If the blood does not clot for any reason, such as hemophilia (see p.424), or because of *anticoagulant* or *antithrombotic* drugs, bleeding will not stop.

Stopping severe bleeding

In a minor wound, bleeding usually stops by itself after a short time. In a severe wound, blood may flow so freely that it cannot clot before spurting from the body. The goal of first aid is therefore to stop the flow of blood as quickly as possible.

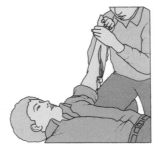

1 Lay the victim down and if possible raise the injured part. This will reduce the flow of blood out of the wound.

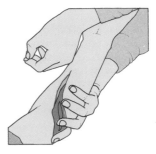

2 Pick out any visible and easily removable objects such as glass or metal, but do not probe for anything embedded in the wound.

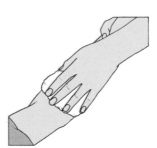

3 Press hard on the wound until visible bleeding stops with a pad that is as clean as possible. If the wound is gaping, hold its edges firmly together. If there is anything in the wound, exert pressure around it, not over it.

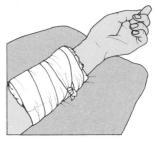

4 Take a firm pad and bind it tightly over the whole wound so that pressure is maintained. If no proper dressing is available, use an item of clean clothing.

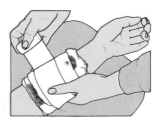

5 If blood oozes through the bandage, do not remove the dressing. Instead put more padding over the wound and bandage this tightly.

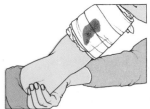

6 If direct pressure fails to slow down or stop the bleeding, you may be able to control it more effectively by pressing on a particular pressure point (see Box).

Arterial pressure points

If direct pressure on the wound is not effective, or if the wound is too extensive for direct pressure, there is another way to stop bleeding. Apply pressure to a major artery, at a point between the wound and the heart where the artery can be compressed against a bone.

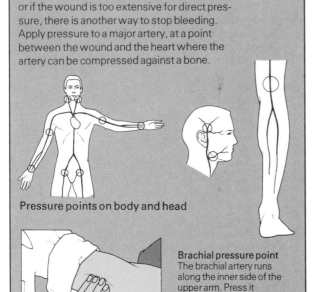

Pressure points on body and head

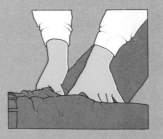

Brachial pressure point
The brachial artery runs along the inner side of the upper arm. Press it against the arm bone with your fingertips at a point between the victim's armpit and elbow, in line with the muscle.

Femoral pressure point
The femoral artery runs across the groin before going down the leg. Hold the victim's upper thigh with both hands and press hard in the center of the groin with both thumbs, one on top of the other. See if the bleeding stops.

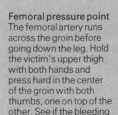

Shock

A person in shock is usually pale, faint and sweating, with a weak, rapid pulse and cold, moist skin. He or she may be thirsty and anxious, and may become drowsy, confused and eventually unconscious. Someone who is in shock requires immediate first aid and urgent medical attention. (For general information, see Shock, p.386.)

GET MEDICAL HELP NOW!

The prevention of shock

Shock can follow any severe injury, particularly if there are severe burns or blood loss. Blood loss can be internal, so you may not see any blood. First-aid treatment after *all* severe injuries should therefore include measures to prevent or at least to minimize shock.

1 Lay the victim down, head low, face forward, and with legs raised 30 cm (about 1 ft), so blood will flow from the legs to the upper body. If the person is unconscious, place in the recovery position (see p.805).

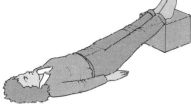

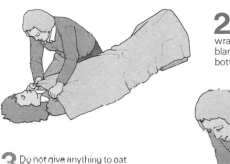

2 Loosen any tight clothing, and prevent heat loss by wrapping the person in a coat or blanket. Do not use hot-water bottles or electric blankets.

3 Do not give anything to eat or drink unless medical help is several hours away. Then you can give a conscious person water or a weak solution of water and salt or baking soda. Offer reassurance and make the person as comfortable as you can.

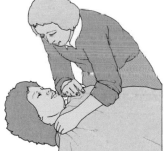

Head injuries

Head injuries nearly always bleed profusely. If you are treating a superficial head wound, apply a clean pad or handkerchief to the wound with steady pressure.

If the patient has a bad head injury (whether actual or suspected), tie a clean pad lightly over the wound. If you apply pressure on the wounded area to stop the bleeding, you may press broken fragments of skull bone or other foreign bodies into the brain.

If a clear, straw-colored fluid (known as cerebrospinal fluid) comes out of an ear, place a clean pad loosely over the ear, but do not try to prevent the fluid from draining.

Treating a severed limb or digit

If a part of the body is cut off, it is vital to get both the victim and the severed part to the emergency room of the nearest hospital immediately. The greater the time lapse, the less chance there is of successfully rejoining the severed part of the body. It is important to keep the part clean and cool. If possible put it in a plastic bag and then inside another plastic bag packed tightly with ice. If this is impossible, place the part inside any clean container. Take the container with the victim to the hospital and make sure the medical staff know about it at once.

Chest injuries

If the chest wall is penetrated in an accident, air can enter the chest cavity. This reduces the amount of air entering the lungs. You will be able to hear the noise of air being sucked in as the victim inhales, and see blood-stained bubbles around the wound as he or she exhales. *Do not* remove any object that is embedded in the wound, and do not give anything to eat or drink.

1 Press firmly with a clean pad held in the palm of your hand over the site of the wound to make an airtight seal.

2 Lay the person down, with head and shoulders raised and the body leaning slightly toward the injured side.

3 Cover the entire wound with a large dressing. A cloth or sheet of foil will do if no sterile dressing is available.

4 Cover the dressing with a thick pad of cotton and bandage or tape it firmly on, so that the seal remains airtight.

Electric shock

The shock of an electric current entering and leaving the body can knock someone down, cause unconsciousness or stop breathing and heart-beat. The current fans out through the underlying tissues and may cause deep and widespread damage, even though a small mark is all that is visible on the skin where the current entered and exited.

GET MEDICAL HELP NOW!

Dealing with electric shock

First switch off the current if possible, or safely separate the victim from the source of the current with a nonconducting material such as wood or a dry rope. Until this has been done the victim may be electrically "live" and anyone trying to give first aid will also receive a shock. This does not apply to someone who has been struck by lightning; he or she is not "live" and can be given first aid right away.

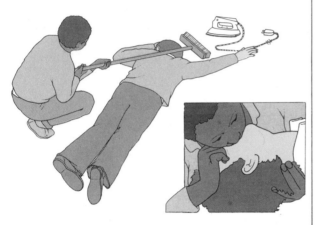

1 Switch off the current, or knock the person away from the source of electricity with a dry, nonconducting object such as a wooden chair or a broom handle.

2 Check breathing and heart-beat. If the person is not breathing, start mouth-to-mouth resuscitation (see p.802).

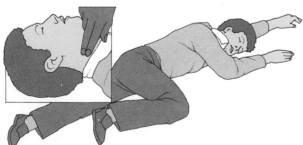

3 If the person's heart is not beating, cardiopulmonary resuscitation (CPR) should be started if you are trained in the procedure.

4 If the person is breathing but unconscious, place in the recovery position (see p.805). Treat any visible burns (right), and have someone get medical help.

Severe burns

Burns may be caused by dry heat, moist heat (steam, hot liquids), electricity, friction, or corrosive chemicals. The severity of a burn depends partly on the area of skin damaged, and partly on the depth of the injury. A severe (third-degree) burn will destroy all the layers of the skin, leaving a relatively painless area that may look white or charred.

GET MEDICAL HELP NOW!

Dealing with severe burns

If someone's clothing is on fire, throw the person to the ground with the burning side uppermost. Smother the flames with whatever is at hand, directing the flames away from the head towards the feet.

Avoid pricking or bursting blisters, and do not breathe or cough over the burned area. Quickly remove anything constricting (shoes, rings, bracelets) from the burned part, because later it will swell and make it difficult to remove them. *Do not* dress the burn with anything fluffy such as cotton, and *do not* apply any lotions or ointments to it.

Note: Nothing but cold water should be put on the burn. If the skin has been burned by corrosive chemicals, it is vital to put the entire area under a steady flow of running water immediately.

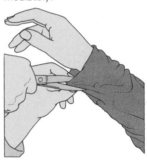

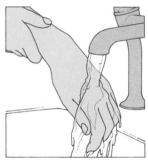

1 Remove clothing that has been soaked in hot fat or boiling water immediately. Do not remove dry, burned clothing or any clothing that is stuck to the burn.

2 Immerse the burned part in cold water for at least ten minutes if possible. If the burned area is extensive, cover it with a folded sheet or towel soaked in cold water.

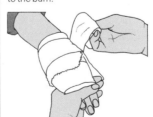

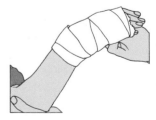

3 Lightly bandage the whole burned area with a clean, dry dressing. If fluid oozes through, cover with another layer. A limb can be protected inside a clean plastic bag.

4 Raise a burned limb to reduce swelling, and give the person frequent small sips of cool water to combat fluid loss, as long as the person is conscious and not vomiting.

Hypothermia

Body temperature is normally constant at 98.6°F (about 37°C). During prolonged exposure to cold, more body heat may be lost than can easily be replaced, so the body temperature may drop. This is known as hypothermia.

In young, healthy people hypothermia occurs only after prolonged physical exertion in cold, windy conditions. In the elderly (see p.723) and the very young, it can occur more easily. Once the stores of energy have been used up, the fall in body temperature causes a gradual physical and mental slowing down, which may pass unnoticed. The person becomes increasingly clumsy, unreasonable, irritable and sleepy. Speech becomes slurred. There is confusion, drowsiness and eventually coma, with slow, weak breathing and heart rate. The condition requires immediate medical attention.

GET MEDICAL HELP NOW!

1 If the victim is unconscious, check breathing. If he or she has stopped breathing regularly, artificial respiration (see p.802) may be necessary.

2 Once breathing is regular, shelter the victim from the cold. If you have to remain outdoors until help arrives, cover the victim's head and insulate him or her from the ground.

3 If possible, change the victim into warm, dry clothes and give warm drinks if the person does not cough or vomit. *Do not* give alcohol.

4 Once help arrives, a healthy adult can be rewarmed gradually in a well-heated room, or more rapidly in a warm (not hot) bath.

Frostbite

Frostbite (see p.412) is a serious condition and needs urgent medical attention. Get the person inside as soon as possible and send for help. Meanwhile shelter the person from the wind, give warm drinks, and cover the frozen part with extra clothing or blankets, or warm it against your body. *Do not* use direct heat and *do not* rub the area. As frostbitten parts warm up, encourage the person to move them gently, but do not let the person walk if the feet are frostbitten.

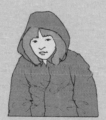

If the hands are frostbitten, tuck them into the person's armpits under the coat or put them in warm water 101°–103°F (about 38°–39°C).

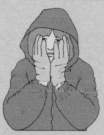

If the face is affected, cover it with dry, gloved hands until normal color returns.

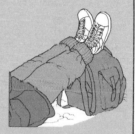

If toes or feet are affected, keep them elevated or immerse them in warm water 101°–103°F (about 38°–39°C).

Heatstroke

Heatstroke usually occurs because of prolonged exposure to very hot conditions. The mechanism in the brain that regulates body temperature stops functioning, and body temperature rises rapidly to 104°F (40°C) or higher. The person is flushed, with hot, dry skin and strong, rapid pulse. He or she quickly becomes confused or unconscious. Anyone who has heatstroke should receive medical attention. First move the person to the coolest available place.

Heat exhaustion

Heat exhaustion occurs when someone who is not used to it is exposed to very hot weather, and does not get enough liquid and salt. The condition is caused by excessive sweating. The person's skin becomes pale and clammy. He or she may feel sick, dizzy and faint. The pulse rate and breathing become rapid and headache or muscle cramps may develop. Heatstroke may follow.

1 Remove clothing and wrap the victim in a cold wet sheet, or sponge with cold or tepid water.

2 Fan the victim, either by hand or with an electric fan or a hair-dryer set to cold.

3 When body temperature drops to about 101°F (38°C), place the victim in the recovery position (see p.805).

4 Cover with a dry sheet and continue to fan. If body temperature starts to rise again, repeat the cooling process.

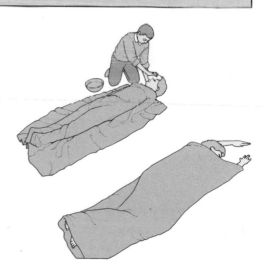

1 Lay the person down in a cool, quiet place, with feet raised a little.

2 Loosen any tight clothing and give water to drink. Add one teaspoonful of salt to each liter (quart).

Fractures and dislocations

Without an *X-ray* it is not always possible to tell if a bone is fractured, or broken, so if you are in doubt, treat an injury as a fracture. Suspect a dislocation or fracture if the person cannot move or put weight on the injured part, or if it is very painful or misshapen (see Fractures, p.534).

GET MEDICAL HELP NOW!

How to treat a broken or dislocated bone

Do not try to force back a dislocated bone yourself. This should be done by a physician. Splint the limb in the position in which you found it, and take the person to a hospital, unless the injury makes walking impossible. In such cases summon medical help and wait until it arrives.

1 Treat any severe bleeding (see p.806). Move the person as little as possible. Movement may further displace broken bones and damage organs. Cover an open wound with a clean dressing.

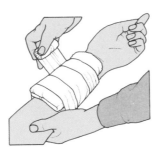

2 Give nothing to eat or drink because a general anesthetic may be given when the bones are set. Keep the person warm and watch for signs of shock (see p.807).

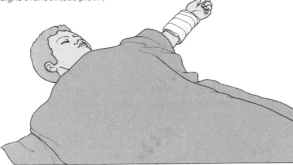

Spinal injuries

If the person has severe pain in the neck or spine, any tingling or loss of feeling or control in the limbs, or any loss of bladder or bowel control, the spinal column may be fractured. In such cases *do not* move the person unless his or her life is in immediate danger or he or she is choking on vomit. If the person must be moved, keep the body straight, do not bend the back or neck, and do not twist the body. Move the body in a straight line, preferably on a rigid surface such as a door or a table.

Applying a splint

Splinting is usually necessary, especially if you have to move the injured person or if there is a long delay before help arrives. Splinting prevents movement, relieves pain and stops the break from becoming any worse. A splint should be rigid and, if possible, long enough to immobilize the joints above and below the injury. Splints can be made with padded pieces of wood, magazines, or even pillows if necessary.

For a broken upper arm or a broken leg, be sure to put some padding between the arm and the torso or between the legs, before splinting the injured limb. Use cloth (bandages, ties, or scarves) to tie the splint in place.

Broken lower arm
Place lower arm at a right angle across the person's chest, with palm facing towards the chest and thumb pointing upward. Put padded splint around lower arm. Splint should reach from the elbow to beyond the wrist.

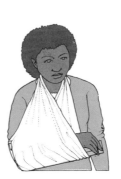

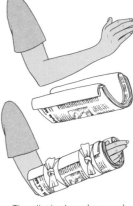

Tie splint in place above and below the break. Support lower arm with a wide sling tied around the neck, so the fingers are slightly higher than the elbow.

Splinting injured leg to uninjured leg
Gently straighten the knee of the injured leg. Place padding between the injured person's legs. Tie the injured leg to the other leg in several places, but not directly over the break.

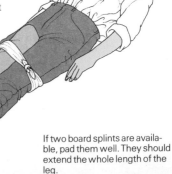

If two board splints are available, pad them well. They should extend the whole length of the leg.

Poisoning

Swallowing is the most usual form of poisoning (including food poisoning and deliberate self-poisoning). Other forms include bites, stings (see p.812) or drugs injected through the skin, inhaled gases such as exhaust fumes (right), and chemicals absorbed through the skin.

GET MEDICAL HELP NOW!

How to deal with a poisoning emergency

First contact a Poison Control Center, a hospital emergency room or a physician for instructions. Tell them the victim's age, the name of the poison, how much was taken and when, whether the victim has vomited, and how far you are from medical help. Follow the instructions you are given exactly. There are two things you may be told to do under certain circumstances: dilute the poison with water or milk; and induce vomiting to eliminate the poison. These things are done only if the victim is conscious.

Do not induce vomiting if you do not know what the victim has swallowed, or if he or she has taken an acid, an alkali or a petroleum product, unless the Poison Control Center specifically tells you to do so. Water, not milk, is given if the person has swallowed a petroleum product.

Poisoning from smoke, chemical or gas fumes

Be extremely careful when rescuing a victim from an area filled with fumes or smoke. If possible, avoid making the attempt alone. Breathe deeply and rapidly two or three times, and take a deep breath and hold it, before entering the area. Remain close to the ground to avoid inhaling hot air and fumes (hot air rises toward the ceiling). If the area is very hot or the fumes are very heavy, you should have an independent source of air. Do not try to do anything except move the victim into the fresh air.

Once you have moved the person away from the smoke or fumes, check to see if he or she is breathing. If the victim is not breathing, follow the steps for mouth-to-mouth resuscitation (see p.802).

Loosen tight clothing. Get medical attention for the victim even if he or she appears to recover completely. Inform rescue personnel about the need for oxygen.

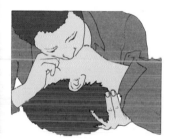

1 If the person is unconscious, check breathing. If he or she is not breathing, start artificial respiration (see p.802).

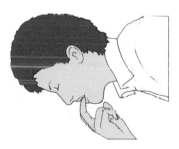

2 If the person is conscious, and the poison is not acid, alkali or a petroleum product, place the person face down and stick your finger down the throat to induce vomiting.

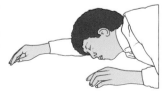

3 If the person is unconscious but breathing or conscious but drowsy, place in the recovery position (see p.805).

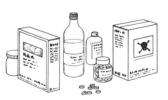

4 Keep any containers that may have held the poison, and a sample of any vomit for the hospital to analyze. Get medical help as soon as possible.

Common household poisons

The following substances are found in most households. If they are swallowed or get into your eyes, they are extremely harmful and possibly even fatal. All such substances should therefore be stored out of reach of small children and in child-proof containers. Also, be sure these items are always correctly labeled.

Alcohol
Cigarettes and tobacco
Aspirin
Drugs of any kind
Bleach
Toilet cleaner
Dishwashing liquid
Laundry detergent
Scouring pads
Oven cleaner
Furniture polish
Weedkiller
Grease remover
Insecticide
Drain cleaner
Paint thinner
Cosmetics

Bites and stings

The injuries that come under this heading are varied, and range from the mild to the extremely serious and possibly fatal. Each geographical area has its own dangers, so make sure that you and your children know about local poisonous plants and insects and dangerous animals in the particular area in which you live.

Insects

Allergic reactions to insect stings

Some people are allergic to stings from certain insects. An allergic reaction to a sting may be life-threatening. The extreme case of a total body allergic reaction is called anaphylactic shock. Symptoms may include severe swelling in parts of the body other than the area of the sting, such as the eyes, lips and tongue; weakness; coughing or wheezing; severe itching; stomach cramps; nausea and vomiting; anxiety; difficulty in breathing; bluish tinge to skin; dizziness; collapse; unconsciousness and/or hives on the body. Many people know that they have such an allergy, and have an emergency kit available. If this is not the case, remove the stinger by scraping it out with a knife or fingernail (do not use tweezers, as you may squeeze more venom out) and apply a light constricting band two to four inches above the sting (right). Make the victim as comfortable as possible, and get medical help at once.

Minor insect bites and stings

Symptoms of a minor insect bite or sting may include pain, swelling at the site, redness, itching, and/or burning. Multiple stings may cause a toxic reaction with headache, muscle cramps, fever, drowsiness or even unconsciousness. A severe toxic reaction may require medical treatment. Remove any stinger without using tweezers. Wash the area with soap and water. Apply an ice pack or cold compresses to the area.

Bees, wasps and hornets Only the honey bee leaves a stinger in the skin. Remove it without using tweezers, to avoid squeezing more venom into the area.

Spiders Bites from poisonous spiders are especially dangerous for young children and the elderly or ill. Three poisonous spiders are found in the United States: black widows; brown recluse, or fiddler, spiders and tarantulas. If you have extreme pain or other symptoms after being bitten by a spider put ice or cold compresses on the bite and go for medical help at once. Take the spider with you if possible.

Scorpions Some scorpions are more poisonous than others. Treat their bite like a spider bite, and get medical help.

Snake bites

If you are bitten by a snake, it is important to know whether or not it is poisonous. There are four major kinds of poisonous snakes in North America: rattlesnakes, copperheads, cottonmouths and coral snakes. You should become familiar with the appearance of these snakes. Try to capture and kill the snake that bit you, or at least be able to describe it.

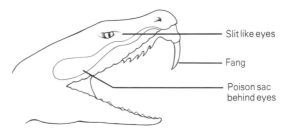

Slit like eyes

Fang

Poison sac behind eyes

Poisonous snakes
The rattlesnake, copperhead and cottonmouth all have slit-like eyes with poison sacs behind them. They also have long fangs. The coral snake has rounded eyes, but has fangs like the other poisonous snakes.

Rattlesnakes have a characteristic rattle on the end of their tails. Cottonmouths, also called water moccasins, have a white lining in their mouths, for which they are named. A coral snake has red, yellow and black rings and a black nose.

Treating a snake bite
The instructions below do not apply if the victim is bitten by a coral snake. In such cases, the victim should be immobilized and medical help obtained at once. In the case of any snake bite, if possible keep the bitten area below the victim's heart.

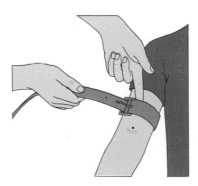

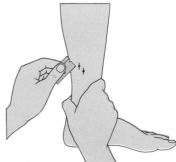

1 If the bite is on an arm or leg, place a light constricting band two to four inches above the bite toward the body. Do not cut off circulation. Leave the band on until medical help arrives. Wash the bite area with soap and water. Immobilize the area. Do not use ice or cold compresses.

2 Immediately make a ¼ inch deep cut with a sterile blade through each fang mark in the direction of the length of the limb. Do not make cross-mark cuts. Draw out venom with suction cups or by sucking. Spit out venom.

Animal bites

Treat superficial bites and scratches the same way as cuts and scrapes (see p.814). Seek immediate medical aid for human bites or any deep bites, especially the puncture wounds of any animal since such bites easily become infected and carry the risk of tetanus. A tetanus injection may be needed. If you are bitten by *any* animal, domestic or wild, the animal should be caught and impounded so it can be checked for rabies immediately. If the animal is dead, it should still be checked. Treatment with anti-rabies serum may be needed (see Rabies, p.564).

Jellyfish stings

Jellyfish stings are seldom dangerous, though they may cause painful burning and swelling. Relieve the symptoms with calamine lotion. The Portuguese Man of War may cause a more serious reaction, with shortness of breath and fainting. Scrape off the stings, which stick to the skin, with dry sand if possible, and get medical help. Place the person in the recovery position (see p.805) and keep him or her warm while waiting for help to arrive.

Foreign object in the ear or nose

Children often stuff small objects such as beans or beads into their ears or noses. Do not try and remove these, but take the child to a physician.

Insect in the ear

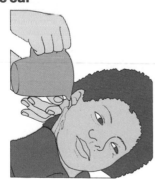

If an insect becomes lodged in the ear, get the person to tilt his or her head with the affected ear up. Then float out the insect by pouring warm (not hot) mineral, olive, or baby oil into the ear. Pull the ear lobe gently backward and upward to straighten the ear canal while you do this. If the insect does not come out, take the person to a physician.

Poisonous plants

Some plants can cause an allergic reaction on the skin of some people. Poison ivy, oak and sumac are three of the most common of these. They may grow anywhere, but are often found in woods and uncultivated fields. An oily substance on the leaves gets on your skin and causes an itchy, oozing rash if you touch the plant. The rash may spread all over your body and cause considerable discomfort.

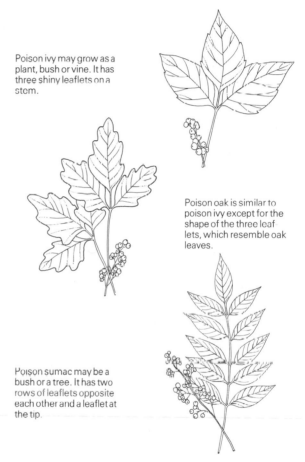

Poison ivy may grow as a plant, bush or vine. It has three shiny leaflets on a stem.

Poison oak is similar to poison ivy except for the shape of the three leaflets, which resemble oak leaves.

Poison sumac may be a bush or a tree. It has two rows of leaflets opposite each other and a leaflet at the tip.

After exposure to any of these plants, remove your clothes as soon as possible and wash the exposed area with soap and water. Then sponge with rubbing alcohol. Wash the clothes also. If you scratch the rash, it may spread and get worse. See a physician if the reaction is severe or if the rash appears on your face or genitals.

Other plants such as nettles can cause temporary irritation and/or local rashes or swelling. The problem should go away within a few hours (see also Eczema and dermatitis, p.253).

Cuts and scrapes

If blood spurts from a wound or flows so heavily that it cannot be stopped after several minutes of pressure, this is severe bleeding (see p.806) and is a medical emergency.

Slight bleeding from a cut or graze usually stops spontaneously within a few minutes. If it does not, press a gauze pad firmly over the wound for about five minutes. Any wound that later becomes tender, inflamed, or appears to contain pus should be seen by a physician.

If the cut is deep or irregular, on the face, or if the edges gape so badly that they cannot easily be drawn together with surgical tape, seek medical aid. Such cuts probably need stitching to aid healing and to prevent scarring. A scrape with dirt or grit embedded beneath the skin should also be properly cleaned and dressed by a physician.

If bleeding from the ear or nose follows a severe blow on the head, the base of the skull may be fractured. Keep the person's neck and back firmly supported and do not bend them. Seek medical help at once. Do not move the person unless absolutely necessary (see Head injuries, p.807).

Puncture wound A deep wound caused by something dirty such as a nail or an animal's tooth is more likely than others to become infected, because dirt is carried deep into the tissues and the wound bleeds very little. Numbness, tingling or weakness in a limb can follow a deep cut or puncture wound. Underlying nerves or tendons may be damaged. Antibiotics and a tetanus injection may be necessary after a deep wound.

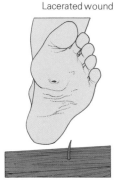

Lacerated wound

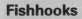

Puncture wound

Bleeding carries dirt out of most wounds, so you only need to clean around a cut. Wipe from the edges of the wound outward, using a clean gauze or cotton pad for each stroke.

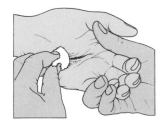

Small cuts heal best if left uncovered. If the edges of the cut gape, however, draw them together and put one or two strips of surgical tape ("butterfly strips") across the gap.

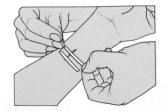

Minor burns and scalds

If a burn or scald damages only the superficial layer of skin over a fairly small area, causing reddening and perhaps blistering, it can be treated at home. Severe burns (see p.808) are a medical emergency. Sunburn is usually only a minor burn.

Superficial burns are very painful, so the goal of first aid is to relieve the pain. If blisters form over a burn, do not break them. If they are on a part of the skin normally rubbed by clothing, cover with a light dressing (see Blisters, next page). Do not put any cream, grease or ointment on a burn, except for a large area of mild sunburn, which can be soothed with calamine lotion.

Plunge the burned area into cold water, or hold it under a cold running tap for ten minutes or until the pain stops or lessens. Do not put ice on a burn because it may injure the tissue.

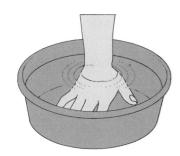

Fishhooks

If the barb of a fishhook becomes embedded in the skin, get a physician to remove it. Only try to remove it yourself if no medical help is available, and consult a physician afterwards because of the high risk of infection.

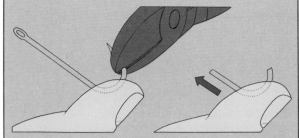

1 Push the hook on through the skin until the barb protrudes. Then cut off either the barb or the shank, close to the skin.

2 Draw the unbarbed portion gently through the skin. Clean the wound and cover it with a dressing.

Splinters

A small splinter projecting from the skin can usually be removed by a gentle pull with a pair of tweezers. To remove a splinter embedded under the skin, slit the skin over one end of the splinter with the tip of a needle that has been sterilized in a flame and allowed to cool for a moment, and lift up the end of the splinter with the needle tip. Then you should be able to remove it with tweezers. If it does not come out easily, do not probe further. Take the person to a physician.

Bruises

Bruises occur when a fall or blow causes bleeding into the tissues beneath the skin. They normally fade slowly, change color as they do, and disappear without any treatment after 10 to 14 days. If any bruise does not fade or disappear, or if you notice bruises appearing for no apparent reason, consult your physician.

Bruises on the head or the shin, where the bone is just beneath the skin, may swell considerably. To reduce pain and swelling, apply an ice pack or wring out a cloth in cold water and lay it over the bruise for about ten minutes with moderate pressure.

Bruising around the eye, known as a "black eye," may swell dramatically. Apply a cool or cold wet cloth to the area for ten minutes. If any disturbance of vision follows a blow to the eye, seek medical aid.

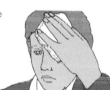

Blisters

Blisters form on the skin because of allergic reactions, or when the skin is damaged by friction or burns. New skin forms beneath the blister, and the fluid in it is gradually absorbed. Eventually the outer layer of skin comes off. No first-aid treatment is needed unless the blister breaks or is likely to be damaged by further friction. In such cases, wash the area with soap and water, and protect it with an adhesive bandage.

Do not prick the blister or try to remove it. This will leave the raw skin beneath painful and open to infection.

Sprains and strains

If a joint or muscle is wrenched beyond its normal range of movement, the joint is said to be sprained (see p.532), the muscle strained (see Pulled muscle, p.532). The symptoms for both types of injury are the same: pain, swelling and bruising. A severe sprain may be indistinguishable from a fracture and should be treated as a fracture, or break (see p.810).

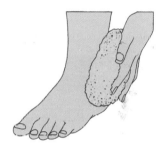

1 Sponge a mild strain or sprain with cold water or apply ice wrapped in a cloth to reduce pain and swelling.

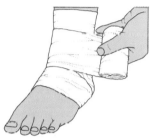

2 Support the joint or muscle with a bandage, and do not put any weight on it for a day or two.

Applying a figure-eight bandage

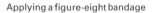

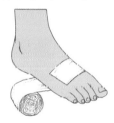

1 Anchor the bandage with one or two circular turns around the foot.

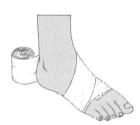

2 Bring the bandage diagonally across the top of the foot and around the ankle. Continue to bring the bandage down across the top of the foot and under the arch.

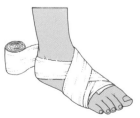

3 Continue figure-eight turns, with each turn overlapping the last one by about three-fourths of its width.

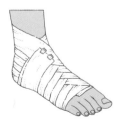

4 Bandage until the foot (not toes), ankle and lower leg are covered. Secure bandage with tape or clips.

Foreign object in the eye

Never try to remove anything that is on the pupil of the eye, or that seems to be stuck or embedded in the white of the eye. In such circumstances, do not let the injured person rub the eye, but cover both eyes with a soft pad to help stop extra eye movements, and seek medical help.

If the foreign object is floating on the white of the eye or on the inside of the eyelid, try to remove it with the corner of a clean cloth, handkerchief, or paper tissue as described below. Do not let the person rub the eye.

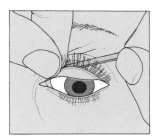

1 Seat the person in a good light. Get the person to look up while you pull the lower lid gently down. If you can see the object, pick it off with the corner of the cloth.

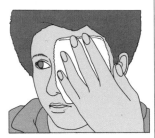

2 If you can see nothing, pull the upper lid down and out over the lower lid and let it slide back. This may be enough to dislodge the object.

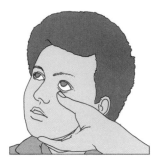

3 If nothing happens, ask the person to look down while you place a toothpick or swab across the upper lid and fold the lid up over it.

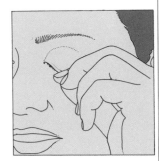

4 If you can see the object, pick it off with the cloth. If not, cover the eye with a soft pad and seek medical help.

Corrosive chemicals in the eye

Chemicals or corrosive fluids splashed in the eye must be washed out quickly by holding the person's opened eye under a gentle flow of running water. Tilt the head toward the injured side so that the chemical is not washed into the uninjured eye. Keep the eyelids apart with your fingers. After ten minutes cover the eye with a pad and get the person to a hospital.

Emergency childbirth

GET MEDICAL HELP NOW!

Sometimes a woman's labor proceeds so fast (especially if the baby is not her first) that there is not enough time to reach a hospital or get medical help before the baby is born. If you are the only person present at such a birth, remember that it is a natural process: interfere as little as possible. Most births are *not* life-threatening emergencies.

Preparing for the birth

Try to make the room or shelter warm, and the mother comfortable with pillows. Put a clean sheet or newspapers underneath her, if possible with a plastic sheet beneath them. If you can, boil a pair of scissors and a length of string to sterilize them.

If the mother seems distressed or in a lot of pain, be calm and reassuring. As the birth proceeds, there may be a lot of blood-stained fluid. This is normal during a birth.

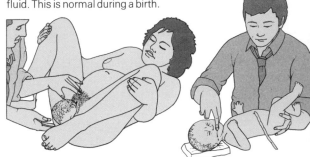

1 When the baby's head is visible in the vagina, birth is imminent. Once the head and shoulders emerge, support the baby by holding the head up. Do not pull. The rest of the baby's body will slide out.

2 Holding the baby with its head lower than its feet, wipe mucus from both nose and mouth. If breathing does not start within one minute of birth, give artificial respiration (see p.802).

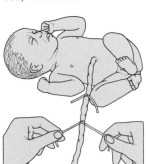

3 Wait until the cord stops pulsating before cutting it. Tie a tight knot with sterilized string at least 13 cm (6 in) away from the baby's navel and another knot 5 cm (2 in) further away. Cut the cord between the two knots.

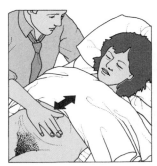

4 Within 20 minutes after the baby the placenta will usually emerge. Do not pull on the cord; it may tear off. If bleeding seems heavy, massage the lower abdomen gently every few minutes until help arrives.

The page numbers in italic type refer to an article or box on the subject. If you have a symptom that you cannot find in this index, turn to the Chartfinder on p.68 to locate an appropriate self-diagnosis symptom chart. For information on a specific drug or a type of drug, look in the Drug index starting on p.776. For fast access to first-aid treatment, see the First-aid index on p.801.

Other indexes include:
**Symptom
chart-finder, p.68**
Drug index, p.776
First-aid index, p.801